KU-018-304

Nutrition in Clinical Practice

LIVERPOOL JMU LIBRARY

3 1111 01490 7677

615.
854

KAT

liverpool
JMU
Learning and Information Services

Accession no	
D 1012222 W	
Supplier DA	Invoice Date
Class no	
Site M	Fund code ELS4

Nutrition in Clinical Practice

A Comprehensive, Evidence-Based Manual for the Practitioner

THIRD EDITION

David L. Katz, MD, MPH, FACPM, FACP
Director, Prevention Research Center
Yale University School of Public Health
Griffin Hospital
Clinical Instructor in Medicine
Yale University School of Medicine
Director, Integrative Medicine Center
Griffin Hospital
President, American College of Lifestyle Medicine
Derby, Connecticut

With

Rachel S.C. Friedman, MD, MHS
Department of Family Medicine
The Permanente Medical Group
Santa Rosa, California
Assistant Clinical Professor
Department of Community and Family Medicine
University of California
San Francisco, California

and

Sean C. Lucan, MD, MPH, MS
Department of Family and Social Medicine
Albert Einstein College of Medicine
Montefiore Medical Center
Bronx, New York

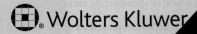

Wolters Kluwer

Philadelphia • Baltimor
Buenos Aires • Hong

Executive Editor: Rebecca Gaertner
Senior Product Development Editor: Kristina Oberle
Production Project Manager: Alicia Jackson
Senior Manufacturing Manager: Beth Welsh
Marketing Manager: Stephanie Manzo
Design Coordinator: Stephen Druding
Production Services: S4Carlisle Publishing Services (P) Ltd.

Copyright © 2015 by Wolters Kluwer

Two Commerce Square

2001 Market Street
Philadelphia, PA 19103 USA
LWW.com

2nd edition, © 2008 by LIPPINCOTT WILLIAMS & WILKINS, a Wolters Kluwer Business
1st edition © 2001 by LIPPINCOTT WILLIAMS & WILKINS

All rights reserved. This book is protected by copyright. No part of this book may be reproduced or transmitted in any form or by any means, including as photocopies or scanned-in or other electronic copies, or utilized by any information storage and retrieval system without written permission from the copyright owner, except for brief quotations embodied in critical articles and reviews. Materials appearing in this book prepared by individuals as part of their official duties as U.S. government employees are not covered by the above-mentioned copyright. To request permission, please contact Wolters Kluwer at Two Commerce Square, 2001 Market Street, Philadelphia, PA 19103, via email at permissions@lww.com, or via our website at lww.com (products and services).

9 8 7 6 5 4 3 2

Printed in China

Library of Congress Cataloging-in-Publication Data

Katz, David L., 1963-author.
  Nutrition in clinical practice : a comprehensive, evidence-based manual for the practitioner /
David L. Katz ; with Rachel S.C. Friedman, Sean C. Lucan. — Third edition.
     p. ; cm.
  Includes bibliographical references and index.
  ISBN 978-1-4511-8664-2 (paperback : alk. paper)
  I. Friedman, Rachel S. C., author.   II. Lucan, Sean C., author.   III. Title.
  [DNLM: 1. Nutritional Physiological Phenomena.   2. Evidence-Based
  Medicine. QU 145]
  RM216
  615.8'54—dc23
                                                                2014015290

Care has been taken to confirm the accuracy of the information presented and to describe generally accepted practices. However, the authors, editors, and publisher are not responsible for errors or omissions or for any consequences from application of the information in this book and make no warranty, expressed or implied, with respect to the currency, completeness, or accuracy of the contents of the publication. Application of this information in a particular situation remains the professional responsibility of the practitioner; the clinical treatments described and ~~nded~~ may not be considered absolute and universal recommendations.

~~rted~~ every effort to ensure that drug selection and ~~ce~~ with the current recommendations and practice ~~of~~ ongoing research, changes in government regu-~~n~~ relating to drug therapy and drug reactions, the ~~t~~ for each drug for any change in indications and ~~ons.~~ This is particularly important when the recom-~~loyed~~ drug.

~~n~~ this publication have Food and Drug Administration ~~cted~~ research settings. It is the responsibility of the ~~status~~ of each drug or device planned for use in his or

New York • London
Hong Kong • Sydney • Tokyo

RRS1509

To our patients, and yours.
They are the reason.

David L. Katz, MD, MPH, FACPM, FACP, is the founding (1998) director of Yale University's Yale-Griffin Prevention Research Center. He received his BA from Dartmouth College (1984; magna cum laude); his MD from the Albert Einstein College of Medicine (1988); and his MPH from the Yale University School of Public Health (1993). He is a two-time diplomate of the American Board of Internal Medicine, a board-certified specialist in preventive medicine/public health, and a clinical instructor in medicine at the Yale School of Medicine.

Dr. Katz is the editor-in-chief of the journal *Childhood Obesity*, president of the American College of Lifestyle Medicine, founder and president of the nonprofit Turn the Tide Foundation, and medical director for the Integrative Medicine Center at Griffin Hospital in Derby, Connecticut. He is the principal inventor of the NuVal nutritional guidance system, currently in more than 2,000 US supermarkets in more than 30 states, coast to coast. He holds five US patents on other inventions, with several patents currently pending.

Dr. Katz has published nearly 200 scientific articles and textbook chapters, innumerable blogs and columns, nearly 1,000 newspaper articles, and authored or coauthored 15 books to date, including multiple editions of textbooks in both nutrition and preventive medicine.

Dr. Katz has been extensively involved in medical education. He was a founding director of one of the nation's first combined residency training programs in internal medicine and preventive medicine (Griffin Hospital, Derby, Connecticut); and served as director of medical studies in public health at the Yale University School of Medicine for a span of 8 years. He has led classes and given lectures for Yale students in medicine, public health, nursing, the physician assistants program, and undergraduates as well as medical residents and faculty.

Dr. Katz is the recipient of many awards for his contributions to public health and medical education. He has been named one of America's top physicians in preventive medicine three times by the Consumer's Research Council of America and serves as a judge of best diets for the annual ranking published by *US News & World Report*. In 2009, he was a widely supported nominee for the position U.S. Surgeon General. He was named one of the 25 most influential people in the lives of children by *Children's Health Magazine*. In 2012, he was cited by Greatist.com as one of the 100 most influential people in health and fitness (no. 19: http://greatist.com/health/most-influential-health-fitness-people/), and recognized again in 2013, moving up to no. 13 (http://greatist.com/health/most-influential-health-fitness-people). He has been honored for career accomplishments by numerous organizations including the Association of Yale Alumni in Public Health; the Academy of Nutrition and Dietetics; and the American College of Preventive Medicine. In 2013, he was awarded an honorary doctorate by the University of Bridgeport in Connecticut for his contributions to public health and patient care.

Dr. Katz has an extensive media portfolio, having worked for ABC News/Good Morning America as an on-air contributor, a writer for the *New York Times* syndicate, and a columnist to *O, the Oprah Magazine*. Currently, he is a blogger/medical review board member for the *Huffington Post*, a health contributor to *US News & World Report*, one of the original 150 "thought leader" Influencer bloggers for LinkedIn, a blogger and columnist for *TIME* magazine, and a contributing health writer on childhood obesity for About.com.

Dr. Katz speaks routinely at conferences and meetings throughout the United States, and around the world, and has delivered addresses in at least seven countries. He is a recognized thought leader in nutrition, chronic disease prevention/health promotion, weight management, and integrative medicine. Widely recognized as a gifted public speaker, he has been acclaimed by peers as the "poet laureate of health promotion."

Dr. Katz and his wife Catherine live in Connecticut; they have five children.

Rachel Summer Claire Friedman, MD, MHS, is a practicing family physician in Santa Rosa, California, at Kaiser Permanente Medical Center, where she cares for a socioeconomically diverse population ranging from newborns to nonagenarians, with a strong focus on holistic approaches and preventive care, utilizing creativity and innovation to provide optimal support for patients in pursuing healthy lifestyles and optimal health. She received a BA in History of Medicine from Harvard University (2001; magna cum laude, Phi Beta Kappa) and MD and MHS degrees from Yale School of Medicine (2008). While in medical school, she worked with Dr. Katz to edit the 2nd edition of this textbook and update his innovative *Nutrition Detectives* curriculum. She personally taught the curriculum to more than 600 schoolchildren in Connecticut from 2005 to 2008. She completed her family medicine residency training at the Santa Rosa Family Medicine Residency, a UCSF affiliate, where she also completed fellowship training in integrative/holistic medicine. Believing in the power of music and whimsy to support health and disease management, she coauthored a full-length educational play, *Diabetes: The Musical* (HYPERLINK "http://www.diabetesthemusical.com" www.diabetesthemusical.com), which has been featured at several local and national medical conferences. She has cocreated a food system leadership curriculum, training physicians how to counsel patients toward sustainable healthy food choices, and she has conducted a randomized clinical trial assessing the effects on fruit and vegetable consumption when at-risk low-income pregnant women are prescribed farmers market vouchers by their personal physicians. She has been recognized as a leader in the field of family medicine as a Pisacano Leadership Foundation Scholar, and her work connecting community clinics to local food banks and farmers markets and conducting supermarket visits with her patients has been published by local and national family medicine organizations as well as NPR. She is a contributor and editorial board member of the award-winning peer-reviewed medical publication *Sonoma Medicine*. She lives in Sonoma County with her son and her husband, who is head winemaker for their small family winery Orpheus Wines.

Sean C. Lucan, MD, MPH, MS, is a practicing family physician in Bronx, New York, caring for predominantly low-income, minority patients at a federally qualified health center. Much of his clinical time is spent counseling patients on nutrition and managing diet-related diseases. Sean received his MD and MPH degrees from Yale. He subsequently earned an MS in health policy research from the University of Pennsylvania. His current research focuses on how different aspects of local food environments may influence what people eat, and what the implications are for obesity and chronic diseases, particularly in vulnerable communities. Sean has published more than 40 papers in the scientific literature, given more than 50 presentations at national and international science meetings, and has given invited talks around the country on his work. He has received several national awards, including the 2006 AAFP/BMS Award for Excellence in Graduate Medical Education, the 2008 Resident Scholar Award from the AAFP Commission on Sciences, and the 2010 STFM Distinguished Research Paper Award. His research on food environments and nutrition disparities has been recognized with four consecutive contracts from the NIH Loan Repayment Program in Health Disparities. He has been a Pisacano Leadership Foundation Scholar, a Robert Wood Johnson Foundation Clinical Scholar, an Einstein Men's Division Scholar, and is currently a fellow (honorary distinction) in The Obesity Society. He is on the editorial board at *American Journal of Health Promotion*, reviews for 14 other journals on nutrition, public health, and family medicine, and has coauthored a textbook on epidemiology, biostatistics, preventive medicine, and public health.

CONTRIBUTING AUTHORS

Ather Ali, ND, MPH, MHS
Associate Research Scientist, Department
of Pediatrics
Integrative Medicine Specialist,
Yale Stress Center
Director, Integrative Medicine at Yale
Yale University School of Medicine
New Haven, Connecticut

Michelle M. Chen
Senior Medical Student
Yale University School of Medicine
New Haven, Connecticut

Kimberly N. Doughty, MPH
Doctoral Candidate in Nutrition
University of Massachusetts Amherst
Research Associate
Yale-Griffin Prevention Research Center
New Haven, Connecticut

Asiri S. Ediriwickrema
Senior Medical Student
Yale University School of Medicine
New Haven, Connecticut

Kofi D. Essel, MD
Senior Pediatric Resident—Community
Health Track
Children's National Medical Center
Washington, District of Columbia

Jonathan Fu, MD, MHS
Department of Emergency Medicine
University of California San Francisco
Medical Center
San Francisco, California

Richard Joseph, BS
MD/MBA Candidate
Stanford University School of Medicine
Stanford, California

Stacey Kallem, MD
Resident Physician
Children's Hospital of Philadelphia
Philadelphia, Pennsylvania

Dhruv Khullar
Senior Medical Student
Yale School of Medicine
New Haven, Connecticut

Jessica J. Kim, MD
Department of Family Practice and Surgery
Contra Costa Regional Medical Center
Martinez, California

Ashley Maltz, MD, MPH
Assistant Professor, Clinician Educator Track
University of New Mexico School of Medicine
Department of General Internal Medicine
Albuquerque, New Mexico

Stephanie M. Meller
Senior Medical Student
Yale University School of Medicine
New Haven, Connecticut

David Merrick, MD
Resident Physician in Internal Medicine
University of Pennsylvania
Philadelphia, Pennsylvania

Lindsay Moyer, MS, RD
Washington, DC

Maria F. Nardell
Senior Medical Student
Yale University School of Medicine
New Haven, Connecticut

Valentina Vinante, MD, MPH
Resident in Obstetrics and Gynaecology
Frauenklinik Fontana Chur, Switzerland

Ming-Chin Yeh, PhD, MEd, MS
Associate Professor
Nutrition Program
CUNY School of Public Health
Hunter College, City University of New York
New York, New York

There are two prior editions of *Nutrition in Clinical Practice*, and thus two prior prefaces. That argues for brevity this time around, and I gladly concede.

That there is an opportunity for a third addition is testimony to the success of the first two. I find that gratifying, of course, but it is credit we share. This endeavor was always about practice more than theory; reading and application, more than writing. I am grateful so many colleagues recognize the relevance of nutrition to their practices and patients. It is upon that shared conviction that the rationale for this effort rests.

That there is need for a new edition is likely self-evident. The medical literature is not only vast, but growing at an ever accelerating pace. The nearly 10,000 citations in this third edition testify to how salient nutrition research is in that formidable flow of information. This new edition updates both content and citations, while reaffirming those fundamentals of nutrition that have stood the test of time. Those, too, are salient.

At the outset, we had thought to add many new chapters, but found that much of the new content situated itself comfortably into existing chapters. When it wasn't broken, we decided not to fix it. Many chapters thus have new sections, and all have been comprehensively revised; but the basic structure of the book and sequence of chapters is much as it was. My hope is that familiarity in this case will breed only accessibility and user-friendliness.

We did add a section on current, and controversial, topics in clinical nutrition. This section cannot, of course, be comprehensive; nor can it promise to be entirely current at the time of publication, let alone some number of months or years after that. The preoccupation with nutrition and diet in popular culture shifts rapidly, if redundantly, over time. This section is, more than anything, an acknowledgment of that preoccupation; of its relevance to clinical practice and counseling; and of the important opportunity to approach such topics with the same dispassionate review of evidence germane to all other subjects in this diverse space. Those principles should remain reliably current.

Perhaps most importantly, the third edition is the beneficiary of a wonderful hybrid vigor, courtesy of my diverse team of associate and assistant authors. Associate authors, Drs. Friedman and Lucan, bring to the project well cultivated knowledge of nutrition and a pragmatism born of regular clinical practice. The larger group of assistant authors encompasses medical students, dietitians, public health professionals, naturopathic physicians, and nutritional epidemiologists—all committed to the same goal of reconciling the robust evidence base underlying nutrition and health with the constraints of clinical practice, for the benefit of provider and patient alike.

The captain, we know, goes down with the ship; but he (historically) or she cannot generally sail it alone. A book like this is much the same. And so it is that I am indebted to the team without whom I would have found this update an oppressive venture at best, but must personally accept responsibility for any lapses in our seaworthiness. Should there prove to be any important omissions or inadvertent misrepresentations, I am accountable for them. I am hopeful there will be few, if any.

We have worked hard to bring you a distillation of the current evidence in nutrition, enriched by relevant theory, but devoted to practice. And so it is that we go once more into the breach, together, in an effort to translate what we know about nutrition and health into what we do. A succession of editions is all well and good, but the true measure of our collective success is the years this body of knowledge can add to the lives of our patients, and the life it can add to their years. May those metrics reward us all.

—*David L. Katz*

While compiling this text, I have been as committed to what it excludes as to what it includes. Excellent, comprehensive textbooks, even encyclopedias, of nutrition have been written. I have made use of a good many of them in this effort. But as it may, in fact, be considered true that we "are" what we eat, such books cover a vast array of topics in agonizing details. Agonizing, that is, for the clinician seeking the answers to clinical questions but quite appropriate for the nutritional biochemist.

First among the principles to which this text is devoted is *clinical relevance*. If material seemed likely to be of use to the clinician interacting with a patient, even occasionally, it was included. If such an application seemed far-fetched, or if the material did not support an understanding that would enhance such an exchange, it was left out. The range of nutrition topics germane to clinical care is quite expansive. Thus, a fairly selective inclusion process resulted in leaving quite a lot still to be said.

The second principle governing the compilation of this text is *consistency of application*. Only in books do states of health and disease, and the underlying factors that promote them, stay neatly in their own columns and rows. In reality, these states coexist in single patients, often in complex abundance. Therefore, mutually exclusive, disease-specific nutrition recommendations are apt to be of limited clinical utility. Conversely, if dietary recommendations never change in accommodation to varying states of health and clinical objectives, a book of many chapters seems an excessive effort to portray this set of uniform guidelines. I have sought the middle ground between the subtle applications of nutritional management that pertain to the occasional disease or risk factor and the unifying features of diet that may be universally applied to promote health.

The third principle governing this effort is that to be of use, material intended for clinical application must be described in terms of the extent, consistency, and quality, of *the underlying evidence*. This may be considered a text of evidence-based medicine, with the literature reviewed for each chapter considered to represent preliminary, suggestive, or definitive evidence of any association described.

I strove to be consistent in the application of such terms, but found myself sometimes using, for example, "conclusive" rather than "definitive." Despite such variation, the character of the evidence base should generally be clear. Associations supported by animal or in vitro or observational evidence only were considered *preliminary*; associations supported by a combination of basic science studies as well as observational studies in humans, or by limited interventional studies in humans, were considered *suggestive*; and associations subtended by the results of either large-scale human intervention trials (particularly randomized, controlled trials), or the aggregation of consistent results from numerous less rigorous studies were considered *definitive*.

The fourth principle, related to the third, is that for a subject of scrutiny to be well understood, it must be *viewed in its entirety* (or some approximation thereof). There is a risk (although certainly, too, a benefit) when each of many experts elaborates one particular aspect of nutrition as it pertains to health. That risk was perhaps never better expressed than in the allegorical poem, *The Blind Men and the Elephant*, by John Godfrey Saxe. I in no way wish to suggest that the expert authors of detailed chapters in the standard nutrition texts suffer any semblance of blindness, but rather that something of the overall character of nutrition and health is missed when only a small part is examined in great detail. I have become convinced, for example, that nominal n-3 fatty acid deficiency is likely widespread in the United States and contributing to adverse health outcomes. This conclusion is reached less on the basis of definitive evidence in any one area and more on the basis of remarkably consistent and voluminous evidence in the aggregate, across the expanse of many subjects. Only one author, struggling through each of many chapters in turn, may infuse the characterization of each topic with understanding derived from the others. As I cannot dispute the potential disadvantages of solo authorship, I have sought instead to capitalize fully on any potential advantages. I have therefore freely shared what insights I have gained in the sequential review of so many topics, endeavoring at all times to be clear about the sources of my opinion and the nature of the evidence.

The final principle to which this text is devoted is the notion that there should be a *theoretical model* in which the complex interplay of human behavior, food, and health outcomes is decipherable. In much the same way that unifying threads of evidence have led me to specific recommendations for nutrition management, I have come through this labor convinced of the utility of the *evolutionary biology model* of human dietary behavior. This argument is elaborated in Chapter 39. The behavior and physiology of all animals are largely governed by the environments to which they adapted; there is both reason and evidence to suggest that, with regard to nutrition, the same is true of us.

While there is some interpretation offered in this text, it is only that which a devotee and teacher of evidence-based principles of medicine could abide and not avoid. In the inescapable need to convey to you my interpretations, I have endeavored to cleave as close and consistently to fact as possible. In the time-honored medical tradition of blending the best of available science with just the requisite art, I submit this work to you as a platform for the clinical practice of nutrition.

Following the introduction, a concise but comprehensive overview of dietary influences on the organ system or pathology under discussion is provided. The overview is generally divided into the influence of the overall dietary pattern (*Diet*) and the influence of specific nutrient (*Nutrients/Nutriceuticals*). As indicated, other topics are included in the overview, such as pathophysiology, epidemiology, and other issues of clinical relevance and/or general interest. The overview section uses the scheme above to rate the available evidence for each practice. Unpublished and non–peer-reviewed literature has been accessed as required to facilitate preparation of this text, but the assessment of evidence is based only on the peer-reviewed literature; references are to be found at the end of each chapter. Following the overview, other *Topics of Interest* not related directly to dietary management are provided as indicated (e.g., surgical management of severe

obesity). Chapters conclude with *Clinical Highlights*, a summary of those nutritional interventions of greatest clinical utility and for which the evidence is decisive, convincing, or suggestive. Each chapter is cross-referenced with other chapters and with pertinent *Nutrient/Nutriceutical Reference Tables* and other *Nutrition Resource Materials* in Section III.

Claims, Disclaimers, and Acknowledgments

Solo authorship of a text on nutrition may seem an act of either brash imprudence or unpardonable hubris. At times, poring over references and painstakingly compiling chapters, I have been tempted to think it both. But, please accept my assurances that it is neither. There is very definitely method in the potential madness of this project.

I am a clinician with an active practice in primary care internal medicine. Every day in the office I am confronted by the abiding interest of my patients in their own nutritional practices and by the innumerable attendant questions. And to be of use to my patients, to offer guidance when guidance is needed, I must have the answers at hand. I can certainly refer to a dietitian for counseling in support of clinical goals, but hardly as a means of answering each question that comes along.

So the clinician in practice, encountering what I in my practice encounter every day, must be able to answer a range of questions about nutrition and health, nutrition and disease. If unable to do so, the clinician misses a crucial opportunity to influence favorably the role of dietary behavior in the mitigation of chronic disease. On the list of the leading causes of death in the United States, dietary practices rank number 2, just behind smoking.

My nutrition expertise, cultivated by training, research, and teaching over the past 15 years, is appropriate for this project. But I certainly cannot claim to have the consummate knowledge in each of the diverse content areas of this text that is owned by that field's luminaries. To those experts, far too numerous to mention here, I owe a monumental debt. I have endeavored to make their work accessible to an audience of clinicians, but, in doing so, I have traveled the many trails they so painstakingly blazed.

My legitimacy, or perhaps my excuse, then, is not so much my claim to expertise in everything from lipid metabolism to ergogenic aids, but rather my dual devotion to nutrition and to clinical practice. The experts to whom I am indebted have made their contributions to the literature, yet the accessibility of that literature to the busy practitioner is suspect. This text is as much translation as original work, the translation of current nutrition knowledge into a form useful to the clinician. This text of nutrition is both by, and for, the practicing clinician. If any one practitioner is to access all of this information and apply it to clinical practice, it is only reasonable that one clinician has been able to write it.

And so that is why I have written this text and justified the interminable hours of effort to myself. To those whose work has guided me, I offer thanks. For any omissions, or worse still, misrepresentations, I accept full responsibility (who else could I blame?). Yet even this solo effort has depended, and greatly benefited, from the direct and indirect contributions of many individuals. I owe debts of gratitude; I have little hope to repay to those who made this book possible.

—*David L. Katz*

ACKNOWLEDGMENTS

First, and perhaps foremost, I am grateful to the panoply of researchers whose work is cited throughout this text. The effort of writing this book seemed considerable, but is of course vanishingly trivial in comparison to compiling the evidence on which it is based. This text is principally a distillation of evidence, and inclines with the vast weight of it. The many who have contributed to that mass of information are my teachers, my mentors, and in some cases, my heroes. I am indebted to this community of scholarship.

I owe thanks to my literary agent, Rick Broadhead, who helped navigate all of us—ably, as ever—from aspiration to collaboration. I very much appreciate the timely, supportive, and always professional contributions of our editors at Wolters Kluwer Health–Lippincott Williams & Wilkins, in particular Sonya Seigafuse, Rebecca Gaertner, and Kristina Oberle. My thanks as well to others involved in the many ancillary efforts critical to completion of a book, from graphic art for the cover to careful proofing, production, and marketing.

I was delighted to work again with my friend and colleague, Dr. Rachel Friedman, and to add to the mix my friend and colleague, Dr. Sean Lucan. The project is the better for both of their contributions. I am grateful to Dr. Lucan particularly for helping out when the new demands of motherhood put Rachel in the bind of choosing between our timeline, or maybe getting an occasional hour of sleep. We came through as a team, and I am grateful.

I am grateful as well to the other members of our expanded team, the assistant authors who helped us divvy up and update these many chapters. The basic obligations unified us, but the diversity of backgrounds and perspectives undoubtedly fortified us as well. My thanks, and congratulations, to the expanded team that worked harmoniously throughout the process and brought the product to its timely completion.

Thanks, as ever, to my administrative assistant, Helen Day, who gets me where I need to be when competing demands on my time—including those involved in writing a book— make me a bit dizzy.

Lastly, and most intimately, I acknowledge the debt I owe my family for the love and support that is inevitably the sustenance for such endeavors as this. That they remain both covetous of time with me and willing to forgo it unbegrudgingly when duty calls is a source of pride and appreciation, love and humility. I imagine my coauthors have similar debts, and similar sentiments. Writing books means many hours alone—but it is the larger something of which we are, alone, just a part that makes books and writing matter. So thank you, too.

CONTENTS

Nutrition in
Clinical Practice

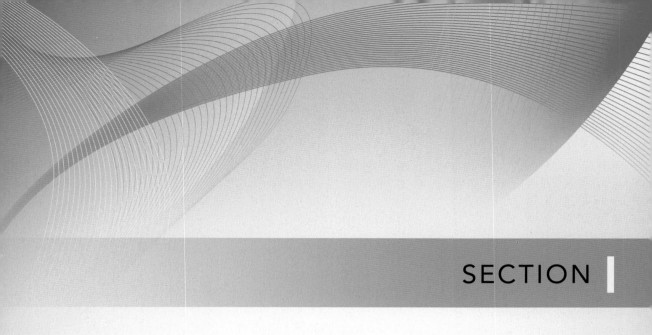

Clinically Relevant Nutrient Metabolism

CHAPTER 1

Clinically Relevant Carbohydrate Metabolism

Carbohydrate represents the predominant form of all living matter and is thus the principal dietary source of energy for humans in virtually every culture. Plants are composed principally of carbohydrate, the bulk of which consists of starch, the carbohydrate energy reserve in plants, and cellulose, which makes up cell walls. Generally between 50% and 70% of calories are derived from carbohydrate among human populations, with higher amounts prevailing in less developed countries.

The main metabolic function of dietary carbohydrate is to provide energy. Carbohydrate metabolism is principally directed toward the maintenance, utilization, and storage of carbohydrate energy reserves, in the form of circulating glucose and tissue-bound glycogen. Glucose in plasma is the most readily available energy source for cells, and thus homeostatic mechanisms for the maintenance of relatively stable blood glucose levels must be robust, absent pathology (see Chapter 6). Glycogen acts as a storage carbohydrate in animal cells, analogous to the role of starch in plants. From culinary and gustatory perspectives, carbohydrates contribute significantly to the palatability of food, most notably when conferring sweetness. Unlike protein, which provides essential amino acids, and fat, which provides essential fatty acids, the carbohydrate nutrient class does not, *a priori*, denote a specific group of essential nutrients; however, it serves as the principal dietary source of vitamins and minerals for many people. Furthermore, because fiber is classified as carbohydrate (see Section VIIE), dietary fiber intake is derived primarily from carbohydrate-rich foods. Dietary fiber can be classified as viscous (pectin, β-glucan, guar gum) and nonviscous (cellulose, lignin, hemicellulose). Carbohydrates are so named because their chemical structure, $C_n(H_2O)_n$, consists of carbon and water molecules in a 1:1 ratio. Digestible carbohydrates include polysaccharides and the sugars of the monosaccharide and disaccharide classes (see Table 1-1). In structural terms, the polysaccharide macromolecules are "complex" carbohydrate and the mono- and disaccharides are "simple" carbohydrate. Polysaccharides include cellulose and starches, of which only starch is digestible. The starches that predominate in the human diet, amylose and amylopectin, are glucose polymers. Starch is sequestered in plant cells behind a robust cell wall, rendering it relatively resistant to digestion until the cell wall is disrupted by heat and moisture during cooking. There are several categories of "resistant starch," which remains inaccessible to digestion despite exposure to heat (1). In the typical Western diet, approximately 2% to 5% of ingested starch is resistant. Resistant starches stimulate the growth of colonic bacteria that in turn ferment the starches into short-chain fatty acids.

Disaccharides include sucrose, a molecule composed of glucose and fructose; lactose, a molecule composed of glucose and galactose; and maltose, two molecules of glucose. Monosaccharides of dietary importance include glucose, which is derived principally from the hydrolysis of dietary starch, fructose, and galactose. The five-carbon monosaccharides, ribose and deoxyribose, are synthesized endogenously for the production of nucleic acids. Sorbitol is the alcohol of glucose. The alcohol of xylose, xylitol, is used as a sweetener in the food industry.

Carbohydrate can be absorbed only in the form of monosaccharides. Therefore, all complex carbohydrates must undergo hydrolysis in the gut. This process begins in the mouth with the release of salivary amylase, which disrupts the α-1,4-glucosidic bonds of amylose, a straight chain glucose polymer, breaking it down to maltose and

TABLE 1.1

The Classification of Carbohydrate as Simple or Complex, Based on Structural and Functional Properties[a]

		Function	
		Simple	Complex
Structure	*Simple*	Monosaccharides (glucose, galactose, fructose) and disaccharides (maltose, sucrose, lactose) added to foods or beverages in processing or present in foods low in other, more complex, carbohydrate, especially fiber	Monosaccharides or disaccharides packaged in foods that contain fiber, complex starch, and/or protein or fat
		Representative foods: sugar-sweetened soft drinks, sugary breakfast cereals	Representative foods: fruits, vegetables, yogurt
	Complex	Polysaccharide starch, amylopectin	Polysaccharide starch, amylase, celluloses, gums, pectins (fibers)
		Representative foods: white rice	Representative foods: whole grain wheat, beans, lentils

[a]See pages 7–9 for further discussion.

oligosaccharides. Amylopectin, the other primary constituent of plant starch that constitutes 80% of ingested polysaccharide, contains a branched α-1,6-glucosidic bonds that are resistant to amylase and is instead digested by isomaltase in the intestinal brush border.

The glucose linkages in cellulose are derived from a β-1,4 bond for which no enzyme is available, accounting for the indigestibility of cellulose. The products of the action of salivary and pancreatic amylase are maltose and maltotriose from amylose; and maltose, maltotriose, limit dextrin (a composite of 1,4-α and 1,6-α glucose molecules), and glucose from amylopectin. Structurally, amylopectin is more complex than amylose; however, serum glucose levels rise more rapidly after the ingestion of amylopectin than amylose, suggesting that functionally, amylose is the more complex starch (2). This discrepancy between structure and bioavailability highlights the difficulty in reliably distinguishing between simple and complex carbohydrate (see pages 7–9).

Starches in whole foods, such as grains and legumes, are packaged together with proteins and fiber that can interfere with digestion by acting as a physical barrier to amylase. Thus, the efficiency with which starch is converted to glucose depends not only on the structure of the starch itself but also on the overall composition of the food of which it is a part (3).

When carbohydrate intake is very high, the glucose load can be handled in one of two ways. Excess glucose can be taken into cells and stored as glycogen or fat, as is the case in nondiabetic individuals. If the carbohydrate load cannot be taken up into cellular storage, excess glucose builds up in the blood stream, resulting in the development of diabetes mellitus (see Chapter 06). The liver and muscle are the primary depots for glucose, where it is stored in the form of glycogen.

Increasing plasma glucose levels result in energy release and oxidative phosphorylation generating adenosine triphosphate (ATP) and citrate via the citric acid cycle, an enzymatic cascade used by all aerobic organisms to generate ATP from the products of glycolysis. The citric acid cycle is initiated via the action of pyruvate dehydrogenase and citrate synthase, which initiate entry of pyruvate into the citric acid cycle. High levels of ATP provide negative feedback on the enzyme phosphofructokinase to decrease glycolysis, resulting in accumulation of the intermediate product fructose-6-phosphate. Fructose-6-phosphate is converted to fructose-2,6-biphosphate, which reactivates phosphofructokinase.

The marked rises in ATP and citrate produced by aerobic metabolism result in buildup of citric acid cycle substrates, including oxaloacetic acid and acetyl CoA, which act as potent stimulators of fatty acid synthesis. Consequently, a large dietary carbohydrate load results in body fat deposition as a means of preventing hyperglycemia. Some studies suggest that excess quantities of carbohydrate-rich foods such as high-fructose corn syrup can promote uric acid formation (4,5), leading to alkalinization of the urine and formation of ammonium acid urate kidney stones. Calories in excess of need, from any macronutrient source, are stored as body fat once glycogen stores are filled. The prototypical 70 kg adult can store approximately 300 g of glycogen, for a total carbohydrate energy reserve of approximately 1,200 kcal. When that reserve is filled, surplus calories from any macronutrient source are preferentially stored as fat (6).

The rate of glycolysis can be altered by as much as 90-fold in response to the metabolic needs of working muscle. Abundant carbohydrate intake induces glycolysis and inhibits gluconeogenesis, whereas fasting stimulates the inverse processes. Energy stores within the cell are carefully monitored by proteins that can send signals to influence metabolism in response to changes in energy levels. When ATP levels are high, the tricarboxylic acid cycle is slowed, and glycolysis is inhibited. Conversely, high levels of adenosine diphosphate (ADP) and adenosine monophosphate (AMP) induce glycolysis to regeneration of ATP.

Anaerobic glucose metabolism in muscle leads to the production of pyruvate, which can be further metabolized to CO_2 in muscle or transported to the liver. During vigorous physical activity, oxygen levels decrease, and the muscle tissue is unable to support the metabolism of pyruvate to CO_2. Anaerobic metabolism ensues to reoxidize nicotinamide adenine dinucleotide (NADH) formed during glycolysis, resulting in the production of lactate. The accumulation of lactic acid during vigorous activity is potentially responsible for the muscle pain that often develops, although this theory has been contested (7).

Carbohydrate in the cytosol plays an essential role in protein glycosylation and is tightly regulated by cellular enzymes. When blood glucose levels are abnormally high, however, abnormal glycosylation, or glycation, can occur outside the cell. Proteins in tissues continuously exposed to the circulating glucose are particularly vulnerable, including the glomerular basement membrane, the vascular endothelium, and the lens of the eye. Glucose and galactose are metabolized in the lens of the eye, and elevated serum levels of either are associated with cataract formation. Thus, both diabetes mellitus and galactosemia are risk factors for cataract formation.

Glycation constitutes an important cumulative injury to cells that is associated with aging, linking high consumption of sugar to premature or accelerated aging of cells (see Chapter 31). Fructose glycates nearly 10 times as efficiently as glucose. However, even at high intake, the fructose level in blood is only about 10% that of glucose. Thus, fructose may contribute equally to glycation as glucose when intake is high.

Several potential replacement sweeteners are in development, including the sugar D-tagatose, which demonstrates a significantly lower lever of glycation compared with glucose (8). Starch is degraded upon exposure to pancreatic amylase and intestinal brush border enzymes in the upper and middle portions of the jejunum. Brush border enzymes include isomaltase, sucrase, and lactase (in some adults; see Chapter 24). An excess of enzyme is available for most oligosaccharide digestion, with the exception of lactose. Lactase availability limits the rate at which lactose is cleaved to glucose and galactose. Brush border enzymes are inhibited as levels of monosaccharides rise in the intestinal lumen, preventing an accumulation of sugars that could result in osmotic diarrhea. Dietary sucrose induces the enzymes sucrase and maltase. Lactase levels, however, are not influenced by the quantity of dietary lactose.

Starches resistant to enzymatic digestion are fermented by bacteria in the large bowel, which liberate 50% to 80% of the available energy in the form of fatty acids and release carbon dioxide and methane as byproducts. The fatty acids produced in the large bowel include butyric, isobutyric, propionic, and acetic acids. Cells of the large bowel derive energy from butyric acid and isobutyric acid in particular, and these molecules may play an important role in protecting the bowel mucosa from carcinogens.

Monosaccharides are absorbed by simple diffusion, facilitated diffusion, and active transport. The L-isomers of glucose and galactose are absorbed exclusively by passive diffusion. Ingestion of a 50 g load of any of these sugars will exceed the rate of absorption through passive diffusion, resulting in gastrointestinal (GI) discomfort. Passive diffusion is slowed by the movement of water into the gut lumen produced by the osmotic effect of ingested sugars. The D-stereoisomers of glucose and galactose are absorbed through protein cannels by active transport, facilitating more rapid uptake into the blood than passive diffusion. Fructose, a monosaccharide derived from sucrose, is absorbed via facilitated diffusion. Osmotic diarrhea is induced by the acute ingestion of approximately 100 g of fructose; more sugar is tolerated if ingested as sucrose, because digestion of the disaccharide shows the rate of absorption.

Lactase deficiency, the most common enzyme deficiency affecting carbohydrate metabolism, is present in approximately half of all adults worldwide. Besides humans, milk ingestion is typically limited to infancy in most animal; therefore, the lactase gene is expressed predominantly in infancy and deactivated thereafter. Lactose ingestion in adulthood favored the selection of genetic mutations that preserved lactase production into adulthood. Variation in adult lactose tolerance by ethnic background appears to correlate with the practice of dairying over millennia, although a causal association has not been elucidated. Lactose-intolerant adults can generally tolerate about 5 g of lactose (equal to approximately 100 mL [3.4 oz] of milk) without symptoms (see Chapter 24). Lactose tolerance can be assessed by administering 50 g of lactose and measuring the serum glucose. If glucose rises more than 1.4 mmol per L, the lactose has been efficiently hydrolyzed.

Glucose is the principal source of nutrient energy. It is metabolized to carbon dioxide and water via the tricarboxylic acid cycle. Alternatively, glucose can be stored as glycogen or converted to fatty acids for deposition in adipose tissue. Approximately 5% of the available energy from oxidation is lost when glucose is converted to glycogen, and more than 25% is lost when glucose is stored as fat. Glycogen stores in muscle and the liver account for approximately 300 g, or 1,200 kcal, sufficient to meet the energy needs of a fasting adult on a 2,000 kcal diet for approximately 14 hours. Nearly 100 times as much energy, or 120,000 kcal, is stored in the adipose tissue of a lean adult. However, only a small portion of this energy is readily available, generally enough to support energy needs for up to 10 days. Once glycogen stores are full, excess dietary carbohydrate is converted to fatty acids and stored in adipose tissue. The efficiency with which different sugars are converted to fat is variable.

As an energy source, carbohydrate is intermediate between fat and protein with regard to both energy density and satiety induction. Carbohydrate provides roughly 4 kcal per g, which is slightly more than that of protein. The satiety index of carbohydrate—meaning the degree to which a given "dose," measured in calories, induces a sense of fullness—is higher than that of fat and lower than that of protein (see Chapter 38). Complex carbohydrate is more satiating than simple carbohydrate, due largely to the fiber content. Viscous fibers have been shown to reduce appetite more readily than nonviscous fibers by slowing the emptying of the stomach and acting as a physical barrier that shields carbohydrates from digestive enzymes (9). Fiber adds volume but not calories to food, and soluble fiber may contribute to satiety by other mechanisms as well (see Chapter 38 and Section VIIE).

After carbohydrate ingestion, most of the glucose in the circulation escapes hepatic first-pass removal, whereas most fructose is absorbed by the liver, where it is used to produce glucose, lipid, or lactate. Fructose ingestion raises serum levels of both lactic acid and uric acid. Galactose is metabolized principally in the liver and the rate of metabolism can serve as a marker of liver function. Galactose rises in serum in proportion to the dose ingested, although serum levels of galactose are blunted by concomitant administration of glucose, either orally or intravenously.

Most tissues utilize a variety of nutrients for fuel, but the brain and red blood cells rely solely on glucose, except in periods of prolonged fasting, during which they can covert to ketone-body metabolism. Congenital deficiency of the enzyme glucose-6-phosphate dehydrogenase principally affects the red blood cells, occurring in populations with historical exposure to malaria. These individuals are susceptible to hemolysis in the presence of drugs that disrupt glutathione reduction, such as sulfonamides.

The adult brain requires approximately 140 g of glucose per day, accounting for 560 kcal. Glucose needs increase during pregnancy and lactation, during which glucose is used in the production of lactose. Both amino acids and triglycerides can be used to synthesize glucose. Gluconeogenesis can produce approximately 130 g of glucose per day in the absence of carbohydrate ingestion if other nutrients are abundant. Although the glucose deficit can be compensated by ketone-body metabolism, fat oxidation also requires glucose. Once glycogen stores are depleted, therefore, a minimal intake of 50 g of glucose in any form appears to be necessary. Glucose can be produced endogenously, and it is thus not considered an essential nutrient. However, the recognition that a balanced diet requires carbohydrate has resulted in the establishment of a recommended dietary allowance (RDA) for adults of 130 g of sugar or starch daily (10).

A diet rich in fructose (20% to 25% of total energy intake) results in elevated serum triglycerides and LDL, although levels tend to normalize over a period of weeks in lean individuals, whereas a diet rich in glucose has the opposite effect (11). Conversely, a high-glucose diet results in elevated serum glucose and insulin levels, which are unaffected by a high-fructose diet (12). High-carbohydrate diets lower levels of high-density lipoproteins, especially when compounded with high-fructose intake. Consequently, a diet high in sucrose has deleterious effects on the lipid profile, whereas these effects are partially mitigated in a diet containing predominantly complex carbohydrates (13). Polyunsaturated fat in the diet also blunts the fasting triglyceride rise induced by sucrose, and decreases LDL (14,15). Individuals with hypertriglyceridemia tend to have a particularly brisk rise in triglycerides in response to high-carbohydrate intake.

CARBOHYDRATE METABOLISM AND THE ENDOCRINE SYSTEM

Glucose levels in the blood are primarily regulated by the action of insulin and glucagon, released from the beta-cells of the pancreas. The main role of insulin is to promote energy entry and storage in cells when blood glucose levels are high, which is accomplished via several mechanisms: translocation of GLUT-4 glucose transporters to the plasma membrane, which facilitates glucose entry into liver, skeletal muscle, and adipose tissues; stimulation of glycogen and fat formation; inhibition of fat utilization for energy via suppression of glucagon release; inhibition of gly-coneogenesis by the liver. Glucagon is released when blood glucose levels fall, and its actions are directly opposite of those produced by insulin, promoting glycogen breakdown to release glucose and synthesis of new glucose via gluconeogenesis in the liver and kidney.

The gut has emerged as a major regulator of carbohydrate metabolism with discovery of the role of incretins, peptide hormones released from the intestinal L cell in response to the presence of nutrients in the lumen of the small intestine. GLP-1, one of the most well characterized incretins, acts to lower blood glucose via stimulation of insulin release, increasing insulin sensitivity in the tissues, promoting beta-cell mass, suppression of glucagon secretion, delaying gastric emptying, and increasing satiety in the brain.

The adrenal gland also plays a role in glucose homeostasis via release of epinephrine, which stimulate glycogenolysis in the liver. Epinephrine also stimulates glycogenolysis in skeletal muscle, whereas glucagon does not.

THE COMPLEXITY OF CARBOHYDRATE

Despite widespread use of the terminology, clear definitions of "complex" and "simple" carbohydrate are elusive, in part because such definitions rely on structural or functional classifications. According to the National Library of Medicine's *Medical Encyclopedia* (16), a simple carbohydrate is composed of mono- or disaccharides, while complex carbohydrates are composed of units containing three or more sugar molecules (see Table 1-1). This definition is structural rather than functional, and is oversimplifed in several important ways. For example, whole grain bread is commonly classified as a complex carbohydrate and, table sugar, a simple carbohydrate, the reality is that breads and other products labeled as "whole grain" may contain varying amounts of whole grain, varying amounts of refined grain, and, often, additions of sugar. Thus, the actual food item is a mix of simple and complex carbohydrates based on a structural definition. Many fruits contain the monosaccharide fructose, and many vegetables contain the disaccharide maltose, facilitating a functionally misleading classification of fruits and vegetables as "simple" carbohydrates based solely on the structural definition.

A functional definition of carbohydrate complexity is based on the metabolic fate of ingested items. Foods that engender a brisk rise in blood glucose, and consequently blood insulin, are considered simple carbohydrates from a functional perspective. Foods that induce low and slow postingestive increases in glucose and insulin are functionally complex carbohydrates. In such a scheme, fruits and vegetables would be considered sources of complex, rather than simple, carbohydrate, which conforms better to prevailing views on their place in a healthful diet. This would not refute the presence in such foods of structurally simple carbohydrate but would take into account how nutrients are packaged in such foods and base characterization on the overall influence of the food on metabolic response rather than on the chemical structure of a given constituent.

A functional rather than structural approach to the characterization of carbohydrate complexity is generally quite consistent with glycemic load (GL) values and less so with glycemic index (GI) values (17) (see The Glycemic Index and Glycemic Load on pages 8–9, Tables 1-2 and 1-3). Given the increasing evidence that low-GL diets may offer diverse health benefits (18–32; see Chapters 5 and 6), this would seem to lend support for functional categorization.

TABLE 1.2

The Glycemic Index of Some Common Foods

Food Group	Food	Glycemic Index
Breads	White bread[a]	100
	Whole wheat bread	99
	Pumpernickel	78
Cereal products	Cornflakes	119
	Shredded wheat	97
	Oatmeal	85
	White rice	83
	Spaghetti	66
	Bulgur wheat	65
	Barley	31
Fruit	Raisins	93
	Bananas	79
	Oranges	66
	Grapes	62
	Apples	53
	Cherries	32
Vegetables	Parsnips	141
	Baked potato	135
	Carrots	133
	Corn	87
	Boiled potato	81
	Peas	74
	Yams	74
Legumes	Lima beans	115
	Baked beans	60
	Chick peas	49
	Red lentils	43
	Peanuts	19
Dairy products	Yogurt	52
	Ice cream	52
	Milk	49
Sugar	Sucrose	86

[a]Reference standard. In some applications, sucrose rather than white bread is used as the reference standard, and given a value of 100.

Source: Adapted from Jenkins DJA, Jenkins AL. The glycemic index, fiber, and the dietary treatment of hypertriglyceridemia and diabetes. *J Am Coll Nutr* 1987;6:11–17

TABLE 1.3

The Glycemic Index and Glycemic Load of Some Common Foods[a]

Food/Portion	Carbohydrate (g)	Glycemic Index	Glycemic Load
Potato/1 each, 170 g	43	85	37
Carrots/0.5 c, 78 g[b]	8	47	4
Apple/each, 154 g	22	38	8
Apple juice/1 cup	29	40	12
Soft drink/20 fl oz	68	63	43
Milk/1 cup	12	27	3
Lentils/0.5 cup, 99 g	20	29	6
Peanuts/3 T, 30 g	5	14	1
Instant rice/0.75 cup, 124 g	26	91	24
Spaghetti/0.75 cup, 105 g	30	44	13

[a]For the GI and GL scores for an extensive list of foods, see American Journal of Clinical Nutrition. *Revised international table of GI values.* Available at http://www.ajcn.org/cgi/content/full/76/1/5#SEC2; accessed 9/18/07.

[b]Note that although carrots and soft drinks have rather comparable GI scores, their GL scores differ by more than an order of magnitude.

Source: Adapted from Foster-Powell K, Holt SH, Brand-Miller JC. International table of glycemic index and glycemic load values. *Am J Clin Nutr* 2002;76:5–56.

Another wrinkle in the definition of carbohydrate complexity is the manner in which foods package nutrients. While sugar added to a whole grain breakfast cereal is structurally similar to that added to a candy bar, its metabolic fate is influenced by the company it keeps. Fiber in grain products, in particular soluble fiber (see Section VIIE), slows the entry of glucose (and lipids) from the GI tract into the bloodstream, attenuating postprandial glycemia, lipemia, and insulinemia (18,33–36). Fiber added to food during processing, including inulin, polydextrose, and maltodextrin, share some laxative properties with natural fibers; however, their effect on blood glucose and cholesterol are quite modest (37).

For this reason, there is a practical rationale for classifying foods as sources of simple or complex carbohydrate based on their overall nutritional composition and the metabolic fate of the carbohydrate they provide. Because the chemical classification of carbohydrate as simple or complex does not adequately reflect metabolic responses to different foods, nomenclature in this area is a matter of considerable dispute (38,39).

While this dispute plays out, the clinician is encouraged to consider whole grains, vegetables, fruits, beans, and legumes as sources of complex carbohydrate based on the metabolic implications of their dietary intake (40). Products in which added sugar and/or refined (white) flour are principal ingredients as well as grain products low in fiber content should be considered, from a functional perspective, simple carbohydrate sources.*

CARBOHYDRATE RESTRICTION FOR WEIGHT LOSS

The popularity of carbohydrate restriction as a weight loss aid peaked since the first edition of *Nutrition in Clinical Practice* was published; the trend has subsequently lost considerable momentum (41,42). In general, the wholesale rejection of a macronutrient class may facilitate weight loss in the short term by restricting choice and thus calories but is at odds with the nutrient balance required for optimal health and the dietary balance required for pleasure and sustainability (43). Long-term carbohydrate

*A grain product—bread, cereal, cracker, etc.—providing less than 2 g fiber per 100 calories is relatively low in fiber, generally highly processed, and apt to have a high GL; therefore, such foods are functionally simple carbohydrate sources. An exception is whole grains such as brown rice, which are intrinsically lower in fiber than other grains commonly consumed. The GI, and load, of low-fiber grains tends to be higher than that of high-fiber grains; see Tables 1-2 and 1-3.

restriction has not been shown to be superior to other dietary patterns for weight loss, and may actually precipitate adverse health outcomes (42). The practice of wholesale carbohydrate restriction therefore not encouraged, while selective restriction of sugar and simple carbohydrate certainly is. The restriction of simple sugars has been associated with improvements in nonalcoholic fatty liver (44). The topic of carbohydrate restriction is addressed in greater detail in Chapters 5 and 45.

NONNUTRITIVE SWEETENERS

Nonnutritive sweeteners, often referred to as "artificial sweeteners," have been in use for the past century to confer an appetizing sweet taste without contributing to the caloric content of food. The FDA has granted approval for five nonnutritive sweeteners: acesulfame potassium, aspartame, neotame, saccharin, and sucralose, and a naturally occurring low-calorie sweetener stevia (45). Nonnutritive sweeteners bind sweet taste receptors by mimicking the structural motifs of natural carbohydrates; however, they elicit an effective sweetness response 200 to 600 times stronger than table sugar. Because of this, they can be added to food in such small quantities as to negate their caloric contribution (46). For decades, nonnutritive sweeteners were considered an effective method of reducing caloric intake without sacrificing palatability of food and drink, however recent studies have produced evidence that their use may actually contribute to obesity in adults and children via dysregulation of energy balance (47–51).

Several hypotheses have emerged to explain the paradoxical association of nonnutritive sweeteners and weight gain. For example, nonnutritive sweeteners may alter the gut microbiological flora, triggering an inflammatory process that promotes insulin resistance and weight gain (52). Another potential mechanism suggests that the GI tract utilizes sweet taste as a means of predicting a high-calorie meal, and will alter its absorptive properties to compensate (53). Finally, the recent discovery of sweet taste receptors in the GI tract has provoked a new hypothesis that nonnutritive sweeteners inappropriately activate sugar receptors in the gut, leading to GLP-1 release and insertion of glucose transporters in intestinal epithelia (54–56).

THE GLYCEMIC INDEX AND GLYCEMIC LOAD

The GI, first developed by Dr. David Jenkins et al. (57) at the University of Toronto and initially used for diabetic exchange lists, entered into the popular lexicon with the advent of "low-carbohydrate" dieting in the 1990s (see Chapter 5). The GI is defined as the area under the two-hour postprandial curve for blood glucose values, relative to a reference standard (often white bread or table sugar) and based on a fixed dose of carbohydrate. Recently, the GL has gained increased popularity as a tool for dietary guidance and has been implicated in regulating food reward and cravings (58). The GL is the GI of a food multiplied by the amount of carbohydrate per serving. For example, while the GI would require a comparison between a small amount of ice cream and a very large serving of carrots to "fix" the dose of carbohydrate at the same value in each case, the GL would be based on the amount of carbohydrate in a typical serving of carrot or ice cream (see Tables 1-2 and 1-3).

There is mounting evidence that a low-GL diet is generally healthful and of particular value in ameliorating insulin resistance or impaired glycemic responses (59). As well, a low-GL diet has been associated with decreased risk of cancer (60,61), cardiovascular disease (62), and hypertension (63); however, the importance of applying GI or GL measures to the diets of healthy individuals has been questioned (64), and some of the health implications of low versus high GI/GL foods remain unresolved (60,65).

As a practical matter, guiding patients toward a less processed diet abundant in vegetables, fruits, and whole grains, along with healthful oils from plant sources and lean protein, as is clearly warranted on general principles (see Chapter 45), will also direct them toward a diet relatively low in overall GL. The converse is likely to be true as well (i.e., guidance toward a low-GL diet will result in increased intake of vegetables, fruits, and whole grains), but it need not be. Advice to consume "carbohydrate foods" with a low-GL will correspond closely with advice to eat more whole grains, vegetables, and fruits. However, foods high in fat, including saturated fat, but low in sugar or starch will also have a low-GL but not necessarily warrant a prominent place in a healthful diet. Thus, the clinician is encouraged to offer guidance to patients in terms of foods and their place in a health-promoting diet (see Chapters 45 and 47) rather than based on some isolated property of a food or food group.

REFERENCES

1. Keim NL, Levin RJ, Havel PJ. Carbohydrates. In: Shils ME, Shike M, Ross AC, Caballero B, Cousins RJ, eds. *Modern nutrition in health and disease*, 10th ed. Philadelphia, PA: Lippincott Williams & Wilkins, 2006:64–65.
2. van Amelsvoort JMM, Westrate JA. Amylose–amylopectin ratio in a meal affects postprandial values in male volunteers. *Am J Clin Nutr* 1992;55:712–718.
3. Gray GM. Digestion and absorption of carbohydrate. In: Stipanuk MH, ed. *Biochemical and physiological aspects of human nutrition*. Philadelphia, PA: Saunders, 2000:91–106.
4. Stirpe F, Della CE, Bonetti E, et al. Fructose-induced hyperuricaemia. *Lancet* 1970;2:1310–1311.
5. Nakagawa T, Hu HB, Zharikov S, et al. A causal role for uric acid in fructose-induced metabolic syndrome. *Am J Physiol Renal Physiol* 2006;290:F625–F631.
6. McGrane MM. Carbohydrate metabolism—synthesis and oxidation. In: Stipanuk MH, ed. *Biochemical and physiological aspects of human nutrition*. Philadelphia, PA: Saunders, 2000:158–210.
7. Cheung K, Hume P, Maxwell L. Delayed onset muscle soreness: treatment strategies and performance factors. *Sports Med* 2003;33:145–164.
8. Kim P. Current studies on biological tagatose production using L-arabinose isomerase: a review and future perspective. *Appl Microbiol Biotechnol* 2004;65:243–249.
9. Wanders AJ, van den Borne JJ, de Graaf C, et al. Effects of dietary fibre on subjective appetite, energy intake and body weight: a systematic review of randomized controlled trials. *Obes Rev* 2011;12:724–39.
10. Panel on Macronutrients, Food and Nutrition Board, Institute of Medicine of the National Academies of Science. Dietary carbohydrates: sugars and starches. In: *Dietary reference intakes for energy, carbohydrate, fiber, fat, fatty acids, cholesterol, protein, and amino acids*. Washington, DC: National Academy Press, 2002:265–338.
11. Angelopoulos TJ, Lowndes J, Zukley L, et al. The effect of high-fructose corn syrup consumption on triglycerides and uric acid. *J Nutr* 2009;139:1242S–1245S.
12. Schaefer EJ, Gleason JA, Dansinger ML. Dietary fructose and glucose differentially affect lipid and glucose homeostasis. *J Nutr* 2009;139(6):1257S–1262S.
13. Jiménez-Gómez Y, Marín C, Peérez-Martínez P, et al. A low-fat, high-complex carbohydrate diet supplemented with long-chain (n-3) fatty acids alters the postprandial lipoprotein profile in patients with metabolic syndrome. *J Nutr* 2010;140(9):1595–1601.
14. Roche HM, Gibney MJ. Effect of long-chain n-3 polyunsaturated fatty acids on fasting and postprandial triacylglycerol metabolism. *Am J Clin Nutr* 2000;71(1 suppl):232S–237S.
15. Mensink RP, Katan MB. Effect of dietary fatty acids on serum lipids and lipoproteins. A meta-analysis of 27 trials. *Arterioscler Thromb* 1992;12(8):911–919.
16. National Library of Medicine. *Medical encyclopedia.* Available at http://www.nlm.nih.gov/medlineplus/ency/article/002469.htm; accessed 9/4/06.
17. Buyken AE, Dettmann W, Kersting M, et al. Glycaemic index and glycaemic load in the diet of healthy schoolchildren: trends from 1990 to 2002, contribution of different carbohydrate sources and relationships to dietary quality. *Br J Nutr* 2005;94:796–803.
18. McMillan-Price J, Petocz P, Atkinson F, et al. Comparison of 4 diets of varying glycemic load on weight loss and cardiovascular risk reduction in overweight and obese young adults: a randomized controlled trial. *Arch Intern Med* 2006;166:1466–1475.
19. Liu S. Lowering dietary glycemic load for weight control and cardiovascular health: a matter of quality. *Arch Intern Med* 2006;166:1438–1439.
20. Hu Y, Block G, Norkus EP, et al. Relations of glycemic index and glycemic load with plasma oxidative stress markers. *Am J Clin Nutr* 2006;84:70–76.
21. Murakami K, Sasaki S, Takahashi Y, et al. Dietary glycemic index and load in relation to metabolic risk factors in Japanese female farmers with traditional dietary habits. *Am J Clin Nutr* 2006;83:1161–1169.
22. Wolever TM, Brand-Miller JC. Influence of glycemic index/load on glycemic response, appetite, and food intake in healthy humans. *Diabetes Care* 2006;29:474–475.
23. Pittas AG, Das SK, Hajduk CL, et al. A low-glycemic load diet facilitates greater weight loss in overweight adults with high insulin secretion but not in overweight adults with low insulin secretion in the CALERIE trial. *Diabetes Care* 2005;28:2939–2941.
24. Liese AD, Schulz M, Fang F, et al. Dietary glycemic index and glycemic load, carbohydrate and fiber intake, and measures of insulin sensitivity, secretion, and adiposity in the Insulin Resistance Atherosclerosis Study. *Diabetes Care* 2005;28:2832–2838.
25. Lajous M, Willett W, Lazcano-Ponce E, et al. Glycemic load, glycemic index, and the risk of breast cancer among Mexican women. *Cancer Causes Control* 2005;16:1165–1169.
26. Ebbeling CB, Leidig MM, Sinclair KB, et al. Effects of an ad libitum low-glycemic load diet on cardiovascular disease risk factors in obese young adults. *Am J Clin Nutr* 2005;81:976–982.
27. Pereira MA, Swain J, Goldfine AB, et al. Effects of a low-glycemic load diet on resting energy expenditure and heart disease risk factors during weight loss. *JAMA* 2004;292:2482–2490.
28. Ludwig DS. Glycemic load comes of age. *J Nutr* 2003;133:2695–2696.
29. Ebbeling CB, Leidig MM, Sinclair KB, et al. A reduced-glycemic load diet in the treatment of adolescent obesity. *Arch Pediatr Adolesc Med* 2003;157:773–779.
30. Pawlak DB, Ebbeling CB, Ludwig DS. Should obese patients be counselled to follow a low-glycaemic index diet? Yes. *Obes Rev* 2002;3:235–243.
31. Slyper A, Jurva J, Pleuss J, et al. Influence of glycemic load on HDL cholesterol in youth. *Am J Clin Nutr* 2005;81:376–379.
32. Davis MS, Miller CK, Mitchell DC. More favorable dietary patterns are associated with lower glycemic load in older adults. *J Am Diet Assoc* 2004;104:1828–1835.

33. Dahl WJ, Lockert EA, Cammer AL, et al. Effects of flax fiber on laxation and glycemic response in healthy volunteers. *J Med Food* 2005;8:508–511.

34. Wolf BW, Wolever TM, Lai CS, et al. Effects of a beverage containing an enzymatically induced-viscosity dietary fiber, with or without fructose, on the postprandial glycemic response to a high glycemic index food in humans. *Eur J Clin Nutr* 2003;57:1120–1127.

35. Nishimune T, Yakushiji T, Sumimoto T, et al. Glycemic response and fiber content of some foods. *Am J Clin Nutr* 1991;54:414–419.

36. Jenkins DJ, Jenkins AL. Dietary fiber and the glycemic response. *Proc Soc Exp Biol Med* 1985;180:422–431.

37. Raninen K, Lappi J, Mykkänen H, et al. Dietary fiber type reflects physiological functionality: comparison of grain fiber, inulin, and polydextrose. *Nutr Rev* 2011; 69(1):9–21.

38. Complex carbohydrates: the science and the label. *Nutr Rev* 1995;53:186–193.

39. Asp NG. Classification and methodology of food carbohydrates as related to nutritional effects. *Am J Clin Nutr* 1995;61(4 suppl):930s–937s.

40. Aller EE, Abete I, Astrup A, et al. Starches, sugars and obesity. *Nutrients* 2011;3(3):341–369.

41. Hellmich N. *Atkins: have we had our fill? USA Today.* January 08, 2005. Available at http://www.usatoday.com/news/health/2005-08-01-atkins_x.htm; accessed 9/4/06.

42. Frigolet ME, Ramos Barragán VE, Tamez González M. Low-carbohydrate diets: a matter of love or hate. *Ann Nutr Metab* 2011;58(4):320–334.

43. Katz DL. Competing dietary claims for weight loss: finding the forest through truculent trees. *Annu Rev Public Health* 2005;26:61–88.

44. Carvalhana S, Machado MV, Cortez-Pinto H. Improving dietary patterns in patients with nonalcoholic fatty liver disease. *Curr Opin Clin Nutr Metab Care* 2012;15(5):468–73.

45. Pepino MY, Bourne C. Non-nutritive sweeteners, energy balance, and glucose homeostasis. *Curr Opin Clin Nutr Metab Care* 2011;14(4):391–395.

46. Magnuson BA, Burdock GA, Doull J, et al. Aspartame: a safety evaluation based on current use levels, regulations, and toxicological and epidemiological studies. *Crit Rev Toxicol* 2007;37(8):629–727.

47. Sylvetsky A, Rother KI, Brown R. Artificial sweetener use among children: epidemiology, recommendations, metabolic outcomes, and future directions. *Pediatr Clin North Am* 2011;58(6):1467–1480.

48. Yang Q. Gain weight by "going diet?" Artificial sweeteners and the neurobiology of sugar cravings: neuroscience 2010. *Yale J Biol Med* 2010;83(2):101–108.

49. Mattes RD, Popkin BM. Nonnutritive sweetener consumption in humans: effects on appetite and food intake and their putative mechanisms. *Am J Clin Nutr* 2009;89(1):1–14.

50. Fowler SP, Williams K, Resendez RG, et al. Fueling the obesity epidemic? Artificially sweetened beverage use and long-term weight gain. *Obesity* (Silver Spring) 2008;16:1894–1900.

51. Dhingra R, Sullivan L, Jacques PF, et al. Soft drink consumption and risk of developing cardiometabolic risk factors and the metabolic syndrome in middle-aged adults in the community. *Circulation* 2007;116:480–488.

52. Vijay-Kumar M, Aitken JD, Carvalho FA, et al. Metabolic syndrome and altered gut microbiota in mice lacking Toll-like receptor 5. *Science* 2010;328:228–231.

53. Swithers SE, Davidson TL. A role for sweet taste: calorie predictive relations in energy regulation by rats. *Behav Neurosci* 2008;122:161–173.

54. Jang HJ, Kokrashvili Z, Theodorakis MJ, et al. Gut-expressed gustducin and taste receptors regulate secretion of glucagon-like peptide-1. *Proc Natl Acad Sci USA* 2007;104:15069–15074.

55. Margolskee RF, Dyer J, Kokrashvili Z, et al. T1R3 and gustducin in gut sense sugars to regulate expression of Na^+-glucose cotransporter 1. *Proc Natl Acad Sci USA* 2007;104:15075–15080.

56. Mace OJ, Affleck J, Patel N, et al. Sweet taste receptors in rat small intestine stimulate glucose absorption through apical GLUT2. *J Physiol* 2007;582:379–392.

57. Jenkins DJ, Wolever TM, Taylor RH, et al. Glycemic index of foods: a physiological basis for carbohydrate exchange. *Am J Clin Nutr* 1981;34:362–366.

58. Lennerz BS, Alsop DC, Holsen LM, et al. Effects of dietary glycemic index on brain regions related to reward and craving in men. *Am J Clin Nutr* 2013;98(3):641–647.

59. Wolever TM, Mehling C. Long-term effect of varying the source or amount of dietary carbohydrate on postprandial plasma glucose, insulin, triacylglycerol, and free fatty acid concentrations in subjects with impaired glucose tolerance. *Am J Clin Nutr* 2003;77:612–621.

60. Hu J, La Vecchia C, Augustin LS, et al; the Canadian Cancer Registries Epidemiology Research Group. Glycemic index, glycemic load and cancer risk. *Ann Oncol* 2013;24(1): 245–251.

61. Romieu I, Ferrari P, Rinaldi S, et al. Dietary glycemic index and glycemic load and breast cancer risk in the European Prospective Investigation into Cancer and Nutrition (EPIC). *Am J Clin Nutr* 2012;96(2):345–355.

62. Dong JY, Zhang YH, Wang P, et al. Meta-analysis of dietary glycemic load and glycemic index in relation to risk of coronary heart disease. *Am J Cardiol* 2012;109(11):1608–1613.

63. Lin PH, Chen C, Young DR, et al. Glycemic index and glycemic load are associated with some cardiovascular risk factors among the PREMIER study participants. *Food Nutr Res* 2012;56.

64. Mayer-Davis EJ, Dhawan A, Liese AD, et al. Towards understanding of glycaemic index and glycaemic load in habitual diet: associations with measures of glycaemia in the Insulin Resistance Atherosclerosis Study. *Br J Nutr* 2006;95:397–405.

65. Giles GG, Simpson JA, English DR, et al. Dietary carbohydrate, fibre, glycaemic index, glycaemic load and the risk of postmenopausal breast cancer. *Int J Cancer* 2006;118: 1843–1847.

SUGGESTED READING

Gray GM. Digestion and absorption of carbohydrate. In: Stipanuk MH, ed. *Biochemical and physiological aspects of human nutrition*. Philadelphia, PA: Saunders, 2000:91–106.

Keim NL, Levin RJ, Havel PJ. Carbohydrates. In: Shils ME, Shike M, Ross AC, Caballero B, Cousins RJ, eds. *Modern nutrition in health and disease*, 10th ed. Philadelphia, PA: Lippincott Williams & Wilkins, 2006:62–82.

Lewis BA. Structure and properties of carbohydrates. In: Stipanuk MH, ed. *Biochemical and physiological aspects of human nutrition.* Philadelphia, PA: Saunders, 2000:3–22.

Lupton JR, Trumbo PR. Dietary fiber. In: Shils ME, Shike M, Ross AC, Caballero B, Cousins RJ, eds. *Modern nutrition in health and disease,* 10th ed. Philadelphia, PA: Lippincott Williams & Wilkins, 2006:83–91.

Lupton JR, Turner ND. Dietary fiber. In: Stipanuk MH, ed. *Biochemical and physiological aspects of human nutrition.* Philadelphia, PA: Saunders, 2000:143–154.

McGrane MM. Carbohydrate metabolism—synthesis and oxidation. In: Stipanuk MH, ed. *Biochemical and physiological aspects of human nutrition.* Philadelphia, PA: Saunders, 2000:158–210.

Panel on Macronutrients, Food and Nutrition Board, Institute of Medicine of the National Academies of Science. Dietary carbohydrates: sugars and starches. In: *Dietary reference intakes for energy, carbohydrate, fiber, fat, fatty acids, cholesterol, protein, and amino acids.* Washington, DC: National Academy Press, 2002:265–338.

Panel on Macronutrients, Food and Nutrition Board, Institute of Medicine of the National Academies of Science. Dietary, functional, and total fiber. In: *Dietary reference intakes for energy, carbohydrate, fiber, fat, fatty acids, cholesterol, protein, and amino acids.* Washington, DC: National Academy Press, 2002:339–421.

Watford M, Goodridge AG. Regulation of fuel utilization. In: Stipanuk MH, ed. *Biochemical and physiological aspects of human nutrition.* Philadelphia, PA: Saunders, 2000:384–407.

CHAPTER 2

Clinically Relevant Fat Metabolism

Lipids are categorized broadly as compounds that are soluble in organic solvents but not in water, and are derived from both plant and animal products. Cholesterol, an important constituent of cell membranes and myelin, is found exclusively in animal tissues. Cholesterol is utilized in the production of adrenal and gonadal steroid hormones and bile acids.

Dietary fat serves as a source of energy and precursors in prostaglandin metabolism, and it contributes essential structural components of cells. Polyunsaturated fatty acids (PUFAs) are precursors of eicosanoids, including prostaglandins, thromboxanes, and leukotrienes.

Most of the fat energy in the diet is derived from triglycerides, molecules formed by linkage via ester bonds of three fatty acid molecules to a molecule of glycerol. Among the three principal classes of macronutrients (carbohydrate, protein, and fat), lipids provide the greatest energy density—approximately 9 kcal per g. In addition to providing concentrated energy, dietary lipids enhance the palatability and absorption of fat-soluble micronutrients, such as vitamins A, D, E, and K (see Chapter 4).

The three major classes of naturally occurring fats are saturated, monounsaturated, and polyunsaturated. Fat molecules containing no double bonds between adjacent carbon atoms are classified as *saturated* because available carbon bonds are maximally occupied by hydrogen atoms, while molecules containing one or more double bonds are *unsaturated*. Trans fats are a clinically significant subset of monounsaturated fats that are produced by conversion of the carbon double bond to the trans isomer form. Recent research has revealed two major sources of dietary trans fats (or trans fatty acids [TFAs]): iTFAs, which are produced through partial hydrogenation (i.e., using hydrogen to saturate available carbon binding sites) of naturally polyunsaturated fats, and rTFA, which are formed from the biohydrogenation of ruminants (e.g., vaccenic acid and linoleic acid (1–4). iTFAs have adverse health effects that may considerably exceed those of saturated fat (5) and are a topic of intense interest in public health nutrition and food policy (6). Some epidemiological studies report that rTFAs, found primarily in dairy products and meat, do not increase the risk of coronary heart disease but may actually reduce it.

Along with its high energy density, dietary fat has a low satiety index, meaning that calorie for calorie, it is less filling than the other macronutrient classes (7–10). This is consistent with a preponderance of evidence linking relatively high-fat diets and foods with a high energy density to weight gain (11–14) (see Chapter 5), although this topic remains a matter of some debate (15,16).

ABSORPTION AND TRANSPORT

Lipases produced by the tongue and stomach act on triglycerides in the upper gastrointestinal tract; both require an acid environment. For the most part, lipases are active at the 1- and 3-ester bonds in a triglyceride molecule, but not at the 2 linkage. The transport of hydrophobic lipids in an aqueous medium is accomplished through emulsification, the dispersal of fat into tiny droplets, which is achieved by mechanical churning of stomach contents against a partially closed pylorus. In the duodenum, bile salts contribute to the stabilization of lipid micelles, preventing them from reaggregating. In addition to fatty acids, micelles are rich in 2-monoglycerides because of the resistance of the fatty acid at the 2 position in glycerol to lipolysis.

Emulsification and chemical digestion of fat are accelerated in the duodenum; mechanical digestion in the stomach serves to decrease droplet size and increase exposed surface area. The presence of fatty acids and amino acids and the secretion of hydrochloric acid in the stomach trigger the release of cholecystokinin-pancreozymin as well as secretin. The acidity of the gastric chyme is reversed by the buffering effects of the duodenal mucosa, the secretin-induced release of bicarbonate from the pancreas, and the release of alkaline bile from the gall bladder induced by cholecystokinin.

In the upper small bowel, pancreatic lipase acts on emulsified fat droplets once it is activated in the alkaline environment. Lipase is held to the droplets by colipase, which is secreted concurrently from the pancreas. Pancreatic lipase also cleaves fatty acids at the 1 and 3 positions of a triglyceride, producing two molecules of free fatty acid and one of monoglyceride (i.e., a fatty acid bound to glycerol in the 2 carbon position). Fat absorption then occurs predominantly in the proximal portion of the small bowel.

Free fatty acids and monoglycerides are readily absorbed in the upper small intestine. Short-chain fatty acids are absorbed into portal blood, bound to albumin, and transported to the liver. Longer-chain fatty acids and cholesterol are reesterified to triglycerides, and then packaged into chylomicrons that are transported via lymph.

Bile salts separate from the lipid droplets at the mucosa and are ultimately reabsorbed in the lower small bowel as part of the enterohepatic circulation. Bile acid sequestrants lower cholesterol by interrupting this circulation, causing bile acids to

be lost in stool and depleted; their reconstitution requires consumption of cholesterol. Phytosterols and stanols, cholesterol-like compounds in plants, similarly result in cholesterol loss in stool by direct inhibition of its absorption in the small bowel (17).

Absorption of ingested triglycerides is facilitated by phospholipid, which is present in the diet in much smaller quantities. Phospholipids serve to emulsify triglycerides in the stomach. They are structurally important in separating hydrophobic lipids from water in the cell membrane.

Fatty acids and monoglycerides are absorbed almost completely, whereas cholesterol is absorbed from 30% to 70%. Fatty acids can be used as an energy source by most cells, erythrocytes and cells of the central nervous system being notable exceptions. The brain uses glucose exclusively for fuel unless the supply is depleted, at which time ketone bodies produced from the catabolism of fatty acids can serve as an alternative energy source. The mitochondrial transport of long-chain fatty acids requires a carrier, carnitine transferase. The fixed metabolic needs for fat can be met with an intake level of as little as 20 to 25 g per day.

Energy consumed in excess of need is stored principally as triglycerides in adipose tissue, predominantly as palmitic (saturated) and oleic (monounsaturated) acids (see Table 2-1). The fatty acid composition of food influences the fatty acid composition of adipose tissue (18). The energy reserves in body fat even in lean individuals are generally 100-fold greater than glycogen stores,

TABLE 2.1

Classes of Fat and Fatty Acids of Dietary Significance

Fatty Acid	Class[a]			
	Saturated	Monounsaturated	Polyunsaturated	Essential
Myristic acid	C14:0			
Palmitic acid	C16:0			
Stearic acid	C18:0			
Oleic acid		C18:1, ω-9		
Linoleic acid			C18:2, ω-6	✓
γ-Linolenic acid			C18:3, ω-6	
Arachidonic acid			C20:4, ω-6	✓
Linolenic acid			C18:3, ω-3	✓
Eicosapentaenoic acid			C20:5, ω-3	
Docosahexaenoic acid			C22:6, ω-3	

[a]Fatty acids are designated by C, followed by the number of carbon atoms per molecule and then a second number to signify the number of double bonds (unsaturated sites). ω is used to signify the position of the first (or only) double bond in an unsaturated fatty acid, relative to the "ω" carbon, which is the carbon farthest from the terminal carboxyl group.

providing a depot of approximately 120,000 kcal. Often overlooked in discussions of obesity is the important role of body fat deposition as a survival mechanism for a species long subject to cycles of feast and famine (see Chapter 44).

The longer the chain length of fatty acids, the less readily they are absorbed. There are virtually no short-chain fatty acids (with 2 to 4 carbons) of nutritional significance. Medium-chain triglycerides, which have 6 to 12 carbons, are absorbed more readily than longer-chain triglycerides because of their more efficient emulsification and greater water solubility. They also tend to be absorbed (i.e., bound to albumin without reesterification by enterocytes) directly into the portal circulation, whereas the micelles are absorbed via lymphatics. There is interest in the use of medium-chain triglycerides, both enterally and parenterally, as an energy source in various clinical states associated with fat malabsorption, including premature birth, AIDS, and pancreatic insufficiency (19–23). Recent evidence suggests that dietary medium-chain triglycerides may contribute a therapeutic advantage of preserving insulin sensitivity in patients with metabolic syndrome (24).

Portal flow is considerably faster than lymphatic flow. Thus, medium-chain triglycerides are relatively unaffected by deficiencies of bile salts, require minimal pancreatic lipase activity, are relatively unaffected by impaired enterocyte function, and are absorbed far faster than long-chain triglycerides (see Chapter 18). Long-chain triglycerides of the omega-3 (ω-3) variety from marine sources are more readily absorbed than saturated or monounsaturated fatty acids of comparable length.

Cholesterol in the bowel, whether of endogenous or exogenous origin, is incompletely absorbed. There is debate regarding the upper limit of cholesterol absorption in adults; efficiency is thought to vary between 20% and 80% (25). Although some authorities believe it to be maximal at approximately 500 mg per day, others believe 40% of up to 2 g of intestinal cholesterol will be absorbed daily. Ingested cholesterol affects serum cholesterol, but to a limited extent in part because of limited absorption and in part because of the importance of endogenous cholesterol biosynthesis. A high cholesterol intake may raise serum cholesterol by as much as 15%, although accumulating evidence suggests that this may depend on the overall pattern of dietary intake (26–28). When intake of saturated and trans fat is low,

cholesterol in the diet is less clearly linked to serum cholesterol levels or to the risk of coronary heart disease (29). The bacterial degradation of unabsorbed cholesterol in the large bowel may contribute to the increased risk of colon cancer associated with diets high in animal fat (30–32).

Average stool fat in adults is in the range from 4 to 6 g per day. With very high fat intake, fat absorption continues more distally in the small bowel. Of note, human infants have a similar capacity to absorb fat when fed human milk because of the presence of lipase in human milk. Lipase is absent from bovine milk, and bottle-fed infants are subject to some degree of fat malabsorption (see Chapters 27 and 29).

Adults have a reserve capacity to absorb as much as twice the amount of fat typically present in even high-fat diets. Although neonates have low levels of bile salts and thus have a limited ability to form micelles, the lipase present in human milk can cleave even the fatty acid at the 2 position in glycerol, producing free fatty acids that are relatively readily absorbed, independent of micelle formation. Capacity for fat absorption tends to decline with age in older adults. Vitamin D deficiency appears to be one consequence of clinical importance.

Partial gastric resections tend to produce some degree of fat malabsorption, with fecal fat increasing from 4 to 6 g up to 15 g per day; this effect may contribute to the weight loss observed after gastric bypass surgery (see Chapter 5). Exocrine pancreatic insufficiency results in fat malabsorption. Disease or resection of the ileum may result in bile acid deficiency, which leads to fat malabsorption.

LIPOPROTEIN METABOLISM

Triglycerides are the principal source of fuel from fat and the principal source of energy stored in adipose tissue. Cholesterol and phospholipids act primarily as membrane constituents. In the fasting state, fatty acids for energy production are derived from adipose tissue stores. In the fed state, fatty acids are available from chylomicrons and very-low-density lipoprotein (VLDL); the extraction of triglycerides from these particles is mediated by the enzyme lipoprotein lipase. Most fat is transported via triglycerides resynthesized in enterocytes.

Fatty acids with chain lengths shorter than 14 carbons are bound to albumin and transported directly to the liver via the portal vein. Endothelial cells can take up lipoprotein particles, as well as free fatty acid bound to albumin; triglyceride from lipoprotein particles is the predominant delivery source.

Triglycerides are packaged in chylomicrons, which contain unesterified cholesterol in the outer layer and esterified cholesterol in the core. There is some evidence that the ingestion of fat of any type stimulates endogenous production of primarily saturated fatty acids, which are released into the circulation along with the fat from exogenous sources.

Enterocytes package ingested fat into chylomicrons and VLDL, both of which contain apoprotein B_{48}. High-density lipoprotein (HDL), manufactured in the liver and rich in apoproteins C (apo C) and E (apo E), interacts with the lipoproteins of intestinal origin. HDL transfers apo C and apo E to chylomicrons. Apo C serves as a cofactor that activates lipoprotein lipase, whereas apo E in the chylomicron remnant core facilitates the particle's uptake by hepatocytes.

The activity of lipoprotein lipase is stimulated by heparin and insulin. The hypertriglyceridemia, seen in poorly controlled diabetes mellitus, is associated with reduced insulin action, which leadings to reduced lipoprotein lipase activity (see Chapter 6). Niacin activates lipoprotein lipase, which explains its utility in treating hypertriglyceridemia. Lipoprotein lipase is inhibited by glucagon, thyroid-stimulating hormone, catecholamines, and adrenocorticotrophic hormone; these hormones generally also stimulate the release of free fatty acids from adipose tissue reserves.

Free fatty acids are used to produce ATP in muscle and adipose tissue; if not used immediately for energy generation, they are reesterified to triglycerides. This process requires the enzyme glycerol-3-phosphate, which necessitates both glucose and insulin for synthesis. Therefore, carbohydrate feeding has the tendency to drop the concentration of free fatty acids in circulation by augmenting the availability of glucose and the levels of insulin. Insulin action promotes reesterification of free fatty acids into triglycerides and opposes lipolysis. Free fatty acid taken up from plasma by the liver is predominantly incorporated into VLDL. High levels of VLDL production in the liver lead to hypertriglyceridemia, a characteristic feature of hyperinsulinemic and insulin-resistant states (33,34) (see Chapter 6).

Fatty acids from chylomicrons and VLDL are used for fuel by the heart, smooth muscle, red muscle fibers, kidneys, and platelets in particular. In addition, they serve as substrate for the formation and function of biomembranes. The fatty acid composition of lipid particles formed by enterocytes influences cellular and subcellular membrane integrity and function, as well as the synthesis of prostaglandins and leukotrienes (see Chapters 11 and 33). Fatty acids extracted from lipoprotein particles of intestinal origin contribute to the energy stored in adipose tissue. The fatty acid composition of VLDL synthesized by the liver is influenced by dietary fat composition, which influences the composition of adipose tissue. Both VLDL and the low-density lipoprotein (LDL) produced when VLDL is acted on by lipoprotein lipase are atherogenic and are taken up by macrophages and subendothelial smooth muscle cells.

Uptake of HDL by the liver is influenced by the interaction of apo E and its receptor. There are several isoforms of apo E, encoded by various mutations in the apo E allele. Apo EII is associated with the accumulation of chylomicrons and VLDL in blood due to impaired hepatic uptake. Although the concentration of HDL in plasma is lower than that of LDL, HDL particles are present in larger numbers. HDL particles exchange apoproteins and surface lipids with chylomicrons and VLDL. Cholesterol acquired by HDL is esterified by the enzyme lecithin cholesterol acyltransferase. The esterified cholesterol moves to the core of the HDL particle, facilitating additional uptake of cholesterol from other lipoprotein particles. HDL is largely taken up by the liver, as well as other tissues with high cholesterol requirements, including the adrenal glands and ovaries.

Virtually all human tissues can synthesize cholesterol from acetate. The rate-limiting step in cholesterol biosynthesis involves the enzyme β-hydroxy-β-methylglutaryl coenzyme A (HMG-CoA) reductase. HMG-CoA reductase is stimulated by insulin and inhibited by glucagon. The class of drugs now referred to as "statins" are HMG-CoA reductase inhibitors, and they work by inhibiting the rate-limiting enzyme in cholesterol biosynthesis. High cholesterol feeding can inhibit endogenous cholesterol synthesis, whereas gastrointestinal loss of cholesterol, such as that induced by bile acid sequestrant drugs, can actually stimulate endogenous production.

When LDL receptors are deficient, as in familial hyperlipidemia type IIA, rising levels of LDL do not inhibit cholesterol biosynthesis, as they do normally. Under conditions of homeostasis, an adult in a Western country may consume a daily average of 335 mg of cholesterol. An additional 800 mg per day is synthesized endogenously. Approximately 400 mg is lost daily in bile acids, another 600 mg in biliary cholesterol, and 50 mg in the production of steroid hormones, and 85 mg is excreted as sterols from skin. Thus, 1,135 mg of cholesterol is exchanged daily. Most cholesterol in circulation is in the esterified form, produced through the action of lecithin cholesterol acyltransferase, which is manufactured by the liver. Esterification of cholesterol is also mediated by acyl-CoA cholesterol acyltransferase, particularly in the liver. The esterifying enzymes have different preferences for fatty acid substrate.

FATTY ACIDS

Fatty acids, carbon chains with the basic formula $CH_3(CH_2)_nCOOH-$, are short, medium, or long chain, and they are saturated, monounsaturated, or polyunsaturated. Short-chain fatty acids have fewer than 6 carbons; medium-chain fatty acids have 6 to 10; and long-chain fatty acids have 12 or more. Saturated fatty acids contain no carbon-to-carbon double bonds, whereas monounsaturates contain one and polyunsaturates contain more than one. PUFAs are further divided into those with the initial double-bond 3 carbons from the methyl terminus of the molecule (n-3 or ω-3 fatty acids), those with the initial double-bond 6 carbons from the methyl terminus (n-6 or ω-6 fatty acids), and other varieties. The synthesis of cholesterol, saturated fatty acids, and unsaturated fatty acids from acetyl coenzyme A occurs endogenously; thus, none of these nutrients is essential in the diet. Certain PUFAs cannot be synthesized endogenously and therefore are considered essential (see Table 2-1). Naturally occurring fatty acids tend to have even numbers of carbons, to be unbranched, and to be in the cis configuration relative to double bonds. The industrial process of partially hydrogenating polyunsaturated oils results in the production of a preponderance of now rather notorious trans stereoisomers of monounsaturated fat (35–37), a formulation with favorable commercial properties but decidedly adverse effects on health.

The trans configuration allows for tighter packing of the molecules, with resultant heat resistance. The melting point of a triglyceride is the product of carbon chain length of its constituent fatty acids, the configuration of the fatty acids (cis or trans), and the position of the fatty acid with regard to the glycerol molecule. Saturation of fatty acids raises the melting point and decreases water solubility. While providing the favorable properties to industry of longer shelf life and higher melting point, the physiologic effects of trans fat are more comparable to (and more adverse than) those of saturated fats than to those of monounsaturates in the cis configuration (see Chapter 7).

Conjugated linoleic acid, a family of isomers of an 18-carbon PUFA found in meat and dairy, has generated interest as a potential aid in weight loss. At present, despite some promising findings in animal studies, human evidence is at best mixed (38–45), and adverse health effects of this group of fats cannot be excluded with confidence.

ESSENTIAL FATTY ACIDS

Most fatty acids can be synthesized endogenously from excess energy of any source or from other fatty acids; those that are required for metabolic functions and cannot be synthesized endogenously are essential nutrients. Certain fatty acids of the n-3 and n-6 polyunsaturated classes are referred to as essential fatty acids (EFAs) (see Table 2-1 and Section VIIE). Fatty acid synthesis occurs primarily in the liver. Enzymes involved in fatty acid synthesis have a high affinity for fatty acids of the n-3 PUFA class, with successively lesser affinity for fatty acids of the n-6, n-9 and n-7 PUFA classes. Affinity in general is greater the less saturated the fatty acid. The composition of fatty acids in cell membranes can provide evidence of EFA deficiency, as the end products of fatty acid metabolism vary with the substrate. EFAs of the n-3 and n-6 classes are substrates for the lipoxygenase and cyclooxygenase enzymes. The products of EFA metabolism are referred to collectively as eicosanoids.

The eicosanoid products of EFA metabolism clearly vary with the distribution of n-3 and n-6 fatty acids in the diet, with implications for immune function, hemostasis, and metabolism, as discussed in more detail elsewhere (see Chapters 9 and 11). Deficiency of EFAs is associated with impaired growth, abnormal skin, and infertility.

EFAs of the n-3 class are preferentially incorporated into the brain and the retina. The requirement for n-3 fatty acid is not reliably known, but various lines of evidence support greater proportional intake of n-3 fatty acids than the Western diet generally provides (see Chapters 7, 11, 29, and 44). Long-chain n-3 PUFAs have been shown to reduce obesity in rodent models via suppression of appetite, enhanced fat oxidation and energy expenditure, and reduced fat deposition; however, evidence in humans is limited (46). Two important n-3 PUFAs, eicosapentaenoic acid (EPA) and docosahexaenoic acid (DHA), have been directly associated with reduced inflammation (47) and cardiac risk (48,49); however, this benefit remains controversial (50,51; also 52, p. e6698). There are three important n-3 PUFAs. As noted at the start, not all of them are found in fish—two of the three are. The ratio of n-3 to n-6 fatty acids in the diet may be an important determinant of eicosanoid ratios, with implications for immune system function and inflammation (53) (see Chapters 11 and 20). Anthropologists suggest that the "native" ratio of n-3 to n-6 fatty acids in the human diet is roughly from 1:1 to 1:4; the corresponding ratio in the typical modern American diet is between 1:11 and 1:20 (54). This preponderance of n-6 to n-3 fatty acids exerts a proinflammatory influence (see Chapter 11). Consumption of a diet with a high n-3 to n-6 ratio has been associated with decreased risk of breast cancer (55) and diabetes (56); however, one observational study noted an association between increased n-3 fatty acid intake and prostate cancer (57). Despite the apparent relevance of the n-3 to n-6 ratio, there is growing consensus that the total amount of n-6 and n-3 fatty acids in the diet may be more important than the ratio per se (58,59). High intake of saturated or trans fat increases requirements for EFAs.

Animals and humans are deficient in an enzyme needed to convert oleic acid to linoleic acid and therefore require linoleic acid, an ω-6 fatty acid, in the diet. Linoleic acid can be converted to the 20-carbon arachidonic acid, also an ω-6. Therefore, arachidonic acid is essential in the diet only when linoleic acid intake is inadequate. Thus, one n-6 fatty acid is truly essential, whereas a second is conditionally essential. The third polyunsaturate considered essential is α-linolenic acid (ALA), an 18-carbon ω-3. The importance of ω-3 fatty acids to homeostasis and a variety of physiologic states is discussed throughout the text (see especially Chapters 7, 9, 11, and 20). Linolenic acid can be metabolized to DHA (22 carbons, n-3) or EPA

(20 carbons, n-3) (see Table 2-1), both of which are important constituents of cell membranes and are particularly abundant in the retina and brain. The longer-chain n-3 fatty acids may be obtained directly from the consumption of fish and seafood, as well as certain algae. The efficiency with which humans convert ALA to DHA or EPA is variable and unpredictable.

PUFAs of the n-6 class are particularly important in cell and subcellular membranes throughout the body; both linoleic and arachidonic acid are abundant in structural phospholipids. In addition, as noted, polyunsaturates of both n-6 and n-3 classes are important eicosanoid precursors. As discussed elsewhere (see Chapters 9, 11, and 20), the relative abundance of each class of EFA in the diet influences the distribution of prostaglandins and leukotrienes, with important implications for platelet function and inflammatory reactions. In general, the n-6 fatty acids promote both platelet aggregation and inflammatory activity, whereas the n-3 fatty acids are inhibitory. Consumption of excessive n-6 eicosanoids, found primarily in vegetable oils, has been associated with arthritis, inflammation, and cancer (60–62). At present, intake of linoleic acid not less than 1% to 2% of total daily calories (3 to 6 g per day for an adult) is recommended, as is intake of ALA (or other n-3 fatty acids) at not less than 25% the level of n-6 fatty acids. As of the 2002 *Dietary Reference Intakes* (63), RDA had not been established for either n-6 or n-3 EFAs. RDAs (recommended dietary allowance) require scientific evidence indicating the level of nutrient intake required to meet the needs of nearly all individuals in a given age and gender group. When this standard cannot be met, the adequate intake (AI) level may be provided instead. The AI for linoleic acid (n-6) is 17 g per day for men and 12 g per day for women. The AI for ALA (n-3) is 1.6 g per day for men and 1.1 g per day for women. The evidence standards used in determining the various measures of the *Dietary Reference Intakes* are detailed online at http://www.nap.edu/books/0309085373/html/20.html.

CURRENT INTAKE PATTERNS AND RECOMMENDATIONS

Dietary fat constitutes as little as 10% of total ingested energy in some Asian countries, as much as 45% in some European countries, and between 30% and 40% in the United States. The National

Health and Nutrition Examination Surveys suggest that fat ingestion as a proportion of total calories is declining in the United States, from more than 40% to a current level of approximately 34% (64,65). However, total fat intake has remained relatively constant, because of an increase in total energy consumption (66). Principal sources of fat in the US diet include red meat, other meats, and dairy products. The proportion of fat contributed by vegetable oils has increased in recent years because of consumption of fast foods cooked with such oils, as well as dressings, spreads, condiments, and processed foods that incorporate vegetable fat.

The health effects of dietary fat in the United States are predominantly those of excess rather than those of deficiency, although the contributions of relative n-3 fatty acid deficiency to chronic disease may be considerable. Saturated fat and trans fat in the diet are the principal exogenous determinants of serum cholesterol levels, which in turn influence risk of cardiovascular events (see Chapter 7). Dietary cholesterol may contribute as well to serum cholesterol, but this association is increasingly suspect, as noted previously, and cholesterol is consumed in milligram rather than in gram amounts; it therefore contributes relatively less to serum levels than to dietary fat, even when the association is valid (see Chapter 7 and the Hegsted and Keys equations in Section VIIA).

Conventional recommendations regarding dietary fat are that the total not exceed 30% of calories, saturated fat intake not exceed 10% of calories, and cholesterol intake not exceed 300 mg per day. There is ongoing debate, however, about both optimal quantity and distribution of dietary fat (67–70). On the basis of confluent lines of evidence, recommendations may be made for approximately 25% of total calories from fat; less than 5% of total calories derived from the combination of saturated and trans fat; approximately 10% to 15% of calories from polyunsaturated fat, divided between n-6 and n-3 fatty acids in a ratio of between 4:1 and 1:1; and the remaining 10% to 15% of calories from monounsaturated fat (see Chapters 7 and 45). Of note, the requirement for vitamin E and other antioxidants rises with consumption of polyunsaturated fat, as fatty acids with double bonds are particularly subject to oxidation and rancidification.

Saturated fats derived from both animal and plant sources constitute approximately 12% of calories in the prevailing US diet. Most naturally occurring oils and fats contain a variety of fatty acids. Butter fat, beef fat, and coconut oil are all highly saturated, although the distribution of saturated fatty acids is considerably variable (see Section VIF). Tropical oils—coconut oil, palm oil, and palm kernel oil—are among the few predominantly saturated oils of plant origin (71). These oils were used to replace much of the animal fat in the US food supply several decades ago and were in turn substantially replaced by partially hydrogenated oils (trans fat).

The average intake of trans fatty acid in the United States, from processed and snack foods, spreads, and dressings, is approximately 2.5% to 3% of calories and has been increasing until recently; pressure on the food industry to eliminate trans fats is now considerable. On December 2006, New York City's Board of Health voted to ban trans fats in restaurants, making this the first mayor city to strictly limit trans fats. Philadelphia city council passed a ban on February 2007, followed by proposed legislation in San Francisco, Chicago, and Massachusetts. In July 2008, California became the first to pass a statewide ban on trans fats in restaurants. The fast-food chain KFC had announced elimination of trans fat use nationwide. Because of the desirable commercial properties of saturated and trans fats, but with trans fat labeling requirements in place, some in the food industry have begun to explore several alternatives, including novel hydrogenation procedures using metal catalysts that reduce the formation of trans stereoisomers (72); selective plant breeding and genetic engineering to create edible seed oils with modified fatty acid composition; interesterification, a process that involves hydrolysis and reformation of the ester bond between fatty acid and glycerol to produce fats with a wide range of melting points; and a return to the use of tropical oils, including palm oil and coconut oil. The fatty acid profile of tropical oils may not be as adverse to health as once thought, and is a matter of ongoing investigation (73–75).

A potential hazard of efforts to reduce fat intake is that visible fat in oils may be eliminated, resulting in the fat hidden in processed foods accounting for a higher percentage of total fat intake. Oils (and some spreads) are apt to be the main sources of EFAs, whereas the fat added during food processing is predominantly either saturated or trans and thus most apt to exert an adverse influence on health.

Triglycerides, the principal dietary fat, are composed of three fatty acid molecules esterified with one glycerol molecule. The diverse combinations of fatty acids with glycerol result in a great variety of dietary fat. Fatty acids in the saturated class include stearic (18 carbons), palmitic (16 carbons), myristic (14 carbons), lauric (12 carbons), and medium-chain fatty acids (8 to 10 carbons). The principal dietary monounsaturate derived from nature is oleic acid (18 carbons, cis configuration), whereas the trans stereoisomer elaidic acid is derived primarily from industrial hydrogenation of fat. PUFAs include the n-6 linoleic acid (18 carbons) and the n-3 fatty acids linolenic (18 carbons), eicosapentaenoic (20 carbons), and docosahexaenoic (22 carbons).

In the US diet, the major saturated fatty acids are palmitic and stearic acids. The predominant monounsaturated fatty acid is oleic acid. The principal sources of polyunsaturates in the diet are plants, which provide predominantly linoleic acid (18-carbon, n-6 fatty acid) and linolenic acid (18-carbon, n-3), and seafood, which are rich in EPA and DHA.

Of note, there is increasing appreciation for variability in the health effects of saturated fatty acids. Whereas myristic acid (14 carbons) and palmitic acid (16 carbons) are both thought to be atherogenic, stearic acid (18 carbons) does not seem to increase the risk of atherogenesis, and is thus not included among the list of recommended restricted intake saturated fats from the 2010 Dietary Guidelines Advisory Committee (76) (see Chapters 7 and 39). This is generally thought to have limited implications for dietary guidance at present because of the correlation between stearic acid and atherogenic fats in most foods (77). Whether stearic acid might prove useful in the formulation of oils with favorable properties for both health and commerce remains to be seen. The relevance of stearic acid to the health effects associated with consumption of dark chocolate is addressed in Chapter 39. Lauric acid, a short-chain (12-carbon) saturated fat, constitutes about half of the fatty acid content in coconut oil, laurel oil, and palm kernel oil. Consumption of lauric acid, similar to many other saturated fats, has been shown to increase total cholesterol (78); however, lauric acid specifically raises HDL, producing a more favorable cholesterol ratio (79), which may reduce the risk of atherosclerotic disease (80). However, results of a meta-analysis of dietary fat composition on HDL/LDL ratio suggest that the effects of consumption of lauric acid on coronary artery disease remain uncertain (81).

Linoleic acid is found in a variety of commonly used vegetable oils, including corn, sunflower, and safflower. Evening primrose oil provides γ-linolenic acid, a form that bypasses an intermediate metabolic step. Plant sources particularly rich in linolenic acid (n-3) include flaxseed, soy, rapeseed (canola), and walnuts. Long-chain n-3 fatty acids are abundant in salmon, mackerel, sardines, and scallops. Farm-raised fish may provide less n-3 fatty acid than does wild fish, as the source of n-3 PUFAs in fish is the vegetation and plankton on which they feed. Similarly, the flesh of wild ungulates contains n-3 PUFAs in appreciable amounts, whereas the flesh of domesticated feed animals does not.

EFAs are derived from either vegetable sources or the flesh of herbivorous animals consuming plant matter that contains these nutrients. EFAs modified during processing, with resultant formation of trans isomers or movement of double bonds, may act as metabolic competitors of the EFAs in their native state. During processing of vegetables for the production of vegetable oils, much of the sterols and phospholipids are removed. Sterols interfere with cholesterol absorption; for this reason, cholesterol absorption may increase as a result of processed vegetable oil in the diet. The plant sterol β-sitosterol has been used to lower serum cholesterol modestly by interfering with cholesterol absorption. Phosphatidylcholine, a phospholipid, also interferes with cholesterol absorption. Plant stanols and sterols are being incorporated into more and more "functional" foods that may be of use in lipid lowering. Reductions in serum lipids between 10% and 15% have been observed with intake of 2 g of phytosterols/stanols per day.

REFERENCES

1. US Food and Drug Administration. *Revealing trans fats.* Available at http://publications.usa.gov/epublications/reveal-fats/reveal-fats.htm accessed 11/26/06.
2. Gebauer SK, Chardigny JM, Jakobsen MU, et al. Effects of ruminant trans fatty acids on cardiovascular disease and cancer: a comprehensive review of epidemiological, clinical, and mechanistic studies. *Adv Nutr* 2011;2(4):332–354.
3. Bakalar N. WELL; vital signs | nutrition: trans fat limits show benefits in New York. *New York Times,* July 24, 2012. Available at http://query.nytimes.com/gst/fullpage.html?res=9D0DE5DB1E3EF937A15754C0A9649D8B63&ref=transfattyacids

4. Strom S. Local laws fighting fat under siege. *New York Times*, June 30, 2011. Available at http://www.nytimes.com/2011/07/01/business/01obese.html?ref=transfattyacids&_r=0

5. Ascherio A, Willett WC. Health effects of trans fatty acids. *Am J Clin Nutr* 1997;66(4 suppl):1006s–1010s.

6. Nichols M. New York trans fat ban wins backing at hearing. *MSNBC*, October 31, 2006. Available at http://www.msnbc.msn.com/id/15488824/; accessed 11/26/06.

7. Holt SH, Miller JC, Petocz P, et al. A satiety index of common foods. *Eur J Clin Nutr* 1995;49:675–690.

8. Poppitt SD, Prentice AM. Energy density and its role in the control of food intake: evidence from metabolic and community studies. *Appetite* 1996;26:153–174.

9. Blundell JE, Stubbs RJ. High and low carbohydrate and fat intakes: limits imposed by appetite and palatability and their implications for energy balance. *Eur J Clin Nutr* 1999;53(suppl 1):s148–s165.

10. Rolls BJ, Miller DL. Is the low-fat message giving people a license to eat more? *J Am Coll Nutr* 1997;16:535–543.

11. Astrup A. The role of dietary fat in obesity. *Semin Vasc Med* 2005;5:40–47.

12. Bray GA, Paeratakul S, Popkin BM. Dietary fat and obesity: a review of animal, clinical and epidemiological studies. *Physiol Behav* 2004;83:549–555.

13. Shikany JM, Vaughan LK, Baskin ML, et al. Is dietary fat fattening? A comprehensive research synthesis. *Crit Rev Food Sci Nutr* 2010;50(8):699–715.

14. Melanson EL, Astrup A, Donahoo WT. The relationship between dietary fat and fatty acid intake and body weight, diabetes, and the metabolic syndrome. *Ann Nutr Metab* 2009;55(1–3):229–243.

15. Westerterp-Plantenga MS. Fat intake and energy-balance effects. *Physiol Behav* 2004;83:579–585.

16. Willett WC. Dietary fat plays a major role in obesity: no. *Obes Rev* 2002;3:59–68.

17. Ostlund RE Jr. Phytosterols and cholesterol metabolism. *Curr Opin Lipidol* 2004;15:37–41.

18. Plakke T, Berkel J, Beynen AC, et al. Relationship between the fatty acid composition of the diet and that of the subcutaneous adipose tissue in individual human subjects. *Hum Nutr Appl Nutr* 1983;37:365–372.

19. Wanten GJ, Naber AH. Cellular and physiological effects of medium-chain triglycerides. *Mini Rev Med Chem* 2004;4:847–857.

20. Craig GB, Darnell BE, Weinsier RL, et al. Decreased fat and nitrogen losses in patients with AIDS receiving medium-chain-triglyceride-enriched formula vs those receiving long-chain-triglyceride-containing formulas. *J Am Diet Assoc* 1997;97:605–611.

21. Wanke CA, Pleskow D, Degirolami PC, et al. A medium chain triglyceride-based diet in patients with HIV and chronic diarrhea reduces diarrhea and malabsorption: a prospective, controlled trial. *Nutrition* 1996;12:766–771.

22. Caliari S, Benini L, Sembenini C, et al. Medium-chain triglyceride absorption in patients with pancreatic insufficiency. *Scand J Gastroenterol* 1996;31:90–94.

23. Rego Costa AC, Rosado EL, Soares-Mota M. Influence of the dietary intake of medium chain triglycerides on body composition, energy expenditure and satiety: a systematic review. *Nutr Hosp* 2012;27(1):103–108.

24. Nagao K, Yanagita T. Medium-chain fatty acids: functional lipids for the prevention and treatment of the metabolic syndrome. *Pharmacol Res* 2010;61(3):208–212.

25. Otten JJ, Hellwig JP, Meyers LD, eds., for the Institute of Medicine. *Dietary reference intakes: the essential guide to nutrient requirements*. Washington, DC: National Academy Press, 2006:140–143.

26. Hu FB, Stampfer MJ, Rimm EB, et al. A prospective study of egg consumption and risk of cardiovascular disease in men and women. *JAMA* 1999;281:1387–1394.

27. Herron KL, Lofgren IE, Sharman M, et al. High intake of cholesterol results in less atherogenic low-density lipoprotein particles in men and women independent of response classification. *Metabolism* 2004;53:823–830.

28. Constance C. The good and the bad: what researchers have learned about dietary cholesterol, lipid management and cardiovascular disease risk since the Harvard Egg Study. *Int J Clin Pract Suppl* 2009;(163):9–14, 27–43.

29. Kratz M. Dietary cholesterol, atherosclerosis and coronary heart disease. *Handb Exp Pharmacol* 2005;170:195–213.

30. Tlaskalová-Hogenová H, Štěpánková R, Kozáková H, et al. The role of gut microbiota (commensal bacteria) and the mucosal barrier in the pathogenesis of inflammatory and autoimmune diseases and cancer: contribution of germ-free and gnotobiotic animal models of human diseases. *Cell Mol Immunol* 2011;8(2):110–120.

31. Wong JM, de Souza R, Kendall CW, et al. Colonic health: fermentation and short chain fatty acids. *J Clin Gastroenterol* 2006;40(3):235–243.

32. Hu J, La Vecchia C, de Groh M, et al. Dietary cholesterol intake and cancer. *Ann Oncol* 2012;23(2):491–500.

33. Al-Mahmood A, Ismail A, Rashid F, et al. Isolated hypertriglyceridemia: an insulin-resistant state with or without low HDL cholesterol. *J Atheroscler Thromb* 2006;13:143–148.

34. Moro E, Gallina P, Pais M, et al. Hypertriglyceridemia is associated with increased insulin resistance in subjects with normal glucose tolerance: evaluation in a large cohort of subjects assessed with the 1999 World Health Organization criteria for the classification of diabetes. *Metabolism* 2003;52:616–619.

35. Ascherio A, Katan MB, Zock PL, et al. Trans fatty acids and coronary heart disease. *N Engl J Med* 1999;340:1994–1998.

36. Valenzuela A, Morgado N. Trans fatty acid isomers in human health and in the food industry. *Biol Res* 1999;32:273–287.

37. Oomen CM, Ocke MC, Feskens EJ, et al. Association between trans fatty acid intake and 10-year risk of coronary heart disease in the Zutphen Elderly Study: a prospective population-based study. *Lancet* 2001;357:746–751.

38. Larsen TM, Toubro S, Astrup A. Efficacy and safety of dietary supplements containing CLA for the treatment of obesity: evidence from animal and human studies. *J Lipid Res* 2003;44:2234–2241.

39. Riserus U, Smedman A, Basu S, et al. CLA and body weight regulation in humans. *Lipids* 2003;38:133–137.

40. Belury MA, Mahon A, Banni S. The conjugated linoleic acid (CLA) isomer, t10c12-CLA, is inversely associated with changes in body weight and serum leptin in subjects with type 2 diabetes mellitus. *J Nutr* 2003;133:257s–260s.

41. Westerterp-Plantenga MS. Fat intake and energy-balance effects. *Physiol Behav* 2004;83:579–585.

42. Plourde M, Jew S, Cunnane SC, et al. Conjugated linoleic acids: why the discrepancy between animal and human studies? *Nutr Rev* 2008;66(7):415–421.

43. Dilzer A, Park Y. Implication of conjugated linoleic acid (CLA) in human health. *Crit Rev Food Sci Nutr* 2012;52(6):488–513.

44. McCrorie TA, Keaveney EM, Wallace JM, et al. Human health effects of conjugated linoleic acid from milk and supplements. *Nutr Res Rev* 2011;24(2):206–227.

45. Onakpoya IJ, Posadzki PP, Watson LK, et al. The efficacy of long-term conjugated linoleic acid (CLA) supplementation on body composition in overweight and obese individuals: a systematic review and meta-analysis of randomized clinical trials. *Eur J Nutr* 2012;51(2):127–134.

46. Buckley JD, Howe PRC. Long-chain omega-3 polyunsaturated fatty acids may be beneficial for reducing obesity—a review. *Nutrients.* 2010; 2(12): 1212–1230.

47. Calder PC. The role of marine omega-3 (n-3) fatty acids in inflammatory processes, atherosclerosis and plaque stability. *Mol Nutr Food Res* 2012;56(7):1073–1080.

48. Gruppo Italiano per lo Studio della Sopravvivenza nell' Infarto miocardico. Dietary supplementation with n-3 polyunsaturated fatty acids and vitamin E after myocardial infarction: results of the GISSI-Prevenzione trial. *Lancet* 1999;354:447–455. [Errata in: *Lancet* 2001;357:642].

49. Tavazzi L, Maggioni AP, Marchioli R, et al. Effect of n-3 polyunsaturated fatty acids in patients with chronic heart failure (the GISSI-HF trial): a randomised, double-blind, placebo-controlled trial. *Lancet* 2008;372:1223–1230.

50. Kromhout D, Giltay EJ, Geleijnse JM. n-3 Fatty acids and cardiovascular events after myocardial infarction. *N Engl J Med* 2010;363:2015–2026.

51. Kwak SM, Myung SK, Lee YJ, et al. Efficacy of omega-3 fatty acid supplements (eicosapentaenoic acid and docosahexaenoic acid) in the secondary prevention of cardiovascular disease: a meta-analysis of randomized, double-blind, placebo-controlled trials. *Arch Intern Med* 2012;172(9):686–694.

52. Chowdhury R, Stevens S, Gorman D, et al. Association between fish consumption, long chain omega 3 fatty acids, and risk of cerebrovascular disease: systematic review and meta-analysis. *BMJ* 2012;345:e6698.

53. Browning LM. n-3 polyunsaturated fatty acids, inflammation and obesity-related disease. *Proc Nutr Soc* 2003;62:447–453.

54. Simopoulos AP. Evolutionary aspects of omega-3 fatty acids in the food supply. *Prostaglandins Leukot Essent Fatty Acids.* 1999;60:421–429

55. Zheng JS, Hu XJ, Zhao YM, et al. Intake of fish and marine n-3 polyunsaturated fatty acids and risk of breast cancer: meta-analysis of data from 21 independent prospective cohort studies. *BMJ* 2013;346:f3706.

56. Zheng JS, Huang T, Yang J, et al. Marine N-3 polyunsaturated fatty acids are inversely associated with risk of type 2 diabetes in Asians: a systematic review and meta-analysis. *PLoS One* 2012;7(9):e44525.

57. Brasky TM, Darke AK, Song X, et al. Plasma phospholipid fatty acids and prostate cancer risk in the SELECT trial. *J Natl Cancer Inst* 2013;105(15):1132–1141.

58. Harris WS. The omega-6/omega-3 ratio and cardiovascular disease risk: uses and abuses. *Curr Atheroscler Rep* 2006;8:453–459.

59. Wijendran V, Hayes KC. Dietary n-6 and n-3 fatty acid balance and cardiovascular health. *Annu Rev Nutr* 2004;24:597–615.

60. Simopoulos AP. The importance of the ratio of omega-6/omega-3 essential fatty acids. *Biomed Pharmacother* 2002;56 (8):365–379.

61. Emily S, Ericson, U, Gullberg B, et al. Do both heterocyclic amines and omega-6 polyunsaturated fatty acids contribute to the incidence of breast cancer in postmenopausal women of the Malmö diet and cancer cohort? *Int J Cancer* 2008;123(7):1637–1643.

62. Berquin IM, Min Y, Wu Ruping, et al. Modulation of prostate cancer genetic risk by omega-3 and omega-6 fatty acids. *J Clin Invest* 2007;117 (7):1866–1875.

63. Institute of Medicine. *Dietary reference intakes for energy, carbohydrate, fiber, fat, fatty acids, cholesterol, protein, and amino acids (macronutrients).* Washington, DC: National Academy Press, 2002. Available at http://www.nap.edu/books/0309085373/html/336.html; accessed 9/18/07.

64. MMWR. Daily dietary fat and total food-energy intakes–Third National Health and Nutrition Examination Survey, phase 1, 1988–1991. *MMWR* 1994;43:116.

65. Katz DL, Brunner RL, St. Jeor ST, et al. Dietary fat consumption in a cohort of American adults, 1985–1991: covariates, secular trends, and compliance with guidelines. *Am J Health Promot.* 1998;12:382.

66. Kennedy ET, Bowman SA, Powell R. Dietary-fat intake in the US population. *J Am Coll Nutr* 1999;18:207.

67. Connor WE, Connor SL. Should a low-fat, high-carbohydrate diet be recommended for everyone? The case for a low-fat, high-carbohydrate diet. *N Engl J Med* 1997;337:562.

68. Katan MB, Grundy SM, Willett WC. Should a low-fat, high-carbohydrate diet be recommended for everyone? Beyond low-fat diets. *N Engl J Med* 1997;337:563.

69. Aranceta J, Pérez-Rodrigo C. Recommended dietary reference intakes, nutritional goals and dietary guidelines for fat and fatty acids: a systematic review. *Br J Nutr* 2012;107(suppl 2):S8–S22.

70. Hooper L, Summerbell CD, Thompson R, et al. Reduced or modified dietary fat for preventing cardiovascular disease. *Cochrane Database Syst Rev* 2012;5:CD002137.

71. Council on Scientific Affairs. Saturated fatty acids in vegetable oils. *JAMA* 1990;263:3146–3148.

72. Tarrago-Trani MT, Phillips KM, Lemar LE, et al. New and existing oils and fats used in products with reduced transfatty acid content. *J Am Diet Assoc* 2006;106(6):867–880.

73. Cox C, Sutherland W, Mann J, et al. Effects of dietary coconut oil, butter and safflower oil on plasma lipids, lipoproteins and lathosterol levels. *Eur J Clin Nutr* 1998;52: 650–654.

74. Pehowich DJ, Gomes AV, Barnes JA. Fatty acid composition and possible health effects of coconut constituents. *West Indian Med J* 2000;49:128–133.

75. McNamara DJ. Palm oil and health: a case of manipulated perception and misuse of science. *J Am Coll Nutr* 2010;29(suppl 3):240S–244S.

76. Aro A, Jauhiainen M, Partanen R, et al. Stearic acid, trans fatty acids, and dairy fat: effects on serum and lipoprotein lipids, apolipoproteins, lipoprotein(a), and lipid transfer proteins in healthy subjects. *Am J Clin Nutr* 1997;65:1419–1426.

77. Hu FB, Stampfer MJ, Manson JE, et al. Dietary saturated fats and their food sources in relation to the risk of coronary heart disease in women. *Am J Clin Nutr* 1999;70: 1001–1008.

78. Micha R, Mozaffarian D. Saturated fat and cardiometabolic risk factors, coronary heart disease, stroke, and diabetes: a fresh look at the evidence. *Lipids* 2010;45(10):893–905.

79. Mensink RP, Zock PL, Kester ADM, et al. Effects of dietary fatty acids and carbohydrates on the ratio of serum total to HDL cholesterol and on serum lipids and apolipoproteins: a meta-analysis of 60 controlled trials. *Am J Clin Nutr* 2003;77(5):1146–1155.

80. Thijssen MA, Mensink RP. Fatty acids and atherosclerotic risk. In von Eckardstein A, ed. *Atherosclerosis: diet and drugs*. Berlin, Germany: Springer, 2005:171–172.

81. Mensink RP, Zock PL, Kester ADM, et al. Effects of dietary fatty acids and carbohydrates on the ratio of serum total to HDL cholesterol and on serum lipids and apolipoproteins: a meta-analysis of 60 controlled trials1,2,3. *Am J Clin Nutr* 2003;77(5):1146–1155.

SUGGESTED READING

National Research Council. *Recommended dietary allowances*, 10th ed. Washington, DC: National Academy Press, 1989.

CHAPTER 3

Clinically Relevant Protein Metabolism

Protein represents one of three principal classes of macronutrients; the other classes are carbohydrate and fat. Dietary protein is required as a source of amino acids, both essential and nonessential, for use in the synthesis of structural and functional body proteins. The need for amino acids is driven by the constant turnover of body tissues; the demands of growth and development; anabolism induced by muscle use; and tissue repair. In its function as a source of fuel, protein is the least energy-dense of the macronutrient classes, providing between 3 and 4 kcal per g, although it closely approximates the energy density of carbohydrate. Calorie for calorie, it is the most satiating, a property of increasing significance and interest at a time of epidemic obesity (see Chapter 5).

Protein is unique among the macronutrient classes for containing nitrogen. The metabolism of amino acids in the body encompasses synthesis and degradation. Amino acids are synthesized to be incorporated into body proteins or to contribute to the body store of free amino acids for subsequent use in anabolism. Amino acids are degraded to produce other products of use and/or to generate energy. Protein represents the second largest energy store in the body after fat. When catabolized to produce energy, protein yields carbon dioxide and water through the tricarboxylic acid (TCA) cycle, also known as the Krebs, or citric acid, cycle. Nitrogenous waste is generated, which is metabolized to urea for excretion. Nitrogenous intermediates, such as ammonia, are toxic, and are accumulated when hepatic (see Chapter 17) or renal (see Chapter 16) function is impaired. For this reason, protein restriction is often warranted in states of hepatic and/or renal insufficiency.

Ingested proteins are broken down by pepsin in the stomach and further by pancreatic enzymes activated on release into the duodenum. Pancreatic enzyme release is stimulated by the presence of protein in the stomach and inhibited when the level of trypsin, a protein-directed pancreatic enzyme, exceeds the available protein to which it can bind. Unbound trypsin inhibits the release of trypsinogen, a precursor to trypsin. Trypsin and other pancreatic proteases, or enzymes that break down protein, are specific to peptide bonds adjacent to particular amino acids or amino acid classes (see Table 3-1). Amino acids and dipeptides are absorbed through the mucosa of the small bowel. The amount of protein absorbed daily is derived from that ingested, as well as the protein from gastrointestinal secretions and the sloughing of gastrointestinal cells into the bowel lumen.

Once absorbed, amino acids are transported to the liver via the portal vein. The liver is the principal site of catabolism for all the essential amino acids, except those with branched chains. The branched-chain amino acids are catabolized principally in muscle and kidney, which provides a rationale for their use in selected cases of advanced liver disease (see Chapter 17).

The liver responds to varying levels of intake of the essential amino acids by inducing or inhibiting specific enzymatic pathways. Metabolism of essential amino acids consumed in excess of need is accelerated to eliminate the excess. The degree of regulation is less strict for nonessential amino acids, the metabolism of which is roughly proportional to the amount ingested. The synthetic functions of the liver relying on metabolized protein as substrate vary over time according to the availability of amino acids from the circulation. While nutrition texts at one time asserted the need for all essential amino acids to be ingested concomitantly for anabolism to occur, this is now known to be false. Such metabolic fastidiousness

TABLE 3.1

Amino Acids of Importance in Human Metabolism, Categorized as Essential, Conditionally Essential, or Nonessential

Amino Acid Classification	Structural Category[a]
Essential	
Histidine	Aromatic
Isoleucine	Neutral (branched chain)
Leucine	Neutral (branched chain)
Lysine	Basic
Methionine	Sulfur containing
Phenylalanine	Aromatic
Threonine	Neutral
Tryptophan	Aromatic
Valine	Neutral (branched chain)
Conditionally Essential[b]	
Cysteine	Sulfur containing
Tyrosine	Aromatic
Nonessential	
Alanine	Neutral
Arginine	Basic
Aspartic acid	Acidic
Asparagine	Acidic
Glutamic acid	Acidic
Glutamine	Acidic
Glycine	Neutral
Proline	Cyclic
Serine	Neutral

[a]Amino acids are categorized based on their molecular structure as neutral, sulfur containing, cyclic, aromatic, basic, and acidic (amino acids and amides). Leucine, isoleucine, and valine are also referred to as branched-chain amino acids.

[b]Required in diet if precursor from column 1 is consumed in inadequate quantity.

Source: Matthews DE. Proteins and amino acids. In: Shils M, Shike M, Ross AC, et al., eds. *Modern nutrition in health and disease*, 10th ed. Philadelphia, PA: Lippincott Williams & Wilkins, 2006:23–61.

would certainly have posed a survival threat to our nutritionally challenged forebears. We now know that as long as the full panoply of essential amino acids is consumed over a reasonable span of time, certainly up to 24 hours, anabolism proceeds apace (1–5).

Plasma levels of amino acids are influenced by dietary intake to varying degrees. The liver controls the release of specific amino acids into the peripheral circulation, but the levels of some amino acids rise as intake exceeds metabolic demand. Conversely, levels in plasma fall as intake falls, but only as low as the level needed to satisfy the demand of body tissues. At that level, called the point of inflection, plasma levels are maintained as intake falls, barring frank deficiency, by turnover of protein stores. This level has been used to determine the dietary requirements for certain amino acids, although it is not a reliable index for all of them.

Carbohydrate ingestion stimulates insulin release, and insulin facilitates the entry of amino acids into muscle. Because insulin is involved in protein metabolism, ingestion of a mixed meal containing protein and carbohydrate typically induces a more brisk insulin response than does ingestion of carbohydrate alone, a point obscured in recent years by proponents of low-carbohydrate diets (see Chapters 5 and 6).

The levels of branched-chain amino acids, in particular, fall after a carbohydrate meal, with attendant insulin release. Branched-chain amino acids (leucine, isoleucine, and valine) compete with tryptophan for uptake by brain cells. Thus, a carbohydrate meal inducing a brisk insulin response will result in preferential uptake of tryptophan by the brain by reducing plasma levels of competitive amino acids. Tryptophan is used in the production of serotonin, which is thought to be both soporific and mood enhancing. Selective serotonin reuptake inhibitors (SSRI) antidepressants work by raising serotonin levels in the brain (6). Tryptophan is rate-limiting in the synthesis of serotonin, and thus serotonin levels depend largely on hepatic regulation of protein degradation and the release of tryptophan and its uptake by the brain.

During a fast, the prototypical 70-kg adult loses approximately 50 g of protein per day from skeletal muscle, the largest depot in the body. The principal amino acids released from muscle are alanine and glutamine, which are the main carriers of nitrogen from muscle to the liver. Alanine is transported directly to the liver, whereas glutamine is transported to the intestine and transaminated to alanine before reaching the liver through the portal circulation.

In the liver, the carbon chain of alanine is used in gluconeogenesis, whereas the amino group is metabolized to urea or recycled to other amino acids. Under carefully controlled conditions, 3-methylhistidine, a product of protein catabolism in muscle, can be measured in urine to assess the extent of amino acid release from muscle to the liver.

The most readily accessible, and therefore measurable, pool of proteins is that circulating in plasma. Plasma proteins are predominantly glycoproteins and albumin. The levels of plasma proteins fall and rise with nutritional status. Albumin levels decline with significant malnutrition, but they are relatively insensitive to minor or short-term aberrations in dietary intake. Prealbumin and retinol-binding protein are better indicators of short-term deficits of dietary protein or energy (see Chapter 26).

For a 70-kg adult, daily dietary protein intake in the United States is approximately 100 g, augmented by approximately 70 g secreted or sloughed into the bowel. Roughly 160 of these 170 g are absorbed as amino acids or dipeptides, and 10 g are lost in stool. Approximately 300 g of protein is synthesized each day, utilizing nearly 200 g of recycled protein in addition to the 100 g ingested. Recycled proteins are derived from intestinal secretions and cells, plasma proteins, muscle, and senescent blood cells. A 100-g pool of free amino acids, predominantly nonessential, is maintained as well. A total of 400 g of amino acids is exchanged daily. Protein intake is 100 g, and 300 g of protein is derived daily from body-tissue turnover. Of this pool, 300 g is used for protein synthesis, and 100 g is consumed in catabolism.

Dietary protein provides amino acids for the synthesis of cells in all body tissues. Amino acids are essential if they cannot be synthesized endogenously. There are nine essential amino acids in humans: histidine, isoleucine, leucine, lysine, methionine, phenylalanine, threonine, tryptophan, and valine. Two other amino acids, cysteine and tyrosine, become essential if intake of their precursors, methionine and phenylalanine, respectively, is limited. The nonessential amino acids include arginine, alanine, aspartic acid, asparagine, glutamic acid, glutamine, glycine, proline, and serine. Other amino acids are derived from these 20 (see Table 3-1).

Ingested amino acids serve one of four purposes. They are used in the synthesis of tissue proteins, catabolized to meet energy needs, incorporated into energy stores as glycogen or adipose tissue, or used to synthesize other nitrogen-containing moieties, such as other amino acids, catecholamines, or purine bases. Amino acid degradation in the liver results in the formation of urea, most of which is secreted into urine. In the gut, about 20% of urea is converted to ammonia, which in turn is cleared by the liver via the enterohepatic circulation.

Amino acids are used in the synthesis of the purine bases, adenine and guanine, and the pyrimidine bases, uracil and cytosine. These ribonucleotides serve as precursors for DNA synthesis. Glutamine is important in the biosynthesis of purines. The initial step in pyrimidine biosynthesis involves carbamoyl phosphate, which also serves as a substrate for urea synthesis. When arginine intake is deficient, or in individuals with a deficiency of ornithine-carbamoyl transferase, excessive carbamoyl phosphate is diverted to the pyrimidine synthesis pathway. The result is the spillage of orotic acid in the urine, which is therefore a marker of arginine deficiency.

Arginine and glycine are metabolized in the kidney and liver to produce creatine. Creatine is transported to muscle, where it is stored as creatine and creatine phosphate. A dehydration reaction in muscle converts creatine and creatine phosphate to creatinine, which is released from muscle into the pool of total body water. Slightly less than 2% of creatine in the body is converted to creatinine each day. The quantity of urinary creatinine is a product of muscle mass, the concentration of creatine in muscle, and dietary intake of creatine in meat.

Ammonia is formed in the kidney as an end product of glutamine metabolism. The glutamine ultimately is metabolized to α-ketoglutarate, which is used in gluconeogenesis during a protracted fast. Acidosis and starvation accelerate ammonia production.

Protein metabolism is linked to carbohydrate and fat metabolism. In the fasted state, insulin levels are low and glucagon levels are elevated. Lipases in adipose tissue release fatty acids and glycerol. Glycogen stores in the liver are consumed to meet energy needs for the first 12 to 18 hours of fasting. With more protracted fasting, energy needs are met by the release of protein from muscle and intestine, serving as a substrate for gluconeogenesis in the liver. The gluconeogenic amino acids are alanine, glutamine, glycine, serine, and threonine. Free fatty acids are used in the liver to produce ketone bodies. Muscle uses free fatty acids, and subsequently ketone bodies, as an alternative fuel to glucose. Lysine and leucine are ketogenic, whereas isoleucine, phenylalanine, threonine, tryptophan, and tyrosine are potentially both ketogenic and gluconeogenic.

With feeding, insulin levels rise and glucagon levels subside. Glucose is carried into the liver and muscle, both to reconstitute glycogen and to be used as fuel. Insulin suppresses the action of lipases in adipose tissue and inhibits the release of fatty acids.

NITROGEN BALANCE

Nitrogenous wastes are removed from the body in urine as urea, ammonia, uric acid, and creatinine and in stool as unabsorbed proteins. Minor losses occur through skin and in the form of shed integument and the secretions of mucous membranes. Ordinarily, urea accounts for approximately 80% of the nitrogenous waste in urine. During a protracted fast, the proportion of urine nitrogen lost in the form of ammonia rises, particularly in response to acidosis.

Proteins typically contain approximately 16% nitrogen; therefore, 1 g of nitrogen corresponds to 6.25 g of total protein. Nitrogen balance (B) is measured as the difference between intake (I) and all losses, including urine (U), feces (F), skin (S), and miscellaneous minor losses (M):

$$B = I - (U + F + S + M)$$

B may be positive, negative, or zero. (For additional pertinent formulas, see Section VIIA.)

Nitrogen balance is affected by total energy intake. When ingested calories exceed need, protein needs fall, and nitrogen balance remains positive. When energy intake falls to near or below requirements, protein needs rise, and nitrogen balance tends to become negative unless protein intake increases substantially. Amino acid requirements in men have been estimated to range from 0.5 g/kg/day when energy intake is high (57 kcal/kg/day) to over 1 g/kg/day when energy intake is low (40 kcal/kg/day). Even with high intake of energy, however, essential amino acid consumption below required levels will result in negative nitrogen balance. In a state of normal health and dietary adequacy in an adult, nitrogen balance is maintained, with intake matching losses.

DIETARY PROTEIN REQUIREMENTS

Protein requirements have been estimated on the basis of replacing obligate nitrogen losses (i.e., those losses that persist on a protein-free diet) and on the basis of maintaining healthy adults in nitrogen balance. For children, estimates have been based on the maintenance of optimal growth. Requirements during pregnancy and lactation have been estimated on the basis of optimal fetal and neonatal growth.

Obligate nitrogen losses on a protein-free diet have been estimated at approximately 54 mg per kg. To replace this amount of nitrogen, 340 mg of protein is required (nitrogen is multiplied by 6.25 to give an average relative protein mass). Therefore, 0.34 g/kg/day of protein is required to replenish obligate losses of sedentary adults. The World Health Organization increases that value to 0.45 g/kg/day to account for individual variation. Replacement studies have further demonstrated that as protein is replenished, the efficiency of its utilization declines as intake approaches requirements. This inefficiency adds 30% to required intake, increasing the estimate for adults to 0.57 g/kg/day. Where energy intake is not clearly in excess of need, this estimate is further raised to 0.8 g/kg/day.

In the United States, the average daily requirement for total protein has been estimated at 0.6 g/kg/day, given the availability of both abundant nutrient energy for most of the population and of protein of high biologic quality. This figure was increased by two standard deviations to 0.75 g/kg/day and then rounded up to 0.8 g/kg/day to establish the RDA (recommended dietary allowance) for adult men and women in the United States. Pregnancy adds approximately 10 g to daily protein needs, and lactation adds nearly 15 g for the first 6 months, then in the range of 12 g thereafter. Rapid growth in early childhood results in substantially higher needs for protein. The RDA for infants up to 6 months of age is 2.2 g/kg/day; between 6 months and 1 year, it is 1.2 g/kg/day; and by age 7, it declines to approximately 1.0 g/kg/day (see Table 3-2). The adult RDA of 0.8 g/kg/day pertains beginning at age 15 in females and 19 in males. Higher intake levels may be indicated with vigorous physical activity (see Chapter 32).

Estimates are available of the required daily intake of each of the essential amino acids for both children and adults (see Section VIIE). The proportion of daily protein intake that must be made up of essential amino acids declines from over 40% in infancy, to approximately 35% in children, and further to 20% in adults. When protein losses attributable to acute illness or injury are being made up during the convalescent period, protein

TABLE 3.2

Recommended Dietary Allowance of Protein Based on Age and Sex, Pregnancy, and Lactation

Population Group	RDA for Protein in g/kg/day
Infants, 0 to 6 months	1.52[a]
Infants, 7 to 12 months	1.2
Boys and girls, 1 to 3 years	1.05
Boys and girls, 4 to 8 years	0.95
Boys and girls, 9 to 13 years	0.95
Boys and girls, 14 to 18 years	0.85[b]
Men and women, 19 to >70 years	0.80[b]
Pregnant women	1.1
Lactating women	1.3

[a]The AI, or adequate intake, rather than the RDA; an RDA value is not available.

[b]Whereas the recommended protein intake per kilogram body weight is the same for males and females in these age groups, the absolute protein intake recommended differs due to prevailing differences in body mass.

Source: Adapted from Panel on Macronutrients, Food and Nutrition Board, Institute of Medicine of the National Academies of Science. Protein and amino acids. In: *Dietary reference intakes for energy, carbohydrate, fiber, fat, fatty acids, cholesterol, protein, and amino acids*. Washington, DC: National Academy Press; 2005:589–768.

with 35% to 40% essential amino acids is generally favored. Protein restriction is required during acutely decompensated hepatic insufficiency (see Chapter 17) and uremia (see Chapter 16).

For protein synthesis to occur, all essential amino acids must be available simultaneously; they need not be ingested simultaneously, however. Essential amino acids can be mobilized from tissue stores to support anabolism. Thus, an adequate intake of complete protein over time, rather than at any one time, is vital. There is some evidence to suggest that the ingestion of essential amino acids in temporal proximity to exercise may foster muscle protein synthesis (7–20) (see Chapter 32).

If there is a prevailing deficit in any of the essential amino acids, its generation to permit protein synthesis will require catabolism. Thus, the ingestion of balanced protein is necessary to prevent negative nitrogen balance. Protein synthesis may be accelerated within the first several postprandial hours; nonetheless, the ingestion of incomplete but complementary protein meals over a day supports protein synthesis

comparably to the ingestion of balanced protein during a single meal.

High doses of single amino acids may be toxic; this is particularly true for methionine and tyrosine. Antagonism, in which high doses of an amino acid interfere with the metabolism of another, may also occur; this is true for the branched-chain amino acids (valine, leucine, and isoleucine). An imbalance in amino acids refers to situations in which tissue growth is impaired due to limiting amounts of one or more amino acids, despite adequate total protein intake.

PROTEIN QUALITY/BIOLOGIC VALUE

The quality of dietary protein refers to the array of amino acids provided. The more completely food protein provides essential amino acids, the greater its biologic quality. A variety of methods have been used to gauge the biologic value of protein, the favored of which is to determine the proportion of a protein used in metabolism without raising nitrogen losses. A formula used to indicate the degree to which ingested nitrogen is retained is a common measure of protein quality, or biologic value:

$$\text{Biologic value} = [\text{Food N} - (\text{Fecal N} + \text{Urinary N})]/(\text{Food N} - \text{Fecal N})$$

The value for egg albumin, which represents a complete source of amino acids, is 100; other proteins are compared with this reference standard. Alternative measures of protein quality are also in use; the biologic value of protein may be expressed as the ratio of the limiting amino acid per gram of a particular food to its quantity per gram of egg. Lysine, sulfur-containing amino acids (cysteine, methionine), and tryptophan tend to be limiting.

Proteins used more completely in metabolism are considered to be of higher biologic value. In general, meat and eggs provide protein of high biologic value, as do dairy products, whereas protein of plant origin tends to be of lower quality because it meets amino acid requirements less completely. However, soybean and other legumes (e.g., lentils), certain beans, and nuts provide very high biologic quality protein (see Table 3-3, and Section VIIF). Furthermore, consuming a diet containing protein primarily derived from plant sources as opposed to animal sources may help reduce the risk of coronary artery disease and stroke (21,22). The higher the biologic quality of ingested protein, the less of it is required to meet metabolic needs and vice versa. Of note, balanced vegetarian diets readily meet protein requirements because of the complementary amino acid profiles of various plant foods and because amino acids ingested at one time can be banked in body tissues for later use in anabolism.

Plants contain a wide variety of amino acids not used in protein synthesis in humans, some of which are actually toxic. The biologic value of plant protein may be modified further by other constituents that interfere with digestion. The soybean, for example, contains an inhibitor of trypsin, although it is inactivated by cooking. Whereas egg, dairy products, and meats provide protein of high biologic value when consumed alone, other foods do so in combinations. Vegetables combined with legumes or beans and cereal grains combined with nuts, seeds, or legumes, comprise complete protein sources (e.g., rice and beans, peanut butter on whole-grain bread). Generally, a well-balanced diet in the United States provides ample protein of high biologic value. Vegans need to be particularly attentive to food combinations to be assured of optimal protein intake (see Chapter 43), but these combinations suffice when they are achieved over time; they need not pertain strictly to individual meals.

Table 3-3 lists foods and food combinations that are good sources of protein, offering all or nearly all essential amino acids.

PROTEIN DEFICIENCY

Malnutrition develops when protein needs are not met. In the developing world, protein-deficiency typically occurs when children are weaned from breast milk, resulting in a condition known as kwashiorkor. Infants and children with kwashiorkor are bloated and edematous. Their rotund bellies tend to misrepresent their severe malnourishment. Conversely, there is no mistaking a condition of wasting and emaciation due to a deficit of total calories (protein and other). This condition is known as marasmus.

In the United States during the 1970s, the use of very-low-calorie liquid diets that did not provide adequate protein was associated with sudden cardiac death due to the leaching of amino acids from viscera, including the heart. Susceptibility to this effect may be greater during such diets than during complete starvation because of other metabolic effects of total starvation (see Chapter 26). During starvation, approximately 25% of structural proteins can be turned over before life is threatened—often enough to sustain a fast for as long as 30 to 50 days. Very-low-calorie

TABLE 3.3	
Foods and Food Combinations That Provide Complete Protein (i.e., All Essential Amino Acids)	
Food or Food Combination	Comment
Eggs	The amino acid profile of egg albumin is virtually ideal for satisfying human need and is used as the reference standard in some measures of protein quality.
Meat, poultry, fish, seafood	Animal products provide the complete array of essential amino acids in varying proportions. There are, however, other important differences among meat sources, including the quantity and variety of fat and cholesterol content.
Dairy	Human breast milk is, ipso facto, an optimal protein source in infancy. Milk of other origins approximates, but does not exactly match, the amino acid profile of human milk.
Soy	Raw soy contains an enzyme that inhibits the action of trypsin on protein digestion; the enzyme is inactivated by cooking. Thus, cooked soy is a source of complete protein, but raw soy is not.
Grains and beans Grains and dairy Grains and legumes Nuts or seeds and legumes	Many simple and popular dishes, such as wheat cereal with milk, peanut butter on bread, and rice and beans provide plant-food pairings that offer complete protein.

Note: There are various measures for the quality of a protein source, and some include terms for digestibility, bioavailability, and other properties, along with the complement of amino acids.

liquid diets now provide complete protein, to allow for a so-called protein-sparing modified fast (see Chapter 5), considerably mitigating the risks involved.

SATIETY INDEX OF PROTEIN

Calorie-for-calorie, protein is the most satiating (filling) of the nutrient classes (23), followed by complex carbohydrate, then simple carbohydrate, and, finally, fat (24–28). This means it takes more calories from fat than from either carbohydrate or protein to feel comparably full. Because fat is the least satiating of the nutrient classes, high-fat foods can readily contribute to overconsumption of calories (29–36).

Because protein is the most filling of the nutrient classes, increasing protein intake—as is recommended in some popular diets—may be of some use in weight control (37–41). However, the available evidence generally indicates that simply adjusting the levels of various macronutrients in the diet is unlikely to exert a significant influence on total calories consumed over time (28,42–45).

FOOD PROCESSING

Heating food can reduce the availability of lysine in particular. If exposed to high heat, proteins can denature and potentially become less readily digestible. In some cases, however, heat actually enhances the protein quality of a food. As has been mentioned, soy contains an inhibitor of trypsin that interferes with protein digestion; it is inactivated when soy is cooked. Oxidation may deplete methionine.

Many processed meats contain high levels of sodium, phosphorus, and nitrites. Consumption of processed meat has been associated with an increased risk of type 2 diabetes (45–48), chronic obstructive pulmonary disease (COPD) (49), colon cancer (50,51), pancreatic cancer (52).

REFERENCES

1. Matthews DE. Proteins and amino acids. In: Shils ME, Shike M, Ross AC, Caballero B, Cousins RJ, eds. *Modern nutrition in health and disease*, 10th ed. Philadelphia, PA: Lippincott Williams & Wilkins, 2006:23–61.
2. Panel on Macronutrients, Food and Nutrition Board, Institute of Medicine of the National Academies of Science. Protein and amino acids. In: *Dietary reference intakes for energy, carbohydrate, fiber, fat, fatty acids, cholesterol, protein, and amino acids*. Washington, DC: National Academy Press, 2002:589–768.
3. McNurlan MA, Garlick PJ. Protein synthesis and degradation. In: Stipanuk MH, ed. *Biochemical and physiological aspects of human nutrition*. Philadelphia, PA: Saunders, 2000:211–232.
4. Stipanuk MH, Watford M. Amino acid metabolism. In: Stipanuk MH, ed. *Biochemical and physiological aspects of human nutrition*. Philadelphia, PA: Saunders, 2000:233–286.
5. Fuller MF. Protein and amino acid requirements. In: Stipanuk MH, ed. *Biochemical and physiological aspects of human nutrition*. Philadelphia, PA: Saunders, 2000:287–304.
6. Shabbir F, Patel A, Mattison C, et al. Effect of diet on serotonergic neurotransmission in depression. *Neurochem Int* 2013;62(3):324–329.
7. Tipton KD, Gurkin BE, Matin S, et al. Nonessential amino acids are not necessary to stimulate net muscle protein synthesis in healthy volunteers. *J Nutr Biochem* 1999;10:89–95.
8. Tipton KD, Ferrando AA, Phillips SM, et al. Postexercise net protein synthesis in human muscle from orally administered amino acids. *Am J Physiol* 1999;276:E628–E634.
9. Volpi E, Kobayashi H, Sheffield-Moore M, et al. Essential amino acids are primarily responsible for the amino acid stimulation of muscle protein anabolism in healthy elderly adults. *Am J Clin Nutr* 2003;78:250–258.
10. Tipton KD, Elliott TA, Cree MG, et al. Ingestion of casein and whey proteins results in muscle anabolism after resistance exercise. *Med Sci Sports Exerc* 2004;36:2073–2081.
11. Borsheim E, Tipton KD, Wolf SE, et al. Essential amino acids and muscle protein recovery from resistance exercise. *Am J Physiol Endocrinol Metab* 2002;283:E648–E657.
12. Paddon-Jones D, Sheffield-Moore M, Zhang XJ, et al. Amino acid ingestion improves muscle protein synthesis in the young and elderly. *Am J Physiol Endocrinol Metab* 2004;286:E321–E328.
13. Tipton KD, Rasmussen BB, Miller SL, et al. Timing of amino acid–carbohydrate ingestion alters anabolic response of muscle to resistance exercise. *Am J Physiol Endocrinol Metab* 2001;281:E197–E206.
14. Tipton KD, Borsheim E, Wolf SE, et al. Acute response of net muscle protein balance reflects 24-h balance after exercise and amino acid ingestion. *Am J Physiol Endocrinol Metab* 2003;284:E76–E89.
15. Bohe J, Low A, Wolfe RR, et al. Human muscle protein synthesis is modulated by extracellular, not intramuscular amino acid availability: a dose–response study. *J Physiol* 2003;552:315–324.
16. Pitkanen HT, Nykanen T, Knuutinen J, et al. Free amino acid pool and muscle protein balance after resistance exercise. *Med Sci Sports Exerc* 2003;35:784–792.
17. Lemon PW, Berardi JM, Noreen EE. The role of protein and amino acid supplements in the athlete's diet: does type or timing of ingestion matter? *Curr Sports Med Rep* 2002;1:214–221.
18. Wolfe RR. Effects of amino acid intake on anabolic processes. *Can J Appl Physiol* 2001;26:S220–S227.
19. Drummond MJ, Dreyer HC, Fry CS, et al. Nutritional and contractile regulation of human skeletal muscle protein synthesis and mTORC1 signaling. *J Appl Physiol* 2009;106(4):1374–1384.
20. Walker DK, Dickinson JM, Timmerman KL, et al. Exercise, amino acids, and aging in the control of human

muscle protein synthesis. *Med Sci Sports Exerc* 2011; 43(12):2249–2258.

21. Hu FB. Plant-based foods and prevention of cardiovascular disease: an overview. *Am J Clin Nutr* 2003;78(3 suppl): 544S–551S.

22. Pan A, Sun Q, Bernstein AM, et al. Red meat consumption and mortality: results from 2 prospective cohort studies. *Arch Intern Med* 2012; 172(7):555–563.

23. Anderson GH, Moore SE. Dietary proteins in the regulation of food intake and body weight in humans. *J Nutr* 2004;134:974S–979S.

24. Stubbs J, Ferres S, Horgan G. Energy density of foods: effects on energy intake. *Crit Rev Food Sci Nutr* 2000;40:481–515.

25. Crovetti R, Porrini M, Santangelo A, et al. The influence of thermic effect of food on satiety. *Eur J Clin Nutr* 1998;52: 482–488.

26. Holt SH, Miller JC, Petocz P, et al. A satiety index of common foods. *Eur J Clin Nutr* 1995;49:675–690.

27. Westerterp-Plantenga MS, Rolland V, Wilson SA, et al. Satiety related to 24 h diet-induced thermogenesis during high protein/carbohydrate vs high fat diets measured in a respiration chamber. *Eur J Clin Nutr* 1999;53:495–502.

28. Raben A, Agerholm-Larsen L, Flint A, et al. Meals with similar energy densities but rich in protein, fat, carbohydrate, or alcohol have different effects on energy expenditure and substrate metabolism but not on appetite and energy intake. *Am J Clin Nutr* 2003;77:91–100.

29. Green SM, Wales JK, Lawton CL, et al. Comparison of high-fat and high-carbohydrate foods in a meal or snack on short-term fat and energy intakes in obese women. *Br J Nutr* 2000;84:521–530.

30. Green SM, Burley VJ, Blundell JE. Effect of fat- and sucrose-containing foods on the size of eating episodes and energy intake in lean males: potential for causing overconsumption. *Eur J Clin Nutr* 1994;48:547–555.

31. Blundell JE, Burley VJ, Cotton JR, et al. Dietary fat and the control of energy intake: evaluating the effects of fat on meal size and postmeal satiety. *Am J Clin Nutr* 1993;57:772S–777S.

32. Blundell JE, MacDiarmid JI. Fat as a risk factor for overconsumption: satiation, satiety, and patterns of eating. *J Am Diet Assoc* 1997;97:S63–S69.

33. Golay A, Bobbioni E. The role of dietary fat in obesity. *Int J Obes Relat Metab Disord* 1997;21:S2–S11.

34. Rolls BJ. Carbohydrates, fats, and satiety. *Am J Clin Nutr* 1995;61:960S–967S.

35. Blundell JE, Lawton CL, Cotton JR, et al. Control of human appetite: implications for the intake of dietary fat. *Annu Rev Nutr* 1996;16:285–319.

36. Saris WH. Sugars, energy metabolism, and body weight control. *Am J Clin Nutr* 2003;78:850S–857S.

37. Westerterp-Plantenga MS, Lejeune MP, Nijs I, et al. High protein intake sustains weight maintenance after body weight loss in humans. *Int J Obes Relat Metab Disord* 2004;28:57–64.

38. Poppitt SD, McCormack D, Buffenstein R. Short-term effects of macronutrient preloads on appetite and energy intake in lean women. *Physiol Behav* 1998;64:279–285.

39. Wycherley TP, Moran LJ, Clifton PM, et al. Effects of energy-restricted high-protein, low-fat compared with standard-protein, low-fat diets: a meta-analysis of randomized controlled trials. *Am J Clin Nutr* 2012;96(6):1281–1298.

40. Westerterp-Plantenga MS, Lemmens SG, Westerterp KR. Dietary protein—its role in satiety, energetics, weight loss and health. *Br J Nutr* 2012;108 (suppl 2):S105–S112.

41. Halford JC, Harrold JA. Satiety-enhancing products for appetite control: science and regulation of functional foods for weight management. *Proc Nutr Soc* 2012;71(2):350–362.

42. Jequier E. Pathways to obesity. *Int J Obes Relat Metab Disord* 2002;26:S12–S17.

43. Gerstein DE, Woodward-Lopez G, Evans AE, et al. Clarifying concepts about macronutrients' effects on satiation and satiety. *J Am Diet Assoc* 2004;104:1151–1153.

44. Vozzo R, Wittert G, Cocchiaro C, et al. Similar effects of foods high in protein, carbohydrate and fat on subsequent spontaneous food intake in healthy individuals. *Appetite* 2003;40:101–107.

45. Marmonier C, Chapelot D, Louis-Sylvestre J. Effects of macronutrient content and energy density of snacks consumed in a satiety state on the onset of the next meal. *Appetite* 2000;34:161–168.

46. Pan A, Sun Q, Bernstein AM, et al. Red meat consumption and risk of type 2 diabetes: 3 cohorts of US adults and an updated meta-analysis. *Am J Clin Nutr* 2011;94:1088–1096.

47. Fretts AM, Howard BV, McKnight B, et al. Associations of processed meat and unprocessed red meat intake with incident diabetes: the Strong Heart Family Study. *Am J Clin Nutr* 2012;95:752–758.

48. Song Y, Manson JE, Buring JE, et al. A prospective study of red meat consumption and type 2 diabetes in middle-aged and elderly women: the women's health study. *Diabetes Care* 2004;27:2108–2115.

49. Schulze MB, Manson JE, Willett WC, et al. Processed meat intake and incidence of Type 2 diabetes in younger and middle-aged women. *Diabetologia* 2003;46:1465–1473.

50. Varraso R, Jiang R, Barr RG, et al. Prospective study of cured meats consumption and risk of chronic obstructive pulmonary disease in men. *Am J Epidemiol* 2007;166(12): 1438–1445.

51. Miller PE, Lazarus P, Lesko SM, et al. Meat-related compounds and colorectal cancer risk by anatomical subsite. *Nutr Cancer* 2013;65(2):202–226.

52. Aune D, Chan DS, Vieira AR, et al. Red and processed meat intake and risk of colorectal adenomas: a systematic review and meta-analysis of epidemiological studies. *Cancer Causes Control* 2013; 24(4):611–627.

53. Larsson SC, Wolk A. Red and processed meat consumption and risk of pancreatic cancer: meta-analysis of prospective studies. *Br J Cancer* 2012;106(3):603–607.

Overview of Clinically Relevant Micronutrient Metabolism

Needs for nutrient energy are met by the macronutrient classes discussed in Chapters 1 through 3. Macronutrients—protein, carbohydrate, and fat—are consumed in quantities measured in grams and are plainly visible to the naked eye. In contrast, specific metabolic needs are met by various classes of micronutrients that are typically consumed in milligram or microgram amounts.

Micronutrients include vitamins and vitamin-like substances, minerals, and specific subclasses of macronutrients essential for survival. This chapter provides an overview of clinically relevant micronutrients and micronutrient classes. More detailed information for specific nutrients of interest can be found in the nutrient reference tables in Section VIIE.

VITAMINS

By definition, vitamins are organic compounds the body requires in small amounts for metabolic processes but cannot produce endogenously. In some instances, some endogenous production does occur but either is inadequate for metabolic demand or requires ingestion of a precursor. The consumption of provitamin A carotenoids is an example of the latter; vitamin D production in the skin can be an example of the former.

Vitamins are divided into water-soluble and fat-soluble groups. In addition, there are vitamin-like compounds—nutrients that meet some but not all of the defining criteria for vitamins. Some of these compounds are subject to reclassification if and when their essential role in metabolism is established. Historically, this has been predicated upon identifying a deficiency syndrome.

The letter designations of vitamins are something of an anachronism, reflecting the sequence in which essential dietary "factors" were discovered in the early part of the twentieth century.

The essential functions of vitamin B, for example, came over time to be attributed to a variety of nutrients that then took on numeric designations as well. In some instances, the numeric designations came into wide use (e.g., vitamins B_6 and B_{12}), whereas in other instances, the chemical name supplanted the alphanumeric. Further subdivisions have been identified over time, so that each of certain vitamins (e.g., vitamins A, D, and B_6) comprises a group of related compounds. Therefore, although the chemical name is preferred in most instances, the alphanumeric designation retains value in reference to a group of compounds with a shared biologic function.

Water-Soluble Vitamins

Water-soluble vitamins are generally readily available in the food supply, are well absorbed, and are stored to a very limited extent in the body. The water-soluble vitamins include the B complex—thiamine (B_1), riboflavin (B_2), niacin (B_3), pantothenic acid (B_5), pyridoxine (B_6), folate, biotin, cyanocobalamin (B_{12})—and ascorbic acid, or vitamin C. Vitamins included in the B complex are not chemically related to one another, but rather represent discrete nutrients initially (1910 to 1920) thought to be a single water-soluble vitamin.

Thiamine (B_1)

Thiamine functions as a cofactor in the decarboxylation of keto acids and interconversion of sugars; it plays a role in the pentose phosphate pathway and Krebs cycle, essentially serving to generate accessible energy. Because thiamine releases energy from ingested macronutrients, requirements vary with total energy intake.

Overt deficiency manifests as beriberi and occurs at an intake below 0.12 mg per 1,000 kcal in adults. Beriberi manifests in adults in two forms, either dry or wet beriberi. Dry beriberi presents with symmetrical peripheral sensory and motor neuropathies, and wet beriberi presents as neuropathy with cardiac involvement. Deficiency of thiamine often occurs in alcoholism and manifests as the Wernicke-Korsakoff syndrome. The administration of dextrose to thiamine-deficient patients can further deplete thiamine and induce an acute encephalopathic state; therefore, alcoholics seen for acute care should receive thiamine before dextrose. Additionally, alcoholics should receive thiamine supplementation to prevent Wernicke-Korsakoff syndrome from chronic malnutrition.

With an RDA (recommended dietary allowance) of 0.5 mg per 1,000 kcal, or 1.2 mg per day for men, 1.1 mg per day for women, and 1.4 mg per day during pregnancy and lactation, thiamine is innocuous in high doses. Paleolithic intake is estimated to have been nearly 4 mg per day in adults. Thiamine is widely found in foods but is abundant in relatively few, including pork, and grains and seeds with intact bran. Of note, heat during food preparation may affect thiamine function. Several studies have shown potential therapeutic applications for thiamine in treating diabetic retinopathy and nephropathy. In vitro studies have demonstrated that thiamine decreases apoptosis induced by high-glucose-conditioned extracellular matrix in human retinal pericytes, and a pilot study supported high-dose thiamine as a potential treatment for end-stage diabetic nephropathy (1,2).

Riboflavin (B₂)

Riboflavin catalyzes oxidation-reduction reactions in intermediate metabolism as a component of flavin mononucleotide and flavin adenine dinucleotide. The metabolic functions of vitamin B_6 and niacin require adequate riboflavin. Riboflavin deficiency most often occurs along with deficiencies of other water-soluble vitamins; reduced absorption from gastrointestinal conditions, insufficient intake with protein-calorie malnutrition, and increased excretion of riboflavin with antibiotics and systemic infections may also contribute specifically to deficiency. Riboflavin deficiency manifests as pathology of the skin and mucous membranes, particularly glossitis and stomatitis. Previous data support efficacy of high-dose riboflavin treatment (400 mg per day) for migraine prophylaxis (3,4). Several case reports have also demonstrated resolution of lactic acidosis induced by nucleoside reverse-transcriptase inhibitors when treated with riboflavin (50 mg per day) (5). The RDA for riboflavin is 0.6 mg per 1,000 kcal, or 1.3 mg per day for men, 1.1 mg per day for women, 1.4 mg per day during pregnancy, and 1.6 mg per day during lactation. Higher intake is not associated with known toxicity. Paleolithic intake is estimated to have been upward of 6 mg per day. Riboflavin is naturally abundant in meat and dairy products and in grain products in the United States as a result of fortification.

Niacin (B₃)

Niacin refers to both nicotinic acid and nicotinamide. The vitamin functions in glycolysis, cellular respiration, and fatty acid metabolism as a component of nicotinamide adenine dinucleotide (NAD) and nicotinamide adenine dinucleotide phosphate (NADP). Niacin can be synthesized from the amino acid tryptophan; therefore, niacin ingestion is not essential when tryptophan is available in sufficient amount. However, conditions requiring increased demand for tryptophan, including carcinoid syndrome, isoniazid therapy, and Hartnup disease, can present with niacin deficiency. The efficiency with which tryptophan is converted to niacin is enhanced by the action of estrogens. In general, approximately 60 mg of tryptophan can be used to produce 1 mg of niacin; therefore, either is considered one niacin equivalent (NE).

Overt deficiency of niacin manifests as pellagra, a syndrome comprised of dermatitis (manifested as skin rash on sun-exposed areas), diarrhea (with abdominal pain and vomiting), and, when advanced, dementia. Pellagra is most common in patients suffering from alcoholism, anorexia nervosa, or malabsorptive disease. The RDA for niacin is 16 mg NE for adult males and 14 mg NE for adult females, with increased needs for females during pregnancy and lactation (18 and 17 mg NE, respectively). High-dose niacin (1.5 to 3 g per day) is used pharmacologically to treat hyperlipidemia and is associated with prostaglandin-induced vasodilation and flushing. Niacin may cause insulin resistance and has potential for hepatic toxicity in high doses; special attention should therefore be given to patients with diabetes and the monitoring of liver enzymes during niacin treatment. A paleolithic intake estimate is not available. Niacin is widely distributed in nature and is especially abundant in meat, dairy products, eggs, nuts, and fortified grain products.

Pantothenic Acid (B₅)

Pantothenic acid is a component of coenzyme A and the acyl carrier protein of fatty acid synthetase, which is integrated with the Krebs cycle and biotin dependent processes. As such, the vitamin is vital to the metabolism of, and energy release from, carbohydrate, protein, and fat. It plays a role in the synthesis of acetylcholine, functions in cholesterol and steroid hormone biosynthesis, and is required for protoporphyrin production.

Deficiency induced under experimental conditions leads to a wide range of manifestations, but a naturally occurring deficiency syndrome is not known to exist. Malnourished prisoners of war have been known to develop paresthesias of the feet (burning foot syndrome) relieved by administration of pantothenic acid. An adequate intake (AI) for pantothenic acid has been set at 5 mg per day for adults, 6 mg per day during pregnancy, and 7 mg per day during lactation; this is based on data about usual intakes for US adults, as insufficient information is available for setting a true RDA. An estimate of paleolithic intake is not available. High doses of pantothenic acid are apparently safe but can cause diarrhea. Pantothenic acid is found in fish and poultry, organ meats, eggs, tomato products, broccoli, legumes, and whole grains; it can also be produced by colonic bacteria.

Pyridoxine (B₆)

Vitamin B_6 refers to pyridoxine, pyridoxal, and pyridoxamine, which function in transamination reactions. Vitamin B_6 is therefore of fundamental importance to amino acid metabolism, and B_6 requirements rise as protein intake rises. It also functions as a coenzyme in pathways of gluconeogenesis, heme, sphingolipid, and neurotransmitter biosynthesis. Overt deficiency manifests as dermatitis, anemia, depression, and seizures. The RDA for vitamin B_6 is 0.016 mg per g of protein, resulting in a recommendation of 1.3 mg per day for most adults between 19 and 50 years old. The RDA for females 51 years and older is 1.5 mg per day and for males it is 1.7 mg per day. Additionally, the RDA during pregnancy is 1.9 mg per day and 2 mg per day during lactation. An estimate of paleolithic intake is not available. High doses well above the RDA, generally used for treating

neuropathies, are relatively safe but may induce a transient dependency and may be neurotoxic (6). Numerous drugs, including isoniazid, L-dopa, and theophylline, alter vitamin B_6 status such that adjuvant supplementation may be advised. Genetic syndromes, including homocystinuria, cystathioninuria, and xanthurenic aciduria, can mimic vitamin B_6 deficiency; pyridoxine is used to treat homocystinuria. Pyridoxine has also been shown to improve mild to moderate nausea during pregnancy, and can be taken with doxylamine succinate, an antihistamine, for improved efficacy (7–9). Fish, poultry, and other meats are good sources of B_6, and other common sources in the US food supply include fortified cereals, soy products, and noncitrus fruits.

Folic Acid

Folate is converted to the biologically active tetrahydrofolic acid, which functions as a coenzyme in the transfer of 1-carbon units. Folate is essential in the metabolism of many amino acids and in the biosynthesis of nucleic acids. All rapidly dividing tissues are dependent on folate for viability.

Deficiency, which is common in developing countries, but may also be more common in developed countries than previously believed, manifests as macrocytic anemia, gastrointestinal disturbances, and glossitis. Folate deficiency has been identified as the most common nutrient deficiency in the United States, and is often seen in the elderly, alcoholics, and infants drinking goat's milk instead of cow's milk. It is also associated with certain drug use including trimethoprim, methotrexate, and phenytoin.

The RDA for folate has been set at 400 μg per day for all adults. The recognition that higher folate intake at the time of conception greatly reduces the risk of neural tube defects has resulted in mandated fortification of grain products since 1998 in the United States; data suggest that the rate of neural tube defects dropped by 25% within 2 years of fortification (3). Females of reproductive age are therefore advised to take supplements or eat folate-enriched foods. Current recommendations advise taking 400 to 800 μg per day one month before conception and during the first trimester (10,11). Afterwards, the RDA has increased to 600 μg per day for pregnant females and 500 μg per day during lactation (12). The approximation of this higher intake by the estimated paleolithic intake of 380 to 420 μg per day is noteworthy. Women with epilepsy may need higher folate supplementation since antiepileptic drugs have been known to alter folate metabolism and increase the risk of neural tube defects. The American College of Obstetricians and Gynecologists recommends taking 4 mg per day prior to conception (13,14). During pregnancy, monitoring folate and α-fetoprotein is important, and a folate level of at least 4 mg per mL may be necessary to ensure proper organogenesis (15).

Folate supplementation may serve to lower levels of blood homocysteine; the importance of this to cardiovascular risk is controversial (see Chapter 7). The principal risk of high-dose intake of folate is the masking of B_{12} deficiency. Folate is abundant in fruits and vegetables, particularly green leafy vegetables, and in fortified grains.

Biotin

Biotin functions as a component of several enzymes involved in the transfer of carboxyl units. These enzymes participate in fatty acid synthesis, gluconeogenesis, and the citric acid cycle. Biotin deficiency is unusual but can be induced by the ingestion of sufficient raw egg albumin, which contains avidin, a biotin antagonist. Deficiency is characterized by alopecia, seborrheic dermatitis, nausea and vomiting, depression, glossitis, and lethargy. Biotin is utilized for treating multiple carboxylase deficiency.

The RDA for biotin is not established, but the National Research Council has recommended intake in the range from 30 to 100 μg per day in adults. Paleolithic intake has not been estimated. High doses are not associated with any known toxicity. Good sources of biotin include yeast, soybeans, eggs (yolk), peanut butter, and mushrooms.

Vitamin B_{12}

Vitamin B_{12} refers to a group of cobalamin-containing compounds; the commercially available form is cyanocobalamin. Vitamin B_{12} is required to produce the active form of folate and participates in most aspects of folate metabolism. In addition, vitamin B_{12} is necessary for the conversion of methylmalonyl CoA to succinyl CoA. Methylmalonyl CoA accumulates when B_{12} is deficient; this deficiency impairs myelin formation and results in neuropathy. Methylmalonic acid is used as a screening marker to distinguish B_{12} deficiency from folate deficiency.

Unlike other water-soluble vitamins, which are replenished frequently from diverse dietary sources, B_{12} is stored in the liver in reserves that can last up to 30 years. Therefore, deficiency results when either dietary intake is deficient for protracted periods or absorption is impaired. The former situation occurs rarely and is usually due to veganism (strict vegetarianism), while the latter is more common, arising from gastric atrophy, *Helicobacter pylori* infection, chronic proton pump inhibitor use, and lack of intrinsic factor, a protein required for B_{12} absorption (see Chapter 43).

Deficiency of B_{12} due to lack of intrinsic factor is known as pernicious anemia. The deficiency syndrome consists of macrocytic anemia, a myelopathic syndrome known as subacute combined degeneration, and neuropathy consisting of paresthesias and/or deficits of memory and cognition. Sufficient folate intake can overcome the effects of B_{12} deficiency on the bone marrow but not the nervous system. The RDA for adults is 2.4 μg per day, 2.6 μg per day during pregnancy, and 2.8 μg per day during lactation. Paleolithic intake of B_{12} has not been estimated. There is no known toxicity associated with high doses. Vitamin B_{12} is found in meats, dairy products, shellfish, and eggs; it is naturally absent in all plant foods but is contained in fortified breakfast cereals.

Vitamin C (Ascorbic Acid)

Vitamin C is a cofactor in hydroxylation reactions that are particularly important in the production of collagen. Diverse roles of the nutrient suggest that it is of importance in immune function, wound healing, and possibly allergic reactions. Vitamin C functions as a potent antioxidant, generating interest in its potential to combat disease and retard the aging process. The serum level of vitamin C peaks at an intake in the range of 150 mg per day.

The RDA, previously set at 60 mg per day for adults, has been revised upward to 90 mg per day as the importance of antioxidants to health has become increasingly clear. Currently, the RDA is 90 mg per day for men, 75 mg per day for women, 85 mg per day during pregnancy, and 120 mg per day during lactation. Patients who smoke are recommended to add an additional 35 mg per day. High doses of vitamin C are relatively innocuous, but toxic effects, particularly gastrointestinal discomfort, at doses in excess of 500 mg per day have been reported. Overt deficiency manifests as scurvy and occurs at an intake level of approximately 10 mg per day in adults. Paleolithic intake of vitamin C is estimated to have been slightly above 600 mg per day. Ascorbate is abundant in fruits, especially citrus fruits, and a variety of vegetables.

Fat-Soluble Vitamins

In general, fat-soluble vitamins are stored in the body in sufficient reserves so that daily intake is not required. The fat-soluble vitamins include A, D, E, and K. Deficiencies in fat-soluble vitamins are associated with fat malabsorption which is present in several diseases, including cystic fibrosis, celiac disease, cholestatic liver disease, small bowel Crohn's disease, and pancreatic disease. Additionally, bariatric surgery can predispose patients to fat malabsorption and, therefore, patients will likely need postsurgical supplementation of fat-soluble vitamins (16).

Vitamin A

Vitamin A refers to a group of compounds known as retinoids with varying degrees of vitamin A activity; the predominant compound is retinol. Active vitamin A can be synthesized endogenously from carotenoid precursors. More than 500 carotenoids are known, but only approximately 10% of them have provitamin A activity. Among that 10% are β-carotene, α-carotene, and cryptoxanthin.

Vitamin A is incorporated into the rod and cone cells of the retina; in the rods, it is a structural constituent of rhodopsin and functions in night vision, whereas in the cones, it is utilized to produce iodopsin. Vitamin A also functions in the generation of epithelial cells, in the growth of bones and teeth, in reproduction (by several mechanisms), and in immune function.

Deficiency of vitamin A, due to malnutrition or fat malabsorption, results in night blindness and, in more extreme cases, more severe eye injury and visual impairment resulting from drying of the eye, or xerophthalmia. Deficiency is also associated with increased susceptibility to infectious disease. The RDA for vitamin A is measured in retinol activity equivalents (RAE), so called because of the various nutrients that can be used to produce active vitamin A. One RAE is equal to 1 μg of all-trans retinol, 12 μg of food-based all-trans-β-carotene, or 24 μg of other all-trans

provitamin A carotenoids. An intake of 900 RAE is recommended daily for adult males and 700 RAE for adult females, 770 RAE during pregnancy, and 1,300 RAE during lactation. Retinoids have therapeutic uses in certain diseases including measles, certain skin disorders, and acute promyelocytic leukaemia.

Paleolithic intake is estimated to have been three to four times the RDA and approximately twice the current intake among adults in the United States. Symptoms of vitamin A toxicity include headache, vomiting, visual disturbances, elevated cerebrospinal fluid pressure, desquamation, liver damage, and birth defects. Symptoms may result from single doses greater than 100,000 RAE in adults or 60,000 RAE in children. The upper limit has been set at 3,000 RAE vitamin A per day for adults. Toxicity does not result from the ingestion of provitamin A carotenoids. However, preformed vitamin A is efficiently absorbed in the small intestine and can lead to toxicity. Preformed vitamin A is found in organ meats, especially liver, and in fish, egg yolks, and fortified milk. Carotenoids are abundant in brightly colored fruits and vegetables. Vitamin A is potentially teratogenic in high doses, and thus prenatal vitamins generally provide lower levels than do standard supplements (see Chapter 27).

Vitamin D

Vitamin D refers to calciferol and related chemical compounds. Unique among vitamins, vitamin D is essential in the diet only when the skin is not exposed to sufficient ultraviolet light, which acts to produce vitamin D from a precursor stored in skin. Melanin in skin impedes vitamin D synthesis, so that dark-skinned people in temperate climates are particularly subject to deficiency without adequate dietary intake. The development of pale skin is now thought to be the result of a single, discrete genetic mutation that favored survival among peoples migrating northward out of Africa as a result of enhanced vitamin D production (4,5). After synthesis or ingestion, vitamin D undergoes two hydroxylation reactions, one each in the liver and the kidney, to the metabolically active 1,25-dihydroxycholecalciferol, or calcitriol. Calcitriol functions as a hormone that regulates the metabolism of calcium and phosphorus. Fundamentally, vitamin D promotes the intestinal absorption of calcium. Vitamin D is closely regulated by parathyroid hormone, as well as estrogen, placental growth hormone, and prolactin, which play a role in meeting increased demands during pregnancy and lactation. In addition to bone mineral homeostasis, vitamin D also plays a key role in various other organ systems. Both the vitamin D receptor and 1-α-hydroxylase have been found in neurons and glial cells, and vitamin D deficiency has been associated with brain health (17,18). Vitamin D deficiency is common in patients with Alzheimer's disease, depression, and lower cognitive function (19). However, a recent trial found no effect of vitamin D supplementation on patients with depression and low vitamin D levels (20). Additionally, vitamin D deficiency is associated with pancreatic beta cell dysfunction, insulin resistance, atherosclerosis, coronary artery disease, malignancies, and immune dysfunction (21). A recent study demonstrated that vitamin D deficiency, especially 25-hydroxyvitamin D concentrations lower than 30 nanomolar per L, was associated with increased mortality from all causes, cardiovascular diseases, cancer, and respiratory diseases (22).

Deficiency occurs with inadequate dietary intake and inadequate sun exposure, manifesting as rickets in children and osteomalacia in adults. Vitamin D in childhood may be important not only for bone health but also for the prevention of chronic diseases such as cancer, cardiovascular disease, and autoimmune disorders (6). When sun exposure is abundant, there is no requirement for dietary vitamin D; therefore, the recommended intake is predicated on the inconsistency of population exposure to sunlight. The AI developed for vitamin D is 15 μg (600 IU) daily during childhood, adolescence, and early adulthood; AI increases to 15 and 20 μg daily for adults ages 51 to 70 and 70 and older, respectively, and 15 μg daily during pregnancy and lactation. The new recommendations were established while assuming minimal sunlight exposure. Vitamin D supplementation is required in infants who are exclusively breast-fed due to low content of vitamin D in human milk. Patients receiving steroids will require increased vitamin D supplementation due to the steroid's inhibitory effect on vitamin D absorption in the gut. An estimate of paleolithic intake is unavailable. Sun exposure cannot result in vitamin D toxicity, but high-dose supplements can. The recommended safe upper limit is no more than 4,000 IU per day; intake greater than this may cause vitamin D intoxication, characterized by soft tissue calcification, kidney stones, and hypercalcemia. Vitamin D is found in fatty fish, but the principal source in the United States is milk, which is generally fortified with 100 IU per cup.

Vitamin E

Vitamin E refers to a group of compounds collectively known as tocopherols and tocotrienols. The most abundant and biologically active is α-tocopherol. Vitamin E functions as a lipid antioxidant, protecting and preserving the integrity of cellular and subcellular membranes. Overt deficiency is rare because of the distribution of vitamin E in the food supply. Deficiency is thought to manifest as muscle weakness, hemolysis, ataxia, and impaired vision.

The RDA is expressed in α-tocopherol equivalents (TE) and is 15 mg (equivalent to 22.5 IU) per day for adults. Higher intakes are required when the diet is rich in polyunsaturated fatty acids (PUFAs) that are subject to rancidification. Vitamin E is found in vegetable oils, so intake tends to rise with intake of PUFAs. The recommended upper limit for vitamin E is 1,500 IU from natural sources and 1,100 IU of synthetic vitamin E for adults without fat malabsorption.

A variety of health benefits have been claimed for doses between 200 and 800 IU daily; however, most recent trials have generated negative results (see Chapter 7 and Section VIIE). Vitamin E interferes somewhat with vitamin K metabolism and therefore can prolong the prothrombin time at high doses. High-dose supplementation in patients on anticoagulants or platelet-inhibiting drugs is apt to be particularly hazardous. Vitamin E supplements are racemic and have a fraction of the activity; however, all isomers can contribute to potential adverse effects (23). Supplemental vitamin E is primarily α-tocopherol, but natural forms have high amounts of γ-tocopherol, which can provide unique health benefits (24). Of note, several trials showing negative results of high-dose vitamin E used primarily α-tocopherol supplementation. Paleolithic intake is estimated to have been approximately 33 mg per day, approximately twice the current RDA. Vitamin E is found in vegetable oils and seeds. Due to its distribution in fat, high dietary intake is unusual and not recommended.

Vitamin K

Vitamin K refers to a group of compounds derived from naphthoquinone that are essential in the production of prothrombin; clotting factors VII, IX, and X; and proteins C and S. Vitamin K appears to have other functions as well, particularly related to bone and kidney metabolism. Vitamin K activity is related to its requirement as a cofactor for proteins with carboxyglutamic acid residues. Proteins involved in bone mineralization that require vitamin K include osteocalcin and matrix Gla protein. However, studies observing effects of vitamin K supplementation for treating osteoporosis has provided conflicting results. Limited amounts of vitamin K are stored in the body. Needs are met partly but not completely by synthesis of the vitamin by intestinal bacteria. Of interest, high doses of vitamins A and E may decrease vitamin K absorption and activity.

Deficiency of vitamin K, such as that induced by oral anticoagulant treatment, results in coagulopathy. Warfarin-induced coagulopathies can often be reversed by vitamin K supplementation. Newborns, who are particularly susceptible to deficiency due to a lack of intestinal flora, receive a prophylactic parenteral dose soon after birth. The RDA for an adult male is 120 μg per day and for an adult female is 90 μg per day. An estimate of paleolithic intake is not available. There is no particular toxicity associated with high-dose vitamin K. The vitamin is abundant in green leafy and cruciferous vegetables.

VITAMIN-LIKE SUBSTANCES

Certain organic nutrients for which a true requirement remains uncertain have vitamin-like properties. The nutrients listed here, and others, could come to be considered vitamins if and when an essential biologic function is identified, along with a need for dietary intake.

Choline

Choline is a water-soluble amine that functions as a key component of phosphatidylcholine (lecithin), sphingomyelin, and acetylcholine, all molecules that are vital to the structural integrity of biologic membranes and lipoprotein particles. Although humans can synthesize choline endogenously in the presence of adequate supplies of serine, methionine, vitamin B_{12}, and folate, the ION Food and Nutrition board established a recommended AI in 1998 of 550 mg per day for adult males and 425 mg per day for adult females.

A deficiency syndrome in humans has not been identified, however, decreased choline intake is thought to be associated with liver disease, muscle damage, atherosclerosis, and possible neurologic disease (25). Choline is critical during fetal development as well, and can influence spinal cord structure and function and impact memory development (26). Choline is widely distributed in the food supply.

Taurine

Taurine, an amino acid, functions in a variety of metabolic activities, including neuromodulation, stabilization of cell membranes, and osmotic regulation. Its influence on osmotic regulation, which occurs primarily in the brain and kidneys, can be beneficial in epilepsy, congestive heart failure, hypertension, and diabetes (27). Recent studies are investigating the role of taurine in cardiovascular disease due to its protective role in reperfusion injury and oxidation, as well as its antihypertensive and antiatherogenic properties (28). It is required for the production of certain bile salts. Taurine is not considered an essential nutrient because it can be synthesized from cysteine or methionine. However, because dietary taurine is thought to be essential during infant development, taurine is currently added to all infant formulas. There is no clear evidence of a deficiency syndrome or evidence of toxicity associated with high doses; nevertheless, it should be used with caution in patients with a history of hemostatic disorders. Taurine is relatively abundant in meat and seafood.

Carnitine

Carnitine is a nitrogenous compound synthesized from lysine and methionine in the liver and kidney. It functions in transesterification reactions and in the transport of long-chain fatty acids into mitochondria. Synthesis is adequate in the adult but may not be in newborns. Carnitine supplementation becomes important in preterm infants and hemodialysis patients. Certain drugs, including valproic acid, and stress states associated with sepsis, trauma, and organ failure can require increased demand for carnitine as demonstrated in humans and animals (29–31). Whereas human milk delivers adequate carnitine, the same may not be true of formula.

Deficiency in humans has been established, generally resulting from inborn errors of metabolism. Deficiency is predominantly manifest as muscle weakness, cardiomyopathy, and hypoglycemia. Supplementation is inconsistently beneficial in deficiency syndromes. Carnitine is abundant in meats and dairy products.

Inositol

Inositol is an alcohol, structurally similar to glucose. It functions as a constituent of phospholipids in biologic membranes and has been found to be essential for the replication of many human cell lines. To date, human deficiency has not been established. Inositol is found in cereal grains and can be synthesized from glucose. Current studies have shown multiple anticancer effects of inositol, and one pilot clinical study showed promise in using inositol to treat breast cancer (32).

Bioflavonoids

Bioflavonoids are water soluble, brightly colored phenolic compounds found in plants. They are believed to influence capillary permeability and fragility. Bioflavonoids are found in wine, beer, cocoa, and tea, and particularly in citrus fruits. A deficiency has not been defined in humans. Evidence of health benefit from this class of antioxidants is accumulating (see Chapters 7, 39, and 45).

Lipoic Acid

Lipoic acid is fat soluble and related to B vitamins. It functions as a coenzyme, transferring acyl groups, specifically, it is involved in enzyme complexes associated with glucose metabolism like pyruvate dehydrogenase. Lipoic acid is currently being investigated for its potential to limit oxidative damage resulting in diabetic neuropathy, improve glucose utilization, block viral transcription, and treat glaucoma and cataracts (33–35). A deficiency state is not known to exist in humans.

Coenzyme Q (Ubiquinone)

Coenzyme Q refers to a group of lipid-like compounds, structurally related to vitamin E. Members of the group all contain an isoprenoid side chain off a quinone ring; the number of units in the side chain varies from 6 to 10. Coenzyme Q_{10}, the group member of greatest interest to date, is the variety native to human mitochondria.

Coenzyme Q functions in mitochondrial electron transport. The highest cellular concentration of ubiquinone is in the inner membrane of the mitochondrion. Due to its role in energy metabolism, the highest tissue concentrations of ubiquinone reside in the heart, liver, and kidneys. Coenzyme Q is widely distributed in the food supply, and a true deficiency state has not been established. Interest in the potential benefits of higher doses than are generally provided by diet is considerable (see Section VIIE). Of particular interest is its potential to prevent atherosclerosis and cardiovascular disease. Statin drugs and some β-blockers, including propranolol, can reduce endogenous production of ubiquinone by as much as 40% (36). There are limited studies demonstrating the efficacy of coenzyme Q supplementation with statin use; however, a 150 to 200 mg per day supplement is recommended (37–39).

ANTIOXIDANTS

Multiple epidemiologic studies have demonstrated that diets with high amounts of fruit, vegetables, and nuts reduced the risk of developing multiple chronic conditions, including cancer, cardiovascular disease (CVD), and chronic obstructive pulmonary disease (COPD). Specifically, antioxidant nutrients within these food sources, including vitamin C, vitamin E, carotenoids, flavonoids, and selenium, impede atherogenesis and carcinogenesis by preventing oxidative damage of DNA, lipids, and proteins. Several observational studies have shown that patients with high occurrence of CVD, cancer, and COPD usually have decreased plasma levels of several antioxidants. However, multiple prospective studies have not clearly demonstrated a decreased risk of CVD, cancer, or COPD, with supplementation of either a single or combination of antioxidant nutrients (40). Of note, the Alpha-Tocopherol, Beta Carotene Cancer Prevention Study Group in 1994 showed that vitamin E supplementation was associated with an increase in hemorrhagic stroke mortality, and β-carotene was associated with increased incidence of cerebral hemorrhage (41). A meta-analysis conducted in 2007 actually showed that treatment with high dose β-carotene, vitamin A, and vitamin E may increase mortality (42). Antioxidant supplementation is not recommended for prevention of chronic disease in the general public, and needs to be evaluated carefully before recommendations are given for other patient groups.

MINERALS AND TRACE ELEMENTS

Although the term *mineral* is often applied to essential dietary inorganic elements, some of this group are not minerals, and *elements* is the proper designation. Nonetheless, those elements found most abundantly in human tissue are minerals and, given their abundance, are referred to as dietary macrominerals. They include calcium, phosphorus, magnesium, potassium, sodium, chloride, and sulfur. These substances are present in the body in amounts above 100 mg, up to as much as hundreds of grams. In contrast, trace elements are present in the body in milligram or even microgram quantities. Trace elements essential to human health include iron, copper, zinc, cobalt, molybdenum, selenium, manganese, iodine, chromium, fluoride, silicon, nickel, boron, arsenic, tin, and vanadium.

Macrominerals

Calcium

Healthy adults store more than 1 kg of calcium in the body, predominantly in bones and teeth. Calcium, a vital structural component of the skeleton, is essential for muscular contraction and participates in a variety of other biologic processes, including coagulation. Calcium deficiency results in osteopenia, with the skeletal depot serving to maintain serum levels under most circumstances. The RDA for calcium varies throughout the life cycle, with peak requirements in adolescents and the elderly; 1,200 mg per day is adequate for most adults. During pregnancy and lactation, the RDA for calcium is 1,300 mg per day for 14 to 18-year-old women, and 1,000 mg per day for 19 to 50-year-old women (43). A recent study by the U.S. Preventive Task Force reported that evidence was insufficient for recommending daily calcium supplementation in asymptomatic postmenopausal women for prevention of fractures (44). Paleolithic intake is estimated to have been nearly 2 g per day, more than twice the typical intake in the United States. Excessive intake accompanied by vitamin D supplementation may lead to

dyspepsia, constipation, soft tissue calcification, and hypercalcemia, although these outcomes are not associated with high intake from whole-food sources. Supplementation of greater than 500 mg per day should be divided due to a plateau in calcium absorption. Further, high protein intake can cause hypercalciuria due to decreased renal calcium reabsorption, and will require increased calcium intake (45). Dairy products, including milk, cheese, and yogurt, are the best dietary source of readily bioavailable calcium, providing approximately 300 mg per serving. Other sources of calcium include dark green vegetables, nuts, breads, and cereals.

Phosphorus

Phosphorus is primarily incorporated along with calcium into the hydroxyapatite of bones and teeth. Phosphorus also functions in the synthesis of nucleic acids and phospholipids and in the formation of high-energy phosphate bonds in ATP. Phosphorus intake should approximate calcium intake, and the RDA for the two nutrients is matched. Phosphorus deficiency is rare but can occur in patients with chronic alcoholism or those recovering from diabetic ketoacedosis. Symptoms of deficiency include muscle weakness, paresthesias, seizures, hemolytic anemia, impaired white blood cell function, and tissue hypoxia due to shifting of the oxygen–hemoglobin dissociation curve. Paleolithic intake has not been estimated but likely corresponds with the higher calcium intake. Excess dietary phosphorus, exceeding the calcium intake by more than two-fold, can lead to hypocalcemia and possibly secondary hyperparathyroidism. Foods rich in protein are generally rich in phosphorus as well; thus, meat and dairy products are good sources.

Magnesium

The 20 to 30 g of magnesium stored in an adult body are principally in bone and muscle. Magnesium is vital to the structural integrity of the mitochondrial membrane, nucleic acids, ribosomes, and functions as a cofactor in diverse metabolic pathways involving more than 300 enzymes (46). Specifically, magnesium is involved in hormone receptor binding, calcium channel gating, cellular membrane function, neuronal activity, muscular contraction and excitability (47). It is used as an antiseizure and an antihypertensive agent during eclampsia and preeclampsia, and a tocolytic during labor. Magnesium has also been shown to be beneficial for treating acute myocardial infarctions by providing protection against ischemia, reperfusion injury, and arrhythmias, while also improving contractility in stunned myocytes. The LIMIT-2 trial, a double-blind randomized trial, observed a reduction in 28-day mortality, incidence of left ventricular failure, and reduction in long-term mortality in patients receiving magnesium sulfate after an acute myocardial infarction (48). However, later trials including the ISIS-4 and MAGIC trials, failed to demonstrate efficacy in using magnesium to treat acute myocardial infarction leading to controversy in its clinical use (49,50). Severe deficiency, generally the result of malabsorption, diabetes, or alcoholism, is manifest as anorexia, irritability, psychosis, and seizures. Accumulating evidence suggests that chronic mild magnesium deficiency may contribute to the development of hypertension, coronary artery disease, arrhythmias, metabolic syndrome, type 2 diabetes, preeclampsia, and osteoporosis (51). A recent case-control study and meta-analysis suggests that increased magnesium intake is associated with lower risks of colorectal cancer (52). The RDA is 420 mg per day for adult males and 320 mg per day for adult females. Hypomagnesemia is rare; however, it is estimated that 75% of Americans do not meet the RDA for magnesium. This is predominantly due to mineral depletion in soil and water and consequently in food sources, reduced vegetable and whole grain intake, and medication use (53). Paleolithic intake has not been estimated. Excess intake of magnesium appears to be dangerous only in individuals with impaired renal function; toxicity is manifest as nausea, vomiting, and hypotension. Severe hypermagnesemia is life threatening. Mild elevations in serum magnesium concentrations may result in hypotension, cutaneous flushing, nausea, and vomiting. Higher serum magnesium levels can cause neuromuscular dysfunction, including drowsiness or even respiratory dysfunction. Severe hypermagnesemia may also lead to bradycardia, complete heart block, atrial fibrillation, and asystole (47). Dietary sources of magnesium include green vegetables, grains, beans, and seafood.

Potassium

Potassium is the principal cation of the intracellular space. It functions in osmotic regulation,

acid–base balance, and muscle cell depolarization. The cardiac muscle is particularly sensitive to potassium concentrations. Dietary deficiency of potassium is uncommon, but conditions producing fluid shifts, such as surgery, or metabolic imbalances such as diabetic ketoacidosis, can produce life-threatening derangements of the serum potassium. Potassium deficiency manifests with muscular weakness, paralysis, and confusion. Low dietary potassium is associated with increased risk of hypertensive crises and stroke (54). Deficiency is usually associated with increased gastrointestinal or urinary losses, most commonly due to vomiting diarrhea, laxative abuse, or diuretics. High dietary potassium intake is not associated with toxicity when renal function is normal. There is no RDA for potassium, but a daily intake by adults of at least 3 g per day is advised. Paleolithic intake is estimated to have been more than 10 g per day, exceeding current intake levels by a factor of four. Potassium is abundant in grains, legumes, vegetables, and fruits. Citrus fruits, raisins, and bananas are particularly good sources.

Sodium

Sodium is the major extracellular cation. The body of an adult stores approximately 100 g of sodium; more than half is in the extracellular space, and much of the remainder is in bone. Sodium functions to regulate the distribution of water in the body, regulate acid–base balance, and maintain transmembrane potential. Sodium deficiency, which results in hyponatremia, causes weakness, fatigue, anorexia, and confusion; if severe, hyponatremia can cause seizures and be life threatening.

There is no RDA for sodium, but a daily intake of at least 115 mg is thought to be essential, and an intake of at least 500 mg is advised. Excess intake may play a role in hypertension and osteoporosis, and is associated with CVD and stroke. Intake should be limited to not more than 2,400 mg per day; typical daily intake in the United States is nearly 4,000 mg. Paleolithic intake of sodium is estimated to have been less than 1,000 mg per day. Of note, potassium intake exceeded sodium intake by a factor of more than 10 in the prehistoric diet of humans, whereas in the modern diet of developed countries, sodium intake exceeds that of potassium by a factor of 2. Sodium is abundant in foods of animal origin, but it is present in the food supply principally as a seasoning or preservative added to processed foods.

Chloride

Chloride is distributed with sodium in the extracellular fluid, where it functions to maintain fluid and acid–base balance. Chloride functions in digestion as a constituent of hydrochloric acid in the stomach. Chloride deficiency does not generally occur under normal circumstances, but it can accompany sodium deficiency in the context of volume depletion or result from metabolic derangements. Chloride deficiency results in alkalosis and impaired cognition. The RDA for chloride has not been established; dietary deficiency is not considered a health threat. Chloride toxicity has not been reported. Paleolithic intake has not been estimated to date, but it likely corresponds to the lower sodium intake. Dietary chloride is derived largely from salt, with the same sources as for sodium.

Sulfur

Sulfur is present in all cells, principally as a component of the amino acids cystine, cysteine, methionine, and taurine. Cysteine is the rate-limiting substrate in glutathione synthesis, which is an antioxidant and involved in drug metabolism. Sulfur functions in collagen synthesis and in energy transfer. A deficiency syndrome has not been described. Sulfur is derived in the diet from the amino acids in which it is incorporated; therefore, intake corresponds with the quality and quantity of protein intake.

Trace Elements

Iron

Approximately 4 g of iron is stored in the body of a typical adult male and slightly less than 3 g in the body of a typical adult female. The primary function of iron is to transport oxygen as a component of hemoglobin, and the bulk of stored iron is in red blood cells. Iron is also incorporated in myoglobin, mitochondrial cytochromes, and several enzyme systems such as peroxidase and catalase. Iron-containing enzyme systems generally function in oxidation reactions.

Iron deficiency manifests in sequence as depleted ferritin, impaired erythropoiesis, and then microcytic hypochromic anemia, and it develops over time because of blood losses or inadequate intake. Iron deficiency is associated with impaired immunity and impaired cognition in children, and is the most common nutritional deficiency worldwide. Behavioral symptoms of iron deficiency include apathy, lethargy, and pica. The RDA for iron is 10 mg per day for adult males and 15 mg per day for adult females, with variations over the life cycle. During pregnancy the RDA for iron is 27 mg per day, and during lactation, the RDA for iron is 10 mg per day (55). Paleolithic intake is estimated to have been nearly 90 mg per day, which is six- to nine-fold higher than the RDA.

Toxicity from dietary iron in healthy individuals is virtually unknown, although a role in oxidative injury to cells has been proposed. Ferrous sulfate can be lethal at a dose of 3,000 mg in children and 200 to 250 mg per kg in adults. In individuals with hemochromatosis, a genetic disease resulting in enhanced iron absorption, iron accumulates to toxic levels, producing multiorgan system failure. Iron is absorbed in the upper small intestine. Absorption is enhanced by ascorbic acid and impaired by fiber, phytates, and oxalates in plant foods. Heme iron in meat is more readily absorbed than nonheme iron in plants. Good sources of iron include beef, lamb, and liver, and the dark meat of poultry. Beans, peas, broccoli, nuts and seeds, and green leafy vegetables are good sources of nonheme iron.

Copper

The store of copper—approximately 50 to 120 mg—in an adult body functions in at least 15 enzyme systems, largely those involved in oxidation and energy production. Copper participates in enzymes influencing immune cell function, collagen and elastin synthesis, and neurotransmitter generation. Dietary intake of copper generally readily exceeds requirements, and deficiency is rare. However, deficiency may occur in premature infants, and patients with malabsorption from celiac disease, cystic fibrosis, or Crohn's disease. Copper deficiency may also occur in patients with nephrotic syndrome or prior gastric surgery (56). Manifestations of copper deficiency include abnormal hair, skin depigmentation, myeloneuropathy, microcytic hypochromic anemia, neutropenia, and bone demineralization.

Excess zinc intake, which may occur with supplementation for treatment of the common cold and other conditions, can chelate ingested copper, prevent its absorption, and consequently cause deficiency (56,57). The RDA for copper is 900 μg per day for adults. An estimate of paleolithic intake is not available.

Copper toxicity from whole-food ingestion is unknown. Copper toxicity can occur with supplement ingestion in the range from 10 to 30 mg; symptoms include vomiting, diarrhea, and liver damage. Severe neurocognitive effects of copper toxicity are seen in Wilson's disease, a recessive genetic defect in copper metabolism. Copper is found in shellfish, legumes, nuts, seeds, and liver.

Zinc

The amount of zinc stored in the adult human body, approximately 2 to 2.5 g, resides primarily in bone, but it is distributed to all body tissues. Zinc functions in nearly 100 enzyme systems, plays prominent roles in CO_2 transport and digestion, and maintaining protein structure and nuclear stability. Zinc also influences DNA and RNA synthesis, immune function, collagen synthesis, olfaction, and taste. Zinc deficiency can manifest as anorexia, impaired growth and sexual maturation, impaired immune function, impaired wound healing and skin lesions, impotence, hypogonadism, oligospermia, alopecia, night blindness, and ageusia. Dermatologic changes associated with zinc deficiency primarily manifest in the extremities or around body orifices.

Although overt deficiency is rare in the absence of malnutrition, mild deficiency may be prevalent in the United States, particularly among the elderly. Zinc absorption may be impaired in pancreatic disease, and zinc, copper, and iron may all compete for absorption in the gut. Diabetes is associated with increased zinc excretion in the urine; however, supplementation may be associated with worsening glucose intolerance. Symptoms of deficiency include skin lesions and alopecia, as well as growth retardation in children with insufficient zinc. The RDA for zinc is 11 mg per day for adult males and 8 mg per day for adult females. Paleolithic intake is estimated to have been three to four times the RDA. High-dose zinc supplementation can result in vomiting; over time, zinc supplementation can interfere with copper metabolism. Supplementation in excess of 15 mg per day is controversial. Zinc supplements, including intranasal zinc, have been associated with anosmia (58). Zinc is found in meat, shellfish (especially oysters), legumes, nuts, and, to a lesser extent, grains.

Cobalt

Cobalt is an integral component of vitamin B_{12}, and a normal adult body contains approximately 1 mg of the element. Toxicity, manifesting as cardiomyopathy, has been observed in heavy drinkers of beer to which cobalt was added to improve foaming. There is no RDA for cobalt. Seafood represents the best dietary source.

Molybdenum

Molybdenum is a component of several enzyme systems that function in uric acid formation and in fluoride, iron, copper, and sulfur metabolism. Deficiency under natural conditions is unknown, but it has been observed in individuals with inborn errors of metabolism and following long-term total parenteral nutrition lacking the element. Manifestations of deficiency are principally neurocognitive, including irritability and eventually coma. The recommended daily intake for adults is 45 μg. An estimate of paleolithic intake is not available. Toxicity occurs at intakes in the range from 10 to 15 mg per day and manifests as diarrhea, anemia, and gout. High intake of molybdenum interferes with copper metabolism and possibly copper absorption. Molybdenum is found in dairy products, cereal grain, and legumes; concentration in food varies with concentration in soil.

Selenium

Selenium is a constituent of glutathione peroxidase, an important antioxidant, and enzyme systems involved in the synthesis of thyroid hormones. Selenium deficiency is associated with two diseases endemic to areas of China with low soil selenium content: Keshan disease is a cardiomyopathy, and Kashin–Beck syndrome is an inflammatory arthritis. Overt selenium deficiency in the United States is unknown. Low selenium intake, however, is suspected to increase the risk of atherosclerotic heart disease and several cancers, and may cause impaired immune function, macrocytosis, and whitened nail beds. Multiple studies suggest a benefit of selenium supplementation in HIV and Crohn's disease (59–61). The RDA is 70 μg per day for adult males, 55 μg per day for adult females, and 20 μg per day for children. Estimates of paleolithic intake of selenium have not been reported.

Toxicity can occur at high doses (well above 200 μg per day) and manifests as nausea, diarrhea, fatigue, neuropathy, loss of hair and nails, and potentially cirrhosis. The Nutritional Prevention of Cancer Trial found that selenium supplementation in patients with prior nonmelanoma skin cancer were at greater risk for developing squamous cell carcinoma and total nonmelanoma skin cancer (62). Selenium is widely distributed in the food supply, with concentrations varying with soil content. Brazil nuts are the most concentrated source, containing 544 μg per ounce of nut.

Manganese

Approximately 12 to 20 mg of manganese is stored in the body of an adult, with most found in bone, liver, and the pituitary gland. Manganese is concentrated in mitochondria. It functions as a component of numerous enzyme systems involved in connective tissue formation, urea synthesis, and energy release. Manganese deficiency has not been observed in humans under natural conditions. Although, a study examining the effects of manganese depletion in young men suggested that manganese deficiency may result in the development of scaly dermatitis and dyslipidemia (63). The RDA has not been established, but an intake of 2 to 5 mg per day is recommended for adults. Estimates of paleolithic intake have not been reported. Toxicity due to ingestion is rare; dementia and psychosis have been seen in manganese miners with heavy inhalation exposure. Manganese absorption is increased in iron deficiency, formula feeding, biliary obstruction, and long-term total parenteral nutrition. Dietary sources of manganese include nuts, grains, shellfish, coffee, and tea.

Iodine

The adult body contains approximately 20 to 50 mg of iodine, virtually all of which is incorporated into thyroid hormones (thyroxine and triiodothyronine). Iodine deficiency, common in regions with low soil iodine and lack of food supply fortification, results in endemic goiter. Maternal iodine deficiency during pregnancy and deficiency in infancy are associated with the syndrome of cretinism. Iodine metabolism is impeded by goitrogens contained in cabbage, cassava, and peanuts. Dietary pattern can influence susceptibility to goiter.

The RDA is 150 μg per day for adults, 220 μg per day during pregnancy, and 290 μg per day during lactation. In the United States, this level is met through fortification of salt. Paleolithic intake of iodine has not been reported. Dietary iodine intake in excess of the RDA is rarely toxic. Supplementation in excess of 50 mg per day can interfere with thyroid function and lead to an acne-like skin condition termed iododerma. Fish and shellfish are good sources of iodine, although fortified salt is the most reliable dietary source.

Chromium

The adult body contains 6 to 10 mg of chromium that is widely distributed throughout the body. The principal function of chromium is as a component of glucose tolerance factor, a complex that apparently facilitates binding of insulin to its receptors. Chromium supplementation may be of therapeutic benefit in insulin resistance (see Chapter 6). Chromium also functions in macronutrient oxidation and lipoprotein metabolism. Deficiency is associated with glucose intolerance, peripheral neuropathy, and, if severe, encephalopathy. Absorption in the small intestine is decreased with higher levels of zinc and iron; additionally, antacids and nonsteroidal anti-inflammatory drugs may also reduce absorption. In contrast, vitamin C has been shown to increase chromium uptake. The RDA for chromium has not been established, but the Food and Nutrition Board has advised an intake of 25 to 35 μg per day for adults. Estimates of paleolithic intake of chromium have not been reported. Toxicity from dietary sources is unknown primarily because of poor oral bioavailability. Sources include yeast, grains, nuts, prunes, potatoes, and seafood.

Fluoride

An adult body contains less than 1 g of fluoride, virtually all of which is in the bones and teeth. Definitive evidence that fluoride is an essential nutrient is lacking, but a role for fluoride in preventing dental caries and strengthening bone is well established. Fluoride deficiency is associated with increased susceptibility to dental caries and osteoporosis. The RDA has not been established, but an intake range from 1.5 to 4.0 mg per day for adults is recommended by the Food and Nutrition Board. The recommended intake for infants and children ranges from 0.01 to 3 mg per day, depending on age and weight. These recommendations are also based on the level of fluoridation of the drinking water. Children should not receive additional fluoride supplementation if the fluoride level in the drinking water is greater than 0.6 mg per L (64). In developed countries, fluoride intake and urinary excretion is no longer dependent on the level of drinking water fluoridation as fluoride toothpaste comprises a significant proportion of ingested fluoride (65). Estimates of paleolithic intake have not been reported.

Fluoride intake in the range of 2 to 8 mg/kg/day in childhood can produce mottling of the teeth known as fluorosis. Intake of 20 to 80 mg per day in adults can adversely affect bone, muscle, kidney, and nerve tissue. Increased fluoride uptake into bone may increase bone density, but can also increase risk of fracture. Acute fluoride toxicity can cause gastrointestinal disturbances like pain, nausea, vomiting, and diarrhea. Severe cases may progress to renal and cardiac dysfunction, which can ultimately lead to death. Fluoride is ubiquitous in the food supply, but in very small amounts, varying with the concentration in soil and ground water. The principal source in the Unites States is supplemented water supplies.

Silicon

Silicon is present in all tissues in trace amounts, functioning in calcification, cell growth, and mucopolysaccharide formation. Deficiency in humans has not been established. There is no RDA, and optimal intake is unknown. Good dietary sources include barley and oats.

Nickel

Approximately 10 mg of nickel is widely distributed in the adult body. Nickel appears to play a role in nucleic acid metabolism. A deficiency state in humans has not been elucidated, although deficiency is well established in animal models. Intake of approximately 30 μg per day for adults is thought to be appropriate. Recent reports discussed cases of nickel toxicity presenting with abdominal pain, nausea, polycythemia, and proteinuria (66). Cereal grains and most vegetables contain nickel.

Boron

Boron is thought to influence calcium and estrogen metabolism, vitamin D inactivation, and, consequently, to play a role in bone mineralization. Boron may also function in cell membrane formation. An overt deficiency state has not been defined, but low levels are associated with osteoporosis in particular. An RDA has not been established, but expert opinion supports an intake of approximately 1 mg per day for adults. Toxicity due to supplementation apparently occurs at levels above 50 mg per day and manifests as nausea, vomiting, diarrhea, dermatitis, and cognitive impairment. Boron is found in beans, nuts, vegetables, beer, and wine.

Arsenic

The adult body is thought to contain approximately 20 mg of arsenic, widely distributed in all tissues and concentrated in skin, hair, and nails. Several animal studies have demonstrated that arsenic may be essential for amino acid metabolism and regulation of gene expression; however, clear evidence for its importance in human nutrition is lacking (67,68). No RDA exists, but an intake of 12 to 15 μg per day is thought to be appropriate for adults. Toxicity from food sources is unknown; arsenic toxicity results from ingestion of concentrated arsenic or industrial exposure and has become a known problem in Bangladesh and West Bengal, India, where long-term ingestion of inorganic arsenic from drinking wells led to arsenicosis in hundreds of thousands. Manifestations of toxicity include a burning sensation in the mouth, abdominal pain, nausea, vomiting, and diarrhea. Hepatotoxicity and encephalopathy can occur with higher doses, and chronic arsenic exposure can cause multiple health consequences, including increased risk for developing multiple forms of cancer, diabetes, skin disease, and chronic cough. Additionally, chronic arsenic exposure has been shown to be toxic to renal, hepatic, cardiovascular, and neuronal function (69). There have been several reports demonstrating greater than expected amounts of arsenic in common food sources. Seafood is the richest source of dietary arsenic. A recent consumer report has shown elevated arsenic levels in multiple food groups including various rice and cereal products. People who consumed multiple rice dishes had a 44% higher level of urinary arsenic (70). There are also concerns that organic brown rice syrup, a common alternative sweetener to high-fructose corn syrup, may add significant amounts of arsenic into the diet. For instance, milk formula containing brown rice syrup was determined to contain arsenic concentrations greater than six times the safe drinking water limit (71). Another review examined the total arsenic in young chicken from data obtained by the Food Safety and Inspection Service from 1994 to 2000, and found arsenic levels in chicken that were three to four times greater than other meat sources. Therefore, average levels of arsenic intake may have been underestimated in people consuming mostly chicken (72).

Tin

Approximately 14 mg of tin is widely distributed in the tissues of adult humans, although none is found in brain tissue. Tin is thought to function in oxidation-reduction reactions, but its exact role is unknown. Tin deficiency in humans has not been elucidated. The RDA has not been established, and the range of optimal intake is unknown. Tin is thought to be minimally toxic, as it is poorly absorbed. Tin is widely distributed in the food supply, but in very small amounts. Dietary intake rises as much as 30-fold when food stored in tin cans is eaten frequently.

Vanadium

Approximately 25 mg of vanadium is widely distributed in the tissues of adult humans. The element is concentrated in serum, bones, teeth, and adipose tissue. Vanadium appears to influence several important enzyme systems, including that of ATPase and enzymes associated with blood glucose regulation. Vanadium stimulates glycolysis via glucokinase and phosphofructokinase and may decrease gluconeogenesis by decreasing the activity of glucose-6-phosphatase. Due to its contributions to glucose regulation, vanadium is purported to have beneficial effects in patients with diabetes (73). Additionally, vanadium may inhibit cholesterol biosynthesis. Deficiency in humans has not been established. There is no RDA, and optimal intake levels are unknown. Toxicity is low and is due to poor absorption, but inhalation of vanadium dust in industrial settings may lead to abdominal cramps, diarrhea, hemolysis, hypertension, and fatigue. Shellfish, mushrooms, and several spices, including pepper and dill, are relatively rich sources of vanadium.

Other

Restrictions of dietary cadmium, lead, and lithium have produced abnormalities in laboratory animals, but there is as yet no evidence of human requirements.

ESSENTIAL AMINO ACIDS

Dietary proteins are composed predominantly of a group of 20 amino acids. Of these, humans can readily synthesize 11. The remaining nine—histidine, isoleucine, leucine, lysine, methionine, phenylalanine, threonine, tryptophan, and valine—must be ingested to meet metabolic demand and therefore are referred to as essential (see Chapter 3). An absolute dependence on dietary histidine in adults is uncertain. Infants may also require dietary arginine. Cysteine and tyrosine are synthesized endogenously from methionine and phenylalanine, respectively, and therefore are semi-essential. The need for dietary intake varies inversely with the ingestion of their precursors.

The RDA for protein in adults has been established at or near 0.8 g/kg/day. Paleolithic intake is thought to have been much higher, in the range from 2.5 to 3.5 g/kg/day. Essential amino acid needs are met when protein of high biologic value is consumed. The four least abundant essential amino acids—lysine, methionine/cysteine, threonine, and tryptophan—are used to gauge the quality of dietary protein. Sources of high-quality protein include egg white, milk, meat, soybeans, beans, and lentils. These issues are addressed in more detail in Chapter 3.

ESSENTIAL FATTY ACIDS

The PUFAs required for normal metabolism that cannot be synthesized endogenously are essential dietary nutrients. Two such fatty acids, linoleic acid (C18, ω-6) and α-linolenic acid (C18, ω-3), are unconditionally essential, whereas arachidonic acid (C20, ω-6), which can be synthesized from linoleic acid, is essential when supplies of its precursor are deficient. Essential fatty acids participate in a wide variety of metabolic functions, including eicosanoid synthesis and biomembrane development.

Overt deficiency of essential fatty acids has not been observed in free-living adults, but its manifestations, including hair loss, desquamative dermatitis, and impaired wound healing, are known from cases of deficient parenteral nutrition. The RDA has not been established for essential fatty acids, but an intake of linoleic acid at 1% to 2% of total calories is advised. Of note, the ω-6:ω-3 ratio in the typical US diet is more than 10:1, whereas the ratio estimated for the paleolithic diet is between 4:1 and 1:1.

Dietary sources of linoleic acid include most vegetable oils; evening primrose oil is a particularly rich source. Sources of α-linolenic acid include linseeds and flaxseeds and their oils, and marine foods, especially salmon, mackerel, sardines, scallops, and oysters. The ω-3 content of fish is derived from phytoplankton and algae, so farmed fish are generally lower in ω-3 than their free-living counterparts. For further details, see Chapter 2 and Section VIIE.

MULTIVITAMINS

Multivitamin supplementation consists of taking a combination of vitamins and minerals at amounts greater than the level of recommended daily intake. US nutrient intake is typically lower than recommended, and both caloric and nutritional intake decreases with age, and therefore, providing a strong rationale for recommending multivitamin supplementation. However, there has not been clear evidence for recommending multivitamin supplementation as a preventative measure. A recent study demonstrated a significant albeit small reduction in risk for total cancer in males with daily multivitamin supplementation, but did not reduce major cardiovascular events, myocardial infarctions, strokes, or CVD mortality (74,75). In contrast, there have been studies suggesting that supplementation is not completely benign. The risks of high-dose antioxidant supplementation was discussed earlier, and another study demonstrated an increased in total mortality risk in older woman using dietary multivitamin supplements (76). Although specific nutrient supplementation may be indicated to prevent certain diseases, including osteoporosis in the elderly, multivitamin supplementation is primarily recommended for treating nutritional deficiency and not for specific disease prevention.

WHOLE-FOOD BASED SUPPLEMENTS

Whole-food supplements are extracts from food sources that maintain the original context of nutrients found in food. These substances are more complex than vitamin supplements but can still be delivered in pill form. The extracts used to construct these supplements, consisting of variety of nutrients, enzymes, coenzymes, antioxidants, trace elements, and other factors, are expected to work synergistically as they do in their original food source toward providing the desired health benefits. For example, regular consumption of fruits and vegetables are beneficial for a several reasons including their antioxidant properties. However, vitamin C alone only accounts for 0.4% of the total antioxidant activity in an apple, and additional phytochemicals found in fruits may therefore be essential for providing the desired health benefits (77). New studies are beginning to examine whole-food rather than single nutrient interventions for addressing etiologies and possible therapies for certain diseases. A whole-food intervention demonstrated that tomato sauce constituents significantly decreased leukocyte oxidative damage in patients with prostate cancer (78). Lycopene is considered the primary antioxidant constituent in tomato extracts and has shown to have antitumor effects; however, a study in rats demonstrated that whole tomato and broccoli interventions were superior in reducing tumor weight than lycopene alone (79). Whole-food based supplementation may prove superior to conventional approaches to nutrient supplementation by preserving the native context of nutrients; research in this area is on-going.

REFERENCES

1. Rabbani N, Alam S, Riaz S, et al. High-dose thiamine therapy for patients with type 2 diabetes and microalbuminuria: a randomised, double-blind placebo-controlled pilot study. *Diabetologia* 2009;52(2):208–12. doi:10.1007/s00125-008-1224-4.
2. Beltramo E, Nizheradze K, Berrone E, et al. Thiamine and benfotiamine prevent apoptosis induced by high glucose-conditioned extracellular matrix in human retinal pericytes. *Diabetes Metab Res Rev* 2009;25(7):647–656. doi:10.1002/dmrr.1008.
3. Schoenen J. Effectiveness of high-dose riboflavin in migraine prophylaxis. A randomized controlled trial. *Neurology* 1998;50(2):466–470.
4. Boehnke C, Reuter U, Flach U, et al. High-dose riboflavin treatment is efficacious in migraine prophylaxis: an open study in a tertiary care centre. *Eur J Neurol* 2004;11(7):475–477.
5. Luzzati R, Del Bravo P, Di Perri G, et al. Riboflavine and severe lactic acidosis. *Lancet* 1999;353(9156):901–902.
6. Schaumburg H, Kaplan J, Windebank A, et al. Sensory neuropathy from pyridoxine abuse. *N Eng J Med* 1983;309(8):445–448. doi:10.1056/NEJM198308253090801.
7. Koren G, Maltepe C. Pre-emptive therapy for severe nausea and vomiting of pregnancy and hyperemesis gravidarum. *J Obstet Gynaecol* 2004;24(5):530–533. doi:10.1080/01443610410001722581.
8. Matthews A, Dowswell T, Haas DM, et al. Interventions for nausea and vomiting in early pregnancy. *Cochrane Database Syst Rev* 2010;(9):CD007575. doi:10.1002/14651858.CD007575.pub2.

9. Niebyl JR, Goodwin TM. Overview of nausea and vomiting of pregnancy with an emphasis on vitamins and ginger. *Am J Obstet Gynecol* 2002;186(5 suppl understanding): S253–S255.

10. U.S. Preventive Services Task Force. Folic acid for the prevention of neural tube defects: U.S. Preventive services task force recommendation statement. *Ann Intern Med* 2009;150(9):626–31.

11. Wolff T, Witkop CT, Miller T, et al. Folic acid supplementation for the prevention of neural tube defects: an update of the evidence for the U.S. Preventive services task force. *Ann Intern Med* 2009;150(9):632–639.

12. National Research Council. *Dietary reference intakes for thiamin, riboflavin, niacin, vitamin B6, folate, vitamin B12, pantothenic acid, biotin, and choline.* Washington, DC: National Academies Press; 1998

13. Committee on Educational Bulletins of the American College of Obstetricians and Gynecologists. ACOG educational bulletin: seizure disorders in pregnancy: number 231, December 1996. *Int J Gynecol Obstet* 1997;56(3): 279–286. doi:10.1016/S0020-7292(97)83388-7.

14. National Guideline Clearinghouse. *Neural tube defects.* Rockville, MD: Agency for Healthcare Research and Quality (AHRQ). June 09, 2013. Available at http://www.guideline.gov/content.aspx?id=3994.

15. Ogawa Y, Kaneko S, Otani K, et al. Serum folic acid levels in epileptic mothers and their relationship to congenital malformations. *Epilepsy Res* 1991;8(1):75–78.

16. Fujioka K. Follow-up of nutritional and metabolic problems after bariatric surgery. *Diabetes Care.* 2005;28(2): 481–484. doi:10.2337/diacare.28.2.481.

17. Eyles DW, Smith S, Kinobe R, et al. Distribution of the vitamin D receptor and 1 alpha-hydroxylase in human brain. *J Chem Neuroanat* 2005;29(1):21–30. doi:10.1016/j.jchemneu.2004.08.006.

18. Holmoy T, Moen SM. Assessing vitamin D in the central nervous system. *Acta Neurol Scand* 2010;122(suppl s190):88–92. doi:10.1111/j.1600-0404.2010.01383.x.

19. Balion C, Griffith LE, Strifler L, et al. Vitamin D, cognition, and dementia: a systematic review and meta-analysis. *Neurology* 2012;79(13):1397–1405. doi:10.1212/WNL.0b013e31826c197f.

20. Kjaergaard M, Waterloo K, Wang CE, et al. Effect of vitamin D supplement on depression scores in people with low levels of serum 25-hydroxyvitamin D: nested case-control study and randomised clinical trial. *Br J Psychiatry* 2012;201(5):360–368. doi:10.1192/bjp.bp.111.104349.

21. Overton E, Yin M. The rapidly evolving research on vitamin D among HIV-infected populations. *Curr Infect Dis Rep* 2011;13(1):83–93. doi:10.1007/s11908-010-0144-x.

22. Schottker B, Haug U, Schomburg L, et al. Strong associations of 25-hydroxyvitamin D concentrations with all-cause, cardiovascular, cancer, and respiratory disease mortality in a large cohort study. *Am J Clin Nutr* 2013;97(4):782–793. doi:10.3945/ajcn.112.047712.

23. Food and Nutrition Board, Institute of Medicine. *Dietary reference intakes for vitamin C, vitamin E, selenium, and carotenoids.* Washington, DC: National Academies Press, 2000:95–185.

24. Reiter E, Jiang Q, Christen S. Anti-inflammatory properties of α- and γ-tocopherol. *Mol Aspects Med* 2007;28 (5–6):668–691. doi:10.1016/j.mam.2007.01.003.

25. Zeisel SH, Da Costa K-A. Choline: an essential nutrient for public health. *Nutr Rev* 2009;67(11):615–623. doi:10.1111/j.1753-4887.2009.00246.x.

26. Zeisel SH. Choline: critical role during fetal development and dietary requirements in adults. *Annu Rev Nutr* 2006;26(1): 229–250. doi:10.1146/annurev.nutr.26.061505.111156.

27. Ghandforoush-Sattari M, Mashayekhi S, Krishna CV, et al. Pharmacokinetics of oral taurine in healthy volunteers. *J Amino Acids* 2010;2010. doi:10.4061/2010/346237.

28. Xu YJ, Arneja AS, Tappia PS, et al. The potential health benefits of taurine in cardiovascular disease. *Exp Clin Cardiol* 2008;13(2):57–65.

29. Dare AJ, Phillips ARJ, Hickey AJR, et al. A systematic review of experimental treatments for mitochondrial dysfunction in sepsis and multiple organ dysfunction syndrome. *Free Radic Biol Med* 2009;47(11):1517–1525. doi:10.1016/j.freeradbiomed.2009.08.019.

30. Lheureux P, Penaloza A, Zahir S, et al. Science review: carnitine in the treatment of valproic acid-induced toxicity–what is the evidence? *Crit Care* 2005;9(5):431.

31. Lheureux PE, Hantson P. Carnitine in the treatment of valproic acid-induced toxicity. *Clin Toxicol* 2009; 47(2):101–11.

32. Bacic I, Druzijanic N, Karlo R, et al. Efficacy of IP6 + inositol in the treatment of breast cancer patients receiving chemotherapy: prospective, randomized, pilot clinical study. *J Exp Clin Cancer Res* 2010;29:12.

33. Ametov AS, Barinov A, Dyck PJ, et al. The sensory symptoms of diabetic polyneuropathy are improved with α-lipoic acid. *Diabetes Care* 2003;26(3):770–776. doi:10.2337/diacare.26.3.770.

34. Head K. Natural therapies for ocular disorders part two: cataracts and glaucoma. *Altern Med Rev* 2001;6(2):141–166.

35. Suzuki YJ, Aggarwal BB, Packer L. α-Lipoic acid is a potent inhibitor of NF-κB activation in human T cells. *Biochem Biophys Res Commun* 1992;189(3):1709–1715.

36. Plotnikoff GA, Dusek J. Hypertension. In: Rakel D, ed. *Integrative medicine*, 3rd ed. Philadelphia, PA: Saunders, 2012: 208–216.

37. Bookstaver DA, Burkhalter NA, Hatzigeorgiou C. Effect of coenzyme Q10 supplementation on statin-induced myalgias. *Am J Cardiol* 2012;110(4):526–529. doi:10.1016/j.amjcard.2012.04.026.

38. Caso G, Kelly P, McNurlan MA, et al. Effect of coenzyme q10 on myopathic symptoms in patients treated with statins. *Am J Cardiol* 2007;99(10):1409–1412. doi:10.1016/j.amjcard.2006.12.063.

39. Young JM, Florkowski CM, Molyneux SL, et al. Effect of coenzyme Q(10) supplementation on simvastatin-induced myalgia. *Am Journal Cardiol* 2007;100(9):1400–1403. doi:10.1016/j.amjcard.2007.06.030.

40. Stanner S, Hughes J, Kelly C, et al. A review of the epidemiological evidence for the 'antioxidant hypothesis'. *Public Health Nutr* 2004;7(03):407–422. doi:10.1079/PHN2003543.

41. The effect of vitamin E and beta carotene on the incidence of lung Cancer and other cancers in male smokers. *N Engl J Med* 1994;330(15):1029–1035. doi:10.1056/NEJM199404143301501.

42. Bjelakovic G, Nikolova D, Gluud LL, et al. Mortality in randomized trials of antioxidant supplements for primary and secondary prevention: systematic review and meta-analysis. *JAMA* 2007;297(8):842–857.

43. Ross AC, Taylor CL, Yaktine AL, et al., eds. *Dietary reference intakes for calcium and vitamin D*. Washington, DC: National Academies Press, 2011.

44. Moyer VA. Vitamin D and calcium supplementation to prevent fractures in adults: U.S. Preventive Services Task Force recommendation statement. *Ann Intern Med*. 2013;158(9):691–696 doi:10.7326/0003-4819-158-9-201305070-00603. PubMed PMID: 23440163.

45. Linkswiler HM, Zemel MB, Hegsted M, et al. Protein-induced hypercalciuria. *Fed Proc*. 1981;40(9):2429–2433

46. Fawcett W, Haxby E, Male D. Magnesium: physiology and pharmacology. *Br J Anaesth* 1999;83(2):302–320.

47. Jahnen-Dechent W, Ketteler M. Magnesium basics. *Clin Kidney J* 2012;5(suppl 1):i3–i14. doi:10.1093/ndtplus/sfr163.

48. Woods KL, Fletcher S, Roffe C, et al. Intravenous magnesium sulphate in suspected acute myocardial infarction: results of the second Leicester Intravenous Magnesium Intervention Trial (LIMIT-2). *Lancet* 1992;339(8809):1553–1558.

49. ISIS-4 (Fourth International Study of Infarct Survival) Collaborative Group. ISIS-4: a randomised factorial trial assessing early oral captopril, oral mononitrate, and intravenous magnesium sulphate in 58,050 patients with suspected acute myocardial infarction. *Lancet* 1995;345(8951):669–685.

50. Magnesium in Coronaries (MAGIC) Trial. Early administration of intravenous magnesium to high-risk patients with acute myocardial infarction in the Magnesium in Coronaries (MAGIC) Trial: a randomised controlled trial. *Lancet* 2002;360(9341):1189–1196.

51. Geiger H, Wanner C. Magnesium in disease. *Clin Kidney J* 2012;5(suppl 1):i25–i38. doi:10.1093/ndtplus/sfr165.

52. Wark PA, Lau R, Norat T, et al. Magnesium intake and colorectal tumor risk: a case-control study and meta-analysis. *Am J Clin Nutr* 2012;96(3):622–631. doi:10.3945/ajcn .111.030924.

53. Guerrera MP, Volpe SL, Mao JJ. Therapeutic uses of magnesium. *Am Fam Physician* 2009;80(2):157–162.

54. Green DM, Ropper AH, Kronmal RA, et al. Serum potassium level and dietary potassium intake as risk factors for stroke. *Neurology* 2002;59(3):314–320. doi:10.1212/wnl.59.3.314.

55. Food and Nutrition Board, Institute of Medicine. *Dietary reference intakes for vitamin A, vitamin K, arsenic, boron, chromium, copper, iodine, iron, manganese, molybdenum, nickel, silicon, vanadium, and zinc*. Washington, DC: National Academies Press, 2001.

56. Koppel B. Nutritional and alcohol-related neurologic disorders. In: Goldman L, Schafer A, eds. *Goldman's Cecil medicine*, 24th edn. New York, NY: Elsevier, 2011:2382–2386.

57. Willis MS, Monaghan SA, Miller ML, et al. Zinc-induced copper deficiency: a report of three cases initially recognized on bone marrow examination. *Am J Clin Pathol* 2005;123(1):125–131. doi:10.1309/v6gvyw2qtyd5c5pj.

58. Alexander TH, Davidson TM. Intranasal zinc and anosmia: the zinc-induced anosmia syndrome. *Laryngoscope*. 2006;116(2):217–220 doi:10.1097/01.mlg .0000191549.17796.13.

59. Hurwitz BE, Klaus JR, Llabre MM, et al. Suppression of human immunodeficiency virus type 1 viral load with selenium supplementation: a randomized controlled trial. *Arch Intern Med*. 2007;167(2):148–154

60. Ringstad J, Kildebo S, Thomassen Y. Serum selenium, copper, and zinc concentrations in Crohn's disease and ulcerative colitis. *Scand J Gastroenterol* 1993;28(7):605–608. doi:10.3109/00365529309096096.

61. Rannem T, Ladefoged K, Hylander E, et al. Selenium status in patients with Crohn's disease. *Am J Clin Nutr* 1992;56(5):933–937.

62. Duffield-Lillico AJ, Slate EH, Reid ME, et al. Selenium supplementation and secondary prevention of nonmelanoma skin cancer in a randomized trial. *J Natl Cancer Inst*. 2003;95(19):1477–1481

63. Friedman BJ, Freeland-Graves JH, Bales CW, et al. Manganese balance and clinical observations in young men fed a manganese-deficient diet. *J Nutr* 1987;117(1):133–143.

64. Food and Nutrition Board, Institute of Medicine. *Dietary reference intakes for calcium, phosphorus, magnesium, vitamin D, and fluoride*. Washington, DC: National Academies Press, 1997.

65. Maguire A, Zohouri FV, Hindmarch PN, et al. Fluoride intake and urinary excretion in 6- to 7-year-old children living in optimally, sub-optimally and non-fluoridated areas. *Community Dent Oral Epidemiol* 2007;35(6):479–488. doi:10.1111/j.1600-0528.2006.00366.x.

66. Fuentebella J, Kerner JA. Nickel toxicity presenting as persistent nausea and abdominal pain. *Dig Dis Sci*. 2010;55(8):2162–2164

67. Cooney CA. Dietary selenium and arsenic affect DNA methylation. *J Nutr* 2001;131(6):1871.

68. Uthus EO. Evidence for arsenic essentiality. *Environ Geochem Health*. 1992;14(2):55–58

69. Vahter ME. Interactions between arsenic-induced toxicity and nutrition in early life. *J Nutr* 2007;137(12): 2798–2804.

70. ConsumerReportsorg. *Arsenic in your food*. November 2012. Available at http://consumerreports.org/cro/magazine/2012/11/arsenic-in-your-food/index.htm

71. Jackson BP, Taylor VF, Karagas MR, et al. Arsenic, organic foods, and brown rice syrup. *Environ Health Perspect* 2012;120(5):623–626. doi:10.1289/ehp.1104619. PubMed PMID: 22336149.

72. Lasky T, Sun W, Kadry A, et al. Mean total arsenic concentrations in chicken 1989–2000 and estimated exposures for consumers of chicken. *Environ Health Perspect* 2004;112(1):18–21.

73. Badmaev V, Prakash S, Majeed M. Vanadium: a review of its potential role in the fight against diabetes. *J Altern Complement Med* 1999;5(3):273–291.

74. Gaziano J, Sesso HD, Christen WG. Multivitamins in the prevention of cancer in men: the physicians' health study II randomized controlled trial. *JAMA* 2012:1–10. doi:10.1001/jama.2012.14641.

75. Sesso HD, Christen WG, Bubes V, et al. Multivitamins in the prevention of cardiovascular disease in men: the physicians' health study II randomized controlled trial. *JAMA* 2012;308(17):1751–1760. doi:10.1001/jama.2012.14805.

76. Mursu J, Robien K, Harnack LJ, et al. Dietary supplements and mortality rate in older women: the Iowa women's health study. *Arch Intern Med* 2011;171(18):1625–1633. doi:10.1001/archinternmed.2011.445.

77. Liu RH. Health benefits of fruit and vegetables are from additive and synergistic combinations of phytochemicals. *Am J Clin Nutr*. 2003;78(3):517S–520S

78. Chen L, Stacewicz-Sapuntzakis M, Duncan C, et al. Oxidative DNA damage in prostate cancer patients consuming tomato sauce-based entrees as a whole-food intervention. *J Natl Cancer Inst* 2001;93(24):1872–1879. doi:10.1093/jnci/93.24.1872.

79. Canene-Adams K, Lindshield BL, Wang S, et al. Combinations of tomato and broccoli enhance antitumor activity in Dunning R3327-H prostate adenocarcinomas. *Cancer Res* 2007;67(2):836–43. doi:10.1158/0008-5472.can-06-3462.

■ SUGGESTED READING

Otten JJ, Hellwig JP, Meyers LD, eds. *Dietary reference intakes. The essential guide to nutrient requirements.* Washington, DC: National Academy Press, 2006.

Standing Committee on the Scientific Evaluation of Dietary Reference Intakes, Food and Nutrition Board, Institute of Medicine. *Dietary reference intakes for calcium, phosphorus, magnesium, vitamin D, and fluoride.* Washington, DC: National Academies Press, 1997.

Nutritional Management in Clinical Practice: Diet, in Sickness and in Health

CHAPTER 5

Diet, Weight Regulation, and Obesity

The United States is the epicenter of a global obesity pandemic. Driven by advances in food production that have made palatable, economical calories in excess of need readily available to almost the entire population almost all the time and by comparable advances in labor-saving technologies, obesity and overweight now engulf over two-thirds of adults in the United States, besides nearly one-third of children (1,2). With rates rising to unprecedented levels with each passing year, obesity is rightly referred to as an epidemic and is, arguably, the most poorly controlled and potentially dire health threat facing the United States. Obesity is the major modifiable risk factor for type 2 diabetes (itself now epidemic) and a major contributor to most predominant causes of premature death and disability, including but not limited to cardiovascular disease, cancer, stroke, obstructive pulmonary disease, and degenerative arthritis. Secular trends are similar in most other developed countries. Cultural transitions in developing countries are associated with a rapid rise in the rate of obesity as well, even while historical public health scourges such as microbial diseases persist. Obesity thus constitutes a global health crisis. At the International Congress on Obesity in Sydney, Australia, in September 2006, it was announced that for the first time in history, the planetwide population of overweight (over 1 billion) outnumbered the hungry (roughly 600 to 700 million) (3).

An inability to curtail the spread of obesity has resulted in a tendency to exaggerate the complexities, if not the difficulties, of the challenges involved. While the investigation of obesity rightly subsumes metabolism, genetics, lipidology, endocrinology, and even newly emerging disciplines such as nutrigenomics, it must be conceded that human physiology is much the same as it ever was and thus cannot house the explanation for suddenly skyrocketing obesity rates. That answer resides in an environment that is not the same as it was before, rendering human adaptations to a world of caloric scarcity and a high demand for physical exertions largely obsolete. In short, our patients (and we) are getting fat in record numbers for the simple reason that they (and we) can do so—for the first time in history. It is scarcely an exaggeration to say that human intelligence, since it first evolved, has been dedicated to making obesity possible by establishing a reliable supply of palatable food and by inventing technologies to reduce the physical ardors required for survival. We have become, in the fullness of time, victims of our own resourcefulness and success.

But while accounting for the obesity epidemic is simple, reversing it will be anything but easy—and from this derives the false and even harmful perspective that complexity impedes our progress. This view is false because a reduction in caloric intake to the level required for maintenance of a healthful weight is all that is universally needed for weight control. This view is harmful because it shifts attention and resources from the demanding but potentially rewarding task of pursuing what we know to the often-frivolous task of parsing what we do not. The role of clinicians in contending with this challenge is itself a subject of debate. The U.S. Preventive Services Task Force recommends that although behavioral counseling has small-to-moderate benefits in improving diet, such counseling should be done in selected patients rather than routinely (4).

Being less bound by the constraints of applied evidence, if no less respectful of them, I can point out the potential fallacy in this guidance. An analogy best serves.

Imagine that a landslide traps a hiker behind a mound of boulders. Then imagine that rescue workers each try, one at a time, to move the boulders. Because no one of them can do so, the conclusion is reached that efforts to move boulders are probably futile and best abandoned. Or, minimally, the evidence may be insufficient to recommend for or against attempts to move boulders. This tack abandons the hiker to his or her fate as well, of course.

The fallacy here is that while no one person can move a boulder, several people working together perhaps can. We are accustomed in medical research to some degree of reductionism, the study of active ingredients. Thus, when obesity interventions are studied, they are generally examined discretely, independently of societal trends. When such interventions fail to make appreciable differences in the outcome(s) of interest—generally some measure of weight—we conclude that they are ineffective. Or, at best, we fail to conclude that they are effective.

But the "mass" against which we are working is daunting. The world is powerfully, and ever more, obesigenic. Even interventions that apply an effective counterforce may fail to move this massive and ever-accumulating resistance. The implications are that for there to be any hope of curtailing the obesity epidemic, we must apply all reasonable countermeasures concurrently. In fact, a 2012 report issued by the Institute of Medicine (IOM) acknowledges that there is no one panacea for the obesity epidemic and that a broad, integrated approach is needed to curtail the epidemic (5).

Clinical counseling is among these countermeasures, and it is a potentially vital element. Schools, families, industry, media, policy makers, and public health practitioners have roles to play, too, and we may accomplish little until such efforts align (6,7). But in pursuit of that alignment, who better than we to lead? Certainly it would be shameful to merely follow, and it would be disgraceful to get out of the way.

Sufficient research evidence is available to inform rational and promising approaches to weight control counseling in clinical settings (see Chapters 46 and 47). When such efforts are adopted, evaluated, refined, and combined with the mobilization of other antiobesity programs, policies, and resources, we may at last come to find that we can move boulders, and even mountains, after all.

OVERVIEW

Definitions of Overweight and Obesity and Measures of Anthropometry

The predominant measure used to characterize weight at the population level is body mass index (BMI), generally expressed as weight (mass), in kilograms, divided by the height, in meters squared (kg per m^2). This measure of weight adjusted for height offers the benefits of simplicity and convenience for assessing weight in large populations and for monitoring trends over time. BMI, however, is a notoriously crude measure of adiposity (body fat stores) and anthropometry (the distribution of those fat stores), both of which are of more importance to health than weight, per se. BMI cannot distinguish between fat and muscle mass, nor between peripherally versus centrally distributed fat mass.

Despite its limitations when applied to an individual, BMI performs well at the population level for several reasons. BMI trends reflect trends in adiposity, not muscularity. There is nothing to suggest that increasing legions of the muscular and fit are responsible for consistent increases in BMI in the United States and other countries; there is much to suggest that rising BMI is indicative of increasing adiposity. The distinction between excess body fat and muscularity is easily made at the individual level, and thus the use of the BMI is unlikely to generate clinically relevant confusion (8–10). Finally, such crude measures as the BMI, and even casual inspection, correlate fairly well with costly and sophisticated measures of adiposity (11–14).

Overweight in adults is defined as BMI at or above 25 kg per m^2 (15). Adult obesity is defined in grades. Stage I obesity is a BMI of 30 to 34.9; stage II obesity is a BMI of 35 to 39.9; and stage III obesity is a BMI of 40 or higher (see Table 5-1). A BMI of 25 to 29.9 is "overweight." Stage III obesity was formerly known as "morbid obesity." (1) The name change is appropriate and important for two reasons. First, although a BMI of 40 is quite high, it is not invariably associated with morbidity. Second, and of greater

TABLE 5.1

Current Definitions of Overweight and Obesity in Adults

BMI	Category
<18	Underweight
18 to <25	Healthy weight
25 to <30	Overweight
30 to <35	Stage I obesity
35 to <40	Stage II obesity
≥40	Stage III obesity (formerly "morbid" obesity)

importance epidemiologically, morbidity is often induced by obesity at a BMI well below 40. The risks of complications of excess adiposity may, in general, be considered low, moderate, and high as BMI rises through overweight to stage III obesity, but the actual risk in an individual will vary (16–19). The correspondence between BMI and common measures of height and weight is shown in Table 5-2, and a BMI calculator is displayed in Table 5-3. Children are classified as obese if they are at or above the 95th percentile for age- and sex-adjusted BMI (based on a historical reference population from 1971) and as overweight if they are at or above the 85th percentile (20).

TABLE 5.2

Weights that Correspond to Overweight and the Three Stages of Obesity for Men and Women of Average Height and Frame

Gender	Average Height	Weight Corresponding to BMI of 25 (Overweight) (lb)	Weight Corresponding to BMI of 30 (Stage I Obesity) (lb)	Weight Corresponding to BMI of 35 (Stage II Obesity) (lb)	Weight Corresponding to BMI of 40 (Stage III Obesity) (lb)
Female	5'4"	145	174	203	233
Male	5'9"	169	203	237	270

TABLE 5.3

BMI Based on Measures of Height and Weight[a]

	Height in Feet and Inches									
Weight in Pounds	4'10"	5'	5'2"	5'4"	5'6"	5'8"	5'10"	6'	6'2"	6'4"
	2	20	18	<18	<18	<18	<18	<18	<18	<18
110	23	21.5	20	19	<18	<18	<18	<18	<18	<18
120	25	23.5	22	21	19	18	<18	<18	<18	<18
130	27	25	24	22	21	20	19	<18	<18	<18
140	29	27	26	24	23	21	20	19	18	<18
150	31	29	27.5	26	24	23	22	20	19	18
160	33.5	31	29	27.5	26	24	23	22	20.5	19.5
170	36	33	31	29	27.5	26	24	23	22	21
180	38	35	33	31	29	27	26	24.5	23	22
190	40	37	35	33	31	29	27	26	24.5	23
200	>40	39	37	34	32	30	29	27	26	24
210	>40	41	38	36	34	32	30	28.5	27	26
220	>40	>40	40	38	36	33	32	30	28	27
230	>40	>40	>40	40	37	35	33	31	30	28
240	>40	>40	>40	>40	39	37	34.5	33	31	29
250	>40	>40	>40	>40	40	38	36	34	32	30.5
260	>40	>40	>40	>40	>40	40	37	35	33	32
270	>40	>40	>40	>40	>40	>40	39	37	35	33
280	>40	>40	>40	>40	>40	>40	40	38	36	34
290	>40	>40	>40	>40	>40	>40	>40	39	37	35
300	>40	>40	>40	>40	>40	>40	>40	41	39	37

[a]Height in feet and inches is shown across the top, and weight in pounds is shown in the left-hand column. Each entry in the table represents the BMI for a particular combination of height and weight. BMIs that represent the transition points from lean to overweight, from overweight to obese, and from one stage of obesity to the next are shown in bold. BMI values are close approximations due to rounding. BMI values in the recommended, or "healthiest," range are shaded in gray. Note that if a patient is very slight, or very muscular, that person's BMI might fall above or below the shaded area and still be consistent with excellent health. An online BMI calculator is available at http://www.nhlbisupport.com/bmi/bmicalc.htm.

Source: Katz DL, Gonzalez MH. *The way to eat.* Naperville, IL: Sourcebooks, 2002.

Alternatives to BMI for classifying obesity vary in complexity and suitability for the clinical setting. Of most potential value is the waist circumference, which has supplanted the waist-to-hip ratio (WHR) over recent years. This measure requires looping a tape measure about the waist at the narrowest point, generally corresponding to the level of the umbilicus and the posterior superior iliac crests. In general, a waist circumference above 40 inches (approximately 102 cm) is of concern in an adult man, and above 34 inches (88 cm) is elevated for a woman (21). An elevated waist circumference is a hallmark of central adiposity, and it is a risk factor for insulin resistance (see Chapter 7).

Men are generally more subject to central or abdominal obesity (therefore also known as android obesity) than women; this anthropometric pattern is referred to descriptively as the "apple" pattern of obesity. An elevated BMI with a normal waist circumference is consistent with peripheral obesity, also referred to as gynoid obesity, or the "pear" pattern. Although in general men are more subject to abdominal obesity and women to peripheral obesity, the patterns are not gender specific. Following menopause in particular, women are increasingly subject to abdominal obesity (22,23).

Abdominal obesity is distinct from peripheral obesity with regard to its physiology and complications. Central obesity correlates with the accumulation of visceral adipose tissue. This body habitus is linked to insulin-resistance syndrome and diabetes risk (see Chapter 6). As a result, there is a strong association between central obesity and cardiovascular disease risk (24) (see Chapters 6 and 7); this association is much less apparent for peripheral obesity. One mediating mechanism of cardiovascular risk in central obesity appears to be an association with high sympathetic tone (25–30). This, in turn, may be related to the density of adrenergic receptors in centrally distributed and visceral adipose tissue. Although associated with metabolic complications of obesity, central fat tissue tends to be more readily mobilized than peripheral fat, in part because adrenergic receptors facilitate fat oxidation during catabolism. Thus, the frequently reported complaint of women that men lose weight more readily is often valid.

Of note, not even all centrally distributed fat is of comparable metabolic importance. Work by Després et al. (31) suggested that some individuals accumulate central fat predominantly in the subcutaneous layer, whereas others have a particular predilection for accumulating visceral fat. Visceral fat, and specifically fat accumulation in the liver, is the particular arbiter of cardiometabolic implications of excess adipose tissue. Visceral fat in even relatively modest excess appears to induce metabolic perturbations, notably insulin resistance (see Chapters 6 and 7). There is apparent ethnic as well as inter-individual variation in the propensity to deposit fat in the liver; Asian populations consistently show evidence of insulin resistance at BMI levels considered normal in the United States.

Other anthropometric measures, such as skin-fold thickness, bioelectrical impedance, dual-energy x-ray absorptiometry (DEXA), and hydrostatic weighing are unlikely to be of use in the clinical practice setting. Each of these techniques can be used to calculate or directly measure lean body mass and adipose tissue mass, with varying degrees of time, trouble, cost, and accuracy. Body density can also be measured by the administration of "heavy" (tritiated) water, with evaluation of adiposity based on the volume of distribution (32). Underwater weighing permits assessment of body density as well. Bioelectrical impedance also is used to calculate fat mass. DEXA or dual-photon absorptiometry may be the best available method for measuring total body fat. Computed tomography and magnetic resonance imaging may be used to quantify body fat, with particular utility for visualizing and quantifying visceral fat (33,34). Although such sophisticated techniques offer advantages in research settings, there is satisfactory evidence that even simple observation is a fairly reliable gauge of excess body fat in the clinical setting.

Along with fat tissue distribution, adipocyte size versus number has implications for the health effects of obesity (17). An excess of adipose tissue can result from enlargement of existing adipocytes, the generation of additional adipocytes, or some combination of these. Weight gain attributable to enlargement of existing adipocytes is termed "hypertrophic" obesity, and it is the predominant mechanism for the storage of excess fat weight gained in adulthood. Extreme weight gain in adults will induce the generation of new adipocytes. When excess fat weight is gained in early childhood and near puberty, there is a particular predisposition to generate new adipocytes;

weight gain in this pattern is termed "hyperplastic" obesity.

As is true of virtually all cell types, adipocytes have a characteristic size range. Adipocytes exert an influence on the central nervous system, via chemical messengers such as leptin (see appetite, below, and Chapter 38), to remain within their normal size range. Once an excess number of adipocytes has been generated, the only way an individual can achieve thinness is by reducing this population of cells to below normal size. This is something the cells seem to resist with considerable vigor. There is apparently less resistance to attempts at reducing overly enlarged adipocytes to a smaller size within the standard range.

The implications of these patterns and their effects on weight regulation are that predominantly hyperplastic obesity is uniquely resistant to weight loss and control efforts relative to predominantly hypertrophic obesity. This suggests that weight gain early in life will compound the difficulty involved in achieving weight control. In light of this physiologic mechanism, the dangers of ever-earlier-onset obesity and the rising prevalence of childhood obesity are clear. Sustainable weight loss is notoriously difficult even when overweight first occurs in adulthood; it may be all but impossible for those subject to obesity from early childhood. The importance of childhood obesity-prevention strategies is thus self-evident.

Weight Trends and the Epidemiology of Obesity

In the United States, obesity is not only epidemic but arguably the gravest and most poorly controlled public health threat of our time (35–37). Over two-thirds of the adults in the United States are overweight or obese. The most recent data available suggest that the prevalence of obesity may have plateaued over the past few years (1,2). While this may offer a glimmer of hope, there are less sanguine interpretations of the data. A plateau in any trend is inevitable as the limits of its range are approximated. Further, the prevalence of overweight and obesity does not adequately reflect the distribution of actual weights in the population.

There is evidence that the more extreme degrees of obesity are increasing in prevalence faster than overweight (38). This suggests that the minority in the population that has resisted

the tendency toward excessive weight gain thus far may remain resistant and not contribute to the ranks of the overweight and obese. Those, however, who have already succumbed to obesity trends may remain vulnerable to increasing weight gain over time, thus transitioning through overweight to progressively severe degrees of obesity. This implies that even if the cumulative prevalence of overweight and obesity were to stabilize at current levels, the health effects of obesity may well continue to worsen.

Trends in Children

The rate of childhood obesity has tripled in the past two decades (39). Over 30% of children in the US population at large are considered overweight or obese. In some ethnic minority groups, this figure rises to 40% (2).

Recent studies indicate that obesity is occurring at ever-younger ages. A marked rise in the prevalence of overweight among infants and toddlers has been documented both in the United States and globally (40,41). As in adults, BMI is a crude indicator of adiposity and fat distribution in children. Data indicate that waist circumference has been rising in tandem with BMI in children, which is of concern since abdominal adiposity has worse health implications (42).

Global Trends

The increasingly global economy has rendered obesity an increasingly global problem, with the United States the putative epicenter of an obesity pandemic (43–45). Worldwide, an estimated 1.4 billion adults are overweight or obese (46). Rates of obesity are already high and rising in most developed countries, and they are lower but rising faster in countries undergoing a cultural transition (47). In China, India, and Russia, the constellation of enormous population, inadequate control of historical public health threats such as infectious disease, and the advent of epidemic obesity and attendant chronic disease represent an unprecedented challenge (48–50). In countries undergoing a time of even more rapid cultural transition and development, the effects on obesity and chronic disease are astonishing. For example, in Qatar, the rates of obesity and diabetes are even higher than those in the United States, with 75% of adults overweight or obese and 17% of adults with type 2 diabetes (51). Obesity control is among the current priorities of the World Health Organization. Universal dietary preferences (see Chapter 44) evidently predominate over cultural patterns as nutrient-dilute, energy-dense foods become available (52,53). At the 10th International Congress on Obesity held in Sydney, Australia, in September 2006, World Health Organization data were reported, indicating that for the first time in history, there are more overweight than hungry people on the planet.

The fundamental health implications of obesity appear to be universal. Appropriate threshold values for the definition of overweight and obesity, however, should likely vary with ethnicity and associated anthropometry. As noted, Asian populations appear to have a predilection for central, and visceral, fat deposition and thus a vulnerability to insulin resistance at a BMI deemed normal and innocuous for most occidental populations. There are noteworthy variations in BMI, waist circumference, and lean body mass among diverse ethnic groups. As addressed in Chapter 44, genetic variability in the susceptibility to obesity and its metabolic sequelae is quite pronounced.

Obesity and Morbidity

The health consequences of obesity are in general well characterized, as is the economic toll (54–62). The toll of the epidemic is most starkly conveyed by the impact on children. In the past two decades, due to childhood obesity, type 2 diabetes has been transformed from a condition occurring almost exclusively at or after middle age into a pediatric epidemic affecting children as young as 6 (63). Less than a generation ago, type 2 diabetes was routinely referred to as "adult onset" diabetes.

The National Cholesterol Education Program (NCEP) Adult Treatment Panel issues guidance for the identification and management of cardiovascular risk factors in adults. The guidance for management of hyperlipidemia with lifestyle or pharmacotherapy varies on the basis of other risk factors. The potent influence of diabetes on cardiovascular risk is indicated by the fact that recommendations for the management of hyperlipidemia in diabetic patients are the same as for patients with established coronary disease (64). In essence, diabetes is taken to be a forme fruste of coronary atherosclerosis.

There is no reason to think the implications of diabetes for vascular disease should differ between adult and pediatric populations. That there is not a "Pediatric Treatment Panel" of the NCEP is attributable to the historical rarity of significant cardiovascular risk factors in children. There is also little reason to think that chronic diseases are tethered to chronological age, from which biological age can differ markedly. That "adult onset" diabetes has migrated down the age curve to become an increasingly common diagnosis among the ranks of the under-10-year-olds is a potentially ominous portent for the evolution of other chronic diseases. To some extent, obesity early in life may be seen as accelerating the aging process itself.

On our current trajectory, the prevalence of type 2 diabetes will quadruple by 2050, with the rate of growth outpacing that of type 1 diabetes (65). While the actual percentage of children subject to type 2 diabetes is still low (66) (see Chapter 6), even that may change as obesity develops at ever earlier ages. When "adult onset" diabetes occurs in 7- and 8-year-olds, we may expect to begin seeing cardiovascular events in 17- and 18-year-olds who by that age will have been diabetic for a decade. Personal communication suggests that such cases, though thankfully still rare, do already occur. The rate of overweight is rising among even infants and toddlers, and a rise in waist circumference in children seems to bode ill for future trends in insulin resistance (67) (see Chapter 7). The Centers for Disease Control and Prevention (CDC) currently projects that one in three individuals born in the United States in the year 2000 or later will develop diabetes in his or her lifetime, and for African Americans, the figure is one in two.

Data from the National Center for Health Statistics (68) indicate that children growing up in the United States today will ultimately suffer more chronic disease and premature death due to poor dietary habits and lack of physical activity than from exposure to tobacco, drugs, and alcohol combined. These data also suggest that current trends in the United States could translate into shorter life expectancy for children than for their parents, although such projections are complicated by a host of countervailing influences, including advances in medical technologies (69).

Obesity is an often important step along the causal pathway to most prevalent chronic diseases in developed countries. The link between obesity and diabetes is especially strong, with rising obesity rates directly responsible for epidemic type 2 diabetes in adults and children alike. Obesity, at least when distributed centrally, engenders a plethora of cardiac risk factors and is thus an important contributor to cardiovascular disease (see Chapter 7). An observational cohort study conducted by the American Cancer Society (70) representing more than 15 million person years of observation has demonstrated a link between obesity and most cancers. Obesity is associated with asthma, sleep apnea, osteoarthritis, and gastrointestinal disorders as well. More detailed discussion of these associations is provided in Chapters 6 to 8, 12, 15, and 18.

Obesity in children has been linked to increased risk of developing hypertension (71–74), hypercholesterolemia (75,76), hyperinsulinemia (75), insulin resistance (77,78), hyperandrogenemia (77,78), gallstones (79–81), hepatitis and fatty liver (82–85), sleep apnea (86–90), orthopedic abnormalities (e.g., slipped capital epiphyses) (91–95), and increased intracranial hypertension (96–101). Obesity during adolescence increases rates of cardiovascular disease (102–106) and diabetes (103,107) in adulthood, in both men and women. In women, adolescent obesity is associated with completion of fewer years of education, higher rates of poverty, and lower rates of marriage and household income (103). In men, obesity in adolescence is associated with increased all-cause mortality and mortality from cardiovascular disease and colon cancer (103,108). Adults who were obese as children have increased mortality and morbidity, independent of adult weight (103,109–112). Childhood obesity appears to be accelerating the onset of puberty in girls and may delay puberty in boys (113).

Reports that weight cycling may be associated with morbidity or mortality, independently of obesity, are of uncertain significance (111,114–116). There is evidence that when other risk factors are adequately controlled in the analysis, weight cycling does not predict mortality independently of obesity (117–119). There is also evidence that cardiovascular risk factors are dependent on the degree of obesity and fat accumulation over time rather than weight regain following loss (120,121). The benefits of weight loss are thought to override any potential hazards of weight regain (122); therefore, efforts at weight loss generally should be encouraged even in obese individuals with a prior history of weight cycling (123). However, repeated cycles of weight loss and regain may render subsequent weight loss more difficult by affecting body composition and metabolic rate, although this is an area of some controversy. For this reason, among others, weight-loss efforts should be predicated on sustainable adjustments to diet and lifestyle, whenever possible, rather than extreme modifications over the short term.

Psychological Sequelae of Obesity and Weight Bias

Often overlooked but of clear relevance to office-based dietary counseling is the relationship between obesity and mental health. Body image, adversely affected and even distorted by obesity, is important to self-esteem (124,125). Thus, poor self-esteem is a common consequence of obesity (the converse often also being true, with poor self-esteem adversely affecting diet; see Chapter 34) (126). This has important implications for dietary modification efforts (see Chapters 46 and 47). Repeated cycles of weight loss and regain may have particularly adverse effects on psychological well-being, although research in this area is limited (114,127,128).

Evidence consistently and clearly indicates that obesity engenders antipathy, resulting in stigma, social bias, and discrimination (124,129,130). Obese children suffer from poor self-esteem (126,131,132) and are subjected to teasing, discrimination, and victimization (109,133,134). Bullying and weight status can develop into a vicious cycle in which the stress of being teased may make the child more likely to seek out comfort food, thus further hindering the chance of achieving a healthy weight. The topic of weight bias is of ever-increasing concern as the worsening epidemic of obesity directs increasing societal attention to the topic.

The severity of prejudice against obesity is startling. Studies among school children consistently indicate a strong and nearly universal distaste for obesity as compared to other and equally noticeable variations in physiognomy.

In addition to its obvious implications for the overall well-being of obese persons, weight bias has implications for public policy. There is some evidence to suggest that the routine measurement of student BMI by schools, with reports home to parents, may enhance awareness of, and responses to, childhood obesity. This intervention has been implemented successfully in Arkansas and is thought to have contributed to the apparent turnaround in childhood obesity trends in Arkansas (135). Nonetheless, there is considerable opposition to this strategy, due largely to its potential for stigmatizing obese children and vilifying their parents (136). The solution to weight bias, however, cannot be to deny the problem of obesity. Rather, obesity and prejudice must both be confronted. And when the problem of obesity is attacked, it must be consistently and abundantly clear that the attack is against the condition and its causes, not its victims. All clinicians share in the responsibility for highlighting this distinction.

As is true of the metabolic effects of obesity, psychosocial sequelae of the condition tend to vary with its severity (137).

Economic Toll of Obesity

Overweight and obesity are thought to add an estimated $113 billion to national health-related expenditures in the United States each year or fully 5% to 10% of the nation's medical bill (138). Obesity has been a major driver of increased Medicare expenditures over the past decade (139). Compared to medical spending on healthy weight adults, medical spending on obese adults may be as much as 100% higher (56). Additionally, if the current childhood obesity epidemic is not halted, researchers forecast that from 2030 to 2050, there will be an additional $254 billion of obesity-related costs from both direct medical costs and loss of productivity (140).

There is also evidence to suggest that obesity results in personal financial disadvantage; poverty is predictive of obesity, and obesity is also predictive of less upward financial mobility (141–143). Thorpe et al. (139) have attributed to obesity alone 12% of the increase in healthcare spending in the United States over recent years (144,145). Obesity-related expenditures by private insurers purportedly increased 10-fold between 1987 and 2002.

A report in the American Journal of Health Promotion (146) indicates that obesity increases healthcare and absenteeism-related costs by $460 to $2,500 per worker per year. Roughly one-third of this cost is induced by higher rates of absenteeism, and two-thirds are induced by healthcare expenditures. These costs are distributed to lean workers as well, who pay higher healthcare premiums as a result, and to the employer, who experiences higher operating costs.

But some may actually profit from obesity, notably those in businesses responsible for selling the excess calories that make weight gain possible. In a provocative piece in the Washington Post, Michael Rosenwald (147) suggested that obesity is an integral aspect of the American economy, influencing industries as diverse as food, fitness, and healthcare. The trade-off between obesity-related profits and losses has been considered elsewhere (148). Costs and benefits are often a matter of perspective, and what is good finance for the seller may be bad for the buyer. Close and Schoeller (149) have pointed out that bargain pricing on oversized fast-food meals and related products actually increases net cost to the consumer, largely as a consequence of weight gain. The higher costs over time relate to adverse health effects of obesity as well as increased food intake by larger persons. (Note the paradox here: In order to sustain the market for the excess calories that contribute to obesity, obesity is necessary, as it drives up the calories required just to maintain weight; obesity depends on an excess of calories, and the effective peddling of that excess of calories depends on obesity.) Another cost of obesity is reduced fuel efficiency when driving and carrying more weight. Stated bluntly, the "all-you-can-eat" buffet is not much of a bargain both because excess calories resulting in excess weight lead to increased costs of living and because most beneficiaries of discounted dietary indulgences wind up willing to spend a fortune to lose weight they gained at no extra charge. There may be some utility in pointing this out to patients.

Obesity and Mortality

One of the most contentious and controversial aspects of the obesity epidemic has been a reliable accounting of the mortality toll. Recent debate of this issue has been particularly intense, precipitated by competing projections made by CDC scientists (150,151). However, this area has a history of controversy.

In 1993, McGinnis and Foege (152) identified the combination of dietary pattern and sedentary lifestyle as the second leading cause of preventable, premature death in the United States, accounting for some 350,000 deaths per year. Obesity contributes to the majority of these deaths and was considered to be directly or indirectly responsible for approximately 300,000 annual deaths (153).

Calle et al. (154) reported a linear relationship between BMI and mortality risk, based on an observational cohort of more than 1 million subjects followed for 14 years. In this cohort, high BMI was less predictive of mortality risk in blacks than in whites. Manson et al. (155) found a linear relationship between BMI and mortality risk in women from the Nurses' Health Study; the lowest risk of all-cause mortality occurred in women with a BMI 15% below average with stable weight over time. Including women with a smoking history in the analysis yielded a J-shaped mortality curve, with a higher mortality rate among the leanest women. In a study of over 2 million men and women, Engeland et al. (156) also found a J- or U-shaped mortality curve with the lowest rate of death at a BMI between 22.5 and 25. In a study of over half a million adults by Adams et al. (157), after controlling for smoking status and initial health, both overweight and obesity was associated with an increased risk of death. Most recently, a highly publicized meta-analysis by Flegal et al. (158) found that while obesity was associated with a higher all-cause mortality relative to normal weight, overweight was associated with a significantly *lower* all-cause mortality rate.

Data supporting the relationship between obesity and mortality risk come from a variety of sources and generally are consistent (159,160). There is evidence that obesity in adolescence, at least in males, is predictive of increased all-cause mortality (108). Data from the Iowa Women's Health Study suggested that WHR (now supplanted by waist circumference) might be a superior predictor of mortality risk to BMI in women. Whereas BMI produced a J-shaped curve, WHR and mortality were linearly related (161). This issue remains important but is often neglected in the obesity/mortality debate: Not all obesity is created equal in terms of cardiometabolic risk. Although earlier studies often demonstrated a J-shaped relationship between BMI and mortality, in the largest cohort studies, the relationship is linear (162). It is unsurprising that people thin due to serious illness have a high rate of mortality. Studies that assessed participants for chronic illness and excluded them in various ways yielded a straightening of the BMI/mortality curve over virtually its entire length, as noted previously (162,157).

Partly on the basis of this new evidence, a National Institutes of Health (NIH) consensus conference was held in 1998 to revisit the definition of overweight then in common use. It was at that time that the now prevailing definitions (see Table 5-1) of overweight and obesity were established. Because the prior threshold for overweight had been higher (BMI 27.2 in women, 27.8 in men), the sardonic observation was made that more than 10 million people who had gone to bed lean one day woke up overweight the next.

The revised definitions of obesity, revised mortality curves, and increasing prevalence of obesity all contributed to a heightened concern for the mortality toll of overweight. The data published in 1993 by McGinnis and Foege that had established tobacco as the leading, modifiable root cause of premature death in the United States were perceived to have contributed to societal efforts to curtail the harms of smoking. It was in this context that Mokdad et al. (150) made extrapolations from population data to suggest in 2004 that some 400,000 premature deaths each year in the United States were attributable to obesity and that obesity would soon overtake tobacco as the leading cause of premature death.

The most ardent rebuttal to this claim was made by Flegal et al. (151), who used data from the National Health and Nutrition Examination Surveys (NHANES) to extrapolate the mortality toll of obesity. Contending that Mokdad et al. had failed to adjust appropriately for age distribution, Flegal et al. reported a much weaker association between BMI and mortality, with as few as 100,000 to 150,000 premature deaths ensuing. Most provocatively, Flegal et al. (158) reported both in this study and a subsequent meta-analysis that overweight in middle-aged adults, a BMI between 25 and 30, was actually associated with a lower mortality rate than so-called ideal weight.

A related controversy is the likely impact of obesity on life expectancy in the future. The claim has been made that due to epidemic obesity, we are now raising the first generation of children with a shorter projected life expectancy than that of their parents (69,163). This view, too, has been refuted, with claims that life expectancy will continue to rise into the future.

There is now a rich litany of arguments on both sides of the obesity/mortality divide, with arguments for and against a high mortality toll now (164–167) and in the future (see Figure 5-1). The CDC has officially addressed the controversy on more than one occasion, with much of

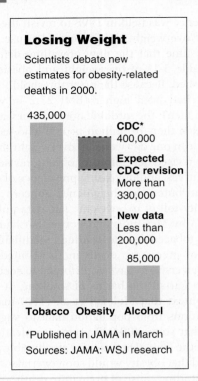

Losing Weight

Scientists debate new
estimates for obesity-related
deaths in 2000.

435,000

CDC*
400,000

**Expected
CDC revision**
More than
330,000

New data
Less than
200,000

85,000

Tobacco Obesity Alcohol

*Published in JAMA in March
Sources: JAMA: WSJ research

FIGURE 5.1. How many Americans die each year
from obesity?

Source: Mckay B. *Wall Street Journal* December 3, 2004:A15.

the debate spilling over into the popular press
(150,151,153,168–194).

Fortunately, there is no need to reach absolute
consensus on the death toll of obesity to appreciate the threat it represents. It may be that obesity
is killing fewer people than projected because of
advances in tertiary care. Certainly the means of
compensating for chronic diseases in advanced
states improve with each passing year. But compensation for chronic disease by such means as
endovascular procedures, polypharmacy, and/
or surgery is not nearly as good as, and is vastly
more expensive than, preserving good health.
That obesity accounts for an enormous burden of
chronic disease is beyond dispute; it lies on the
well-established causal pathways toward virtually
all of the leading causes of premature death and
disability in industrialized countries, including
diabetes, cardiovascular disease, cancer, degenerative arthritis, stroke, and, to a lesser extent,
obstructive pulmonary disease. Thus, while the
number of years obesity may be taking out of life
is debatable, there is no argument that it is taking
life out of years.

Of note, the Flegal meta-analysis (158) focused on mortality and did not take examine the
impact of obesity on morbidity. Moreover, when
people become ill, they generally lose weight;
however, the study did not exclude those who
were thin due to illness. Additionally, the study
did not exclude individuals who were thin for
other reasons, for example, anorexia nervosa,
severe depression, cocaine use, all of which may
cause increased mortality in healthy weight individuals as compared to overweight individuals.

While the arguments about the impact of
obesity on mortality are based on statistical
subtleties and projections from relatively small
samples, the American Cancer Society data are
based on an observational cohort study involving
nearly 1 million people now followed for nearly
20 years. This robust sample, cited in neither the
Mokdad nor Flegal papers, demonstrates a linear
association between BMI and mortality. This association is clear and unencumbered by contentious
statistics (195,196).

There is, finally, a simple logic about the association between obesity and mortality. Obesity
contributes mightily to the prevalence of diabetes, cancer, heart disease, and, to a lesser extent,
stroke. These, in turn, are the leading proximal
causes of death in the United States. It would
seem far-fetched that a condition contributing to
all the leading causes of death is entirely unimpli-
cated itself in the causation of death.

Less far-fetched is the lack of a direct association. Death certificates rarely cite obesity as cause
of death because it is generally a distal, or "upstream," factor. Obesity contributes to chronic
diseases, which in turn contribute to acute events
that contribute directly to death. Standard data-
gathering mechanisms may simply be blind, or
nearly so, to the contributions of obesity to mortality. This is especially probable in light of the
relative neglect of obesity in the standard medical
history. A prototypical causal pathway is shown
in Figure 5-2, with indications of the causes of
death certain, likely, and unlikely to appear on a
death certificate.

Another important consideration is that BMI,
as noted previously, is a relatively poor index of
health at the level of any given individual. A low
or normal BMI attributable to a healthful diet and
regular physical activity is obviously quite distinct from a normal or low BMI attributable to
depression, isolation, chronic illness, or an eating

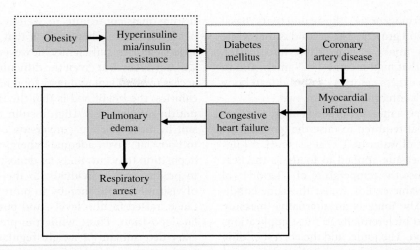

FIGURE 5.2. Obesity is a distal, "upstream," factor in premature death from multiple causes. Because of its distance from the actual precipitating events at the time of death, obesity is unlikely to be identified on a death certificate. The solid black bars enclose what is certain to be listed on a typical death certificate as cause of death, the solid gray bars enclose what is likely to be listed as the underlying cause of death, and the dashed bars enclose information that is unlikely to appear on the death certificate at all.

disorder. Similarly, an elevated BMI due to fitness and muscularity has health implications opposite those of excess adiposity. Finally, even excess adiposity differs in its effects on health on the basis of fat distribution, as discussed previously. In each case, these factors would bias assessment of the obesity/mortality association toward the null. The waist circumference appears to be a far better predictor of morbidity and mortality than the BMI (197–200), in much the same way that low-density lipoprotein (LDL) and the LDL:HDL ratio (the ratio between low- and high-density lipoprotein) discriminate cardiovascular risk far more reliably than does total cholesterol.

The implications of this line of reasoning are that obesity is a major contributor to premature mortality, but that generating an accurate and precise body count attributable to obesity per se will long remain elusive. The attribution of significant morbidity to obesity is far less challenging and is a sufficient basis in its own right to treat epidemic obesity as a bona fide clinical and public health imperative.

Energy Balance and the Pathogenesis of Obesity

The relentlessly increasing global prevalence of obesity (see Global Trends) has engendered understandable frustration among policy makers, public health practitioners, and health care providers alike. Attendant upon this frustration has been a tendency to see obesity as complex. It is anything but. While resolving the modern obesity epidemic may indeed prove as complex as it is challenging, explaining the epidemic is easy. People who gain excess weight over time are in a state of positive energy balance. The longer that state persists, and the greater the imbalance, the more weight is gained.

The balance referred to in "energy balance" is between energy units (typically, but not necessarily, measured in kilocalories or kilojoules) taken into the body and energy units expended by the body. Because the relationship between energy and matter is governed by fundamental laws of physics referable back to Sir Isaac Newton, the implications of energy balance are substantially self-evident. When more energy is taken into the body than is consumed by all energy-expending processes, the surplus is converted into matter. When energy expenditure exceeds energy intake, matter must be converted into energy to make up the deficit. Thus, positive energy balance increases a body's matter, and negative energy balance decreases it. When energy intake and output are matched, matter—body mass in this case—remains stable.

Several details of clinical interest complicate this otherwise simple construct. The first is that while energy intake is limited to a single activity, eating, energy output is expressed in several ways, including thermogenesis, physical activity, basal metabolism, and growth. The second is that while excess energy intake is convertible into matter, the nature of that matter can vary. Namely, and in simple terms, excess calories can build lean body tissue, fat, or a combination of the two.

The calorie is a measure of food energy and represents the heat required to raise the temperature of 1 g, or cm³, of water by 1°C at sea level. A kilocalorie, the measure applied to foods, is the heat required to raise the temperature of 1 kg or L, of water by the same extent, under the same conditions (201). The joule is an alternative measure of energy used preferentially in most applications other than food. The joule, and the corresponding kilojoule, is 4.184 times smaller than the calorie and kilocalorie, respectively.

There has been some recent controversy asking the question "is a calorie, a calorie?" (202). However, as already stated, a calorie is simply a unit of energy, and as such, 1 cal will always equal 1 cal (just as 1 m will always equal 1 m). Where the difference truly lies is that some foods are better for us than others, and one of the many virtues of better-for-us foods is that they tend to help us feel full on fewer calories and thus can tip the balance in the calories in, calories out equation (203).

Calories consumed ("in") is at least conceptually relatively simple: food. As noted, calories expended ("out") is the more complicated combination of resting energy expenditure (REE), basal metabolic rate (BMR), physical activity, and thermogenesis. The formula includes energy dedicated to linear growth in children, which contributes to basal requirements. There is a limited literature to suggest an association between relatively greater protein intake and relatively higher REE at a given body mass than that associated with other macronutrient classes (see discussion of macronutrient classes, page 74). Thermogenesis is influenced by sympathetic tone and leptin, which in turn may be influenced by insulin (see Chapter 6) and, therefore, to some degree, by macronutrient distribution. A comparable number of calories from different macronutrient sources almost certainly will not be comparably satiating (see Chapter 42), so macronutrient distribution may influence satiety and, thereby, subsequent energy intake.

If an individual is genetically predisposed to insulin resistance, high levels of postprandial insulin may contribute to weight gain, all else being equal (see Chapter 6). If that individual restricts calories sufficiently, however, weight gain will not occur. But given the difficulty people with access to abundant and tasty food have restricting calories, the likelihood is that the individual will not do so effectively. High insulin levels may result in more efficient conversion of food energy to body fat, given adequate energy intake for fat deposition to occur. Body fat deposition will lead, in predisposed individuals, to the accumulation of visceral fat and thereby to more insulin resistance, raised insulin levels, and potentially more fat deposition. Thus, while the predominant dietary determinant of weight regulation is clearly total energy intake, macronutrient distribution, endocrine factors, and diverse genetic predispositions may contribute important mitigating influences at any given level of calorie consumption.

In essence, then, the pathogenesis of obesity involves the complex details of a very simple energy balance formula: When calories in exceed calories out, weight rises and vice versa. Specifically, whenever caloric intake exceeds caloric expenditure by roughly 3,500 to 4,000 kcal, a pound of body fat will be generated. Theoretically, a pound of fat stores 4,086 kcal (9 kcal per g of fat, multiplied by the 454 g in a pound). However, a pound of living tissue is not actually just fat but must also contain the various structures and fluids required for the viability of that fat, such as blood, blood vessels, neurons, etc. By convention, an excess of 3,500 kcal is used to approximate the energy requirement for a pound of weight gain. By the same convention, a deficit of 3,500 kcal relative to expenditure will translate into a pound of body fat lost. For this reason, a daily caloric deficit of roughly 500 kcal is generally advised to achieve weight loss at the modest and sustainable pace of 1 lb per week.

The complexity underlying the energy balance formula is reflected in a wide range of genetic, physiologic, psychological, and sociologic factors implicated in weight gain. Efforts to control weight, prevent gain, or facilitate loss must address energy balance to be successful. Control of body weight relies on achieving a stable balance between energy input and energy consumption at a desired level of energy storage.

Working against this goal is the natural tendency of the body to accumulate fat. The storage of energy in the form of adipose tissue is adaptive

LIVERPOOL JOHN MOORES UNIVERSITY LEARNING SERVICES

in all species with variable and unpredictable access to food. In humans, only about 1,200 kcal of energy is stored as glycogen in the prototypical 70 kg adult, enough to support a fast of 12 to 18 hours at most. A human's ability to survive a more protracted fast depends on energy reserves in body fat, which average 120,000 kcal in a 70 kg adult. The natural tendency to store available energy as body fat persists, although the constant availability of nutrient energy has rendered this tendency maladaptive, whereas it once was, and occasionally still is, vital for survival.

The development of obesity appears to be related to an increase in both the size and number of adipocytes. Excess energy intake in early childhood and adolescence leads more readily to increases in fat cell number. In adults, excess energy consumption leads initially to increases in adipocyte size and only with more extreme imbalance to increased number (see Definitions of Overweight and Obesity and Measures of Anthropometry, page 56). Childhood obesity does not lead invariably to adult obesity, as the total number of adipocytes in a lean adult generally exceeds the number in an obese child. Thus, correction for early energy imbalance can restore the number of adipocytes to the normal range. However, childhood obesity is a strong predictor of obesity, and its complications, in adulthood (204).

In general, lesser degrees of obesity are more likely to be due to increased fat cell size, whereas more severe obesity often suggests increased fat cell number as well. Obesity due exclusively to increased adipocyte size is hypertrophic, whereas that due to increased fat cell number is hyperplastic. Weight loss apparently is more difficult to maintain in hyperplastic as compared to hypertrophic obesity because it requires reducing an abnormally high number of total adipocytes down to an abnormally low size. Adipocytes may actively regulate their size so that it is maintained within the normal range. Such signaling involves various chemical messengers released from adipose tissue, including angiotensinogen, tissue necrosis factor, and others, along with leptin. Adipocytes also produce lipoprotein lipase, which acts on circulating lipoprotein particles, especially very-low-density lipoprotein, to extract free fatty acids, which then are stored in the adipocyte as triglyceride.

The imbalance between energy consumption and expenditure that leads to excess weight gain can be mediated by either and generally is mediated by both. Relative inactivity and abundantly available calories both contribute. As noted previously, energy expenditure is composed of BMR, the thermic effect of food, and physical activity (Table 5-1). On average, BMR accounts for up to 70% of total energy expenditure, thermogenesis approximately 15%, and physical activity approximately 15%. The contribution of physical activity to energy expenditure is, of course, quite variable. REE can be measured by various methods, with the doubly labeled water method representing the prevailing standard in research settings (201,205).

In clinical settings, basal energy requirements for weight maintenance can be estimated by use of the Harris-Benedict Equation (see Section VIIA). A rough estimate of calories needed to maintain weight at an average level of activity is derived by multiplying the ideal weight of a woman (in pounds) by 12 to 14 and that of a man by 14 to 16. BMR is lower in women than in men when matched for height and weight due to the higher body fat content in women; muscle imposes a higher metabolic demand than fat at equal mass. A strong genetic component to the BMR results in familial clustering as well as clustering within ethnic groups predisposed to obesity (206–210) (see Chapter 44). BMR is largely explained by lean body mass, but among subjects matched for lean body mass, age, and sex, a variation of as much as 30% may be seen. This explains, at least in part, why comparable energy intake will produce obesity in some individuals but not in others. There is a clear implication in this for clinicians committed to compassionate weight-management counseling: What patients contend about predisposition to weight gain may very well be true (see Chapter 47). (The occasional patient tells me they only need to smell food to gain weight, and I think, compassion notwithstanding, it reasonable to remain a bit dubious about such claims.)

Total body weight generally correlates inversely with BMR at the population level but correlates positively with BMR in an individual, as weight loss reduces BMR, and weight gain increases it (211). The notion that larger people require more calories at rest than smaller people to maintain their weight should be all but self-evident, as is the fact that the maintenance calories of a horse are greater than those of a mouse.

BMR may fall by as much as 30% with dieting, although sustained reductions tend to be smaller, which explains why the maintenance of weight loss becomes increasingly difficult over time after initial success. The phenomenon of the "weight-loss plateau" is attributable to the equilibration of lower caloric intake with lower energy requirements resulting from reduced body mass. While both predictable and understandable, this phenomenon is often intensely frustrating for patients. Weight-management counseling should anticipate and address this universal tendency.

Reductions in BMR may contribute as well to increasing difficulty in losing weight after successive attempts (212), although this concept is debated (213–215). A plausible mechanism is that both fat mass and lean body mass are reduced when calories are restricted, whereas weight regain due to caloric excess will result in an increase in fat mass preferentially. Thus, cycles of weight loss and regain have the potential to increase the percentage of body fat and thereby lower calorie requirements for maintenance at any given weight.

When exercise is used as a mainstay in weight loss or maintenance efforts, this mechanism is forestalled. Resistance training that builds muscle can increase BMR, both by increasing total body mass and/or by increasing the percentage of lean body mass. As muscle is more metabolically active than fat, the conversion of body mass from fat to muscle at a stable weight will increase BMR. This pattern may frustrate patients who rely on a scale to gauge weight loss success, but in fact a reduction in fat mass and an increase in lean body mass clearly is a weight management success and should be regarded as such, despite the unmoving dial on a bathroom scale. There is consensus among authorities that in those experiencing cardiometabolic complications of obesity, a weight reduction of 10% is often conducive to clinically important risk reduction. Less well described, but certainly plausible, is similar improvement in those who lower weight less but redistribute weight from fat to lean.

Energy expenditure per unit body mass peaks in early childhood due to the metabolic demands of growth. Total energy expenditure generally peaks in the second decade, and energy intake often does as well. Thereafter, energy requirements decline with age, as does energy consumption. Energy expenditure tends to decline more than energy intake so that weight gain and, increasing, adiposity are characteristic of aging (see Chapter 31).

It is of interest that the capacity of the body to store excess calories in an energy reserve composed of adipose tissue is adaptive in any environment imposing cyclical caloric deprivation. This tendency becomes maladaptive only when an excess of calories is continuously available. Also of note, the adaptive capacity for weight gain is generally variable among individuals and populations, and it is somewhat systematically variable between men and women.

Men are far more prone than premenopausal women to accumulate excess fat at the belly and within the abdominal viscera, rendering them more susceptible to cardiometabolic sequelae of obesity. As mentioned earlier, the central pattern of obesity, known colorfully as the "apple" pattern, is referred to as android. In contrast, the "pear," or peripheral, pattern of obesity is gynoid.

There is a potential explanation for the tendency of women of reproductive age to store body fat more innocuously than men in evolutionary biology. Namely, reproduction depends on a woman's ability to meet both her own caloric needs and those of a developing fetus (see Chapter 27). The capacity to create a large enough energy reserve to help ensure a successful pregnancy may be a critical, and of course uniquely female, adaptation. A final contribution to this admittedly speculative construct is made by the effects in women of reducing body fat content below a critical threshold. Menses ceases, and a state of infertility ensues. This effect is most commonly observed in young female athletes as well as girls with eating disorders, in whom it represents a threat of irreversible osteopenia (see Chapters 14 and 25).

Thermogenesis

Food ingestion increases sympathetic tone, raising levels of catecholamines as well as insulin. Brown adipose tissue, concentrated in the abdomen and present in varying amounts, functions principally in the regulation of energy storage and wastage by inducing heat generation in response to stimulation by catecholamines, insulin, and thyroid hormone. The increase in sympathetic tone postprandially results in thermogenesis (heat generation), which may consume up to 15% of ingested calories. Some researchers even suggest targeting thermogenesis for antiobesity efforts (216,217). A reduced thermic effect of food may contribute to the development of obesity, although this is controversial (218,219). Approximately 7% to 8%

of total energy expenditure is accounted for by obligatory thermogenesis, but up to an additional 7% to 8% is facultative and may vary between the lean and obese.

Insulin resistance may be associated with reduced postprandial thermogenesis. However, obesity apparently precedes reduced thermogenesis, suggesting that impaired thermogenesis is unlikely as an explanation for susceptibility to obesity. Thermogenesis is related to the action of β_3-adrenergic receptors, the density of which varies substantially. Reduced thermogenesis may contribute to weight gain with aging, as thermogenesis apparently declines with age, at least in men (220,221).

Physical Activity

Energy consumption generally has risen in industrialized countries over recent decades as both the energy density of the diet and portion sizes have increased. During the same period, energy expenditure generally has fallen, largely due to changes in the environment and the patterns of work and leisure activity. According to the most recent data from the CDC, a majority of Americans do not meet the physical activity recommendations of 30 minutes of moderate-intensity activities at least 5 days per week (222). A reduction in exercise-related energy expenditure contributes to energy imbalance and weight gain. The attribution of weight gain to physical inactivity is compounded by the associations between sedentary behavior and poor diet (223). For example, data from the *Behavioral Risk Factor Surveillance System* indicate that relative inactivity correlates with a high dietary fat intake (224).

Although there is consensus that physical activity is essential to long-term weight maintenance, the mechanisms of benefit remain controversial. Evidence that physical activity reduces food intake or results in extended periods of increased oxygen consumption is lacking, and there is evidence to the contrary. Exercise has the potential to increase the BMR by increasing muscle mass. Energy consumption during exercise can help maintain energy balance. For example, a pound of weight loss per week requires a daily deficit of approximately 500 kcal; at a constant level of dietary intake, such a deficit could be achieved by 45 minutes of jogging or 75 minutes of brisk walking per day (see Table 5-4). The efficiency for linking energy consumption to physical work of contracting muscle

is approximately 30%; 70% of the available energy is wasted as heat. There is little evidence that the efficiency of work-related energy metabolism differs between the lean and obese.

Currently, there is a strong national emphasis on the health benefits of physical activity, as evidenced by First Lady Michelle Obama's *Let's Move!* campaign (225) and President Obama's *The Presidents Challenge* (226). Overall, however, little progress has been made toward *Healthy People 2020* objectives in this category (227). Although the utility of physical activity per se in promoting weight loss is uncertain, lifetime physical activity apparently mitigates age-related weight gain and clearly is associated with important health benefits (228–231). Moreover, the argument that physical activity does not promote weight loss is flawed. Physical activity can indeed promote weight loss and burn fat but only if we engage in enough of it and do not then overeat. The problem is that even those of us who exercise daily are relatively sedentary by historical standards. In the obesigenic environment of the modern world, we are more prone to excessive energy intake and inadequate energy expenditure than any previous generation (232,233).

The issue of whether physical activity and attendant fitness are more important to health than weight control has generated some controversy. Some authors have argued that fitness is more important than fatness, while others have defended the alternative view (80,234–254).

This dispute may be more distracting than helpful. At the population level, most fit people are at least relatively lean, while relative fatness and lack of fitness similarly correlate. While "fit" might trump "fat" in terms of health effects, only an estimated 9% of the population resides in this category of both fit and fat (see Table 5-5) (255).

Evidence from large cohort studies suggests that fitness and fatness are independent predictors of health outcomes. The combination of fit and lean is clearly preferable over all others. Of the two, it appears that weight may influence outcomes slightly more strongly than fitness level (238).

Evidence from the National Weight Control Registry suggests that regular physical activity may be an important element in lasting weight control (256,257). Physical activity is among the best predictors of long-term weight maintenance (258–263). It has been estimated that the expenditure of approximately 12 kcal per kg body weight per day in physical activity is the

TABLE 5.4

Energy Expenditure of Some Representative Physical Activities[a]

Activity	METs[b] (multiples of RMR)	kcal/min
Resting (sitting or lying down)	1.0	1.2–1.7
Sweeping	1.5	1.8–2.6
Driving (car)	2.0	2.4–3.4
Walking slowly (2 mph)	2.0–3.5	2.8–4
Bicycling slowly (6 mph)	2.0–3.5	2.8–4
Horseback riding (walk)	2.5	3–4.2
Playing volleyball	3.0	3.5
Mopping	3.5	4.2–6.0
Golfing	4.0–5.0	4.2–5.8
Swimming slowly	4.0–5.0	4.2–5.8
Walking moderately fast (3 mph)	4.0–5.0	4.2–5.8
Playing baseball	4.5	5.4–7.6
Bicycling moderately fast (12 mph)	4.5–9.0	6–8.3
Dancing	4.5–9.0	6–8.3
Skiing	4.5–9.0	6–8.3
Skating	4.5–9.0	6–8.3
Walking fast (4.5 mph)	4.5–9.0	6–8.3
Swimming moderately fast	4.5–9.0	6–8.3
Playing tennis (singles)	6.0	7.7
Chopping wood	6.5	7.8–11
Shoveling snow	7.0	8.4–12
Digging	7.5	9–12.8
Cross-country skiing	7.5–12	8.5–12.5
Jogging (10 to 12-minute-mile pace)	7.5–12	8.5–12.5
Playing football	9.0	9.1
Playing basketball	9.0	9.8
Running (8-minute-mile pace)	15	12.7–16.7
Running (4-minute-mile pace)	30	36–51
Swimming (crawl stroke) fast	30	36–51

[a]All values are estimates and based on a prototypical 70 kg male; energy expenditure is generally lower in women and higher in larger individuals. MET and kcal values derived from different sources may not correspond exactly.

[b]A MET is the rate of energy expenditure at rest, attributable to the resting (or basal) metabolic rate (RMR). Although resting energy expenditure varies with body size and habitus, a MET is generally accepted to equal approximately 3.5 mL/kg/min of oxygen consumption. The energy expenditure at one MET generally varies over the range from 1.2 to 1.7 kcal/min. The intensity of exercise can be measured relative to the RMR in METs.

Source: Data from Ensminger AH, et al. The concise encyclopedia of foods and nutrition. In: Wilmore JH, Costill DL, eds. *Physiology of sport and exercise. Human kinetics.* Champaign, IL: publisher, 1994; American College of Sports Medicine. *Resource manual for guidelines for exercise testing and prescription,* 2nd ed. Philadelphia, PA: Williams & Wilkins, 1993; Burke L, Deakin V, eds. *Clinical sports nutrition.* Sydney, Australia: McGraw-Hill Book Company, 1994; McArdle WD, Katch FI, Katch VL. *Sports exercise nutrition.* Baltimore, MD: Lippincott Williams & Wilkins, 1999.

minimum protective against increasing body fat over time (264). The contribution of physical activity to weight maintenance may vary among individuals on the basis of genetic factors that are as yet poorly understood (265,266).

Over recent years, there has been accumulating and encouraging evidence that lifestyle activity, as opposed to structured aerobic exercise, may be helpful in both achieving and maintaining weight loss (267,268). Such unobtrusive

TABLE 5.5

Combinations of Fatness and Fitness[a]

Weight	Fitness	
	High	Low
Lean	+/+ (a)	+/− (b)
Overweight	+/− (c)	− (d)

[a]At the population level, cells a and d predominate over cells b and c. A + sign indicates a favorable influence, and a − sign indicates a negative one.

physical activity may be more readily accepted by exercise-averse patients.

Macronutrient Metabolism

There is some degree of metabolic control over the consumption and distribution of macronutrients. Cortisone, galanin, and endogenous opioid peptides stimulate the medial hypothalamus to promote fat intake. Dopamine has antagonistic effects, suppressing desire for fat intake. Amphetamines act as dopamine precursors and thereby tend to reduce fat intake. Drugs such as neuroleptics (e.g., phenothiazines) that antagonize dopamine often are associated with excess fat intake and weight gain. Endogenous opioid peptides and growth hormone-releasing factor may play a role in the regulation of protein intake.

Carbohydrate intake and craving is mediated by effects of γ-aminobutyric acid, norepinephrine, neuropeptide Y, and cortisol on the paraventricular nucleus of the medial hypothalamus. Activity of this system tends to be high when serum glucose and/or glycogen stores are low. Suppression of carbohydrate craving apparently is mediated by serotonin (see Chapters 34 and 38) and cholecystokinin. Insulin resistance may be associated with carbohydrate craving due to elevations of norepinephrine, cortisone, and neuropeptide Y. The interactions of appetite signaling with macronutrients are further discussed in Chapter 38. The role of macronutrient distribution in weight control efforts is addressed on page 74.

Sociocultural Factors

The imbalance between energy intake and energy expenditure fundamental to obesity is largely the product of an interaction between physiologic traits and sociocultural factors. Human metabolism is the product of some 6 million years of natural selection (see Chapter 44), the overwhelming majority of which occurred in an environment demanding vigorous physical activity and providing access to a largely nutrient-dense but energy-dilute diet (269). In such an environment characterized by cyclical feast and famine, metabolic efficiency would be favored, as would a capacity to store nutrient energy in the body against the advent of famine (270).

Such an environment likely would shape behavioral responses as well. The tendency to binge eat, characteristic of modern-day hunter-gatherers and many animal species, is adaptive when food is occasionally abundant but often deficient; therefore, such a tendency may be nearly universal in humans (269). The increasing frequency of binge eating disorder (see Chapter 25) likely represents the convergence of this widespread native tendency, with the ever-increasing opportunities to indulge it to harmful excess. Even in the absence of pathology, the constant and abundant availability of tasty food in conjunction with this tendency constitutes a formula for excess energy consumption.

An innate preference for sweet foods has been well documented in humans and other animals (271). Such a preference would likely be adaptive in a primitive environment, as naturally sweet foods (e.g., fruit, honey) provide readily metabolizable energy and are rarely toxic. There is evidence of a strong pleasure response to dietary fat, mediated in part by opioid receptors (272). A strong affinity for dietary fat would have been adaptive in an environment where dietary fat was scarce yet represented a source of concentrated energy and essential nutrients. Similarly, the need for a range of micronutrients and the potential difficulty in consistently finding a variety of foods would likely have cultivated a strong preference for dietary variety. This trait, sensory-specific satiety, becomes maladaptive in an environment providing food in ·constant variety as well as abundance, favoring excessive intake (273) (see Chapter 38).

The imbalance between energy intake and expenditure is compounded by modern conveniences that have led to a decline in physical activity associated with daily activities (131). The global spread of modern technology is associated with the emergence of obesity as a global public health problem (274). Prevailing patterns of behavior, including use of convenience devices that minimize physical activity (e.g., elevators, remote control devices) and consumption of an energy-dense diet, are generally reinforced at the societal level, often taking on culturally normative implications (275). Sociocultural influences are powerful determinants of both activity and dietary patterns (276,277) and, in the modern context, of obesity.

Both obese and lean individuals generally underreport calorie intake, but the degree of underreporting is greater in the obese. Generally, calorie consumption is higher in obese than in lean individuals (278,279), as would be expected.

Other Factors

Endocrinopathy, such as Cushing's syndrome or hypothyroidism, is a rare cause of obesity. Relatively few obese patients have hypothyroidism, and most previously lean patients with hypothyroidism do not become obese as a result of the thyroid disease.

An association has been noted between variations in the microbiota (endogenous commensal flora) of the human colon and obesity. A similar association has been cited between adenovirus exposure and obesity (280). These associations may be of a causal nature or may be statistical flukes. But even if causal, they still have the potential to divert attention from the more important and painfully obvious causes of epidemic obesity: caloric excess and relative inactivity. While the novel associations may tantalize, they should not be exaggerated. When a prevailing excess of calories and prevailing deficiency of physical activity have been eliminated from the formula, if there is any obesity left to explain, the day of the novel theory will have arrived. It will be most welcome.

Genetic Influences on Energy Balance and Weight

There is a strong genetic contribution to obesity, mediated along several important pathways. Genes influence REE, thermogenesis, lean body mass, and appetite. There is, thus, an important potential genetic influence on both energy intake and expenditure. Overall, genetic factors are thought to explain roughly 40% of the variation in BMI. Adoption studies demonstrating an association between obesity in a child and the biological parents, despite rearing by surrogate parents, and twin studies showing anthropometric correspondence between identical twins reared apart are particularly useful sources of insight in this area (281–284).

Genetic factors are of clinical importance as they help explain individual vulnerability to weight gain and its sequelae. Minimally, an appreciation for genetic factors in energy balance should foster insight and compassion relevant to clinical counseling. Maximally, elucidation of genetic contributions to obesity may illuminate novel therapeutic options over time.

Dozens of genes have been implicated as candidates for explaining, at least partly, susceptibility to obesity in different individuals; gene–gene interactions are highly probable in most cases (285–289). Only in rare instances is a monogenic explanation invoked. Of these, the most common appears to be a mutation in the melanocortin-4 receptor gene (MC4R), which interferes with satiety signals mediated by α-melanocyte-stimulating hormone. This mutation may account for up to 4% of severe obesity in humans. A variety of mutations may interfere with leptin signaling, and some of these may prove to be monogenic causes of obesity. One hundred and twenty-seven candidate genes for obesity-related traits were listed in the most recent update from the Human Obesity Gene Map (290).

Leptin, produced in adipose tissue, binds to receptors in the hypothalamus, providing information about the state of energy storage and affecting satiety (291,292). Binding of leptin inhibits secretion of neuropeptide Y, which is a potent stimulator of appetite.

The Ob gene was originally identified in mice, and Ob/Ob mice are deficient in leptin and obese (293). The administration of leptin to Ob/Ob mice results in weight loss. In humans, obesity is associated with elevated leptin levels (294). Nonetheless, the administration of leptin to obese humans has been associated with modest weight loss (295), suggesting that leptin resistance rather than deficiency may be an etiologic factor in some cases of human obesity (296). Leptin is the primary chemical messenger that signals adipocyte repletion to the hypothalamus; leptin resistance thus has the potential to delay or preclude satiety. The importance of leptin to the epidemiology of obesity has recently been reviewed (297–300).

Much of the genetic influence on weight regulation may be mediated by variation in REE (301), and appetite/satiety, addressed in Chapter 38 (302).

While the contribution of genes to obesity deserves both recognition and respect, it should not distract from the ultimate hegemony of environmental influences. Genes help explain varied susceptibility to, and expression of, obesity under any given set of environmental conditions. Stated another way, genes help explain the expanse of the "bell curve" characterizing the distribution of weight in a given population at a given time. Isolating the effects of genes on obesity from obesigenic elements in the environment is a considerable challenge (303); thinking of obesity as a product of gene–environmental interaction in most cases may be the best means of meeting this challenge at present (304,305).

Environmental factors better explain the position of that entire bell curve relative to a range of potential distributions. The genetic profile of US residents today, for example, may be quite similar to the profile 60 years ago, while the weight distributions for those two populations differ dramatically. The explanation for this divergence over time has much more to do with environmental change than with genetic change. The related topic of nutrigenomics is addressed briefly in Chapter 45.

The Gut Microbiome and Obesity

Recent advances have allowed scientists to identify the micro-organisms making up the human intestinal tract. Initial research done in mouse models (306–308) followed by subsequent studies in humans (309–311) have demonstrated distinct gut microbiota in obese as compared to lean individuals. Moreover, studies suggest that these differences in gut microbiota may influence energy balance and thus obesity (312). Interestingly, the effects of the microbiome on obesity seems to be transmissible. In mouse models, "transplantation" of gut microbes from obese mice to normal mice results in greater increases in total body fat as compared to those receiving microbes from lean mice (313). Although more research needs to be conducted before becoming a mainstay of treatment, alterations of the gut microbiome through probiotics, antibiotics, and fecal transplantation open intriguing new pathways for the treatment of obesity (314,315).

Environmental Obesigenicity

The term "obesigenic" has been coined to characterize the constellation of factors in the modern environment that contribute to weight gain. Obesigenicity ensues from any influence that contributes to a relative increase in energy intake or a relative decline in energy expenditure. Weight gain and eventually obesity result whenever habitual energy intake exceeds habitual energy expenditure.

Obesigenic elements in modern societies encompass labor-saving technology; energy-dense, low-cost, ubiquitous food; food marketing; reliance on cars; suburban sprawl; time demands that preclude food preparation at home; school policies that curtail physical education; and more.

When contending with obesity and weight control at the level of an individual patient or family, the clinician is well advised to consider the contributory forces at the social level that render obesity so prevalent and relentless. An appreciation for environmental obesigenicity fosters realistic perspectives on the causes and solutions for obesity and protects against the temptation to "blame the victim." The evolutionary context that best highlights the obesigenicity of the modern environment is the subject of Chapter 44. Implications for effective obesity control are addressed in Chapter 47.

Dieting, Dietary Pattern, and Weight Management

Energy intake varies with the macronutrient composition of the diet. Each gram of dietary carbohydrate releases 4 kcal of energy when metabolized, each gram of protein releases slightly less than 4 kcal, and each gram of fat releases approximately 9 kcal on average. There is, of course, variation around these average values among the diverse food sources within each macronutrient category.

Despite significant variability in basal metabolism, it is possible to estimate energy requirements. Several formulas are available to approximate energy needs based on age, body mass, and state of health. The most widely cited of these are the Harris-Benedict Equation and simplifications of it (see Section VIIA). Such formulas typically are used to determine the caloric requirements of inpatients receiving total parenteral nutrition, but they are equally applicable to the ambulatory setting. Although it is relatively straightforward to estimate caloric needs, the utility of doing so in the outpatient setting is debatable. Unless a patient is willing to carefully count calories, there is likely to be a substantial discrepancy between a formulaic recommendation and actual practice.

The availability of software—and more recently, smartphone apps—for tracking calorie intake may render determination of energy needs more useful.

Because approximately 70% of calories are spent on basal metabolism, even vigorous physical activity may be insufficient to control weight when caloric intake substantially exceeds the needs of REE. Although the number of calories required to maintain weight varies substantially among individuals, the degree of caloric restriction, relative to habitual intake, required to produce weight loss is more predictable. Each pound of body fat represents a repository of approximately 4,000 kcal, as noted previously. To lose a pound of fat requires that energy expenditure be increased by 4,000 kcal or that intake be restricted by a comparable amount. To reduce caloric intake by 4,000 kcal over a week requires a daily restriction of between 500 and 600 kcal. In a 2,000 kcal diet, this represents a 25% reduction in total calorie intake. Therefore, whatever the baseline calorie intake required to maintain weight, a reduction of 500 to 600 kcal per day will generally result in approximately 1 lb of weight loss per week initially. As basal metabolism declines, further reductions may be required to sustain the weight loss (see Chapter 47).

Successful dietary approaches to weight loss involve either restricting overall calories or restricting specific foods or macronutrient classes. There is an intuitive rationale for restricting dietary fat in efforts to control weight: It is the most calorically dense macronutrient and the least satiating per calorie (see Table 5-6). Per gram, fat contains at least twice as much energy as protein or carbohydrate. The fiber, protein, and water content of foods all contribute to their satiating effects, facilitating fullness with fewer calories, whereas fat produces the opposite effect, increasing the calories required to feel satisfied (316). Consequently, every gram of fat removed from the diet would need to be replaced with twice the mass of these other macronutrients to replace the lost calories. In addition, because carbohydrate sources in particular are apt to contain at least some fiber that is noncaloric, the volume differential between fat and carbohydrate to achieve the same calorie load is even greater than the mass difference. At a certain point, volume becomes limiting in calorie intake (this topic is addressed in Chapter 38).

However, there is evidence that fat restriction has important limitations in achieving weight control. Although NHANES III data suggest that the proportion of total calories consumed as

---

TABLE 5.6

Properties of the Macronutrient Classes Germane to Energy Balance

Macronutrient Class	Energy Density	Satiety Index[a]	Comments
Fat	Highest; 9 kcal/g	Lowest	The notion seems to prevail that fat is filling, but on a calorie-for-calorie basis, it is the least satiating of the macronutrient classes.
Simple carbohydrate	4 kcal/g	Intermediate; lower than for complex carbohydrate	The satiety threshold for sugar is higher than that for other nutrients, thus making sugar an important contributor to caloric excess in most people.
Complex carbohydrate	<4 kcal/g	Intermediate; higher than for simple carbohydrate	Sources of complex carbohydrate—whole grains, fruits, and vegetables—are rich in water and fiber, both of which increase food volume and contribute to satiety yet provide no calories.
Protein	3–4 kcal/g	Highest	Protein is generally more filling, calorie-for-calorie, than other food classes, although this may not be true when compared to complex carbohydrates very high in fiber and/or water content.

[a]The satiety index is a measure of how filling a food is based on comparison of isoenergetic servings.

fat has declined over recent years in the United States, total fat intake has been stable due to increases in the intake of calories from other macronutrient sources, particularly carbohydrate (317). Roughly 49% of calories in the typical American diet come from carbohydrate, roughly 15% from protein, 34% from fat, and 2% from alcohol (a concentrated source of calories, at 7 kcal per g; see Chapter 40).

There is evidence that, in general, portion sizes have been increasing in the United States for several decades at least, leading to an increase in total calories consumed, regardless of the source. The still-booming low-fat and nonfat food industry capitalized on the expectation of the public that fat restriction would facilitate weight control and promote health. For many, the result has been excessive intake of nutrient-poor foods that are high in simple sugars and low in fiber. Although these foods are less calorically dense than their higher-fat predecessors, they are often consumed in excess due to the ostensible "guiltlessness" of the consumer and possibly to lesser effects on satiety; SnackWells cookies are prototypical. Overindulgence in fat-reduced but energy-dense foods composed principally of simple carbohydrate, and the inevitable effects on weight contributed mightily to the dawn of the recent "low-carb" dieting era. In contrast to the patterns that prevailed, however, the guidance offered regarding low-fat eating always emphasized naturally low-fat foods, such as vegetables and fruits, rather than highly processed snack and dessert items. Such misapplication of dietary guidance appears to be a generalizable vulnerability when guidance is offered in terms of nutrient classes rather than foods (318).

In response to the accelerating obesity pandemic, competing weight-loss diets have propagated; those touting carbohydrate restriction have recently been most in vogue, although this trend has clearly crested (319,320) and is waning, although still the subject of at least intermittent interest (321).

There are numerous reviews on the subject of diet for weight loss (45,322–338). In the aggregate, this literature lends strongest support to sensible, balanced diets abundant in fruits, vegetables, whole grains, and lean protein sources, with some restriction in total fat, simple sugars, and refined starches. Weight-loss approaches popular over recent years include fat-restricted diets, carbohydrate-restricted diets (included the Paleo diet), low-glycemic diets, and Mediterranean and other largely plant-based diets. Each of these is considered in turn.

Fat-Restricted Diets

High dietary fat intake has historically been a powerful predictor of weight gain (339). Epidemiological studies have consistently shown that increasing dietary fat is associated with increased prevalence of obesity (340). Transcultural comparisons dating back at least to the work of Ancel Keys suggest that higher intake of dietary fat is associated with higher rates of obesity and chronic disease (341–343). Most authorities concur that high intake of dietary fat contributes to obesity at the individual and population levels. The theoretical basis for weight loss through dietary fat restriction is strong, given the widely acknowledged primacy of calories in weight governance and the energy density of fat (344). Dietary fat is the most energy dense and least satiating of the macronutrient classes (345–347) (see Table 5-6).

When fat restriction is in accord with prevailing views on nutrition (i.e., achieved by shifting from foods high in fat to naturally low-fat foods), the results are consistently favorable with regard to energy balance and body weight. A review of the results from 28 clinical trials showed that a reduction of 10% in the proportion of energy from fat was associated with a decrease in weight of 16 g per day (348). A 2-year randomized weight-loss trial comparing a very low-fat vegan diet to a more moderate low-fat diet found that both diets led to weight loss, but the subjects on the vegan diet incurred significant weight loss at both 1 year (4.9 vs. 1.8 kg) and 2 years out (3.1 vs. 0.8 kg) (349).

Despite the extensive literature supporting dietary fat restriction for weight loss and control, there are dissenting voices (350). For the most part, dissent is predicated on the failure of dietary fat restriction to achieve population-level weight control in the United States. Recent trends in the United States suggest that fat intake over recent decades has held constant, not been reduced, and that intake of total calories has risen to dilute the percentage of food energy derived from fat; increased consumption of highly processed, fat-reduced foods is the principal basis for these trends (351). Thus, the failure of dietary fat restriction to facilitate weight control is likely more a problem of how the guidance has been applied than any errancy in the guidance itself (352).

In response to the public's interest in fat restriction, the food industry generated a vast array of low-fat, but not necessarily low-calorie, foods over the past two decades. The increase in calories was driven by increased consumption of calorie-dense, nutrient-dilute, fat-restricted foods, contemporaneous with a trend toward increasing portion sizes in general (316,353–356). Lowering the fat content of processed foods while increasing consumption of simple sugars and starch is not consistent with the long-standing recommendations of nutrition authorities to moderate intake of dietary fat. Yet it is this distorted approach to dietary fat "restriction" that best characterizes secular trends in dietary intake at the population level and that subtends the contention that dietary fat is unrelated to obesity.

Carbohydrate-Restricted Diets

Although the popularity of carbohydrate-restricted diets for weight loss appears to be waning, these diets have been so in vogue over recent years that they have reshaped the US food supply. While recent preoccupation with this dietary practice has been particularly intense and widespread, it is worth noting that interest in carbohydrate restriction for weight loss is not new; Atkins' *Diet Revolution* was first published in 1972 (357). In 1978, Rabast et al. (358) used isocaloric formula diets to compare fat- and carbohydrate-restricted approaches to weight loss in 45 obese adults. Carbohydrate restriction resulted in greater weight loss (14 ± 7.2 kg vs. 9.8 ± 4.5 kg) at 30 days.

Review of low-carbohydrate diets to date suggests that short-term weight loss is consistently achieved, but that neither weight-loss sustainability nor long-term effects on overall health has yet been determined (359–364). Brehm et al. (365) examined weight loss, cardiac risk factors, and body composition in 53 obese women randomly assigned to a very-low-carbohydrate diet or a calorie-restricted, balanced diet with 30% of calories from fat. Subjects assigned to the very-low-carbohydrate diet group lost more weight (8.5 ± 1.0 vs. 3.9 ± 1.0 kg; $p < 0.001$) and more body fat (4.8 ± 0.67 vs. 2.0 ± 0.75 kg; $p < 0.01$) than those assigned to the calorie-restricted, balanced diet group; cardiac risk measures improved

comparably in both groups at 6 months. Sondike et al. ran a 12-week weight-loss trial comparing low-carbohydrate to moderately fat-restricted diets in 30 overweight adolescents. There was significantly greater weight loss with the low-carbohydrate assignment. However, LDL cholesterol levels improved with fat restriction but not with carbohydrate restriction (366). A systematic review published in *Lancet* in 2004 found that weight loss achieved while on low-carbohydrate diets was associated with the duration of the diet and restriction of energy intake but not with restriction of carbohydrates per se (367).

Carbohydrate restriction does appear to improve satiety and decrease hunger, perhaps lending to its greater success in short-term weight loss. One study investigating carbohydrate and fat restriction effects on hunger perception in overweight premenopausal women suggested that a greater decrease in hunger perception may lead to a greater weight loss observed in the carbohydrate-restriction group (368). A recent systematic review of RCTs of low-carbohydrate diets did find that across the board there was a higher attrition rate in the low-fat groups compared to low-carbohydrate groups (369), supporting this theory.

However, the anorexic effect of a lower-carbohydrate diet may in fact be related to the increased protein content, not the restriction of carbohydrates; protein is noteworthy for its high satiety index (370,371). In 1999, Skov et al. (372) reported an interesting variation on the low-carbohydrate diet theme by comparing two fat-restricted (30% of calories) diets, one high in carbohydrate (58% of calories) and the other high in protein (25% of calories). The researchers followed 65 overweight adults for 6 months and gave them diets strictly controlled with regard to nutritional composition but unrestricted in calories. More weight was lost with high protein (8.9 kg) intake than with high carbohydrate (5.1 kg) intake; no weight loss occurred in a control group. Furthermore, a recent meta-analysis comparing isocaloric low-fat diets differing only in proportion of carbohydrates and protein have found increased weight loss with high-protein, lower-carbohydrate diets than with high-carbohydrate, lower-protein diets. (372,373).

While interest in the Atkins and South Beach diet has slowed, new interest in the so-called Paleolithic diet and the plant-based "eco-Atkins" diets (374) have brought new popularity to the high-protein, lower-carbohydrate approach. These diets emphasize consumption of foods found in the supposed "native" human environment—plants, nuts, seeds, legumes, eggs, and in the case of the Paleo diet, fish and lean meats—while eschewing all grains and sugar. While evidence is limited, one small 3-month pilot study of patients with type 2 diabetes found improved glycemic control and increased weight loss when subjects adhered to the Paleo diet compared to a conventional diabetes diet (375). Recent hype aside, benefits likely increase when adherents use it as guidance away from high carbohydrate, processed foods. Weight loss will likely follow the same pattern seen in many of the existing low-carbohydrate studies (376), with unclear health benefits unless following the equally "Paleo" practices of our Stone Age ancestors of consuming as much as 100 g fiber daily and burning up to 4,000 calories per day through vigorous activity.

Two studies of low-carbohydrate diets that received widespread attention are those by Samaha et al. (377) and Foster et al. (378), published in the same issue of the *New England Journal of Medicine* in 2003. Samaha et al. compared a very-low-carbohydrate diet (<30 g carbohydrate per day) to a fat- and calorie-restricted diet in 132 adults with BMI of 35 or above over a 6-month period. The carbohydrate-restricted diet resulted in greater weight loss at 6 months than the low-fat diet, but was also associated with a far greater reduction in daily calorie intake (a mean reduction of 271 kcal per day for the low-fat diet and 460 kcal for the low-carbohydrate diet). Foster et al. compared the Atkins diet, as described in *Dr. Atkins' New Diet Revolution* (379), to a fat- and calorie-restricted diet in 63 obese adults followed for 12 months. The low-carbohydrate diet produced significantly greater weight loss at 6 months but not 12 months. Calorie intake was not reported. In both studies, attrition and recidivism were high; Samaha et al. noted that their trial was unblinded, whereas Foster et al. made no mention of blinding. Foster published a follow-up study in 2010 again comparing a low-carbohydrate diet to a low-fat diet, this time for 2 years. The low-carbohydrate diet produced just slightly greater weight loss at 12 months, with no difference compared to the low-fat diet by year 2 year of follow-up (380).

In a widely publicized study comparing the effectiveness and adherence rates of four popular weight-loss diets among overweight subjects with hypertension, dyslipidemia, or fasting hyperglycemia, Dansinger et al. (381) found no significant difference in mean weight loss between groups at 1 year. Predictably, the study reported no significant differences in mean total calorie reduction between groups, lending support to the widely accepted notion that total calorie consumption, regardless of macronutrient content, is of prime importance in weight-loss efforts. All diet groups (Atkins, Weight Watchers, Ornish, and Zone) had poor adherence rates, with no significant difference between groups. In all diet groups, greater adherence to the diet resulted in improved weight outcomes; participants in the top tertile of adherence had a mean loss of 7% body weight. No significant differences in cardiac risk factors were noted across groups; in each group, the amount of weight loss predicted improvements in several risk factors.

Fairly similar results were seen in a study by Gardner et al. (320) published in 2007. These investigators randomized just over 300 premenopausal women to one of four diets: the Atkins diet, the Zone diet, the Ornish diet, or the LEARN cognitive behavioral therapy program. At 12 months, weight loss was greatest in the Atkins group, differing significantly only from the Zone diet. Cardiac risk factors assessed included lipids, blood pressure, insulin, and glucose and were fairly similar across treatment categories. Media attention to the study was intense and generally ignored several salient limitations. First, weight loss was limited in all four diet groups; the Atkins group lost a mean of roughly only 10 lb in a year. Second, the Atkins group was gaining back weight faster than the other groups at the 12-month mark. Third, the two treatment assignments that differed most in outcomes (Atkins and Zone diets) differed least in dietary composition, obviating any simple conclusions about the association between macronutrient profile and weight loss.

In a 6-month noncontrolled trial, Westman et al. (364) assessed the effects of a very-low-carbohydrate diet among 51 overweight or obese adults. Carbohydrate intake of less than 25 g per day was recommended to start and was increased to 50 g upon achievement of 40% of target weight loss. Mean daily calorie consumption at follow-up was 1447 ± 350 but was not measured at baseline.

Calorie restrictions were not prearranged; however, subjects were instructed to eat only until hunger was relieved. All subjects available for follow-up developed ketonuria; levels were used to verify self-reported carbohydrate intake. Subjects lost a mean of 10.3% ± 5.9% body weight. Significant decreases in total cholesterol, LDL, and triglyceride levels as well as increases in HDL were reported.

Yancy et al. (382) compared a low-carbohydrate diet plus nutritional supplementation to a low-fat diet with calorie deficit of 500 to 1,000 calories per day among 120 overweight, hyperlipidemic subjects. Both groups received exercise recommendations and attended group meetings. The low-fat diet group lost significantly less weight than the low-carbohydrate diet group at 6 months (mean change, −12.9% vs. −6.7%; $p < 0.001$). Reductions in fat mass were similar between groups. The low-carbohydrate group had lower attrition, yet the low-fat group appeared to have better adherence to the diet.

Brinkworth et al. (383) compared the effectiveness at 68 weeks of two calorie- and fat-controlled 12-week diets: a standard protein group (15% protein, 55% carbohydrate) and a high-protein group (30% protein, 40% carbohydrate). Results indicated no significant difference in weight loss between groups; however, neither group had high compliance with the diet. Both diets significantly increased HDL cholesterol concentrations ($p < 0.001$) and decreased fasting insulin, soluble intercellular adhesion molecule-1 (sICAM-1), and C-reactive protein (CRP) levels ($p < 0.05$).

In a small group of obese patients with type 2 diabetes that consumed habitual diets for 7 days followed by a low-carbohydrate diet for 14 days, Boden et al. (384) found that the two-week low-carbohydrate diet resulted in spontaneous reduction in energy intake by almost one-third, from 3,111 kcal per day to 2,164 kcal per day; weight loss during this period was completely accounted for by reduced caloric intake. This study highlighted the calorie reduction associated with carbohydrate restriction that, while providing an obvious mechanism for inducing weight loss, is frequently left unmentioned (385). Several other studies comparing low-carbohydrate to low-fat or conventional diets with durations ranging from 6 to 12 weeks were reviewed. Studies using comparable energy intake among subjects across groups consistently reported comparable weight loss, regardless of the target population (386–390).

Another study examining isocaloric diets differing only in carbohydrate composition came to similar results. Golay et al. (388) assigned 68 overweight adults to approximately isocaloric low- (25% of calories) and moderate- (45% of calories) carbohydrate diets for 12 weeks; they observed comparable losses of weight, waist circumference, and body fat in both groups. For the most part, metabolic indices were favorably and comparably influenced by both diets as well.

Poppitt et al. (391) achieved significant weight loss among 46 adult subjects with metabolic syndrome followed for 6 months by substituting carbohydrate for fat. Complex carbohydrate substitution for fat was associated with both weight loss and amelioration of the lipid profile; the substitution of simple carbohydrate for fat did not result in weight gain.

The recent preoccupation with carbohydrate restriction appears to be reactionary to the recent era during which fat restriction was prioritized. The popular press and media reports suggest that the public feels misled by promises that fat restriction would lead to weight loss. In particular, the widely known U.S. Department of Agriculture (USDA) food guide pyramid came under attack as a contributor to worsening obesity rates (392) and has now been replaced by MyPlate (393), which some have still criticized as vague, not representative of the best available evidence, and influenced by special interest groups (394). The adulteration of messages in the pyramid under the influence of special interest groups is the subject of a book (395). The competition between low-fat and low-carbohydrate diets for weight loss has in some ways polarized debate beyond the point of reason or utility (385,396). There is little to suggest that the selective vilification of a macronutrient class is prudent or useful in the pursuit of sustainable weight loss.

Low-Glycemic Diets

Advocates of low-carbohydrate diets often share a common rationale pertaining to minimizing the glycemic index (GI) or glycemic load (GL) of the diet. The GI of a food is a measure of how much its ingestion raises blood glucose levels postprandially, measured as the area under the glucose curve (397). Carbohydrate-containing foods can be ranked according to the typical postprandial glycemic response they induce (398). The GI, developed by Dr. David Jenkins et al. (399) at the

University of Toronto in 1981, compares foods on the basis of a fixed and equal dose of intrinsic carbohydrate, customarily 50 g. This fixed-dose comparison is a weakness of the index when it is applied to dietary guidance. Nearly 10 medium-sized carrots are required to produce a 50-g dose of carbohydrate, as compared to 1 cup of vanilla ice cream. Ice cream consequently has a markedly lower GI than carrots (see Table 5-7). This deficit led to the development of the GL. Taking both GI and standard serving sizes into account, the GL is the weighted average GI of a food multiplied by the percentage of energy from carbohydrate (400,401) and is believed to better predict the glycemic impact of foods under real-world conditions (398).

The relationship between weight and BMI is roughly analogous to the relationship between GI and GL. Weight may be high, but a person may still be lean if he or she is tall. Similarly, the GI may be high, but the glycemic effect of that food may be modest if the carbohydrate content is relatively dilute. An expansive table of GI and GL values of common foods, published in 2002, is available at www.ajcn.org (402). A few foods representing the range of potential divergence between GI and GL are shown in Table 5-8.

A recent review suggests that low-GL diets are associated with marked weight benefits and loss of adiposity in ad libitum studies in overweight or obese adults and children (403). Some studies suggest that the primary mechanisms by which low-GI foods may facilitate weight loss is through their ability to increase satiety and reduce subsequent food intake (404,405).

A trial by Ebbeling et al. (406) reveals some of the potential distortions introduced when means of improving dietary intake pattern are considered as mutually exclusive of one another. This group of investigators compared a diet reduced in GL, with 30% to 35% of calories from fat, to a diet termed "conventional" in which fat was restricted to 25% to 30% of calories, but the quality of the carbohydrate choices was unaddressed. The reduced-GL diet resulted in slightly greater weight loss and control of insulin resistance than the control diet in the 16 obese adolescents followed. What seems most noteworthy, however, is that the range of fat intake for the low-fat and low-GL diets was actually contiguous. Thus, this study actually compared two diets that differed little with regard to fat content, one in which GL was controlled, the other in which it was not. This is very much like comparing complex to simple carbohydrate and finding that complex carbohydrate has preferable health effects. Regrettably, in the rush to defend competing dietary claims, this simple message is obscured.

Overall evidence to date suggests that with regard to weight loss, both high- and low-GI or GL diets will produce equivalent weight loss over 6 months, assuming equivalent dietary fat and carbohydrate intake. Two recent short-term trials investigating the role of GI on energy intake, weight, and risk factors for chronic disease found no significant differences between

TABLE 5.7

Glycemic Index of Some Common Foods

Food Group	Food	Glycemic Index
Breads	White bread[a]	100
	Whole wheat bread	99
	Pumpernickel	78
Cereal products	Cornflakes	119
	Shredded wheat	97
	Oatmeal	85
	White rice	83
	Spaghetti	66
	Bulgur wheat	65
	Barley	31
Fruit	Raisins	93
	Bananas	79
	Oranges	66
	Grapes	62
	Apples	53
	Cherries	32
Vegetables	Parsnips	141
	Baked potato	135
	Carrots	133
	Corn	87
	Boiled potato	81
	Peas	74
	Yams	74
Legumes	Lima beans	115
	Baked beans	60
	Chick peas	49
	Red lentils	43
	Peanuts	19
Dairy products	Yogurt	52
	Ice cream	52
	Milk	49
Sugar	Sucrose	86

[a]Reference standard.

Source: Adapted from Jenkins DJ, Jenkins AL. The glycemic index, fiber, and the dietary treatment of hypertriglyceridemia and diabetes. *J Am Coll Nutr* 1987;6:11–17.

TABLE 5.8

Glycemic Index and Glycemic Load of a Few Foods that Demonstrate How the Values May Diverge[a]

Food	GI	Serving Size	Carbohydrate Dose (g)	GL
Chickpeas	51	150 g	30	11
Vanilla ice cream	54	50 g	9	3
Strawberries	57	120 g	3	1
Orange	69	120 g	11	5
Whole wheat bread	73	30 g	13	7
Orange juice	81	250 mL	26	15
Coca Cola	90	250 mL	26	16
Plain bagel	103	70 g	35	25
Doughnut	108	47 g	23	17
Carrots	131	80 g	6	5

[a]The foods are listed from lowest to highest GI.

Source: Data from Foster-Powell K, Holt SH, Brand-Miller JC. International table of glycemic index and glycemic load values: 2002. Am J Clin Nutr 2002;76:5–56.

groups in energy intake, body weight, or fat mass (407,408). The primacy of calories in weight control is reaffirmed.

Low-GL diets may support children in obesity prevention. In 2000, Spieth et al. (409) reported the results of a retrospective cohort study comparing a low-GI diet to a low-fat diet for weight loss in 107 obese children. Greater reduction in the BMI was observed at approximately 4 months in the low-GI group (–1.53 kg per m^2 [95% CI, –1.94 to –1.12]) than in the low-fat diet group (–0.06 kg per m^2 [–0.56 to +0.44], $p < 0.001$).

While low-GL diets may not have any unique bearing on weight loss compared to other approaches, they do appear to have positive benefits on metabolic markers and glycemic control. In a 2002 study by Heilbronn et al. (410) 45 overweight subjects with type 2 diabetes were randomly assigned to either a high- or low-GI diet following 4 weeks of a high-saturated-fat diet. All diets were energy restricted. Weight loss did not differ between treatments; however, a significantly greater reduction in LDL was observed on the low-GI diet. A 6 month trial of Asian, nondiabetic women with a history of gestational diabetes randomized into a high-GI or low-GI group; significant reductions in body weight, BMI, and WHR were observed only in the low-GI group ($p < 0.05$), as were significant improvements in glucose tolerance (411).

A recent review suggests that low-GL diets are associated with marked weight benefits and loss of adiposity in ad libitum studies in overweight or obese adults and children (412). Some studies

suggest that the primary mechanisms by which low-GL foods may facilitate weight loss is through their ability to increase satiety and reduce subsequent food intake (404,405).

Few authors have explicitly addressed the fact that there are various means of achieving a diet with a low GL overall. McMillan-Price et al. (413) did so in a randomized trial of roughly 130 overweight adults. Two diets relatively high in carbohydrate and two diets relatively high in protein (and thus, lower in carbohydrate) were compared on the basis of differing GLs. The study showed, as most do, that restricting calorie intake by any means led to roughly comparable weight loss in the short term, although trends hinted at a benefit of low GL. The percentage of subjects achieving a weight reduction of at least 5% was significantly greater on the low-GL diets – both high-carbohydrate and high-protein – than on their higher-GL counterparts. Similarly, body fat loss was enhanced, at least among women, by the low-GL diets. Whereas LDL cholesterol decreased significantly on the high-carbohydrate, low-GL diet, it actually increased on the high-protein, low-GL diet.

Aggregated, these findings point strongly toward the importance of food choices, rather than choices among macronutrient categories, as a major arbiter of cardiac risk. A low-GL diet can be achieved by minimizing carbohydrate intake, but this approach is apt to toss out the baby with the bathwater. High-carbohydrate foods such as most whole grains, beans, legumes, vegetables, and even fruits can contribute to a low-GL dietary pattern. Such foods also provide a diversity of micronutrients of potentially great importance to overall health, and cardiovascular health specifically, antioxidant flavonoids and carotenoids noteworthy among them.

By demonstrating that a high-carbohydrate, low-GL diet may offer particular cardiac benefit, this study points toward a diet in which choice within macronutrient categories is given at least as much consideration as choice among those categories. This perspective is concordant with a large volume of research suggesting that cardiac risk may be mitigated by reducing dietary fat and by shifting fat intake from saturated and trans-fatty acids to monounsaturates and polyunsaturates. Cardiac health at the population level will likely be well served when dietary guidance is consistently cast in terms of healthful, wholesome foods rather than competition among the three macronutrient classes from which a diet is composed.

Mediterranean Diets

The Mediterranean diet differs from the typical US diet in the quantity and quality of fat and the quantity of unrefined grains, vegetables, fruit, and lean protein sources (414). The Mediterranean dietary pattern is low in saturated fat and high in monounsaturated fatty acids, high in antioxidants including vitamins C and E, and high in fiber and folic acid. Olive oil is the dominant fat source, and consumption of fruits and vegetables, grains, fish, and legumes are moderate to high. Wine is commonly served with meals (415). Although there is variation in the Mediterranean diet, depending on country and region due to cultural, ethnic, religious, economic, and agricultural production differences (414,416–418), the dietary characteristics common to the region have been consistently associated with good health and longevity. Of note, many of the Mediterranean populations enjoying good health have traditionally high rates of physical activity compared to Western societies (419), potentially confounding comparisons based on dietary pattern.

The Mediterranean diet is relatively high in total fat. Some have expressed concerns that adherence to this diet may promote weight gain (420). However, because of the overall pattern of foods in this diet, i.e., its emphasis on whole foods and vegetarian protein sources, it is not based largely on energy-dense foods as most higher-fat diets tend to be. Data from a population-based study of 23,597

adult men and women suggest that adherence to a traditional Mediterranean diet is unrelated to BMI in both sexes, after adjusting for total energy intake. Rising obesity rates observed in Mediterranean populations have been ascribed to falling levels of physical activity in conjunction with new dietary influences from the United States, contributing to increased energy intake (421).

Evidence from cross-sectional studies generally supports a beneficial association between weight status and the traditional Mediterranean dietary pattern (422,423). Based on a sample of more than 3,100 Spanish men and women, Schroder et al. found that obesity risk decreased in men and women with increasing adherence to the traditional Mediterranean dietary pattern ($p = 0.01$ and $p = 0.013$, respectively) (422).

The evidence is convincing that energy-dense foods generally contribute to weight gain. However, it is also clear that when energy restriction can be achieved on a diet relatively high in fat content, weight loss is achieved (424). A Mediterranean diet, which is high in monounsaturated fatty acids but not predominantly composed of energy-dense foods, may be more effective at long-term weight loss than a diet based predominantly on restriction of total fat because it may be more palatable and therefore better sustained.

McManus et al. (425) evaluated a calorie-controlled, moderate-fat Mediterranean diet compared to a standard low-fat diet (also calorie controlled). The Mediterranean diet resulted in superior long-term participation and adherence, leading to greater weight loss. The moderate-fat group lost a mean of 4.1 kg, reduced BMI by 1.6 kg per m^2, and lowered waist circumference by 6.9 cm, compared to increases in the low-fat group of 2.9 kg, 1.4 kg per m^2, and 2.6 cm, respectively, at 18 months ($p < 0.001$) (425). A 2004 study by Flynn et al. (426) demonstrated weight loss along with a reduction in cholesterol levels and increased feelings of well-being among 115 postmenopausal women after 15 months on a Mediterranean diet. The intervention involved a weekly cooking class for 1 year, with professional chefs providing training in the correct use of natural ingredients of traditional Mediterranean cuisine.

Esposito et al. followed 3,000 women and 3,600 men for 4 years as half adhered to a Mediterranean-style diet and half to a low-fat diet based on AHA guidelines. At year 1, subjects in the Mediterranean arm had lost significantly more weight than their low-fat dieting counterparts (-6.2 vs. -4.2 kg). This difference was attenuated by the end of the 4 year study (427). One important limitation of this study and others is that diet was self-reported.

There is some evidence that in addition to facilitating weight loss, a moderately hypocaloric Mediterranean diet may also improve body composition and health outcomes among obese subjects, improving metabolic profile and preventing loss of fat-free mass (428). A recent meta-analysis of 20 RCTs evaluating different dietary approaches to weight loss in people with type 2 diabetes found that the Mediterranean diet had the greatest effect on glycemic control of any dietary approach, and along with a low-carbohydrate diet led to the greatest weight loss in subjects (429). Another recent meta-analysis found that Mediterranean diets appear to be more effective than low-fat diets in improving cardiovascular risk factors such as high blood pressure, dyslipidemia, and inflammatory markers (430).

It is worth noting that although many studies have demonstrated successful weight control and health improvements with adoption of the Mediterranean diet (425,428), some have included supports such as cooking classes to ensure that participants learn how to correctly use the natural ingredients of traditional Mediterranean cuisine (426). More research is needed to determine whether the Mediterranean diet can be realistically and reliably implemented and sustained among free-living populations in the United States, given the current state of ubiquitous access to, and American affinity for, energy-dense snacks and fast foods. Continuing to eat oversized servings of french fries, but adorning them with olive oil, does not qualify as a healthful application of the Mediterranean diet.

Weight-Loss Diets and Body Composition

One of the most tantalizing claims of popular weight-loss diets is that weight loss can be achieved or facilitated by means other than energy restriction. Deemphasizing calories is, in fact, quite characteristic of popular weight-loss approaches. Proponents of carbohydrate restriction contend that limiting intake of carbohydrate allows for weight loss, regardless of calorie intake (431). At least one study reported at the 2003 meeting of the North American Association for the Study of Obesity (432) suggested greater weight loss over a 12-week period among subjects on a low-carbohydrate diet than among those on

a low-fat diet, despite 300 more calories per day on the carbohydrate-restricted assignment.

However, only limited data are available to date on the effects of carbohydrate restriction on body composition. There is clear evidence of a dehydrating effect of very-low-carbohydrate diets, and of ketosis, in the short term (45); thus, some of the early weight loss on low-carbohydrate diets is almost certainly water. This may explain why low-carbohydrate diets consistently show increased weight loss in the short term, yet long-term trials fail to show persistent differences in weight loss compared to low-fat or Mediterranean diets (429). An association between increasing dietary fat and increasing body fat has been noted (421). Nelson et al. (433) reported a positive association between dietary fat and body fat and negative associations with body fat for both total and complex carbohydrate.

Hays et al. (434) recently reported that a diet rich in complex carbohydrate resulted in an increase in lean body mass and a decrease in body fat among 34 subjects with impaired glucose tolerance. Similar results have been observed by other groups (435). Volek et al. (436), however, reported a loss of body fat and an increase in lean body mass with carbohydrate restriction in 12 volunteers followed for 6 weeks. The effects of physical activity on body composition are, of course, clear and noncontroversial, with increased activity leading to relative increases in lean body mass at the expense of body fat (437,438).

Recent focus in the specific metabolic properties of fructose has led to vilification of fructose, especially high-fructose corn syrup, for its role in the obesity epidemic (439). Indeed, Americans consume too much sugar, and added dietary sugar has been linked to weight gain (440). There may be important physiologic distinctions in the way fructose is metabolized in the liver compared to sucrose (441). However, available evidence suggests that similar decreases in weight and body fat result from hypocaloric diets whether the primary sugar content is fructose or glucose (442), arguing against claims that the replacement of sucrose with high-fructose corn syrup is the biggest contributor to the rise in obesity. Furthermore, fructose as found naturally in whole fruit, in typical dietary consumption, has been shown to support weight loss and reduction of cardiovascular risk factors (443). Recommendations should therefore focus on reducing all refined sugar and processed simple carbohydrates, not replacing fructose with glucose or developing novel products such as "fructose-free" soda (441).

Overall, there is little evidence to support a claim that loss of body fat is achieved preferentially by redistributing macronutrients at isoenergetic levels (341,444). Worth noting, once again, is that a pound of body fat represents an energy reserve of over 4,000 kcal; a pound of muscle, a reserve of roughly 1,800 kcal; and a pound of water, no latent energy whatsoever. While each weighs a pound, each requires a markedly different energy deficit to be lost; water can be lost with no energy deficit. Thus, until proved otherwise, the most plausible explanation for enhanced weight loss at any given level of energy intake is the loss of body compartments that represent lesser energy reserves. Such losses of water and muscle protein are undesirable.

Popular Diets

A search on Amazon.com using the terms "diet," "weight loss," and "weight control" yields bibliographies of 87,670; 85,269; and 36,622, respectively (445). The same terms entered into web search on Google yield 134 million; 326 million; and 219 million sites, respectively (446). Thus, it is far beyond the scope of this or any other text—or even plausibility—to characterize even a representative sample of weight-loss diets, programs, and products being promoted to the general public.

The best that can be done to characterize these myriad claims on the basis of evidence is to apply a process of exclusion. In a systematic review of the obesity-prevention and obesity-control literature (447), strategies that emerge as most promising with regard to lasting weight control involve achieving an energy-controlled and balanced diet along with regular physical activity. Fundamentally, claims for virtually any other approach to sustainable weight loss are unsubstantiated. There is little or no scientific evidence to support the contentions of the most popular diets, including those based on carbohydrate restriction (e.g., the Atkins diet), those based on food combination or food proportioning (e.g., the Zone diet), or those based on the GI (e.g., the South Beach diet, the GI diet) (444). There is, of course, no shortage of anecdotal support and testimonials for virtually all the popular diets.

Worth noting is that a modest proportion of the books on the subject of diet address not so much the *what* of weight loss as the *how*, describing strategies for achieving a diet and lifestyle that

evidence indicates to be associated with both lasting weight control and good health. Among the offerings in this category are approaches based on energy density (448,449), water and fiber content (450), and the array of skills and strategies needed to navigate through the modern, "toxic" nutritional environment (451). Related to these are books dedicated to the same goal for children and/or families (452).

Potential Hazards of Popular Weight-Loss Diets

There is little to suggest that dietary fat restriction as a weight-loss or weight-control method poses any likelihood of harm, even if restriction of total fat is other than optimal. Perhaps because societies subject to high rates of obesity also tend to consume excessive quantities of harmful fats, the literature generally indicates that restriction of dietary fat is both conducive to weight loss and health promoting (453,454). Many cultures recognized for good health and longevity have native diets very low in fat (53); few free-living societies adhere to dietary patterns low in carbohydrate. The worst that can be said of fat restriction for weight loss is that if extreme, it may not be optimal for health (455). Even critics of dietary fat restriction appear to agree that low-fat diets offer health benefits relative to the typical American diet, which is high in saturated and trans fats.

Carbohydrate restriction, in contrast, when extreme, is actually or potentially linked to an array of adverse health effects (45). These adverse effects stem from wholesale reductions in carbohydrate intake and do not pertain to shifting calories within the carbohydrate class from sugars and refined grains to whole grains, fruits, and vegetables, a practice with widespread support.

There is evidence that weight loss attributable to carbohydrate restriction is in part body water loss. Gluconeogenesis consumes water along with glycogen, and ketone bodies cause increased renal excretion of sodium and water (456). Studies indicate that dizziness, fatigue, and headache are common side effects of ketosis (457).

Ketosis is potentially harmful, with possible long-term sequelae, including hyperlipidemia, impaired neutrophil function, optic neuropathy, osteoporosis, and protein deficiency, as well as alterations in cognitive function. Children on ketogenic diets as part of an antiseizure regimen have developed dehydration, constipation, and kidney stones. In response to ketosis, renal calcium excretion increases. To make up for the loss of calcium in urine, it is mobilized from bone to circulation (456). One study of adolescents on a ketogenic diet showed decreased bone mineral density after just 3 months, despite vitamin D and calcium supplementation (457). Sustained ketosis causes bone resorption, suggesting a risk for osteoporosis (458).

A comparison of eight high-protein, low-carbohydrate diets indicates that the Atkins diet had the highest level of total fat, saturated fat, and cholesterol (457). Consuming a diet high in saturated fat may raise total and LDL cholesterol levels, both of which contribute to cardiovascular disease. A significant increase in LDL has been reported among subjects on the Atkins diet, although this finding is inconsistent and is often accompanied by a potentially countervailing rise in HDL. An increase in CRP on the Atkins diet has been observed, suggesting an inflammatory response. A high intake of saturated fat generally increases the risk of insulin resistance (457), contradicting the contention of low-carbohydrate diet proponents that carbohydrates are to blame for insulin resistance (431). High-fat diets may also predispose to cancer (459).

High protein intake may negatively affect renal function in healthy individuals, and it certainly accelerates renal disease in diabetes. In patients with renal dysfunction on a high-protein diet, there is glomerular damage causing spillage of plasma proteins and resultant tubular injury and fibrosis (457). Urinary calcium excretion is also increased, and hypercalciuria may ensue, predisposing to calcium stone formation (458). High protein intake imposes a metabolic burden on both the liver and kidneys, requiring additional excretion of urea and ammonia (460).

Extreme carbohydrate restriction is potentially associated with increased risk of dysthymia, if not depression, through a serotonergic mechanism (461). The production of serotonin in the brain requires delivery and uptake of tryptophan, which is influenced by both the availability of tryptophan and the actions of insulin. With very low carbohydrate intake and blunted insulin release, tryptophan delivery to the brain is impaired, serotonin production is limited, and mood instability has been reported to ensue (462); the public health significance of this mechanism remains uncertain.

Finally, high-protein, low-carbohydrate diets simply do not allow for adequate intake of fruits (and to a lesser extent, vegetables), restricting nutrient and fiber-rich foods shown to be protective against a wide array of chronic diseases (463–466). Soluble fiber lowers cholesterol, reducing the risk for cardiovascular disease, and lowers insulin secretion after meals by slowing nutrient absorption (457,467). By several mechanisms, fiber is thought to contribute to satiety and calorie control. Fruit and vegetable intake has long been, and remains, well below recommended levels in the United States (468,469).

The known and potential hazards of extreme carbohydrate restriction are summarized in Table 5-9.

Weight Loss Sustainability

As opposed to most people who commit a lifetime to sequential dieting, the literature on long-term weight loss success is thin; frequency of dieting is a negative predictor of lasting weight control (470). The best available data are from observational studies (471), transcultural comparisons, and the National Weight Control Registry (472). The Registry was established to characterize the behavioral patterns of individuals successful at long-term maintenance of considerable weight loss (an average loss of 30 kg maintained for over 5 years).

Registry data indicate that a relatively low-fat, and therefore energy-dilute, diet is a mainstay of successful weight maintenance, as is regular physical activity (473–476). Fundamentally, people successful at lasting weight control tend to subscribe to a pattern of behaviors highly concordant with prevailing recommendations for overall good health (257,473–475,477–479). Limited time spent watching television is also characteristic of long-term weight control (480). There is nothing to suggest that any other approach to weight loss, no matter the apparent advantages at the start, can compete with a healthful, balanced diet and regular physical activity in the long run.

Dietary Pattern and Health

In the Diabetes Prevention Program, a low-calorie, low-fat diet coupled with moderately intense physical activity for at least 150 minutes per week reduced the incidence of type 2 diabetes by 58% (481). Similarly, the DASH Collaborative Research Group has shown that hypertension can be prevented and treated by reducing intake of saturated and total fat and adopting a diet rich

TABLE 5.9

Known and Potential Adverse Effects of Extreme Restriction of Dietary Intake of Carbohydrate

Adverse Effect	Mechanism
Constipation	An established effect attributable to low intake of dietary fiber.
Dehydration	Gluconeogenesis consumes water along with glycogen, and ketone bodies cause increased renal excretion of sodium and water.
Depression/dysthymia	A theoretical risk due to impaired delivery of tryptophan to the brain and impaired serotonin production.
Halitosis	An established effect of ketosis.
Hepatic injury	A potential sequela of high protein intake over time.
Increased cancer risk	A potential sequela of increased consumption of animal products and decreased consumption of grains and fruit.
Increased cardiovascular disease risk	A potential sequela of increased consumption of animal products and decreased consumption of grains and fruit.
Nausea	An established side effect of ketosis.
Nephropathy	A potential consequence of high intake of protein over time.
Osteopenia	An established effect of ketosis. Hypercalciuria is induced by high intake of dietary protein.
Renal calculi	A known sequela of ketosis. Risk is increased by dehydration.

Source: Adapted from Pagano-Therrien J, Katz DL. The low-down on low-carbohydrate diets: responding to your patients' enthusiasm. *The Nurse Practitioner* 2003;28:5,14.

in fruits, vegetables, grains, and low-fat dairy (482,483). Cardiovascular disease prevention has been demonstrated with both low-fat (484) and Mediterranean dietary patterns (485). Weight loss is a common element in all of these successful interventions.

Reviews of diet for optimal health do not necessarily demonstrate complete accord on all points but are nonetheless substantially confluent with regard to fundamentals (158). Diets comprised primarily of unprocessed, whole foods, rich in fruits, vegetables, and whole grains; restricted in animal fats and trans fat from processed foods; limited in refined starches and added sugar; providing protein principally from lean sources; and offering fat principally in the form of monounsaturated and polyunsaturated oils are linked to good health (194,486–492). With regard to diet and optimal health, debate is substantially limited to variations on this basic theme rather than any fundamental departures from it. This topic is addressed at greater length in Chapter 45.

Health Implications of the "Native" Human Diet

A noteworthy contribution is made to considerations of dietary pattern and human health by the anthropology literature. Quite distinct from biomedical research, a fairly extensive body of work characterizes what is and is not known about the native nutritional habitat of our species. While there is debate about many details, there is general consensus that humanity adapted over eons to an environment in which calories were relatively scarce and physical activity demands were high (493). Saturated and trans fat intake were low and negligible, respectively; micronutrient intake was high; and protein intake was from lean sources (267,494).

The traditional human diet was of course low in both starch and sugar, but it was rich in complex carbohydrate from a variety of plant foods (267). Many, but not all, anthropologists suggest that we were more gatherers than hunters and that meat likely contributed less to our subsistence than did the gathering of diverse plant foods (495,496). That this should be relevant to human health requires nothing more than acknowledging that human beings are creatures. For all other species under our care, epitomized by zoological parks, the diet we provide is an adaptation of the diet consumed in the wild. The "native" human diet appears to have provided roughly 25% of calories from fat, 20% to 25% of calories from protein, and the remainder from complex carbohydrate (267); this pattern is remarkably confluent with that demonstrating compelling health benefit in clinical trials (481,482).

Dietary Guidelines for Weight Control, Health Promotion, or Both

On the basis of its review of evidence linking dietary pattern to health outcomes, the U.S. Preventive Services Task Force advises clinicians to endorse to all patients over the age of 2 a nutrient-dense diet low in saturated fats, added sugars, and sodium, while abundant in fruits, vegetables, and whole grains (497,498). These recommendations are highly concordant with those of the National Heart, Lung, and Blood Institute at the NIH (499).

In 2010, the IOM released updated dietary guidelines reiterating its recommendations for 45% to 65% of calories from carbohydrate, 20% to 35% from fat, and 10% to 35% from protein, in conjunction with 60 minutes each day of moderately intense physical activity (500). The IOM guidelines further emphasize the restriction of saturated and trans fat and their replacement with monounsaturated and polyunsaturated fat. The American College of Preventive Medicine has formally adopted a position in support of dietary recommendations within the IOM ranges since 2002 (501).

The Dietary Guidelines for Americans were last updated in 2010 (502). The main tenets of the newly released guidelines, issued by the U.S. Departments of Health and Human Services (HHS) and Agriculture (USDA) (258), are to choose a variety of nutrient-dense foods and beverages and to limit intake of saturated and trans fats, cholesterol, added sugars, salt, and alcohol. The dietary guidelines are represented schematically in the new MyPlate graphic, shown in Figure 5-3 (502).

The Centers for Disease Control has partnered with the nonprofit Produce for Better Health Foundation to develop the Fruit & Veggies—More Matters initiative to encourage Americans to increase fruit and vegetable consumption (503), similar to the National Cancer Institute's "5-a-day" program encouraging fruit and vegetable intake and endorses dietary guidelines (504). The American Heart Association offers dietary guidelines that call for balancing caloric intake and physical activity to maintain healthy body weight, with a diet rich in vegetables and fruits, whole grains, omega-3 rich fish, and a limited intake of saturated fat (<7% of total calories) and minimal to no trans fat (505). Both the American Dietetic Association and the American Diabetes Association support the USDA/IOM dietary guidelines and

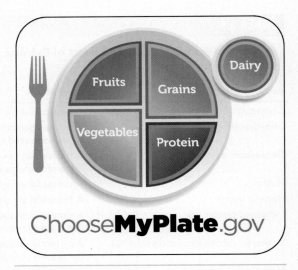

FIGURE 5.3. MyPlate illustrates the five food groups that make up a healthy diet. Use the image to help build a healthy plate at every meal.

Source: http://www.choosemyplate.gov/.

both recommends an emphasis on whole grains, at least five servings of fruits and vegetables daily, restriction of saturated fat and cholesterol, and limited sugar and sweet consumption (506,507). Differing only in detail, all these recommendations are substantially congruent.

Both health and weight control appear to be facilitated by a mixed, balanced diet that is based on healthful, wholesome foods within each nutrient class rather than by choosing a nutrient class to abandon (Table 5-10) (508–510).

CLINICAL INTERVENTIONS FOR OBESITY: LIFESTYLE COUNSELING, PHARMACOTHERAPY, MEDICALLY SUPERVISED DIETS, AND BARIATRIC SURGERY

Lifestyle Counseling

The primary clinical intervention for weight management is lifestyle counseling, addressed more fully in Chapter 47.

The case for universal weight-management counseling in clinical care has not yet been made on the basis of evidence. The U.S. Preventive Services Task Force recommends intensive dietary counseling for patients with overt cardiovascular risk factors and routine screening for obesity, but it concludes that evidence is insufficient to

TABLE 5.10

Comparison of Diets Recommended for Health Promotion

	Low-carbohydrate	Low-fat/ Vegetarian/Vegan	Low-glycemic	Mediterranean	Mixed/balanced	Paleolithic
Health benefits relate to:	Emphasis on restriction of refined starches and added sugars in particular.	Emphasis on plant foods direct from nature; avoidance of harmful fats.	Restriction of starches, added sugars; high fiber intake.	Foods direct from nature; mostly plants; emphasis on healthful oils, notably monounsaturates.	Minimization of highly processed energy-dense foods; Emphasis on wholesome foods in moderate quantities.	Minimization of processed foods. Emphasis on natural plant foods and lean meats.
Compatible elements:	Limited refined starches, added sugars, processed foods; limited intake of certain fats; emphasis on whole plant foods, with or without lean meats, fish, poultry, seafood.					
And all potentially consistent with:	Food, not too much, mostly plants.[a,b,c]					

[a]Pollan M. 2007. Unhappy meals. *New York Times Mag.* Jan 28. http://www.nytimes.com/2007/01/28/magazine/28nutritionism.y.html?pagewanted=all

[b]Portion control may be facilitated by choosing better-quality foods which have the tendency to promote satiety with fewer calories.

[c]While neither the low-carbohydrate nor Paleolithic diet need be "mostly plants," both can be.

Source: Katz DL, Meller S. Can we say what diet is best? *Ann Rev Pub Health.* 2013; in press.

support routine dietary or weight-management counseling for adults without known hypertension, hyperlipidemia, cardiovascular disease, or diabetes (497,498,511). Relatively few interventions have been conducted that aim to introduce such counseling into the native environments of clinical practice, and even fewer have demonstrated efficacy of low-intensity interventions, such as brief counseling sessions with the primary care clinician (512). There are exceptions, however (513), with more attention thus far to physical activity than to diet (514–518).

But relative absence (paucity) of evidence is not evidence of absence, and the history of medicine is populated by actions that anticipated rather than followed evidence of effect. The tendency to act first and validate after is particularly justified in times of crisis, when inaction is, itself, a noteworthy hazard. Obesity is such a crisis and thus warrants action on the basis of informed judgment if scientific evidence falls somewhat short of current need.

There is suggestive evidence that physician counseling of overweight patients is supportive of weight loss and of the use of appropriate methods to achieve such weight loss (519). Overall, evidence in support of counseling is limited, largely because such counseling is limited (520); the only effective interventions appear to be those of medium- and high-intensity behavioral counseling (498).

Worth noting in societies such as the United States, which has both highly prevalent obesity and preoccupation with slimness, is a tendency for even normal-weight individuals to "diet." In addition, such injudicious practices as smoking may be used as a means to maintain body weight (521). The clinician should be equally prepared to discourage ill-advised weight control practices as to encourage salutary ones. There is some evidence that patients who discuss weight control with their healthcare providers are more apt to pursue weight loss and control by healthful and prudent means (519,522). Also noteworthy is increasing recognition of the need to reform clinical practice patterns on the basis of both available evidence and professional judgment. A regional plan for obesity control in the New England states, developed by the New England Coalition for Health Promotion (NECON) includes guidance for physician counseling based on such considerations (523).

Theories of behavior modification and their adaptation into the primary care setting for the promotion of healthful eating, physical activity, and weight control are addressed in Chapter 46. Several salient principles warrant particular emphasis. First, given the prevalence of obesity, counseling for weight control should be universal. Second, given the popularity of weight-loss approaches that diverge from well-established practice for health promotion, the principal focus of weight control efforts should, in fact, be health. As noted earlier in this chapter, the best available evidence links dietary and activity patterns conducive to health with long-term maintenance of weight. Third, given that obesity is epidemic in both adults and children, the unit to which counseling should be aimed is the family or household rather than the individual patient. Adult patients have a responsibility to engage their children in healthful lifestyle practices, and they will find lifestyle change easier and more sustainable for themselves when the effort involves household-wide solidarity. Finally, weight control efforts should be directed toward long-term sustainability rather than the fast start that seems perennially tantalizing to patients.

Technology for Lifestyle Intervention

Preliminary evidence suggests that interactive computer-based interventions for weight loss can be effective (524). A recent small randomized clinical trial examined the effects of adding mobile technology to usual care in lifestyle intervention for weight loss on 69 overweight or obese patients at an outpatient clinic. Individuals in the "+mobile" intervention group received personal digital assistants to self-monitor diet and exercise, as well as added phone coaching sessions; at the end of 12 months, the +mobile group sustained an increased average weight loss of 3.9 kg over the control group (525).

Pharmacotherapy

Noradrenergic agents and serotonergic agents have received Food and Drug Administration (FDA) approval for weight loss, principally by means of suppressing appetite (526,527). Selective serotonin reuptake inhibitors, such as fluoxetine, as well as compounds such as caffeine, ephedrine, and amphetamines are not FDA approved for weight loss but have been used for that purpose. Ephedrine was banned by the FDA after highly publicized reports of toxicity.

Fenfluoramine stimulates the release and inhibits the reuptake of serotonin, whereas phentermine stimulates the release of norepinephrine (526). Although both drugs were FDA approved for the treatment of obesity, the combination, "Fen-Phen," was never approved per se but was widely used until 1997, when an association with valvular heart disease was reported (528). The use of fenfluoramine, or dexfenfluoramine, is more convincingly associated with a risk of pulmonary hypertension when therapy continues beyond 3 months, although the occurrence is rare (526). The use, apparent toxicity, and withdrawal of Fen-Phen focused attention on the inappropriate use of pharmacotherapy to achieve cosmetic outcomes in mild obesity; under such circumstances, the potential toxicity of even fairly safe medication may well outweigh the benefits (529).

Phentermine has recently returned to the market in combination with topiramate. This combo drug was approved by the FDA in 2012 for the treatment of obesity. Topiramate, previously approved for treatment of convulsive disorders and migraines, has generated interest as an antiobesity drug ever since weight loss was noted as a common side effect (530). Early evidence from clinical trials suggest phentermine/topiramate to be effective at weight loss, as approximately 75% of subjects achieved 5% weight loss and nearly half lost 10% of their initial body weight (531,532). Of note, phentermine/topiramate is classified as pregnancy category X as it has teratogenic properties, limiting its utility in women of child-bearing age (533).

Also FDA approved as of 2012 is lorcaserin, a reuptake inhibitor of serotonin, dopamine, and norepinephrine. Evidence to date shows lorcaserin to cause mean body weight loss of approximately 5.8 kg compared to 2.2 kg from placebo (534,535). Side effects include headache, depression, anxiety, and suicidal thoughts. In 2013, lorcaserin was withdrawn from the European market out of concern for increased risk of cancer with long-term use (536).

Orlistat, FDA approved for obesity and available over-the-counter as of 2007 (537), works by inhibiting lipases in the gastrointestinal tract (538). In clinical trials, orlistat has been shown to induce clinically significant, modest weight loss (539) and improve glycemic control in diabetics (540,541). The drug must be taken in advance of meals containing fat and is limited by gastrointestinal side effects related to fat malabsorption.

Sibutramine, a reuptake inhibitor of both serotonin and norepinephrine, was FDA approved until 2010 for the treatment of obesity, but it was then withdrawn from the market due to concern over increased cardiovascular events and strokes. The limiting side effect associated with use of sibutramine is hypertension, mediated by the effects on norepinephrine levels. In randomized trials, sibutramine is clearly effective in facilitating modest weight loss up to 12 months, but weight is regained if the drug is discontinued, and data on long-term use are not available (542). Sibutramine facilitates weight loss by suppressing appetite (inducing satiety) and increasing energy expenditure by augmenting thermogenesis, and it appears to induce a preferential loss of visceral fat (543).

Rimonabant, an endocannabinoid receptor blocker (544–548), demonstrated great promise as a new drug for obesity as of the last edition of this textbook. The drug appears to attenuate a pathway fundamental to diverse addictions and tolerances and thus was hoped to offer benefit for behavior modification efforts addressing diet, tobacco, and other substances. Preliminary clinical trial data suggested a significant contribution to weight loss, along with amelioration of carbiometabolic risk indices (549–551). However, a large-scale, double-blind placebo-controlled trial of rimonabant in 18,695 patients across 42 countries was prematurely discontinued in 2010 because of serious concerns by health regulators of increased neuropsychiatric effects with rimonabant compared to placebo (232 [2.5%] vs. 120 [1.3%]) (552). Four people in the rimonabant group committed suicide, compared to one in the placebo group. The case of rimonabant highlights the need for caution in the development of pharmacotherapy for obesity; even an increased risk of 1% of a serious side effect could cause great morbidity given the millions of overweight and obese patients who might be candidates for such intervention.

A 2007 meta-analysis of placebo-controlled trials of obesity drugs found that sibutramine is associated with an average weight loss of 4.3 kg (9.55 lb; CI 3.6 to 4.7 kg) and orlistat with an average weight loss of 2.9 kg (6.44 lb; 2.5 to 3.2 kg) compared to placebo (553). A 2012 meta-analysis of 94 studies on orlistat, sibutramine, and/or rimonabant concluded that the latter two drugs, which have been withdrawn from the market due to concerns over side effects, were the most effective at weight loss; the authors concluded that promising future therapies might therefore involve physiologically similar drugs to sibutramine and rimonabant formulated to reduce serious side effects (554).

A number of drugs are in various stages of development and testing; reviews on the topic are available (546,555–562). Fixed-dose combination therapy with bupropion/naltrexone shows promise as a new weight-loss drug that can also ameliorate symptoms of depression (563). Liraglutide, a glucagon-like peptide-1 analogue of the hormone incretin is currently approved for treatment of diabetes, and owing to its known weight-loss effects in diabetic patients is currently under phase-III trials for treatment of obesity (564).

Advances in the understanding of the physiology of appetite and satiety, the hormones and cytokines that govern these pathways, and the pathophysiology of obesity, offer the promise of new pharmacologic approaches to its control. Growth hormone secretion is abnormally low in obesity, possibly due to leptin resistance (385). The administration of growth hormone improves body composition in obese subjects during energy restriction and weight loss; therefore, there is interest in the potential therapeutic use of either growth hormone or growth hormone-releasing peptides in the treatment of obesity (385). Other agents under current investigation include GLP-1 receptor agonists and pancreatic lipase inhibitors. β_3-adrenergic receptor agonists, corticotropin-releasing factor-binding protein ligand inhibitor, leptin receptor agonists, and neuropeptide Y receptor antagonists (561,565,566).

Pharmacotherapy is increasingly viewed as a potentially important adjunct to lifestyle interventions in the control of obesity (527,567). As weight generally is regained when pharmacologic agents are discontinued, the need for agents that are safe in the long term and/or robust behavioral interventions that can sustain the weight loss achieved with short-term medication use is clear. Clinicians should be prepared to consider long-term use of pharmacologic agents, as is commonly done with other conditions that are somewhat responsive to diet, such as hypertension and hyperlipidemia. Weight loss during pharmacotherapy should perhaps not be considered an indication for cessation of treatment, any more than the treatment of diabetes, hypertension, or hyperlipidemia to goal levels of glucose, blood pressure, or LDL indicate discontinuation of therapy. However, to apply the same standard in obesity treatment, the long-term safety of pharmacologic agents will need to be assessed. In the meantime, pharmacotherapy generally should be reserved for more severe obesity or obesity associated with metabolic, psychological, or functional complications, so pharmacotherapy is likely to be associated with greater net benefit than risk. The use of prescription pharmacotherapy for purely cosmetic weight control is, on the basis of currently available evidence, generally ill advised.

Despite enthusiasm in some quarters for the potential contributions of pharmacotherapy to weight management, there are reasons for caution and even reticence. The costs of obesity, noted previously, are an already ominous influence on total health-related expenditures in the United States; routine pharmacotherapy for weight management could potentially accelerate the rise of obesity-related costs to intolerable levels. In addition, obesity is a common problem at ever-younger ages; reliance on pharmacotherapy for weight control in children suggests obvious liabilities. Finally, weight gain is a normal, rather than aberrant, physiologic response to positive energy balance. Numerous, overlapping layers of metabolic defense against starvation likely render this mechanism highly resistant to pharmacotherapeutic manipulation. This has led some to conclude that polypharmacy may be required to facilitate weight control (568). The alternative view, to which I subscribe, is that drug treatment of obesity is likely to prove perennially disappointing (569).

Surgery

Bariatric surgery encompasses an array of procedures from banded gastroplasty to Roux-en-Y gastric bypass (570). The procedures induce weight loss by reducing the volume of food tolerated at any given time; inducing some degree of nutrient malabsorption; altering endocrine influences on appetite and satiety, such as ghrelin signaling from the stomach; or a combination of these (571). Generally, the more extensive procedures produce more dramatic weight loss by inducing malabsorption (572), but the effectiveness of banding procedures has been established (573,574). There is evidence to suggest that an intragastric balloon, approved in Europe and Canada but not yet in the United States, may be effective as a short-term treatment of obesity, although concerns linger about potential complications related to obstruction and pressure (575,576).

Overall, bariatric surgery is well established as the most effective treatment for severe (stage III) obesity (577,578). The effectiveness of the procedure, in conjunction with the rising prevalence of obesity in general and severe obesity in particular, has resulted in a rapid increase in the number of procedures performed annually; bariatric surgery is now one of the most common gastrointestinal surgeries performed, with an estimated 340,000 procedures performed globally in 2011 (579,580). The bariatric surgery experience and literature are increasingly encompassing adolescents (581,582) and children (583,584), along with ever-older adults (585–587).

Surgery generally is indicated only for the management of severe obesity, and then only if other therapies have been tried and have proved ineffective (588,589). A BMI greater than 40, previously referred to as "morbid" obesity and preferably referred to as stage III obesity, or "severe" obesity, should raise the consideration of surgical management. Patients with lesser degrees of obesity may be candidates for surgery if refractory to other interventions and experiencing morbidity or reduced quality of life due to the obesity (590–592). A recent widely publicized study found substantially increased weight loss and greater likelihood of type 2 diabetes remission following bariatric surgery compared with conventional medical therapy (593). However, as Ludwig, Ebbeling, and Livingston suggested in a thought provoking *JAMA* article in 2012, there are important study design considerations to address in interpreting the results of studies comparing surgical to nonsurgical interventions; given the morbidity and cost of bariatric surgery, more research is warranted to compare surgical interventions with equivalently intense nonsurgical treatment. Use of low-intensity outpatient diet and exercise prescriptions, they argue, which "have notoriously poor effectiveness," are a poor comparison with the multidisciplinary intensive program surrounding bariatric surgery. A better control arm might instead be a multicomponent lifestyle intervention involving residential

treatment for medically supervised rapid weight loss, prepared meals at home, meetings with a nutritionist and personal trainer, group classes, and more (594).

Bariatric procedures have evolved rapidly in recent years, particularly with the advent of laparoscopic approaches in the mid-1990s (570,590,595–599). The surgical options are generally placed into one of four categories: malabsorptive procedures, malabsorptive/restrictive procedures, restrictive procedures, and other, experimental procedures (597). The jejunoileal bypass is an example of a malabsorptive procedure, now rarely done, as is the duodenal switch; the Roux-en-Y gastric bypass is the prototypical malabsorptive/restrictive procedure and the prevailing technique overall; various approaches to gastric banding are restrictive techniques, including the now popular and relatively simple sleeve gastrectomy which has been used as a standalone restrictive procedure or as a first stage surgery to a more intensive bypass in severely obese patients (600). Transoral gastroplasty (601) and gastric pacing (570,597) exemplify currently experimental approaches. Clear illustrations of the various surgical techniques are provided by the American Academy of Family Physicians (423).

Weight loss of up to 33% has been maintained after gastric bypass surgery for up to 10 years, an outcome superior to nonsurgical approaches (602); loss of 50% or more of excess weight is commonly achieved within the first postoperative year, with up to 65% to 70% average excess weight loss maintained at 3 to 5 years (603). Meta-analyses to date have found weight loss greatest with diversionary procedures like jejunoileal bypass, intermediate with malabsorptive/restrictive procedures, and lowest with banding techniques; however, the less efficacious procedures have fewer adverse effects and morbidity (584,604).

Complications and mortality depend on the procedure performed. Surgical mortality in skilled hands generally is as low as 0.1% to 0.3% (591,602,605), usually related to pulmonary emboli and anastomoses leaks; postoperative complications were as high as 40% in 2001 (606), but recent increases in laparoscopic and banding techniques have reduced serious complication rates to approximately 5% (605).

Candidates for bariatric surgery require thorough preparation for the effects of such surgery on lifestyle and dietary pattern. The benefits of surgery are generally only well maintained in patients who receive supportive behavioral counseling (602). Postoperative challenges include nutrient deficiencies related to malabsorption, psychological adjustment, and alterations in dietary pattern required to accommodate restrictive effects of the procedure (607). These issues indicate the importance of close monitoring by an experienced and multidisciplinary medical team following any bariatric procedure (571,572,603,607,609). Bariatric surgery is generally deemed cost-effective for suitably selected patients (610).

Left gastric artery embolization, a minimally invasive procedure heretofore indicated primarily for gastrointestinal bleeding, has shown promising possibilities as a weight-loss procedure, though current evidence is limited to retrospective analysis (611) and case reports only. The theoretical mechanism is suppression of the appetite-inducing hormone ghrelin, usually supplied by the left gastric artery. Prospective clinical trials are warranted.

Lipectomy and liposuction are generally considered to be of cosmetic benefit only. These procedures do not reliably improve the metabolic complications of obesity, and they impose a non-trivial risk of complications (612–618).

Medically Supervised Diets

Low-calorie diets typically restrict energy intake to between 1,000 and 1,200 kcal per day. Such diets can be constructed to provide balanced nutrition or to be unbalanced in favor of a particular macronutrient class. Evidence of a benefit of unbalanced low-energy diets is, for the most part, lacking, and differences in weight loss are largely attributable to differences in diuresis (619). Evidence for emphasizing a particular macronutrient class is discussed elsewhere in this chapter. Generally, low-calorie diets pose a threat of micronutrient deficiency, and a multivitamin/ mineral supplement is appropriate. As a balanced, energy-restricted diet is compatible with both weight-control and health-promotion goals, such an approach to obesity is widely applicable.

Very-low-energy diets used in the 1970s provided inadequate protein and resulted in visceral protein losses. Cardiac protein mobilization was associated with dysrhythmia and sudden death (619). With attention to the quantity and quality of protein provided, very-low-energy diets can be

administered safely; such diets typically are referred to as "protein-sparing modified fasts" and provide approximately 600 kcal per day (619). Very-low-calorie diets (VLCDs) can be based on a narrow range of proteinaceous solid foods (i.e., lean meat, fish, poultry) or a commercial liquid formula. These diets are indicated only in the management of severe obesity and may be a final noninvasive effort prior to bariatric surgery (620,621).

There is limited evidence of the feasibility of managing VLCDs in primary care practice (622), and there is some evidence of their utility in reducing weight preoperatively in severely obese patients considered at high risk for elective surgery because of their obesity (623). Kansanen et al. (624) reported the effectiveness of VLCD in treating sleep apnea syndrome in a small group of obese adults followed for 3 months. Micronutrient supplementation and extensive behavioral support are required; therefore, such diets should be undertaken only when the requisite supervision and multidisciplinary support are established. Although very-low-energy diets induce substantial weight loss (e.g., 44 lb in 12 weeks), they are generally ineffective at maintaining such losses over the long term (619). Ryttig et al. (625) compared two 24-month weight-loss programs in obese university students, one commencing with a very-low-calorie induction diet and the other relying on a balanced, energy-restricted diet throughout. Although the initial weight loss was substantially greater in the VLCD group, weight loss at 2-year follow-up did not differ. A recent meta-analysis of the effects of various strategies for maintenance of weight loss following a VLCD or low-calorie diet found improved maintenance with antiobesity drugs, meal replacements, and high-protein diets, but no significant improvement with dietary supplements or exercise (626).

Meta-analysis suggests that VLCDs offer only short-term benefit over less severe calorie restriction; the use of liquid meal replacements as part of a strategy to reduce calories more moderately is suggested as a comparably effective, less cumbersome, and costly approach (627).

Commercial Weight-Loss Programs

Overall, there is limited evidence that any commercial weight-loss programs produce sustainable weight loss; a recent systematic review highlights the paucity of research on the topic (628). Only about half of those listed in the National Weight Control Registry report using a commercial weight loss program (629).

In a study of nearly 200 participants in a Sandoz weight-loss program, few had maintained initial weight loss at 3 years (630). Regular physical activity was the best predictor of sustained weight loss. Concerns have been expressed about the costs of commercial programs relative to the sustainable weight loss achieved (631).

Due in part to congressional investigation of the commercial weight-loss industry in the early 1990s, credible programs now generally provide information to prospective clients about results achieved. The industry is evolving as the understanding of obesity advances, and results from older programs may or may not pertain to newer ones. Wadden and Frey (632) reported promising results of a proprietary weight-loss program beginning with a VLCD at 5-year follow-up. A short-term study of a Weight Watchers program also produced favorable results, but with follow-up limited to 4 weeks (633). A study sponsored by Jenny Craig, Inc., suggests that the high relapse rate of commercial weight-loss programs may be an artifact of premature cessation of treatment (634).

Overall, the literature on outcomes in commercial weight-loss programs is sparse (635). A multibillion-dollar industry would doubtless be supporting the generation of publications were there good news to report. However, as programs adopt new methods, they may be contributory to efforts to achieve lasting changes in lifestyle that help control weight.

One promising new arena for medically supervised, commercial weight-loss programs includes those addressed at overweight and obese children and adolescents. Available evidence suggests that weight-loss camps and alternative schools may be highly effective at reducing BMI as well as improving measures of health and fitness (636). Further studies are needed to determine long-term effects.

At present, the clinician is well advised to consider such programs with an open-minded skepticism. Assessment should be based in part on whether the program provides knowledge or skills that will support lifelong efforts to control weight rather than the short-term management of the patient's diet. The limited evidence available offers some support for the Weight Watchers program specifically and self-monitoring in general (628,634,637–642).

RELATED TOPICS OF INTEREST

Nutrients, Nutriceuticals, and Functional Foods

There are, in general, few substantiated claims for micronutrients that can be consumed in conventional or megadoses to facilitate weight loss (643). In spite of this, use of supplements for weight loss is a popular practice (644–646). Clinicians are encouraged to inquire routinely about their patients' practices in this area. The well-publicized toxicity of ephedra (647,648) is a precautionary tale highlighting the potential dangers in reliance on nutriceuticals and botanicals for weight loss. The Federal Trade Commission generated a report highlighting deception in the advertisements for weight-loss products in 2002 (649). While caution and skepticism in this area are warranted, some promising leads in the literature deserve the practitioner's consideration. It may be useful to mentally categorize the plethora of weight-loss products by purported mechanism in order to better advise patients of potential hazards versus benefit.

Increase Energy Expenditure

This category includes the popular but dangerous ephedra alkaloids, as well as caffeine-containing foods and supplements. At safe doses, caffeine and catechins in foods like green tea (650) likely do support some degree of short-term weight loss; however, there is no evidence that they can help in the maintenance phase of weight loss. Caution is advised.

Modulate Carbohydrate Metabolism

Chromium is a cofactor in insulin metabolism, and its supplementation may lower insulin levels in insulin-resistant individuals (see Chapter 6). There is as yet no definitive evidence of a role for chromium in weight management per se, but an argument for supplementation in the insulin-resistant obese patient could be made on theoretical grounds. A recent Cochrane review suggests favorable effects of chromium on weight loss from a small number of trials (651); further research into the effects of chromium picolinate supplementation on insulin sensitization and weight management are thus needed and warrant close attention (652–655).

Increase Satiety

The popularity of natural plant extracts that appear to suppress appetite has skyrocketed in recent years. Examples include Hoodia gordonii (658), a plant chewed by indigenous peoples of the Kalahari Desert, and Garcinia cambogia, made from the tamarind fruit rind. While there is some research to suggest that these effects are plausible (656), the overwhelming evidence thus far does not support most of these plant extract diet supplements as either effective or safe (657). Thus, despite public and media interest (659), use of either of these or other such products for weight management would be premature at best. Studies of safety and efficacy are warranted.

Increase Fat Oxidation or Decrease Fat Synthesis

Conjugated linoleic acid, a family of isomers of an 18-carbon polyunsaturated fatty acid found in meat and dairy, has generated interest as a potential aid in weight loss. At present, despite some promising findings in animal studies, human evidence is at best mixed (659–663); several short-term studies have found reductions in body fat with CLA supplementation, with a theoretical mechanism involving adipocyte apoptosis or increased fat oxidation (664,665). Nevertheless, adverse health effects of this group of fats, including potentially deleterious effects on insulin sensitivity (666), cannot be excluded with confidence.

Block Fat Absorption

Olestra, or sucrose polyester, is a nonabsorbable fat substitute approved by the FDA in 1996 for use as a food additive in snack foods; it is discussed in detail in Chapter 42. To date, there is no convincing evidence that olestra in the food supply leads to sustainable weight loss or prevents weight gain. Its use for purposes of weight control can neither be encouraged nor discouraged with great enthusiasm on the basis of the available evidence (see Chapter 42). The product was not a commercial success; it has been banned in several countries, though remains available in a limited number of snack items in the United States as of this printing.

Calcium

There is a suggestion, now employed in marketing by the Dairy Council of America, that calcium from dairy sources may facilitate weight loss and, in particular, the preferential loss of adipose tissue. The research literature on this topic is far from definitive, with conflicting results to date (667–673). In general, studies sponsored by the dairy industry more commonly demonstrate positive outcomes. There is insufficient evidence to justify reliance on calcium supplementation or dairy to facilitate weight loss, but the inclusion of low- or nonfat dairy in the diet and calcium supplementation are supported by other considerations (see Chapters 8 and 14).

Resveratrol

A phytoestrogen most notably found in grape skins, resveratrol has garnered recent interest as a potent antioxidant. While human studies are lacking, recent promising murine studies point to resveratrol's ability to reduce body weight and hyperglycemia in obese and diabetic animals (674,675). One recent study (676) found that resveratrol supplementation in mice fed a high-fat, adipogenic diet actually induced downregulation of signaling cascades related to inflammation and adipogenesis.

Alcohol

Ethanol provides 7 kcal per g; therefore, it is more energy dense than either carbohydrate or protein and only slightly less so than fat. As a result of this energy density, ethanol consumption may contribute to obesity. There is some evidence that ethanol may increase REE while reducing fat oxidation (677). These effects may contribute preferentially to lipid storage. The role of alcohol in the diet is addressed more fully in Chapter 40.

Soda and Other Soft Drinks

The beverage industry has long disavowed any causal link between soda consumption and obesity. The bias in industry-sponsored research on this topic has recently been highlighted (678), and a systematic review suggests, as does common sense, that calories from soft drinks do, indeed, contribute meaningfully to the risk of weight gain (679). Globally, increasing soft drink consumption appears to correlate with increasing worldwide overweight and obesity (680). Pilot data suggest that reducing soft drink intake facilitates weight loss (681), especially in children and adolescents in whom sugar-sweetened beverages represent an increasing proportion of total calories consumed (682).

Of note, although increased caloric intake from soft drinks may contribute to weight gain, decreasing caloric intake via diet soda may not lead to weight loss. Multiple recent studies have found positive association between diet soda and weight gain for both adults and children (683).

Complementary and Alternative Medicine

In addition to the nutriceuticals described above, limited evidence suggests roles for hypnotherapy and acupuncture (684,685) in the management of obesity. A recent meta-analysis found acupuncture to be an effective treatment for modest weight loss compared to placebo or sham treatments, though more high-quality, long-term studies are needed (686).

Pregnancy

Women with normal weight generally should gain between 16 kg (25 to 35 lb) during pregnancy (687). Normal weight is defined as a BMI between 18.5 and 24.9. The basis of a minimum weight gain recommendation in pregnancy is to reduce the risk of low birth weight in the neonate (687). There is agreement that, in overweight women, weight gain during pregnancy should be of a lesser magnitude. In 2009, the IOM released new gestational weight gain guidelines for the first time in 20 years; the new recommendations suggest that women with a prepregnancy BMI in the overweight range, 25 to 29.9, should gain between 7 and 11.5 kg (15 to 25 lb) (688–691). While some have suggested that in obese women with a prepregnancy BMI of 30 and above no minimum weight gain is necessary (692), the new IOM guidelines recommend a total pregnancy weight gain of 5 to 9 kg (11 to 20 lb) (693). In the United States, each pregnancy is associated with the retention of as much as 5.5 lb; therefore, pregnancies contribute to the development of lifelong obesity in women (694). There is evidence that women who are able to follow the IOM guidelines on gestational weight gain may not incur that risk of long-term weight retention (695). The prevention of excessive pregnancy-related weight gain and its retention in the postpartum period are therefore important to efforts at controlling the rising prevalence of overweight/obesity in women (696).

Pregnant women who are obese have an increased incidence of gestational diabetes (691,697,698), preeclampsia (691,697–701), fetal macrosomia (691,702–706), induction of labor (691,707), primary cesarean (701,698–710), postpartum infection (709–712), and neural tube defects in offspring (713–715). Obesity in pregnancy may increase the risk of preeclampsia and pregnancy-induced hypertension (716,717). Available analyses suggest increased healthcare costs for women who are obese during pregnancy (718); in one small study comparing 89 overweight women with 54 normal-weight women, the cost at care during pregnancy was 3.2 times higher for the severely obese women (697). Hood and Dewan (719) found that hospital stay was longer for obese compared with nonobese women at delivery. Based on data from the 1988 National Maternal and Infant Health Survey, Cogswell et al. (702) reported the incidence of obesity in pregnancy as 17%; slightly lower estimates have been reported by others. Further studies are warranted to explore the effect of lifestyle interventions for overweight and obese pregnant women (720). The topic is more fully addressed in Chapter 27.

Breast-feeding

In addition to its multiple nutritional benefits, protracted breast-feeding may confer weight-related benefits on both mother and baby. Because of its metabolic demands, breast-feeding can reduce postpartum weight retention (721). And, there is evidence from multiple observational trials that protracted breast-feeding may provide some protection against the later development of obesity in the child (627). Unfortunately, prospective clinical trials utilizing interventions to increase exclusive breast-feeding duration have thus far failed to cause significant reductions in childhood obesity prevalence (722,723). The importance of breast-feeding and of establishing judicious dietary patterns early in life are discussed in Chapters 38 and 47.

Obesity Management in Children

Most weight-loss programs available for children are similar to adult treatment programs (110). Long-term weight loss is achieved more successfully in children than in adults (110,724,725). Recent analysis suggests that relatively small amounts of weight loss, or just slowed weight gain, may be all that is needed for overweight or obese children to return to normal weight-for-height growth curves over time (726). Evidence supports the inclusion of dietary change, behavior modification, parental involvement, and follow-up in a pediatric obesity program (727–729). Programs have emphasized both reduction in sedentary behaviors (730) and dietary modification (110). Childhood food preferences are greatly influenced by parents' food choices and eating habits (see Chapters 29 and 38); therefore, family-based approaches are encouraged (109). Recent evidence emphasizes the importance of parental role in childhood obesity; a randomized controlled trial of family-based or parent-only intervention found the parent-only intervention as effective as the family-based treatment of overweight children (731). Another recent study found a "halo effect" on the families of patients undergoing bariatric surgery; obese children were found to have lower BMI at 12 months after their parent had undergone the surgery, emphasizing the characterization of obesity as a familial disease (732). More evidence is needed to determine best approaches to home-based prevention (109,733,734). One small study of snacking in school-age children found that offering a combination of vegetables and cheese compared to either alone or potato chips led to 72% fewer calories consumed during an ad lib snacking session (735). A randomized controlled trial designed to reduce television, videotape, and videogame use among third- and fourth-grade children showed statistically significant decreases in BMI in the intervention group as compared with controls after the 6-month intervention (736). Novel school and camp residential experiences may offer comprehensive, multidisciplinary approaches that give children and adolescents structure and skills to support not only weight loss, but also increased fitness, emotional coping, and self-esteem (737). Experience with pharmacotherapy and surgery for obesity in children is rather limited, but may be appropriate in limited cases where comorbid medical conditions exist and benefits outweigh risks (738,739). Strategies for weight management in children are addressed in Chapter 47.

Summary of Recommended Management Strategies

Evidence that sustainable weight loss is enhanced by means other than caloric restriction is lacking. Whereas short-term weight loss is consistently achieved by any dietary approach to the restriction of choice and thereby calories, lasting weight control is not. Competing dietary claims imply that fundamental knowledge of dietary pattern and human health is lacking; an extensive literature belies this notion. The same dietary and lifestyle pattern conducive to health promotion is consistently associated with weight control. A bird's-eye view of the literature on diet and weight reveals a forest otherwise difficult to discern through the trees. Competing diet claims are diverting attention and resources from what is actually and urgently needed: a dedicated and concerted effort to make the basic dietary pattern known to support both health and weight control more accessible to all.

Against the backdrop of this increasingly acute need, the identification of practical and generalizable solutions to the obesity crisis has proved elusive. From research interventions, to commercial weight loss programs, to supplements, potions, and devices, innumerable approaches to weight loss have been devised. That none of these has yet met the need of the population is clearly reflected in the stubborn epidemiology of obesity.

Obesity is as relevant to prevailing views on beauty, fashion, and body image as it is to public health, and thus it engenders unique preoccupations (740–746). Individuals reluctant to take antihypertensive or lipid-lowering medication for fear of side effects may aggressively pursue pharmacotherapy, or even surgery, for weight control (747–749). The visibility of obesity, the stigma associated with it (750–752) (it is often said that antiobesity sentiment is the last bastion of socially acceptable prejudice), and the difficulty most people experience in their efforts to resist it contribute to its novel influences on attitude and behavior. This widespread state of volatile frustration renders the public susceptible to almost any persuasive sales pitch for a weight-loss lotion, potion, or program.

The natural consequence of acute and substantially unmet need is frustration. This public frustration has created a seemingly limitless market for weight-loss approaches. This same frustration has engendered a prevailing gullibility so that virtually any weight-loss claim is accepted at face value. Dual aphorisms might be considered for characterizing the obesity epidemic. Until recently, organized responses to this degenerating crisis have been tepid at best, suggesting that among public health professionals, familiarity breeds complacency, if not outright contempt. Among members of the general public, desperation breeds gullibility.

It is thus a seller's market for weight-loss wares. The litany of competing claims for effective weight loss is producing increasing confusion among both the public at large and health care professionals (753). In the mix is everything from science to snake oil, with no assurances that science is the more popular choice.

The concept of the "ideal" body weight and efforts to reach it may be both unrealistic and harmful for most overweight patients. The benefits of moderate weight loss are sufficiently clear to justify efforts to induce a loss of 5% to 10% of total weight, which is apt to be much more readily achievable. Perhaps better still is an emphasis on the means of achieving weight loss—namely changes in diet and activity pattern rather than weight per se, as the patient has control over the former but can only indirectly influence the latter. Most adult patients concerned about weight regulation will have made multiple attempts at weight control, with at best transient success. Above all, clinicians must not submit to "blame the victim" temptations in this setting.

Temporary weight loss is no more a definitive resolution of the metabolic factors that promote obesity than transient euglycemia is a resolution of diabetes. Therefore, diets designed for short-term weight loss offer no convincing benefit either in terms of sustained weight loss or health outcomes. Because dietary and lifestyle management of weight must be permanent, it is essential that the dietary patterns applied be compatible with recommendations for health promotion in general. Fad diets promoted for purposes of rapid weight loss are unsubstantiated in the peer-reviewed literature. Even if conducive to weight management over time, such diets would be ill advised unless shown to promote health and prevent disease. There is overwhelming consensus that a diet rich in complex carbohydrates, particularly whole grains, fruits, and vegetables, along with healthful oils and lean protein sources, is conducive to optimal health outcomes (see Chapter 45). So that patients are not offered a choice between health promotion and weight control, a health-promoting diet should be recommended for purposes of weight control. Such a diet is nutrient dense, fiber dense, and relatively energy dilute—all properties supportive of weight loss and maintenance.

Several general modifications of the overall dietary pattern are likely to facilitate weight control. Some benefit may derive from frequent, small meals or snacks rather than the conventional three meals a day. One study examining snacking habits in overweight women enrolled in a weight-loss study found that mid-morning snackers lost more weight than afternoon or evening snackers (754). Physiologically, there is some evidence that distributing the same number of calories in small snacks ("nibbling") rather than larger meals ("gorging") may reduce 24-hour insulin production, at least in insulin-resistant individuals (755) (see Chapter 6). Speechly et al. (756) reported evidence that snacking attenuates appetite relative to larger meals spaced farther apart. A group of seven obese men was provided an ad libitum lunch following a morning "preload" provided as a single meal or multiple snacks with the same total nutrient and energy composition. Subjects ate significantly (27%) less following multiple small meals than after a single larger one. Insulin peaked at higher levels following the single meal and was sustained above baseline for longer with the multiple small meals. Total area under the insulin curves was similar in both groups.

Evidence in support of "snacking" as a means of controlling weight or improving insulin metabolism is preliminary and not undisputed (757,758). However, there is generally a profound psychological component to disturbances of weight regulation, and the distribution of meals and calories may be germane. Most patients trying to control their weight are both tempted by and afraid of preferred foods. Consequently, many such patients resist eating for protracted periods during the day, only to overindulge in a late-day or evening binge. This pattern perpetuates a dysfunctional and tense relationship between the patient and his or her diet.

Patients caught up in this pattern should be advised to bring healthful and calorically dilute foods with them every day (see Chapter 47) and systematically to resist foods made available by others. Patients should be encouraged to eat whenever they want, but only those foods chosen in advance. By having free access to low-calorie foods (e.g., fresh fruits, fresh vegetables, nonfat dairy, dried fruit, whole grain breads or cereals), patients may overcome their fear of needing to "go hungry" for extended periods each day. In addition, frequent snacking during the day obviates the need and desire for a compulsive and binge-like meal at the end of the day. Finally, for many patients, the ideal time for exercise is after work. Overweight patients who have avoided food much of the day may simply be too hungry after work to exercise. A meal at such a time often is prepared impulsively and eaten not only to satisfy energy needs but also to assuage the pent-up frustrations of the day. On questioning, many overweight patients acknowledge that they often eat, and overeat, for reasons having nothing to do with hunger.

There are multiple benefits to physical activity after work and/or prior to the evening meal. Exercise is an effective means of moderating psychological stress (759) and may attenuate the need to resolve such stress with food. In addition, exercise may temporarily suppress appetite and generally enhances self-esteem, both of which are conducive to more thoughtful choices as the evening meal is prepared. Finally, and most evident, is the additional caloric expenditure resulting from the added activity. A meta-analysis of weight-loss studies published in 1997 reveals important limitations in the field of obesity management but suggests that best results to date have been achieved by combining energy-restricted diets with aerobic exercise (760).

In conjunction with redistribution of calories, several other specific recommendations may be made in the context of primary care encounters that may facilitate weight loss. Dietary fat restriction generally should be recommended, with sufficient detail provided to facilitate food choices (see Chapter 47). A recent systematic review of 33 randomized controlled trials and 10 cohort studies found consistent evidence that dietary fat restriction led to small but statistically significant and sustained weight loss (761). The best available evidence indicates that mean intake in the United States is currently 34% of calories (NHANES III). All other evidence aside, the caloric density of fat, not to mention the obvious link between calorie intake and weight control, justifies efforts to moderate dietary fat intake in all efforts at weight loss or maintenance.

Along with fat restriction, patients should be advised to liberalize or increase their intake of fruits and vegetables and whole grain products. In addition to being calorically dilute, these foods tend to be rich in fiber, which is noncaloric yet satiating, at least in the short term (see Chapter 1). Foods such as dried fruits, which are relatively dense in calories, are nonetheless useful in weight loss efforts due to the high fiber content and their capacity to induce satiety with limited intake.

Among the most successful strategies for changing the overall dietary pattern is the substitution of ingredients in otherwise familiar dishes. Familiarity is among the principal factors governing dietary preference, and resistance to changing the diet can be formidable. Attempts at reducing dietary fat intake in the Women's Health Trial were most successfully sustained when they relied on substituting lower-fat ingredients in recipes that preserved the appearance and taste of familiar foods (762). Although this advice can be offered in the primary care setting, patients will need detailed information on ingredient substitutions to implement such recommendations successfully. Referral to a dietitian and referral to appropriate literature are often both necessary (see Section III). Difficulty in treating obesity has led to increased emphasis on the importance of prevention. However, effective and practical methods of prevention have yet to be demonstrated.

The likely reason for this is that no single approach to weight control will be effective at the population level. Weight gain and epidemic obesity are the consequences of a perfect storm of obesigenic influences of our own devising, from fast food to suburban sprawl. Long denizens of a world characterized by a relative scarcity of calories and unavoidably arduous physical exertions, we (and our patients) are victims of our own success. Quite simply, our species has no native defenses against caloric excess or the lure of the couch—because we never needed them before.

So while simple to explain, epidemic obesity will be anything but easy to fix. We must overcome the propensity of our genes, the propulsive force of culture, and some 6 million years of gathering momentum.

Obesity prevention will require a comprehensive system of reforms addressing prevailing knowledge, behavior, policies, and the environment. We need nutrition education and physical education in schools. We need schools that provide nutrition meeting high standards and regular bouts of physical activity. We need physical activity breaks to be a standard part of the work day. Every neighborhood needs to provide recreational facilities and sidewalks, and new neighborhoods should be designed so that it makes sense to get around them by foot rather than car.

We need social engineering to give us back time to prepare food at home or ways to eat out that offer good nutrition at low cost.

We need to make use of stairs rather than elevators the social norm. We need to overhaul the food supply and eliminate the "junk" food category. We need to subsidize the sale of fresh fruits and vegetables. We need truth in advertising, marketing that emphasizes what matters for a healthy life, and controls on food marketing to children. We need to educate families about how to practice good nutrition and good physical activity together. It should once again be possible for children to walk and bike to school.

Clinicians will, in fact, not be *the* solution to the problem of epidemic obesity, as many components of a comprehensive weight-management campaign that would satisfy population needs fall outside the clinical purview. But clinicians have a vital role to play, as both educators and advocates. And given the magnitude and urgency of this crisis, to do otherwise is simply no longer acceptable. We have a choice of being part of the solution or, failing that, being part of a status quo that propagates the problem. As the IOM outlines in its recent report on obesity prevention, we need healthcare providers to adopt standards of practice for prevention, screening, diagnosis, and treatment of overweight and obesity; emphasize prepregnancy counseling on maintenance of a healthy weight before, during, and after pregnancy; and advocate publically for healthy communities that support healthy eating and active living (763).

In the weight-loss literature, interventions achieve caloric restriction by various means, ranging from direct provision of food (764), systems of incentive/disincentive (765), cognitive behavioral therapy (766), fat restriction (767), and the color-coding of food choices based on nutrient density (768). In general, those interventions achieving the most extreme degrees of caloric restriction also produce the greatest initial weight loss. However, a rebound weight gain is typically observed; in general, the more rapid the initial weight loss, the greater and more rapid the subsequent weight gain (769,770). This observation appears to be of generalizable significance, likely due to the fact that the extreme caloric restriction necessary for very rapid weight loss is intrinsically unsustainable. When the means used to achieve initial weight loss are unsustainable, weight regain is consistently observed.

The recent preoccupation with carbohydrate restriction appears to be reactionary to the antecedent era during which fat restriction was prioritized. The popular press and media reports suggest that the public feels misled by promises that fat restriction would lead to weight loss. In particular, the widely known USDA food guide pyramid has come under attack as a contributor to worsening obesity rates (392). The adulteration of messages in the pyramid under the influence of special interest groups is the subject of a recent book (395). The CDC has recently released data indicating that over the past several decades, weight has gone up as carbohydrate consumption has risen (352).

An impassive examination of these trends, and related scientific evidence, paints a rather different picture, however. Dietary guidelines have long emphasized consumption of specific low-fat foods, namely whole grains, vegetables, and fruits. In response to the public's interest in fat restriction, the food industry generated a vast array of low-fat but not necessarily low-calorie foods over the past two decades, prototypical of which is SnackWells cookies and other snacks. Upon close inspection, the CDC data reveal that total fat intake never meaningfully declined; rather, fat as a proportion of total calories was diluted somewhat by an increase in total calorie intake (351,771,772). The increase in calories was driven by increased consumption of calorie-dense, nutrient-dilute, fat-restricted foods, contemporaneous with a trend toward increasing portion sizes in general (316,353–356).

The competition between low-fat and low-carbohydrate diets for weight loss has in some ways polarized debate beyond the point of reason or utility. Lowering the fat content of processed foods while increasing consumption of simple sugars and starch is not consistent with the longstanding recommendations of nutrition authorities to moderate intake of dietary fat. Yet it is this distorted approach to dietary fat "restriction" that best characterizes secular trends in dietary intake at the population level and that subtends the contention that dietary fat is unrelated to obesity. An extensive literature belies this claim.

The theoretical basis for weight loss through dietary fat restriction is strong, given the widely acknowledged primacy of calories in weight governance and the energy density of fat (344).

Also noteworthy are data from the National Weight Control Registry, which indicate that lasting weight loss is consistently attributable to relatively fat-restricted, balanced diets in conjunction with regular physical activity (258). The weight-loss benefit of advice to follow fat-restricted diets is, however, no more enduring than that of advice to restrict calories by any other means (773).

Despite the extensive literature supporting dietary fat restriction for weight loss and control, there are dissenting voices (350). For the most part, dissent is predicated on the failure of dietary fat restriction to achieve population-level weight control in the United States and on the good health of Mediterranean populations with fat intake as high as 40% of calories (774). In addition, the evidence is clear that when energy restriction can be achieved on a diet relatively high in fat content, weight loss is achieved (424), suggesting the primacy of energy intake over macronutrient intake in weight regulation. The principal basis for recommending fat restriction, per se, for weight control is as a healthful means of facilitating reduced energy consumption. To the extent that fast food and highly processed junk foods are also high in fat—especially saturated and trans fats—switching to less processed whole foods naturally lower in these fats is both health promoting and conducive to weight loss. Thus, given the increasing appreciation for the healthful properties of unsaturated oils, however (see Chapters 2, 7, and 45), advice to restrict certain fats (e.g., saturated, trans) in conjunction with other strategies for moderating the energy density of the diet and total caloric intake is more fully concordant with the current state of evidence.

Similarly, advice to limit carbohydrate intake is of some utility if the restrictions are directed preferentially to added sugar and refined grains. Restriction of total carbohydrate intake may facilitate short-term weight loss by limiting dietary variety and choice but is at odds with an abundance of evidence regarding sustainable weight control and overall health (see Chapter 45), and it epitomizes "throwing out the baby with the bathwater." Casting dietary guidance in terms of food choices, rather than macronutrient categories, is clearly warranted to avoid propagating such blunders (775).

Recent trends in the United States suggest that fat intake over recent decades has held constant, not been reduced, and that intake of total calories has risen to dilute the percentage of food energy derived from fat; increased consumption of highly processed, fat-reduced foods is the principal basis for these trends (351). Thus, the failure of dietary fat restriction to facilitate weight control is more a problem of adherence than effectiveness (352). The Mediterranean diet differs from the typical American diet not only in the quantity of fat but also in the type of fat and the quantity of unrefined grains, vegetables, fruit, and lean protein sources (414). Further, many of the Mediterranean populations enjoying good health have traditionally high rates of physical activity compared to Western societies; the effects of physical inactivity and high dietary fat intake may be synergistic with regard to weight gain (419).

There is some evidence to suggest that dietary protein may preserve REE following weight loss (776). This, together with protein's high satiety index, suggests a benefit of protein intake at the high end of the range advisable for overall health as an aid to weight loss and control efforts (372,777).

Although it is clear that a balance between energy intake and energy expenditure is the principal determinant of weight maintenance in an individual, the factors responsible for the wide variations in the set point for that equilibrium are only partly understood. Genetic factors apparently play both direct (i.e., by influencing levels of leptin) and indirect (i.e., by influencing levels of thyroid hormone, the degree of postprandial thermogenesis, the mass of brown fat) roles in establishing the propensity for weight gain or loss in an individual. Environmental influences, such as the prevailing food supply and accessibility of opportunities for physical activity, are comparably important. The rising prevalence of obesity throughout the industrialized world makes clear that far from being a problem of impaired self-restraint in an individual, obesity may be seen as a public health threat mediated by a "toxic" nutritional environment. An appreciation for the public health importance of obesity, its complex pathogenesis, and principles of management are supportive of optimal interventions by clinicians.

CLINICAL HIGHLIGHTS

The majority of patients with weight control problems seen in primary care either will be overweight or have nonsevere obesity (BMI between 25 and 35). Evidence is lacking that pharmacotherapy is beneficial in this group. Clinicians should be prepared to consider long-term use of pharmacologic agents, as is commonly done with other diet-sensitive conditions, such as hypertension and hyperlipidemia, as an adjunct to lifestyle in the management of obesity. Such decisions should be reached in consideration of the degree and duration of obesity, its refractoriness to lifestyle interventions, its physical and/or psychological sequelae, and the risk-to-benefit ratio of pharmacotherapy, to the extent it can be determined. The use of pharmacotherapy for minimal overweight without sequelae is generally not indicated.

There is no evidence that commercial weight-loss programs are successful in the long term, but such programs are modifying their methods over time and may yet prove to be of value. Although the results of dietary counseling are often disappointing, there is suggestive evidence that physician counseling and multidisciplinary behavioral intervention can be an important factor both in achieving weight loss and in encouraging patients to apply safe and appropriate methods. It is noteworthy that obesity may be the single most common condition encountered in primary care, yet it is often not addressed by primary care providers. There is convincing evidence that severe obesity can be managed effectively in the short term with low- and very-low-calorie liquid diets; evidence is little more than suggestive that such benefits can be sustained in the absence of intensive behavioral intervention. Evidence is decisive that surgery is beneficial in carefully selected patients with severe obesity (less than 2% to 3% of the total population of overweight individuals), but intensive behavioral intervention is required to sustain the weight loss achieved, and novel residential programs may be effective as an alternative to surgery for obese children and adolescents.

The evidence favoring fat as well as total energy restriction to achieve and maintain weight loss is convincing, if not definitive. There is limited evidence that, within the context of a fat- and energy-restricted diet, relatively more protein and relatively less carbohydrate may result in lower fasting insulin levels. However, weight loss consistently lowers insulin as well. Further, studies have generally varied carbohydrate and protein content within close proximity to the recommended levels of intake. Thus, there is no meaningful evidence that extreme alterations of the basic mixed, balanced health-promoting diet (see Chapter 45) are indicated to achieve or maintain weight loss. On the contrary, weight loss is promoted by a diet consistent with recommendations for health promotion. Such recommendations include portion control to restrict energy intake; restriction of fat intake to reduce the energy density of the diet; abundant intake of vegetables, fruits, and whole grains; avoidance of sugar-sweetened beverages; and consistent physical activity (see Chapter 45). The advisable dietary pattern is rich in complex carbohydrates, but liberal intake of protein is reasonable and may be advantageous, provided that the protein is from mostly plant-based sources (e.g., beans, legumes, fish, poultry, egg white) and those low in saturated fat. The application of such a diet permits weight loss and the promotion of health to be addressed conjointly; alternative weight-loss diets, whether or not they facilitate short-term weight loss, are not consistent with the long-term dietary pattern advised for health maintenance and the prevention of disease. Physical activity is among the best predictors of long-term weight maintenance. Given the many impediments to long-term compliance with such guidelines (see Chapters 44 to 47), the ultimate control of epidemic obesity almost certainly will require environmental changes that facilitate consistent physical activity and consumption of a nutrient-dense but relatively energy-dilute diet. In the interim, the clinician can and should make a meaningful contribution to any given patient's capacity to resist and defy the obesigenic influences in his or her life. The clinical focus should consistently be placed on the family/household rather than just the individual; on health rather than just weight; and on long-term sustainability. Practical approaches to efficient counseling so these topics may routinely be addressed in the primary care setting are explored in Chapter 47.

■ REFERENCES

1. Flegal KM, Carroll MD, Kit BK, et al. Prevalence of obesity and trends in the distribution of body mass index among US adults, 1999–2010. *JAMA* 2012;307(5):491–497.
2. Ogden CL, Carroll MD, Kit BK, et al. Prevalence of obesity and trends in body mass index among us children and adolescents, 1999–2010. *JAMA* 2012;307(5):483–490.
3. The Associated Press. *Experts at International Congress on Obesity warn of deadly global pandemic.* September 03, 2006. Available at http://www.usatoday.com/news/health/2006-09-03-obesity-conference_x.htm; accessed 9/21/07.

4. U.S. Preventive Services Task Force. *Behavioral counseling interventions to promote a healthful diet and physical activity for cardiovascular disease prevention in adults: U.S. Preventive Services Task Force Recommendation Statement.* AHRQ Publication No. 11-05149-EF-2. June 2012. http://www.uspreventiveservicestaskforce.org/uspstf11/physactivity/physrs.htm

5. Institute of Medicine. *Accelerating progress in obesity prevention: solving the weight of the nation.* Available at: http://iom.edu/Reports/2012/Accelerating-Progress-in-Obesity-Prevention.aspx; accessed 5/15/2012.

6. Nestle M, Jacobson MF. Halting the obesity epidemic: a public health policy approach. *Public Health Rep* 2000;115:12–24.

7. Novak NL, Brownell KD. Obesity: a public health approach. *Psychiatr Clin of North Am* 2011;34(4):895–909.

8. Doll S, Paccaud F, Bovet P, et al. Body mass index, abdominal adiposity and blood pressure: consistency of their association across developing and developed countries. *Int J Obes Relat Metab Disord* 2002;26:48–57.

9. Dalton M, Cameron AJ, Zimmet PZ, et al. Waist circumference, waist–hip ratio and body mass index and their correlation with cardiovascular disease risk factors in Australian adults. *J Intern Med* 2003;254:555–563.

10. Balkau B, Sapinho D, Petrella A, et al. Prescreening tools for diabetes and obesity-associated dyslipidaemia: comparing BMI, waist and waist hip ratio. The D.E.S.I.R. Study. *Eur J Clin Nutr* 2006;60:295–304.

11. Korner A, Gelbrich G, Muller G, et al. Critical evaluation of methods for determination of body fat content in children: back to basic parameters? *Horm Metab Res* 2007;39:31–40.

12. Kontogianni MD, Panagiotakos DB, Skopouli FN. Does body mass index reflect adequately the body fat content in perimenopausal women? *Maturitas* 2005;51:307–313.

13. Turconi G, Guarcello M, Maccarini L, et al. BMI values and other anthropometric and functional measurements as predictors of obesity in a selected group of adolescents. *Eur J Nutr* 2006;45:136–143.

14. Centers for Disease Control and Prevention. *Defining overweight and obesity.* Available at http://www.cdc.gov/nccdphp/dnpa/obesity/defining.htm; accessed 3/18/07.

15. Mokdad AH, Ford ES, Bowman BA, et al. Prevalence of obesity, diabetes, and obesity-related health risk factors, 2001. *JAMA* 2003;289:76–79.

16. Ikeda J, Hayes D, Satter E, et al. A commentary on the new obesity guidelines from NIH. *J Am Diet Assoc* 1999;99:918–919.

17. Weinsier R. Clinical assessment of obese patients. In: Fairburn CG, Brownell KD, eds. *Eating disorders and obesity. A comprehensive handbook.* New York, NY: Guilford, 1995:463–468.

18. Franz MJ. Managing obesity in patients with comorbidities. *J Am Diet Assoc* 1998;98:s39–s43.

19. Guh DP, Zhang W, Bansback N, et al. The incidence of comorbidities related to obesity and overweight: a systematic review and meta-analysis. *BMC Public Health* 2009;9:88.

20. Centers for Disease Control and prevention. *Basics about childhood obesity.* http://www.cdc.gov/obesity/childhood/basics.html

21. World Health Organization. *Waist circumference and waist–hip ratio.* Report of a WHO Expert Consultation, Geneva.

8–11 December 2008 http://whqlibdoc.who.int/publications/2011/9789241501491_eng.pdf.

22. Astrup A. Physical activity and weight gain and fat distribution changes with menopause: current evidence and research issues. *Med Sci Sports Exerc* 1999;31(11 suppl):s564–s567.

23. Polotsky HN, Polotsky AJ. Metabolic implications of menopause. *Semin Reprod Med* 2010;28(5):426–434.

24. Ostchega Y, Hughes JP, Terry A, et al. Abdominal obesity, body mass index, and hypertension in US adults: NHANES 2007–2010. *Am J Hypertens* 2012;25(12):1271–1278.

25. Reaven G, Lithell H, Landsberg L. Hypertension and associated metabolic abnormalities—the role of insulin resistance and the sympathoadrenal system. *N Engl J Med* 1996;334:374–381.

26. Alvarez GE, Beske SD, Ballard TP, et al. Sympathetic neural activation in visceral obesity. *Circulation* 2002:106;2533–2536.

27. Egan B. Neurohumoral, hemodynamic and microvascular changes as mechanisms of insulin resistance in hypertension: a provocative but partial picture. *Int J Obes* 1991;15(suppl 2):133–139.

28. Smith MM, Minson CT. Obesity and adipokines: effects on sympathetic overactivity. *J Physiol* 2012;590(pt 8):1787–1801.

29. Lambert GW, Straznicky NE, Lambert EA, et al. Sympathetic nervous activation in obesity and the metabolic syndrome—causes, consequences and therapeutic implications. *Pharmacol Ther* 2010;126(2):159–172.

30. Grassi G. Sympathetic overdrive and cardiovascular risk in the metabolic syndrome. *Hypertens Res* 2006;29(11):839–847.

31. Després JP. Cardiovascular disease under the influence of excess visceral fat. *Crit Pathw Cardiol* 2007;6:51–59.

32. Pi-Sunyer F. Obesity. In: Shils M, Olson J, Shike M, eds. *Modern nutrition in health and disease*, 8th ed. Philadelphia, PA: Lea & Febiger, 1994.

33. Bray G. Obesity. In: EE Ziegler LF, ed. *Present knowledge in nutrition*, 7th ed. Washington, DC: ILSI Press, 1996.

34. Lee SY, Gallagher D. Assessment methods in human body composition. *Curr Opin Clin Nutr Metab Care* 2008;11(5):566–572.

35. Mascie-Taylor CG, Karim E. The burden of chronic disease. *Science* 2003;302:1921–1922.

36. Tillotson JE. Pandemic obesity: what is the solution? *Nutr Today* 2004;39:6–9.

37. Jeffery RW, Utter J. The changing environment and population obesity in the United States. *Obes Res* 2003;11:12s–22s.

38. Sturm R, Hattori A. Morbid obesity rates continue to rise rapidly in the United States. *Int J Obes* 2013;37(6):889–891.

39. Ogden CL, Carroll MD, Flegal KM. Epidemiologic trends in overweight and obesity. *Endocrinol Metab Clin North Am* 2003;32:741–760.

40. Kim J, Peterson KE, Scanlon KS, et al. Trends in overweight from 1980 through 2001 among preschool-aged children enrolled in a health maintenance organization. *Obesity* (Silver Spring) 2006;14:1107–1112.

41. de Onis M, Blössner M, Borghi E. Global prevalence and trends of overweight and obesity among preschool children. *Am J Clin Nutr* 2010;92(5):1257–1264.

42. Li C, Ford ES, Mokdad AH, et al. Recent trends in waist circumference and waist-height ratio among US children and adolescents. *Pediatrics* 2006;118(5):e1390–e1398.

43. Chopra M, Galbraith S, Darnton-Hill I. A global response to a global problem: the epidemic of overnutrition. *Bull World Health Organ* 2002;80:952–958.

44. Damcott CM, Sack P, Shuldiner AR. The genetics of obesity. *Endocrinol Metab Clin North Am* 2003;32:761–786.

45. Katz DL. Pandemic obesity and the contagion of nutritional nonsense. *Public Health Rev* 2003;31:33–44.

46. World Health Organization. *Obesity and overweight fact sheet*. http://www.who.int/mediacentre/factsheets/fs311/en/index.html.

47. Drewnowski A. Nutrition transition and global dietary trends. *Nutrition* 2000;16:486–487.

48. Silventoinen K, Sans S, Tolonen H, et al. WHO MONICA Project. Trends in obesity and energy supply in the WHO MONICA Project. *Int J Obes Relat Metab Disord* 2004;28:710–718.

49. Misra A, Vikram NK. Insulin resistance syndrome (metabolic syndrome) and obesity in Asian Indians: evidence and implications. *Nutrition* 2004;20:482–491.

50. Jahns L, Baturin A, Popkin BM. Obesity, diet, and poverty: trends in the Russian transition to market economy. *Eur J Clin Nutr* 2003;57:1295–1302.

51. http://www.linkedin.com/today/post/article/2013031515 2612-23027997-qatar-s-cultural-crisis-wealth-health-wisdom-and-opportunity?trk=mp-author-card.

52. Lands W, Hamazaki T, Yamazaki K, et al. Changing dietary patterns. *Am J Clin Nutr* 1990;51:991–993.

53. Drewnowski A, Popkin BM. The nutrition transition: new trends in the global diet. *Nutr Rev* 1997;55:31–43.

54. Thompson D, Wolf AM. The medical-care cost burden of obesity. *Obes Rev* 2001;2:189–197.

55. Thompson D, Edelsberg J, Colditz GA, et al. Lifetime health and economic consequences of obesity. *Arch Intern Med* 1999;159:2177–2183.

56. Hammond RA, Levine R. The economic impact of obesity in the United States. *Diabetes Metab Syndr Obes* 2010;3:285–295.

57. Finkelstein EA, Ruhm CJ, Kosa KM. Economic causes and consequences of obesity. *Annu Rev Public Health* 2005;26(1):239–257.

58. Finkelstein EA, Trogdon JG, Brown DS, et al. The lifetime medical cost burden of overweight and obesity: implications for obesity prevention. *Obesity* (Silver Spring) 2008;16(8):1843–1848.

59. Shamseddeen H, Getty JZ, Hamdallah IN, et al. Epidemiology and economic impact of obesity and type 2 diabetes. *Surg Clin North Am* 2011;91(6):1163–1172,vii.

60. Trasande L, Elbel B. The economic burden placed on healthcare systems by childhood obesity. *Expert Rev Pharmacoecon Outcomes Res* 2012;12(1):39–45.

61. Wang Y, Beydoun MA, Liang L, et al. Will all Americans become overweight or obese? Estimating the progression and cost of the US obesity epidemic. *Obesity* 2008;16(10):2323–2330.

62. Withrow D, Alter DA. The economic burden of obesity worldwide: a systematic review of the direct costs of obesity. *Obes Rev* 2011;12(2):131–141.

63. Aye T, Levitsky LL. Type 2 diabetes: an epidemic disease in childhood. *Curr Opin Pediatr* 2003;15:411–415.

64. National Cholesterol Education Program (NCEP) Expert Panel. Third report of the National Cholesterol Education Program (NCEP) Expert Panel on Detection, evaluation, and treatment of high blood cholesterol in adults (Adult Treatment Panel III) final report. *Circulation* 2002;106:3143–3421.

65. Imperatore G, Boyle JP, Thompson TJ, et al. Projections of type 1 and type 2 diabetes burden in the U.S. population aged <20 years through 2050 dynamic modeling of incidence, mortality, and population growth. *Dia Care* 2012;35(12):2515–2520.

66. Dabelea D, Bell RA, D'Agostino RB Jr, et al. Incidence of diabetes in youth in the United States. *JAMA* 2007;297(24):2716–2724.

67. Lis C, Ford ES, Mokdad AH, et al. Recent trends in waist circumference and waist-height ratio among US children and adolescents. *Pediatrics* 2006;118:1390–1398.

68. Bloom B, Cohen RA, Vickerie JL, et al. Summary health statistics for US children: National Health Interview Survey, 2001. *Vital Health Stat* 10(216). Available at http://www.cdc.gov/nchs/data/series/sr_10/sr10_216.pdf; accessed 1/07.

69. Olshansky SJ, Passaro DJ, Hershow RC et al. A potential decline in life expectancy in the United States in the 21st Century. *NEJM* 2005;352:1138–1145.

70. Calle EE, Thun MJ. Obesity and cancer. *Oncogene* 2004;23:6365–6378.

71. Rames LK, Clarke WR, Connor WE, et al. Normal blood pressure and the evaluation of sustained blood pressure elevation in childhood: the Muscatine study. *Pediatrics* 1978;61:245–251.

72. Figueroa-Colon R, Franklin FA, Lee JY, et al. Prevalence of obesity with increased blood pressure in elementary school-aged children. *South Med J* 1997;90:806–813.

73. Urrutia-Rojas X, Egbuchunam CU, Bae S, et al. High blood pressure in school children: prevalence and risk factors. *BMC Pediatr* 2006;6:32.

74. Sorof J, Daniels S. Obesity hypertension in children: a problem of epidemic proportions. *Hypertension* 2002;40(4):441–447.

75. Falkner B, Michel S. Obesity and other risk factors in children. *Ethn Dis* 1999;9:284–289.

76. Friedland O, Nemet D, Gorodnitsky N, et al. Obesity and lipid profiles in children and adolescents. *J Pediatr Endocrinol Metab* 2002;15(7):1011–1016.

77. Richards GE, Cavallo A, Meyer WJ, et al. Obesity, acanthosis nigricans, insulin resistance, and hyperandrogenemia: pediatric perspective and natural history. *J Pediatr* 1985;107:893–897.

78. Viner RM, Segal TY, Lichtarowicz-Krynska E, et al. Prevalence of the insulin resistance syndrome in obesity. *Arch Dis Child* 2005;90(1):10–14.

79. Friesen CA, Roberts CC. Cholelithiasis. Clinical characteristics in children. Case analysis and literature review. *Clin Pediatr* (Phila) 1989;28:294–298.

80. Holcomb GW Jr, O'Neill JA Jr, Holcomb GW. Cholecystitis, cholelithiasis and common duct stenosis in children and adolescents. *Ann Surg* 1980;191:626–635.

81. Kaechele V, Wabitsch M, Thiere D, et al. Prevalence of gallbladder stone disease in obese children and adolescents: influence of the degree of obesity, sex, and pubertal development. *J Pediatr Gastroenterol Nutr* 2006;42(1):66–70.

82. Kinugasa A, Tsunamoto K, Furukawa N, et al. Fatty liver and its fibrous changes found in simple obesity of children. *J Pediatr Gastroenterol Nutr* 1984;3:408–414.

83. Tominaga K, Kurata JH, Chen YK, et al. Prevalence of fatty liver in Japanese children and relationship to obesity. An epidemiological ultrasonographic survey. *Dig Dis Sci* 1995;40:2002–2009.

84. Tazawa Y, Noguchi H, Nishinomiya F, et al. Serum alanine aminotransferase activity in obese children. *Acta Paediatr* 1997;86:238–241.

85. Schwimmer JB, Deutsch R, Kahen T, et al. Prevalence of fatty liver in children and adolescents. *Pediatrics* 2006;118(4):1388–1393.

86. Silvestri JM, Weese-Mayer DE, Bass MT, et al. Polysomnography in obese children with a history of sleep-associated breathing disorders. *Pediatr Pulmonol* 1993;16:124–129.

87. Marcus CL, Curtis S, Koerner CB, et al. Evaluation of pulmonary function and polysomnography in obese children and adolescents. *Pediatr Pulmonol* 1996;21:176–183.

88. Mallory GB Jr, Fiser DH, Jackson R. Sleep-associated breathing disorders in morbidly obese children and adolescents. *J Pediatr* 1989;115:892–897.

89. Arens R, Muzumdar H. Childhood obesity and obstructive sleep apnea syndrome. *J Appl Physiol* 2010;108(2):436–444.

90. Tauman R, Gozal D. Obesity and obstructive sleep apnea in children. *Paediatr Respir Rev* 2006;7(4):247–259.

91. Kelsey JL. The incidence and distribution of slipped capital femoral epiphysis in Connecticut. *J Chronic Dis* 1971;23:567–578.

92. Kelsey JL, Acheson RM, Keggi KJ. The body build of patients with slipped capital femoral epiphysis. *Am J Dis Child* 1972;124:276–281.

93. Loder RT, Aronson DD, Greenfield ML. The epidemiology of bilateral slipped capital femoral epiphysis. A study of children in Michigan. *J Bone Joint Surg Am* 1993;75:1141–1147.

94. Wilcox PG, Weiner DS, Leighley B. Maturation factors in slipped capital femoral epiphysis. *J Pediatr Orthop* 1988;8:196–200.

95. Manoff EM, Banffy MB, Winell JJ. Relationship between body mass index and slipped capital femoral epiphysis. *J Pediatr Orthop* 2005;25(6):744–746.

96. Scott IU, Siatkowski RM, Eneyni M, et al. Idiopathic intracranial hypertension in children and adolescents. *Am J Ophthalmol* 1997;124:253–255.

97. Durcan FJ, Corbett JJ, Wall M. The incidence of pseudotumor cerebri. Population studies in Iowa and Louisiana. *Arch Neurol* 1988;45:875–877.

98. Corbett JJ, Savino PJ, Thompson HS, et al. Visual loss in pseudotumor cerebri. Follow-up of 57 patients from five to 41 years and a profile of 14 patients with permanent severe visual loss. *Arch Neurol* 1982;39:461–474.

99. Sugerman HJ, DeMaria EJ, Felton WL 3rd, et al. Increased intra-abdominal pressure and cardiac filling pressures in obesity-associated pseudotumor cerebri. *Neurology* 1997;49:507–511.

100. Balcer LJ, Liu GT, Forman S, et al. Idiopathic intracranial hypertension: relation of age and obesity in children. *Neurology* 1999;52(4):870–870.

101. Kesler A, Fattal-Valevski A. Idiopathic intracranial hypertension in the pediatric population. *J Child Neurol* 2002;17(10):745–748.

102. Willett WC, Manson JE, Stampfer MJ, et al. Weight, weight change, and coronary heart disease in women. Risk within the 'normal' weight range (see comments). *JAMA* 1995;273:461–465.

103. Dietz WH. Childhood weight affects adult morbidity and mortality. *J Nutr* 1998;128:411s–414s.

104. Srinivasan SR, Bao W, Wattigney WA, et al. Adolescent overweight is associated with adult overweight and related multiple cardiovascular risk factors: the Bogalusa Heart Study. *Metabolism* 1996;45:235–240.

105. Lauer RM, Clarke WR. Childhood risk factors for high adult blood pressure: the Muscatine Study. *Pediatrics* 1989;84:633–641.

106. Mossberg HO. 40-year follow-up of overweight children. *Lancet* 1989;2:491–493.

107. Morrison JA, Glueck CJ, Horn PS, et al. Childhood predictors of adult type 2 diabetes at 9- and 26-year follow-ups. *Arch Pediatr Adolesc Med* 2010;164(1):53–60.

108. Must A, Jacques P, Dallal G, et al. Long-term morbidity and mortality of overweight adolescents. *N Engl J Med* 1992;327:1350–1355.

109. Strauss R. Childhood obesity. *Curr Probl Pediatr* 1999;29:1–29.

110. Schonfeld-Warden N, Warden CH. Pediatric obesity. An overview of etiology and treatment. *Pediatr Clin North Am* 1997;44:339–361.

111. Lissner L, Odell P, D'Agostino R, et al. Variability of body weight and health outcomes in the Framingham population. *N Engl J Med* 1991;324:1839–1844.

112. Reilly JJ, Kelly J. Long-term impact of overweight and obesity in childhood and adolescence on morbidity and premature mortality in adulthood: systematic review. *Int J Obes* (Lond). 2011;35(7):891–898.

113. Burt Solorzano CM, McCartney CR. Obesity and the pubertal transition in girls and boys. *Reproduction* 2010;140(3):399–410.

114. Brownell K. Effects of weight cycling on metabolism, health, and psychological factors. In: Fairburn CG, Brownell KD, eds. *Eating disorders and obesity. A comprehensive handbook*. New York, NY: Guilford, 1995:56–60.

115. Rzehak P, Meisinger C, Woelke G, et al. Weight change, weight cycling and mortality in the ERFORT Male Cohort Study. *Eur J Epidemiol* 2007;22(10):665–673.

116. Taing KY, Ardern CI, Kuk JL. Effect of the timing of weight cycling during adulthood on mortality risk in overweight and obese postmenopausal women. *Obesity* (Silver Spring). 2012;20(2):407–4133.

117. Iribarren C, Sharp D, Burchfiel C, et al. Association of weight loss and weight fluctuation with mortality among Japanese American men. *N Engl J Med* 1995;333:686–692.

118. Stevens VL, Jacobs EJ, Sun J, et al. Weight cycling and mortality in a large prospective US study. *Am J Epidemiol* 2012;175(8):785–792.

119. Field AE, Malspeis S, Willett WC. Weight cycling and mortality among middle-aged or older women. *Arch Intern Med* 2009;169(9):881–886.

120. Wing R, Jeffery R, Hellerstedt W. A prospective study of effects of weight cycling on cardiovascular risk factors. *Arch Intern Med* 1995;155:1416–1422.

121. Graci S, Izzo G, Savino S, et al. Weight cycling and cardiovascular risk factors in obesity. *Int J Obes Relat Metab Disord* 2004;28(1):65–71.

122. National task force on the prevention and treatment of obesity. Weight cycling. *JAMA* 1994;272:1196–1202.

123. Jeffery RW. Does weight cycling present a health risk? *Am J Clin Nutr* 1996;63:452s–455s.

124. Stunkard A, Sobal J. Psychosocial consequences of obesity. In: Fairburn CG, Brownell KD, eds. *Eating disorders and obesity: a comprehensive handbook.* New York, NY: Guilford, 1995:417–421.

125. Schwartz MB, Brownell KD. Obesity and body image. *Body Image.* 2004;1(1):43–56.

126. Strauss RS. Childhood obesity and self-esteem. *Pediatrics* 2000;105(1):e15.

127. Petroni ML, Villanova N, Avagnina S, et al. Psychological distress in morbid obesity in relation to weight history. *Obes Surg* 2007;17(3):391–399.

128. Marchesini G, Cuzzolaro M, Mannucci E, et al. Weight cycling in treatment-seeking obese persons: data from the QUOVADIS study. *Int J Obes Relat Metab Disord* 2004;28(11):1456–1462.

129. Gortmaker SL, Must A, Perrin JM, et al. Social and economic consequences of overweight in adolescence and young adulthood. *N Engl J Med* 1993;329:1008–1012.

130. Puhl RM, Heuer CA. The stigma of obesity: a review and update. *Obesity* 2009;17(5):941–964.

131. Hill J, Melanson E. Overview of the determinants of overweight and obesity: current evidence and research issues. *Med Sci Sports Exerc* 1999;31:S515–S521.

132. McClure AC, Tanski SE, Kingsbury J, et al. Characteristics associated with low self-esteem among US adolescents. *Acad Pediatr* 2010;10(4):238–244.e2.

133. Griffiths LJ, Wolke D, Page AS, et al. Obesity and bullying: different effects for boys and girls. *Arch Dis Child* 2006;91(2):121–125.

134. Janssen I, Craig WM, Boyce WF, et al. Associations between overweight and obesity with bullying behaviors in school-aged children. *Pediatrics* 2004;113(5):1187–1194.

135. Thompson JW, Card-Higginson P. Arkansas' experience: statewide surveillance and parental information on the child obesity epidemic. *Pediatrics* 2009;124(suppl 1):S73–S82.

136. Nihiser AJ, Lee SM, Wechsler H, et al. BMI measurement in schools. *Pediatrics.* 2009;124(suppl 1):S89–S97.

137. Maddi S, Khoshaba D, Persico M, et al. Psychosocial correlates of psychopathology in a national sample of the morbidly obese. *Obes Surg* 1997;7:397–404.

138. Tsai AG, Williamson DF, Glick HA. Direct medical cost of overweight and obesity in the USA: a quantitative systematic review. *Obes Rev* 2011;12(1):50–61.

139. Thorpe KE, Howard DH. The rise in spending among medicare beneficiaries: the role of chronic disease prevalence and changes in treatment intensity. *Health Aff* (Millwood). 2006;25:378–388.

140. Lightwood J, Bibbins-Domingo K, Coxson P, et al. Forecasting the future economic burden of current adolescent overweight: an estimate of the coronary heart disease policy model. *Am J Public Health* 2009;99(12):2230–2237.

141. Costello D. The price of obesity; beyond the health risks, the personal financial costs are steep, recent studies show. *Los Angeles Times* August 1, 2005.

142. Zagorsky JL. Health and wealth. The late-20th century obesity epidemic in the US. *Econ Hum Biol* 2005;3:296–313.

143. Sturm R. The effects of obesity, smoking, and drinking on medical problems and costs. *Health Aff* (Millwood). 2002;21:245–253.

144. Thorpe KE, Florence CS, Howard DH, et al. The impact of obesity on rising medical spending. *Health Aff* (Millwood) 2004;suppl web exclusives:w4-480–w4-486.

145. Thorpe KE. Factors accounting for the rise in health-care spending in the United States: the role of rising disease prevalence and treatment intensity. *Public Health* 2006;120:1002–1007.

146. Finkelstein E, Fiebelkorn C, Wang G. The costs of obesity among full-time employees. *Am J Health Promot* 2005;20:45–51.

147. Rosenwald MS. Why America has to be fat. A side effect of economic expansion shows up in front. *Washington Post* January 22, 2006:F01.

148. *Wall Street Journal* online. *Cheap food, societal norms and the economics of obesity.* August 25, 2006. Available http://online.wsj.com/public/article/SB115634907472843442_xrNV2M1 Pwf8pAcQYUWEBITP1LQ_20060901.html; accessed 9/21/07.

149. Close RN, Schoeller DA. The financial reality of overeating. *J Am Coll Nutr* 2006;25:203–209.

150. Mokdad AH, Marks JS, Stroup DF, et al. Actual causes of death in the United States, 2000. *JAMA* 2004;291:1238–1245.

151. Flegal KM, Graubard BI, Williamson DF, et al. Excess deaths associated with underweight, overweight, and obesity. *JAMA* 2005;293:1861–1867.

152. McGinnis J, Foege W. Actual causes of death in the United States. *JAMA* 1993;270(18):2207–2212.

153. Allison DB, Fontaine KR, Manson JE, et al. Annual deaths attributable to obesity in the United States. *JAMA* 1999;282:1530–1538.

154. Calle EE, Thun MJ, Petrelli JM, et al. Body-mass index and mortality in a prospective cohort of US adults. *N Engl J Med* 1999;341(15):1097–1105.

155. Manson J, Willett W, Stampfer M, et al. Body weight and mortality among women. *N Engl J Med* 1995;333:677–685.

156. Engeland A, Bjørge T, Selmer RM, et al. Height and body mass index in relation to total mortality. *Epidemiology* 2003;14(3):293–299.

157. Adams KF, Schatzkin A, Harris TB, et al. Overweight, obesity, and mortality in a large prospective cohort of persons 50 to 71 years old. *N Engl J Med* 2006;355(8):763–778.

158. Flegal KM, Kit BK, Orpana H, et al. Association of all-cause mortality with overweight and obesity using standard body mass index categories: a systematic review and meta-analysis. *JAMA* 2013;309(1):71–82.

159. Lee I, Manson J, Hennekens C, et al. Body weight and mortality: a 27-year follow up of middle aged men. *JAMA* 1993;270:2823–2828.

160. Garrison R, Castelli W. Weight and thirty-year mortality of men in the Framingham study. *Ann Intern Med* 1985;103:1006–1009.

161. Folsom A, Kaye S, Sellers T, et al. Body fat distribution and 5-year risk of death in older women. *JAMA* 1993;269:483–487.

162. Manson J, Stampfer M, Hennekens C, et al. Body weight and longevity. A reassessment. *JAMA* 1987;257:353–358.

163. Mizuno T, Shu IW, Makimura H, et al. Obesity over the life course. *Sci Aging Knowledge Environ* 2004;2004:4.

164. Mckay B. Admitting errors, agency expected to revise findings; big health concerns remain. *Wall Street Journal* November 23, 2004:A1.

165. Kolata G. Data on deaths from obesity is inflated, US agency says. *New York Times* November 24, 2004.

166. Mann CC. Public health. Provocative study says obesity may reduce US life expectancy. *Science* 2005;307: 1716–1717.

167. Olshansky SJ, Passaro DJ, Hershow RC, et al. A potential decline in life expectancy in the United States in the 21st century. *N Engl J Med* 2005;352:1138–1145.

168. Ogden CL, Flegal KM, Carroll MD, et al. Prevalence and trends in overweight among US children and adolescents, 1999–2000. *JAMA* 2002;288:1728–1732.

169. Mckay B. Doctors debate how to gauge lifestyle's effect on mortality. *Wall Street J* December 14, 2004:D6.

170. Yee D. CDC fixes error in figuring obesity risk. *Associated Press* January 18, 2005.

171. McKay B. CDC concedes it overstated obesity-linked deaths. *Wall Street J* January 18, 2005.

172. Obesity Death Figures Lowered. *Reuters Health* January 18, 2005.

173. Obesity set "to cut US life expectancy." *Reuters* February 2, 2005.

174. CDC again cuts estimate of obesity-linked deaths. *Associated Press* April 19, 2005.

175. Mark DH. Deaths attributable to obesity. *JAMA* 2005;293(15):1918–1919.

176. Gregg W, Foote A, Erfurt JC, et al. Worksite follow-up and engagement strategies for initiating health risk behavior changes. *Health Educ Quart* 1990;17:455–478.

177. Mokdad AH, Marks JS, Stroup DF, et al. Correction: actual causes of death in the United States, 2000. *JAMA* 2005;293:293–294.

178. Gregg EW, Cheng YJ, Cadwell BL, et al. Secular trends in cardiovascular disease risk factors according to body mass index in US adults. *JAMA* 2005;293:1868–1874.

179. Flegal KM, Williamson DF, Pamuk ER, et al. Estimating deaths attributable to obesity in the United States. *Am J Public Health* 2004;94:1486–1489.

180. Flegal KM, Graubard BI, Williamson DF. Methods of calculating deaths attributable to obesity. *Am J Epidemiol* 2004;160:331–338.

181. Centers for Disease Control and Health. Dangers of being overweight overstated. *Associated Press* April 19, 2005.

182. Kolata G. Some extra heft may be helpful, new study says. *New York Times* April 20, 2005.

183. So is obesity bad for you or not? *Reuters.* April 20, 2005.

184. Kolata G. Why thin is fine, but thinner can kill. *New York Times* April 24, 2005.

185. Flegal KM. Estimating the impact of obesity. *Soz Praventivmed.* 2005;50:73–74.

186. Neergaard L. Risks jump as obesity escalates. *Associated Press* May 1, 2005.

187. Tanner L. Experts say obesity still a health risk. *Associated Press* May 2, 2005.

188. Koplan JP. Attempts to downplay obesity ignore dangers. *Atlanta Journal-Constitution* April 29, 2005.

189. Couzin J. A heavyweight battle over CDC's obesity forecasts how many people does obesity kill? *Science* 2005;5723:770–771.

190. Marchione M. CDC stresses obesity problem, faults study. *Associated Press* June 2, 2005.

191. Hu FB, Willett WC, Stampfer MJ, et al. Calculating deaths attributable to obesity. *Am J Public Health* 2005;95:932–933.

192. Flegal KM, Pamuk ER. Letter. Flegal et al. respond. *Am J Public Health* 2005;95:932–933.

193. Warner M. Striking back at the food police. *New York Times* June 12, 2005.

194. JAMA News Releases. *Being obese, underweight, associated with increased risk of death.* April 19, 2005.

195. Calle EE, Rodriguez C, Walker-Thurmond K, et al. Overweight, obesity, and mortality from cancer in a prospectively studied cohort of US adults. *N Engl J Med* 2003;348:1625–1638.

196. Calle EE, Teras LR, Thun MJ. Obesity and mortality. *N Engl J Med* 2005;353:2197–2199.

197. de Hollander EL, Bemelmans WJ, Boshuizen HC, et al. The association between waist circumference and risk of mortality considering body mass index in 65- to 74-year-olds: a meta-analysis of 29 cohorts involving more than 58 000 elderly persons. *Int J Epidemiol* 2012;41(3): 805–817.

198. Czernichow S, Kengne A-P, Stamatakis E, et al. Body mass index, waist circumference and waist-hip ratio: which is the better discriminator of cardiovascular disease mortality risk?: evidence from an individual-participant meta-analysis of 82 864 participants from nine cohort studies. *Obes Rev* 2011;12(9):680–687.

199. Leitzmann MF, Moore SC, Koster A, et al. Waist circumference as compared with body-mass index in predicting mortality from specific causes. *PLoS ONE* 2011;6(4): e18582.

200. Koster A, Leitzmann MF, Schatzkin A, et al. Waist circumference and mortality. *Am J Epidemiol* 2008;167(12): 1465–1475.

201. Schoeller D. Recent advances from application of doubly labeled water to measurement of human energy expenditure. *J Nutr* 1999;129:1765–1768.

202. http://opinionator.blogs.nytimes.com/2012/03/20/is-a-calorie-a-calorie/

203. http://www.huffingtonpost.com/david-katz-md/calories_b_1369749.html

204. Reilly JJ, Kelly J. Long-term impact of overweight and obesity in childhood and adolescence on morbidity and premature mortality in adulthood: systematic review. *Int J Obes* 2005. 2011;35(7):891–898.

205. Schoeller DA. Insights into energy balance from doubly labeled water. *Int J Obes* (Lond). 2008;32(suppl 7): S72–S75.

206. Rush E, Plank L, Robinson S. Resting metabolic rate in young Polynesian and Caucasian women. *Int J Obes Relat Metab Disord* 1997;21:1071–1075.

207. Ravussin E, Gautier J. Metabolic predictors of weight gain. *Int J Obes Relat Metab Disord* 1999;23:37–41.

208. Luke A, Dugas L, Kramer H. Ethnicity, energy expenditure and obesity: are the observed black/white differences meaningful? *Curr Opin Endocrinol Diabetes Obes* 2007;14(5):370–373.

209. Gannon B, DiPietro L, Poehlman ET. Do African Americans have lower energy expenditure than Caucasians? *Int J Obes Relat Metab Disord* 2000;24(1):4–13.

210. Sun M, Gower BA, Bartolucci AA, et al. A longitudinal study of resting energy expenditure relative to body composition during puberty in African American and white children. *Am J Clin Nutr* 2001;73(2):308–315.

211. Leibel R, Rosenbaum M, Hirsch J. Changes in energy expenditure resulting from altered body weight. *N Engl J Med* 1995;332:621–628.

212. Astrup A, Gotzsche P, Werken KD, et al. Meta-analysis of resting metabolic rate in formerly obese subjects. *Am J Clin Nutr* 1999;69:1117–1122.

213. Weinsier RL, Nagy TR, Hunter GR, et al. Do adaptive changes in metabolic rate favor weight regain in weight-reduced individuals? An examination of the set-point theory. *Am J Clin Nutr* 2000;72(5):1088–1094.

214. Byrne NM, Wood RE, Schutz Y, et al. Does metabolic compensation explain the majority of less-than-expected weight loss in obese adults during a short-term severe diet and exercise intervention? *Int J obes* (Lond). 2012;36(11):1472–1478.

215. Maclean PS, Bergouignan A, Cornier M-A, et al. Biology's response to dieting: the impetus for weight regain. *Am J Physiol Regul Integr Comp Physiol* 2011;301(3): R581–R600.

216. Wijers SL, Saris WH, Van Marken Lichtenbelt WD. Recent advances in adaptive thermogenesis: potential implications for the treatment of obesity. *Obes Rev* 2009;10(2):218–226.

217. Clapham JC, Arch JRS. Targeting thermogenesis and related pathways in anti-obesity drug discovery. *Pharmacol Ther* 2011;131(3):295–308.

218. Stock M. Gluttony and thermogenesis revisited. *Int J Obes Relat Metab Disord* 1999;23:1105–1117.

219. Lowell BB, Bachman ES. β-Adrenergic receptors, diet-induced thermogenesis, and obesity. *J Biol Chem* 2003;278(32):29385–29388.

220. Kerckhoffs D, Blaak E, Baak MV, et al. Effect of aging on beta-adrenergically mediated thermogenesis in men. *Am J Physiol* 1998;274:e1075–e1079.

221. Saely CH, Geiger K, Drexel H. Brown versus white adipose tissue: a mini-review. *Gerontology* 2012;58(1):15–23.

222. Centers for Disease Control and Prevention. *US physical activity statistics*. June 12, 2010. Available at: http://apps.nccd.cdc.gov/PASurveillance/StateSumResultV.asp?CI= &Year=2007&State=0,1#data.

223. Gillman MW, Pinto BM, Tennstedt S, et al. Relationships of physical activity with dietary behaviors among adults. *Prev Med* 2001;32(3):295–301.

224. Simoes E, Byers T, Coates R, et al. The association between leisure-time physical activity and dietary fat in American adults. *Am J Public Health* 1995;85:240–244.

225. *Let's Move*. Available at: http://www.letsmove.gov/about; accessed 12/4/2012.

226. *The President's Challenge*. Available at https://www.presidentschallenge.org; accessed 4/17/2013.

227. *Healthy People 2020*. Available at http://www.healthypeople.gov/2020/topicsobjectives2020/objectiveslist.aspx?topicId=33.

228. Dipietro L. Physical activity in the prevention of obesity: current evidence and research issues. *Med Sci Sports Exerc* 1999;31:s542–s546.

229. Goldberg JH, King AC. Physical activity and weight management across the lifespan. *Annu Rev Public Health* 2007;28:145–170.

230. Jakicic JM, Davis KK. Obesity and physical activity. *Psychiatr Clin North Am* 2011;34(4):829–840.

231. Catenacci VA, Wyatt HR. The role of physical activity in producing and maintaining weight loss. *Nat Clin Pract Endocrinol Metab* 2007;3(7):518–529.

232. http://health.usnews.com/health-news/blogs/eat-run/2012/11/08/exercise-of-math-and-myth.

233. Katz DL. Unfattening our children: forks over feet. *Int J Obes* 2011;35(1):33–37.

234. Christou DD, Gentile CL, DeSouza CA, et al. Fatness is a better predictor of cardiovascular disease risk factor profile than aerobic fitness in healthy men. *Circulation* 2005;111:1904–1914.

235. Eisenmann JC, Wickel EE, Welk GJ, et al. Relationship between adolescent fitness and fatness and cardiovascular disease risk factors in adulthood: the Aerobics Center Longitudinal Study (ACLS). *Am Heart J* 2005;149:46–53.

236. Norman AC, Drinkard B, McDuffie JR, et al. Influence of excess adiposity on exercise fitness and performance in overweight children and adolescents. *Pediatrics* 2005;115:e690–e696.

237. Coakley EH, Kawachi I, Manson JE, et al. Lower levels of physical functioning are associated with higher body weight among middle-aged and older women. *Int J Obes Relat Metab Disord* 1998;22:958–965.

238. Hu FB, Willett WC, Li T, et al. Adiposity as compared with physical activity in predicting mortality among women. *N Engl J Med* 2004;351:2694–2703.

239. Weinstein AR, Sesso HD, Lee IM, et al. Relationship of physical activity vs body mass index with type 2 diabetes in women. *JAMA* 2004;292:1188–1194.

240. Fang J, Wylie-Rosett J, Cohen HW, et al. Exercise, body mass index, caloric intake, and cardiovascular mortality. *Am J Prev Med* 2003;25:283–289.

241. Haapanen-Niemi N, Miilunpalo S, Pasanen M, et al. Body mass index, physical inactivity and low level of physical fitness as determinants of all-cause and cardiovascular disease mortality—16 y follow-up of middle-aged and elderly men and women. *Int J Obes Relat Metab Disord* 2000;24:1465–1474.

242. Martinez ME, Giovannucci E, Spiegelman D, et al. Leisure-time physical activity, body size, and colon cancer in women. Nurses' Health Study Research Group. *J Natl Cancer Inst* 1997;89:948–955.

243. Giovannucci E, Ascherio A, Rimm E, et al. Physical activity, obesity, and risk for colon cancer and adenoma in men. *Ann Intern Med* 1995;122:327–334.

244. Patel AV, Rodriguez C, Bernstein L, et al. Obesity, recreational physical activity, and risk of pancreatic cancer in a large US cohort. *Cancer Epidemiol Biomarkers Prev* 2005;14:459–466.

245. Wei M, Kampert JB, Barlow CE, et al. Relationship between low cardiorespiratory fitness and mortality in normal-weight, overweight, and obese men. *JAMA* 1999;282:1547–1553.

246. Katzmarzyk PT, Janssen I, Ardern CI. Physical inactivity, excess adiposity and premature mortality. *Obes Rev* 2003;4:257–290.

247. Wessel TR, Arant CB, Olson MB, et al. Relationship of physical fitness vs body mass index with coronary artery disease and cardiovascular events in women. *JAMA* 2004;292:1179–1187.

248. Lee DC, Sui X, Blair SN. Does physical activity ameliorate the health hazards of obesity? *Br J Sports Med* 2009;43(1):49–51.

249. Fogelholm M. Physical activity, fitness and fatness: relations to mortality, morbidity and disease risk factors. A systematic review. *Obes Rev* 2010;11(3):202–221.

250. Kwon S, Burns TL, Janz K. Associations of cardiorespiratory fitness and fatness with cardiovascular risk factors among adolescents: the NHANES 1999–2002. *J Phys Act Health* 2010;7(6):746–753.

251. Woo J, Yu R, Yau F. Fitness, fatness and survival in elderly populations. *Age* (Dordrecht, Netherlands). 2013;35(3):973–984.

252. Hainer V, Toplak H, Stich V. Fat or fit: what is more important? *Diabetes Care* 2009;32(suppl 2):S392–397.

253. Suriano K, Curran J, Byrne SM, et al. Fatness, fitness, and increased cardiovascular risk in young children. *J Pediatr* 2010;157(4):552–558.

254. McAuley P, Pittsley J, Myers J, et al. Fitness and fatness as mortality predictors in healthy older men: the veterans exercise testing study. *J Gerontol A Biol Sci Med Sci.* 2009;64A(6):695–699.

255. Duncan GE. The "fit but fat" concept revisited: population-based estimates using NHANES. *Int J Behav Nutr Phys Act.* 2010;7:47.

256. Phelan S, Wyatt HR, Hill JO, et al. Are the eating and exercise habits of successful weight losers changing? *Obesity* 2006;14:710–716.

257. Wing RR, Hill JO. Successful weight loss maintenance. *Annu Rev Nutr* 2001;21:323–341.

258. Zachwieja JJ. Exercise as a treatment for obesity. *Endocrinol Metab Clin North Am* 1996;25:965–988.

259. Doucet E, Imbeault P, Almeras N, et al. Physical activity and low-fat diet: is it enough to maintain weight stability in the reduced-obese individual following weight loss by drug therapy and energy restriction? *Obes Res* 1999;7:323–333.

260. Rippe JM, Hess S. The role of physical activity in the prevention and management of obesity. *J Am Diet Assoc* 1998;98:s31–s38.

261. Saris W. Exercise with or without dietary restriction and obesity treatment. *Int J Obes Relat Metab Disord* 1995;19(suppl 4):s113–s116.

262. Mekary RA, Feskanich D, Hu FB, et al. Physical activity in relation to long-term weight maintenance after intentional weight loss in premenopausal women. *Obesity* 2010;18(1):167–174.

263. Lee I DL. Physical activity and weight gain prevention. *JAMA* 2010;303(12):1173–1179.

264. Saris W. Exercise with or without dietary restriction and obesity treatment. *Int J Obes Relat Metab Disord* 1995;19(suppl 4):s113–s116.

265. Heitmann B, Kaprio J, Harris J, et al. Are genetic determinants of weight gain modified by leisure-time physical activity? A prospective study of Finnish twins. *Am J Clin Nutr* 1997;66:672–678.

266. Graff M, North KE, Monda KL, et al. The combined influence of genetic factors and sedentary activity on body mass changes from adolescence to young adulthood: the National Longitudinal Adolescent Health Study. *Diabetes Metab. Res. Rev* 2011;27(1):63–69.

267. Andersen R, Wadden T, Bartlett S, et al. Effects of lifestyle activity vs structured aerobic exercise in obese women: a randomized trial. *JAMA* 1999;281:335–340.

268. Eaton S, Eaton SB 3rd, Konner M. Paleolithic nutrition revisited: a twelve-year retrospective on its nature and implications. *Eur J Clin Nutr* 1997;51:207–216.

269. Bellisari A. Evolutionary origins of obesity. *Obes Rev* 2008;9(2):165–180.

270. Mennella JA, Beauchamp GK. Early flavor experiences: research update. *Nutr Rev* 1998;56:205–211.

271. Drewnowski A. Why do we like fat? *J Am Diet Assoc* 1997;97:s58–s62.

272. Rolls B. Sensory-specific satiety. *Nutr Rev*1986;44:93–101.

273. James W, Ralph A. New understanding in obesity research. *Proc Nutr Soc* 1999;58:385–393.

274. Nestle M, Wing R, Birch L, et al. Behavioral and social influences on food choice. *Nutr Rev* 1998;56:s50–s64; discussion s64–s74.

275. Glanz K, Basil M, Maibach E, et al. Why Americans eat what they do: taste, nutrition, cost, convenience, and weight control concerns as influences on food consumption. *J Am Diet Assoc* 1998;98:1118–1126.

276. Axelson M. The impact of culture on food-related behavior. *Annu Rev Nutr* 1986;6:6345–6363.

277. Lichtman S, Pisarska K, Berman E, et al. Discrepancy between self-reported and actual caloric intake and exercise in obese subjects. *N Engl J Med* 1992;327:1893–1898.

278. Braam L, Ocke M, Bueno-de-Mesquita H, et al. Determinants of obesity-related underreporting of energy intake. *Am J Epidemiol* 1998;147:1081–1086.

279. Gabbert C, Donohue M, Arnold J, et al. Adenovirus 36 and obesity in children and adolescents. *Pediatrics* 2010;126(4):721–726.

280. Sorensen TI. Genetic epidemiology utilizing the adoption method: studies of obesity and of premature death in adults. *Scand J Soc Med* 1991;19:14–19.

281. Rasmussen F, Kark M, Tholin S, et al. The Swedish Young Male Twins Study: a resource for longitudinal research on risk factors for obesity and cardiovascular diseases. *Twin Res Hum Genet* 2006;9:883–889.

282. Hakala P, Rissanen A, Koskenvuo M, et al. Environmental factors in the development of obesity in identical twins. *Int J Obes Relat Metab Disord* 1999;23:746–753.

283. Koeppen-Schomerus G, Wardle J, Plomin R. A genetic analysis of weight and overweight in 4-year-old twin pairs. *Int J Obes Relat Metab Disord* 2001;25:838–844.

284. Echwald S. Genetics of human obesity: lessons from mouse models and candidate genes. *J Intern Med* 1999;245:653–666.

285. Perusse L, Bouchard C. Genotype-environment interaction in human obesity. *Nutr Rev* 1999;57:s31–s37.

286. Bell CG, Walley AJ, Froguel P. The genetics of human obesity. *Nat Rev Genet* 2005;6(3):221–234.

287. Walley AJ, Asher JE, Froguel P. The genetic contribution to non-syndromic human obesity. *Nat Rev Genet* 2009;10(7):431–442.

288. Cheung WW, Mao P. Recent advances in obesity: genetics and beyond. *ISRN Endocrinol* 2012;2012:1–11.

289. Rankinen T, Zuberi A, Chagnon YC, et al. The human obesity gene map: the 2005 update. *Obesity* 2006;14(4):529–644.

290. Clement K. Leptin and the genetics of obesity. *Acta Paedietr Suppl* 1999;88:51–57.

291. Marti A, Berraondo B, Martinez J. Leptin: physiological actions. *J Physiol Biochem*. 1999;55:43–49.

292. Lonnquist F, Nordfors L, Schalling M. Leptin and its potential role in human obesity. *J Intern Med* 1999;245:643–652.

293. Ronnemaa T, Karonen S-L, Rissanen A, et al. Relation between plasma leptin levels and measures of body fat in identical twins discordant for obesity. *Ann Intern Med* 1997;126:26–31.

294. Heymsfield S, Greenberg A, Fujioka K, et al. Recombinant leptin for weight loss in obese and lean adults: a randomized, controlled, dose-escalation trial. *JAMA* 1999;282:1568–1575.

295. Hamann A, Matthaei S. Regulation of energy balance by leptin. *Exp Clin Endocrinol Diabetes* 1996;104:293–300.

296. Enriori PJ, Evans AE, Sinnayah P, et al. Leptin resistance and obesity. *Obesity* 2006;14:254s–258s.

297. Zhang Y, Scarpace PJ. The role of leptin in leptin resistance and obesity. *Physiol Behav* 2006;88:249–256.

298. Paracchini V, Pedotti P, Taioli E. Genetics of leptin and obesity: a huge review. *Am J Epidemiol* 2005;162:101–114.

299. Oswal A, Yeo G. Leptin and the control of body weight: a review of its diverse central targets, signaling mechanisms, and role in the pathogenesis of obesity. *Obesity* 2010;18(2):221–229.

300. Ravussin E. Energy metabolism in obesity. Studies in the Pima Indians. *Diabetes Care* 1993;16:232–238.

301. Konturek SJ, Konturek JW, Pawlik T, et al. Brain–gut axis and its role in the control of food intake. *J Physiol Pharmacol* 2004;55:137–154.

302. Marti A, Moreno-Aliaga MJ, Hebebrand J, et al. Genes, lifestyles and obesity. *Int J Obes Relat Metab Disord* 2004;28:s29–s36.

303. Bouchard C. Gene–environment interactions in the etiology of obesity: defining the fundamentals. *Obesity* 2008;16(S3):S5–S10.

304. Qi L, Cho YA. Gene-environment interaction and obesity. *Nutrition Reviews* 2008;66(12):684–694.

305. Turnbaugh PJ, Ley RE, Mahowald MA, et al. An obesity-associated gut microbiome with increased capacity for energy harvest. *Nature* 2006;444, 1027–1031.

306. Turnbaugh PJ, Bäckhed F, Fulton L, et al. Diet-induced obesity is linked to marked but reversible alterations in the mouse distal gut microbiome. *Cell Host Microbe* 2008;3(4):213–223.

307. Bäckhed F, Ding H, Wang T, et al. The gut microbiota as an environmental factor that regulates fat storage. *Proc Natl Acad Sci USA.* 2004;101(44):15718–15723.

308. Turnbaugh PJ, Gordon JI. The core gut microbiome, energy balance and obesity. *J Physiol* (Lond) 2009;587(pt 17):4153–4158. doi:10.1113/jphysiol.2009.174136.

309. Turnbaugh PJ, Hamady M, Yatsunenko T, et al. A core gut microbiome in obese and lean twins. *Nature* 2009;457(7228):480–484. doi:10.1038/nature07540.

310. Ley RE. Obesity and the human microbiome. *Curr Opin Gastroenterol* 2010;26(1):5–11.

311. Schwiertz A, Taras D, Schafer K et al. Microbiota and SCFA in lean and overweight healthy subjects. *Obesity* (Silver Spring) 2010;18:190–195.

312. Turnbaugh PJ, Ley RE, Mahowald MA, et al. An obesity-associated gut microbiome with increased capacity for energy harvest. *Nature* 2006;444(7122):1027–1031.

313. Kootte RS, Vrieze A, Holleman F, et al. The therapeutic potential of manipulating gut microbiota in obesity and type 2 diabetes mellitus. *Diabetes Obes Metab* 2012;14(2):112–120.

314. Vrieze A, Holleman F, Serlie MJ et al. Metabolic effects of transplanting gut microbiota from lean donors to subjects with metabolic syndrome. *Diabetologia* 2010;53:S44.

315. Holt SH, Miller JC, Petocz P, et al. A satiety index of common foods. *Eur J Clin Nutr* 1995;49:675–690.

316. Astrup A. The American paradox: the role of energy-dense fat-reduced food in the increasing prevalence of obesity. *Curr Opin Clin Nutr Metab Care* 1998;1:573–577.

317. Pollan M. The age of nutritionism. How scientists have ruined the way we eat. *New York Times Magazine* January 28, 2007; cover story.

318. Warner M. Is the low-carb boom over? *New York Times* December 5, 2004. Available at http://www.nytimes.com/2004/12/05/business/yourmoney/05atki.html?ex=1184212800&en=2a5eee7041084409&ei=5070; accessed 9/21/07.

319. Howard T. Atkins nutritionals files for bankruptcy protection. *USA Today* August 1, 2005.

320. Gardner CD, Kiazand A, Alhassan S, et al. Comparison of the Atkins, Zone, Ornish, and LEARN diets for change in weight and related risk factors among overweight premenopausal women: the A TO Z Weight Loss Study: a randomized trial. *JAMA* 2007;297:969–977.

321. Jebb SA. Dietary strategies for the prevention of obesity. *Proc Nutr Soc* 2005;64:217–227.

322. Moloney M. Dietary treatments of obesity. *Proc Nutr Soc* 2000;59:601–608.

323. Astrup A. Dietary approaches to reducing body weight. *Best Pract Res Clin Endocrinol Metab* 1999;13:109–120.

324. Astrup A, Ryan L, Grunwald GK, et al. The role of dietary fat in body fatness: evidence from a preliminary meta-analysis of ad libitum low-fat dietary intervention studies. *Br J Nutr* 2000;83:s25–s32.

325. Rolls BJ, Ello-Martin JA, Tohill BC. What can intervention studies tell us about the relationship between fruit and vegetable consumption and weight management? *Nutr Rev* 2004;62:1–17.

326. Wadden TA, Butryn ML. Behavioral treatment of obesity. *Endocrinol Metab Clin North Am* 2003;32:981–1003.

327. Plodkowski RA, Jeor STS. Medical nutrition therapy for the treatment of obesity. *Endocrinol Metab Clin North Am* 2003;32:935–965.

328. Bedno SA. Weight loss in diabetes management. *Nutr Clin Care* 2003;6:62–72.

329. Wing RR, Gorin AA. Behavioral techniques for treating the obese patient. *Prim Care* 2003;30:375–391.

330. Vermunt SH, Pasman WJ, Schaafsma G, et al. Effects of sugar intake on body weight: a review. *Obes Rev* 2003;4:91–99.

331. Pirozzo S, Summerbell C, Cameron C, et al. Should we recommend low-fat diets for obesity? *Obes Rev* 2003;4:83–90.

332. Drewnowski A. The role of energy density. *Lipids* 2003;38:109–115.

333. Cheuvront SN. The Zone Diet phenomenon: a closer look at the science behind the claims. *J Am Coll Nutr* 2003;22:9–17.

334. Jequier E, Bray GA. Low-fat diets are preferred. *Am J Med* 2002;113:41s–46s.

335. Katz DL. Competing dietary claims for weight loss: finding the forest through truculent trees. *Annu Rev Public Health* 2005;26:61–88.

336. Hoelscher DM, Kirk S, Ritchie L, et al. Position of the Academy of Nutrition and Dietetics: interventions for the prevention and treatment of overweight and obesity. *J Acad Nutr Diet* 2013;113(10):1375–1394.

337. Bray GA. Lifestyle and pharmacological approaches to weight loss: efficacy and safety. *J Clin Endocronol Metab* 2008;93(11 suppl 1):S81–S88.

338. Jensen MD, Ryan DH, Apovian CM, et al. 2013 AHA/ACC/TOS guideline for the management of overweight and obesity in adults: a report of the American College of Cardiology/American Heart Association Task Force on Practice Guidelines and The Obesity Society. *J Am Coll Cardiol* 2013;pii:S0735-1097(13)06029-4.

339. Schrauwen P, Westerterp KR. The role of high-fat diets and physical activity in the regulation of body weight. *Br J Nutr* 2000;84:417–427.

340. Bray GA, Paeratakul S, Popkin BM. Dietary fat and obesity: a review of animal, clinical and epidemiological studies. *Physiol Behav* 2004;83:549–555.

341. Keys A, Menotti A, Aravanis C, et al. The seven countries study: 2,289 deaths in 15 years. *Prev Med* 1984;13:141–154.

342. Keys A, Aravanis C, Blackburn H, et al. Coronary heart disease: overweight and obesity as risk factors. *Ann Intern Med* 1972;77:15–27.

343. Keys A. Relative obesity and its health significance. *Diabetes* 1955;4:447–455.

344. Katz DL. Clinically relevant fat metabolism. In: Katz DL, ed. *Nutrition in clinical practice*. Philadelphia, PA: Lippincott, Williams & Wilkins, 2001:9–15.

345. Peters JC. Dietary fat and body weight control. *Lipids* 2003;38:123–127.

346. Hill JO, Melanson EL, Wyatt HT. Dietary fat intake and regulation of energy balance: implications for obesity. *J Nutr* 2000;130:284S–288S.

347. Schutz Y. Macronutrients and energy balance in obesity. *Metabolism* 1995;44:7–11

348. Bray G, Popkin B. Dietary fat intake does affect obesity. *Am J Clin Nutr* 1998;68:1157–1173.

349. Turner-McGrievy GM, Barnard ND, Scialli AR. A two-year randomized weight loss trial comparing a vegan diet to a more moderate low-fat diet. *Obesity* (Silver Spring) 2007;15:2276–81.

350. Willett WC, Leibel RL. Dietary fat is not a major determinant of body fat. *Am J Med* 2002;113:47s–59s.

351. Wright JD, Kennedy-Stephenson J, Wang CY, et al. Trends in intake of energy and macronutrients—United States, 1971–2000. *MMWR Morb Mortal Wkly Rep* 2004;53:80–82.

352. Jequier E. Pathways to obesity. *Int J Obes Relat Metab Disord* 2002;26:s12–s17.

353. Rolls BJ, Miller DL. Is the low-fat message giving people a license to eat more? *J Am Coll Nutr* 1997;16:535–543.

354. Harnack LJ, Jeffery RW, Boutelle KN. Temporal trends in energy intake in the United States: an ecologic perspective. *Am J Clin Nutr* 2000;71:1478–1484.

355. McCrory MA, Fuss PJ, Saltzman E, et al. Dietary determinants of energy intake and weight regulation in healthy adults. *J Nutr* 2000;130:276s–279s.

356. Nestle M. Increasing portion sizes in American diets: more calories, more obesity. *J Am Diet Assoc* 2003;103:39–40.

357. Atkins RC. *Dr. Atkins' diet revolution*. New York, NY: Bantam Books, 1972.

358. Rabast U, Kasper H, Schonborn J. Comparative studies in obese subjects fed carbohydrate-restricted and high carbohydrate 1,000-calorie formula diets. *Nutr Metab* 1978;22:269–277.

359. Bravata DM, Sanders L, Huang J, et al. Efficacy and safety of low-carbohydrate diets: a systematic review. *JAMA* 2003;289:1837–1850.

360. Wood RJ. Effect of dietary carbohydrate restriction with and without weight loss on atherogenic dyslipidemia. *Nutr Rev* 2006;64:539–545.

361. Krauss RM, Blanche PJ, Rawlings RS, et al. Separate effects of reduced carbohydrate intake and weight loss on atherogenic dyslipidemia. *Am J Clin Nutr* 2006;83:1025–1031; quiz 1205.

362. Siri PW, Krauss RM. Influence of dietary carbohydrate and fat on LDL and HDL particle distributions. *Curr Atheroscler Rep* 2005;7:455–459.

363. Volek JS, Sharman MJ, Gomez AL, et al. Comparison of a very low-carbohydrate and low-fat diet on fasting lipids, LDL subclasses, insulin resistance, and postprandial lipemic responses in overweight women. *J Am Coll Nutr* 2004;23:177–184.

364. Westman EC, Yancy WS, Edman JS, et al. Effect of 6-month adherence to a very low carbohydrate diet program. *Am J Med* 2002;113:30–36.

365. Brehm BJ, Seeley RJ, Daniels SR, et al. A randomized trial comparing a very low carbohydrate diet and a calorie-restricted low fat diet on body weight and cardiovascular risk factors in healthy women. *J Clin Endocrinol Metab* 2003;88:1617–1623.

366. Sondike SB, Copperman N, Jacobson MS. Effects of a low-carbohydrate diet on weight loss and cardiovascular risk factor in overweight adolescents. *J Pediatr* 2003;142:253–258.

367. Astrup A, Meinert Larsen T, Harper A. Atkins and other low-carbohydrate diets: hoax or an effective tool for weight loss? *Lancet* 2004;364:897–899.

368. Nickols-Richardson SM, Coleman MD, Volpe JJ, et al. Perceived hunger is lower and weight loss is greater in overweight premenopausal women consuming a low-carbohydrate/high-protein vs high-carbohydrate/low-fat diet. *J Am Diet Assoc* 2005;105:1433–1437.

369. Hession M, Rolland C, Kulkarni U, et al. Systematic review of randomized controlled trials of low-carbohydrate vs. low-fat/low-calorie diets in the management of obesity and its comorbities. *Obes Rev* 2009;10(1):36–50.

370. Belza A, Ritz C, Sorensen MQ, et al. Contribution of gastroenteropancreatic appetite hormones to protein-induced satiety. *Am J Clin Nutr* 2013;97(5):980–989.

371. Weigle DS, Breen PA, Matthys CC, et al. A high-protein diet induces sustained reductions in appetite, ad libitum caloric intake, and body weight despite compensatory changes in diurnal plasma leptin and ghrelin concentrations. *Am J Clin Nutr* 2005;85:41–48.

372. Skov A, Toubro S, Ronn B, et al. Randomized trial on protein vs. carbohydrate in ad libitum fat reduced diet for the treatment of obesity. *Int J Obes Relat Metab Disord* 1999;23:528–536.

373. Wycherley TP, Moran LJ, Clifton PM, et al. Effects of energy-restricted high-protein, low-fat compared with standard protein, low-fat diets: a meta-analysis of randomized controlled trials. *Am J Clin Nutr* 2012;96(6):1281–1298.

374. Jenkins DJ, Wong JM, Kendall CW, et al. The effect of a plant-based low-carbohydrate ("Eco-Atkins") diet on body weight and blood lipid concentrations in hyperlipidemic subjects. *Arch Intern Med* 2009;169:1046–1054.

375. Jonsson T, Granfeldt Y, Ahren B, et al. Beneficial effects of a Paleolithic diet on cardiovascular risk factors in type 2 diabetes: a pilot study. *Cardiovasc Diabetol* 2009;8:35.

376. http://www.huffingtonpost.com/david-katz-md/paleo-diet_b_889349.html.

377. Samaha FF, Iqbal N, Seshadri P, et al. A low-carbohydrate as compared with a low-fat diet in severe obesity. *N Engl J Med* 2003;348:2074–2081.

378. Foster GD, Wyatt HR, Hill JO, et al. A randomized trial of a low-carbohydrate diet for obesity. *N Engl J Med* 2003;348:2082–2090.

379. Atkins R. *Atkins' new diet revolution*. New York, NY: M. Evans & Company, 1999.

380. Foster GD, Wyatt HR, Hill JO, et al. Weight and metabolic outcomes after 2 years on a low-carbohydrate versus low-fat diet: a randomized trial. *Ann Intern Med* 2010;153:147–157.

381. Dansinger ML, Gleason JA, Griffith JL, et al. Comparison of the Atkins, Ornish, Weight Watchers, and Zone diets for weight loss and heart disease risk reduction: a randomized trial. *JAMA* 2005;293:43–53.

382. Yancy WS, Olsen MK, Guyton JR, et al. A low-carbohydrate, ketogenic diet versus a low-fat diet to treat obesity and hyperlipidemia: a randomized, controlled trial. *Ann Intern Med* 2004;140:769–777.

383. Brinkworth GD, Noakes M, Keogh JB, et al. Long-term effects of a high-protein, low-carbohydrate diet on weight control and cardiovascular risk markers in obese hyperinsulinemic subjects. *Int J Obes Relat Metab Disord* 2004;28:661–670.

384. Boden G, Sargrad K, Homko C, et al. Effect of a low-carbohydrate diet on appetite, blood glucose levels, and insulin resistance in obese patients with type 2 diabetes. *Ann Intern Med* 2005;142:403–411.

385. Bray GA. Is there something special about low-carbohydrate diets? *Ann Intern Med* 2005;142:469–470.

386. Segal-Isaacson CJ, Johnson S, Tomuta V, et al. A randomized trial comparing low-fat and low-carbohydrate diets matched for energy and protein. *Obes Res* 2004;12:130s–140s.

387. Golay A, Allaz A, Morel Y, et al. Similar weight loss with low- and high-carbohydrate diets. *Am J Clin Nutr* 1996;63:174–178.

388. Golay A, Eigenheer C, Morel Y, et al. Weight-loss with low or high carbohydrate diet? *Int J Obes Relat Metab Disord* 1996;20:1067–1072.

389. Meckling KA, O'Sullivan C, Saari D. Comparison of a low-fat diet to a low-carbohydrate diet on weight loss, body composition, and risk factors for diabetes and cardiovascular disease in free-living, overweight men and women. *J Clin Endocrinol Metab* 2004;89:2717–2723.

390. Miyashita Y, Koide N, Ohtsuka M, et al. Beneficial effect of low carbohydrate in low calorie diets on visceral fat reduction in type 2 diabetic patients with obesity. *Diabetes Res Clin Pract* 2004;65:235–241.

391. Poppitt SD, Keogh GF, Prentice AM, et al. Long-term effects of ad libitum low-fat, high-carbohydrate diets on body weight and serum lipids in overweight subjects with metabolic syndrome. *Am J Clin Nutr* 2002;75:11–20.

392. Willet WC. *Eat, drink, and be healthy*. New York, NY: Simon & Schuster, 2001.

393. US Department of Agriculture, US Department of Health and Human Services. Dietary Guidelines for Americans 2010–Policy Document. Available at http://www.cnpp.usda.gov/DGAs2010-PolicyDocument.htm Updated May 2, 2011; accessed 6/2/11.

394. http://www.hsph.harvard.edu/nutritionsource/plate-replaces-pyramid/.

395. Nestle M. *Food politics*. Berkeley, CA: University of California Press, 2002.

396. Klein S. Clinical trial experience with fat-restricted vs. carbohydrate-restricted weight-loss diets. *Obes Res* 2004;12:141s–144s.

397. Ludwig DS. The glycemic index: physiological mechanisms relating obesity, diabetes, and cardiovascular disease. *JAMA* 2002;287:2414–2423.

398. Colombani PC. Glycemic index and load-dynamic dietary guidelines in the context of disease. *Physiol Behav* 2004;83:603–610.

399. Wikipedia. *Glycemic index*. Available at http://en.wikipedia.org/wiki/Glycemic_index; accessed 9/21/07.

400. Moyad MA. Fat diets and obesity—part II: an introduction to the theory behind low-carbohydrate diets. *Urol Nurs* 2004;24:442–445.

401. Wikipedia. *Glycemic load*. Available at http://en.wikipedia.org/wiki/Glycemic_load; accessed 9/21/07.

402. Foster-Powell K, Holt SH, Brand-Miller JC. *International table of glycemic index and glycemic load values*. July 2002. Available at http://www.ajcn.org/cgi/content-nw/full/76/1/5/T1; accessed 9/21/07.

403. Livesey G. Low-glycaemic diets and health: implications for obesity. *Proc Nutr Soc* 2005;64:105–113.

404. Ludwig DS, Majzoub JA, Al-Zahrani A, et al. High glycemic index foods, overeating, and obesity. *Pediatrics* 1999;103:e26.

405. Warren JM, Henry CJ, Simonite V. Low glycemic index breakfasts and reduced food intake in preadolescent children. *Pediatrics* 2003;112:e414.

406. Ebbeling CB, Leidig MM, Sinclair KB, et al. A reduced-glycemic load diet in the treatment of adolescent obesity. *Arch Pediatr Adolesc Med* 2003;157:773–779.

407. Sloth B, Krog-Mikkelsen I, Flint A, et al. No difference in body weight decrease between a low-glycemic-index and a high-glycemic-index diet but reduced LDL cholesterol after 10-wk ad libitum intake of the low-glycemic-index diet. *Am J Clin Nutr* 2004;80:337–347.

408. Raatz SK, Torkelson CJ, Redmon JB, et al. Reduced glycemic index and glycemic load diets do not increase the effects of energy restriction on weight loss and insulin sensitivity in obese men and women. *J Nutr* 2005;135:2387–2391.

409. Spieth LE, Harnish JD, Lenders CM, et al. A low-glycemic index diet in the treatment of pediatric obesity. *Arch Pediatr Adolesc Med* 2000;154:947–951.

410. Heilbronn LK, Noakes M, Clifton PM. The effect of high-and low-glycemic index energy restricted diets on plasma lipid and glucose profiles in type 2 diabetic subjects with varying glycemic control. *J Am Coll Nutr* 2002;21:120–127.

411. Shyam S, Arshad F, Abdul Ghani R, et al. Low glycaemic index diets improve glucose tolerance and body weight in women with previous history of gestational diabetes: a six month randomized trial. *Nutr J* 2013;12:68

412. Livesey G. Low-glycaemic diets and health: implications for obesity. *Proc Nutr Soc* 2005;64:105–113.

413. McMillan-Price J, Petocz P, Atkinson F, et al. Comparison of 4 diets of varying glycemic load on weight loss and cardiovascular risk reduction in overweight and obese young adults: a randomized controlled trial. *Arch Intern Med* 2006;166:1466–1475.

414. Simopoulos AP. The Mediterranean diets: what is so special about the diet of Greece? The scientific evidence. *J Nutr* 2001;131:3065s–3073s.

415. Kok FJ, Kromhout D. Atherosclerosis—epidemiological studies on the health effects of a Mediterranean diet. *Eur J Nutr* 2004;43:2–5.

416. Kris-Etherton P, Eckel RH, Howard BV, et al. Lyon Diet Heart Study. Benefits of a Mediterranean-style, National Cholesterol Education Program/American Heart Association Step I dietary pattern on cardiovascular disease. *Circulation* 2001;103:1823–1825.

417. Cukur CS, de Guzman MR, Carlo G. Religiosity, values, and horizontal and vertical individualism–collectivism: a study of Turkey, the United States, and the Philippines. *J Soc Psychol* 2004;144:613–634.

418. DeJong MJ, Chung ML, Roser LP, et al. A five-country comparison of anxiety early after acute myocardial infarction. *Eur J Cardiovasc Nurs* 2004;3:129–134.

419. Astrup A. Macronutrient balances and obesity: the role of diet and physical activity. *Public Health Nutr* 1999;2:341–347.

420. Ferro-Luzzi A, James WP, Kafatos A. The high-fat Greek diet: a recipe for all? *Eur J Clin Nutr* 2002;56:796–809.

421. Trichopoulou A, Naska A, Orfanos P, et al. Mediterranean diet in relation to body mass index and waist-to-hip ratio: the Greek European Prospective Investigation into Cancer and Nutrition Study. *Am J Clin Nutr* 2005;82:935–940.

422. Schroder H, Marrugat J, Vila J, et al. Adherence to the traditional Mediterranean diet is inversely associated with body mass index and obesity in a Spanish population. *J Nutr* 2004;134:3355–3361.

423. Shubair MM, McColl RS, Hanning RM. Mediterranean dietary components and body mass index in adults: the peel nutrition and heart health survey. *Chronic Dis Can* 2005;26:43–51.

424. Shah M, Garg A. High-fat and high-carbohydrate diets and energy balance. *Diabetes Care* 1996;19:1142–1152.

425. McManus K, Antinoro L, Sacks F. A randomized controlled trial of a moderate-fat, low-energy diet compared with a low fat, low-energy diet for weight loss in overweight adults. *Int J Obes Relat Metab Disord* 2001;25:1503–1511.

426. Flynn G, Colquhoun D. Successful long-term weight loss with a Mediterranean style diet in a primary care medical centre. *Asia Pac J Clin Nutr* 2004;13:s139.

427. Esposito K, Maiorino MI, Ciotola M et al. Effects of a Mediterranean-style diet on the need for antihyperglycemic drug therapy in patients with newly diagnosed type 2 diabetes: a randomized trial. *Ann Intern Med* 2009;151:306–14.

428. De Lorenzo A, Petroni ML, De Luca PP, et al. Use of quality control indices in moderately hypocaloric Mediterranean diet for treatment of obesity. *Diabetes Nutr Metab* 2001;14:181–188.

429. Ajala O, English P, Pinkney J. Systematic review and meta-analysis of different dietary approaches to the management of type 2 diabetes. *Am J Clin Nutr* 2013;97(3):505–516.

430. Nordmann AJ, Suter-Zimmerman K, Bucher HC, et al. Meta-analysis comparing Mediterranean to low-fat diets for modification of cardiovascular risk factors. *Am J Med* 2011;124(9):841–851.

431. Atkins R. *Dr. Atkins' new diet revolution.* New York, NY: HarperCollins, 2002.

432. Marks JB. Advances in obesity treatment: clinical highlights from the NAASO 2003 annual meeting. *Clin Diabetes* 2004;22:23–26.

433. Nelson LH, Tucker LA. Diet composition related to body fat in a multivariate study of 203 men. *J Am Diet Assoc* 1996;96:771–777.

434. Hays NP, Starling RD, Liu X, et al. Effects of an ad libitum low-fat, high-carbohydrate diet on body weight, body composition, and fat distribution in older men and women—a randomized controlled trial. *Arch Intern Med* 2004;164:210–217.

435. Siggaard R, Raben A, Astrup A. Weight loss during 12 weeks ad libitum carbohydrate-rich diet in overweight and normal weight subjects at a Danish work site. *Obes Res* 1996;4:347–356.

436. Volek JS, Sharman MJ, Love DM, et al. Body composition and hormonal responses to a carbohydrate-restricted diet. *Metabolism* 2002;51:864–870.

437. Racette SB, Schoeller DA, Kushner RF, et al. Effects of aerobic exercise and dietary carbohydrate on energy expenditure and body composition during weight reduction in obese women. *Am J Clin Nutr* 1995;61:486–494.

438. Kirk EP, Jacobsen DJ, Gibson C, et al. Time course for changes in aerobic capacity and body composition in overweight men and women in response to long-term exercise: the Midwest Exercise Trial (MET). *Int J Obes Relat Metab Disord* 2003;27:912–919.

439. Lustig RH. Fructose: it's "alcohol without the buzz." *Adv Nutr* 2013;4(2):226–235.

440. Johnson RK, Appel LJ, Brands M, et al; American Heart Association Nutrition Committee of the Council on Nutrition, Physical Activity, and Metabolism and the Council on Epidemiology and Prevention. Dietary sugars intake and cardiovascular health: a scientific statement from the American Heart Association. *Circulation* 2009;120(11):1011–1020.

441. Ludwig D. Examining the health effects of fructose. *JAMA* 2013;E1–E2.

442. Lowndes J, Kawiecki D, Pardo S, et al. The effects of four hypocaloric diets containing different levels of sucrose or high fructose corn syrup on weight loss and related parameters. *Nutr J* 2012;11:55

443. He FJ, Nowson CA, Lucas M, et al. Increased consumption of fruit and vegetables is related to a reduced risk of

coronary heart disease: metaanalysis of cohort studies. *J Hum Hypertens* 2007;21(9):717–728.

444. Sacks FM, Bray GA, Carey VJ, et al. Comparison of weight-loss diets with different compositions of fat, protein, and carbohydrates. *N Engl J Med* 2009,360:9.

445. Amazon.com. Available at http://www.amazon.com; accessed 12/21/13.

446. Google. Available at http://www.google.com; accessed 12/21/13.

447. Yale-Griffin Prevention Research Center. *Obesity systematic review*. Atlanta, GA: Centers for Disease Control, Grant #U48-CCU115802, 10/00–8/03.

448. Ornish D. *Eat more, weigh less: Dr. Dean Ornish's life choice program for losing weight safely while eating abundantly*. New York, NY: Quill Publishing, 2000.

449. Vartabedian RE, Matthews K. *Nutripoints: the breakthrough point system for optimal health*, 3rd ed. New York, NY: Designs for Wellness Press, 1994.

450. Rolls BJ, Barnett RA. *The volumetrics weight-control plan: feel full on fewer calories*. New York, NY: HarperCollins, 2000.

451. Katz DL, Gonzalez MH. *The way to eat*. Naperville, IL: Sourcebooks, 2002.

452. Sears W. *The family nutrition book: everything you need to know about feeding your children—from birth to age two*. Boston, MA: Little Brown & Company, 1999.

453. Astrup A. The role of dietary fat in the prevention and treatment of obesity. Efficacy and safety of low-fat diets. *Int J Obes Relat Metab Disord* 2001;25:s46–s50.

454. Connor W, Connor S. Should a low-fat, high-carbohydrate diet be recommended for everyone? The case for a low-fat, high-carbohydrate diet. *N Engl J Med* 1997;337:562–563.

455. Katan M, Grundy S, Willett W. Should a low-fat, high-carbohydrate diet be recommended for everyone? Beyond low-fat diets. *N Engl J Med* 1997;337:563–566.

456. Denke M. Metabolic effects of high-protein, low-carbohydrate diets. *Am J Cardiol* 2001;88:59–61.

457. Tapper-Gardzina Y, Cotugna N, Vickery C. Should you recommend a low-carb, high-protein diet? *Nurse Pract* 2002;27:52–57.

458. Eisenstein J, Roberts SB, Dallal G, et al. High-protein weight-loss diets: are they safe and do they work? A review of the experimental and epidemiologic data. *Nutr Rev* 2002;60:189–200.

459. Katz DL. Diet and cancer. In: Katz DL, ed. *Nutrition in clinical practice*. Philadelphia, PA: Lippincott Williams & Wilkins, 2000:114–126.

460. St Jeor S, Howard B, Prewitt E, et al. Dietary protein and weight reduction: a statement for healthcare professionals from the Nutrition Committee of the Council on Nutrition, Physical Activity, and Metabolism of the American Heart Association. *Circulation* 2001;104: 1869–1874.

461. Katz DL. Diet, sleep-wake cycles, and mood. In: Katz DL, ed. *Nutrition in clinical practice*. Philadelphia, PA: Lippincott Williams & Wilkins, 2001:243–247.

462. Benton D. Carbohydrate ingestion, blood glucose and mood. *Neurosci Biobehav Rev* 2002;26:293–308.

463. Terry P, Terry JB, Wolk A. Fruit and vegetable consumption in the prevention of cancer: an update. *J Intern Med* 2001;250:280–290.

464. Van Duyn MA, Pivonka E. Overview of the health benefits of fruit and vegetable consumption for the dietetics professional: selected literature. *J Am Diet Assoc* 2000;100:1511–1521.

465. Weisburger JH. Eat to live, not live to eat. *Nutrition* 2000;16:767–773.

466. Ornish D. Was Dr. Atkins right? *Am J Diet Assoc* 2004;104:537–542.

467. Chandalia M, Garg A, Lutjohann D, et al. Beneficial effects of high dietary fiber intake in patients with type 2 diabetes mellitus. *N Engl J Med* 2000;342:1392–1398.

468. Casagrande SS, Wang Y, Anderson C, et al. Have Americans increased their fruit and vegetable intake? The trends between 1988 and 2002. *Am J Prev Med* 2007;32:257–263.

469. Centers for Disease Control and Prevention. Fruit and vegetable consumption among adults—United States, 2005. *MMWR Morb Mortal Wkly Rep* 2007;56:213–217.

470. Pasman W, Saris W, Westerterp-Plantenga M. Predictors of weight maintenance. *Obes Res* 1999;7:43–50.

471. Mattes RD. Feeding behaviors and weight loss outcomes over 64 months. *Eat Behav* 2002;3:191–204.

472. Thomas JG, Bond DS, Phelan S, et al. Weight-loss maintenance for 10 years in the national weight control registry. *Am J Prev Med* 2014;46(1):17–23.

473. McGuire MT, Wing RR, Klem ML, et al. Long-term maintenance of weight loss: do people who lose weight through various weight loss methods use different behaviors to maintain their weight? *Int J Obes Relat Metab Disord* 1998;22:572–577.

474. Shick SM, Wing RR, Klem ML, et al. Persons successful at long-term weight loss and maintenance continue to consume a low-energy, low-fat diet. *J Am Diet Assoc* 1998;98:408–413.

475. Klem ML, Wing RR, McGuire MT, et al. A descriptive study of individuals successful at long-term maintenance of substantial weight loss. *Am J Clin Nutr* 1997;66:239–246.

476. Champagne CM, Broyles ST, Moran LD, et al. Dietary intakes associated with successful weight loss and maintenance during the Weight Loss Maintenance trial. *J Am Diet* Assoc 2011;111(12):1826–1835.

477. Gorin AA, Phelan S, Wing RR, et al. Promoting long-term weight control: does dieting consistency matter? *Int J Obes Relat Metab Disord* 2004;28:278–281.

478. Wyatt HR, Grunwald GK, Mosca CL, et al. Long-term weight loss and breakfast in subjects in the National Weight Control Registry. *Obes Res* 2002;10:78–82.

479. Klem ML. Successful losers. The habits of individuals who have maintained long-term weight loss. *Minn Med* 2000;83:43–45.

480. Raynor DA, Phelan S, Hill JO, et al. Television viewing and long-term weight maintenance: results from the National Weight Control Registry. *Obesity* 2006;14:1816–1824.

481. Knowler WC, Barrett-Connor E, Fowler SE, et al. Reduction in the incidence of type 2 diabetes with lifestyle intervention or metformin. *N Engl J Med* 2002;346:393–403.

482. Sacks FM, Svetkey LP, Vollmer WM, et al. Effects on blood pressure of reduced dietary sodium and the Dietary Approaches to Stop Hypertension (DASH) diet. DASH-Sodium Collaborative Research Group. *N Engl J Med* 2001;344:3–10.

483. Blumenthal JA, Babyak MA, Hinderliter A, et al. Effects of the DASH diet alone and in combination with exercise and weight loss on blood pressure and cardiovascular biomarkers in men and women with high blood pressure: the ENCORE study. *Arch Intern Med* 2010;170:126–135.

484. Ornish D, Scherwitz LW, Billings JH, et al. Intensive lifestyle changes for reversal of coronary heart disease. *JAMA* 1998;280:2001–2007.

485. de Lorgeril M, Salen P. The Mediterranean-style diet for the prevention of cardiovascular diseases. *Public Health Nutr* 2006;9:118–123.

486. Hu FB, Willett WC. Optimal diets for prevention of coronary heart disease. *JAMA* 2002;288:2569–2578.

487. Hu FB, Manson JE, Willett WC. Types of dietary fat and risk of coronary heart disease: a critical review. *J Am Coll Nutr* 2001;20:5–19.

488. Hu FB. Plant-based foods and prevention of cardiovascular disease: an overview. *Am J Clin Nutr* 2003;78:544S–551S.

489. Katz DL. Dietary recommendations for health promotion and disease prevention. In: Katz DL, eds. *Nutrition in clinical practice*. Philadelphia, PA: Lippincott, Williams & Wilkins, 2001:291–298.

490. Reddy KS, Katan MB. Diet, nutrition and the prevention of hypertension and cardiovascular diseases. *Public Health Nutr* 2004;7:167–186.

491. Mathers JC. Nutrition and cancer prevention: diet-gene interactions. *Proc Nutr Soc* 2003;62:605–610.

492. Key TJ, Schatzkin A, Willett WC, et al. Diet, nutrition and the prevention of cancer. *Public Health Nutr* 2004;7:187–200.

493. Eaton SB, Strassman BI, Nesse RM, et al. Evolutionary health promotion. *Prev Med* 2002;34:109–118.

494. Baschetti R. Paleolithic nutrition. *Eur J Clin Nutr* 1997;51:715–716.

495. Katz DL. Evolutionary biology, culture, and determinants of dietary behavior. In: Katz DL, ed. *Nutrition in clinical practice*. Philadelphia, PA: Lippincott Williams & Wilkins, 2001:279–290.

496. Eaton S, Eaton SB 3rd, Konner M, et al. An evolutionary perspective enhances understanding of human nutritional requirements. *J Nutr* 1996;126:1732–1740.

497. US Preventive Services Task Force. *Guide to clinical preventive services*, 2nd ed. Baltimore, MD: Williams and Wilkins, 1996.

498. Moyer VA. Behavioral counseling interventions to promote a healthful diet and physical activity for cardiovascular disease prevention in adults: a US Preventive Services Task Force Recommendation Statement. *Ann Intern Med* 2012;157:367–372.

499. North American Association for the Study of Obesity. *The practical guide to identification, evaluation, and treatment of overweight and obesity in adults*. Bethesda, MD: National Institutes of Health, National Heart, Lung, and Blood Institute, 2000.

500. Food and Nutrition Board, Institute of Medicine, National Academies of Science. *Dietary reference intakes for energy, carbohydrate, fiber, fat, fatty acids, cholesterol, protein, and amino acids (macronutrients)*. Washington, DC: National Academy Press, 2010.

501. American College of Preventive Medicine. *Diet in the prevention and control of obesity, insulin resistance, and type II diabetes*. Available at http://www.acpm.org/2002-057(F).htm; accessed 12/02.

502. US Department of Agriculture. *Dietary guidelines for Americans 2010*. Available at http://www.cnpp.usda.gov/DGAs2010-PolicyDocument.htm; accessed 12/29/13.

503. *Fruits and veggies—more matters*. Available at http://www.fruitsandveggiesmorematter.org; accessed 12/29/13.

504. National Cancer Institute. *National Cancer Institute dietary guidelines*. Available at http://www.pueblo.gsa.gov/cic_text/food/guideeat/guidelns.html; accessed 9/02.

505. Lichtenstein AH, Appel LJ, Brands M, et al. Diet and lifestyle recommendations revision 2006: a scientific statement from the American Heart Association Nutrition Committee. *Circulation* 2006;114:82–96.

506. American Dietetic Association. Weight management—position of ADA. *J Am Diet Assoc* 2002;102:1145–1155.

507. American Diabetes Association. Nutrition recommendations and interventions for diabetes: A position statement of the American Diabetes Association. *Diabetes Care* 2008;31:S61–S78.

508. Kennedy ET, Bowman SA, Spence JT, et al. Popular diets: correlation to health, nutrition, and obesity. *J Am Diet Assoc* 2001;101:411–420.

509. Hung T, Sievenpiper JL, Marchie A, et al. Fat versus carbohydrate in insulin resistance, obesity, diabetes and cardiovascular disease. *Curr Opin Clin Nutr Metab Care* 2003;6:165–176.

510. Katz DL, Meller S. Can we say what diet is best? *Ann Rev Pub Health* 2014;35:83–103.

511. US Preventive Services Task Force. *Screening and interventions to prevent obesity in adults*. December 2003. Available at: http://www.ahrq.gov/clinic/uspstf/uspsobes.htm; accessed 3/18/07.

512. Lin JS, O'Connor E, Whitlock EP, et al. Behavioral counseling to promote physical activity and a healthful diet to prevent cardiovascular disease in adults: a systematic review for the U.S. Preventive Services Task Force. *Ann Intern Med* 2010;153:736–750.

513. Ockene I, Hebert J, Ockene J, et al. Effect of physician-delivered nutrition counseling training and an office-support program on saturated fat intake, weight, and serum lipid measurements in a hyperlipidemic population: Worcester Area Trial for Counseling in Hyperlipidemia (WATCH). *Arch Intern Med* 1999;159:725–731.

514. Long BJ, Calfas KJ, Wooten W, et al. A multisite field test of the acceptability of physical activity counseling in primary care: project PACE. *Am J Prev Med* 1996;12:73–81.

515. Blackburn DG. Establishing an effective framework for physical activity counseling in primary care settings. *Nutr Clin Care* 2002;5:95–102.

516. Albright CL, Cohen S, Gibbons L, et al. Incorporating physical activity advice into primary care: physician-delivered advice within the activity counseling trial. *Am J Prev Med* 2000;18:225–234.

517. Kerse N, Elley CR, Robinson E, et al. Is physical activity counseling effective for older people? A cluster randomized, controlled trial in primary care. *J Am Geriatr Soc* 2005;53:1951–1956.

518. Petrella RJ, Koval JJ, Cunningham DA, et al. Can primary care doctors prescribe exercise to improve fitness? The Step Test Exercise Prescription (STEP) project. *Am J Prev Med* 2003;24:316–322.

519. Nawaz H, Adams M, Katz D. Weight loss counseling by health care providers. *Am J Public Health* 1999;89:764–767.

520. Tham M, Young D. The role of the general practitioner in weight management in primary care—a cross sectional study in general practice. *BMC Fam Pract* 2008;9:66

521. Biener L, Heaton A. Women dieters of normal weight: their motives, goals, and risks. *Am J Public Health* 1995;85:714–717.

522. Nawaz H, Katz D, Adams M. Physician–patient interactions regarding diet, exercise and smoking. *Prev Med.* 2000;31:652–657.

523. NECON. *Strategic plan for prevention and control of overweight and obesity in New England.* Available at http://www.neconinfo.org/02-11-2003_Strategic_Plan.pdf; accessed 9/21/07.

524. Wieland LS, Falzon L, Sciamanna CN, et al. Interactive computer-based interventions for weight loss or weight maintenance in overweight or obese people. *Cochrane Database Syst Rev* 2012;8:CD007675.

525. Spring B, Duncan JM, Janke EA, et al. Integrating technology into standard weight loss treatment: a randomized controlled trial. *JAMA Intern Med* 2013;173(2):105–111.

526. Ryan D. Medicating the obese patient. *Endocrinol Metab Clin North Am* 1996;25:989–1004.

527. Aronne L. Modern medical management of obesity: the role of pharmaceutical intervention. *J Am Diet Assoc* 1998;98:s23–s26.

528. Connolly HM, Crary JL, McGoon MD, et al. Valvular heart disease associated with fenfluramine-phentermine (see comments) (published erratum appears in *N Engl J Med* 1997;337:1783). *N Engl J Med* 1997;337:581–588.

529. Curfman GD. Diet pills redux. *N Engl J Med* 1997;337:629–630.

530. Bray GA, Hollander P, Klein S, et al. A 6-month randomized, placebo-controlled, dose-ranging trial of topiramate for weight loss in obesity. *Obes Res* 2003;11:722–733.

531. Gadde KM, Allison DB, Ryan DH, et al. Effects of low-dose, controlled-release, phentermine plus topiramate combination on weight and associated comorbidities in overweight and obese adults (CONQUER): a randomized, placebo-controlled, phase 3 trial. *Lancet* 2011;377:1341–1352.

532. Garvey WT, Ryan DH, Look M, et al. Two-year sustained weight loss and metabolic benefits with controlled-release phentermine/topiramate in obese and overweight adults (SEQUEL): a randomized, placebo-controlled, phase 3 extension study. *Am J Clin Nutr* 2012;95:297–308.

533. Fleming JW, McClendon KS, Riche DM. New obesity agents: lorcaserin and phentermine/topiramate. *Ann Pharmacother* 2013;47:1007–1016.

534. Smith SR, Weissman NJ, Anderson CM, et al. Behavioral Modification and Lorcaserin for Overweight and Obesity Management (BLOOM) Study Group. Multicenter, placebo-controlled trial of lorcaserin for weight management. *N Engl J Med* 2010;363:245–256.

535. Fidler MC, Sanchez M, Raether B, et al; BLOSSOM Clinical Trial Group. A one-year randomized trial of lorcaserin for weight loss in obese and overweight adults: the BLOSSOM trial. *J Clin Endocrinol Metab* 2011;96:3067–3077.

536. http://www.ema.europa.eu/docs/en_GB/document_library/Medicine_QA/2013/05/WC500143811.pdf.

537. GlaxoSmithKline. *Alli.* Available at http://www.myalli.com; accessed 3/19/07.

538. Hvizdos K, Markham A. Orlistat: a review of its use in the management of obesity. *Drugs* 1999;58:743–760.

539. Sjostrom L, Rissanen A, Andersen T, et al. Randomized placebo-controlled trial of orlistat for weight loss and prevention of weight regain in obese patients. *Lancet* 1998;352:167–173.

540. Leblanc ES, O'Connor E, Whitlock EP, et al. Effectiveness of primary care-relevant treatments for obesity in adults: a systematic evidence review for the U.S. Preventive Services Task Force. *Ann Intern Med* 2011;155:434–447.

541. Padwal R, Li SK, Lau DC. Long-term pharmacotherapy for obesity and overweight. *Cochrane Database Syst Rev* 2004;(3):CD004094.

542. McNeely W, Goa KL. Sibutramine. A review of its contribution to the management of obesity. *Drugs* 1998;56:1093–1124.

543. Gaal LV, Wauters M, Leeuw ID. Anti-obesity drugs: what does sibutramine offer? An analysis of its potential contribution to obesity treatment. *Exp Clin Endocrinol Diabetes* 1998;106:35–40.

544. Patel D, Luckstead E. Sport participation, risk taking, and health risk behaviors. *Adoles Med* 2000;11:141–155.

545. Costa B. Rimonabant: more than an anti-obesity drug? *Br J Pharmacol* 2007;150:535–537.

546. Padwal RS, Majumdar SR. Drug treatments for obesity: orlistat, sibutramine, and rimonabant. *Lancet* 2007;369:71–77.

547. Henness S, Robinson DM, Lyseng-Williamson KA. Rimonabant. *Drugs* 2006;66:2109–2119; discussion 2120–2101.

548. Wierzbicki AS. Rimonabant: endocannabinoid inhibition for the metabolic syndrome. *Int J Clin Pract* 2006;60:1697–1706.

549. Scheen AJ, Finer N, Hollander P, et al. Efficacy and tolerability of rimonabant in overweight or obese patients with type 2 diabetes: a randomised controlled study. *Lancet* 2006;368:1660–1672.

550. Pi-Sunyer FX, Aronne LJ, Heshmati HM, et al. Effect of rimonabant, a cannabinoid-1 receptor blocker, on weight and cardiometabolic risk factors in overweight or obese patients: RIO-North America: a randomized controlled trial. *JAMA* 2006;295:761–775.

551. Despres JP, Golay A, Sjostrom L. Effects of rimonabant on metabolic risk factors in overweight patients with dyslipidemia. *N Engl J Med* 2005;353:2121–2134.

552. Topol EJ, Bousser MG, Fox KA, et al. Rimonabant for prevention of cardiovascular events (CRESCENDO): a randomized, multicenter, placebo-controlled trial. *Lancet* 2010;376(9740):517–523.

553. Rucker D, Padwal R, Li SK, et al. Long-term pharmacotherapy for obesity and overweight: updated meta-analysis (published correction appears in *BMJ* 2007;335[7629]). *BMJ* 2007;335(7631):1194–1199.

554. Gray LJ, Cooper N, Dunkley A, et al. A systematic review and mixed treatment comparison of pharmacological interventions for the treatment of obesity. *Obes Rev* 2012;13(6):483–498.

555. Hofbauer KG, Nicholson JR. Pharmacotherapy of obesity. *Exp Clin Endocrinol Diabetes* 2006;114:475–484.

556. Mancini MC, Halpern A. Pharmacological treatment of obesity. *Arq Bras Endocrinol Metabol* 2006;50:377–389.

557. Halford JC. Clinical pharmacotherapy for obesity: current drugs and those in advanced development. *Curr Drug Targets* 2004;5:637–646.

558. Das SK, Chakrabarti R. Antiobesity therapy: emerging drugs and targets. *Curr Med Chem* 2006;13:1429–1460.

559. Sidhaye A, Cheskin LJ. Pharmacologic treatment of obesity. *Adv Psychosom Med* 2006;27:42–52.

560. Spanswick D, Lee K. Emerging antiobesity drugs. *Expert Opin Emerg Drugs* 2003;8:217–237.

561. Kim GW, Lin JE, Blomain ES, et al. Antiobesity pharmacotherapy: new drugs and emerging targets. *Clin Pharmacol Ther* 2013;95:53–66.

562. Carter R, Mouralidarane A, Ray S, et al. Recent advancements in drug treatment of obesity. *Clin Med* 2012;12: 456–460.

563. Greenway FL, Fujioka K, Plodkowski RA, et al. Effect of naltrexone plus bupropion on weight loss in overweight and obese adults (COR-I): a multicentre, randomised, double-blind, placebo-controlled, phase 3 trial. *Lancet* 2010;376:595–605.

564. Astrup A, Rössner S, Van Gaal L, et al. Effects of liraglutide in the treatment of obesity: a randomised, double-blind, placebo-controlled study. *Lancet* 2009;74:1606–16.

565. Leonhardt M, Hrupka B, Langhans W. New approaches in the pharmacological treatment of obesity. *Eur J Nutr* 1999;38:1–13.

566. Carek P, Dickerson L. Current concepts in the pharmacological management of obesity. *Drugs* 1999;57:883–904.

567. Astrup A, Lundsgaard C. What do pharmacological approaches to obesity management offer? Linking pharmacological mechanisms of obesity management agents to clinical practice. *Exp Clin Endocrinol Diabetes* 1998;106:29–34.

568. Aronne LJ. Therapeutic options for modifying cardiometabolic risk factors. *Am J Med* 2007;120:s26–s34.

569. Katz DL. The scarlet burger. *Wall Street J.* November 19, 2003.

570. Salameh JR. Bariatric surgery: past and present. *Am J Med Sci* 2006;331:194–200.

571. Shah M, Simha V, Garg A. Review: long-term impact of bariatric surgery on body weight, comorbidities, and nutritional status. *J Clin Endocrinol Metab* 2006;91: 4223–4231.

572. Kushner RF, Noble CA. Long-term outcome of bariatric surgery: an interim analysis. *Mayo Clin Proc* 2006;81: s46–s51.

573. Provost DA. Laparoscopic adjustable gastric banding: an attractive option. *Surg Clin North Am* 2005;85:vii, 789–805.

574. Yildiz BD, Bostanoglu A, Sonisik M, et al. Long term efficacy of laparoscopic adjustable gastric banding—retrospective analysis. *Adv Clin Exp Med* 2012;21:615–619.

575. Totte E, Hendrickx L, Pauwels M, et al. Weight reduction by means of intragastric device: experience with the bioenterics intragastric balloon. *Obes Surg* 2001;11:519–523.

576. Genco A, Cipriano M, Bacci V, et al. BioEnterics Intragastric Balloon (BIB): a short-term double-blind, randomized, controlled, crossover study on weight reduction in morbidly obese patients. *Int J Obes* 2006;30:129–33.

577. Maggard MA, Shugarman LR, Suttorp M, et al. Meta-analysis: surgical treatment of obesity. *Ann Intern Med* 2005;142:547–559.

578. Padwal R, Klarenbach S, Wiebe N, et al. Bariatric surgery: a systematic review and network meta-analysis of randomized trials. *Obes Rev* 2011;12:602–621.

579. Smoot TM, Xu P, Hilsenrath P, et al. Gastric bypass surgery in the United States, 1998–2002. *Am J Public Health* 2006;96:1187–1189.

580. Buchwald H, Oien DM. Metabolic/bariatric surgery worldwide 2011. *Obes Surg* 2013;23(4):427–436.

581. Tsai WC, Tsai LM, Chen JH. Combined use of astemizole and ketoconazole resulting in torsade de pointes. *J Formos Med Assoc* 1997;96:144–146.

582. Kelleher DC, Merrill CT, Cottrell LT, et al. Recent national trends in the use of adolescent inpatient bariatric surgery: 2000 through 2009. *JAMA Pediatr* 2013;167:126.

583. Inge TH, Xanthakos SA, Zeller MH. Bariatric surgery for pediatric extreme obesity: now or later? *Int J Obes* 2007;31:1–14.

584. Till H, Blüher S, Hirsch W, et al. Efficacy of laparoscopic sleeve gastrectomy (LSG) as a stand-alone technique for children with morbid obesity. *Obes Surg* 2008;18:1047.

585. Fatima J, Houghton SG, Iqbal CW, et al. Bariatric surgery at the extremes of age. *J Gastrointest Surg* 2006;10:1392–1396.

586. Hazzan D, Chin EH, Steinhagen E, et al. Laparoscopic bariatric surgery can be safe for treatment of morbid obesity in patients older than 60 years. *Surg Obes Relat Dis* 2006;2:613–616.

587. Yermilov I, McGory ML, Shekelle PW, et al. Appropriateness criteria for bariatric surgery: beyond the NIH guidelines. *Obesity* 2009;17:1521.

588. Consensus development conference panel. Gastrointestinal surgery for severe obesity. *Ann Intern Med* 1991;115:956–961.

589. Burguera B, Agusti A, Arner P, et al. Critical assessment of the current guidelines for the management and treatment of morbidly obese patients. *J Endocrinol Invest* 2007;30:844-852.

590. Pentin PL, Nashelsky J. What are the indications for bariatric surgery? *J Fam Pract* 2005;54:633–634.

591. Santry HP, Gillen DL, Lauderdale DS. Trends in bariatric surgical procedures. *JAMA* 2005;294:1909–1917.

592. Yermilov I, McGory ML, Shekelle PW, et al. Appropriateness criteria for bariatric surgery: beyond the NIH guidelines. *Obesity* 2009;17:1521.

593. Mingrone G, Panunzi S, De Gaetano A, et al. Bariatric surgery versus conventional medical therapy for type 2 diabetes. *N Engl J Med* 2012;366(17):1577–1585.

594. Ludwig DS, Ebbeling CB, Livingston EH. Surgical vs lifestyle treatment for type 2 diabetes. *JAMA* 2012;308(10): 981–982.

595. Oria H. Gastric banding for morbid obesity. *Eur J Gastroenterol Hepatol* 1999;11:105–114.

596. Schirmer B. Laparoscopic bariatric surgery. *Surg Endosc* 2006;20:s450–s455.

597. Buchwald H, Buchwald JN. Evolution of operative procedures for the management of morbid obesity 1950–2000. *Obes Surg* 2002;12:705–717.

598. Buchwald H, Williams SE. Bariatric surgery worldwide 2003. *Obes Surg* 2004;14:1157–1164.

599. American Academy of Family Physicians CME Center. *Bulletin.* Available at http://www.aafp.org/online/en/home/

cme/selfstudy/cmebulletin/bariatric/objectives/article. html; accessed 3/20/07.

600. Gagner M, Deitel M, Kalberer TL, et al. The Second International Consensus Summit for Sleeve Gastrectomy, March 19–21, 2009. *Surg Obes Relat Dis* 2009;5:476.

601. Familiari P, Costamagna G, Blero D, et al. Transoral gastroplasty for morbid obesity: a multicenter trial with a 1-year outcome. *Gastrointest Endosc* 2011;74:1248–1258.

602. Greenway F. Surgery for obesity. *Endocrinol Metab Clin North Am* 1996;25:1005–1027.

603. Brethauer SA, Chand B, Schauer PR. Risks and benefits of bariatric surgery: current evidence. *Cleve Clin J Med* 2006;73:993–1007.

604. Colquitt JL, Picot J, Loveman E, et al. Surgery for obesity. *Cochrane Database Syst Rev* 2009;(2):CD003641.

605. Flum DR, Belle SH, King WC, et al. Perioperative safety in the longitudinal assessment of bariatric surgery. *N Engl J Med* 2009;361:445.

606. Encinosa WE, Bernard DM, Du D, et al. Recent improvements in bariatric surgery outcomes. *Med Care* 2009;47:531.

607. McMahon MM, Sarr MG, Clark MM, et al. Clinical management after bariatric surgery: value of a multidisciplinary approach. *Mayo Clin Proc* 2006;81:s34–s45.

608. Miller AD, Smith KM. Medication and nutrient administration considerations after bariatric surgery. *Am J Health Syst Pharm* 2006;63:1852–1857.

609. Lynch RJ, Eisenberg D, Bell RL. Metabolic consequences of bariatric surgery. *J Clin Gastroenterol* 2006;40:659–668.

610. Fang J. The cost-effectiveness of bariatric surgery. *Am J Gastroenterol* 2003;98:2097–2098.

611. Oklu R, Gunn AJ, Hamilton EJ. A catheter to curb your appetite? A novel observation of weight loss following left gastric artery embolization in humans *RSNA* 2013; Abstract SSA23-01.

612. Mauer MM, Harris RB, Bartness TJ. The regulation of total body fat: lessons learned from lipectomy studies. *Neurosci Biobehav Rev* 2001;25:15–28.

613. Hausman DB, Lu J, Ryan DH, et al. Compensatory growth of adipose tissue after partial lipectomy: involvement of serum factors. *Exp Biol Med* (Maywood) 2004;229:512–520.

614. Coleman WP 4th, Hendry SL 2nd. Principles of liposuction. *Semin Cutan Med Surg* 2006;25:138–144.

615. Yoho RA, Romaine JJ, O'Neil D. Review of the liposuction, abdominoplasty, and face-lift mortality and morbidity risk literature. *Dermatol Surg* 2005;31:733–743; discussion 743.

616. Grazer FM, de Jong RH. Fatal outcomes from liposuction: census survey of cosmetic surgeons. *Plast Reconstr Surg* 2000;105:436–446; discussion 447–438.

617. Housman TS, Lawrence N, Mellen BG, et al. The safety of liposuction: results of a national survey. *Dermatol Surg* 2002;28:971–978.

618. Commons GW, Halperin B, Chang CC. Large-volume liposuction: a review of 625 consecutive cases over 12 years. *Plast Reconstr Surg* 2001;108:1753–1763; discussion 1764–1757.

619. Council on Scientific Affairs. Treatment of obesity in adults. *JAMA* 1988;260:2547–2551.

620. Saris W. Very-low-calorie diets and sustained weight loss. *Obes Res* 2001;9:295s–301s.

621. Finer N. Low-calorie diets and sustained weight loss. *Obes Res* 2001;9:290s–294s.

622. Molokhia M. Obesity wars: a pilot study of very low calorie diets in obese patients in general practice. *Br J Gen Pract* 1998;48:1251–1252.

623. Pekkarinen T, Mustajoki P. Use of very low-calorie diet in preoperative weight loss: efficacy and safety. *Obes Res* 1997;5:595–602.

624. Kansanen M, Vanninen E, Tuunainen A, et al. The effect of a very low-calorie diet-induced weight loss on the severity of obstructive sleep apnoea and autonomic nervous function in obese patients with obstructive sleep apnoea syndrome. *Clin Physiol* 1998;18:377–385.

625. Ryttig K, Flaten H, Rossner S. Long-term effects of a very low calorie diet (Nutrilett) in obesity treatment. A prospective, randomized, comparison between VLCD and a hypocaloric diet+behavior modification and their combination. *Int J Obes Relat Metab Disord* 1997;21:574–579.

626. Johansson K, Neovius M, Hemmingsson E. Effects of anti-obesity drugs, diet, and exercise on weight-loss maintenance after a very-low-calorie diet or low-calorie diet: a systematic review and meta-analysis of randomized controlled trials. *Am J Clin Nutr* 2014;99(1):14–23.

627. Gilden Tsai A, Wadden TA. The evolution of very-low-calorie diets: an update and meta-analysis. *Obesity* 2006;14:1283–1293.

628. Tsai AG, Wadden TA. Systematic review: an evaluation of major commercial weight loss programs in the United States. *Ann Intern Med* 2005;142:56–66.

629. Klem ML, Wing RR, McGuire MT, et al. A descriptive study of individuals successful at long-term maintenance of substantial weight loss. *Am J Clin Nutr* 1997;66(2):239–246.

630. Grodstein F, Levine R, Troy L, et al. Three year follow up of participants in a commercial weight loss program. *Arch Intern Med* 1996;156:1302–1306.

631. Spielman A, Kanders B, Kienholz M, et al. The cost of losing: an analysis of commercial weight-loss programs in a metropolitan area. *J Am Coll Nutr* 1992;11:36–41.

632. Wadden T, Frey D. A multicenter evaluation of a proprietary weight loss program for the treatment of marked obesity: a five-year follow-up. *Int J Eat Disord* 1997;22:203–212.

633. Lowe M, Miller-Kovach K, Frye N, et al. An initial evaluation of a commercial weight loss program: short-term effects on weight, eating behavior, and mood. *Obes Res* 1999;7:51–59.

634. Wolfe B. Long-term maintenance following attainment of goal weight: a preliminary investigation. *Addict Behav* 1992;17:469–477.

635. Laddu D, Dow C, Hingle M, et al. A review of evidence-based strategies to treat obesity in adults. *Nutr Clin Pract* 2011;26(5):512–525.

636. Huelsing J, Kanafani N, Mao J, et al. Camp jump start: effects of a residential summer weight-loss camp for older children and adolescents. *Pediatrics* 2010;125: e884–e890.

637. Tsai AG, Wadden TA, Womble LG, et al. Commercial and self-help programs for weight control. *Psychiatr Clin North Am* 2005;28:ix,171–192.

638. Witherspoon B, Rosenzweig M. Industry-sponsored weight loss programs: description, cost, and effectiveness. *J Am Acad Nurse Pract* 2004;16:198–205.

639. Volkmar FR, Stunkard AJ, Woolston J, et al. High attrition rates in commercial weight reduction programs. *Arch Intern Med* 1981;141:426–428.

640. Linde JA, Jeffery RW, French SA, et al. Self-weighing in weight gain prevention and weight loss trials. *Ann Behav Med* 2005;30:210–216.

641. Wing RR, Tate DF, Gorin AA, et al. A self-regulation program for maintenance of weight loss. *N Engl J Med* 2006;355:1563–1571.

642. Brown T, Avenell A, Edmunds LD, et al. Systematic review of long-term lifestyle interventions to prevent weight gain and morbidity in adults. *Obes Rev* 2009;10(6):627–638.

643. Swinburn BA, Woollard GA, Chang EC, et al. Effects of reduced-fat diets consumed ad libitum on intake of nutrients, particularly antioxidant vitamins. *J Am Diet Assoc* 1999;99:1400–1405.

644. Blanck HM, Serdula MK, Gillespie C, et al. Use of nonprescription dietary supplements for weight loss is common among Americans. *J Am Diet Assoc* 2007;107:441–447.

645. Blanck HM, Khan LK, Serdula MK. Use of nonprescription weight loss products: results from a multistate survey. *JAMA* 2001;286:930–935.

646. Nachtigal MC, Patterson RE, Stratton KL, et al. Dietary supplements and weight control in a middle-age population. *J Altern Complement Med* 2005;11:909–915.

647. Shekelle PG, Hardy ML, Morton SC, et al. Efficacy and safety of ephedra and ephedrine for weight loss and athletic performance: a meta-analysis. *JAMA* 2003;289:1537–1545.

648. US Food and Drug Administration. *Sales of supplements containing ephedrine alkaloids (ephedra) prohibited.* Available at http://www.fda.gov/oc/initiatives/ephedra/february2004.

649. Federal Trade Commission. *FTC releases report on weight-loss advertising.* September 17, 2002. Available at http://www.ftc.gov/opa/2002/09/weightlossrpt.shtm; accessed 9/21/07.

650. Jurgens TM, Whelan AM, Killian L, et al. Green tea for weight loss and weight maintenance in overweight or obese adults. *Cochrane Database Syst Rev* 2012;12:CD008650.

651. Tian H, Guo X, Want X, et al. Chromium picolinate supplementation for overweight or obese adults. *Cochrane Database Syst Rev* 2013;11:CD010063.

652. Lukaski HC, Siders WA, Penland JG. Chromium picolinate supplementation in women: effects on body weight, composition, and iron status. *Nutrition* 2007;23:187–195.

653. Bhattacharya A, Rahman MM, McCarter R, et al. Conjugated linoleic acid and chromium lower body weight and visceral fat mass in high-fat-diet-fed mice. *Lipids* 2006;41:437–444.

654. Martin J, Wang ZQ, Zhang XH, et al. Chromium picolinate supplementation attenuates body weight gain and increases insulin sensitivity in subjects with type 2 diabetes. *Diabetes Care* 2006;29:1826–1832.

655. National Institutes of Health Office of Dietary Supplements. *Dietary supplement fact sheet: chromium.* Available at http://ods.od.nih.gov/factsheets/chromium.asp; accessed 9/21/07.

656. Avula B, Wang YH, Pawar RS, et al. Determination of the appetite suppressant P57 in Hoodia gordonii plant extracts and dietary supplements by liquid chromatography/electrospray ionization mass spectrometry (LC-MSD-TOF) and LC-UV methods. *J AOAC Int* 2006;89:606–611.

657. Astell KJ, Mathai ML, Su XQ. Plant extracts with appetite suppressing properties for body weight control: a systematic review of double blind randomized controlled clinical trials. *Complement Ther Med* 2013;21:407–416.

658. Hoodia: lose weight without feeling hungry? *Consum Rep* 2006;71:49.

659. Larsen TM, Toubro S, Astrup A. Efficacy and safety of dietary supplements containing CLA for the treatment of obesity: evidence from animal and human studies. *J Lipid Res* 2003;44:2234–2241.

660. Riserus U, Smedman A, Basu S, et al. CLA and body weight regulation in humans. *Lipids* 2003;38:133–137.

661. Belury MA, Mahon A, Banni S. The conjugated linoleic acid (CLA) isomer, t10c12-CLA, is inversely associated with changes in body weight and serum leptin in subjects with type 2 diabetes mellitus. *J Nutr* 2003;133:257s–260s.

662. Westerterp-Plantenga MS. Fat intake and energy-balance effects. *Physiol Behav* 2004;83:579–585.

663. Silveira MB, Carraro R, Monereo S, et al. Conjugated linoleic acid (CLA) and obesity. *Public Health Nutr* 2007;10:1181–1186.

664. Azain MJ, Hausman DB, Sisk MB, et al. Dietary conjugated linoleic acid reduces rat adipose tissue cell size rather than cell number. *J Nutr* 2000;130:1548–54.

665. Close RN, Schoeller DA, Watras AC, et al. Conjugated linoleic acid supplementation alters the 6-mo change in fat oxidation during sleep. *Am J Clin Nutr* 2007;86:797–804.

666. Castro-Webb N, Ruiz-Narvaez EA, Campos H. Cross-sectional study of conjugated linoleic acid in adipose tissue and risk of diabetes. *Am J Clin Nutr* 2012;96:175–181.

667. Shahar DR, Abel R, Elhayany A, et al. Does dairy calcium intake enhance weight loss among overweight diabetic patients? *Diabetes Care* 2007;30:485–489.

668. Major GC, Alarie F, Dore J, et al. Supplementation with calcium + vitamin D enhances the beneficial effect of weight loss on plasma lipid and lipoprotein concentrations. *Am J Clin Nutr* 2007;85:54–59.

669. Harvey-Berino J, Gold BC, Lauber R, et al. The impact of calcium and dairy product consumption on weight loss. *Obes Res* 2005;13:1720–1726.

670. Zemel MB, Richards J, Milstead A, et al. Effects of calcium and dairy on body composition and weight loss in African-American adults. *Obes Res* 2005;13:1218–1225.

671. Bowen J, Noakes M, Clifton PM. Effect of calcium and dairy foods in high protein, energy-restricted diets on weight loss and metabolic parameters in overweight adults. *Int J Obes* 2005;29:957–965.

672. Zemel MB, Thompson W, Milstead A, et al. Calcium and dairy acceleration of weight and fat loss during energy restriction in obese adults. *Obes Res* 2004;12:582–590.

673. Jones KW, Eller LK, Parnell JA, et al. Effects of a dairy- and calcium-rich diet on weight loss and appetite during energy restriction in overweight and obese adults: a randomized trial. *Eur J Clin Nutr* 2013;67:371–376.

674. Gulvady A, Ciolino H, Cabrera R, et al. Resveratrol inhibits the deleterious effects of diet-induced obesity on thymic function. *J Nutr Biochem* 2013;24:1625–1633.

675. Szkudelska K, Szkudelski T. Resveratrol, obesity and diabetes. *Eur J Pharmacol* 2010;635:1–8.

676. Kim S, Jin Y, Choi Y, et al. Resveratrol exerts anti-obesity effects via mechanisms involving down-regulation of adipogenic and inflammatory processes in mice. *Biochem Pharm* 2011;81:1343–1351.

677. Suter P, Schutz Y, Jequier E. The effect of ethanol on fat storage in healthy subjects. *N Engl J Med* 1992;326:983–987.

678. Lesser LI, Ebbeling CB, Goozner M, et al. Relationship between funding source and conclusion among nutrition-related scientific articles. *PLoS Med* 2007;4:e5.

679. Malik VS, Schulze MB, Hu FB. Intake of sugar-sweetened beverages and weight gain: a systematic review. *Am J Clin Nutr* 2006;84:274–288.

680. Basu S, McKee M, Galea G, et al. Relationship of soft drink consumption to global overweight, obesity, and diabetes: a cross-national analysis of 75 countries. *Am J Public Health* 2013;103:2071–2077.

681. Ebbeling CB, Feldman HA, Osganian SK, et al. Effects of decreasing sugar-sweetened beverage consumption on body weight in adolescents: a randomized, controlled pilot study. *Pediatrics* 2006;117:673–680.

682. Boutelle KN, Libbey H, Neumark-Sztainer D, et al. Weight control strategies of overweight adolescents who successfully lost weight. *J Am Diet Assoc* 2009;109:2029-2035.

683. Yang Q. Gain weight by "going diet?" Artificial sweeteners and the neurobiology of sugar cravings. *Yale J Biol Med* 2010;83:101–108.

684. Mulhisen L, Rogers J. Complementary and alternative modes of therapy for the treatment of the obese patient. *J Am Osteopath Assoc* 1999;99:s8–s12.

685. Abdi H, Abbasi-Parizad P, Zhao B, et al. Effects of auricular acupuncture on anthropometric, lipid profile, inflammatory, and immunologic markers: a randomized controlled trial study. *J Altern Complement Med* 2012;18:668–677.

686. Cho SH, Lee JS, Thabane L, et al. Acupuncture for obesity: a systematic review and meta-analysis. *Int J Obes* 2009;33:183–196.

687. Institute of Medicine. *Nutrition during pregnancy*. Washington, DC: National Academy Press, 1990.

688. Butman M. *Prenatal nutrition: a clinical manual*. Boston, MA: Massachusetts Department of Public Health, 1982.

689. Dimperio D. *Prenatal nutrition. Clinical guidelines for nurses*. White Plains, NY: March of Dimes Birth Defects Foundation, 1988.

690. Bracero L, Byrne D. Optimal weight gain during singleton pregnancy. *Gynecol Obstet Invest* 1998;46:9–16.

691. Edwards LE, Hellerstedt WL, Alton IR, et al. Pregnancy complications and birth outcomes in obese and normal-weight women: effects of gestational weight change. *Obstet Gynecol* 1996;87:389–394.

692. Abrams B, Laros R. Prepregnancy weight, weight gain, and birth weight. *Am J Obstet Gynecol* 1986;155:918.

693. Institute of Medicine. Weight gain during pregnancy: re-examining the guidelines. Report Brief: May 2009.

694. Lovelady CA, Garner KE, Moreno KL, et al. The effect of weight loss in overweight, lactating women on the growth of their infants. *N Engl J Med* 2000;342:449–453.

695. Nehring I, Schmoll S, Beyerlein A, et al. Gestational weight gain and long-term postpartum weight retention: a meta-analysis. *Am J Clin Nutr* 2011;94:1225–1231.

696. Butte N. Dieting and exercise in overweight, lactating women. *N Engl J Med* 2000;342:502–503.

697. Galtier-Dereure F, Montpeyroux F, Boulot P, et al. Weight excess before pregnancy: complications and cost. *Int J Obes Relat Metab Disord* 1995;19:443–448.

698. Ratner RE, Hamner LH 3rd, Isada NB. Effects of gestational weight gain in morbidly obese women: I. Maternal morbidity. *Am J Perinatol* 1991;8:21–24.

699. Tomoda S, Tamura T, Sudo Y, et al. Effects of obesity on pregnant women: maternal hemodynamic change. *Am J Perinatol* 1996;13:73–78.

700. Parker JD, Abrams B. Prenatal weight gain advice: an examination of the recent prenatal weight gain recommendations of the Institute of Medicine. *Obstet Gynecol* 1992;79:664–669.

701. Morin KH. Obese and nonobese postpartum women: complications, body image, and perceptions of the intrapartal experience. *Appl Nurs Res* 1995;8:81–87.

702. Cogswell ME, Serdula MK, Hungerford DW, et al. Gestational weight gain among average-weight and overweight women—what is excessive? *Am J Obstet Gynecol* 1995;172:705–712.

703. Edwards LE, Dickes WF, Alton IR, et al. Pregnancy in the massively obese: course, outcome, and obesity prognosis of the infant. *Am J Obstet Gynecol* 1978;131:479–483.

704. Garbaciak J, Richter M, Miller S, et al. Maternal weight and pregnancy complications. *Am J Ostet Gynecol* 1985;152:238–245.

705. Kliegman R, Gross T, Morton S, et al. Intrauterine growth and postnatal fasting metabolism in infants of obese mothers. *J Pediatr* 1984;104:601–607.

706. Kliegman R, Gross T. Perinatal problems of the obese mother and her infant. *Obstet Gynecol* 1985;66:299–306.

707. Ekblad U, Grenman S. Maternal weight, weight gain during pregnancy and pregnancy outcome. *Int J Gynaecol Obstet* 1992;39:277–283.

708. Crane SS, Wojtowycz MA, Dye TD, et al. Association between pre-pregnancy obesity and the risk of cesarean delivery. *Obstet Gynecol* 1997;89:213–216.

709. Isaacs JD, Magann EF, Martin RW, et al. Obstetric challenges of massive obesity complicating pregnancy. *J Perinatol* 1994;14:10–14.

710. Perlow JH, Morgan MA, Montgomery D, et al. Perinatal outcome in pregnancy complicated by massive obesity. *Am J Obstet Gynecol* 1992;167:958–962.

711. Calandra C, Abell DA, Beischer NA. Maternal obesity in pregnancy. *Obstet Gynecol* 1981;57:8–12.

712. Martens MG, Kolrud BL, Faro S, et al. Development of wound infection or separation after cesarean delivery. Prospective evaluation of 2,431 cases. *J Reprod Med* 1995;40:171–175.

713. Werler MM, Louik C, Shapiro S, et al. Prepregnant weight in relation to risk of neural tube defects (see comments). *JAMA* 1996;275:1089–1092.

714. Shaw GM, Velie EM, Schaffer D. Risk of neural tube defect-affected pregnancies among obese women (see comments). *JAMA* 1996;275:1093–1096.

715. Prentice A, Goldberg G. Maternal obesity increases congenital malformations. *Nutr Rev* 1996;54:146–150.

716. Carter JP, Furman T, Hutcheson HR. Preeclampsia and reproductive performance in a community of vegans. *South Med J* 1987;80:692–697.

717. Baker PN. Possible dietary measures in the prevention of pre-eclampsia and eclampsia. *Clin Obstet Gynecol* 1995;9:497–507.

718. Denison F, Norwood P, Bhattacharya S, et al. Association between maternal body mass index during pregnancy, short-term morbidity, and increased health service costs: a population-based study. *BJOG* 2014;121:72–82.

719. Hood DD, Dewan DM. Anesthetic and obstetric outcome in morbidly obese parturients. *Anesthesiology* 1993;79: 1210–1218.

720. http://www.ncbi.nlm.nih.gov/pubmed/22574949.

721. Baker JL, Gamborg M, Heitmann BL, et al. Breastfeeding reduces postpartum weight retention. *Am J Clin Nutr* 2008;88:1543–1551.

722. Kramer MS, Matush L, Vanilovich I, et al. Effects of prolonged and exclusive breastfeeding on child height, weight, adiposity, and blood pressure at age 6.5 y: evidence from a large, randomized trial. *Am J Clin Nutr* 2007;86:1717–1721.

723. Martin RM, Patel R, Kramer MS, et al. Effects of promoting longer-term and exclusive breastfeeding on adiposity and insulin-like growth factor-I at age 11.5 years: a randomized trial. *JAMA* 2013;309:1005–1013.

724. Epstein LH, Valoski A, McCurley J. Effect of weight loss by obese children on long-term growth. *Am J Dis Child* 1993;147:1076–1080.

725. Epstein LH, Valoski AM, Kalarchian MA, et al. Do children lose and maintain weight easier than adults: a comparison of child and parent weight changes from six months to ten years. *Obes Res* 1995;3:411–417.

726. Goldschmidt AB, Wilfley DE, Paluch RA, et al. Indicated prevention of adult obesity: how much weight change in necessary for normalization of weight status in children? *JAMA Pediatr* 2013;167:21–26.

727. Dietz WH. Therapeutic strategies in childhood obesity. *Horm Res* 1993;39:86–90.

728. Williams CL, Bollella M, Carter BJ. Treatment of childhood obesity in pediatric practice. *Ann N Y Acad Sci* 1993;699:207–219.

729. Bocca G, Corpeleijn E, Stolk RP, et al. Results of a multidisciplinary treatment program in 3-year-old to 5-year-old overweight or obese children: a randomized controlled clinical trial. *Arch Pediatr Adolesc Med* 2012;166:1109–1115.

730. Glenny AM, O'Meara S, Melville A, et al. The treatment and prevention of obesity: a systematic review of the literature. *Int J Obes Relat Metab Disord* 1997;21:715–737.

731. Janicke DM, Sallinen BJ, Perri MG, et al. Comparison of parent-only vs family-based interventions for overweight children in underserved rural settings: outcomes from project STORY. *Arch Pediatr Adolesc Med* 2008;162:119–125.

732. Woodard GA, Encarnacion B, Peraza J, et al. Halo effect for bariatric surgery: collateral weight loss in patients' family members. *Arch Surg* 2011;146:1185–1190.

733. Showell NN, Fawole O, Segal J, et al. A systematic review of home-based childhood obesity prevention studies. *Pediatrics* 2013;132:193–200.

734. Wang L, Dalton WT 3rd, Schetzina KE, et al. Home food environment, dietary intake, and weight among overweight and obese children in Southern Appalachia. *South Med J* 2013;106:550–557.

735. Wansink B, Shimizu M, Brumberg A. Association of nutrient-dense snack combinations with calories and vegetable intake. *Pediatrics* 2013;131:22–29.

736. Robinson TN. Reducing children's television viewing to prevent obesity: a randomized controlled trial. *JAMA* 1999;282:1561–1567.

737. http://health.usnews.com/health-news/blogs/eat-run/2013/01/11/school-over-scalpels.

738. Schonfeld-Warden N, Warden CH. Pediatric obesity. An overview of etiology and treatment. *Pediatr Clin North Am* 1997;44:339–361.

739. Kelly AS, Barlow SE, Rao G, et al. Severe obesity in children and adolescents: identification, associated health risks, and treatment approaches: a scientific statement from the American Heart Association. *Circulation* 2013;128:1689.

740. Stevens J, Kumanyika SK, Keil JE. Attitudes toward body size and dieting: differences between elderly black and white women. *Am J Public Health* 1994;84:1322–1325.

741. Caldwell MB, Brownell KD, Wilfley DE. Relationship of weight, body dissatisfaction, and self-esteem in African American and white female dieters. *Int J Eat Disord* 1997;22:127–130.

742. Neff LJ, Sargent RG, McKeown RE, et al. Black–white differences in body size perceptions and weight management practices among adolescent females. *J Adolesc Health* 1997;20:459–465.

743. Thompson SH, Sargent RG. Black and white women's weight-related attitudes and parental criticism of their childhood appearance. *Women Health* 2000;30:77–92.

744. Anderson LA, Eyler AA, Galuska DA, et al. Relationship of satisfaction with body size and trying to lose weight in a national survey of overweight and obese women aged 40 and older, United States. *Prev Med* 2002;35:390–396.

745. Perez M, Joiner TE Jr. Body image dissatisfaction and disordered eating in black and white women. *Int J Eat Disord* 2003;33:342–350.

746. Akan GE, Grilo CM. Sociocultural influences on eating attitudes and behaviors, body image, and psychological functioning: a comparison of African-American, Asian-American, and Caucasian college women. *Int J Eat Disord* 1995;18:181–187.

747. Ashworth M, Clement S, Wright M. Demand, appropriateness and prescribing of "lifestyle drugs": a consultation survey in general practice. *Fam Pract* 2002;19:236–241.

748. Lexchin J. Lifestyle drugs: issues for debate. *CMAJ* 2001;164:1449–1451.

749. Mitka M. Surgery for obesity: demand soars amid scientific, ethical questions. *JAMA* 2003;289:1761–1762.

750. Puhl R, Brownell KD. Ways of coping with obesity stigma: review and conceptual analysis. *Eat Behav* 2003;4:53–78.

751. Puhl RM, Brownell KD. Psychosocial origins of obesity stigma: toward changing a powerful and pervasive bias. *Obes Rev* 2003;4:213–227.

752. Latner JD, Stunkard AJ. Getting worse: the stigmatization of obese children. *Obes Res* 2003;11:452–456.

753. Kappagoda CT, Hyson DA, Amsterdam EA. Low-carbohydrate-high-protein diets: is there a place for them in clinical cardiology? *J Am Coll Cardiol* 2004;43:725–730.

754. Kong A, Beresford SA, Alfano CM, et al. Associations between snacking and weight loss and nutrient intake among postmenopausal overweight to obese women

in a dietary weight-loss intervention. *J Am Diet Assoc* 2011;111:1898–1903.

755. Jenkins D, Wolever T, Vuksan V, et al. Nibbling versus gorging: metabolic advantages of increased meal frequency. *N Engl J Med* 1989;321:929–934.

756. Speechly D, Rogers G, Buffenstein R. Acute appetite reduction associated with an increased frequency of eating in obese males. *Int J Obes Relat Metab Disord* 1999;23:1151–1159.

757. Bellisle F, McDevitt R, Prentice A. Meal frequency and energy balance. *Br J Nutr* 1997;77:s57–s70.

758. Drummond S, Crombie N, Kirk T. A critique of the effects of snacking on body weight status. *Eur J Clin Nutr* 1996;50:779–783.

759. Fox K. The influence of physical activity on mental well-being. *Public Health Nutr* 1999;2:411–418.

760. Miller W, Koceja D, Hamilton E. A meta-analysis of the past 25 years of weight loss research using diet, exercise or diet plus exercise intervention. *Int J Obes Relat Metab Disord* 1997;21:941–947.

761. Hooper L, Abdelhamid A, Moore HJ, et al. Effect of reducing total fat intake on body weight: systematic review and meta-analysis of clinical trials and cohort studies. *BMJ* 2012;345:e7666.

762. Kristal A, White E, Shattuck A, et al. Long-term maintenance of a low-fat diet: durability of fat-related dietary habits in the Women's Health Trial. *J Am Diet Assoc* 1992;92:553–559.

763. http://www.iom.edu/Reports/2012/Accelerating-Progress-in-Obesity-Prevention.aspx.

764. Wing RR, Jeffery RW. Food provision as a strategy to promote weight loss. *Obes Res* 2001;9:271s–275s.

765. Jeffery RW, Wing RR. Long-term effects of interventions for weight loss using food provision and monetary incentives. *J Consult Clin Psychol* 1995;63:793–796.

766. Rapoport L, Clark M, Wardle J. Evaluation of a modified cognitive-behavioural programme for weight management. *Int J Obes Relat Metab Disord* 2000;24:1726–1737.

767. Harvey-Berino J. The efficacy of dietary fat vs. total energy restriction for weight loss. *Obes Res* 1998;6:202–207.

768. Epstein LH. Family-based behavioural intervention for obese children. *Int J Obes Relat Metab Disord* 1996;20:s14–s21.

769. Torgerson JS, Lissner L, Lindroos AK, et al. VLCD plus dietary and behavioural support versus support alone in the treatment of severe obesity. A randomised two-year clinical trial. *Int J Obes Relat Metab Disord* 1997;21:987–994.

770. Wadden T, Foster G, Letizia K. One-year behavioral treatment of obesity: comparison of moderate and severe caloric restriction and the effects of weight maintenance therapy. *J Consult Clin Psychol* 1994;62:165–171.

771. Chanmugam P, Guthrie JF, Cecilio S, et al. Did fat intake in the United States really decline between 1989–1991 and 1994–1996? *J Am Diet Assoc* 2003;103:867–872.

772. Heitmann BL, Lissner L, Osler M. Do we eat less fat, or just report so? *Int J Obes Relat Metab Disord* 2000;24:435–442.

773. Pirozzo S, Summerbell C, Cameron C, et al. Advice on low-fat diets for obesity. *Cochrane Database Syst Rev* 2002;CD003640.

774. Kok FJ, Kromhout D. Epidemiological studies on the health effects of a Mediterranean diet. *Eur J Nutr* 2004;43:12–15.

775. Pollan M. The age of nutritionism: How scientists have ruined the way we eat. *The New York Times Magazine* 2007. Available at http://www.nytimes.com/2007/01/28/magazine/28nutritionism.t.html?ei=5090&en=...&pagewanted=all.

776. Westerterp-Plantenga MS, Lejeune MP, Nijs I, et al. High protein intake sustains weight maintenance after body weight loss in humans. *Int J Obes Relat Metab Disord* 2004;28:57–64.

777. Katz D. Diet, obesity, and weight regulation. In: Katz DL. *Nutrition in clinical practice*. Philadelphia, PA: Lippincott Williams & Wilkins, 2000:37–62.

CHAPTER 6

Diet, Diabetes Mellitus, and Insulin Resistance

The role of dietary management of both type 1 and type 2 diabetes mellitus has been conclusively established. Although patients with type 1 diabetes require exogenous insulin, their glycemic control and the occurrence of diabetes-related complications are related to dietary factors. Most dietary recommendations for diabetes pertain to both types. The one important difference is the need in type 1 diabetes to maintain a very predictable dietary pattern corresponding to a particular insulin regimen. It has been suggested that Alzheimer's disease represents "type 3 diabetes" (1) and may be due in part to chronic insulin resistance and insulin deficiency in the brain (see Chapter 35). Although type 2 diabetes is not sufficient to cause Alzheimer's disease, it may contribute to its pathogenesis or enhance progression, and diabetes medications may have a therapeutic role for dementia (1).

Of the approximately 26 million cases of diabetes in the United States, 90% of adult cases are type 2 (2), and 90% of those patients are overweight (see Chapter 5). Prevalence of diabetes more than doubled between 1990 and 2011 among adults in every age group (3). Among US adolescents, the prevalence of prediabetes and diabetes combined increased from 9% in 1999–2000 to 23% in 2007–2008 (4). In 2002 to 2003, just 3% of diabetes cases in children ages 5 to 9 were type 2, but this figure increased to 24% among 10- to 14-year-olds and nearly 50% among adolescents ages 15 to 19 (5). Incidence of type 1 diabetes in youth has also increased during the last several years in most parts of the world, though the reasons for this trend are not known (6).

Weight control is a fundamental objective in the dietary management of all overweight diabetic patients (see Chapter 5). Whereas traditional approaches to diabetes have focused on exchange lists, and more recently on the glycemic index (GI) of individual foods, attention is increasingly being focused on the effects of foods in combinations and on the overall dietary pattern. There is emerging consensus that the glycemic load (GL) of the diet is one useful gauge of dietary quality of particular relevance to diabetes management and prevention. The pathogenesis of the insulin-resistance syndrome continues to be investigated, as does debate over its defining characteristics and nomenclature. Nonetheless, there is widespread recognition that insulin resistance is increasingly prevalent, affecting up to 50% of overweight adults and 25% of overweight children and adolescents (see Chapter 5). There is at least suggestive evidence that obesity is necessary, if not sufficient, for the development of the insulin-resistance syndrome in most cases (7). Whether an interaction between genetic susceptibility to insulin resistance and particular dietary patterns leads to obesity is less certain.

Insulin resistance and states of impaired glucose metabolism, including both impaired glucose tolerance (IGT) and impaired fasting glucose (IFG), constitute antecedents to type 2 diabetes. The Diabetes Prevention Program has provided definitive evidence that a lifestyle intervention predicated on healthful diet and regular physical activity can forestall the development of diabetes in the majority of such cases. Perhaps no condition offers better testimony than diabetes to the powerful, potential role of food as medicine.

OVERVIEW

Diagnostic Criteria for Diabetes Mellitus

A fasting blood glucose level of 126 mg per dL or greater defines diabetes mellitus (8). When hyperglycemia occurs in childhood as a result of total or nearly total loss of insulin output, the condition is defined as type 1 diabetes. When hyperglycemia results from inadequate insulin action rather than primary β-cell failure, the condition is defined as type 2 diabetes. There is increasing appreciation for hybrid forms of diabetes that encompass features of both type 1 and type 2 as well (2,9).

Epidemiology of Diabetes Mellitus

In the United States, there are some 25.8 million diabetics, of whom roughly 18.8 million are diagnosed and the remainder undiagnosed (10,11). The ratio of diagnosed to undiagnosed diabetes has declined slightly over recent years among the overweight, apparently in response to heightened awareness of diabetes risk in this group (11). More than 90% of the diagnosed cases and virtually all of the undiagnosed cases of diabetes are type 2. Prediabetes, encompassing both IGT; (a blood sugar level of 140 to 199 mg per dL after a 2-hour oral glucose tolerance test) and IFG; (blood sugar level of 100 to 125 mg per dL after an overnight fast), affects some 79 million Americans (10). The metabolic or insulin-resistance syndrome now affects nearly one-fourth of US adults, (12,13).

The World Health Organization estimates that there were approximately 347 million diabetics worldwide as of 2012, and it projects that diabetes deaths will increase by two thirds between 2008 and 2030 (14). Projections in the United States suggest that nearly 1 in 3 individuals born in the year 2000 or after will develop diabetes in their lifetime, and for Hispanics, the figure is nearly 1 in 2 (15–17).

Pathogenesis of Diabetes Mellitus

Type 1 Diabetes Mellitus
Type 1, or insulin-dependent, diabetes mellitus is due to pancreatic β-cell dysfunction or destruction, generally considered the result of an autoimmune process (18). Although the inciting event or exposure is not known with certainty, there is some, albeit controversial, evidence that early exposure to bovine milk proteins in predisposed individuals may play a role (19–22). Wheat gluten has been proposed as an alternative precipitant, and vitamin D and early childhood immune stimulation by infectious agents have been suggested to be protective (23). In contrast to some

early infectious exposures that may attenuate risk, there is an association between enterovirus infection and increased risk (19). There is general consensus that type 1 diabetes is the product of gene/environment interaction and that control of environmental triggers might prevent the disease. In general, however, there is little to suggest that dietary interventions can be used to prevent type 1 diabetes. While a protective role of breastfeeding is intuitive on the basis of prevailing theories of pathogenesis, the evidence to date is largely inconclusive (19,23–27). Discussed later in this chapter, disruptions in the microbiome may also be contributing factors.

Insulin Resistance and Type 2 Diabetes Mellitus
The fundamental distinction between type 1 and type 2 diabetes, at times blurred, is the preservation of endogenous insulin production in type 2. This distinction results in the susceptibility of type 1, but not type 2, diabetics to ketoacidosis. Severely uncontrolled hyperglycemia in type 2 diabetics generally leads instead to nonketotic, hyperosmolar coma, with ketone body production representing the effect of absent insulin-mediated glucose transport.

The development of type 2 diabetes results from the interplay of genetic susceptibility and environmental factors (28). The responsible genes have not been identified with certainty, although multiple alleles are almost certainly involved, and certain candidate mutations have been under study for some time (29). The clustering of type 2 diabetes in families is well established. Interest in genetic susceptibility to type 2 diabetes dates at least to the early 1960s, when James Neel (30), who went on to head the human genome project, speculated that expression of diabetes was due to the confrontation of a thrifty metabolism designed for dietary subsistence with a world of nutritional abundance. The theory of metabolic thriftiness essentially posits that a brisk insulin release in response to ingestion is advantageous in the utilization and storage of food energy when such energy is only sporadically available. The same brisk response in the context of abundantly available nutrient energy leads to hyperinsulinemia, obesity, insulin resistance, and, ultimately with the advent of β-cell failure, diabetes. The thrifty genotype theory is supported by certain lines of evidence but is far from universally accepted and continues to generate considerable interest and debate (31–36).

Factors associated with expression of the disease include excessive nutrient energy intake with resultant obesity, physical inactivity, and advancing age. These factors contribute to the development of insulin resistance at the receptor, an often key element in the development of type 2 diabetes mellitus. Physical activity appears to protect against the advent of type 2 diabetes mellitus both independently and by preventing and mitigating weight gain and obesity (37). As with type 1 diabetes, the microbiome is currently the subject of much research for its potential role in the pathophysiology of both obesity and type 2 diabetes, and is discussed later in this chapter.

Insulin resistance generally precedes, by an uncertain and probably variable period of time, the development of diabetes, although type 2 diabetes can develop in the absence of insulin resistance (38–40). Diabetes generally occurs when receptor-mediated resistance is compounded by β-cell dysfunction and reduced insulin secretion. Basal insulin production in a healthy, lean adult is roughly 20 to 30 units per 24-hour period. In insulin resistance, that output may be as much as quadrupled to maintain euglycemia. Type 2 diabetes following insulin resistance indicates the failure of β-cells to sustain supraphysiologic output of insulin, a decline of insulin output to below normal levels, and the consequent advent of hyperglycemia (41,42). Whereas type 1 diabetes is associated with nearly absent insulin release (0 to 4 units daily), type 2 diabetes is generally thought to emerge in lean individuals when production falls to approximately 14 units per day.

An association between weight gain and the development of diabetes is supported by prospective cohort studies (43–45), although insulin resistance may contribute to the development of obesity as well, so that causality may be bidirectional (46). Data from such sources suggest that weight loss is protective against the development of diabetes. The currently worsening epidemic of obesity in the United States suggests that the prevalence of diabetes will likely rise and that efforts to combat obesity, if ultimately successful, will translate into reduced rates of diabetes as well (see Chapter 5).

The incidence of type 2 diabetes in the pediatric population parallels the increase in pediatric obesity (47). Less than a generation ago,

type 2 diabetes was called "adult-onset" diabetes to distinguish it from "juvenile onset" diabetes. In the span of less than a generation, what was a chronic disease of midlife has become an increasingly routine pediatric diagnosis (48–50).

The Adult Treatment Panel of the National Cholesterol Education Program essentially equates diabetes with established coronary disease in its guidance for cardiac risk factor management (51). With adult-onset diabetes now seen in children younger than age 10, we may anticipate the emergence of cardiovascular disease (CVD) in ever younger individuals (52,53) (see Chapters 5 and 7).

The development and manifestations of insulin resistance relate to the principal actions of insulin. In the liver, insulin inhibits gluconeogenesis, inhibits glycogenolysis, and promotes glycogen production (54). In muscle and adipose tissue, insulin facilitates the uptake of glucose, as well as its use and storage. Insulin exerts important influences on protein and lipid metabolism as well.

The fundamental role of insulin is to coordinate the use and storage of food energy. This requires regulation of both carbohydrate and fat metabolism, as total body glycogen and glucose stores in a healthy adult approximate 300 g. At 4 kcal per g, this represents an energy reserve of 1,200 kcal, enough to support a fast of approximately 12 to 18 hours. Energy stored as triglyceride in adipose tissue in a lean adult totals nearly 120,000 kcal, or 100 times the carbohydrate reserve. Thus, release of energy stores from adipose tissue can protect vital organs during a protracted fast.

In the fed state, the entry of amino acids and monosaccharides into the portal circulation stimulates release of proinsulin from pancreatic β-cells. Insulin is cleaved from the connecting ("C") protein to generate active insulin. Insulin transports both amino acids and glucose into the liver, where it stimulates glycogen synthesis, protein synthesis, and fatty acid synthesis, while suppressing glycogenolysis and gluconeogenesis, as well as proteolysis and lipolysis. Insulin carries both glucose and amino acids into skeletal muscle, and it carries glucose into adipose tissue. Insulin facilitates glycogen synthesis and glycolysis in muscle, and it facilitates fatty acid synthesis in adipose tissue. Insulin also stimulates the synthesis of lipoprotein lipase in capillaries, facilitating the extraction of fatty acids from circulation, and promotes hepatic very-low-density lipoprotein (VLDL) synthesis.

During a fast, insulin levels decline, as levels of glucagon, a product of the pancreatic α-cells, rise. Falling insulin levels promote glycogenolysis, followed by gluconeogenesis, in the liver. In adipose tissue, low insulin levels stimulate lipolysis, releasing fatty acids for use as fuel; ketones are generated in the process of hepatic fatty acid oxidation. High levels of circulating fatty acids inhibit insulin action. Reduced insulin action at skeletal muscle stimulates proteolysis.

In the insulin-resistant state, insulin levels are high, but receptors, particularly those on skeletal muscle, are relatively insensitive to insulin action (55,56). High levels of insulin presumably compensate for receptor-mediated resistance. High insulin levels promote fatty acid synthesis in the liver. The accumulation and circulation of free fatty acids and triglycerides packaged in VLDL aggravate insulin resistance, driving insulin levels higher. Thus, the metabolic derangements are self-perpetuating, generating in the process the manifestations of the insulin-resistance syndrome associated with cardiovascular risk, until the β-cells fail and diabetes develops. With β-cell failure, the resultant low levels of circulating insulin mimic conditions during a fast. The metabolic derangements that distinguish diabetes from fasting include pathologically low insulin levels and, of course, high levels of circulating glucose. Hepatic gluconeogenesis compounds the hyperglycemia, with excess glucose leading to tissue damage through glycosylation. Glycosylation of hemoglobin is routinely used as a measure of the extent of prevailing glycemia (i.e., HgbA1c). High ambient levels of glucose lead to the production of sugar alcohols (e.g., sorbitol, fructose) in many tissues, which in turn can cause cellular distention. The accumulation of such polyols in the lens is causally implicated in the blurred vision that often occurs with poorly controlled diabetes.

In studies of the Pima Indians, a tribe of Native Americans particularly subject to the development of obesity and diabetes mellitus (see Chapter 44), Lillioja et al. (7) showed that insulin resistance is an antecedent of diabetes. During the phase of insulin resistance, serum glucose is normal but insulin levels are abnormally elevated, both in the fasting and postprandial states. The development of obesity appears to be of particular importance in the development of IGT secondary to insulin resistance. A modest degree of hyperglycemia may occur during the period of insulin resistance, acting as a signal to the endocrine pancreas that insulin action is impaired and stimulating more insulin release. Ultimately, both protracted hypersecretion and hyperglycemia may contribute to β-cell dysfunction and overt diabetes.

In a longitudinal study of Pima Indians, Lillioja et al. (57) characterized steps in the pathogenesis of type 2 diabetes. More than 200 nondiabetic subjects were followed for an average of over 5 years, undergoing body composition measures, glucose tolerance testing, and hyperinsulinemic–euglycemic clamp testing to assess insulin action and glucose disposal. The single, strongest predictor of the development of diabetes was impaired insulin action, with a relative risk of over 30; this remained significant after adjustment for body fat. Percentage of body fat and impaired suppression of hepatic gluconeogenesis were also significant predictors of diabetes. The authors concluded that impaired insulin action, or insulin resistance, was the strongest single predictor of impending diabetes, while impaired suppression of hepatic gluconeogenesis was likely to be a secondary event. The factors responsible for β-cell failure, possibly including glucose toxicity and/or "fatigue" secondary to hyperfunction over time, are uncertain. The possibility exists, however, that the pathogenesis of type 2 diabetes is variable in different populations; β-cell failure may occur independently of insulin resistance (58). Noteworthy with regard to the Pima Indians is evidence that restoration of their traditional diet, low in fat and simple sugar and high in fiber from various desert plants, particularly mesquite, ameliorates their tendency toward diabetes and obesity (59). That the habitual nutritional environment should have salutary effects is perhaps supportive of the "thrifty genotype" theory and certainly is supportive of the application of the evolutionary biology model to human nutrition.

Reaven et al. (59) reported that a substantial proportion of cases of hypertension may be related to insulin resistance. While noting that hypertension may occur independently of insulin resistance, and vice versa, the authors note that insulin resistance stimulates the sympathetic nervous system. Under normal fasting conditions, low serum glucose and insulin levels stimulate the activity of an inhibitory pathway from the ventromedial hypothalamus to sympathetic centers in the brainstem. With sustained elevations of both glucose and insulin, the inhibitory pathway remains suppressed, with resultant augmentation of sympathetic tone. Invoking this model, the authors suggest that amelioration of insulin resistance, with diet, weight loss, or pharmacotherapy, may be more important to the reduction of cardiovascular risk in certain hypertensive patients than blood pressure control per se (60).

Thus, the development of type 2 diabetes often is preceded by a protracted period of insulin resistance manifested as the "metabolic syndrome" of obesity, dyslipidemia, and hypertension. Abdominal obesity and hypertriglyceridemia may be particularly early markers of the syndrome and represent a readily detectable indicator of risk for diabetes (61). Of note, the defining features of the insulin-resistance syndrome, and the nomenclature applied, have of late been matters of contention. The American Heart Association supports diagnostic criteria for the metabolic syndrome (62) (see Table 6-1), while the American Diabetes Association has questioned the utility of defining a syndrome at all (63).

Regardless of the terminology applied to the various manifestations of the insulin-resistant state, interventions to treat the condition, particularly

---

TABLE 6.1

American Heart Association Criteria for the Metabolic Syndrome

The American Heart Association and the National Heart, Lung, and Blood Institute recommend that the metabolic syndrome be identified as the presence of three or more of these components:

Elevated waist circumference	Men—Equal to or greater than 40 inches Women—Equal to or greater than 35 inches
Elevated triglycerides	Equal to or greater than 150 mg/dL
Reduced HDL ("good") cholesterol	Men—Less than 40 mg/dL Women—Less than 50 mg/dL
Elevated blood pressure	Equal to or greater than 130/85 mm Hg
Elevated fasting glucose	Equal to or greater than 100 mg/dL

Source: National Cholesterol Education Program. *Adult treatment panel III guidelines.* Available at http://www.americanheart.org/presenter.jhtml?identifier=4756; accessed 3/20/13.

---

supervised weight loss, may both mitigate associated cardiovascular risk and prevent the evolution of diabetes. The Diabetes Prevention Program has provided definitive evidence that intervention with either lifestyle modification or pharmacotherapy can prevent type 2 diabetes in a significant proportion of at-risk individuals (64). In individuals with diagnosed type 2 diabetes, the Look AHEAD trial has demonstrated that intensive lifestyle intervention can improve glucose control and reduce CVD risk factors and medication use (65,66).

There is now definitive evidence in type 1 diabetes (67,68) and strongly suggestive evidence in type 2 diabetes (69,70) that control of serum glucose levels to within the physiologic range delays the development of complications. There is consensus that nutritional management is an essential component in efforts to achieve and maintain good glycemic control. On the other hand, there is some evidence that very aggressive glycemic control may have adverse effects on mortality (71). Such findings are not entirely consistent across studies and are therefore insufficient to dictate clinical practice standards. However, the possibility of adverse effects of stringent glycemic control, along with patient history and individual characteristics, should be considered when determining target values for blood glucose and HbA1c. Other goals of dietary therapy include regulation of serum lipids, weight control, and targeted management of incipient or advancing complications and concomitants of diabetes, such as hypertension, renal insufficiency, and coronary artery disease.

Although essential to the optimal management of diabetes, nutritional interventions are only rarely sufficient. Judicious combinations of dietary/lifestyle and pharmacologic treatment are generally indicated. Sulfonylureas increase insulin production; α-glucosidase inhibitors such as acarbose delay glucose absorption; biguanides such as metformin reduce hepatic gluconeogenesis; thiazolidinediones such as troglitazone enhance peripheral insulin receptor sensitivity; and incretin mimetics, such as exenatide, apparently ameliorate glycemic control by multiple mechanisms of action (72,73). Each class of medication, alone and in combination with others as well as insulin, offers distinct advantages and disadvantages. Excellent reviews of pharmacotherapy are available (74–76).

Dietary Management

Overview

The dietary management of diabetes has varied considerably over the course of the past century. The mainstay of treatment in the early decades of this century was carbohydrate restriction. Dietary fat intake was high to compensate for low caloric intake from carbohydrate. The role of carbohydrate restriction entered its modern era with the development of the GI by Jenkins et al. (77). The GI typically uses a slice of white bread as a reference standard, with a value of 100, and indicates the postprandial rise in serum glucose (and consequently insulin) for fixed portions of specified foods.

However, as shown in Table 6-2, the GI does not provide information that is readily translated into clinical advice. Common perceptions about the simple sugar content of foods do not allow one to predict the glycemic response evoked, as exemplified by the relatively low GI of ice cream and the high GI of certain fruits and vegetables. Similarly, variations in the glycemic responses to different polysaccharides are minimal when these sugars are consumed in the context of a meal. Consequently, attention has turned increasingly to overall meal and diet composition.

Foods with a high GI, such as pasta and bread, need not elicit a postprandial spike in glucose and insulin if such an effect is blunted by other foods consumed concurrently. Foods rich in soluble fiber (see Chapter 1 and Section VIIE) are particularly effective at attenuating such a response. There is some evidence that the distribution of foods may be as important as their GI in the glucose and insulin responses they evoke. Comparing identical diets distributed as either three daily meals or multiple daily snacks, Jenkins et al. (78) reported that frequent snacking, or "nibbling," resulted in significant reductions in insulin release, although there is limited corroborating study of this contention.

As noted in Chapter 5, the GL is increasingly supplanting the GI in both research and clinical practice applications. The GL accounts for both the presence of sugar in foods and its concentration (see Table 6-3). The GL may be applied to meals and even to the overall diet. Studies of low-GL diets show promise for management of insulin resistance, diabetes, obesity, and cardiometabolic risk (79–86), although more study of long-term effects is clearly warranted (87). As noted

TABLE 6.2

Glycemic Index of Some Common Foods

Food Group	Food	Glycemic Index
Breads	White bread[a]	100
	Whole wheat bread	99
	Pumpernickel	78
Cereal products	Cornflakes	119
	Shredded wheat	97
	Oatmeal	85
	White rice	83
	Spaghetti	66
	Bulgur wheat	65
	Barley	31
Fruit	Raisins	93
	Bananas	79
	Oranges	66
	Grapes	62
	Apples	53
	Cherries	32
Vegetables	Parsnips	141
	Baked potato	135
	Carrots	133
	Corn	87
	Boiled potato	81
	Yams	74
	Peas	74
Legumes	Lima beans	115
	Baked beans	60
	Chick peas	49
	Red lentils	43
	Peanuts	19
Dairy products	Yogurt	52
	Ice cream	52
	Milk	49
Sugar	Sucrose	86

[a]Reference standard.

Source: Adapted from Jenkins DJA, Jenkins AL. The glycemic index, fiber, and the dietary treatment of hypertriglyceridemia and diabetes. *J Am Coll Nutr* 1987;6:11–17.

elsewhere in the chapter, comparison of various means of achieving a low-GL dietary pattern is an area in particular need of further study (88).

The principal goals of nutritional management of diabetes are to maintain a normal or near-normal serum glucose level, to prevent or reverse lipid abnormalities, and to thereby mitigate the potential complications of diabetes. Nutritional management of insulin resistance, or prediabetes, if identified as such before the advent of diabetes, is aimed at the prevention of progression to diabetes. Insulin resistance is apt to be detected in the context of the insulin-resistance syndrome,

TABLE 6.3

Glycemic Index and Glycemic Load of a Few Foods that Demonstrate How the Values May Diverge[a]

Food	GI	Serving Size	Carbohydrate Dose (g)	GL
Chickpeas	51	150 g	30	11
Vanilla ice cream	54	50 g	9	3
Strawberries	57	120 g	3	1
Orange	69	120 g	11	5
Whole wheat bread	73	30 g	13	7
Orange juice	81	250 mL	26	15
Coca-Cola	90	250 mL	26	16
Plain bagel	103	70 g	35	25
Doughnut	108	47 g	23	17
Carrots	131	80 g	6	5

[a]The foods are listed from lowest to highest GI.

Source: Data from Foster-Powell K, Holt SH, Brand-Miller JC. International table of glycemic index and glycemic load values. Am J Clin Nutr 2002;76:5–56.

as discussed previously (see also Chapter 5). The combination of elevated serum triglycerides and obesity may be an early indication of insulin resistance (89); postprandial hypertriglyceridemia may be an even earlier indicator.

The utility of a prudent, balanced, health-promoting dietary pattern, in conjunction with moderate physical activity and resultant weight loss, in the prevention of diabetes has been clearly established by the Diabetes Prevention Program (64). In this trial, more than 3,000 adults with prediabetes were randomly assigned to usual care, treatment with 850 mg per day of metformin, or a lifestyle intervention comprised of guidance toward a healthful dietary pattern and 150 minutes of physical activity per week. The trial was concluded early, at 4 years, due to significant treatment effects. Pharmacotherapy reduced the incidence of diabetes by 30%, while the lifestyle intervention was nearly twice as effective, reducing the incidence of diabetes by 58%. Ten years after randomization, diabetes incidence rates were similar between groups, but cumulative incidence of diabetes remained lowest in the lifestyle group (90). The potency of the lifestyle intervention in the Diabetes Prevention Program corresponds very closely to the 60% reduction in the incidence of diabetes reported with use of rosiglitazone in the DREAM trial (91). Evaluation of the Diabetes Prevention Program generally suggests the lifestyle intervention to be an acceptably

cost-effective strategy for diabetes prevention in high-risk individuals (92–94).

Dietary guidelines for the management of diabetes have evolved over the 20th century in light of advances in understanding of nutritional physiology and in an effort to synthesize recommendations for health promotion and disease management apt to pertain simultaneously to individual patients. As of 1986, dietary guidelines for diabetes management were made to resemble the recommendations of the American Heart Association, partly due to the correspondence of heart disease and diabetes in the population. These guidelines have since been modified to accommodate the variable needs and responses of individual patients to nutritional interventions (95).

The American Diabetes Association's (ADA) nutrition recommendations for the prevention of type 2 diabetes emphasize weight loss without endorsing any particular dietary pattern (96). Reducing calorie intake and fat intake are two suggested strategies for achieving weight loss. Lowering dietary GL is recognized as an unproven approach to diabetes prevention; however, consumption of low-GI foods that are nutrient-dense and rich in fiber is encouraged. For the management of existing diabetes, ADA recommendations include an overall healthful dietary pattern that is not excessive in calories, carbohydrate monitoring, and possibly the use of GI and load. Saturated fat intake should be limited to <7% of total calories, and cholesterol intake should be limited to <200 mg daily; however, the latter recommendation is based on weaker evidence. Of note, consuming a diet of foods with higher NuVal™ scores has been associated with a 14% reduction in risk of diabetes (97). The NuVal™ nutritional scoring system uses the Overall Nutritional Quality Index (ONQI) algorithm, which incorporates more than 30 dietary components, including saturated fat, fiber, micronutrients, energy density, and GL.

Macronutrient Distribution

In general, the protein intake recommended for healthy adults, approximately 0.8 g/kg/day, is appropriate in both insulin-resistant states and in diabetes. Protein restriction may be indicated if renal insufficiency develops (see Chapter 16), but protein restriction to prevent the development of renal insufficiency is not clearly indicated. Excessive protein intake may accelerate the development of renal insufficiency, however. Because the long-term effects of diets with more than 20% of energy from protein are not yet clear, the ADA does not recommend high-protein diets for individuals with diabetes, and advises against protein intakes greater than 0.8 g/kg/day in patients with kidney disease (98). Popular books advocating high-protein diets for weight loss and control of insulin release (99–102) are of dubious merit for healthy individuals and are to be avoided in the management of diabetes. That said, a relatively high-protein (i.e., 25% of calories) but low-GL diet may well be preferable to a diet with a high GL (103). As noted earlier, the quality of any dietary pattern is best measured in terms of the specific foods of which it is comprised rather than merely its macronutrient distribution.

Dietary fat restriction in diabetes, resulting in relatively high carbohydrate intake, has been associated with dyslipidemia, specifically hypertriglyceridemia and low high-density lipoprotein (HDL) (95). High carbohydrate intake apparently increases serum triglycerides by stimulating increased hepatic synthesis of VLDL particles (103,104) rather than by inhibiting the activity of lipoprotein lipase or hepatic lipase. Elevated triglycerides in turn may exacerbate insulin resistance both by stimulating insulin release and by interfering with insulin action (105,106). This experience has led to interest in liberalized fat intake, with attention to the source of fat calories. Comparisons of low-fat and low-carbohydrate diets in diabetic patients have yielded somewhat mixed results, perhaps owing to other differences in the prescribed diets within and among studies.

The substitution of monounsaturated fatty acids (MUFAs) for carbohydrate in the diet has been found to improve glycemic control, while lowering triglycerides, raising HDL, and preserving low-density lipoprotein (LDL) levels (107,108). Guldbrand and colleagues reported improvements in HbA1c and HDL concentrations in patients following a low-carbohydrate diet, but no significant change in patients following a low-fat diet (109). Insulin dose also decreased in the low-carbohydrate group relative to the low-fat group. The favorable effects of the low-carbohydrate diet occurred despite similar weight loss in both groups. On the other hand, Davis and colleagues reported similar weight loss in type 2 diabetics following either a low-fat or low-carbohydrate diet after 1 year, but no significant change in hemoglobin A1c or blood pressure in either group (110).

The lipid perturbations seen with high carbohydrate intake may be due, in part or in whole, to ingestion of processed carbohydrate with relatively low fiber content and a high GL. Therefore, the most appropriate comparisons of diets varying in fat content should include a low-fat diet that is also high in fiber. Several such studies have been completed in recent years, with somewhat mixed results. Some studies have found low-fat diets that are high fiber and/or low GI to be comparable or even superior to diets lower in carbohydrates and higher in MUFAs (111–113), whereas others have found a diet moderate in fat to be more beneficial (114,115).

For example, in a comparison of low-fat and high-MUFA diets where mean fiber intake was significantly higher in the low-fat group (36.1 g vs. 24.6 g, $p < 0.05$), Gerhard et al. observed greater weight loss in the low-fat group and no differences in blood lipids or glycemic control between groups (113). In a randomized trial, Milne et al. (111) found both glycemic and lipid control to be comparably, favorably influenced by either a high-carbohydrate, high-fiber diet or a diet in which monounsaturated fat was substituted for carbohydrate. Similarly, Luscombe et al. (112) found both a high-monounsaturated-fat diet and a high-carbohydrate diet with low glycemic properties to be superior to a high-glycemic, high-carbohydrate diet with regard to HDL levels; with regard to other outcomes, all three diets were comparable. Of note, subjects in this study all consumed at least 30 g per day of fiber. Barnard et al. found that a low-fat, high-carbohydrate vegan diet improved glycemia and lipid concentrations significantly more than a diet based on the 2003 recommendations of the ADA (116). Although carbohydrate intake was higher in the vegan diet group, intakes of fiber, fruits, and vegetables were also higher. The results of this study highlight the importance of food choices over macronutrient distribution.

On the other hand, Shai and colleagues reported differential effects of low-fat, low-carbohydrate, and Mediterranean diets in 322 moderately obese adults (114). In this study, weight loss over a 24-month period was greater in the low-carbohydrate and Mediterranean diet groups than in the low-fat group, and lipid profile improvements were greater in the low-carbohydrate group than in the low-fat group. In subgroup analysis of 36 participants with type 2 diabetes, the Mediterranean diet significantly reduced fasting glucose and insulin relative to the low-fat group. Of note, the Mediterranean diet group also consumed the most fiber. In a 2010 study, Elhayany et al. also found that a traditional Mediterranean diet (TM) improved glycemic control, measured by HbA1c, compared with an ADA diet (115). However, a low-carbohydrate Mediterranean diet (LCM) improved glycemic control more than both the TM and ADA diets. It was also the only diet to increase HDL concentrations over time. The ADA and TM diets had the same macronutrient distribution: 50 to 55% carbohydrates, 30% fat, and 15 to 20% protein. The LCM diet was 35% carbohydrates, 45% fat (50% MUFA), and 20% protein.

The current ADA nutrition guidelines do not include specific targets for percentage of calories from carbohydrates, protein, total fat, polyunsaturated fatty acids (PUFAs), or MUFAs (96). The ADA does recommend limiting saturated fat to less than 7% of total calories and minimizing intake of trans fat. High-protein diets (>20% of calories) are not advised because of unknown long-term effects on patients with diabetes. However, some lines of evidence (see Chapters 7 and 45) suggest that maximal metabolic and cardiovascular benefit may be achieved with restriction of saturated and trans fat in combination to below 10% of energy and preferably below 5%; allocation of between 10% and 15% of calories to polyunsaturated fat, but with a 1:4 or higher

ratio of n-3 to n-6 fatty acids; and allocation of approximately 15% of calories to monounsaturated fat. Such a pattern is enhanced further by ensuring that the 50% or more of calories from carbohydrate are derived predominantly from complex carbohydrates with an abundance of fiber, especially soluble fiber. Diets with as much as 50 g per day of fiber have been well tolerated, although they typically require a period of gradual acclimation. Whereas high-carbohydrate, low-fiber diets may elevate triglycerides, high-fiber diets generally lower both fasting and postprandial triglycerides. Further research will be required to elucidate the relative advantages and disadvantages, with regard to weight regulation, glycemic control, lipid metabolism, and cardiovascular risk, of diets varying in fat and carbohydrate composition (117). To date, there have been few if any direct comparisons of the several variations on the theme of healthful eating—notably, a Mediterranean diet rich in unsaturated fat, a diet relatively rich in protein from lean sources, and a low-GL diet rich in complex carbohydrate—that might reasonably compete as best suited for the management and prevention of diabetes. Such trials are eagerly anticipated. Small trials examining dietary variations have, to date, generally focused on some isolated nutritional property as opposed to the overall dietary pattern (118–120).

Exchange Lists

Historically, exchange lists have been a useful, if potentially tedious, tool in dietary management of diabetes. The lists, published at intervals by the American Dietetic Association, generally represent collaborations between the Academy of Nutrition and Dietetics, formerly the American Dietetic Association, and the ADA. Foods are grouped by category, with serving sizes that provide comparable amounts of energy and each class of macronutrient indicated. Thus, foods within a category may be substituted, or "exchanged," for one another with preservation of a particular nutritional composition for that meal or day. A particular emphasis is generally placed on the quantity and quality of carbohydrate ingested (121). The range of foods included on the lists supports compliance with dietary recommendations over a wide range of dietary options. The general approach to exchange list use calls for estimating the appropriate number of total daily calories; dividing those calories into macronutrient classes; and establishing how many calories from each class of macronutrient should be consumed each day. Pi-Sunyer et al. (122) reported results of a randomized, multicenter trial in which consistent use of exchange lists was as effective as a prepared meal program in improving a range of pertinent outcome measures in type 2 diabetic men and women. More recently, Ziemer et al. (123) showed that an emphasis on healthful dietary pattern might serve as an alternative to use of exchange lists, with potential advantages in low-literacy populations. The most recent iteration of the exchange lists was published in 2007 and can be purchased at the Academy of Nutrition and Dietetics website (124).

Special Considerations

The management of diabetes varies to some degree with the circumstances of care for a particular patient. Diabetes management in children must incorporate attention to the maintenance of appropriate growth and invariably should be a collaboration between one or more clinicians (pediatrician or family practitioner and endocrinologist) and a dietitian. Pregnancy induces a sharp decline in insulin requirements during the first trimester, due to glucose uptake by the embryo and placenta. Insulin requirements rise markedly in the third trimester, due to high counterregulatory hormone levels. The management of diabetes during pregnancy should best involve obstetrician, endocrinologist, and dietitian (see Chapter 27). The maintenance of strict glycemic control during pregnancy, both in established and gestational diabetes, is crucial to a good pregnancy outcome and requires intensive and multidisciplinary care. Although complicated by cravings and aversions and increased energy requirements, the principles of nutritional management of diabetes during pregnancy are essentially the same as those applied under other conditions. The benefits of strict glycemic control have been conclusively demonstrated for both type 1 (125) and type 2 (126–129) diabetes.

Hypoglycemia is a potential complication of tight glycemic control in diabetes. Some evidence suggests that a combination of foods with varying glycemic indices can mitigate the risk of hypoglycemia (130). Eating a nutrition bar containing sucrose, protein, and cornstarch results in a "triphasic" glucose release and may be helpful to hypoglycemia-prone diabetics (131). Strict glycemic control in a type 1 diabetic inevitably increases the risk of hypoglycemic episodes. Some studies have suggested that a snack bar at night containing uncooked corn starch may help forestall such episodes, but others have suggested that only pharmacotherapy is a reliable defense (132–134).

Weight Loss and Energy Balance

A mainstay of dietary management of both type 2 diabetes mellitus in the overweight patient and of insulin resistance is weight loss (see Chapters 5 and 47). Clear clinical benefit of even fairly modest weight loss has been demonstrated (95,135–138). Significant amelioration of cardiometabolic risk is generally seen with loss of 7% to 10% of body weight in the obese (137). The amount of weight loss required to induce favorable metabolic effects likely varies with anthropometry, however. Individuals with a predilection for not only central but visceral fat deposition are most subject to the adverse metabolic effects of weight gain, and they also appear to be most responsive to the beneficial effects of even very modest weight loss (138–143). The adverse effects of intra-abdominal fat accumulation explain why some ethnic groups, notably various populations in Southeast Asia, are subject to adverse metabolic effects of obesity at lower BMI values than are generally deemed harmful in the United States (144–146).

Independent of its impact on weight, negative energy balance could possibly play a role in mitigating insulin resistance. In bariatric surgery patients, hepatic insulin sensitivity is normalized within days of surgery, before any considerable weight loss can be achieved (147). In their study, Jazet and colleagues found that just 2 days of a very low-calorie diet significantly reduced basal endogenous glucose production in a small sample of obese type 2 diabetic patients (148). However, during hyperinsulinemia, endogenous glucose production was unchanged. Whole body glucose disposal and lipolysis were not affected in the basal or hyperinsulinemic conditions.

Bariatric surgery can have dramatic effects on weight and glycemic control, reversing diabetes in many cases. In one study, diabetes remission was achieved in 75% of bariatric surgery patients over 2 years (149). In contrast, conventional medical therapy resulted in no remissions and only small improvements in glycemic control. Medical therapy was associated with an 8% reduction in

HbA1c, whereas gastric bypass and biliopancreatic diversion led to reductions of 25% and 43%, respectively. BMI also decreased by approximately 33 kg per m^2 in both bariatric groups, compared with a decrease of 4.7 kg per m^2 in the medical therapy group. Although studies like this one would appear to clearly demonstrate the effectiveness of bariatric surgery in the treatment of type 2 diabetes in severely obese patients, some have suggested that study designs that do not include a truly intensive lifestyle intervention as a comparison treatment are biased toward the surgical intervention (150). The modest weight loss that occurred in the medical therapy group in the Mingrone et al. study is an indication that the diet and lifestyle intervention was not sufficiently intensive. It has been suggested that an appropriate lifestyle intervention would involve residential treatment over several weeks and in-home treatment for several months afterward (150). Provision of prepared meals is recommended initially and regular visits with nutritionists and exercise specialists thereafter.

Glycemic Index and Glycemic Load

The GI, developed by Jenkins et al. (77,151), characterizes the postprandial glucose response to various foods relative to a reference standard, typically white bread; sucrose is an alternative referent. The area under the postprandial glucose curve for a test food is divided by the area under the curve for white bread with an equal amount of carbohydrate (50 g) and multiplied by 100 to establish the GI for the test food.

Complex carbohydrate containing starch initially was thought to induce less of a rise in postprandial glucose than simple carbohydrate, but this has been refuted. The GI of foods is somewhat unpredictable on the basis of the apparent complexity of the carbohydrate content (see Chapter 1), as shown in Table 6-2 (152), as it is influenced by fiber content, processing, and the ratio of amylose to amylopectin (152).

Jenkins and Jenkins (152) suggested that dietary fiber may serve as a surrogate measure of the GI of foods, with high fiber content, particularly the amount of soluble fiber, lowering the glycemic response. Noteworthy is that sucrose has a lower GI than white bread, carrots, baked potato, and lima beans. Bantle et al. (153) studied healthy individuals, as well as type 1 and type 2 diabetics, and found virtually no differences in glycemic or insulin responses to test meals containing fixed amounts of total carbohydrate as glucose, fructose, sucrose, potato starch, or wheat starch. The authors interpreted their data to indicate that sucrose consumption in the context of balanced meals need not be restricted in diabetes other than under specific circumstances, such as during intentional weight loss. In general, the weight of evidence indicates that the sucrose content of the diet is not a reliable indicator of glycemic control, and sucrose restriction in diabetes is not specifically indicated to control the serum glucose (154).

A study by Liljeberg et al. (155) provides one potential explanation for the limited utility of focusing on the glycemic indices of individual foods for the overall control of glucose metabolism. The investigators found that varying the fiber content of breakfast altered the glucose response to foods with a high GI at lunch in a group of healthy subjects (154).

Taking into account both GI and standard serving sizes, the GL is the weighted average GI of a food multiplied by the percentage of energy from carbohydrate (156,157) and is believed to better predict the glycemic impact of foods under real-world conditions (158). The relationship between weight and BMI is roughly analogous to the relationship between GI and GL. Weight may be high, but a person may still be lean if tall. Similarly, the GI may be high, but the glycemic effect of that food may be modest if the carbohydrate content is relatively dilute. An expansive table of GI and GL values of common foods was published in 2002 (159). A few foods representing the range of potential divergence between GI and GL are shown in Table 6-3.

To date, no randomized trials have directly compared the effects of low-GL diets to those of low-GI diets. Therefore, little is known about the relative utility of these measures. The two measures are sometimes grouped together in systematic reviews and meta-analyses. However, there appears to be benefit for both low-GI and low-GL dietary patterns. In a 2008 meta-analysis of 37 prospective cohort studies, Barclay and colleagues reported significant positive associations between diets with higher GI or GL and risks of type 2 diabetes, coronary heart disease (CHD), gallbladder disease, breast cancer, and all diseases combined (160). The effect was strongest for type 2 diabetes; diets in the highest quintile for GI or GL were associated with a 40% increased risk, compared with diets in the lowest quintile. Although both GI and GL were associated with greater risk of chronic disease, the GI had a stronger effect than the GL. In another cross-sectional study, a low-GI diet was associated with improved insulin sensitivity and blood lipid levels, and lower levels of high-sensitivity C-reactive protein (161). GL was not significantly associated with these measures.

Several recent trials have investigated the effects of a low-GI or low-GL diet on weight loss, insulin sensitivity, and cardiovascular risk factors (162,163). In 2007, a Cochrane review summarized the results of six randomized controlled trials of low-GI or low-GL diets (164). The results of the included studies suggest that a low-GI/GL diet may enhance weight loss and decrease total cholesterol and LDL. No differences in HDL, fasting glucose or insulin, or blood pressure were observed. A number of trials have been completed since this review. In the CALERIE study (165), there were no differences between groups randomized to a high-GL or low-GL diet in body composition, metabolic rate, or diet adherence throughout a 12-month intervention period. It is worth noting that the low-GL diet was also lower in carbohydrates (40% of total energy vs. 60% in the high-GL group) and higher in protein (30% vs. 20%) and fat (30% vs. 20%), so the effect of GL per se was not isolated. Philippou and colleagues conducted a series of trials to compare the effects of a low-GI diet to a high-GI diet of comparable macronutrient distribution in overweight men and women, with somewhat mixed results. In a 12-week study, only the low-GI group experienced significant weight loss (163). This group also had significantly lower 24-hour area under the curve (AUC) values for glucose compared with the high-GI group. There were no differences in serum lipid concentrations. In a separate study in middle-aged men with at least one CHD risk factor, a low-GI diet significantly reduced fasting insulin and HOMA-IR, and resulted in significantly greater reductions in total cholesterol and 24-hour ambulatory blood pressure compared with a high-GI diet (165). The low-GI diet was also associated with significant reductions in carotid–femoral pulse wave velocity, LDL, and triglycerides. These effects occurred independently of weight loss, which was not significantly different between groups. In contrast to the findings of this study, Philippou et al. found no effect of

dietary GI on anthropometric measures, blood lipids, or measures of insulin sensitivity in men and women during a 4-month weight maintenance period following weight loss (166).

An important issue often overlooked is that a low GL may be achieved in various ways. The importance of this was beautifully demonstrated by McMillan-Price et al. (88) in a randomized trial of roughly 130 overweight adults. Two diets relatively high in carbohydrate and two diets relatively high in protein (and thus lower in carbohydrate) were compared on the basis of differing GLs. The study showed, as most do, that restricting calorie intake by any means led to roughly comparable weight loss in the short term, although trends hinted at a benefit of low GL. The percentage of subjects achieving an at least 5% weight reduction was significantly greater on the low-glycemic-load diets whether they were high carbohydrate or high protein than on their higher-GL counterparts. Similarly, body fat loss was enhanced, at least among women, by the low-GL diets. Whereas LDL cholesterol decreased significantly on the high-carbohydrate, low-GL diet, it actually increased on the high-protein, low-GL diet.

There are regrettably few trials like those described above, and more are needed. The findings suggest the importance of food choices rather than choices among macronutrient categories, as a major arbiter of cardiac risk. A low-GL diet can be achieved by minimizing carbohydrate intake, but this approach may toss out the baby with the bathwater. High-carbohydrate foods such as most whole grains, beans, legumes, vegetables, and even fruits can contribute to a low-GL dietary pattern. Such foods also provide a diversity of micronutrients of potential importance to overall health, and cardiovascular health specifically, antioxidants flavonoids and carotenoids noteworthy among them. By demonstrating that a high-carbohydrate, low-GL diet may offer particular cardiac benefit, this study points toward a diet in which choice within macronutrient categories is given at least as much consideration as choice among those categories. This perspective is concordant with a large volume of research suggesting that cardiac risk may be mitigated by reducing dietary fat, as well as by shifting fat intake from saturated and trans fatty acids to monounsaturates and polyunsaturates. Cardiac health at the population level will likely be well served when dietary guidance is consistently cast in terms of healthful, wholesome foods rather than competition among the three macronutrient classes from which a diet is composed (see Chapter 45).

Nutrients, Nutriceuticals, and Functional Foods

Nuts and Peanuts

Nut consumption has been consistently associated with reduced risk of CVD and cardiovascular risk factors, particularly serum lipids, but the effect of nuts on diabetes risk and management is less clear (167). Although nuts vary in their nutritional composition, as a whole, they have a favorable nutrient profile; they are rich in monounsaturated and PUFAs, fiber, protein, micronutrients, and polyphenols while containing relatively small amounts of saturated fatty acids and carbohydrates (168). Because of their high fat and fiber content and low carbohydrate content, the inclusion of nuts in the diet may help to improve glycemic control in type 2 diabetes and metabolic syndrome or prevent these conditions from developing.

In the Nurses' Health Study (NHS) cohort, women who consumed nuts at least five times per week had a 27% reduced risk of developing type 2 diabetes compared with those who rarely or never consumed nuts (169). A small but significant reduced risk was also observed for women who consumed peanut butter five or more times per week. However, these findings were not replicated in the Iowa Women's Health Study (170). A more recent analysis of the NHS and NHS II cohorts confirmed the results of the first analysis, also finding that consumption of total nuts (including peanuts, walnuts, and other nuts) or tree nuts five or more times per week was associated with an approximately 15% reduced risk of type 2 diabetes; though these associations were explained by BMI (171). Interestingly, women who ate just two or more servings per week of walnuts had a 24% reduced risk of diabetes compared with those who never or rarely ate walnuts, even after controlling for BMI and other relevant confounders ($p = 0.002$).

Clinical trials have generally not found that the addition of nuts to the diets of individuals with type 2 diabetes or metabolic syndrome improves glycemic control (168). One trial reported reduced fasting insulin and HOMA among participants with metabolic syndrome assigned to an intervention of 30 g per day mixed nuts and healthy diet advice compared to healthy diet advice alone (172). Another study reported greater reduction in fasting insulin in type 2 diabetes patients assigned to a walnut-enriched (30 g per day) low-fat diet compared to an isocaloric low-fat diet without walnuts (173). However, two trials reported increased fasting glucose with the addition of walnuts or cashews to the diet (174,175). The remaining four studies did not find any significant differences in glycemia-related outcomes between intervention and control groups. However, one study published since this review found that the inclusion of 2 oz of mixed nuts daily for 3 months was associated with significant reductions in HbA1c in type 2 diabetics, compared with an isocaloric portion of muffins, or a half dose each of nuts and muffins (176). The results of this study suggest that both the dose of nuts and the foods they replace in the diet may be important determinants of their effects on glycemic control. Additional studies assessing the dose-response effect of nut consumption are needed.

Although a beneficial effect of nuts on glycemic control has not been clearly demonstrated, the documented improvements in cardiovascular risk associated with nut consumption are highly relevant to the diabetic population. A study from the author's own lab found that a walnut-enriched ad libitum diet led to significant improvements in endothelial function, serum total cholesterol, and serum LDL concentrations compared with an ad libitum diet without walnuts in type 2 diabetic individuals (174). Despite the high energy density of nuts, high intake of nuts does not appear to be associated with weight gain or obesity in observational studies or experimental trials (168). Given the strong likelihood of cardiovascular benefits and the low likelihood of adverse effects, the inclusion of nuts in the diet can be recommended to individuals with type 2 diabetes and those at risk.

Sugar, Fructose, and High-Fructose Corn Syrup

White sugar, usually in the form of granulated sugar, is purified sucrose, the crystals of which are naturally white. Brown sugar is less refined and so still contains some molasses from sugar cane. Alternatively, manufacturers may add back molasses to purified sucrose in order to control the ratio and the color. Nutritionally, the differences between white and brown sugar are fairly trivial. When matched on the basis of volume, brown sugar has more calories because it tends to pack more densely; one cup of brown sugar provides 829 calories, while a cup of white granulated sugar provides 774 calories. However, when matched by weight, brown sugar has slightly fewer calories due to the presence of water in the molasses; 100 g of brown sugar contains 373 calories, as opposed to 396 calories in white sugar (177). Sugar crystals provide no nutrients other than sucrose, but molasses adds enough calcium, iron, and potassium to distinguish brown sugar from white sugar, although not enough to make it an important source of any of these nutrients.

Fructose (see Chapter 1), referred to as fruit sugar, is a monosaccharide that does not require insulin for its metabolism. Fructose in the diet comes from honey and fruit; from sucrose, which is made up of fructose and glucose; and from the use of high-fructose corn syrup as a sweetener in soft drinks and processed foods (178–181). Fructose intake reduces postprandial glucose relative to other sugars and starches (182), but it has been conditionally associated with increased triglycerides in type 2 diabetics (183). Fructose restriction in diabetes is not indicated, but substitution of fructose for sucrose does not appear to confer benefit and is not recommended. Ingested fructose is largely cleared by the liver, where it is a substrate for triglyceride production; ingestion of fructose is associated with postprandial hypertriglyceridemia. It is worth noting that high intake of fruit, a concentrated source of fructose, is not associated with adverse effects; this may be attributable to the slow digestion rate of whole fruit (184). An emphasis on limiting ingestion of fructose, per se, is not warranted. Rather, the evidence-based approach is to focus on reducing consumption of refined carbohydrates, including starches and all added sugars.

High-fructose corn syrup (HFCS), produced industrially through a series of enzymatic reactions on corn syrup, is widely used as a sweetener in the US food supply (179,180,185). There is unresolved debate about the relative contributions of HFCS, as compared to sucrose, to weight gain and diabetes risk. The inconclusive nature of this literature, reviewed previously in the *New York Times* (186), suggests that HFCS is, at present, best considered roughly comparable to other forms of added sugar in terms of adverse metabolic effect. In a recent review, White contends that, at levels typically consumed in the United States, fructose is unlikely to elicit the metabolic consequences observed in feeding trials (187). A study by Stanhope and Havel supports White's view; in this trial, postprandial triglyceride concentrations increased similarly after consumption of beverages sweetened with fructose, HFCS, or sucrose (188). However, corn subsidies in the United States make HFCS a particularly inexpensive sweetener, leading to its use in a startling variety of foods and often in surprisingly copious amounts. (The author has identified, for example, popular commercial brands of marinara sauce with more added sugar in the form of HFCS than chocolate fudge ice cream topping, matched for calories.) The ubiquity and abundance of HFCS likely makes it a particular and noteworthy dietary hazard, a contention supported by recent reviews linking soft drink consumption to obesity (189–192) the importance of sugar in any form in the etiology of type 2 diabetes is the subject of ongoing research and much debate. A well-publicized ecologic study of 175 countries by Basu and colleagues (193) has drawn renewed attention to the potential contribution of sugar consumption to the rising worldwide prevalence of type 2 diabetes. The study concluded that for every 150 kcal/person/day increase in sugar availability, there was a 1.1% increase in type 2 diabetes prevalence; an association that was not accounted for by obesity. The findings of this study prompted some to declare sugar "toxic" and the primary villain in the diabetes epidemic, relegating obesity to at least the runner-up position (194). This proclamation is misguided. Although added sugars may contribute to diabetes risk, an ecological study cannot provide evidence of a causative relationship.

Other Sweeteners

Nutritive sweeteners, including corn syrup, honey, molasses, and fruit juice concentrates, appear to offer no advantage to sucrose in the management or prevention of diabetes. Nonnutritive sweeteners (see Chapter 42), such as aspartame, sucralose, and saccharin, confer sweetness without calories and do not raise serum glucose. Such sweeteners may be of some benefit in efforts to control serum glucose and facilitate or maintain weight loss, but evidence is lacking of sustainable benefit in either case. Although fructose does not induce an insulin release, this may actually be disadvantageous with regard to effects on satiety (195).

Aspartame, marketed as Equal and Nutrasweet, is made by linking two amino acids together. While it contains no sugar, it is roughly 200 times as sweet as sugar. Aspartame does contain some calories, but it is used in small amounts due to its intense sweetness, so the calories it adds to the diet are negligible. There is ongoing controversy about health effects of aspartame, but claims that it can cause brain tumors or neurological disease are not considered credible by the FDA. Because aspartame lacks bulk and is not heat stable, it cannot be used in baked goods.

Sucralose, marketed as Splenda, is made by modifying the structure of sugar molecules through the addition of chlorine atoms. It is marketed in the United States as a no-calorie sweetener, but it actually contains 96 calories per cup, about one-eighth the calories of sugar. Splenda contains roughly 2 calories per teaspoon, but FDA regulations allow a product to be labeled as free of calories if it contains fewer than 5 calories per standard serving. Sucralose is up to 1,000 times as sweet as sugar, so Splenda contains relatively small amounts of sucralose combined with fluffed dextrose or maltodextrin to give it bulk for use in baking.

Stevia is a sweetener made by purifying extracts from a group of herbs by the same name that grow in Central and South America. Due to some early controversy about the safety of the extracts, called stevioside and rebaudioside, stevia was available only as a dietary supplement in the United States for some time. The FDA now considers the use of highly refined stevia extracts to be Generally Recognized as Safe (GRAS) when used in nonnutritive sweeteners, foods, and beverages (196). Stevia has been widely used in foods in Japan for the past several decades, without any apparent adverse effects. Stevia provides 30 to 300 times the sweetness of sugar, but it can produce a slightly bitter aftertaste.

While there is much made of the potential toxicity of artificial sweeteners in the blogosphere (as of July 2013, approximately 160,000 blogs addressed the topic), the evidence that these compounds directly cause disease is not strong. However, the evidence that they serve to reduce calories or weight or offer other benefits is not conclusive. Research on artificial sweeteners does not show convincingly that they take calories out of the diet over time; they may simply cause calories to be displaced. Given that these sweeteners are as much as 1,000 times as sweet as sugar, it is possible that they could raise the preference threshold for sweet and contribute to the consumption of processed foods with significant, and arguably superfluous, additions of sugar, typically in the form of HFCS.

Several animal studies have reported weight gain in rats exposed to saccharin or aspartame relative to glucose or sucrose, with (197,198) or without (199) accompanying increases in caloric intake. Prospective cohort studies in humans somewhat corroborate the findings of animal trials; many have reported associations between intake of artificial sweeteners, often in diet sodas, and weight gain or obesity-related chronic disease (200). However, reverse causality and residual confounding are important potential sources of bias. Observational studies that are less prone to reverse causality have reported small, nonsignificant associations (201). Studies in animal models, though essential to clinical research, are not always directly translatable to humans. In particular, the doses of artificial sweeteners typically provided to study rats are not comparable to levels that humans are commonly exposed to. As an example, the amount of aspartame fed to rats in a recent study was approximately 0.27 to 0.4 g per kg body weight per day (199). To consume this much aspartame, a 150-lb person would need to drink more than 100 12-oz cans of diet soda every day (202).

The majority of short-term experimental human trials have found that artificial sweeteners do not increase appetite or energy intake relative to sucrose (203). Of five trials with longer intervention duration (3 to 19 weeks) included in a 2007 review, four noted a beneficial effect of aspartame-sweetened foods or beverages on body weight relative to sucrose-sweetened products. The fifth study reported no differences between groups (204). Because long-term randomized controlled trials are still sparse, the safety and efficacy of artificial sweeteners remains a controversial topic, and more research is needed before their effects can be fully understood. In the meantime, the positions of the American Heart Association, the ADA, and the Academy of Nutrition and Dietetics, all support the use of artificial sweeteners in place of sugar as a means to reduce intake of calories and refined carbohydrates in the context of an otherwise healthful, calorically-restricted diet (205,206). Given that there is little evidence that the use of nonnutritive sweeteners is helpful for weight loss, reducing all sweeteners in the diet may be the optimal strategy for individuals with type 2 diabetes and others.

Fiber

A daily intake of approximately 30 g of dietary fiber from a variety of food sources is recommended to the general public for health promotion and in the management of diabetes (see Chapters 1 and 45). There is evidence that soluble fiber in particular may be of benefit in controlling both glucose and lipid levels in diabetes (207,208). However, the levels of fiber intake required to achieve significant improvements in fasting and postprandial glucose levels have been considered too high for practical application. In a study of men with type 2 diabetes, Anderson et al. (209) reported significant improvements in both serum lipids and glucose with twice daily psyllium totaling 10 g, for a period of 8 weeks. Of note, our Paleolithic ancestors were thought to have consumed nearly 100 g of fiber daily, and this pattern persists among rural peoples in the developing world (210). Fruits, oats, barley, and legumes are particularly good sources of soluble fiber (see Section VIIE). Fiber intake of up to 40 g per day is advocated by the ADA; average fiber intake by US adults ranges between 12 and 18 g per day.

Ethanol

Ethanol consumption independent of other food intake can result in hypoglycemia by transiently interfering with hepatic gluconeogenesis. Therefore, diabetics, particularly those treated with insulin or sulfonylureas, should be advised to consume alcohol only with food. Excessive alcohol intake may contribute to hypertriglyceridemia and deterioration of glucose control. Moderate alcohol intake in diabetes is generally without known adverse effects. The potential cardiovascular benefits of moderate alcohol consumption are discussed in Chapters 7 and 40.

Caffeine

Whether caffeine has beneficial or adverse effects on the cardiometabolic health of individuals with diabetes remains uncertain. In cohort studies, regular coffee consumption has been associated with significantly reduced risk of type 2 diabetes (211). However, there appears to be a similar relationship between consumption of both tea and decaffeinated coffee and diabetes risk, (212) so caffeine may not be the primary component of coffee that contributes to a protective effect. Furthermore, caffeine may actually have adverse effects on glucose metabolism in individuals who already have diabetes. A recent review of randomized controlled trials found that caffeine increased plasma glucose and insulin levels and decreased insulin sensitivity in individuals with type 2 diabetics (213). However, the trials included in this review generally tested single doses of caffeine that were relatively large (200 to 500 mg), and assessed only acute effects on glycemic control when consumed with an oral glucose load. Therefore, the generalizability of these findings to typical caffeine consumption patterns is limited. Of note, one uncontrolled pilot study in 12 coffee drinkers with type 2 diabetes found that abstinence from caffeine was associated with significant reductions in HbA1c after 3 months (214). Long-term trials of caffeine consumption in diabetics, at doses and frequencies that represent typical consumption, are needed before conclusions can be made. The health effects of coffee are discussed in more detail in Chapter 41.

Chromium

Chromium is established as an essential nutrient, with roles in lipid and carbohydrate metabolism (see Chapter 4). Known to function as an insulin cofactor, chromium may bind to a carrier molecule and thereby activate the insulin receptor kinase (215). Chromium may stimulate expression of insulin receptors in skeletal muscle as well (216). Evidence of improved glycemic control with chromium supplementation has been reported (217), but there are conflicting reports in the literature (218–222). Discordant findings to date may relate to varied utility of chromium among the various populations studied; efforts to identify specific populations in which chromium may prove of certain therapeutic benefit are ongoing. Daily supplementation with as much as 8 μg/kg/day is apparently safe and potentially beneficial. A National Institutes of Health-funded trial of chromium picolinate in insulin resistance at doses of 500 μg and 1,000 μg per day, completed in the author's lab, did not find a benefit of either dose on measures of glucose tolerance, insulin resistance, or endothelial function in insulin-resistant individuals (223). However, some studies suggest that individuals with diagnosed type 2 diabetes may benefit from chromium supplementation, (220,224) and particularly those with poorer glycemic control (225).

Vanadium

Vanadium is an ultratrace element. Evidence of a potentially therapeutic role of vanadium in disorders of glucose metabolism has been reported (226). A review of vanadium suggests potential benefit as a cofactor in insulin metabolism in both type 1 and type 2 diabetes (227). The therapeutic window for inorganic vanadium is very narrow. Efforts to improve the safety of vanadium are proceeding concurrently with research into its mechanisms of action (228). Research on vanadium is severely limited. A 2008 review identified only five very small studies of poor methodological quality (229). All studies reported a high incidence of gastrointestinal side effects. Until further progress is made in each of these endeavors, therapeutic applications of vanadium cannot be encouraged.

n-3 Fatty Acids (Fish Oil)

Fish oil is used in the treatment of refractory hypertriglyceridemia, typically when treatment with fibric acid derivatives is incompletely effective. A meta-analysis by Hartweg et al. indicates that n-3 fatty acid supplementation consistently lowers triglycerides by a mean of 25%, with no untoward effects on glucose control in diabetes (230). The same analysis revealed a modest elevation of LDL in response to fish oil therapy. The authors concluded that fish oil may be an appropriate means of managing the dyslipidemia commonly seen in diabetes. There is some evidence to suggest that n-3 fatty acids stimulate hepatic gluconeogenesis and thereby can degrade glycemic control. Thus, their role in routine diabetes management remains uncertain. While reviews to date fail to define a clear role for n-3 fatty acids in diabetes management per se (231,232), a role for fish oil in the attenuation of certain cardiac risks is better substantiated (see Chapters 2 and 7). Thus, fish oil supplementation in diabetes as one among many strategies to mitigate cardiovascular risk may be considered. A standard dose is 1 g once to twice daily.

MUFAs

Improvements in glycemic control and insulin metabolism have been seen in numerous trials that increased the proportion of calories from monounsaturated fats (233–242). A relatively generous intake of monounsaturated fat is now widely recognized among the salient features of a healthful dietary pattern and is addressed further in Chapters 2, 7, and 45. Beneficial effects of MUFA intake on metabolic and cardiovascular risk factors may be responsible for some of the favorable outcomes associated with a Mediterranean diet pattern, discussed elsewhere in this chapter.

Cocoa/Flavonoids

A quickly burgeoning literature suggests beneficial effects of dark chocolate on glycemic control and insulin sensitivity (243–247); the dense concentration of bioflavonoid antioxidants in cacao is the purported "active" ingredient. There are as yet no clear guidelines for the dosing of dark chocolate as a functional food, although efforts to generate such guidance are under way. The topic is further addressed in Chapter 39.

Other Dietary Supplements

Interest in the use of complementary and alternative medicine (CAM) supplements is high among diabetic patients. Approximately one-third of type 1 and type 2 diabetics reported current use of CAM supplements in a 2011 study (248). It is important for clinicians to be able to provide guidance to patients on the evidence regarding the safety and efficacy of dietary supplements.

α- Lipoic acid (ALA) is an endogenously produced antioxidant that may ameliorate symptoms of diabetic neuropathy (249) According to a 2012 meta-analysis, intravenous administration of α-lipoic acid at 600 mg per day is effective in reducing peripheral neuropathy in diabetic patients; however, the effectiveness of oral supplementation has not been demonstrated (250).

Cinnamon has also been evaluated for its potential glucose-lowering effects. Although promising results have been obtained from animal studies, randomized trials in humans have not been conclusive. Some, but not all, supplementation trials have reported modest glucose-lowering effects in patients with type 2 diabetes or insulin resistance (251). In a 2012 pooled analysis, there were no statistically significant differences in measures of glycemic control between intervention groups receiving oral cinnamon preparations with a mean dose of 2 g daily and control groups

(252). This review included studies in patients with type 1 or type 2 diabetes.

New Considerations: Genomics and the Microbiome

Interactions between nutrition and the human genome and microbiome are emerging areas of research in diabetes. Genome-wide association studies (GWAS) have identified at least 44 gene variants associated with type 2 diabetes (253). However, approximately 90% of genetic heritability remains unaccounted for, suggesting that many additional genes with small effect sizes contribute to risk. As a result, incorporating genetic variants into risk prediction models does not significantly improve predictive value. Although the continued identification of additional genes may improve the power to predict diabetes risk, the value of this approach is uncertain; placing added emphasis on the genetic basis of type 2 diabetes may adversely affect patients' attitudes toward prevention and treatment (254). On the other hand, genetic testing might increase motivation to adopt lifestyle changes and adhere to medication regimens among individuals identified as "high risk" (255). A randomized controlled trial testing the effects of genetic testing on BMI, insulin resistance, and health behaviors in primary care patients is currently underway (256).

While effective, widespread use of genetic testing to predict type 2 diabetes may be several decades away; the identification of factors in the environment that influence the expression of diabetes-promoting genes is immediately applicable to practice. In diabetic rats, energy restriction prevents hyperglycemia and alters the expression of hundreds of genes related to glucose or lipid metabolism and signaling pathways in insulin-sensitive tissues (i.e., pancreatic islets, skeletal muscle, and liver) (257). In human subjects with IGT, the Pro12Ala polymorphism of the peroxisome proliferator-activated receptor-gamma 2 (PPAR-γ2) isoform gene has been associated with increased diabetes risk, particularly among less obese individuals (258). However, this effect was only observed in individuals randomized to a control condition and not in individuals assigned to an intensive diet and exercise intervention. The results of this study provide an example of the potential modulating effect of diet and physical activity on the association between a genotype and diabetes. The microorganisms inhabiting the human gut, or the microbiome, may represent an important link between genes, the environment, and risk of type 1 and type 2 diabetes. Although the mechanisms by which intestinal microbiota influence the pathophysiology of type 1 diabetes have not been fully elucidated, it appears likely that different species of bacteria have varying effects on the integrity of the intestinal epithelium and immunity (259). For example, in vitro studies suggest that species of *Bifidobacteria* may protect intestinal epithelial cells from gliadin, a glycoprotein found in gluten that is known to cause intestinal inflammation and permeability (260,261). On the other hand, *Escherichia coli* or *Shigella* may exacerbate gliadin's effects (262). It is not known whether alteration of intestinal microbiota by probiotic supplementation can influence diabetes risk, but a study is currently underway in Finland to determine the effects of probiotic supplements on type 1 diabetes-associated autoantibodies in genetically susceptible children (263).

A 2010 review by Musso et al. summarized the current evidence on the relationship between the microbiome and obesity and diabetes (264). There is now evidence from animal studies to suggest that the composition of the microbiome may mediate obesity through effects on energy absorption from food and energy expenditure via fatty acid oxidation (265). However, the development of obesity in mice also appears to change gut microbiota, favoring the Firmicutes phylum at the expense of Bacteroidetes; this alteration increases the efficiency of energy extraction from food. The same effect is observed when mice are fed a Western (high-fat, high-sugar) diet, and is reversed when a standard (low-fat, high-polysaccharide) diet is resumed. Transplanting gut microbiota from obese mice to lean mice leads to increased energy extraction from food and increased body fat mass. Several small studies in humans have had similar results: obese subjects have a higher proportion of Firmicutes in the gut compared with lean subjects and reduced bacterial diversity, and weight loss increases the proportion of Bacteroidetes. However, these findings have not been consistently replicated in humans. Significant differences have been observed between the gut microbiota compositions of diabetic and nondiabetic individuals, and one study found that probiotic supplementation in pregnant women reduced the risk of gestational diabetes. However, this area of research is still in its infancy; more long-term studies are necessary to determine the safety and efficacy of supplementation with prebiotics or probiotics (264). In the meantime, a healthy diet and weight loss when necessary may promote a favorable composition of gut microbiota.

CLINICAL HIGHLIGHTS

The literature guiding the management and prevention of diabetes is voluminous, complex, and evolving. Pharmacotherapy is, of course, a mainstay in the management of all varieties of diabetes mellitus, the details of which are beyond the scope of this chapter. There are excellent recent reviews covering type 1 and type 2 diabetes, as well as gestational diabetes and diabetes prevention (265–275).

Nutritional and lifestyle therapy is, however, comparably important in effective diabetes management, and it offers far greater promise for diabetes prevention at the population level. Placed in the context of nutritional principles pertinent to the management of related conditions, including obesity, CVD, hypertension, and renal insufficiency, a cohesive approach to the dietary management of both insulin resistance and diabetes emerges.

For the majority of diabetic patients, weight loss and maintenance are mainstays of clinical management. Complex topics in their own right (see Chapters 5, 44, and 47), weight loss and maintenance are best achieved by restriction of nutrient energy in combination with consistent exercise; the Diabetes Prevention Program has clearly demonstrated the value of this approach in the prevention of diabetes in high-risk individuals. Both weight loss and exercise have demonstrated independent benefit in the control of diabetes and its sequelae.

In conjunction with efforts at weight control, diabetes warrants attention to all three classes of macronutrients. Protein intake generally should be maintained at or near 0.8 g/kg/day, with restrictions below this level as required only with the advent of renal insufficiency (see Chapter 16); slightly higher protein intake, up to 25% of calories, is among the strategies highlighted for reducing the dietary GL.

Although controversies persist regarding optimal levels of carbohydrate and fat, the literature on this and other topics generally supports a carbohydrate intake of approximately 55% of calories, with fat comprising 25% to 30%. Carbohydrate should be complex and, perhaps even more importantly, should provide at least 30 g per day of fiber, preferably more. Sources of soluble fiber of particular metabolic benefit include fruits, grains, and legumes. The combination of saturated and trans fat ideally should be restricted to below 5%, and certainly below 10%. Although benefits of n-3 fatty acids remain uncertain, other lines of evidence support allocating roughly 10% of total calories to polyunsaturated fat, with an approximately 1:4 ratio of n-3 to n-6 PUFAs. This pattern is achieved by using unsaturated vegetable oils, eating nuts and seeds, and either including fish routinely in the diet or taking a fish oil supplement. The remaining, approximately 15%, of calories should be allocated to monounsaturated fat. Monounsaturated fat is derived from olive oil, canola oil, olives, avocado, nuts, and seeds in particular.

Given the benefits attached to soluble fiber, a particular effort should be made to increase its intake. Oatmeal, apples, and berries are concentrated sources, readily worked into any health-promoting dietary pattern. Beans and lentils are excellent sources as well, and, if used on occasion as alternative protein sources to meat, offer the additional potential advantage of reducing saturated fat intake. The economy of beans and lentils is also noteworthy in light of the often-heard, if questionable, lament that healthful eating is prohibitively expensive.

Exchange lists, available from the American Dietetic Association, may be of use to both clinicians and patients in efforts to translate such guidelines into actual dietary practice. However, there has been declining reliance on exchange lists over recent years and increasing attention to a potentially more convenient emphasis on healthful foods close to nature. Consultation of a dietitian should be routine in diabetes care and should facilitate the development of meal plans to accommodate clinical recommendations.

Multivitamin/mineral supplementation can be argued on general principles and may be of benefit in diabetes. Chromium is well established as a cofactor in insulin metabolism, although evidence of a beneficial role in either diabetes management or prevention is at present suggestive but not conclusive. Daily supplementation with chromium picolinate, 400 μg twice daily, is apparently safe and potentially beneficial.

Weight control, physical activity, and adjustments of both macronutrient and micronutrient intake should be judiciously combined with carefully selected pharmacotherapy to optimize the control and clinical outcomes of diabetes and to achieve optimal rates of diabetes prevention. In overweight patients with insulin resistance or diabetes, marked benefit may be expected with a 7% to 10% weight loss. The weight loss required for appreciable metabolic benefit likely varies markedly with anthropometry and ethnicity, but population-specific guidelines are as yet unavailable.

REFERENCES

1. de la Monte SM, Wands JR. Alzheimer's disease is type 3 diabetes—evidence reviewed. *J Diabetes Sci Technol* 2008;2(6):1101–1113.

2. Donath MY, Ehses JA. Type 1, type 1.5, and type 2 diabetes: not the diabetes we thought it was. *Proc Natl Acad Sci USA* 2006;103:12217–12218.

3. Centers for Disease Control and Prevention. *Percentage of civilian, noninstitutionalized population with diagnosed diabetes, by age, United States, 1980–2011.* Available at http://www.cdc.gov/diabetes/statistics/prev/national/figbyage.htm; accessed 9/18/13.

4. May AL, Kuklina EV, Yoon PW. Prevalence of cardiovascular disease risk factors among US adolescents, 1999–2008. *Pediatrics* 2012;129(6):1035–1041.

5. Dabelea D, Bell RA, D'Agostino RB Jr, et al. Incidence of diabetes in youth in the United States. *JAMA* 2007;297(24):2716–2724.

6. Tuomilehto J. The emerging global epidemic of type 1 diabetes. *Curr Diab Rep* 2013;13(6):795–804.

7. Lillioja S, Mott D, Howard B, et al. Impaired glucose tolerance as a disorder of insulin action. *N Engl J Med* 1988;318:1217–1225.

8. American Diabetes Association. *Diagnosing Diabetes and Learning About Prediabetes.* Available at http://www.diabetes.org/diabetes-basics/diagnosis/; accessed 4/3/14.

9. Chaparro RJ, Konigshofer Y, Beilhack GF, et al. Nonobese diabetic mice express aspects of both type 1 and type 2 diabetes. *Proc Natl Acad Sci USA* 2006;103:12475–12480.

10. Centers for Disease Control and Prevention. *National diabetes fact sheet, United States 2011.* Available at http://www.cdc.gov/diabetes/pubs/factsheet11.htm; accessed 2/28/13.

11. Gregg EW, Cadwell BL, Cheng YJ, et al. Trends in the prevalence and ratio of diagnosed to undiagnosed diabetes according to obesity levels in the US. *Diabetes Care* 2004;27:2806–2812.

12. Ford ES, Giles WH, Mokdad AH. Increasing prevalence of the metabolic syndrome among US adults. *Diabetes Care* 2004;27:2444–2449.

13. Reaven G, Abbasi F, McLaughlin T. Obesity, insulin resistance, and cardiovascular disease. *Recent Prog Horm Res* 2004;59:207–223.

14. World Health Organization. *Diabetes programme: diabetes fact sheet.* Available at http://www.who.int/mediacentre/factsheets/fs312/en/index.html; accessed 2/28/13.

15. Engelgau MM, Geiss LS, Saaddine JB, et al. The evolving diabetes burden in the United States. *Ann Intern Med* 2004;140:945–950.

16. Narayan KM, Boyle JP, Thompson TJ, et al. Lifetime risk for diabetes mellitus in the United States. *JAMA* 2003;290:1884–1890.

17. Honeycutt AA, Boyle JP, Broglio KR, et al. A dynamic Markov model for forecasting diabetes prevalence in the United States through 2050. *Health Care Manag Sci* 2003;6:155–164.

18. Haller MJ, Atkinson MA, Schatz D. Type 1 diabetes mellitus: etiology, presentation, and management. *Pediatr Clin North Am* 2005;52:1553–1578.

19. Akerblom HK, Vaarala O, Hyoty H, et al. Environmental factors in the etiology of type 1 diabetes. *Am J Med Genet* 2002;115:18–29.

20. Atkinson M, Ellis T. Infants' diets and insulin-dependent diabetes: evaluating the "cows' milk hypothesis" and a role for anti-bovine serum albumin immunity. *J Am Coll Nutr* 1997;16:334.

21. Vaarala O, Knip M, Paronen J, et al. Cow's milk formula feeding induces primary immunization to insulin in infants at genetic risk for type 1 diabetes. *Diabetes* 1999;48:1389–1394.

22. Patelarou E, Girvalaki C, Brokalaki H, et al. Current evidence on the associations of breastfeeding, infant formula, and cow's milk introduction with type 1 diabetes mellitus: a systematic review. *Nutr Rev* 2012;70(9):509–519.

23. Barbeau WE, Bassaganya-Riera J, Hontecillas R. Putting the pieces of the puzzle together—a series of hypotheses on the etiology and pathogenesis of type 1 diabetes. *Med Hypotheses* 2007;68:607–619.

24. Samuelsson U, Johansson C, Ludvigsson J. Breastfeeding seems to play a marginal role in the prevention of insulin-dependent diabetes mellitus. *Diabetes Res Clin Pract* 1993;19:203–210.

25. Meloni T, Marinaro AM, Mannazzu MC, et al. IDDM and early infant feeding. Sardinian case-control study. *Diabetes Care* 1997;20:340–342.

26. Sadauskaite-Kuehne V, Ludvigsson J, Padaiga Z, et al. Longer breastfeeding is an independent protective factor against development of type 1 diabetes mellitus in childhood. *Diabetes Metab Res Rev* 2004;20:150–157.

27. Perez-Bravo F, Oyarzun A, Carrasco E, et al. Duration of breast feeding and bovine serum albumin antibody levels in type 1 diabetes: a case-control study. *Pediatr Diabetes* 2003;4:157–161.

28. Lebovitz H. Type 2 diabetes: an overview. *Clin Chem* 1999;45:1339–1345.

29. Drong AW, Lindgren CM, McCarthy MI. The genetic and epigenetic basis of type 2 diabetes and obesity. *Clin Pharmacol Ther* 2012;92(6):707–715.

30. Neel J. Diabetes mellitus: a "thrifty" genotype rendered detrimental by "progress"? *Am J Hum Genet* 1962;14:353–362.

31. Benyshek DC, Watson JT. Exploring the thrifty genotype's food-shortage assumptions: a cross-cultural comparison of ethnographic accounts of food security among foraging and agricultural societies. *Am J Phys Anthropol* 2006;131:120–126.

32. Prentice AM. Early influences on human energy regulation: thrifty genotypes and thrifty phenotypes. *Physiol Behav* 2005;86:640–645.

33. Prentice AM, Rayco-Solon P, Moore SE. Insights from the developing world: thrifty genotypes and thrifty phenotypes. *Proc Nutr Soc* 2005;64:153–161.

34. Chakravarthy MV, Booth FW. Eating, exercise, and "thrifty" genotypes: connecting the dots toward an evolutionary understanding of modern chronic diseases. *J Appl Physiol* 2004;96:3–10.

35. Speakman JR. Thrifty genes for obesity and the metabolic syndrome—time to call off the search? *Diab Vasc Dis Res* 2006;3:7–11.

36. Dulloo AG, Jacquet J, Seydoux J, et al. The thrifty "catch-up fat" phenotype: its impact on insulin sensitivity during growth trajectories to obesity and metabolic syndrome. *Int J Obes (Lond)* 2006;30:S23–S35.

37. Allen DB, Nemeth BA, Clark RR, et al. Fitness is a stronger predictor of fasting insulin levels than fatness in overweight male middle-school children. *J Pediatr* 2007;150:383–387.

38. Goldfine AB, Bouche C, Parker RA, et al. Insulin resistance is a poor predictor of type 2 diabetes in individuals with no family history of disease. *Proc Natl Acad Sci USA* 2003;100:2724–2729.

39. Kadowaki T. Insights into insulin resistance and type 2 diabetes from knockout mouse models. *J Clin Invest* 2000;106:459–465.

40. Cavaghan MK, Ehrmann DA, Polonsky KS. Interactions between insulin resistance and insulin secretion in the development of glucose intolerance. *J Clin Invest* 2000;106: 329–333.

41. Riddle MC, Genuth S. *Metabolism, II Type 2 diabetes mellitus.* ACP Medcine Online. Available at http://www.medscape.com/viewarticle/548768?rss; accessed 12/28/07.

42. Meece J. Pancreatic islet dysfunction in type 2 diabetes: a rational target for incretin-based therapies. *Curr Med Res Opin* 2007;23:933–944.

43. Colditz GA, Willett WC, Rotnitzky A, et al. Weight gain as a risk factor for clinical diabetes mellitus in women [see comments]. *Ann Intern Med* 1995;122:481–486.

44. Ford E, Williamson D, Liu S. Weight change and diabetes incidence: findings from a national cohort of US adults. *Am J Epidemiol* 1997;146:214.

45. Biggs ML, Mukamal KJ, Luchsinger JA, et al. Association between adiposity in midlife and older age and risk of diabetes in older adults. *JAMA* 2010;303(24):2504–2512.

46. Lazarus R, Sparrow D, Weiss S. Temporal relations between obesity and insulin: longitudinal data from the normative aging study. *Am J Epidemiol* 1998;147: 173–179.

47. Aye T, Levitsky LL. Type 2 diabetes: an epidemic disease in childhood. *Curr Opin Pediatr* 2003;15:411–415.

48. Fagot-Campagna A, Pettitt DJ, et al. Type 2 diabetes among North American children and adolescents: an epidemiologic review and a public health perspective. *J Pediatr* 2000;136:664–672.

49. Pontiroli AE. Type 2 diabetes mellitus is becoming the most common type of diabetes in school children. *Acta Diabetol* 2004;41:85–90.

50. Wiegand S, Maikowski U, Blankenstein O, et al. Type 2 diabetes and impaired glucose tolerance in European children and adolescents with obesity—a problem that is no longer restricted to minority groups. *Eur J Endocrinol* 2004;151:199–206.

51. Expert Panel on Detection Evaluation and Treatment of High Blood Cholesterol in Adults. Executive summary of the third report of the National Cholesterol Education Program (NCEP) Expert Panel on detection, evaluation, and treatment of high blood cholesterol in adults (Adult Treatment Panel III). *JAMA* 2001;285:2486–2497.

52. Apedo MT, Sowers JR, Banerji MA. Cardiovascular disease in adolescents with type 2 diabetes mellitus. *J Pediatr Endocrinol Metab* 2002;15:519–523.

53. Steinberger J, Daniels SR. Obesity, insulin resistance, diabetes, and cardiovascular risk in children: an American Heart Association scientific statement from the Atherosclerosis, Hypertension, and Obesity in the Young Committee (Council on Cardiovascular Disease in the Young) and the Diabetes Committee (Council on Nutrition, Physical Activity, and Metabolism). *Circulation* 2003;107:1448–1453.

54. Moller D, Flier J. Insulin resistance—mechanisms, syndromes, and implications. *N Engl J Med* 1991;325:938–948.

55. Ye J. Role of insulin in the pathogenesis of free fatty acid-induced insulin resistance in skeletal muscle. *Endocr Metab Immune Disord Drug Targets* 2007;7:65–74.

56. Sesti G. Pathophysiology of insulin resistance. *Best Pract Res Clin Endocrinol Metab* 2006;20:665–679.

57. Lillioja S, Mott D, Spraul M, et al. Insulin resistance and insulin secretory dysfunction as precursors of non-insulin-dependent diabetes mellitus. *N Engl J Med* 1993;329:1988–1992.

58. Pimenta W, Mitrakou A, Jensen T, et al. Insulin secretion and insulin sensitivity in people with impaired glucose tolerance. *Diabet Med* 1996;13:s33–s36.

59. Reaven GM, Lithell H, Landsberg L. Hypertension and associated metabolic abnormalities—the role of insulin resistance and the sympathoadrenal system. *N Engl J Med* 1996;334:374–381.

60. Cowen R. Seeds of protection. *Sci News* 1990;137:350–351.

61. Grundy S. Hypertriglyceridemia, insulin resistance, and the metabolic syndrome. *Am J Cardiol* 1999;83:25f–29f.

62. American Heart Association. *Metabolic syndrome.* Available at http://www.americanheart.org/presenter.jhtml?identifier= 4756; accessed 3/20/13.

63. Kahn R, Buse J, Ferrannini E, et al; for the American Diabetes Association and the European Association for the Study of Diabetes. The metabolic syndrome: time for a critical appraisal (ADA statement). *Diabetes Care* 2005;28:2289–2304.

64. Knowler WC, Barrett-Connor E, Fowler SE, et al. Reduction in the incidence of type 2 diabetes with lifestyle intervention or metformin. *N Engl J Med* 2002;346:393–403.

65. Look AHEAD Research Group, Pi-Sunyer X, Blackburn G, et al. Reduction in weight and cardiovascular disease risk factors in individuals with type 2 diabetes: one-year results of the look AHEAD trial. *Diabetes Care* 2007;30(6):1374–1383.

66. Look AHEAD Research Group, Wing RR. Long-term effects of a lifestyle intervention on weight and cardiovascular risk factors in individuals with type 2 diabetes mellitus: four-year results of the Look AHEAD trial. *Arch Intern Med* 2010;27;170(17):1566–1575.

67. Genuth S. Insights from the diabetes control and complications trial/epidemiology of diabetes interventions and complications study on the use of intensive glycemic

treatment to reduce the risk of complications of type 1 diabetes. *Endocr Pract* 2006;12(suppl 1):34–34.

68. The Diabetes Control and Complications Trial Research Group. The effect of intensive treatment of diabetes on the development and progression of long-term complications in insulin-dependent diabetes mellitus. *N Engl J Med* 1993;329:977–986.

69. Clark CM Jr, Adlin V, eds. Risks and benefits of intensive management in non-insulin-dependent diabetes mellitus. The Fifth Regenstrief Conference. *Ann Intern Med* 1996;124:81–186.

70. Brown A, Reynolds LR, Bruemmer D. Intensive glycemic control and cardiovascular disease: an update. *Nat Rev Cardiol* 2010;7(7):369–375.

71. Mitka M. Aggressive glycemic control might not be best choice for all diabetic patients. *JAMA* 2010;303(12):1137–1138.

72. Schnabel CA, Wintle M, Kolterman O. Metabolic effects of the incretin mimetic exenatide in the treatment of type 2 diabetes. *Vasc Health Risk Manag* 2006;2:69–77.

73. Stonehouse AH, Holcombe JH, Kendall DM. Management of type 2 diabetes: the role of incretin mimetics. *Expert Opin Pharmacother* 2006;7:2095–2105.

74. Krentz AJ, Bailey CJ. Oral antidiabetic agents: current role in type 2 diabetes mellitus. *Drugs* 2005;65:385–411.

75. Inzucchi SE. Oral antihyperglycemic therapy for type 2 diabetes: scientific review. *JAMA* 2002;287:360–372.

76. Bennett WL, Maruthur NM, Singh S, et al. Comparative effectiveness and safety of medications for type 2 diabetes: an update including new drugs and 2-drug combinations. *Ann Intern Med* 2011;154(9):602–613.

77. Jenkins D, Wolever T, Taylor R, et al. Glycemic index of foods: a physiological basis for carbohydrate exchange. *Am J Clin Nutr* 1981;34:362–366.

78. Jenkins D, Wolever T, Vuksan V, et al. Nibbling versus gorging: metabolic advantages of increased meal frequency. *N Engl J Med* 1989;321:929–934.

79. Ludwig DS. Clinical update: the low-glycaemic-index diet. *Lancet* 2007;369:890–892.

80. Ebbeling CB, Leidig MM, Sinclair KB, et al. Effects of an ad libitum low-glycemic load diet on cardiovascular disease risk factors in obese young adults. *Am J Clin Nutr* 2005;81:976–982.

81. Pereira MA, Swain J, Goldfine AB, et al. Effects of a low-glycemic load diet on resting energy expenditure and heart disease risk factors during weight loss. *JAMA* 2004;292:2482–2490.

82. Buyken AE, Dettmann W, Kersting M, et al. Glycaemic index and glycaemic load in the diet of healthy schoolchildren: trends from 1990 to 2002, contribution of different carbohydrate sources and relationships to dietary quality. *Br J Nutr* 2005;94:796–803.

83. Shikany JM, Thomas SE, Henson CS, et al. Glycemic index and glycemic load of popular weight-loss diets. *MedGenMed* 2006;8:22.

84. Livesey G. Low-glycaemic diets and health: implications for obesity. *Proc Nutr Soc* 2005;64:105–113.

85. Schulz M, Liese AD, Mayer-Davis EJ, et al. Nutritional correlates of dietary glycaemic index: new aspects from a population perspective. *Br J Nutr* 2005;94:397–406.

86. Olendzki BC, Ma Y, Culver AL, et al. Methodology for adding glycemic index and glycemic load values to 24-hour dietary recall database. *Nutrition* 2006;22:1087–1095.

87. Kelly S, Frost G, Whittaker V, et al. Low glycaemic index diets for coronary heart disease. *Cochrane Database Syst Rev* 2004;4:CD004467.

88. McMillan-Price J, Petocz P, Atkinson F, et al. Comparison of 4 diets of varying glycemic load on weight loss and cardiovascular risk reduction in overweight and obese young adults: a randomized controlled trial. *Arch Intern Med* 2006;166:1466–1475.

89. Zavaroni I, Bonora E, Pagliara M, et al. Risk factors for coronary artery disease in healthy persons with hyperinsulinemia and normal glucose tolerance. *N Engl J Med* 1989;320:702–707.

90. Diabetes Prevention Program Research Group. 10-year follow-up of diabetes incidence and weight loss in the Diabetes Prevention Program Outcomes Study. *Lancet* 2009; 374(9702):1677–1686.

91. DREAM (Diabetes Reduction Assessment with ramipril and rosiglitazone Medication) Trial Investigators, Gerstein HC, Yusuf S, et al. Effect of rosiglitazone on the frequency of diabetes in patients with impaired glucose tolerance or impaired fasting glucose: a randomised controlled trial. *Lancet* 2006;368:1096–1105.

92. Diabetes Prevention Program Research Group. Within-trial cost-effectiveness of lifestyle intervention or metformin for the primary prevention of type 2 diabetes. *Diabetes Care* 2003;26:2518–2523.

93. Eddy DM, Schlessinger L, Kahn R. Clinical outcomes and cost-effectiveness of strategies for managing people at high risk for diabetes. *Ann Intern Med* 2005;143:251–264.

94. Herman WH, Hoerger TJ, Brandle M, et al. The cost-effectiveness of lifestyle modification or metformin in preventing type 2 diabetes in adults with impaired glucose tolerance. *Ann Intern Med* 2005;142:323–332.

95. Horton E, Napoli R. Diabetes mellitus. In: Ziegler E, Filer FJ, eds. *Present knowledge in nutrition*, 7th ed. Washington, DC: ILSI Press, 1996:445–455.

96. American Diabetes Association, Bantle JP, Wylie-Rosett J, et al. Nutrition recommendations and interventions for diabetes: a position statement of the American Diabetes Association. *Diabetes Care* 2008;(suppl 1):S61–S78.

97. Chiuve SE, Sampson L, Willett WC. The association between a nutritional quality index and risk of chronic disease. *Am J Prev Med* 2011;40(5):505–513.

98. American Diabetes Association. Nutrition recommendations and interventions for diabetes: a position statement of the American Diabetes Association. *Diabetes Care* 2008;31(suppl 1):S61–S78.

99. Steward H, Bethea M, Andrews S, et al. *Sugar busters! Cut sugar to trim fat.* New York, NY: Ballantine Books, 1998.

100. Heller R, Heller R. *The carbohydrate addict's lifespan program.* New York, NY: Plume, 1998.

101. Atkins DR. *Atkins' new diet revolution.* New York, NY: M. Evans & Company, 1999.

102. Sears B, Lawren B. *Enter the zone.* New York, NY: Regan Books, 1995.

103. Blades B, Garg A. Mechanisms of increase in plasma triacylglycerol concentrations as a result of high carbohydrate intakes in patients with non-insulin-dependent diabetes mellitus. *Am J Clin Nutr* 1995:996–1002.

104. Lewis G, Steiner G. Acute effects of insulin in the control of VLDL production in humans. *Diabetes Care* 1996;19:390–393.

105. DeFronzo R, Prato SD. Insulin resistance and diabetes mellitus. *J Diabetes Complications* 1996;10:243–245.

106. Boden G, Tataranni P, Baier L, et al. Role of lipids in development of noninsulin-dependent diabetes mellitus: lessons learned from Pima Indians. *Lipids* 1996;31: s267–s270.

107. Garg A, Bonamome A, Grundy S, et al. Comparison of a high-carbohydrate diet with a high-monounsaturated-fat diet in patients with non-insulin-dependent diabetes mellitus. *N Engl J Med* 1988;319:829–843.

108. Garg A, Bantle J, Henry R, et al. Effects of varying carbohydrate content of diet in patients with non-insulin-dependent diabetes mellitus. *JAMA* 1994;271:1421–1428.

109. Guldbrand H, Dizdar B, Bunjaku B, et al. In type 2 diabetes, randomisation to advice to follow a low-carbohydrate diet transiently improves glycaemic control compared with advice to follow a low-fat diet producing a similar weight loss. *Diabetologia* 2012;55(8):2118–2127.

110. Davis NJ, Tomuta N, Schechter C, et al. Comparative study of the effects of a 1-year dietary intervention of a low-carbohydrate diet versus a low-fat diet on weight and glycemic control in type 2 diabetes. *Diabetes Care* 2009;32(7):1147–1152.

111. Milne R, Mann J, Chisholm A, et al. Long-term comparison of three dietary prescriptions in the treatment of NIDDM. *Diabetes Care* 1994;17:74–80.

112. Luscombe N, Noakes M, Clifton P. Diets high and low in glycemic index versus high monounsaturated fat diets: effects on glucose and lipid metabolism in NIDDM. *Eur J Clin Nutr* 1999;53:473–478.

113. Gerhard GT, Ahmann A, Meeuws K, et al. Effects of a low-fat diet compared with those of a high-monounsaturated fat diet on body weight, plasma lipids and lipoproteins, and glycemic control in type 2 diabetes. *Am J Clin Nutr* 2004; 80(3):668–673.

114. Shai I, Schwarzfuchs D, Henkin Y, et al. Weight loss with a low-carbohydrate, Mediterranean, or low-fat diet. *N Engl J Med* 2008;359(3):229–241

115. Elhayany A, Lustman A, Abel R, et al. Of note, all three diets improved body composition, glycemic control, and blood lipids. A low carbohydrate Mediterranean diet improves cardiovascular risk factors and diabetes control among overweight patients with type 2 diabetes mellitus: a 1-year prospective randomized intervention study. *Diabetes Obes Metab* 2010;12(3):204–209.

116. Barnard ND, Cohen J, Jenkins DJ, et al. A low-fat vegan diet and a conventional diabetes diet in the treatment of type 2 diabetes: a randomized, controlled, 74-wk clinical trial. *Am J Clin Nutr* 2009;89(5):1588S-1596S.

117. Roche H. Dietary carbohydrates and triacylglycerol metabolism. *Proc Nutr Soc* 1999;58:201–207.

118. Sargrad KR, Homko C, Mozzoli M, et al. Effect of high protein vs high carbohydrate intake on insulin sensitivity, body weight, hemoglobin A1c, and blood pressure in patients with type 2 diabetes mellitus. *J Am Diet Assoc* 2005;105:573–580.

119. Heilbronn LK, Noakes M, Clifton PM. The effect of high- and low-glycemic index energy restricted diets on plasma lipid and glucose profiles in type 2 diabetic subjects with varying glycemic control. *J Am Coll Nutr* 2002;21: 120–127.

120. Storm H, Thomsen C, Pedersen E, et al. Comparison of a carbohydrate-rich diet and diets rich in stearic or palmitic acid in NIDDM patients. Effects on lipids, glycemic control, and diurnal blood pressure. *Diabetes Care* 1997;20:1807–1813.

121. Gillespie S, Kulkarni K, Daly A. Using carbohydrate counting in diabetes clinical practice. *J Am Diet Assoc* 1998;98:897–905.

122. Pi-Sunyer F, Maggio C, McCarron D, et al. Multicenter randomized trial of a comprehensive prepared meal program in type 2 diabetes. *Diabetes Care* 1999;22:191–197.

123. Ziemer DC, Berkowitz KJ, Panayioto RM, et al. A simple meal plan emphasizing healthy food choices is as effective as an exchange-based meal plan for urban African Americans with type 2 diabetes. *Diabetes Care* 2003;26:1719–1724.

124. Academy of Nutrition and Dietetics. *Choose your foods: exchange lists for diabetes.* Available at https://www.eatright. org/shop/product.aspx?id=4962; accessed 03/24/13.

125. Nathan DM, Cleary PA, Backlund JY, et al. Intensive diabetes treatment and cardiovascular disease in patients with type 1 diabetes. *N Engl J Med* 2005;353:2643–2653.

126. UK Prospective Diabetes Study (UKPDS) Group. Effect of intensive blood-glucose control with metformin on complications in overweight patients with type 2 diabetes (UKPDS 34). *Lancet* 1998;352:854–865.

127. UK Prospective Diabetes Study (UKPDS) Group. Intensive blood-glucose control with sulphonylureas or insulin compared with conventional treatment and risk of complications in patients with type 2 diabetes (UKPDS 33). *Lancet* 1998;352:837–853.

128. Clarke PM, Gray AM, Briggs A, et al. Cost-utility analyses of intensive blood glucose and tight blood pressure control in type 2 diabetes (UKPDS 72). *Diabetologia* 2005;48:868–877.

129. Davidson JA. Treatment of the patient with diabetes: importance of maintaining target HbA(1c) levels. *Curr Med Res Opin* 2004;20:1919–1927.

130. Bell S, Forse R. Nutritional management of hypoglycemia. *Diabetes Educ* 1999;25:41–47.

131. Kalergis M, Schiffrin A, Gougeon R, et al. Impact of bedtime snack composition on prevention of nocturnal hypoglycemia in adults with type 1 diabetes undergoing intensive insulin management using lispro insulin before meals: a randomized, placebo-controlled, crossover trial. *Diabetes Care* 2003;26:9–15.

132. Dyer-Parziale M. The effect of extend bar containing uncooked cornstarch on night-time glycemic excursion in subjects with type 2 diabetes. *Diabetes Res Clin Pract* 2001;53:137–139.

133. Raju B, Arbelaez AM, Breckenridge SM, et al. Nocturnal hypoglycemia in type 1 diabetes: an assessment of preventive bedtime treatments. *J Clin Endocrinol Metab* 2006;91:2087–2092.

134. Tsalikian E, Mauras N, Beck RW, et al. Impact of exercise on overnight glycemic control in children with type 1 diabetes mellitus. *J Pediatr* 2005;147:528–534.

135. Pi-Sunyer FX. How effective are lifestyle changes in the prevention of type 2 diabetes mellitus? *Nutr Rev* 2007;65:101–110.

136. Coughlin CC, Finck BN, Eagon JC, et al. Effect of marked weight loss on adiponectin gene expression and plasma concentrations. *Obesity (Silver Spring)* 2007;15:640–645.

137. Aronne LJ. Therapeutic options for modifying cardiometabolic risk factors. *Am J Med* 2007;120:s26–s34.

138. Lee M, Aronne LJ. Weight management for type 2 diabetes mellitus: global cardiovascular risk reduction. *Am J Cardiol* 2007;99:68b–79b.

139. Mathieu P, Pibarot P, Despres JP. Metabolic syndrome: the danger signal in atherosclerosis. *Vasc Health Risk Manag* 2006;2:285–302.

140. St-Pierre J, Lemieux I, Perron P, et al. Relation of the "hypertriglyceridemic waist" phenotype to earlier manifestations of coronary artery disease in patients with glucose intolerance and type 2 diabetes mellitus. *Am J Cardiol* 2007;99:369–373.

141. Despres JP, Lemieux I. Abdominal obesity and metabolic syndrome. *Nature* 2006;444:881–887.

142. Blackburn P, Despres JP, Lamarche B, et al. Postprandial variations of plasma inflammatory markers in abdominally obese men. *Obesity (Silver Spring)* 2006;14:1747–1754.

143. Després JP. Intra-abdominal obesity: an untreated risk factor for Type 2 diabetes and cardiovascular disease. *J Endocrinol Invest* 2006;29:77–82.

144. Rush EC, Goedecke JH, Jennings C, et al. BMI, fat and muscle differences in urban women of five ethnicities from two countries. *Int J Obes (Lond)* 2007;31:1232–1239.

145. He M, Tan KC, Li ET, et al. Body fat determination by dual energy x-ray absorptiometry and its relation to body mass index and waist circumference in Hong Kong Chinese. *Int J Obes Relat Metab Disord* 2001;25:748–752.

146. Deurenberg-Yap M, Schmidt G, van Staveren WA, et al. The paradox of low body mass index and high body fat percentage among Chinese, Malays and Indians in Singapore. *Int J Obes Relat Metab Disord* 2000;24:1011–1017.

147. Taylor R. Pathogenesis of type 2 diabetes: tracing the reverse route from cure to cause. *Diabetologia* 2008;51(10):1781–1789.

148. Jazet IM, Pijl H, Frolich M, et al. Two days of a very low calorie diet reduces endogenous glucose production (EGP) in obese type 2 diabetic patients despite the withdrawal of blood glucose-lowering therapies including insulin. *Metabolism* 2005;54(6):705–712.

149. Mingrone G, Panunzi S, De Gaetano A, et al. Bariatric surgery versus conventional medical therapy for type 2 diabetes. *N Engl J Med* 2012;366(17):1577–1585.

150. Ludwig DS, Ebbeling CB, Livingston EH. Surgical vs lifestyle treatment for type 2 diabetes. *JAMA* 2012;308(10):981–982.

151. Jenkins D, Wolever T, Jenkins A. Starchy foods and glycemic index. *Diabetes Care* 1988;11:149–159.

152. Jenkins D, Jenkins A. The glycemic index, fiber, and the dietary treatment of hypertriglyceridemia and diabetes. *J Am Coll Nutr* 1987;6:11–17.

153. Bantle J, Laine D, Castle G, et al. Postprandial glucose and insulin responses to meals containing different carbohydrates in normal and diabetic subjects. *N Engl J Med* 1983;309:7–12.

154. American Dietetic Association. Nutrition recommendations and principles for people with diabetes mellitus. *Diabetes Care* 1994;17:519–522.

155. Liljeberg H, Akerberg A, Bjorck I. Effect of the glycemic index and content of indigestible carbohydrates of cereal-based breakfast meals on glucose tolerance at lunch in healthy subjects. *Am J Clin Nutr* 1999;69:647–655.

156. Moyad MA. Fad diets and obesity—part II: an introduction to the theory behind low-carbohydrate diets. *Urol Nurs* 2004;24:442–445.

157. Wikipedia. *Glycemic load.* Available at http://en.wikipedia.org/wiki/Glycemic_load; accessed 10/8/07.

158. Colombani PC. Glycemic index and load-dynamic dietary guidelines in the context of disease. *Physiol Behav* 2004;83:603–610.

159. Foster-Powell K, Holt SHA, Brand-Miller JC. International table of glycemic index and glycemic load values: 2002. *Am J Clin Nutr* 2002;76:5–56. Available at http://www.ajcn.org/cgi/content-nw/full/76/1/5/T1; accessed 10/8/07.

160. Barclay AW, Petocz P, McMillan-Price J, et al. Glycemic index, glycemic load, and chronic disease risk—a meta-analysis of observational studies. *Am J Clin Nutr* 2008;87(3):627–637.

161. Du H, van der A DL, van Bakel MM, et al. Glycemic index and glycemic load in relation to food and nutrient intake and metabolic risk factors in a Dutch population. *Am J Clin Nutr* 2008;87(3):655–661.

162. Das SK, Gilhooly CH, Golden JK, et al. Long-term effects of 2 energy-restricted diets differing in glycemic load on dietary adherence, body composition, and metabolism in CALERIE: a 1-y randomized controlled trial. *Am J Clin Nutr* 2007;85(4):1023–1030.

163. Philippou E, McGowan BM, Brynes AE, et al. The effect of a 12-week low glycaemic index diet on heart disease risk factors and 24 h glycaemic response in healthy middle-aged volunteers at risk of heart disease: a pilot study. *Eur J Clin Nutr* 2008;62(1):145–149.

164. Thomas DE, Elliott EJ, Baur L. Low glycaemic index or low glycaemic load diets for overweight and obesity. *Cochrane Database Syst Rev* 2007;(3):CD005105.

165. Philippou E, Bovill-Taylor C, Rajkumar C, et al. Preliminary report: the effect of a 6-month dietary glycemic index manipulation in addition to healthy eating advice and weight loss on arterial compliance and 24-hour ambulatory blood pressure in men: a pilot study. *Metabolism* 2009;58(12):1703–1708.

166. Philippou E, Neary NM, Chaudhri O, et al. The effect of dietary glycemic index on weight maintenance in overweight subjects: a pilot study. *Obesity* (Silver Spring) 2009;17(2):396–401.

167. Nash SD, Westpfal M. Cardiovascular benefits of nuts. *Am J Cardiol* 2005;95(8):963–965.

168. Kendall CWC, Josse AR, Esfahani A, et al. Nuts, metabolic syndrome, and diabetes. *Br J Nutr* 2010;104:465–473.

169. Jiang R, Manson JE, Stampfer MJ, et al. Nut and peanut butter consumption and risk of type 2 diabetes in women. *JAMA* 2002;288(20):2554–2560.

170. Parker ED, Harnack LJ, Folsom AR. Nut consumption and risk of type 2 diabetes. *JAMA* 2003;290(1):38–39.

171. Pan A, Sun Q, Manson JE, et al. Walnut consumption is associated with lower risk of type 2 diabetes in women. *J Nutr* 2013;143(4):512–518.

172. Casas-Agustench P, Lopez-Uriarte P, Bullo M, et al. Effects of one serving of mixed nuts on serum lipids, insulin resistance and inflammatory markers in patients with the metabolic syndrome. *Nutr Metab Cardiovasc Dis* 2011;21(2):126–135.

173. Tapsell LC, Batterham MJ, Teuss G, et al. Long-term effects of increased dietary polyunsaturated fat from

walnuts on metabolic parameters in type II diabetes. *Eur J Clin Nutr* 2009;63(8):1008–1015.

174. Ma Y, Njike VY, Millet J, et al. Effects of walnut consumption on endothelial function in type 2 diabetic subjects: a randomized controlled crossover trial. *Diabetes Care* 2010;33(3):227–232.

175. Mukuddem-Petersen J, Oosthuizen SW, Jerling JC, et al. Effects of a high walnut and high cashew nut diet on selected markers of the metabolic syndrome: a controlled feeding trial. *Br J Nutr* 2007;97(6):1144–1153.

176. Jenkins DJ, Kendall CW, Banach MS, et al. Nuts as a replacement for carbohydrates in the diabetic diet. *Diabetes Care* 2011;34(8):1706–1711.

177. Nutrient Data Laboratory. *USDA national nutrient database for standard reference*. Available at http://www.nal.usda.gov/fnic/foodcomp/search/; accessed 10/8/07.

178. McGrane MM. Carbohydrate metabolism—synthesis and oxidation. In: Stipanuk MH, ed. *Biochemical and physiological aspects of human nutrition*. Philadelphia, PA: Saunders, 2000:158–210.

179. Kleim NL, Levin RJ, Havel PJ. Carbohydrates. In: Shils ME, Shike M, Ross AC, et al., eds. *Modern nutrition in health and disease*, 10th ed. Philadelphia, PA: Lippincott Williams & Wilkins, 2006:62–82.

180. Melanson KJ, Zukley L, Lowndes J, et al. Effects of high-fructose corn syrup and sucrose consumption on circulating glucose, insulin, leptin, and ghrelin and on appetite in normal-weight women. *Nutrition* 2007;23:103–112.

181. Bray GA, Nielsen SJ, Popkin BM. Consumption of high-fructose corn syrup in beverages may play a role in the epidemic of obesity. *Am J Clin Nutr* 2004;79:537–543.

182. Cozma AI, Sievenpiper JL, de Souza RJ, et al. Effect of fructose on glycemic control in diabetes: a systematic review and meta-analysis of controlled feeding trials. *Diabetes Care* 2012;35(7):1611–1620.

183. Sievenpiper JL, Carleton AJ, Chatha S, et al. Heterogeneous effects of fructose on blood lipids in individuals with type 2 diabetes: systematic review and meta-analysis of experimental trials in humans. *Diabetes Care* 2009; 32(10):1930–1937.

184. Ludwig DS. Examining the health effects of fructose. *JAMA* 2013;310(1):33–34.

185. Wikipedia. *High fructose corn syrup*. Available at http://en.wikipedia.org/wiki/High_fructose_corn_syrup; accessed 4/15/07.

186. Warner M. A sweetener with a bad rap. *New York Times*. July 2, 2006. Available at http://www.nytimes.com/2006/07/02/business/yourmoney/02syrup.html?ex=1176782400&en=3b6e4ecd253953a4&ei=5070; accessed 10/8/07.

187. White JS. Challenging the fructose hypothesis: new perspectives on fructose consumption and metabolism. *Adv Nutr* 2013;4: 246–256.

188. Stanhope KL, Havel PJ. Endocrine and metabolic effects of consuming beverages sweetened with fructose, glucose, sucrose, or high-fructose corn syrup. *Am J Clin Nutr* 2008;88(6):1733S–1737S.

189. Malik VS, Schulze MB, Hu FB. Intake of sugar-sweetened beverages and weight gain: a systematic review. *Am J Clin Nutr* 2006;84:274–288.

190. Schulze MB, Manson JE, Ludwig DS, et al. Sugar-sweetened beverages, weight gain, and incidence of type 2 diabetes in young and middle-aged women. *JAMA* 2004;292:927–934.

191. O'Connor TM, Yang SJ, Nicklas TA. Beverage intake among preschool children and its effect on weight status. *Pediatrics* 2006;118:e1010–e1018.

192. Vartanian LR, Schwartz MB, Brownell KD. Effects of soft drink consumption on nutrition and health: a systematic review and meta-analysis. *Am J Public Health* 2007;97:667–675.

193. Basu S, Yoffe P, Hills N, et al. The relationship of sugar to population-level diabetes prevalence: an econometric analysis of repeated cross-sectional data. *PLoS One* 2013;8(2):e57873.

194. Bittman M. It's the sugar, folks. *The New York Times*. February 27, 2013. Available at http://opinionator.blogs.nytimes.com/2013/02/27/its-the-sugar-folks/?ref=todayspaper&_r=0; accessed 07/23/13.

195. Bantle JP. Is fructose the optimal low glycemic index sweetener? *Nestle Nutr Workshop Ser Clin Perform Programme* 2006;11:83–91.

196. U.S. Food and Drug Administration. *GRN No. 287. GRAS Notice Inventory*. Available at http://www.accessdata.fda.gov/scripts/fcn/fcnDetailNavigation.cfm?rpt=grasListing&id=287; accessed 03/24/13.

197. Swithers SE, Sample CH, Davidson TL. Adverse effects of high-intensity sweeteners on energy intake and weight control in male and obesity-prone female rats. *Behav Neurosci* 2013;127(2):262–274.

198. Swithers SE, Martin AA, Davidson TL. High-intensity sweeteners and energy balance. *Physiol Behav* 2010;100(1):55–62.

199. Feijó Fde M, Ballard CR, Foletto KC, et al. Saccharin and aspartame, compared with sucrose, induce greater weight gain in adult Wistar rats, at similar total caloric intake levels. *Appetite* 2013;60(1):203–207.

200. Yang Q. Gain weight by "going diet?" Artificial sweeteners and the neurobiology of sugar cravings. *Yale J Biol Med* 2010;83:101–108.

201. Hu FB, Malik VS. Sugar-sweetened beverages and risk of obesity and type 2 diabetes: epidemiologic evidence. *Physiol Behav* 2010;100(1):47–54.

202. http://www.nutrasweet.com/articles/article.asp?Id=47.

203. Raben A, Richelsen B. Artificial sweeteners: a place in the field of functional foods? Focus on obesity and related metabolic disorders. *Curr Opin Nutr Metab Care* 2012;15:597–604.

204. Bellisle F, Drewnowski A. Intense sweeteners, energy intake, and the control of body weight. *Eur J Clin Nutr* 2007;61:691–700.

205. Gardner C, Wylie-Rosett J, Gidding SS, et al. Nonnutritive sweeteners: current use and health perspectives: a scientific statement from the American Heart Association and the American Diabetes Association. *Diabetes Care* 2012;35(8):1798–1808.

206. Fitch C, Keim KS; Academy of Nutrition and Dietetics. Position of the Academy of Nutrition and Dietetics: use of nutritive and nonnutritive sweeteners. *J Acad Nutr Diet* 2012;112(5):739–758.

207. Nuttall F. Dietary fiber in the management of diabetes. *Diabetes* 1993;42:503–508.

208. Chandalia M, Garg A, Lutjohann D, et al. Beneficial effects of high dietary fiber intake in patients with type 2 diabetes mellitus. *N Engl J Med* 2000;342:1392–1398.

209. Anderson J, Allgood L, Turner J, et al. Effects of psyllium on glucose and serum lipid responses in men with type 2 diabetes and hypercholesterolemia. *Am J Clin Nutr* 1999;70:466–473.

210. Eaton S, Konner M. Paleolithic nutrition revisited: a twelve-year retrospective on its nature and implications. *Eur J Clin Nutr* 1997;51:207–216.

211. van Dam RM, Hu FB. Coffee consumption and risk of type 2 diabetes: a systematic review. *JAMA* 2005;294(1): 97–104.

212. Huxley R, Lee CM, Barzi T, et al. Coffee, decaffeinated coffee, and tea consumption in relation to incident type 2 diabetes mellitus: a systematic review with meta-analysis. *Arch Intern Med* 2009;169(22):2053–2063.

213. Whitehead N, White H. Systematic review of randomised controlled trials of the effects of caffeine or caffeinated drinks on blood glucose concentrations and insulin sensitivity in people with diabetes mellitus. *J Hum Nutr Diet* 2013;26:111–125.

214. Lane JD, Lane AJ, Surwit RS, et al. Pilot study of caffeine abstinence for control of chronic glucose in type 2 diabetes. *J Caffeine Res* 2012; 2(1):45–47.

215. Vincent J. Mechanisms of chromium action: low-molecular-weight chromium-binding substance. *J Am Coll Nutr* 1999;18:6–12.

216. McCarty M. Complementary measures for promoting insulin sensitivity in skeletal muscle. *Med Hypotheses* 1998;51:451–464.

217. Anderson R. Chromium, glucose intolerance and diabetes. *J Am Coll Nutr* 1998;17:548–555.

218. Kleefstra N, Houweling ST, Bakker SJ, et al. Chromium treatment has no effect in patients with type 2 diabetes mellitus in a Western population: a randomized, double-blind, placebo-controlled trial. *Diabetes Care* 2007;30: 1092–1096.

219. Broadhurst CL, Domenico P. Clinical studies on chromium picolinate supplementation in diabetes mellitus— a review. *Diabetes Technol Ther* 2006;8:677–687.

220. Singer GM, Geohas J. The effect of chromium picolinate and biotin supplementation on glycemic control in poorly controlled patients with type 2 diabetes mellitus: a placebo-controlled, double-blinded, randomized trial. *Diabetes Technol Ther* 2006;8:636–643.

221. Trumbo PR, Ellwood KC. Chromium picolinate intake and risk of type 2 diabetes: an evidence-based review by the United States Food and Drug Administration. *Nutr Rev* 2006;64:357–363.

222. Martin J, Wang ZQ, Zhang XH, et al. Chromium picolinate supplementation attenuates body weight gain and increases insulin sensitivity in subjects with type 2 diabetes. *Diabetes Care* 2006;29:1826–1832.

223. Ali A, Ma Y, Reynolds J, et al. Chromium effects on glucose tolerance and insulin sensitivity in persons at risk for diabetes mellitus. *Endocr Pract* 2011;17(1):16–25.

224. Sharma S, Agrawal RP, Choudhary M, et al. Beneficial effect of chromium supplementation on glucose, HbA1C and lipid variables in individuals with newly onset type-2 diabetes. *J Trace Elem Med Biol* 2011;25(3):149–153.

225. Cefalu WT, Rood J, Pinsonat P, et al. Characterization of the metabolic and physiologic response to chromium supplementation in subjects with type 2 diabetes mellitus. *Metabolism* 2010;59(5):755–762.

226. Thompson K. Vanadium and diabetes. *Biofactors* 1999:43–51.

227. Badmaev V, Prakash S, Majeed M. Vanadium: a review of its potential role in the fight against diabetes. *J Altern Complement Med* 1999;5:273–291.

228. Thompson KH, Orvig C. Vanadium in diabetes: 100 years from phase 0 to phase I. *J Inorg Biochem* 2006;100:1925–1935.

229. Smith DM, Pickering RM, Lewith GT. A systematic review of vanadium oral supplements for glycaemic control in type 2 diabetes mellitus. *QJM.* 2008;101(5):351–358.

230. Hartweg J, Perera R, Montori V, et al. Omega-3 polyunsaturated fatty acids (PUFA) for type 2 diabetes mellitus. *Cochrane Database Syst Rev* 2008;(1):CD003205.

231. Farmer A, Montori V, Dinneen S, et al. Fish oil in people with type 2 diabetes mellitus. *Cochrane Database Syst Rev* 2001;3:CD003205.

232. Montori VM, Farmer A, Wollan PC, et al. Fish oil supplementation in type 2 diabetes: a quantitative systematic review. *Diabetes Care* 2000;23:1407–1415.

233. Ros E. Dietary cis-monounsaturated fatty acids and metabolic control in type 2 diabetes. *Am J Clin Nutr* 2003;78: 617s–625s.

234. Wright J. Effect of high-carbohydrate versus high-monounsaturated fatty acid diet on metabolic control in diabetes and hyperglycemic patients. *Clin Nutr* 1998;17:35–45.

235. Garg A. Dietary monounsaturated fatty acids for patients with diabetes mellitus. *Ann N Y Acad Sci* 1993;683: 199–206.

236. Donaghue KC, Pena MM, Chan AK, et al. Beneficial effects of increasing monounsaturated fat intake in adolescents with type 1 diabetes. *Diabetes Res Clin Pract* 2000;48:193–199.

237. Mann JI, De Leeuw I, Hermansen K, et al. Evidence-based nutritional approaches to the treatment and prevention of diabetes mellitus. *Nutr Metab Cardiovasc Dis* 2004;14:373–394.

238. Strychar I, Ishac A, Rivard M, et al. Impact of a high-monounsaturated-fat diet on lipid profile in subjects with type 1 diabetes. *J Am Diet Assoc* 2003;103:467–474.

239. Martinez-Gonzalez MA, Bes-Rastrollo M. The cardio-protective benefits of monounsaturated fatty acid. *Altern Ther Health Med* 2006;12:24–30.

240. Kris-Etherton PM. AHA science advisory. Monounsaturated fatty acids and risk of cardiovascular disease. *Circulation* 1999;100:1253–1258.

241. Vaughan L. Dietary guidelines for the management of diabetes. *Nurs Stand* 2005;19:56–64.

242. Rodriguez-Villar C, Perez-Heras A, Mercade I, et al. Comparison of a high-carbohydrate and a high-monounsaturated fat, olive oil-rich diet on the susceptibility of LDL to oxidative modification in subjects with type 2 diabetes mellitus. *Diabet Med* 2004;21:142–149.

243. Tomaru M, Takano H, Osakabe N, et al. Dietary supplementation with cacao liquor proanthocyanidins prevents elevation of blood glucose levels in diabetic obese mice. *Nutrition* 2007;23:351–355.

244. Hollenberg NK. Vascular action of cocoa flavonols in humans: the roots of the story. *J Cardiovasc Pharmacol* 2006;47:s99–s102; discussion s119–s121.

245. Fraga CG. Cocoa, diabetes, and hypertension: should we eat more chocolate? *Am J Clin Nutr* 2005;81:541–542.

246. Grassi D, Necozione S, Lippi C, et al. Cocoa reduces blood pressure and insulin resistance and improves endothelium-dependent vasodilation in hypertensives. *Hypertension* 2005;46:398–405.

247. Grassi D, Lippi C, Necozione S, et al. Short-term administration of dark chocolate is followed by a significant increase in insulin sensitivity and a decrease in blood pressure in healthy persons. *Am J Clin Nutr* 2005;81: 611–614.

248. Fabian E, Töscher S, Elmadfa I, et al. Use of complementary and alternative medicine supplements in patients with diabetes mellitus. *Ann Nutr Metab.* 2011;58(2):101–108.

249. Golbidi S, Badran M, Laher I. Diabetes and alpha lipoic acid. *Front Pharmacol* 2011;2:69.

250. Mijnhout GS, Kollen BJ, Alkhalaf A, et al. Alpha lipoic acid for symptomatic peripheral neuropathy in patients with diabetes: a meta-analysis of randomized controlled trials. *Int J Endocrinol* 2012;2012:456279.

251. Kirkham S, Akilen R, Sharma S, et al. The potential of cinnamon to reduce blood glucose levels in patients with type 2 diabetes and insulin resistance. *Diabetes Obes Metabolism* 2009;11(12):1100–1113.

252. Leach MJ, Kumar S. Cinnamon for diabetes mellitus. *Cochrane Database Syst Rev* 2012;9:CD007170.

253. Wheeler E, Barroso I. Genome-wide association studies and type 2 diabetes. *Brief Funct Genomics* 2011;10(2): 52–60.

254. Davies LE, Thirlaway K. The influence of genetic explanations of type 2 diabetes on patients' attitudes to prevention, treatment and personal responsibility for health. *Public Health Genomics* 2013;16(5):199–207.

255. Grant RW, Hivert M, Pandiscio JC, et al. The clinical application of genetic testing in type 2 diabetes: a patient and physician survey. *Diabetologia* 2009;52(11):2299–2305.

256. Cho AH, Killeya-Jones LA, O'Daniel JM, et al. Effect of genetic testing for risk of type 2 diabetes mellitus on health behaviors and outcomes: study rationale, development and design. *BMC Health Serv Res* 2012;12:16.

257. Colombo M, Kruhoeffer M, Gregersen S, et al. Energy restriction prevents the development of type 2 diabetes in Zucker diabetic fatty rats: coordinated patterns of gene expression for energy metabolism in insulin-sensitive tissues and pancreatic islets determined by oligonucleotide microarray analysis. *Metabolism* 2006;55(1):43–52.

258. Lindi VI, Uusitupa MI, Lindström J, et al. Association of the Pro12Ala polymorphism in the PPAR-gamma2 gene with 3-year incidence of type 2 diabetes and body weight change in the Finnish Diabetes Prevention Study. *Diabetes* 2002;51(8):2581–2586.

259. Boerner BP, Sarvetnick NE. Type 1 diabetes: role of intestinal microbiome in humans and mice. *Ann N Y Acad Sci* 2011;1243:103–118.

260. Laparra JM, Sanz Y. Bifidobacteria inhibit the inflammatory response induced by gliadins in intestinal epithelial cells via modifications of toxic peptide generation during digestion. *J Cell Biochem* 2010;109(4):801–807.

261. Olivares M, Laparra M, Sanz Y. Influence of Bifidobacterium longum CECT 7347 and gliadin peptides on intestinal epithelial cell proteome. *J Agric Food Chem* 2011;59(14):7666–7671.

262. Cinova J, De Palma G, Stepankova R, et al. Role of intestinal bacteria in gliadin-induced changes in intestinal mucosa: study in germ-free rats. *PLoS One* 2011;6(1): e16169.

263. Ljungberg M, Korpela R, Ilonen J, et al. Probiotics for the prevention of beta cell autoimmunity in children at genetic risk of type 1 diabetes—the PRODIA study. *Ann N Y Acad Sci* 2006;1079:360–364.

264. Musso G, Gambino R, Cassader M. Obesity, diabetes, and gut microbiota: the hygiene hypothesis. *Diabetes Care* 2010;33(10):2277–2284.

265. Mukhopadhyay P, Chowdhury S. Drug therapy in prediabetes. *J Indian Med Assoc* 2005;103:603–605, 608.

266. Petersen JL, McGuire DK. Impaired glucose tolerance and impaired fasting glucose—a review of diagnosis, clinical implications and management. *Diab Vasc Dis Res* 2005;2:9–15.

267. Irons BK, Mazzolini TA, Greene RS. Delaying the onset of type 2 diabetes mellitus in patients with prediabetes. *Pharmacotherapy* 2004;24:362–371.

268. Anderson DC Jr. Pharmacologic prevention or delay of type 2 diabetes mellitus. *Ann Pharmacother* 2005;39: 102–109.

269. Abuissa H, Bel DS, O'keefe JH Jr. Strategies to prevent type 2 diabetes. *Curr Med Res Opin* 2005;21:1107–1114.

270. Sicat BL, Morgan LA. New therapeutic options for the management of diabetes. *Consult Pharm* 2007;22:45–56.

271. Ceglia L, Lau J, Pittas AG. Meta-analysis: efficacy and safety of inhaled insulin therapy in adults with diabetes mellitus. *Ann Intern Med* 2006;145:665–675.

272. Joy SV, Rodgers PT, Scates AC. Incretin mimetics as emerging treatments for type 2 diabetes. *Ann Pharmacother* 2005;39:110–118.

273. Vivian EM, Olarte SV, Gutierrez AM. Insulin strategies for type 2 diabetes mellitus. *Ann Pharmacother* 2004;38: 1916–1923.

274. Metzger BE. Diet and medical therapy in the optimal management of gestational diabetes mellitus. *Nestle Nutr Workshop Ser Clin Perform Programme* 2006;11:155–165.

275. Langer O. Management of gestational diabetes: pharmacologic treatment options and glycemic control. *Endocrinol Metab Clin North Am* 2006;35:53–78.

SUGGESTED READING

American Diabetes Association. Evidence-based nutrition principles and recommendations for the treatment and prevention of diabetes. *Nutr Clin Care* 2003;6:115–119.

American Diabetes Association Task Force for Writing Nutrition Principles and Recommendations for the Management of Diabetes and Related Complications. American Diabetes Association position statement: evidence-based nutrition principles and recommendations for the treatment and prevention of diabetes and related complications. *J Am Diet Assoc* 2002;102:109–118.

Anderson JW. Diabetes mellitus: medical nutrition therapy. In: Shils ME, Shike M, Ross AC, et al., eds. *Modern nutrition in health and disease*, 10th ed. Philadelphia, PA: Lippincott Williams & Wilkins, 2006:1043–1066.

Anderson JW, Geil PB. Nutritional management of diabetes mellitus. In: Shils ME, Olson JA, Shike M, eds. *Modern nutrition in health and disease*, 8th ed. Philadelphia, PA: Lea & Febiger, 1994.

Bailey C. Insulin resistance and antidiabetic drugs. *Biochem Pharmacol* 1999;58:1511–1520.

Beletate V, El Dib RP, Atallah AN. Zinc supplementation for the prevention of type 2 diabetes mellitus. *Cochrane Database Syst Rev* 2007;1:CD005525.

Brand-Miller JC, Colagiuri S. Evolutionary aspects of diet and insulin resistance. *World Rev Nutr Diet* 1999;84:74–105.

Costacou T, Mayer-Davis EJ. Nutrition and prevention of type 2 diabetes. *Annu Rev Nutr* 2003;23:147–170.

Cunningham JJ. Micronutrients as nutriceutical interventions in diabetes mellitus. *J Am Coll Nutr* 1998;17:7–10.

DeFronzo R. Pharmacologic therapy for type 2 diabetes mellitus. *Ann Intern Med* 1999:281–303.

Fernandez-Real J, Ricart W. Insulin resistance and inflammation in an evolutionary perspective: the contribution of cytokine genotype/phenotype to thriftiness. *Diabetologia* 1999;42:1367–1374.

Feskens EJ, Loeber JG, Kromhout D. Diet and physical activity as determinants of hyperinsulinemia: the Zutphen elderly study. *Am J Epidemiol* 1994;140:350–360.

Fox C, Esparza J, Nicolson M, et al. Is a low leptin concentration, a low resting metabolic rate, or both the expression of the "thrifty genotype"? Results from Mexican Pima Indians. *Am J Clin Nutr* 1998;68:1053–1057.

Garg A, Bantle JP, Henry RR, et al. Effects of varying carbohydrate content of diet in patients with non-insulin-dependent diabetes mellitus. *JAMA* 1994;271:1421–1428.

Garg A, Grundy SM, Koffler M. Effect of high carbohydrate intake on hyperglycemia, islet cell function, and plasma lipoproteins in NIDDM. *Diabetes Care* 1992;15:1572–1580.

Gilden JL. Nutrition and the older diabetic. *Clin Geriatr Med* 1999;15:371–390.

Ginsberg H, Plutzky J, Sobel B. A review of metabolic and cardiovascular effects of oral antidiabetic agents: beyond glucose-level lowering. *J Cardiovasc Risk* 1999;6: 337–346.

Grundy SM. Does the metabolic syndrome exist? *Diabetes Care* 2006;29:1689–1692.

Grundy SM. Does a diagnosis of metabolic syndrome have value in clinical practice? *Am J Clin Nutr* 2006;83:1248–1251.

Grundy SM. Metabolic syndrome: connecting and reconciling cardiovascular and diabetes worlds. *J Am Coll Cardiol* 2006;47:1093–1100.

Grundy SM. A constellation of complications: the metabolic syndrome. *Clin Cornerstone* 2005;7:36–45.

Grundy SM. Metabolic syndrome: therapeutic considerations. *Handb Exp Pharmacol* 2005;170:107–133.

Grundy SM. The optimal ratio of fat-to-carbohydrate in the diet. *Annu Rev Nutr* 1999;19:325–341.

Haller MJ, Atkinson MA, Schatz D. Type 1 diabetes mellitus: etiology, presentation, and management. *Pediatr Clin North Am* 2005;52:1553–1578.

Hansen BC. Obesity, diabetes, and insulin resistance: implications from molecular biology, epidemiology, and experimental studies in humans and animals. *Diabetes Care* 1995;18:a2–a9.

Heilbronn LK, Noakes M, Clifton PM. Effect of energy restriction, weight loss, and diet composition on plasma lipids and glucose in patients with type 2 diabetes. *Diabetes Care* 1999;22:889–895.

Henry RR. Glucose control and insulin resistance in non-insulin-dependent diabetes mellitus. *Ann Intern Med* 1996;124:97–103.

Jeppesen J, Chen YD, Zhou MY, et al. Effect of variations in oral fat and carbohydrate load on postprandial lipemia. *Am J Clin Nutr* 1995;62:1201–1205.

Joffe B, Zimmet P. The thrifty genotype in type 2 diabetes: an unfinished symphony moving to its finale? *Endocrine* 1998;9:139–141.

Leiter LA, Ceriello A, Davidson JA, et al. Postprandial glucose regulation: new data and new implications. *Clin Ther* 2005;27:s42–s56.

Lillioja S. Impaired glucose tolerance in Pima Indians. *Diabetic Med* 1996;13:s127–s132.

Lindstrom J, Ilanne-Parikka P, Peltonen M, et al. Sustained reduction in the incidence of type 2 diabetes by lifestyle intervention: follow-up of the Finnish Diabetes Prevention Study. *Lancet* 2006;368:1673–1679.

Lipkin E. New strategies for the treatment of type 2 diabetes. *J Am Diet Assoc* 1999;99:329–334.

Liu S, Willett WC, Stampfer MJ, et al. A prospective study of dietary glycemic load, carbohydrate intake, and risk of coronary heart disease in US women. *Am J Clin Nutr* 2000;71:1455–1461.

Luscombe ND, Noakes M, Clifton PM. Diets high and low in glycemic index versus high monounsaturated fat diets: effects on glucose and lipid metabolism in NIDDM. *Eur J Clin Nutr* 1999;53:473–478.

Mathers JC, Daly ME. Dietary carbohydrates and insulin sensitivity. *Curr Opin Clin Nutr Metab Care* 1998;1:553–557.

Milne RM, Mann JI, Chisholm AW, et al. Long-term comparison of three dietary prescriptions in the treatment of NIDDM. *Diabetes Care* 1994;17:74–80.

Neel J. The "thrifty genotype" in 1998. *Nutr Rev* 1999;57:s2–s9.

Neff LM. Evidence-based dietary recommendations for patients with type 2 diabetes mellitus. *Nutr Clin Care* 2003;6: 51–61.

Pittas AG. Nutrition interventions for prevention of type 2 diabetes and the metabolic syndrome. *Nutr Clin Care* 2003;6:79–88.

Rao S, Bethel M, Feinglos M. Treatment of diabetes mellitus: implications of the use of oral agents. *Am Heart J* 1999; 138:334–337.

Reaven GM. Metabolic syndrome: definition, relationship to insulin resistance, and clinical utility. In: Shils ME, Shike M, Ross AC, et al., eds. *Modern nutrition in health and disease*, 10th ed. Philadelphia, PA: Lippincott Williams & Wilkins, 2006:1004–1012.

Riccardi G, Capaldo B, Vaccaro O. Functional foods in the management of obesity and type 2 diabetes. *Curr Opin Clin Nutr Metab Care* 2005;8:630–635.

Rosenbloom Al, Joe JR, Young RS, et al. Emerging epidemic of type 2 diabetes in youth. *Diabetes Care* 1999;22: 345–354.

Ryden L, Standl E, Bartnik M, et al. Guidelines on diabetes, pre-diabetes, and cardiovascular diseases: executive summary. The Task Force on Diabetes and Cardiovascular Diseases of the European Society of Cardiology (ESC) and of the European Association for the Study of Diabetes (EASD). *Eur Heart J* 2007;28:88–136.

Scheen AJ, Lefebvre PJ. Insulin action in man. *Diabetes Metab* 1996;22:105–110.

Sharma A. The thrifty-genotype hypothesis and its implications for the study of complex genetic disorders in man. *J Mol Med* 1998;76:568–571.

Shulman GI. Cellular mechanisms of insulin resistance in humans. *Am J Cardiol* 1999;84:3J–10J.

Sjoholm A, Nystrom T. Inflammation and the etiology of type 2 diabetes. *Diabetes Metab Res Rev* 2006;22:4–10.

Spelsberg A, Manson J. Physical activity in the treatment and prevention of diabetes. *Compr Ther* 1995;21:559–564.

Wareham NJ, Franks PW, Harding AH. Establishing the role of gene–environment interactions in the etiology of type 2 diabetes. *Endocrinol Metab Clin North Am* 2002;31: 553–566.

Wood FC, Bierman EL. Is diet the cornerstone in management of diabetes? *N Engl J Med* 1986;315:1224–1227.

CHAPTER 7

Diet, Atherosclerosis, and Ischemic Heart Disease

A therosclerosis starts early in life and clinically manifests as coronary artery disease, cerebrovascular disease, or peripheral vascular disease. It is a leading cause of morbidity and mortality for both men and women. The evidence for associations between both macronutrients and micronutrients and the pathogenesis of coronary artery disease is decisive, deriving from multiple, large observational studies, randomized trials, and in vitro studies.

Risk factors for atherosclerosis include hyperlipidemia, hypercholesterolemia, hypertension, poor lifestyle habits (i.e., smoking and obesity), and physical inactivity. It has been known for over 50 years that total dietary fat intake is linked to hyperlipidemia and coronary disease. Recently, however, evidence has been mounting that although intake of trans fat should be restricted, intake of saturated fat may not be as bad as once believed, and intake of monounsaturated fatty acids (MUFA) and polyunsaturated fatty acids (PUFA)—specifically n-3 PUFA (see Chapter 2)— perhaps should be liberalized. The Mediterranean dietary pattern is noteworthy for its cardioprotective influences and is characterized by a fairly generous intake of total dietary fat overwhelmingly composed of MUFA and PUFA, among other features. Enthusiasm for liberalizing total dietary fat intake in the United States, however, must be tempered by any potential contributions an energy-dense diet might make to obesity risk (see Chapters 2, 5, and 38), especially in the context of other characteristics of a Western diet.

There is decisive evidence of an inverse association between dietary fiber, notably soluble or viscous fiber, and serum lipid levels. Dietary pattern and specific nutrients can influence blood pressure (see Chapter 8), hemostatic tendencies and platelet aggregability (see Chapter 9), adiposity (see Chapter 5), insulin sensitivity and glucose metabolism (see Chapter 6), inflammation (see Chapter 11), oxidation and endothelial function (see Chapter 11), and, by these and other mechanisms, atherogenesis.

The American Dietetic Association recommends combining medical nutrition therapy and lifestyle changes before adding pharmacotherapy (1). When tailored specifically for the purpose, diet offers the lipid-lowering power of statin drugs (2), albeit by means not easily adopted or maintained by most patients. As addressed in Chapter 8, the blood pressure lowering potency of diet can also approximate that of pharmacotherapy (3). Further, lifestyle intervention has been shown to lead to lower cumulative rates of diabetes over time compared to treatment with metformin (4).

The aggregate effect of dietary pattern on cardiovascular risk is formidable (5). In conjunction with other lifestyle practices, such as tobacco avoidance and regular physical activity, judicious dietary practices could contribute to an estimated 80% reduction in cardiac disease rates (6). Conversely, adverse dietary patterns have much to do with the hyperendemicity of cardiovascular disease (CVD) in the United States, other industrialized nations, and developing countries as they undergo cultural transitions (4).

Evidence for the role of nutrition in primary, secondary, and tertiary prevention of acute coronary events is definitive. Dietary counseling (see Chapter 47) is thus an essential component in the primary prevention of heart disease and in the clinical management of all patients with established coronary disease, as well as in the mitigation of virtually all known cardiac risk factors. Clinician support is important for people to achieve their dietary goals. Emerging methods reflect the technology-filled world we live in and include web- and mobile-based nutrition tools to increase dietary compliance (7).

The National Cholesterol Education Program Adult Treatment Panel (NCEP ATP-III) refers to the use of diet and lifestyle as a targeted strategy for cardiac risk reduction as "therapeutic lifestyle changes (TLC)" (8). Table 7-1 shows the low-density lipoprotein (LDL) values on which decisions to initiate TLC or pharmacotherapy are based. Table 7-2 provides an overview of the nutrient distribution that the NCEP recommends. Table 7-3 provides an overview of foods to prioritize in order to achieve the nutrient distribution characterized in Table 7-2.

TABLE 7.1

LDL Cholesterol Goals and Cutpoints for TLC and Drug Therapy in Different Risk Categories

Risk Category	LDL Goal	LDL Level at Which to Initiate TLC	LDL Level at Which to Consider Drug Therapy
CHD or CHD Risk Equivalents			
(10-year risk > 20%)	<100 mg/dL	≥100 mg/dL	≥130 mg/dL (100–129 mg/dL: drug optional)[a]
2+ Risk Factors			
(10-year risk ≤ 20%)	<130 mg/dL	≥130 mg/dL	10-year risk 10% to 20%: ≥130 mg/dL 10-year risk <10%: ≥160 mg/dL
0 or 1 risk factor[b]	<160 mg/dL	≥160 mg/dL	≥190 mg/dL (160–189 mg/dL: LDL-lowering drug optional)

[a]Some authorities recommend use of LDL-lowering drugs in this category if an LDL cholesterol <100 mg/dL cannot be achieved with TLC. Others prefer use of drugs that primarily modify triglycerides and HDL, e.g., nicotinic acid or fibrate. Clinical judgment also may call for deferring drug therapy in this category.

[b]Almost all people with 0 or 1 risk factor have a 10-year risk <10%, thus 10-year risk assessment in people with 0 or 1 risk factor is not necessary.

Source: Reproduced with permission from National Institutes of Health. *Detection, evaluation, and treatment of high blood cholesterol in adults (adult treatment panel III).* Bethesda, MD: National Institutes of Health, 2001: Table 5. Available at http://www.nhlbi.nih.gov/guidelines/cholesterol/atp3xsum.pdf; accessed 10/8/07.

TABLE 7.2

Nutrient Composition of the TLC Diet

Nutrient	Recommended Intake
Saturated fat[a]	Less than 7% of total calories
Polyunsaturated fat	Up to 10% of total calories
Monounsaturated fat	Up to 20% of total calories
Total fat	25%–35% of total calories
Carbohydrate[b]	50%–60% of total calories
Fiber	20–30 g/day
Protein	Approximately 15% of total calories
Cholesterol	Less than 200 mg/day
Total calories (energy)[c]	Balance energy intake and expenditure to maintain desirable body weight/prevent weight gain

[a]Trans-fatty acids are another LDL-raising fat that should be kept at a low intake.

[b]Carbohydrate should be derived predominantly from foods rich in complex carbohydrates, including grains, especially whole grains, fruits, and vegetables.

[c]Daily energy expenditure should include at least moderate physical activity (contributing approximately 200 kcal/day).

Source: Reproduced with permission from National Institutes of Health. *Detection, evaluation, and treatment of high blood cholesterol in adults (adult treatment panel III).* Bethesda, MD: National Institutes of Health, 2001: Table 6. Available at http://www.nhlbi.nih.gov/guidelines/cholesterol/atp3xsum.pdf; accessed 1/6/13.

TABLE 7.3

Recommended Foods and Overall Dietary Pattern to Meet Nutritional Recommendations of the NCEP/ATP III

Food Group	Foods to Choose[a]
Whole grains	Choose 6 oz per day of whole grain breads, cereals, and grains having 3 g or more of fiber per serving. Include oatmeal, oat bran, brown and wild rice varieties, semolina and whole wheat pasta, couscous, barley, and bulgur wheat.
Fruits	Choose 2 cups per day from a rainbow of colors, especially deep yellow, orange, and red: all berries, apples, oranges, apricots, melons, mangos, etc. Select from fresh, frozen, canned packed in juice, and dried varieties. Buy locally grown in season whenever possible.
Vegetables	Choose 2½ cups per day from a rainbow of colors, especially deep yellow, orange, red, and leafy green, such as yellow, red, and green bell peppers; squash; carrots; tomatoes; spinach; sweet potatoes; broccoli; kale; Swiss chard; Brussels sprouts; eggplant; and so on. Select from fresh, frozen, and canned varieties but be mindful of the higher sodium content of canned. Buy locally grown in season whenever possible.
Beans and legumes	Include 3–4 times per week. These can be eaten instead of meat. Include all varieties of beans: black, red, kidney, white, cannellini, garbanzo (chick pea), navy, pinto, lentils, split peas, black-eyed peas, soy, and tofu.
Fish[b]	Include 3–4 times per week, especially the good sources of ω-3 fatty acids: tuna, salmon, mackerel, and cod.
Chicken and turkey[b]	Include up to 1 or 2 times per week. Skinless breast meat is preferred.
Lean beef, pork, and lamb[b]	If desired, include no more than 3–4 times per month. The loin and round cuts are the leanest.
Milk and cheese[b]	Choose at least 2 cups per day from fat-free, skim, or low-fat versions.
Vegetable oils and other added fats	Choose monounsaturated sources daily but use in small amounts: olive oil, canola oil, olives, avocados, almond butter, and peanut butter.
Nuts and seeds	Include 4–5 times per week in *small amounts* of unsalted raw or dry-roasted types: almonds, walnuts, pistachios, peanuts, pecans, cashews, soy nuts, sunflower seeds, pumpkin seeds, and sesame seeds. Mix 1 tablespoon of ground flaxseed daily into other cooked foods.
Eggs[b]	2 egg yolks per week. Choose an ω-3 fatty acid–enriched brand.
Sweets	In moderation. Choose low or nonfat varieties whenever reasonable.

[a]Optional items. Well-balanced vegetarian and vegan diets are wholly compatible with the dietary recommendations of the National Cholesterol Education Program. Note that fish is recommended for particular health benefits; flaxseeds, and/or an ω-3 fatty acid supplement is especially recommended for those who don't eat fish.

[b]See http://www.choosemyplate.gov/supertracker-tools/daily-food-plans.html for guidance on age- and calorie intake-specific guidelines for food group targets linked to the 2010 Dietary Guidelines for Americans.

Source: Adapted from Katz DL, Gonzalez MH. *The way to eat.* Naperville, IL: Sourcebooks, 2002, and based in part on US Department of Health and Human Services. *Dietary guidelines for Americans, 2010.* Available at www.cnpp.usda.gov/dietaryguidelines.htm/; accessed 1/6/12.

OVERVIEW

Diet

CVD remains the leading cause of death in the United States among both men and women, although cancer deaths (see Chapter 12) may exceed heart disease deaths by approximately the year 2020 if present trends continue. This is due largely to a decline in cardiovascular deaths related to advanced technologies and pharmacotherapy rather than to primary prevention (9).

Transcultural studies, such as the Seven Countries study (10–12) and, in particular, migration studies such as Ni-Ho-San (13–15), have long established the powerful role of environmental, cultural, and lifestyle factors in the epidemiology of heart disease. Even within the United Kingdom, diet variations between Wales, Scotland, Northern Ireland, and England are associated with differences in chronic disease mortality rates (16). The increasing capacity to identify genetic susceptibility to heart disease (17) does nothing to diminish the primacy of lifestyle influences. Migration studies reveal marked variation in the epidemiology of heart disease associated with environmental variation, against a backdrop of genetic constancy.

Diet influences the pathogenesis of coronary artery disease in a variety of ways. The initial development of fatty streaks in coronary arteries is associated with high serum lipid levels and free-radical oxidation, both of which are modified by nutrients (18). Progression of coronary lesions is affected by serum lipids, hypertension (see Chapter 8), hyperinsulinemia (see Chapter 6), adiposity (see Chapter 5), and oxidation and inflammation (see Chapter 11), all of which are mediated by both macronutrient and micronutrient intake. Once coronary artery atherosclerosis is established, diet plays a role in determining both progression of plaque deposition and the reactivity of the endothelium, both of which may be predictive of cardiac events (19–21). Interestingly, salt intake is associated with left ventricular hypertrophy and heart failure, independent of blood pressure; thus, dietary salt alterations may be just as protective in addition to weight loss and blood pressure-lowering medications. Dietary manipulations have been shown to modify all the known, modifiable coronary risk factors (22–24) and, when extreme, to induce regression of established lesions (25,26). The role of diet in the management of coronary disease and risk factors is determined by the efficacy of dietary interventions and their complementarity with pharmacologic interventions of proven benefit.

The link between diet and heart disease has been apparent since at least the 1930s, when food shortages in the United States due to the Great Depression were observed to reduce the incidence of cardiovascular events. Similar observations were made in Western Europe during World War II. These "natural experiments" were found to be consistent with global patterns of dietary fat intake and served to establish a link between dietary fat and heart disease risk. Original evidence of the strong association between diet and coronary artery disease derived from transcultural studies and natural experiments.

Since the 1950s, an ever-expanding pool of data derived from a wide variety of study types has overwhelmingly linked dietary pattern to atherosclerotic disease of the coronary arteries and the risk of cardiovascular morbidity and

mortality. The seminal work of Ancel Keys (27) in the 1960s revealed a linear relationship between the total mean per capita fat intake of a country and the incidence of cardiovascular events. Keys's work has since been criticized for not including all the countries originally surveyed and for retaining only those that most supported the proposed association. In retrospect, the data then, as now, suggested a strong association between saturated fats and heart disease but an inverse association for unsaturated fats.

Work over recent years has been focused increasingly on the contribution of specific dietary fats to the atherogenic process. The relative cardiovascular benefits of total fat restriction versus modifying diet to promote monounsaturated and PUFA intake relative to saturated (and trans) fat intake is an area of particular interest (28–32). While debate over the relative merits of restricting versus revising dietary fat intake is protracted and intense (33–36), the practical utility of the discord is suspect. Relative to prevailing dietary patterns in the United States and other Western countries, both dietary fat restriction and the substitution of unsaturated for saturated fats would likely offer advantages. There is evidence of cardiac risk reduction with either approach (29–32,37). Of potentially far greater practical importance than the relative benefits of fat restriction versus improving fat quality are the means by which either pattern is achieved and the cultural context housing the dietary pattern. In Mediterranean countries, a so-called Mediterranean diet abundant in unsaturated oils is coupled to a traditional lifestyle that includes many energy-dilute, nutrient-rich foods and plenty of walking. In this context, the energy density of healthful oils does not contribute to obesity. For example, the consumption of fried foods in Spain is not associated with CAD or mortality and this is likely because the food is cooked with olive or sunflower oil, rather than canola or vegetable oil (38). Studies in the United States and other Western countries, however, show a fairly consistent relationship between dietary energy density and obesity risk (see Chapter 5) (32,39–43). Even putatively healthful oils may confer net harm rather than benefit if they contribute to weight gain and obesity. By reducing the energy density of foods, restricting dietary fat intake may facilitate energy balance and lead to weight loss (44).

Similar caveats pertain to dietary fat restriction. The advent of the "low-carb" diet era (see

Chapter 5) owes much to the failings of dietary fat restriction as a strategy for health promotion and especially weight control. These failings, however, reside more in the application of the guidance than in the guidance itself. Traditional Asian societies and vegetarian groups such as Seventh-Day Adventists (see Chapter 43) with very low-fat dietary patterns predicated on natural, unprocessed foods have excellent health profiles and very low rates of either obesity or CVD (45–47). Uptake of the "low-fat" dietary guidance in the cultural context of the United States, however, resulted in high intake of fat-reduced processed foods, perhaps best epitomized by SnackWells cookies. This adulteration of advice to restrict dietary fat, in which the food industry and the public colluded, may have obscured genuine merit in the advice. There is little, if any, health benefit in substituting refined starches and simple sugars in highly processed foods for atherogenic fats; the metabolic pathways for harmful effects may differ, but the effects themselves may be much the same (see Chapter 6). Similar trends have been seen with the advent of "low-carb" dieting; energy-dense, highly processed foods that could claim to be low in carbohydrate but otherwise had little to recommend them rapidly proliferated. Indeed, a diet lower in carbohydrates but high in protein and fat may portend worse peripheral artery endothelial function and promote atherosclerosis (48,49). Trading between low-fat and low-carbohydrate junk food is of little use in the pursuit of meaningful public health goals.

Studies of carbohydrate-restricted, high-fat diets have generally resulted in modest decreases in LDL and increases in *high-density lipoprotein* (HDL) cholesterol, with a beneficial effect on the LDL:HDL ratio (50–54). Whether these effects represent a net cardiovascular benefit is as yet undetermined by outcome studies, and it may depend on other, perhaps unmeasured, influences of diet on overall vascular health. For example, diets rich in both saturated and MUFAs may raise HDL, but the former may compound, and the latter ameliorate, other cardiac risk factors, including insulin resistance, inflammation, and platelet aggregation (55).

At present, there is evidence to support both dietary fat restriction and fat substitution, along with restriction of refined starches and added sugars in processed foods and their replacement with natural carbohydrate sources, including

vegetables, fruits, whole grains, and legumes. For the most part, direct comparison of dietary patterns low in total fat or abundant in unsaturated fats, with both based on an optimal array of pertinent foods, is very limited; available data suggest comparable benefits of reducing total dietary fat and improving the distribution of dietary fat, provided that both approaches emphasize wholesome food choices (56). Even more deficient are data regarding the reliability with which these alternative patterns may be adopted and maintained, in true accord with the guidance for food choices on which they are based, in real-world settings subject to diverse cultural influences. Such translational research is much needed and eagerly awaited. Thus far, advice to restrict dietary fat or carbohydrate has translated, at the population level, into very questionable dietary practices.

The role of total caloric intake in CVD is somewhat less clear than is the role of obesity (see Chapter 5). When caloric expenditure is high, caloric intake is not thought to represent a cardiac risk factor. However, total calorie intake may have implications for senescence (see Chapter 31), and degradation of cardiovascular health is typically an age-dependent phenomenon. Caloric intake in excess of caloric expenditure results in weight gain, and obesity is associated with heart disease risk (see Chapters 5 and 10). A calorie-restricted diet has been consistently associated with longevity in laboratory animals, including primates (see Chapter 31). Reduced oxidative stress in the arterial wall with calorie restriction may contribute to antithrombogenicity (57). The benefits of calorie restriction, if relevant to humans, apply to a wide variety of diseases, as well as aging, rather than to cardiovascular risk in particular. In contrast, an "empty calorie" diet does not appear to offer any advantages.

Weight loss is of clear and potentially profound cardiac benefit to overweight and obese patients; the topic is addressed extensively in Chapter 5. The National Heart, Lung, and Blood Institute (NHLBI) recommends a loss of roughly 5% to 10% body weight over 6 months to achieve meaningful improvement in the cardiac risk profile (58). The best way to lose weight is slowly, i.e., 0.5 to 1 lb per week. However, this advice presupposes that all obesity is equal with regard to cardiac risk, which is not the case. As addressed in Chapter 5, body fat distribution has important implications for health effects. Central, visceral adiposity is of special concern for cardiac health. In such patients, loss of much less than 10% body weight may confer dramatic cardiac benefit, whereas weight loss may be of little or no clear cardiovascular benefit in patients with peripheral adiposity (59–63). Of note, an average 7% weight loss produced a 58% reduction in the incidence of diabetes in the Diabetes Prevention Program (see Chapter 6) (64). Interestingly, this association may be stronger in women (65). Further, weight loss leads to reduced systolic and diastolic blood pressures (66).

Intake of fruits, vegetables, and cereal grains is inversely correlated with cardiovascular risk, as is total fiber intake (67). The intake of soluble fiber in particular appears to have cardiovascular benefits attributable at least to a hypolipidemic effect (68); hypotensive effects have also been described (see Chapter 8), as have potentially important influences on glycemic and insulinemic responses (see Chapter 6). On a population basis, separating the effects of soluble and insoluble fiber, fruit, vegetable, cereal, and fat intake is complicated by the tendency of dietary behaviors to cluster (69,70). Diets low in atherogenic fat tend to be relatively high in fiber of both types, and vice versa. Nonetheless, convincing epidemiologic associations exist between both low-fat, predominantly vegetarian diets and the MUFA-rich Mediterranean diet and a low incidence of cardiovascular events. The several mechanisms of cardiac risk mitigation attributable to soluble fiber make a strong case for specific benefit; concentrated food sources include oats, beans, lentils, apples, and berries (see Chapter 1 and Section VIIE). A recent study in Europe demonstrated that each 10 g per day intake of fiber was associated with a 15% lower risk of ischemic heart disease mortality regardless of the fiber source (e.g., cereal, fruit, vegetables) (71).

Among the important characteristics apparently common to heart-healthy dietary patterns is a relatively low glycemic load (see Chapters 5 and 6) (72–74). There is persuasive support at present for both low-fat and Mediterranean dietary patterns, derived from both observational and intervention studies. In both cases, cardiovascular benefit is clearly dependent on dietary details. For example, a low-fat diet might be based predominantly on highly processed snack foods or on natural foods such as vegetables, fruits,

beans, grains, and so on; the implications for cardiovascular and overall health differ markedly. McMillan-Price et al. (73) have demonstrated the importance of the specific means by which any given nutritional objective is met; both high- and low-carbohydrate dietary patterns may be adopted to achieve a low glycemic load, and the former may offer cardiovascular advantages. It has also been demonstrated that there is an increased risk of heart disease in proportion to increasing glycemic index in both Caucasians and African Americans without diabetes; however, this may not be true for patients with diabetes, suggesting that the glucose metabolism is as important as the dietary glycemic load (75).

For now, an emphasis on cardioprotective foods may be more helpful than undue preoccupation with macronutrient distribution. With both the NCEP guidelines (see Table 7-2) and the IOM reference ranges providing both meaningful guidance and considerable latitude (76), a diet emphasizing fruits, vegetables, whole grains, nuts, seeds, fish, beans, and lentils—and consequently an abundance of fiber, antioxidants, unsaturated oils, and lean protein and a relative paucity of refined carbohydrate, added sugar, and atherogenic fats—may be recommended with confidence (see Table 7-3). The inclusion of low- or nonfat dairy may offer particular benefits for blood pressure control (see Chapter 8). The OMNI Heart study looked at the cardioprotective benefits of heart healthy food choices. (77). This clinical trial was conducted to determine the influence of macronutrient intake on adiponectin levels, which is a hormone specific to fat cells that has been linked to high levels of HDL cholesterol and lower rates of insulin resistance. The study found that a diet rich in monounsaturated fatty acids, even without weight loss, was associated with higher levels of adiponectin compared with carbohydrate or protein-rich diets, suggesting that incorporation of MUFAs may be helpful for those with high cholesterol and diabetes (78).

An intermediate pattern between competing low-fat and Mediterranean diets is moderate in total fat, while emphasizing healthful oils, and could offer practical advantages such as facilitation of calorie control. This intermediate pattern is rather concordant with the evolutionary biology literature characterizing the "native" human diet; a small trial assessing the effects of such a diet on multiple cardiac risk factors (79) found that eating a contemporary induces an acidotic state within the body compared with retrojected ancestral preagricultural diets, suggesting that our current diets do not provide the genetically determined nutritional requirements for optimal acid–base status and confirm that our bodies are better adapted physiologically to the diets eaten by our ancestors (80).

Along with the role of diet in mitigating overall heart disease risk, diet may be applied effectively in a manner tailored to particular cardiac risk factors. Dietary prevention and management of hypertension can contribute to the prevention of CVD; this topic is discussed in Chapter 8. Chapter 9 covers diet and hemostasis. The effects of diet on peripheral vascular disease and cerebrovascular disease are discussed in Chapter 10. Other topics pertinent to the link between nutrition and CVD risk include obesity (see Chapter 5) and diabetes (see Chapter 6).

Dietary Fat
Total Fat

Excess intake of certain dietary fats produces predictable elevations in serum cholesterol and lipoproteins (Hegsted and Keys equations; see Section VIIA), which translate into fairly predictable increases in the risk of cardiac events (81). Dietary guidelines in the United States (82,83) have been based, in large measure, on evidence linking diet to heart disease. The current guideline for total fat intake is 20% to 35% of total calories for adults ages 19 and older, and excess fat intake has been defined relative to this reference. There is no dietary recommendation for saturated fats as the body makes enough of these on its own.

Dietary fat contributes to atherogenesis primarily by inducing a rise in serum lipid levels, and in this regard, as noted earlier, not all fat is created equal. The principal mechanism by which fat and cholesterol ingestion translate into increased cardiovascular risk is the induced elevation of serum lipoproteins, especially LDL. Intake of saturated fatty acids is associated with increased cholesterol levels. Consuming less than 10% of calories from saturated fatty acids and replacing them with polyunsaturated and monounsaturated fatty acids is associated with lower blood cholesterol. Elevations of LDL result in saturation of the receptor-mediated uptake by hepatocytes (84,85) and the consequent uptake

of LDL by tissue-fixed macrophages. This process of so-called "foam cell" formation is accelerated by the oxidation of LDL. The ingestion of certain PUFAs, notably of the n-6 class, although not associated with elevations of serum lipids, has been implicated in the promotion of lipoprotein oxidation; n-3 PUFAs are apparently protective. The deposition of foam cells in the coronary intima and media induces smooth muscle cell hyperplasia and the growth of obstructing lesions (86,87).

In addition to the chronic effects of fat intake on atherogenesis, there is some evidence that the acute ingestion of a meal high in saturated fat content may represent a cardiac stressor (88). An interest in postprandial atherogenesis dates to at least the 1970s (89). Although the postprandial rise in triglycerides may contribute to the progression of coronary atherosclerosis, the magnitude of lipid changes seems insufficient to explain the observed increase in events; there are a variety of concomitant metabolic responses (90). The acute ingestion of particularly, and perhaps exclusively, saturated or trans fat may destabilize coronary plaque and impair endothelial function (88,91). Evidence is now considerable that endothelial function is a fundamental index of cardiac risk, and it is modified in response to a variety of nutritional influences (92–96).

At present, as noted previously, there is little evidence directly implicating total dietary fat in CVD risk. Rather, the association between increased dietary fat intake and increased cardiovascular risk observed in industrialized countries actually illuminates a link between heart disease and specific categories of fat. Imbalance in PUFA intake, with a relative excess of proinflammatory ω-6 fats (97) and a relative deficiency of anti-inflammatory ω-3 fats, may contribute as well (see Chapters 2 and 11). In societies prone to excess caloric intake and obesity, mediated in part by energy-dense processed foods, total dietary fat may contribute indirectly to heart disease risk.

The optimal dose of dietary fat has been a matter of debate for some time (98,99). The beneficial effects of MUFAs, and certain PUFAs, specifically n-3 fatty acids, on cardiovascular health may be sufficiently strong that an intake of total fat in excess of 30% of calories is desirable, provided that the fat is predominantly of these types (100). Of note to primary care providers is that either the recommended reduction in total fat intake or the consumption of predominantly MUFA and n-3 PUFA both represent significant dietary changes for most patients seen in the United States (101,102).

In a review of the diets of preagricultural humans, one study (103) suggested that the diet to which humans adapted during millions of years of evolution be used as an arbiter until or unless disputes about optimal macronutrient intake can be resolved in prospective intervention trials (see Chapter 44). The Stone Age is divided into Paleolithic, Mesolithic, and Neolithic periods; the Paleolithic began approximately 2.5 million years ago, when our ancestors first started to use rough stone implements, and lasted until approximately 8000 B.C., thereby constituting the major portion of human evolution; the use of more refined stone implements ushered in the Mesolithic period; the use of finely polished stone implements ushered in the Neolithic period. The flesh of wild animals, although containing markedly less total fat than the flesh of domestic cattle, is notably richer in n-3 fatty acids, suggesting that our ancestors consumed this class of nutrient in relative abundance (103). A modest degree of total dietary fat restriction, in conjunction with an emphasis on a salutary distribution of fats, might offer advantages over either approach alone.

Saturated Fat

Saturated fatty acids, those with no carbon–carbon double bonds (see Chapter 2), in particular raise total cholesterol and LDL; although as we learn more about different lipoprotein subtypes, it seems that saturated fats may only raise levels of large buoyant LDL particles—thought to be antiatherogenic—as opposed to the small, dense, atherogenesis-promoting variety (104). Foods rich in saturated fatty acids include the flesh of most domestic mammals raised for human consumption, dairy products, and several vegetable oils, notably coconut, palm, and palm kernel. Evidence linking diets high in saturated fats to cardiovascular events is limited by difficulties in conducting long-term studies requiring assignment of subjects to dietary interventions. A recent 10-year study in over 5,000 people, looked at the influence of different saturated fats on CVD (105). After adjustment for demographics, lifestyle, and dietary confounders, a higher intake of dairy saturated fats was associated with lower CVD risk, while a higher intake of meat saturated fatty acids was associated with greater risk.

Current recommendations call for reducing the intake of saturated fat to 7% or less of calories (8) in those with cardiac risk factors. Average US adult intake of these fats is approximately 13% to 14%. Prehistoric adaptations may be informative; paleolithic intake of saturated fat was approximately 5% to 12% of calories (103,106). There is nothing to suggest a disadvantage in advocating this lower level of saturated fat intake, unless saturated fats are replaced with proinflammatory n-6 PUFAs (107). Nonetheless, a recent review of randomized controlled trials showed that replacing saturated fatty acids with PUFAs (n-3 and n-6 and presumably in a favorable ratio) actually reduced the risk of coronary heart disease (CHD) (108).

Meta-analysis of Siri-Tarino et al. reported no association between dietary saturated fat intake and CVD (109). To clear up the saturated fat controversy, it is necessary to accept that not all saturated fats are the same. Saturated fats represent a group of distinct fats with different properties and evidence for disease association.

The evidence that excessive intake of saturated fat, specifically C14 myristic and C16 palmitic acids, raises serum lipids and promotes atherogenesis is decisive (see Chapter 2). Apparently unique among the highly saturated fatty acids, stearic acid, C18, is neutral with regard to serum lipids and, apparently, cardiac risk—this may just be because stearic acid is absorbed by the body less efficiently (110). This fat is relatively abundant in beef, and particularly so in dark chocolate. Notably, the 2010 Dietary Guidelines Advisory Committee recommended restricting saturated fat intake, not including stearic acid. For further discussion of stearic acid, see Chapters 2 and 39. Likewise, lauric acid—a very short saturated fat molecule, C12, which predominates in coconut oil—is also probably not harmful.

In counseling patients to modify intake of saturated fat, a consideration of all sources of such fat in the diet is essential. The prevailing notion that dietary fat, and saturated fat in particular, derives predominantly from red meat is only partly true. The primary source of dietary fat and saturated fat in the diets of American men is red meat; in the diets of American children, it is milk; and in the diets of American women, it is a combination of dairy products, including cheese, and processed foods (111,112). Studies demonstrate that even subjects educated to be fat averse, in attempting to reduce dietary fat intake in general and saturated fat intake in particular, tend to substitute fat from one source (e.g., meat) with comparable fat from another source (e.g., dairy) (112); however, a recent long-term study found that people who substituted meat saturated fats with dairy saturated fats significantly lowered their risk of heart disease (105). A recent meta-analysis suggests that the danger may actually lie within processed meat rather than red meat, which has been shown to have no association with CHD in some studies (113).

Of note, even the societal trend toward "low-fat" dieting did not actually reduce total fat intake; data from the National Health and Nutrition Examination Survey (NHANES) suggest that total fat consumption remained fairly constant, while total calorie intake was driven up by more consumption of processed carbohydrate foods. Fat intake thus declined as a percentage of total calories, but only because total calories increased (114).

When counseling patients in an effort to reduce saturated (or total) fat intake, a reasonably detailed dietary history is thus essential (see Chapter 47). The contribution to total fat intake of often-overlooked and unreported constituents of diet, such as sauces, dressings, and spreads, can be substantial (112). Assertions by patients that they are eating a diet low in saturated fat because they have reduced or eliminated red meat is generally unreliable.

Cholesterol

The relative contribution of dietary cholesterol to serum lipids is confounded to some extent by the highly correlated distribution of saturated fat and cholesterol in the diet. The meat of domestic mammals, dairy products, and organ meats are all rich in nutrients and associated with elevated serum lipids. The independent contribution of dietary cholesterol to serum cholesterol and cardiovascular risk is increasingly in doubt, however (115). Eggs are a concentrated source of cholesterol, but not fat, and there is accumulating evidence that egg consumption is unrelated to cardiovascular risk (116–118). Shellfish, also relatively high in cholesterol content but low in total and saturated fat, are not convincingly linked to an increase in cardiovascular risk.

Conversely, coconut, palm, and palm kernel oils are highly saturated but are derived from vegetable sources free of cholesterol. These oils have been linked to increased cardiac risk, although the evidence for coconut oil in particular is inconclusive in this regard (119,120) (see Chapter 2). Of note, cholesterol is a constituent of cell membranes and is found only in animal products; the common "cholesterol free" on the label of processed foods or oils not of animal origin is therefore a given and presumably presented to imply a health benefit.

The Keys and Hegsted equations (see Section VIIA) indicate that cholesterol contributes relatively less to serum lipids than does saturated fat intake, in part because while fat intake is measured in grams, cholesterol intake is measured in milligrams. Even so, these equations were devised when support for a role of dietary cholesterol in hyperlipidemia was far stronger than it is now. The recommended intake of cholesterol is up to 300 mg per day in general, with the NCEP advising restrictions below 200 mg in patients with hyperlipidemia (LDL > 100 mg per dL) or established coronary disease (8). A large egg contains about 71% of the recommended 300 mg of cholesterol intake per day. To comply with this recommendation, patients must eliminate or minimize their intake of egg yolks and restrict their intake of red meat, deli meats, cheese, and whole milk and its products. The need for patients at risk for, or even with, heart disease to restrict egg and shellfish intake is far from certain, and guidelines in this area are likely to change as ongoing and new studies conclude (121). Barraj et al. recently reported that for most American adults, consuming one egg per day accounts for <1% of their CHD risk so the significance of these recommendations may be minimal (122).

Trans-fatty Acids

Modern food preparation techniques have greatly increased human exposure to trans-fatty acids, which occur naturally in small quantities in milk. These are called "natural" or "ruminant" trans-fatty acids. It is important to remember that trans fats are not essential. The atherogenicity of artificial trans-fatty acids appears to be much greater than that of their naturally occurring counterparts, attributed in part to their LDL-raising effects (123,124). Some trans fats are produced commercially by bombarding partially unsaturated fatty acids (i.e., fatty acids with some preserved carbon–carbon double bonds; see Chapter 2). The hydrogenation process saturates most of the double bonds in PUFAs in order to make the fats solid at room temperature. The trans isomeric configuration around the remaining double bond results in molecules that pack tightly together, limiting the fluidity of the fat and producing a higher melting point. The stability of these fats at room temperature results in products that retain their shape (e.g., margarine in stick form as opposed to liquid vegetable oil) and increases product shelf life. Although they are advantageous to the food industry, trans fats influence serum lipids similarly to saturated fats (125). (Stated somewhat glibly: In general, dietary fats that reliably extend the shelf life of food products tend to shorten the lives of the people consuming those products.)

Recent evidence has made a compelling case for uniquely harmful effects of trans fats, suggesting that they contribute far more on a per-gram basis to heart disease risks than the saturated fats they were designed to replace. The intake of trans fats is strongly associated with CVD, but the lack of randomized controlled studies has resulted in weaker associations with diabetes and metabolic syndrome (126). Regardless, legislation to remove trans fat from restaurants is increasingly popular (127), and many food manufacturers are removing it from their product lines. Trans fat has been entirely removed from the food supply of at least one country: Denmark (128).

Since 2006, the level of synthetic trans-fatty acids in the US food supply have dramatically decreased; however, presently, many processed foods still contain trans fats; they can be detected on labels by looking for "partially hydrogenated" oils. Commonly hydrogenated oils are soy, cottonseed, and corn. As of January 2006, FDA regulations required that trans fat be listed on the nutrition facts panel. However, when a product contains 0.5 g or less of trans fat per single serving (which may be, and often is, unrealistically small), the FDA allows a "no trans fat" claim on the front of the package (129). When several servings of such a product are consumed, however, the total trans fat dose may be significant. Thus, patients should be encouraged to avoid any product containing hydrogenated or partially hydrogenated oil.

The recommended intake of artificial trans fats is less than 1% of total calories (130), and preferably nil, and thus the upper limit of advisable intake for saturated fat actually should encompass the cumulative intake of saturated and trans fat. Roughly 2.6% of calories in the typical American

diet are derived from trans fat, although this figure may already be declining in response to food industry reformulations.

To replace trans fats, the food production industry has either reverted to natural saturated fats without cholesterol (e.g., palm oil) or produced newer interesterified oils. Interesterification involves moving around the fatty acids within or among the fat molecules to alter the way the compound responds to changes in temperature. Interesterified fats have been used in shortenings and margarine, as well as in parenteral, enteral, and infant feeding to improve the stability of fats. Evidence is lacking regarding the influence of interesterified fats on digestibility or energy balance in adult humans, though benefits have been seen in animals and human infants (131). There are few definitive comparison studies, but it appears that interesterified fats may offer a slightly reduced atherogenic risk compared with hydrogenated fats (132). In two randomized crossover trials, Berry et al. concluded that interesterification of palm oil does not result in adverse postprandial changes in lipids or insulin (133). Other studies have revealed negative impacts on cholesterol (reduced HDL and increased LDL) with both interesterified and trans-fat diets (134,135). Compared with natural palm oil, chemically and enzymatically interesterified palm oil have been found to increase fat deposition and triglycerides levels in animals.

Another altered fat, conjugated linoleic acid, has been suggested as preventative of CVD, but definitive evidence is lacking. Conjugated linoleic acid refers to a mixture of positional and geometric isomers of linoleic acid, characterized as having conjugated double bonds in several positions. The beneficial effects of conjugated linoleic acid consumption are often associated with reductions in cardiac risk factors (i.e., decreased cholesterol and triglyceride levels) (136) however, other studies suggest that conjugated linoleic acid may have negative effects. For example, one study found that conjugated linoleic acid consumption in mice had no effect on atherosclerosis and actually caused adverse changes in lipoprotein and liver lipid metabolism (137). Clinical trials in humans have yielded ambiguous results with both positive and negative effects on cardiac biomarkers found as well as no effects. These discrepancies are due to the lack of standardization in the studies, similar to other clinical nutritional studies in humans (138). In patients with a cardiac history, a recent large clinical trial found that substituting dietary ω-6 linoleic acid in place of saturated fats may even increase mortality (139). At this point, it does not appear that supplementation with dietary conjugated linoleic acid should be recommended.

Polyunsaturated Fat

The two essential fatty acids in the human diet, linoleic (18:2, n-6) and 2-linolenic (18:3, n-3) fatty acids (see Chapter 2), are both polyunsaturated. Humans and other mammals share the capacity to synthesize saturated fatty acids, as well as unsaturated fatty acids of the n-9 and n-7 series, but lack the requisite enzymes to manufacture n-6 and n-3 polyunsaturates. The metabolism of these fats is discussed in greater detail in Chapter 2. Linoleic acid serves as a precursor to arachidonic acid, whereas α-linolenic acid (ALA) serves as a precursor for eicosapentaenoic acid [EPA (20:6, n-3)] and docosahexaenoic acid [DHA (22:5, n-3)].

Collectively, the products of essential fatty acid metabolism are known as eicosanoids, and they include prostaglandins, thromboxanes, and leukotrienes. The optimal intake of n-3 fatty acids is a topic of considerable interest across a wide array of health issues. The n-3, or "ω-3," fatty acids are PUFAs with the first double bond after the third carbon molecule (see Chapter 2). An extensive literature has developed linking high intakes of n-3 polyunsaturates, particularly from marine sources, to low rates of heart disease and blood pressure (140–144).

Whereas n-6 polyunsaturates are readily available in commonly consumed vegetable oils, including soybean, safflower, sunflower, and corn, n-3 fatty acids are less widely distributed. Oils rich in n-3 fatty acids include flaxseed, linseed, marine oils, and, to a lesser degree, canola oil (142). Whereas fish and seafood provide EPA and DHA, the plant sources of n-3 PUFAs generally contain ALA. The distinctive benefits of n-3s are associated with EPA and DHA, and thus the substitution of ALA is of less convincing benefit. The manufacture of EPA and DHA apparently occurs with variable efficiency (see Chapter 2).

Fat-restricted diets may result in relative, if not overt, deficiency of n-3 intake, as well as less-than-optimal intake of MUFA (98,145–147). A diet rich in n-3 fatty acids has been linked to reduced levels of serum triglycerides, reduced

platelet aggregation, and lower blood pressure; the evidence to date for a protective role of n-3 fatty acids against sudden cardiac death is decisive (148), and a general cardioprotective role is strongly suggested (5).

The GISSI–Prevenzione Trial lends strong support to the practice of n-3 fatty acid supplementation. In a factorial design trial of more than 11,000 patients post-myocardial infarction (MI), nearly 3,000 patients received fish oil capsules containing approximately 850 mg EPA and approximately twice the dose of DHA, and another nearly 3,000 patients received matching placebo. At 42-month follow-up, n-3 PUFA supplementation had significantly reduced the cardiovascular event and mortality rates and all-cause mortality (145–147). Data from the GISSI trial demonstrate a clear benefit of fish oil for the prevention of sudden cardiac death in individuals post-MI, with benefit apparently greatest among those with impaired left ventricular function (149–152). A recent randomized clinical trial on n-3 PUFA supplementation in elderly men at high cardiovascular risk showed a nonsignificant reduction in all-cause mortality, but the results are limited by a small sample size (153). An observational study conducted in China (1,154 males and females) found that serum levels of n-3 PUFA were inversely associated with a diagnosis of hypertension, indicating that these fatty acids may be protective against high blood pressure (144). Even when foods traditionally lacking n-3 PUFA (i.e., tomato juice) are enriched with the molecules, consumption can ameliorate cardiovascular risk factors (154).

On the other hand, the Alpha Omega Trial investigated the effects of 400 mg of EPA + DHA and 2 g of ALA on the secondary prevention of CVD in 4,837 people with a history of a MI. Low-dose supplementation did not significantly reduce the rate of major CVD but in women, ALA as compared with placebo and EPA-DHA alone, was associated with a lower risk. In a post-hoc analysis, there was a significant rate reduction in major cardiovascular events in the EPA+DHA group, as compared with ALA alone and placebo, most of which were arrhythmia-related events (155). Though this further supports the notion that the beneficial effects of n-3 PUFA may be antiarrhythmic in nature, a recent meta-analysis showed that n-3 PUFAs do not prevent postoperative or recurrent atrial fibrillation (156) (see broader cardiovascular effects).

Further, the benefits of n-3 PUFA may be related to restoring a balance with n-6 PUFA to achieve our native dietary state. While our native diet consisted of n-3 and n-6 fats in a ratio between 1:1 and 1:4 (with a slight excess of n-6 PUFAs), our modern diet provides us with these fats in a ratio of 1:20 (with a massive excess of n-6s). Evidently, prospective randomized trials have yielded inconsistent results with regards to the association of PUFA with CVD. According to recent meta-analyses, PUFAs do not appear to confer any protection in regards to all-cause or cardiovascular mortality, stroke, or MI (157,158). PUFAs may, however, improve left ventricular remodeling and reduce the risk of heart failure, especially in those with preexisting cardiac disease (159,160). Thus, it is sensible to conclude that we should increase our intake of n-3 PUFA to provide balance.

Monounsaturated Fat

Studies in the 1960s suggested that monounsaturates were neutral with regard to serum lipids, resulting in greater interest in the potential health benefits of polyunsaturates. The cardioprotective effects of MUFAs have come to light largely through cross-cultural epidemiologic studies. Rates of heart disease are low in populations with high consumption of MUFA, even when total fat intake is consequently high, leading to interest in the so-called Mediterranean diet (161–165). There is convincing evidence that monounsaturates' apparent neutral effects on serum cholesterol are due to reductions in LDL and concomitant elevations of HDL, both of which reduce cardiovascular risk (166–169). A meta-analysis in 1995 suggested that the effects of monounsaturates and polyunsaturates on HDL are comparable (170), but subsequent study has generally refuted this contention, suggesting particularly beneficial effects on the LDL:HDL ratio in association with MUFA intake (171). Along with having favorable effects on the LDL:HDL ratio, MUFAs may attenuate atherogenesis by inhibiting LDL oxidation (172–177). Olive oil, a predominant source of MUFA, also contains phenolic compounds with antioxidant properties.

Monounsaturates are abundant in traditional diets of the countries bordering the Mediterranean Sea. There is abundant research on the Mediterranean diet, but comparatively less for MUFAs per se. The Mediterranean diet, consisting of fresh fruit and vegetables, olives, olive oil, wine, fish, and grains, particularly wheat in the form of pasta, has received increasing attention as a means of lowering cardiovascular risk (37,178–184). In a 2-year randomized trial, Shai and colleagues compared the effects of a low-carbohydrate, low-fat, and Mediterranean-style diet on body mass index, glycemic control, and serum lipids in 322 moderately obese adults (185). They demonstrated that although all diets were safe and effective for weight loss, the Mediterranean and low-carbohydrate diets had more favorable effects on glycemic control and lipids, respectively, than the low-fat diet. The Mediterranean diet was particularly effective in reducing fasting blood glucose and insulin in diabetic subjects. These findings suggest that the optimal diet for any individual may be dependent on his or her risk factors and personal preferences. Results of the OMNI-Heart trial provide some support for a Mediterranean-type diet (186), though this trial had a shorter 6-week intervention period. The randomized crossover study assessed the effects of three diets: rich in carbohydrates, MUFA, or protein. The diet rich in MUFA was associated with higher levels of adiponectin compared to the other two diets. Several meta-analyses of prospective cohort studies and/or clinical trials have been carried out in recent years (187–189). In these studies, adherence to the Mediterranean diet was associated with reduced overall mortality, cardiovascular mortality, cancer incidence and mortality, and neurodegenerative diseases; (189) and was inversely associated with components of the metabolic syndrome (187). Just one meta-analysis included randomized trials comparing the Mediterranean diet to a low-fat diet (188). That meta-analysis concluded that the Mediterranean diet produced modestly more favorable effects on body weight, blood lipids, blood pressure, fasting plasma glucose, and C-reactive protein, compared with a low-fat diet. However, in two of the trials, the low-fat diet group also had significantly lower intakes of fiber, protein, and fruits and vegetables; and higher intakes of energy and saturated fat (190,191).

Various aspects of the Mediterranean diet may contribute to its cardioprotective properties. As discussed earlier, n-3 PUFA in fish may favorably affect serum lipids and inhibit platelet aggregation. Alcohol, discussed later (and in Chapter 40), favorably influences serum lipids and raises endogenous tissue plasminogen activator (192).

Fruit and vegetable consumption, discussed later, is likely to be cardioprotective by a variety of mechanisms, as is consumption of grains, seeds, and certain nuts (193). Finally, the effects of polyphenols in olive oil (194) and nuts (195) cannot be disentangled from those of MUFAs. Therefore, the studies completed to date are inadequate to provide decisive evidence of the isolated benefits of monounsaturates but clearly convey the cardioprotective influence of the traditional Mediterranean dietary pattern.

Further evidence supporting a role for monounsaturates in modifying cardiovascular risk derives from intervention studies. Garg et al. (196,197) showed that the Mediterranean diet results in greater improvements in glycemic control than does a diet rich in carbohydrate. One small study identified a positive, linear relationship between proportion of MUFAs relative to saturated fatty acids in a meal and postprandial insulin sensitivity and beta cell function (198). The area under 24-hour insulin curves is known to correlate with cardiac risk. Decreased levels of insulin in patients with manifestations of the insulin-resistance syndrome (truncal obesity, hypertension, hypertriglyceridemia) may result in reduced cardiovascular risk by several mechanisms, including modification of the lipid profile and declines in norepinephrine levels (199–201). The Lyon Diet Heart Study, a controlled trial in patients following a first MI, showed convincing evidence of event reduction with a Mediterranean diet (202–204).

A variety of nuts and seeds are rich in monounsaturates, including walnuts, almonds, peanuts, and sesame seeds. Olives and avocados, both fruits, are excellent sources. The NCEP ATP-III guidelines call for up to 20% of calories from MUFA (8) (see Table 7-3).

Dietary Fats Summary

The optimal level of dietary fat intake for primary prevention of heart disease, or for the management of established heart disease, remains somewhat controversial. Opinion is divided between total fat restriction and more liberal intake of n-3 PUFAs and MUFAs (205–207). The weight of evidence appears to be accumulating in support of the latter (208–210), although they need not be fully mutually exclusive.

Prehistoric human diets may have provided anywhere from 20% to 39% of calories from fat, with about 7.5% to 12% from saturated and naturally occurring trans fat, and the remainder a combination of MUFA and PUFA (106,211). Whereas estimates of the contribution of total and saturated fat to the paleolithic diet vary substantially, and likely varied with geographical location, there is more agreement about the contribution of MUFAs and PUFAs, which was significantly higher than in typical modern diet. The ratio of n-6 to n-3 PUFA, which is approximately 11:1 in the United States and western European diets, was between 2:1 and 8:1 for our ancestors. (106,211). Until or unless intervention studies such as OMNI-Heart (212,213) further elucidate the optimally cardioprotective diet (an eventuality potentially obviated, as noted earlier, by excessive focus on macronutrient distribution and insufficient attention to the foods contributing to each macronutrient category), recommendations consistent with both current evidence and evolutionary theory are appropriate. Saturated fat should be restricted to below 7% of total calories in all cardiac patients; this guideline is appropriate for primary prevention in willing patients as well (214). Trans fats should be minimized in the diets of all individuals. Intake of fish, nuts, soy, olives, avocados, seeds, olive oil, canola oil, and linseed oil should be encouraged to raise n-3 PUFA and MUFA intake. However, these items should substitute in the diet for other sources of fat to avoid raising total fat and/or calorie intake. Dietary fat and cholesterol reduction is best achieved by restricting intake of nonpastured or factory-farmed red meats; processed meats; whole-fat dairy products, especially cheese; cheese- and cream-based sauces and dressings; fatty spreads; and processed foods. Particular attention to detail is necessary to prevent substitution of lipid-raising fats from one source for fats from other sources. Foods rich in cholesterol but low in fat, notably eggs, may not impose any cardiac risk, although opinion in this area is still evolving. NCEP guidelines are still to limit dietary cholesterol to 200 mg per day, commensurate with roughly one egg.

Optimal management of dietary fat intake appears capable of lowering LDL by as much as 20% and total cholesterol by as much as 30%, although lesser reductions are usually seen. Even greater reductions are possible when extreme dietary adjustments specifically tailored to lipid lowering are made (2). Although dietary manipulation produces benefits other than lipid lowering, more aggressive lipid lowering than can be readily achieved by diet alone is indicated for virtually all hyperlipidemic patients with coronary disease. Statin drugs can lower LDL by up to 60%; the effects of these agents are enhanced by dietary therapy.

Finally, the means by which dietary fat is titrated matter as much as the intake levels achieved. The substitution of processed carbohydrate foods for fatty foods substitutes one adverse cardiac influence for another. Objectives related to dietary fat intake should be met within the context of a dietary pattern that places an emphasis on whole foods, providing good nutrition within each of the three macronutrient classes.

Carbohydrate

Interest in carbohydrate restriction was propagated initially by claims regarding facilitated weight loss (see Chapter 5). Concerns about the potential cardiac hazards of low-carbohydrate, high-fat diets led to numerous studies that examined effects on lipids as well as weight. For the most part, such intervention trials suggest that higher-fat weight-loss diets tend to lower LDL modestly while preserving HDL cholesterol levels. On the other hand, lower-fat weight-loss diets tend to reduce both of these lipoprotein levels (215–220) (see Chapter 5). However, increases in LDL have been associated with long-term adherence to a very-low-carbohydrate diet (221). Of potentially greater relevance is the salutary influence of carbohydrate restriction on triglyceride levels and insulin responses (185,212). Overall, the cardiac risk profile has generally improved with low-carbohydrate diets, with benefits largely or perhaps entirely attributable to weight loss but not offset by any potential disadvantages of the dietary pattern (222,223). However, there are no trials of sufficient duration to show that these influences of carbohydrate restriction translate into a reduced risk of actual cardiac events (219).

The liability in thinking in terms of "carbohydrate restriction," however, is that carbohydrate encompasses a large and very diverse array of foods, including fruits, vegetables, and whole grains. As addressed in Chapters 1, 5, 6, and 45, the distinctions among food choices within the carbohydrate category may be of far greater importance to health than alterations in total carbohydrate intake. Health benefits, including cardiovascular benefits, of diets rich in vegetables, fruits, beans and legumes, and,

to only a slighter lesser extent, whole grains, are well established. Conversely, diets high in processed foods, refined starches, and added sugars are disadvantageous in terms of cardiac risk and overall health. There is almost certainly cardiac benefit from adopting a low-glycemic-load diet, but this can be achieved at either relatively low or high carbohydrate intake, and the latter may be preferable (73). Many trials have simply emphasized the relative quantity of one macronutrient class versus another rather than the quality of choices within each class, and thus may obscure this important issue (212). This failing now pertains particularly to the assessment of carbohydrate restriction, but it recapitulates the oversight that has long bedeviled advice regarding dietary fat intake. The liabilities in proffering dietary guidance in the form of macronutrients rather than foods were artfully characterized by Michael Pollan in the *New York Times Magazine* (224).

Overall, there does not appear to be any compelling reason for carbohydrate restriction as a means of reducing cardiac risk, provided that carbohydrate-rich foods are well chosen; to the contrary, dietary patterns associated with long-term health benefits are generally rich in wholesome, high-carbohydrate foods. That said, variation in carbohydrate intake across the range advocated as reasonable by the Institute of Medicine—from 45% to 65% of calories (225)—accommodates similar variation across the range of fat intake discussed previously. Dietary patterns ranging from relatively rich in unsaturated oils and at the lower end of the recommended carbohydrate intake or quite restricted in total fat and at the higher end of the recommended carbohydrate intake appear comparably consistent with cardiac health—provided that the food choices within the macronutrient classes are prudent. Of note, natural and minimally processed foods tend to be less energy dense and more nutrient dense than highly processed counterparts, allowing for a greater intake of an array of beneficial nutrients at any given calorie level appropriate for healthy weight maintenance.

Fruit and Vegetable Intake

Whereas the nutrients responsible for the health-promoting properties of fruits and vegetables are a source of ongoing investigation and controversy, the cardioprotective influence of fruit and vegetable intake is compelling. Population-based studies consistently demonstrate health benefits of high fruit and vegetable intake (64) (see Chapter 43). This dietary pattern is strongly associated with a reduced cancer risk as well (see Chapter 12). The cardioprotective benefits of produce may derive from their vitamins, minerals, antioxidants, soluble and insoluble fibers; the combined effects of several of these components acting in concert and with other components of the diet; or the effect of displacing less-healthy foods (e.g., refined grains, simple sugars, processed meats) that might otherwise be consumed. Favoring the latter two possibilities, the evidence for specific nutrient effects is less convincing than is evidence for the effect of a produce-rich dietary pattern.

The extreme expression of fruit and vegetable intake is a strict vegetarian or vegan diet. Whereas some vegetarians exclude only meat (i.e., lacto-ovo vegetarians), vegans exclude all animal products, including dairy and eggs. The latter group may be at risk for certain micronutrient deficiencies, especially some B vitamins. B vitamins are not fat-soluble. The association between deficiency of vitamin B12, which occurs naturally only in animal foods, and elevated levels of homocysteine raises concern that this dietary pattern might be associated with increased cardiovascular risk, although the significance of homocysteine levels to cardiac risk remains in question. According to a recent Cochrane review, interventions to lower homocysteine levels have not been shown to prevent cardiovascular events (226). To date, population-based studies suggest that vegetarianism is associated with less-than-average cardiovascular risk in developed countries (227–229). For a variety of reasons, vegetarians should become knowledgeable about dietary sources of both macronutrients and micronutrients of importance to ensure proper balance. Taking a daily multivitamin may be a prudent practice for some vegetarians. Vegetarianism is discussed in greater detail in Chapter 43.

NUTRIENTS, NUTRICEUTICALS, AND FUNCTIONAL FOODS

Antioxidants (Vitamins E and C, Carotenoids, and Flavonoids)

Evidence linking antioxidation to a reduced risk of CVD is convincing; evidence in support of specific antioxidant nutrients or compounds is generally not better than suggestive (230). This may be because antioxidants are most effective in as-yet-unidentified combinations or because other nutrient-mediated reactions are equally important. The principal mechanism by which antioxidants confer cardiovascular benefit is thought to be inhibition of LDL oxidation (231,232), although protection of nitric oxide is of nearly comparable interest (233). A diet rich in fruits and vegetables typically provides abundant antioxidants, including carotenoids, tocopherols, flavonoids, and ascorbate, and has been decisively linked to reduced cardiac risk.

A variety of antioxidants have been studied for cardioprotective effects (234). The overall weight of evidence does not support a protective role for β-carotene, although observational studies suggest that foods rich in β-carotene are almost certainly protective (235,236). The literature to date is supportive of protective effects of bioflavonoids, found particularly in dark chocolate/cocoa, tea, red wine, and grape juice, as well as the skins of many fruits and vegetables (237–239). There currently is no convincing evidence of a cardioprotective effect of vitamin C, although diets naturally high in ascorbate appear to be protective (240,241). One potential explanation for the inability to elucidate an independent benefit of vitamin C is that its mechanism of action may require interaction with fat-soluble antioxidants (242). Timimi et al. (243) reported a beneficial effect of acute vitamin C infusion on endothelial function in diabetic subjects. Plotnick et al. (88) reported prevention of dietary fat–induced endothelial dysfunction with concomitant vitamin C and E supplementation in healthy subjects. Such findings tend to perpetuate interest in the potential cardioprotective role of vitamin C despite the paucity of clear evidence to date.

Data from the Cambridge Heart Antioxidant Study suggested a benefit of supplemental vitamin E in the prevention of second MI, although evidence of a mortality benefit was not found (244,245). Beneficial effects of acute vitamin E supplementation on endothelial function have been reported (88). However, in the GISSI–Prevenzione Trial, patients with recent MI (n = 11,324) randomly assigned to vitamin E supplementation (300 mg) did no better than those assigned to placebo with regard to MI or death (246). Similarly, the HOPE trial demonstrated a significant benefit of angiotensin-converting enzyme inhibition with regard to both MI and death in high-risk coronary patients, whereas vitamin E (400 IU) failed to reveal such benefit (247,248). Sesso and colleagues also found no benefit of long-term supplementation (mean follow-up of 8 years) with vitamin E (400 IU every other day) or vitamin C (500 mg daily) on the risk of major cardiovascular events among middle-aged men (249). Thus, the most definitive trials to date fail to support a cardioprotective role of supplemental vitamin E, at least as an isolated intervention. The HOPE and GISSI trials further suggest that excessive intake of vitamin E may confer net harm (250,251). Vitamin E actually constitutes a family of compounds, encompassing tocopherols and tocotrienols (see Chapter 4), but studies have generally used α-tocopherol exclusively. Whether lack of benefit is a reliable finding or the result of using the wrong formulation and/or wrong dose of vitamin E is as yet unknown. A recent meta-analysis of antioxidant supplements reached the same conclusion (252). Isolated antioxidant supplementation cannot be recommended as a cardioprotective strategy at present; consumption of a diet naturally rich in antioxidants certainly can be.

B Vitamins

Accumulating evidence has pointed to the importance of elevations of serum homocysteine in up to one-third of all patients with coronary artery disease (253). Hyperhomocysteinemia is particularly likely to be seen in patients with coronary disease and normal serum lipids (254). Vitamins B_6 and B_{12} and folate participate in the metabolism of methionine. Specific metabolic steps beyond the production of homocysteine are dependent on several B-complex vitamins. Folate levels are apparently most likely to contribute to elevated homocysteine (255). There is some evidence that intake of B vitamins above levels currently recommended may offer protection against CVD (253). However, despite clear evidence that B vitamin supplementation can lower homocysteine levels, cardiac benefits are uncertain (256–259). It is possible that the effects of supplementation depends on baseline homocysteine levels, and on individual genotype. A meta-analysis of six trials found that folic acid supplementation decreased CVD risk in participants with lower baseline homocysteine levels, but slightly increased risk

in participants with higher homocysteine levels (260). The interaction between the effect of supplementation and baseline homocysteine levels above versus below the overall mean was significant ($p = .03$). Common polymorphisms in the gene for methyltetrahydrofolate reductase (MTHFR) are associated with hyperhomocysteinemia and stroke risk, but these associations appear to be stronger in populations with low folate intakes (261).

B-complex supplementation at or near RDA levels may be beneficial and is unlikely to be harmful (B vitamins are water soluble and excesses are renally cleared). However, recommendations for multivitamin supplementation to all patients attempting to reduce their risk of heart disease are not strongly supported by scientific evidence (262), and there is a suggestion of cardiovascular harm with folate supplementation in those with greater homocysteine levels at baseline (260). Reliance on specific B vitamins for cardioprotective effects is unsubstantiated at present, and supplementation cannot be recommended.

Coenzyme Q₁₀

Coenzyme Q_{10} (CoQ$_{10}$) is a benzoquinone, also known as ubiquinone because of its remarkably widespread distribution in nature. Minute quantities are found in virtually all plant-based foods. CoQ$_{10}$ functions within the mitochondrion, where it facilitates electron transport and oxidative phosphorylation (263–265). Given the fundamental role of this coenzyme in energy metabolism, it is perhaps not surprising that its putative health effects are protean. An overview of the role of CoQ$_{10}$ is provided in Section VIIE.

With regard to CVD, evidence is strongest for a beneficial role of CoQ$_{10}$ in heart failure and cardiomyopathy, where supplementation has been associated with improvement in left ventricular function, quality of life, and functional status (265,266). There is evidence of reduced complications post-MI (267), improved hemodynamics post–bypass grafting (268), and improved functional status and symptom relief in patients with angina (269). CoQ$_{10}$ has been shown to have antihypertensive effects as well (270–273). Some trials have tested the effects of coenzyme Q10 in combination with other antioxidants, making it difficult to determine whether each compound individually is effective (273,274).

Supplementation with CoQ_{10} and selenium has been associated with reduced cardiovascular mortality (274). Antioxidant effects of CoQ_{10} apparently preserve levels of both ascorbate and α-tocopherol, enhancing both extracellular and intracellular antioxidant function (274–277). Finally, supplementation with CoQ_{10} appears to reduce levels of lipoprotein (a) (278) and preserve serum levels depleted by statin therapy (279). There are negative clinical trials in each of these areas as well, although false-negative error is possible due to generally small sample sizes and limited statistical power.

Until recently, there was an absence of adequately powered trials in the literature, possibly due to the nonproprietary nature of the compound and the inability of an industry sponsor of such trials to generate correspondingly large profits as a result. New evidence supports the effectiveness of CoQ_{10} in preventing cardiovascular events and increasing survival among patients with heart failure. In their meta-analysis of 13 randomized controlled trials in patients with congestive heart failure, Fotino and colleagues reported a pooled mean net change of 3.67% in the ejection fraction associated with CoQ_{10} supplementation (280). The individual trials included in the meta-analysis had sample sizes ranging from 6 to 69. In contrast, the Q-SYMBIO trial, presented by Mortensen et al. at the Heart Failure 2013 meeting (281) enrolled 420 patients from nine different countries. Participants were assigned to CoQ_{10} (100 mg 3 times daily) or placebo. After 2 years of follow-up, the CoQ_{10} group had significantly lower rates of major adverse cardiac event (14% vs. 25% in placebo group, $p = 0.03$), cardiovascular mortality ($p = 0.02$), hospitalizations ($p = 0.05$), and all-cause mortality (9% vs. 17% in placebo group, $p = 0.01$). The CoQ_{10} group also experienced greater improvements in functional New York Heart Association class ($p = 0.047$). The results of this trial, though not yet published in the peer-reviewed literature, represent some of the strongest evidence regarding CoQ_{10} supplementation to date.

In the aggregate, the evidence supporting a role for coenzyme Q_{10} in the amelioration of CVD and the modification of risk factors is not conclusive, but highly suggestive (281–283). More widespread use of coenzyme Q_{10} in cardiology and primary care practice appears to warrant serious consideration. The usual doses in trials range from 100 to 300 mg per day, dosed b.i.d. Such doses appear to be safe, with virtually no reports of significant toxicity or side effects.

Alcohol

Epidemiologic evidence, both among and within populations, links moderate alcohol consumption to a reduced risk of CVD (284–286). Results of an observational cohort study in France (1999) suggest that moderate alcohol consumption reduces all-cause mortality (287); evidence of benefit was stronger and more consistent for wine than beer. A 2011 meta-analysis of longitudinal cohort studies conducted in the United States and internationally reported that alcohol consumption, compared with no alcohol consumption, was associated with reductions in relative risks of 25% for CVD mortality, 25% for CHD mortality, and 29% for incident CHD (286). Consumption of ≤ 1 drink per day was most consistently associated with reduced cardiovascular risk. Long-term observational studies in the United States have found observations between light to moderate drinking and reduced risk of MI in men and women (288) and cardiovascular and all-cause mortality among males who had survived a first MI (289). However, not only the amount of drinking but also the pattern of drinking may matter. A meta-analysis published in 2008 showed that while regular heavy drinking reduced CVD risk, irregular or binge drinking increased it (290).

Although there is general consensus that ethanol is partly responsible for the cardioprotective effects of alcoholic beverages, red wine may confer additional benefit due to the polyphenolic compounds in the skin of the grape, with resveratrol receiving particular attention of late (291) (see Chapter 31). A small study in 2000 demonstrated enhanced endothelial function following consumption of dealcoholized red wine, with no improvement following consumption of an equivalent amount of red wine with alcohol (292). In a 2012 trial, reductions in systolic and diastolic blood pressures and increases in plasma nitric oxide were observed among men with cardiovascular risk factors after consumption of dealcoholized red wine (293). Neither consumption of red wine with alcohol or gin was associated with improvements in these measures. However, most studies suggest beneficial effects of ethanol in moderate doses (see Chapter 40). Mechanisms by which alcohol may attenuate cardiovascular risk include elevation of HDL, elevation of tissue plasminogen activator, and inhibition of platelet aggregation. At doses above 30 to 45 g per day, alcohol raises blood pressure and is associated with increased cardiac risk, as well as increased risk of other morbidity and mortality. Consumption of one to at most two drinks per day, preferably red wine, is reasonable with regard to cardiovascular risk reduction. Whether or not the practice should be advocated to a particular patient is dependent on other considerations. Despite the generally consistent evidence of cardiovascular benefit with moderate alcohol consumption, concern regarding the adverse effects of heavier drinking generally mitigates enthusiasm for recommending alcohol consumption for health promotion (294,295). Also, even small amounts of alcohol measurably increase the risk of several cancers (particularly of the respiratory tract, digestive tract, and breast), thus limiting or avoiding alcohol may be advisable for those at risk (e.g., breast cancer survivors or those with strong family histories) (296–298). Nonetheless, a dose of up to roughly one drink per day for women (15 g of ethanol) and two drinks per day for men (30 g of ethanol) is convincingly linked to reduced cardiac risk in men and women with and without overt cardiac risk factors and may be advised for that effect (299–305) (see Chapter 40). Red wine features on a short list of foods in the so-called polymeal combination of foods designed, at least hypothetically, to confer maximal cardiac benefit (306).

Iron

Iron may act as a pro-oxidant, generating speculation that it might contribute to the risk of cardiac disease in men and that its depletion in menstruating women might contribute to risk reduction. Epidemiologic evidence supports a potential role for high iron levels in CVD risk, but the evidence to date is inconclusive (307). Whereas high ferritin levels have been directly associated with mortality in patients with peripheral artery disease (PAD) (308), a randomized controlled trial found that reduction of iron stores with phlebotomy in PAD patients was ineffective in reducing all-cause mortality, MI, or stroke (309). A potential role for iron in CVD received a surge of attention when trials such as HERS and the WHI (227,228) refuted a cardioprotective effect of hormone-replacement therapy (HRT) at menopause, hinting

that something other than hormones might protect premenopausal women from heart disease. There is some concern that our measures of body iron stores are inadequate to gauge the potential pro-oxidant effects of iron. A potential association between iron and heart disease risk remains speculative, and somewhat controversial (310–313) current knowledge would suggest that supplements be avoided barring a clear indication for their use. The American Heart Association formerly offered guidance for dietary iron intake but no longer does, perhaps indicative of the topical state of flux.

Magnesium

Serum magnesium concentrations have been found to be inversely associated with CVD risk (314). However, serum levels may merely be a measure of overall dietary pattern, including intake of fruits and vegetables. Magnesium is known to have antiarrhythmic properties and has corresponding potential therapeutic applications in acute cardiac care beyond the scope of this discussion. Clinical trial data on the role of supplemental magnesium in cardiac risk reduction are by and large equivocal, although evidence of a hypotensive effect is conclusive (306–322). Any beneficial effects of magnesium on CVD risk may be mediated in particular by its association with reduced blood pressure (see Chapter 8), though its anti-inflammatory and antimineralization effects may also be important (323). Magnesium is discussed further in Section VIIE. For most patients, a generous intake of magnesium from dietary sources is to be encouraged, whereas supplementation as a matter of routine, other than at doses incorporated into multivitamin/mineral preparations, need not be.

Calcium and Potassium

Cardiovascular benefit of calcium and potassium is associated with blood pressure–lowering effects in particular, as discussed in Chapter 8 (see also Chapter 4 and Section VIIE).

Cocoa/Dark Chocolate

The cardiovascular effects of dark chocolate consumption are convincingly favorable across a wide array of measures. The topic is addressed in Chapter 39.

Plant Stanols/Sterols

The hypolipidemic effects of plant stanols and sterols are well established (324,325). These naturally occurring compounds are found in small quantities in a large range of plant foods. Stanols and sterols interfere with cholesterol absorption in the gut, both from food and from enterohepatic circulation. A dose of roughly 2 g per day has been shown to induce meaningful reductions in LDL. The inclusion of higher doses of plant stanols as part of a dietary portfolio designed for optimal lipid lowering resulted in effects rivaling those of statins (2). Furthermore, adding plant sterols or stanols to a statin regimen is associated with greater reductions in total cholesterol and LDL compared with statin therapy alone (326). There does not appear to be a significant difference between plant sterols and stanols in their effects on serum lipid levels (327).

Garlic

There has long been interest in potential lipid-lowering and blood pressure–lowering effects of garlic and its putative active ingredient. A 2007 clinical trial refutes a lipid-lowering effect, and the blood pressure–lowering effect is uncertain (328). However, a 2012 Cochrane review concluded that garlic did lower blood pressure in two trials in hypertensive patients, but there was insufficient evidence of a beneficial effect on cardiovascular morbidity and mortality (329). While the inclusion of whole garlic in the diet is healthful, its use in pill form to achieve targeted cardiovascular benefit cannot be recommended on the basis of available evidence.

Walnuts, Almonds, and Other Nuts

Nut intake is convincingly and consistently associated with beneficial effects on cardiac risk factors in intervention studies and with reduced event rates in observational studies (330–335). Despite their energy density, nuts are not clearly associated with risk of weight gain (336–338). Honey-roasted or sugar-coated nuts are likely another story. In one large prospective study in a Mediterranean population, men and women who ate nuts at least twice per week had a 40% reduced risk of weight gain during the 28-month follow-up period, compared with those who did not

eat nuts (339). Other studies have also showed benefits, without weight gain (340) including a reduced risk of mortality (341).

Overall, the evidence for benefits of nuts is greatest for walnuts, which offer a particularly favorable fatty acid profile. Almonds have also been associated with cardiac benefit (342,343) and have been included in the polymeal designed to bundle cardioprotective foods, if only in theory (306). In contrast with the findings of an earlier review (335), a 2009 meta-analysis concluded that almond intake appears to lower total cholesterol, but does not improve LDL, HDL, or triglycerides (344). There is some evidence that a lipid-lowering effect of almonds may be limited to hypercholesterolemic individuals (345).

Interesterified Fats

Interesterified oils are unsaturated oils modified in labs in a process that links them to saturated oils, to give them longer shelf life and more heat tolerance. Like trans fat, interesterifed fats are the product on an industrial process, and these two categories of fat may share adverse health effects as well (129,346). Interesterified fats are not yet in wide use, but are likely to become more prevalent in foods, as manufacturers seek to remove trans fats from their products. Most human intervention studies have reported no difference between interesterified fats and their natural counterparts in their effects on blood lipids (347). On the other hand, at least one study reported unfavorable effects of interesterified fats on the lipid profile and glucose metabolism, compared with unmodified palm olein (346). Research in this area is very limited and consists only of small, short-term studies. Further research is needed before the atherogenicity of interesterified fats can be fully understood. In the meantime, it is wise to limit these fats in the diet at least to the same extent as saturated fats; it may be wiser still to exclude them entirely as they will in all cases be markers of highly processed foods, which are unhealthy for lots of other reasons.

Other

Interest is intense in the development of nutriceutical agents with cardioprotective effect. Among compounds of current interest are bioflavonoids, the herb, hawthorn, red yeast rice extract, and resveratrol, a compound extracted from grape skins, to name a few. Many other compounds and nutrients have received attention in the popular press. Evidence is insufficient to recommend clinical applications of most such compounds at present. Resources for remaining abreast of evolving options in the nutriceutical management of cardiac risk factors are discussed in Section VIIJ. The pace of developments in this area is so rapid that no print text can be fully current.

CLINICAL HIGHLIGHTS

Data and opinions pertaining to the nutritional mitigation of cardiovascular risk are scattered throughout a staggeringly vast literature. Within this body of work is room for diverging opinions, both on the basis of data and the current absence thereof. Nonetheless, diverse lines of research and observation have long converged on a discrete set of dietary recommendations.

The typical American diet suffers from both excesses and deficiencies relative to the ideal diet for cardiovascular health. A total fat intake below 35% of calories is recommended, (348) although maldistribution of fat calories is likely more important. Trans fat should be avoided altogether, but emerging evidence suggests saturated fats are not the problem once believed (214). Polyunsaturated and MUFA in a ratio of between 1:1 and 1:2 may be ideal. PUFA should be divided between n-6 and n-3 fatty acids in a ratio between 4:1 and 1:1 rather than the prevailing ratio of 11:1 (n-6:n-3). In patients consuming relatively little wild game or fish, fish oil supplementation, or consistent use of flaxseed oil may be recommended to supplement n-3 fat (α-linolenic acid). Some controversy persists as to the relative health benefits of short-chain versus long-chain n-3 fatty acid consumption (see Chapters 2, 4, and Section VIIE). The importance of supplementing n-3 fatty acids may be even greater in patients with established coronary disease.

Benefits of dietary fiber are well established, and prevailing intake is deficient. A daily intake of at least 30 g of fiber is appropriate and is readily achievable if whole grains, vegetables, and fruits are the principal sources of food energy. This dietary pattern will similarly serve to raise intake of diverse micronutrients, including antioxidants, while allowing for a low glycemic load despite generous intake of total carbohydrate.

The benefits of specific micronutrients are suggested, while the health advantages and specific cardiovascular benefits of generous intake of whole foods are conclusively established. The most recent, and most definitive, trial data argue against a benefit of high-dose (i.e., >400 IU per day) vitamin E supplementation, at least in established heart disease. The potential preventive effects of combinations of antioxidant supplements before coronary disease are overt remain uncertain but there is reason for concern with many individual agents. Arguments for a variety of other micronutrients and nutriceuticals can be made with available evidence; many of these are discussed elsewhere in the text (see, in particular, the nutrient reference tables in Section VIIE).

Barring alcohol-related health problems or contraindications such as liver disease or personal or family history of specific cancers, moderate alcohol consumption (15 to 30 g per day) appears to confer overall benefit; the lower end of this range is more appropriate for women. Restriction of dietary cholesterol seems unjustified. Eggs and shellfish need not be banished from a heart-healthy diet. Likewise, restriction of dietary sodium is not well supported, although restriction of high-sodium processed foods certainly is. Maintenance of near-optimal weight is of clear cardiovascular benefit, particularly when weight gain is centrally distributed. Given the prevalence of obesity, insulin resistance, and type 2 diabetes, dietary strategies for control of these conditions is fundamental to cardiac risk management (see Chapters 5 and 6).

In general, most dietary recommendations for the primary prevention of CVD in adults appear to be safe and appropriate for children over the age of 2 years (349,350) (see Chapter 29). Application of a heart-healthy dietary pattern is appropriate for primary, secondary, and tertiary prevention of heart disease. This pattern is consistent with prevailing and emerging recommendations for health promotion in general (see Chapter 45) and can be expected to confer noncardiovascular health benefits as well. In conjunction with other health-promoting lifestyle practices, the adoption of a heart-healthy diet reliably ameliorates cardiac risk across a broad array of measures (3).

Dietary guidance to patients should be cast in terms of foods rather than nutrient classes. The wide array of foods that comprise our diets span just three macronutrient classes: carbohydrate, fat, and protein. Thus, the actual composition of diets high or low in any given macronutrient can and does vary markedly. Diets high in carbohydrate, for example, may be based on nutrient-poor, energy-dense processed foods or on fruits, vegetables, and whole grains. Diets relatively high in fat may be based on fast food or on the Mediterranean dietary pattern, which is rich in nuts, seeds, olives, avocado, and fish.

The food-based theme of heart-healthy eating is consistent and clear across a wide expanse of literature: Intake of vegetables, fruits, beans, lentils, whole grains, nuts, seeds, olives, avocado, fish, lean meats, and dairy may be encouraged with confidence. Judicious additions of red wine and dark chocolate are advisable as well. All such foods are advisable in amounts appropriate for dietary balance and maintenance of stable and healthful weight. Variations on this basic theme will doubtless prove rich fodder for research for years to come. The theme, however, has by and large stood the test of time and is unlikely to change appreciably in the foreseeable future.

REFERENCES

1. McCabe-Sellers BJ, Skipper A. Position of the American Dietetic Association: integration of medical nutrition therapy and pharmacotherapy. *J Am Diet Assoc* 2010;110(6): 950–956.
2. Jenkins DJ, Kendall CW, Marchie A, et al. Effects of a dietary portfolio of cholesterol-lowering foods vs lovastatin on serum lipids and C-reactive protein. *JAMA* 2003;290: 502–510.
3. Elmer PJ, Obarzanek E, Vollmer WM, et al. Effects of comprehensive lifestyle modification on diet, weight, physical fitness, and blood pressure control: 18-month results of a randomized trial. *Ann Intern Med* 2006;144:485–495.
4. Knowler WC, Fowler SE, Hamman RF, et al. 10-year follow-up of diabetes incidence and weight loss in the Diabetes Prevention Program Outcomes Study. *Lancet* 2009;374:1677–1686.
5. De Caterina R, Zampolli A, Del Turco S, et al. Nutritional mechanisms that influence cardiovascular disease. *Am J Clin Nutr* 2006;83:421s–426s.
6. World Health Organization. *Cardiovascular disease: prevention and control.* Available at http://www.who.int/dietphysicalactivity/publications/facts/cvd/en/; accessed 5/5/07.
7. Yehle, KS, Chen AM, Mobley AR. A qualitative analysis of coronary heart disease patient views of dietary adherence and web-based and mobile-based nutrition tools. *J Cardiopulm Rehabil Prev* 2012;32(4):203–209.
8. National Institutes of Health. *Detection, evaluation, and treatment of high blood cholesterol in adults (Adult Treatment Panel III).* Available at http://www.nhlbi.nih.gov/guidelines/cholesterol/atp3xsum.pdf; accessed 10/8/07.
9. Fox KA, Steg PG, Eagle KA, et al. Decline in rates of death and heart failure in acute coronary syndromes, 1999–2006. *JAMA* 2007;297:1892–1900.
10. Menotti A, Keys A, Kromhout D, et al. Inter-cohort differences in coronary heart diseasemortality in the 25-year follow-up of the seven countries study. *Eur J Epidemiol* 1993;9:527–536.
11. Verschuren WM, Jacobs DR, Bloemberg BP, et al. Serum total cholesterol and long-term coronary heart disease mortality in different cultures. Twenty-five-year follow-up of the seven countries study. *JAMA* 1995;274:131–136.
12. Keys A, Menotti A, Aravanis C, et al. The seven countries study: 2,289 deaths in 15 years. *Prev Med* 1984;13:141–154.
13. Benfante R. Studies of cardiovascular disease and cause-specific mortality trends in Japanese-American men living in Hawaii and risk factor comparisons with other Japanese populations in the Pacific region: a review. *Hum Biol* 1992;64:791–805.
14. Worth RM, Kato H, Rhoads GG, et al. Epidemiologic studies of coronary heart disease and stroke in Japanese men living in Japan, Hawaii and California: mortality. *Am J Epidemiol* 1975;102:481–490.
15. Robertson TL, Kato H, Rhoads GG, et al. Epidemiologic studies of coronary heart disease and stroke in Japanese men living in Japan, Hawaii and California. Incidence of myocardial infarction and death from coronary heart disease. *Am J Cardiol* 1977;39:239–243.
16. Scarborough P, Morgan RD, Rayner M. Differences in coronary heart disease, stroke and cancer mortality rates between England, Wales, Scotland and Northern Ireland: the role of diet and nutrition. *BMJ Open* 2011;1(1):e000263.
17. McPherson R, Pertsemlidis A, Kavaslar N, et al. A common allele on chromosome 9 associated with coronary heart disease. *Science* 2007;316:1488–1491.
18. Musunuru K. Atherogenic dyslipidemia: cardiovascular risk and dietary intervention. *Lipids* 2010;45:907–914.
19. Anthony D. Diagnosis and screening of coronary artery disease. *Prim Care* 2005;32:931–946.
20. Zieman SJ, Melenovsky V, Kass DA. Mechanisms, pathophysiology, and therapy of arterial stiffness. *Arterioscler Thromb Vasc Biol* 2005;25:932–943.
21. Poredos P. Endothelial dysfunction and cardiovascular disease. *Pathophysiol Haemost Thromb* 2002;32:274–277.
22. McCarron D, Oparil S, Chait A, et al. Nutritional management of cardiovascular risk factors. *Arch Intern Med* 1997;157:169–177.
23. Herder R, Demmig-Adams B. The power of a balanced diet and lifestyle in preventing cardiovascular disease. *Nutr Clin Care* 2004;7:46–55.
24. Kromhout D. Diet and cardiovascular diseases. *J Nutr Health Aging* 2001;5:144–149.
25. Ornish D, Brown S, Scherwitz L. Can lifestyle changes reverse coronary heart disease? The lifestyle heart trial. *Lancet* 1990;336:129–133.
26. Temple N. Dietary fats and coronary heart disease. *Biomed Pharmacother* 1996;50:261–268.
27. Keys A, Aravanis C, Blackburn H, et al. Epidemiological studies related to coronary heart disease: characteristics of men aged 40–59 in seven countries. *Acta Med Scand Suppl* 1966:460:1–392.
28. Chahoud G, Aude YW, Mehta JL. Dietary recommendations in the prevention and treatment of coronary heart

disease: do we have the ideal diet yet? *Am J Cardiol* 2004;94:1260–1267.

29. Schaefer EJ, Gleason JA, Dansinger ML. The effects of low-fat, high-carbohydrate diets on plasma lipoproteins, weight loss, and heart disease risk reduction. *Curr Atheroscler Rep* 2005;7:421–427.

30. Ornish D, Scherwitz LW, Billings JH, et al. Intensive lifestyle changes for reversal of coronary heart disease. *JAMA* 1998;280:2001–2007.

31. de Lorgeril M, Salen P. The Mediterranean diet in secondary prevention of coronary heart disease. *Clin Invest Med* 2006;29:154–158.

32. Jebb SA. Dietary determinants of obesity. *Obes Rev* 2007;8: 93–97.

33. Hu FB, Willett WC. Optimal diets for prevention of coronary heart disease. *JAMA* 2002;288:2569–2578.

34. Hu FB, Manson JE, Willett WC. Types of dietary fat and risk of coronary heart disease: a critical review. *J Am Coll Nutr* 2001;20:5–19.

35. Lichtenstein AH, Kennedy E, Barrier P, et al. Dietary fat consumption and health. *Nutr Rev* 1998;56:s3–s19; discussion s19–s28.

36. Lichtenstein AH. Dietary fat and cardiovascular disease risk: quantity or quality? *J Womens Health* (Larchmt) 2003;12:109–114.

37. Willett WC. The Mediterranean diet: science and practice. *Public Health Nutr* 2006;9:105–110.

38. Guallar-Castillon P, Rodriguez-Artalejo F, Lopez-Garcia E, et al. Consumption of fried foods and risk of coronary heart disease: Spanish cohort of the European Prospective Investigation into Cancer and Nutrition study. *BMJ* 2012;344:e363.

39. Popkin BM. Global nutrition dynamics: the world is shifting rapidly toward a diet linked with noncommunicable diseases. *Am J Clin Nutr* 2006;84:289–298.

40. Bray GA, Paeratakul S, Popkin BM. Dietary fat and obesity: a review of animal, clinical and epidemiological studies. *Physiol Behav* 2004;83:549–555.

41. Peters JC. Dietary fat and body weight control. *Lipids* 2003;38:123–127.

42. Hill JO, Melanson EL, Wyatt HT. Dietary fat intake and regulation of energy balance: implications for obesity. *J Nutr* 2000;130:284s–288s.

43. Astrup A. The role of dietary fat in obesity. *Semin Vasc Med* 2005;5:40–47.

44. Hooper L, Abdelhamid A, Moore HJ, et al. Effect of reducing total fat intake on body weight: systematic review and meta-analysis of randomised controlled trials and cohort studies. *BMJ* 2012;345:e7666.

45. American Dietetic Association, Dietitians of Canada. Position of the American Dietetic Association and Dietitians of Canada: vegetarian diets. *J Am Diet Assoc* 2003;103: 748–765.

46. Key TJ, Appleby PN, Rosell MS. Health effects of vegetarian and vegan diets. *Proc Nutr Soc* 2006;65:35–41.

47. Sabate J. The contribution of vegetarian diets to human health. *Forum Nutr* 2003;56:218–220.

48. Merino J, Kones R, Plana N, et al. Negative effect of a low-carbohydrate, high-protein, high-fat diet on small peripheral artery reactivity in patients with increased cardiovascular risk. *Br J Nutr* 2012:1–7.

49. Kostogrys RB, Franczyk-Zarow M, Maslak E, et al. Low carbohydrate, high protein diet promotes atherosclerosis in apolipoprotein E/low-density lipoprotein receptor double knockout mice (apoE/LDLR(-/-)). *Atherosclerosis* 2012;223(2):327–331.

50. Wood RJ. Effect of dietary carbohydrate restriction with and without weight loss on atherogenic dyslipidemia. *Nutr Rev* 2006;64:539–545.

51. Krauss RM, Blanche PJ, Rawlings RS, et al. Separate effects of reduced carbohydrate intake and weight loss on atherogenic dyslipidemia. *Am J Clin Nutr* 2006;83:1025–1031.

52. Gann D. A low-carbohydrate diet in overweight patients undergoing stable statin therapy raises high-density lipoprotein and lowers triglycerides substantially. *Clin Cardiol* 2004;27:563–564.

53. Siri PW, Krauss RM. Influence of dietary carbohydrate and fat on LDL and HDL particle distributions. *Curr Atheroscler Rep* 2005;7:455–459.

54. Wood RJ, Volek JS, Liu Y, et al. Carbohydrate restriction alters lipoprotein metabolism by modifying VLDL, LDL, and HDL subfraction distribution and size in overweight men. *J Nutr* 2006;136:384–389.

55. Denke MA. Dietary fats, fatty acids, and their effects on lipoproteins. *Curr Atheroscler Rep* 2006;8:466–471.

56. Vincent-Baudry S, Defoort C, Gerber M, et al. The Medi-RIVAGE study: reduction of cardiovascular disease risk factors after a 3-mo intervention with a Mediterranean-type diet or a low-fat diet. *Am J Clin Nutr* 2005;82:964–971.

57. Guo Z, Mitchell-Raymundo F, Yang H, et al. Dietary restriction reduces atherosclerosis and oxidative stress in the aorta of apolipoprotein E-deficient mice. *Mech Ageing Dev* 2002;123(8):1121–1131.

58. National Institutes of Health. *Clinical guidelines on the identification, evaluation, and treatment of overweight and obesity in adults: the evidence report*. Available at http://www.nhlbi.nih.gov/guidelines/obesity/ob_gdlns.pdf; accessed 10/8/07.

59. Mathieu P, Pibarot P, Despres JP. Metabolic syndrome: the danger signal in atherosclerosis. *Vasc Health Risk Manag* 2006;2:285–302.

60. Despres JP, Lemieux I. Abdominal obesity and metabolic syndrome. *Nature* 2006;444:881–887.

61. Despres JP. Intra-abdominal obesity: an untreated risk factor for type 2 diabetes and cardiovascular disease. *J Endocrinol Invest* 2006;29:77–82.

62. Despres JP. Is visceral obesity the cause of the metabolic syndrome? *Ann Med* 2006;38:52.

63. Stanforth PR, Jackson AS, Green JS, et al. Generalized abdominal visceral fat prediction models for black and white adults aged 17–65 y: the HERITAGE Family Study. *Int J Obes Relat Metab Disord* 2004;28:925–932.

64. Knowler WC, Barrett-Connor E, Fowler SE, et al. Reduction in the incidence of type 2 diabetes with lifestyle intervention or metformin. *N Engl J Med* 2002;346:393–403.

65. Ditomasso D, Carnethon MR, Wright FM, et al. The associations between visceral fat and calcified atherosclerosis are stronger in women than men. *Atherosclerosis* 2010;208(2):531–536.

66. Stevens JJ, Chambless LE, Nieto FJ, et al. Associations of weight loss and changes in fat distribution with the remission of hypertension in a bi-ethnic cohort: the

Atherosclerosis Risk in Communities Study. *Prev Med* 2003;36(3):330–339.

67. Rimm EB, Ascherio A, Giovannucci E, et al. Vegetable, fruit, and cereal fiber intake and risk of coronary heart disease among men. *JAMA* 1996;275:447–451.

68. Hunninghake D, Miller V, LaRosa J, et al. Long-term treatment of hypercholesterolemia with dietary fiber. *Am J Med* 1994;97:504–508.

69. Wynder E, Stellman S, Zang E. High fiber intake. Indicator of a healthy lifestyle. *JAMA* 1996;275:486–487.

70. Simoes E, Byers T, Coates R, et al. The association between leisure-time physical activity and dietary fat in American adults. *Am J Public Health* 1995;85:240–244.

71. Crowe FL, Key TJ, et al. Dietary fibre intake and ischaemic heart disease mortality: the European Prospective Investigation into Cancer and Nutrition-Heart study. *Eur J Clin Nutr* 2012;66(8):950–995.

72. Pereira MA, Swain J, Goldfine AB, et al. Effects of a low-glycemic load diet on resting energy expenditure and heart disease risk factors during weight loss. *JAMA* 2004;292:2482–2490.

73. McMillan-Price J, Petocz P, Atkinson F, et al. Comparison of 4 diets of varying glycemic load on weight loss and cardiovascular risk reduction in overweight and obese young adults: a randomized controlled trial. *Arch Intern Med* 2006;166:1466–1475.

74. Ebbeling CB, Leidig MM, Sinclair KB, et al. Effects of an ad libitum low-glycemic load diet on cardiovascular disease risk factors in obese young adults. *Am J Clin Nutr* 2005;81:976–982.

75. Hardy DS, Hoelscher DM, Aragaki C, et al. Association of glycemic index and glycemic load with risk of incident coronary heart disease among Whites and African Americans with and without type 2 diabetes: the Atherosclerosis Risk in Communities study. *Ann Epidemiol* 2010;20(8):610–661.

76. Otten JJ, Hellwig JP, Meyers LD, eds. *Dietary reference intakes*. Washington, DC: National Academies Press, 2006.

77. Carey VJ, Bishop L, Charleston J, et al. Rationale and design of the Optimal Macro-Nutrient Intake Heart Trial to Prevent Heart Disease (OMNI-Heart). *Clin Trials* 2005;2:529–537.

78. Yeung EH, Appel LJ, Miller ER 3rd, et al. The effects of macronutrient intake on total and high-molecular weight adiponectin: results from the OMNI-Heart trial. *Obesity* (Silver Spring) 2010;18:1632–1637.

79. National Institutes of Health. *Paleolithic diet and exercise study*. Available at http://clinicaltrials.gov/show/NCT00360516; accessed 4/24/07.

80. Sebastian A, Frassetto LA, Sellmeyer DE, et al. Estimation of the net acid load of the diet of ancestral preagricultural *Homo sapiens* and their hominid ancestors. *Am J Clin Nutr* 2002;76:1308–1316.

81. Anderson K, Castelli W, Levy D. Cholesterol and mortality: 30 years of follow-up from the Framingham Study. *JAMA* 1987;257:2176–2180.

82. Krauss R, Deckelbaum R, Ernst N, et al. Dietary guidelines for healthy American adults. *Circulation* 1996;94:1795–1800.

83. US Department of Health and Human Services. *Dietary guidelines for Americans, 2005*. Available at http://www.health.gov/dietaryguidelines/dga2005/document/; accessed 10/11/07.

84. Goldstein J, Brown M. The LDL receptor and the regulation of cellular cholesterol metabolism. *J Cell Sci* 1985;3:131–137.

85. Goldstein J, Brown M. Regulation of low-density lipoprotein receptors: implications for pathogenesis and therapy of hypercholesterolemia and atherosclerosis. *Circulation* 1987;76:504–507.

86. Gesquiere L, Loreau N, Minnich A, et al. Oxidative stress leads to cholesterol accumulation in vascular smooth muscle cells. *Free Radic Biol Med* 1999;27:134–145.

87. Stein O, Stein Y. Smooth muscle cells and atherosclerosis. *Curr Opin Lipidol* 1995;6:269–274.

88. Plotnick GD, Corrett M, Vogel RA. Effect of antioxidant vitamins on the transient impairment of endothelium-dependent brachial artery vasoactivity following a single high-fat meal. *JAMA* 1997;278:1682–1686.

89. Zilversmit D. Atherogenesis: a postprandial phenomenon. *Circulation* 1979;60:473–485.

90. Lefebvre P, Scheen A. The postprandial state and risk of cardiovascular disease. *Diabetes Med* 1998;15:s63–s68.

91. Williams M, Sutherland W, McCormick M, et al. Impaired endothelial function following a meal rich in used cooking fat. *J Am Coll Cardiol* 1999;33:1050–1055.

92. Deanfield JE, Halcox JP, Rabelink TJ. Endothelial function and dysfunction: testing and clinical relevance. *Circulation* 2007;115:1285–1295.

93. Desjardins F, Balligand JL. Nitric oxide-dependent endothelial function and cardiovascular disease. *Acta Clin Belg* 2006;61:326–334.

94. Davis N, Katz S, Wylie-Rosett J. The effect of diet on endothelial function. *Cardiol Rev* 2007;15:62–66.

95. Adams MR. Clinical assessment of endothelial function. *Endothelium* 2006;13:367–374.

96. Hayoz D, Mazzolai L. Endothelial function, mechanical stress and atherosclerosis. *Adv Cardiol* 2007;44:62–75.

97. Lai CQ, Corella D, Demissie S, et al. Dietary intake of n-6 fatty acids modulates effect of apolipoprotein A5 gene on plasma fasting triglycerides, remnant lipoprotein concentrations, and lipoprotein particle size: the Framingham Heart Study. *Circulation* 2006;113:2062–2070.

98. Katan M, Grundy S, Willett W. Should a low-fat, high-carbohydrate diet be recommended for everyone? Beyond low-fat diets. *N Engl J Med* 1997;337:563–566.

99. Connor W, Connor S. Should a low-fat, high-carbohydrate diet be recommended for everyone? The case for a low-fat, high-carbohydrate diet. *N Engl J Med* 1997;337:562–563.

100. Oliver M. It is more important to increase the intake of unsaturated fats than to decrease the intake of saturated fats: evidence from clinical trials relating to ischemic heart disease. *Am J Clin Nutr* 1997;980s–986s.

101. Kennedy E, Bowman S, Powell R. Dietary-fat intake in the US population. *J Am Coll Nutr* 1999;18:207–212.

102. Ernst N, Sempos C, Briefel R, et al. Consistency between US dietary fat intake and serum total cholesterol concentrations: the National Health and Nutrition Examination Surveys. *Am J Clin Nutr* 1997;66:965s–972s.

103. Eaton S, Konner M. Paleolithic nutrition revisited: a twelve-year retrospective on its nature and implications. *Eur J Clin Nutr* 1997;51:207–216.

104. Musunuru K. Atherogenic dyslipidemia: cardiovascular risk and dietary intervention. *Lipids* 2010;45:907–914.

105. de Oliveira Otto MC, Mozaffarian D, Kromhout D, et al. Dietary intake of saturated fat by food source and incident cardiovascular disease: the Multi-Ethnic Study of Atherosclerosis. *Am J Clin Nutr* 2012;96(2):397–404.

106. Kuipers RS, Luxwolda MF, Dijck-Brouwer DA, et al. Estimated macronutrient and fatty acid intakes from an East African Paleolithic diet. *Br J Nutr* 2010;104:1666–1687.

107. Ramsden CE, Zamora D, Leelarthaepin B, et al. Use of dietary linoleic acid for secondary prevention of coronary heart disease and death: evaluation of recovered data from the Sydney Diet Heart Study and updated meta-analysis. *BMJ* 2013;346:e8707.

108. Mozaffarian D, Micha R, Wallace S, et al. Effects on coronary heart disease of increasing polyunsaturated fat in place of saturated fat: a systematic review and meta-analysis of randomized controlled trials. *PLoS Med* 2010;7(3):e1000252.

109. Siri-Tarino PW, Sun Q, Hu FB, et al. Meta-analysis of prospective cohort studies evaluating the association of saturated fat with cardiovascular disease. *Am J Clin Nutr* 2010;91:535–546.

110. Kritchevsky D. Stearic acid metabolism and atherogenesis: history. *Am J Clin Nutr* 1994;60(6 suppl):997S–1001S.

111. Drewnowski A. Taste preferences and food intake. *Annu Rev Nutr* 1997;17:237–253.

112. Drewnowski A, Schwartz M. Invisible fats: sensory assessment of sugar/fat mixtures. *Appetite* 1990;14:203–217.

113. Micha R, Wallace SK, et al. Red and processed meat consumption and risk of incident coronary heart disease, stroke, and diabetes mellitus: a systematic review and meta analysis. *Circulation* 2010;121(21):2271–2283.

114. Centers for Disease Control and Prevention. *National health and nutrition examination survey*. Available at http://www.cdc.gov/nchs/nhanes.htm; accessed 10/11/07.

115. Kratz M. Dietary cholesterol, atherosclerosis and coronary heart disease. *Handb Exp Pharmacol* 2005;170:195–213.

116. Hu F, Stampfer M, Rimm E, et al. A prospective study of egg consumption and risk of cardiovascular disease in men and women. *JAMA* 1999;281:1387–1394.

117. Kritchevsky SB. A review of scientific research and recommendations regarding eggs. *J Am Coll Nutr* 2004;23:596s–600s.

118. Katz DL, Evans MA, Nawaz H, et al. Egg consumption and endothelial function: a randomized controlled crossover trial. *Int J Cardiol* 2005;99:65–70.

119. Masterjohn C. The anti-inflammatory properties of safflower oil and coconut oil may be mediated by their respective concentrations of vitamin E. *J Am Coll Cardiol* 2007;49:1825–1826.

120. Amarasiri WA, Dissanayake AS. Coconut fats. *Ceylon Med J* 2006;51:47–51.

121. Harvard Medical School. *Egg nutrition and heart disease*. Available at http://www.health.harvard.edu/press_releases/egg-nutrition.htm; accessed 5/5/07.

122. Barraj L, Tran N, Mink P. A comparison of egg consumption with other modifiable coronary heart disease lifestyle risk factors: a relative risk apportionment study. *Risk Anal* 2009;29(3):401–415.

123. Sun Q, Ma J, Campos H, et al. A prospective study of trans fatty acids in erythrocytes and risk of coronary heart disease. *Circulation* 2007;115:1858–1865.

124. Willett WC, Stampfer MJ, Manson JE, et al. Intake of trans fatty acids and risk of coronary heart disease among women. *Lancet* 1993;341:581–585.

125. Ascherio A, Willett W. New directions in dietary studies of coronary heart disease. *J Nutr* 1995;125:647s–655s.

126. Aronis, KN, Joseph RJ, Blackburn GL, et al. Trans-fatty acids, insulin resistance/diabetes, and cardiovascular disease risk: should policy decisions be based on observational cohort studies, or should we be waiting for results from randomized placebo-controlled trials? *Metabolism* 2011;60(7):901–905.

127. *Ban trans fats*. Available at http://www.bantransfats.com; accessed 5/5/07.

128. tfX: The Campaign Against Trans Fat in Food. Denmark's trans fat law. March 11, 2003. Available at http://www.tfx.org.uk/page116.html; accessed 5/5/07.

129. US Food and Drug Administration. *Questions and answers about trans fat nutrition labeling*. January 1, 2006. Available at http://www.cfsan.fda.gov/~dms/qatrans2.html; accessed 4/25/07.

130. American Heart Association. *Fat*. Available at http://www.americanheart.org/presenter.jhtml?identifier=4582; accessed 4/23/07.

131. Berry SE. Triacylglycerol structure and interesterification of palmitic and stearic acid-rich fats: an overview and implications for cardiovascular disease. *Nutr Res Rev* 2009;22(1): 3–17.

132. Alfinslater RB, Aftergood L, Hansen H, et al. Nutritional evaluation of inter-esterified fats. *J Am Oil Chem Soc* 1966;43:110–112.

133. Berry SE, Woodward R, et al. Effect of interesterification of palmitic acid-rich triacylglycerol on postprandial lipid and factor VII response. *Lipids* 2007;42(4):315–323.

134. Zock PL, Katan MB. Hydrogenation alternatives: effects of trans fatty acids and stearic acid versus linoleic acid on serum lipids and lipoproteins in humans. *J Lipid Res* 1992;33:399–410.

135. McGandy RB, Hegsted DM, Myers ML. Use of semisynthetic fats in determining effects of specific dietary fatty acids on serum lipids in man. *Am J Clin Nutr* 1970;23:1288–1298.

136. Funck LG, Barrera-Arellano D, Block JM. [Conjugated linoleic acid (CLA) and its relationship with cardiovascular disease and associated risk factors]. *Arch Latinoam Nutr* 2006;56(2):123–134.

137. Cooper MH, Miller JR, et al. Conjugated linoleic acid isomers have no effect on atherosclerosis and adverse effects on lipoprotein and liver lipid metabolism in apoE-/- mice fed a high-cholesterol diet. *Atherosclerosis* 2008;200(2):294–302.

138. Agueda M, Zulet MA, Martínez JA. [Effect of conjugated linoleic acid (CLA) on human lipid profile]. *Arch Latinoam Nutr* 2009;59(3):245–252.

139. Ramsden CE, Zamora D, Leelarthepin B, et al. Use of dietary linoleic acid for secondary prevention of coronary heart disease and death: evaluation of recovered data from the Sydney Diet Heart Study and updated meta-analysis. *BMJ* 2013;346:e8707.

140. Leaf A, Kang J, Xiao Y, et al. Dietary n-3 fatty acids in the prevention of cardiac arrhythmias. *Curr Opin Clin Nutr Metab Care* 1998;1:225–228.

141. Horrocks L, Yeo Y. Health benefits of docosahexaenoic acid. *Pharmacol Res* 1999;40:211–225.

142. Simopoulos A. Essential fatty acids in health and chronic disease. *Am J Clin Nutr* 1999;70:560s–569s.

143. Marckmann P, Gronbaek M. Fish consumption and coronary heart disease mortality. A systematic review

of prospective cohort studies. *Eur J Clin Nutr* 1999;53: 585–590.

144. Huang T, Shou T, Cai N, et al. Associations of plasma n-3 polyunsaturated fatty acids with blood pressure and cardiovascular risk factors among Chinese. *Int J Food Sci Nutr* 2012;63(6):667–673.

145. Grundy S. What is the desirable ratio of saturated, polyunsaturated, and monounsaturated fatty acids in the diet? *Am J Clin Nutr* 1997;66:988s–990s.

146. Grundy S. Second International Conference on Fats and Oil Consumption in Health and Disease: how we can optimize dietary composition to combat metabolic complications and decrease obesity. Overview. *Am J Clin Nutr* 1998;67:497s–499s.

147. Grundy S. The optimal ratio of fat-to-carbohydrate in the diet. *Annu Rev Nutr* 1999;19:325–341.

148. Harper CR, Jacobson TA. Usefulness of omega-3 fatty acids and the prevention of coronary heart disease. *Am J Cardiol* 2005;96:1521–1529.

149. Marchioli R, Barzi F, Bomba E, et al. Early protection against sudden death by n-3 polyunsaturated fatty acids after myocardial infarction: time-course analysis of the results of the Gruppo Italiano per lo Studio della Sopravvivenza nell'Infarto Miocardico (GISSI)–Prevenzione. *Circulation* 2002;105:1897–1903.

150. Reiffel JA, McDonald A. Antiarrhythmic effects of omega-3 fatty acids. *Am J Cardiol* 2006;98:50i–60i.

151. Macchia A, Levantesi G, Franzosi MG, et al. Left ventricular systolic dysfunction, total mortality, and sudden death in patients with myocardial infarction treated with n-3 polyunsaturated fatty acids. *Eur J Heart Fail* 2005;7:904–909.

152. Richter WO. Long-chain omega-3 fatty acids from fish reduce sudden cardiac death in patients with coronary heart disease. *Eur J Med Res* 2003;8:332–336.

153. Einvik G, Klemsdal TO, Sandvik K, et al. A randomized clinical trial on n-3 polyunsaturated fatty acids supplementation and all-cause mortality in elderly men at high cardiovascular risk. *Eur J Cardiovasc Prev Rehabil* 2010;17(5):588–592.

154. Garcia-Alonso FJ, Jorge-Vidal V, Ros G, et al. Effect of consumption of tomato juice enriched with n-3 polyunsaturated fatty acids on the lipid profile, antioxidant biomarker status, and cardiovascular disease risk in healthy women. *Eur J Nutr* 2012;51(4):415–424.

155. Kromhout D, Giltay EJ, Geleijnse JM, et al. n-3 Fatty acids and cardiovascular events after myocardial infarction. *N Engl J Med* 2010;363(21):2015–2026.

156. Mariani J, Doval HC, Nul D, et al. N-3 polyunsaturated fatty acids higher doses of PUFA are needed to prevent atrial fibrillation: updated systematic review and meta-analysis of randomized controlled trials. *J Am Heart Assoc* 2013;2:e005033.

157. Kotwal S, Jun M, Sullivan D, et al. Omega 3 fatty acids and cardiovascular outcomes: systematic review and meta-analysis. *Circ Cardiovasc Qual Outcomes* 2012;5:808–818.

158. Rizos EC, Ntzani EE, Bika E, et al. Association between omega-3 fatty acid supplementation and risk of major cardiovascular disease events: a systematic review and meta-analysis. *JAMA* 2012;308:1024–1033.

159. Xin W, Wei W, Li X. Effects of fish oil supplementation on cardiac function in chronic heart failure: a meta-analysis of randomised controlled trials. *Heart* 2012;98: 1620–1625.

160. Djousse L, Akinkuolie AO, Wu JH, et al. Fish consumption, omega-3 fatty acids and risk of heart failure: a meta-analysis. *Clin Nutr* 2012;31:846–853.

161. Lorgeril MD. Mediterranean diet in the prevention of coronary heart disease. *Nutrition* 1998;14:55–57.

162. de Lorgeril M, Salen P. Modified cretan Mediterranean diet in the prevention of coronary heart disease and cancer: an update. *World Rev Nutr Diet* 2007;97:1–32.

163. Schroder H. Protective mechanisms of the Mediterranean diet in obesity and type 2 diabetes. *J Nutr Biochem* 2007;18:149–160.

164. Serra-Majem L, Roman B, Estruch R. Scientific evidence of interventions using the Mediterranean diet: a systematic review. *Nutr Rev* 2006;64:s27–s47.

165. de Lorgeril M, Salen P. The Mediterranean-style diet for the prevention of cardiovascular diseases. *Public Health Nutr* 2006;9:118–123.

166. Thomsen C, Rasmussen O, Christiansen C, et al. Comparison of the effects of a monounsaturated fat diet and a high carbohydrate diet on cardiovascular risk factors in first degree relatives to type-2 diabetic subjects. *Eur J Clin Nutr* 1999;53:818–823.

167. Kris-Etherton P, Pearson T, Wan Y, et al. High-monounsaturated fatty acid diets lower both plasma cholesterol and triacylglycerol concentrations. *Am J Clin Nutr* 1999;70:1009–1115.

168. Kris-Etherton P. AHA science advisory: monounsaturated fatty acids and risk of cardiovascular disease. *J Nutr* 1999;129:2280–2284.

169. Lecerf LM. Fatty acids and cardiovascular disease. *Nutr Rev* 2009;67(5):273–283.

170. Gardner CD, Kraemer HC. Monounsaturated versus polyunsaturated dietary fat and serum lipids. A meta-analysis. *Arterioscler Thromb Vasc Biol* 1995;15: 1917–1927.

171. Bod MB, de Vries JH, Feskens EJ, et al. Effect of a high monounsaturated fatty acids diet and a Mediterranean diet on serum lipids and insulin sensitivity in adults with mild abdominal obesity. *Nutr Metab Cardiovasc Dis* 2010;20(8):591–598.

172. Tsimikas S, Reaven P. The role of dietary fatty acids in lipoprotein oxidation and atherosclerosis. *Curr Opin Lipidol* 1998;9:301–307.

173. Alarcon de la Lastra C, Barranco MD, Motilva V, et al. Mediterranean diet and health: biological importance of olive oil. *Curr Pharm Des* 2001;7:933–950.

174. Binkoski AE, Kris-Etherton PM, Wilson TA, et al. Balance of unsaturated fatty acids is important to a cholesterol-lowering diet: comparison of mid-oleic sunflower oil and olive oil on cardiovascular disease risk factors. *J Am Diet Assoc* 2005;105:1080–1086.

175. Owen RW, Giacosa A, Hull WE, et al. Olive-oil consumption and health: the possible role of antioxidants. *Lancet Oncol* 2000;1:107–112.

176. Perez-Jimenez F, Alvarez de Cienfuegos G, Badimon L, et al. International conference on the healthy effect of virgin olive oil. *Eur J Clin Invest* 2005;35:421–424.

177. Nagyova A, Haban P, Klvanova J, et al. Effects of dietary extra virgin olive oil on serum lipid resistance to oxidation and fatty acid composition in elderly lipidemic patients. *Bratisl Lek Listy* 2003;104:218–221.

178. Trichopoulou A. Mediterranean diet: the past and the present. *Nutr Metab Cardiovasc Dis* 2001;11:1–4.

179. Estruch R, Martinez-Gonzalez MA, Corella D, et al. Effects of a Mediterranean-style diet on cardiovascular risk factors: a randomized trial. *Ann Intern Med* 2006;145:1–11.

180. Simopoulos AP. The Mediterranean diets: what is so special about the diet of Greece? The scientific evidence. *J Nutr* 2001;131:3065s–3073s.

181. Esposito K, Marfella R, Ciotola M, et al. Effect of a Mediterranean-style diet on endothelial dysfunction and markers of vascular inflammation in the metabolic syndrome: a randomized trial. *JAMA* 2004;292:1440–1446.

182. Fung TT, Rexrode KM, Mantzoros CS, et al. Mediterranean diet and incidence of and mortality from coronary heart disease and stroke in women. *Circulation* 2009;119:1093–1100.

183. Perona JS, Covas MI, Fitó M, et al. Reduction in systemic and VLDL triacylglycerol concentration after a 3-month Mediterranean-style diet in high-cardiovascular-risk subjects. *J Nutr Biochem* 2010;21(9):892–898.

184. Martinez-Gonzalez MA, Bes-Rastrollo M, Serra-Majem L, et al. Mediterranean food pattern and the primary prevention of chronic disease: recent developments. *Nutr Rev* 2009;67(suppl 1):S111–S116.

185. Shai I, Schwarzfuchs D, Henkin Y, et al. Weight loss with a low-carbohydrate, Mediterranean, or low-fat diet. *N Engl J Med* 2008;359:229–241.

186. Yeung EH, Appel LJ, Miller ER 3rd, et al. The effects of macronutrient intake on total and high-molecular weight adiponectin: results from the OMNI-Heart trial. *Obesity* 2010;184(8):1632–1637.

187. Kastorini CM, Milionis HJ, Esposito K, et al. The effect of Mediterranean diet on metabolic syndrome and its components: a meta-analysis of 50 studies and 534,906 individuals. *J Am Coll Cardiol* 2011;57(11):1299–1313.

188. Nordmann AJ, Suter-Zimmermann K, Bucher HC, et al. Meta-analysis comparing Mediterranean to low-fat diets for modification of cardiovascular risk factors. *Am J Med* 2011;124(9):841–851.

189. Sofi F, Abbate R, Gensini GF, et al. Accruing evidence on benefits of adherence to the Mediterranean diet on health: an updated systematic review and meta-analysis. *Am J Clin Nutr* 2010;92(5):1189–1196.

190. Esposito K, Pontillo A, Di Palo C, et al. Effect of weight loss and lifestyle changes on vascular inflammatory markers in obese women: a randomized trial. *JAMA* 2003;289(14):1799–1804.

191. Esposito K, Marfella R, Ciotola M, et al. Effect of a mediterranean-style diet on endothelial dysfunction and markers of vascular inflammation in the metabolic syndrome: a randomized trial. *JAMA* 2004;292(12):1440–1446.

192. Criqui M, Ringel B. Does diet or alcohol explain the French paradox? *Lancet* 1994;344:1719–1723.

193. Singh R, Rastogi S, Verma R, et al. Randomized controlled trial of cardioprotective diet in patients with recent acute myocardial infarction: results of one year follow up. *BMJ* 1992;304:1015–1019.

194. Martín-Peláez S, Covas MI, Fitó M, et al. Health effects of olive oil polyphenols: recent advances and possibilities for the use of health claims. *Mol Nutr Food Res* 2013;57(5):760–771.

195. Blomhoff R, Carlsen MH, Andersen LF, et al. Health benefits of nuts: potential role of antioxidants. *Br J Nutr* 2006;96(suppl 2):S52–S60.

196. Garg A, Bonamome A, Grundy S, et al. Comparison of a high-carbohydrate diet with a high-monounsaturated-fat diet in patients with non-insulin-dependent diabetes mellitus. *N Engl J Med* 1988;319:829–843.

197. Garg A, Bantle J, Henry R, et al. Effects of varying carbohydrate content of diet in patients with non-insulin-dependent diabetes mellitus. *JAMA* 1994;271:1421–1428.

198. López S, Bermúdez B, Pacheco YM, et al. Distinctive postprandial modulation of b cell function and insulin sensitivity by dietary fats: monounsaturated compared with saturated fatty acids. *Am J Clin Nutr* 2008;88(3):638–644.

199. Grundy S. Hypertriglyceridemia, insulin resistance, and the metabolic syndrome. *Am J Cardiol* 1999;83:25f–29f.

200. Reaven G, Lithell H, Landsberg L. Hypertension and associated metabolic abnormalities the role of insulin resistance and the sympathoadrenal system. *N Engl J Med* 1996;334:374–381.

201. Kirk EP, Klein S. Pathogenesis and pathophysiology of the cardiometabolic syndrome. *J Clin Hypertens* 2009;11(12):761–765.

202. Lorgeril MD, Salen P, Monjaud I, et al. The "diet heart" hypothesis in secondary prevention of coronary heart disease. *Eur Heart J* 1997;18:13–18.

203. Lorgeril MD, Salen P. What makes a Mediterranean diet cardioprotective? *Cardiol Rev* 1997;14:15–21.

204. Lorgeril MD, Salen P, Martin J-L, et al. Effect of a Mediterranean type of diet on the rate of cardiovascular complications in patients with coronary artery disease. *J Am Coll Cardiol* 1996;28:1103–1108.

205. Katan M. High-oil compared with low-fat, high-carbohydrate diets in the prevention of ischemic heart disease. *Am J Clin Nutr* 1997;66:974s–979s.

206. Heitmann BL, Lissner L. Can adverse effects of dietary fat intake be overestimated as a consequence of dietary fat underreporting? *Public Health Nutr* 2005;8:1322–1327.

207. Shai I, Schwarzfuchs D, Henkin Y. Weight loss with a low-carbohydrate, Mediterranean, or low-fat diet. *N Engl J Med*. 2008;359(3):229–241

208. Siscovick D, Raghunathan T, King I, et al. Dietary intake and cell membrane levels of long chain n-3 polyunsaturated fatty acids and the risk of primary cardiac arrest. *JAMA* 1995;274:1363–1367.

209. Lavie CJ, Milani RV, Mehra MR, et al. Omega-3 polyunsaturated fatty acids and cardiovascular diseases. *J Am Coll Cardiol* 2009;54:585–594.

210. Erkkilä A, de Mello VDF, Risérus U, et al. Dietary fatty acids and cardiovascular disease: an epidemiological approach. *Prog Lipid Res* 2008;47:172–187.

211. Konner M, Eaton SB. Paleolithic nutrition: twenty-five years later. *Nutr Clin Pract* 2010;25(6):594–602.

212. Appel LJ, Sacks FM, Carey VJ, et al. Effects of protein, monounsaturated fat, and carbohydrate intake on blood pressure and serum lipids: results of the Omni Heart randomized trial. *JAMA* 2005;294:2455–2464.

213. Miller ER 3rd, Erlinger TP, Appel LJ. The effects of macronutrients on blood pressure and lipids: an overview of the DASH and OmniHeart trials. *Curr Atheroscler Rep* 2006;8:460–465.

214. American Heart Association Nutrition Committee, Lichtenstein AH, Appel LJ, et al. Diet and lifestyle recommendations revision 2006: a scientific statement from

the American Heart Association Nutrition Committee. *Circulation* 2006;114(1):82–96.

215. Cunningham W, Hyson D. The skinny on high-protein, low-carbohydrate diets. *Prev Cardiol* 2006;9:166–171.

216. Last AR, Wilson SA. Low-carbohydrate diets. *Am Fam Physician* 2006;73:1942–1948.

217. Crowe TC. Safety of low-carbohydrate diets. *Obes Rev* 2005;6:235–245.

218. Bilsborough SA, Crowe TC. Low-carbohydrate diets: what are the potential short- and long term health implications? *Asia Pac J Clin Nutr* 2003;12:396–404.

219. Noble CA, Kushner RF. An update on low-carbohydrate, high-protein diets. *Curr Opin Gastroenterol* 2006;22: 153–159.

220. Nordmann AJ, Nordmann A, Briel M, et al. Effects of low-carbohydrate vs low-fat diets on weight loss and cardiovascular risk factors: a meta-analysis of randomized controlled trials. *Arch Intern Med* 2006;166:285–289.

221. Brinkworth GD, Noakes M, Buckley JD, et al. Long-term effects of a very-low-carbohydrate weight loss diet compared with an isocaloric low-fat diet after 12 mo. *Am J Clin Nutr* 2009;90(1):23–32.

222. Dansinger ML, Gleason JA, Griffith JL, et al. Comparison of the Atkins, Ornish, Weight Watchers, and Zone diets for weight loss and heart disease risk reduction: a randomized trial. *JAMA* 2005;293:43–53.

223. Wood RJ, Volek JS, Davis SR, et al. Effects of a carbohydrate-restricted diet on emerging plasma markers for cardiovascular disease. *Nutr Metab* (Lond) 2006;3:19.

224. Pollan M. The age of nutritionism. *New York Times Magazine* January 28, 2007.

225. Otten JJ, Hellwig JP, Meyers LD, eds; for the Institute of Medicine of the National Academies of Science. *Dietary reference intakes*. Washington, DC: National Academies Press, 2006.

226. Martí-Carvajal AJ, Solà I, Lathyris D, et al. Homocysteine-lowering interventions for preventing cardiovascular events. *Cochrane Database Syst Rev* 2013;1:CD006612.

227. Huang TY, Bin Z, Jusheng L, et al. Cardiovascular disease mortality and cancer incidence in vegetarians: a meta-analysis and systematic review. *Ann Nutr Metab* 2012.

228. Key TJ, Fraser GE, Thorogood M, et al. Mortality in vegetarians and non-vegetarians: a collaborative analysis of 8300 deaths among 76,000 men and women in five prospective studies. *Public Health Nutr* 1998;1(1):33–41.

229. Key TJ, Fraser GE, Thorogood M, et al. Mortality in vegetarians and nonvegetarians: detailed findings from a collaborative analysis of 5 prospective studies. *Am J Clin Nutr* 1999;70(3 suppl):516S–524S.

230. Farbstein D, Kozak-Blickstein A, Levy AP. Antioxidant vitamins and their use in preventing cardiovascular disease. *Molecules* 2010;15:8098–8110.

231. Chopra M, Thurnham D. Antioxidants and lipoprotein metabolism. *Proc Nutr Soc* 1999;58:663–671.

232. Jacob RA, Burri BJ. Oxidative damage and defense. *Am J Clin Nutr* 1996;63:985s–990s.

233. Yetik-Anacak G, Catravas JD. Nitric oxide and the endothelium: history and impact on cardiovascular disease. *Vascul Pharmacol* 2006;45:268–276.

234. Buring J, Gaziano J. Antioxidant vitamins and cardiovascular disease. In: Bendich A, Deckelbaum RJ, eds.

Preventive nutrition: the comprehensive guide for health professionals. Totowa, NJ: Humana Press, 1997:171–180.

235. Tavani A, Vecchia CL. Beta-carotene and risk of coronary heart disease. A review of observational and intervention studies. *Biomed Pharmacother* 1999;53:409–416.

236. Kritchevsky S. Beta-carotene, carotenoids and the prevention of coronary heart disease. *J Nutr* 1999;129:5–8.

237. Kromhout D. Fatty acids, antioxidants, and coronary heart disease from an epidemiological perspective. *Lipids* 1999;34:s27–s31.

238. Lairon D, Amiot M. Flavonoids in food and natural antioxidants in wine. *Curr Opin Lipidol* 1999;10:23–28.

239. Vinson J. Flavonoids in foods as in vitro and in vivo antioxidants. *Adv Exp Med Biol* 1998;439:151–164.

240. Gaziano J, Manson J. Diet and heart disease. The role of fat, alcohol, and antioxidants. *Cardiol Clin North Am* 1996;14:69–83.

241. Hensrud D, Heimburger D. Antioxidant status, fatty acids, and cardiovascular disease. *Nutrition* 1994;10:170–175.

242. Beyer R, Ness A, Powles J, et al. Vitamin C and cardiovascular disease: a systematic review. *J Cardiovasc Risk* 1996;3:513–521.

243. Timimi F, Ting H, Haley E, et al. Vitamin C improves endothelium-dependent vasodilation in patients with insulin-dependent diabetes mellitus. *J Am Coll Cardiol* 1998;31:552–557.

244. Stephens N, Parsons A, Schofield P, et al. Randomized controlled trial of vitamin E in patients with coronary disease: Cambridge Heart Antioxidant Study. *Lancet* 1996;347:781–786.

245. Rimm E, Willett W, Hu F, et al. Folate and vitamin B6 from diet and supplements in relation to risk of coronary heart disease among women. *JAMA* 1998;279:359–364.

246. Investigators G-P. Dietary supplementation with n-3 polyunsaturated fatty acids and vitamin E after myocardial infarction: results of the GISSI–Prevenzione Trial. *Lancet* 1999;354:447–455.

247. The Heart Outcomes Prevention Evaluation Study Investigators. Effects of an angiotensin converting-enzyme inhibitor, ramipril, on cardiovascular events in high-risk patients. *N Engl J Med* 2000;342:145–153.

248. The Heart Outcomes Prevention Evaluation Study Investigators. Vitamin E supplementation and cardiovascular events in high-risk patients. *N Engl J Med* 2000;342:154–160.

249. Sesso HD, Buring JE, Christen WG, et al. Vitamins E and C in the prevention of cardiovascular disease in men: the Physicians' Health Study II randomized controlled trial. *JAMA* 2008;300(18):2123–2133.

250. Marchioli R, Levantesi G, Macchia A, et al. Vitamin E increases the risk of developing heart failure after myocardial infarction: results from the GISSI–Prevenzione Trial. *J Cardiovasc Med* (Hagerstown) 2006;7:347–350.

251. Lonn E, Yusuf S, Hoogwerf B, et al. Effects of vitamin E on cardiovascular and microvascular outcomes in high-risk patients with diabetes: results of the HOPE study and MICRO-HOPE substudy. *Diabetes Care* 2002;25: 1919–1927.

252. Bjelakovic G, Nikolova D, Gluud LL, et al. Mortality in randomized trials of antioxidant supplements for primary and secondary prevention: systematic review and meta-analysis. *JAMA* 2007;297:842–857.

253. Nygard O, Vollset S, Refsum H, et al. Total plasma homocysteine and cardiovascular risk profile. The Hordaland Homocysteine Study. *JAMA* 1995;274:1526–1533.

254. Mittynen L, Nurminen M, Korpela R, et al. Role of arginine, taurine and homocysteine in cardiovascular diseases. *Ann Med* 1999;31:318–326.

255. Verhoef P, Stampfer M, Buring J, et al. Homocysteine metabolism and risk of myocardial infarction: relation with vitamins B_6, B_{12}, and folate. *Am J Epidemiol* 1996;143:845–859.

256. Toole JF, Malinow MR, Chambless LE, et al. Lowering homocysteine in patients withischemic stroke to prevent recurrent stroke, myocardial infarction, and death: the Vitamin Intervention for Stroke Prevention (VISP) randomized controlled trial. *JAMA* 2004;291:565–574.

257. Lonn E, Yusuf S, Arnold MJ, et al. Homocysteine lowering with folic acid and B vitamins in vascular disease. *N Engl J Med* 2006;354:1567–1577.

258. Bonaa KH, Njolstad I, Ueland PM, et al. Homocysteine lowering and cardiovascular events after acute myocardial infarction. *N Engl J Med* 2006;354:1578–1588.

259. Bazzano LA. No effect of folic acid supplementation on cardiovascular events, cancer or mortality after 5 years in people at increased cardiovascular risk, although homocysteine levels are reduced. *Arch Intern Med* 2010;170:1622–1631.

260. Miller ER 3rd, Juraschek S, Pastor-Barriuso R, et al. Meta analysis of folic acid supplementation trials on risk of cardiovascular disease and risk interaction with baseline homocysteine levels. *Am J Cardiol* 2010;106(4):517–527.

261. Holmes MV, Newcombe P, Hubacek JA, Effect modification by population dietary folate on the association between MTHFR genotype, homocysteine, and stroke risk: a meta-analysis of genetic studies and randomised trials. *Lancet* 2011;378(9791):584–94.

262. NIH State-of-the-Science Conference Statement on multivitamin/mineral supplements and chronic disease prevention. *NIH Consens State Sci Statements* 2006;23:1–30.

263. Rauchova H, Drahota Z, Lenaz G. Function of coenzyme Q in the cell: some biochemical and physiological properties. *Physiol Res* 1995;44:209–216.

264. Crane F, Sun I, Sun E. The essential functions of coenzyme Q. *Clin Investig* 1993;71:s55–s59.

265. Baggio E, Gandini R, Plancher A, et al. Italian multicenter study on the safety and efficacy of coenzyme Q_{10} as adjunctive therapy in heart failure. *Mol Aspects Med* 1994;15:s287–s294.

266. Langsjoen H, Langsjoen P, Willis R, et al. Usefulness of coenzyme Q_{10} in clinical cardiology: a long-term study. *Mol Aspects Med* 1994;15:s165–s175.

267. Singh R, Wander G, Rastogi A, et al. Randomized, double-blind placebo-controlled trial of coenzyme Q_{10} in patients with acute myocardial infarction. *Cardiovasc Drugs Ther* 1998;12:347–353.

268. Chello M, Mastroroberto P, Romano R, et al. Protection by coenzyme Q_{10} from myocardial reperfusion injury during coronary artery bypass grafting. *Ann Thorac Surg* 1994;58:1427–1432.

269. Kamikawa T, Kobayashi A, Yamashita T, et al. Effects of coenzyme Q_{10} on exercise tolerance in chronic stable angina pectoris. *Am J Cardiol* 1985;56:247–251.

270. Langsjoen P, Willis R, Folkers K. Treatment of essential hypertension with coenzyme Q_{10}. *Mol Aspects Med* 1994;15:s265–s272.

271. Singh R, Niaz M, Rastogi S, et al. Effect of hydrosoluble coenzyme Q_{10} on blood pressures and insulin resistance in hypertensive patients with coronary artery disease. *J Hum Hypertens* 1999;13:203–208.

272. Digiesi V, Cantini F, Oradei A, et al. Coenzyme Q_{10} in essential hypertension. *Mol Aspects Med* 1994;15:s257–s262.

273. Sander S, Coleman CI, Patel AA, et al. The impact of coenzyme Q10 on systolic function in patients with chronic heart failure. *J Card Fail* 2006;12(6):464–472.

274. Alehagen U, Johansson P, Björnstedt M, et al. Cardiovascular mortality and N-terminal-proBNP reduced after combined selenium and coenzyme Q10 supplementation: a 5-year prospective randomized double-blind placebo-controlled trial among elderly Swedish citizens. *Int J Cardiol* 2013;167(5):1860–1866.

275. Shargorodsky M, Debby O, Matas Z, et al. Effect of long-term treatment with antioxidants (vitamin C, vitamin E, coenzyme Q10 and selenium) on arterial compliance, humoral factors and inflammatory markers in patients with multiple cardiovascular risk factors. *Nutr Metab* (Lond) 2010;7:55.

276. Thomas S, Neuzil J, Stocker R. Inhibition of LDL oxidation by ubiquinol-10. A protective mechanism for coenzyme Q in atherogenesis? *Mol Aspects Med* 1997;18:s85–s103.

277. Niki E. Mechanisms and dynamics of antioxidant action of ubiquinol. *Mol Aspects Med* 1997;18:s63–s70.

278. Singh R, Niaz M. Serum concentration of lipoprotein (a) decreases on treatment with hydrosoluble coenzyme Q_{10} in patients with coronary artery disease: discovery of a new role. *Int J Cardiol* 1999;68:23–29.

279. Bargossi A, Grossi G, Fiorella P, et al. Exogenous CoQ_{10} supplementation prevents plasma ubiquinone reduction induced by HMG-CoA reductase inhibitors. *Mol Aspects Med* 1994;15:s187–s193.

280. Fotino AD, Thompson-Paul AM, Bazzano LA. Effect of coenzyme Q10 supplementation on heart failure: a meta-analysis. *Am J Clin Nutr* 2013;97:268–275.

281. Mortensen SA, Kumar A, Dolliner P, et al. The effect of Coenzyme Q10 on morbidity and mortality in chronic heart failure. Results from the Q-SYMBIO study [abstract no. 440]. *Eur J Heart Fail* 2013;15(S1):S20.

282. Rosenfeldt FL, Haas SJ, Krum H, et al. Coenzyme Q10 in the treatment of hypertension: a meta-analysis of the clinical trials. *J Hum Hypertension.* 2007;21(4):297–306.

283. Ho MJ, Bellusci A, Wright JM. Blood pressure lowering efficacy of coenzyme Q10 for primary hypertension. *Cochrane Database Syst Rev.* 2009;4:CD007435.

284. Flegal K, Cauley J. Alcohol consumption and cardiovascular risk factors. *Recent Dev Alcohol* 1985;3:165–180.

285. Zakhari S, Gordis E. Moderate drinking and cardiovascular health. *Proc Assoc Am Physicians* 1999;111:148–158.

286. Ronksley PE, Brien SE, Turner BJ, et al. Association of alcohol consumption with selected cardiovascular disease outcomes: a systematic review and meta-analysis. *BMJ* 2011;342:d671.

287. Renaud S, Gueguen R, Siest G, et al. Wine, beer, and mortality in middle-aged men from eastern France. *Arch Intern Med* 1999;159:1865–1870.

288. Mukamal KJ, Jensen MK, Grønbaek M, et al. Drinking frequency, mediating biomarkers, and risk of myocardial infarction in women and men. *Circulation* 2005;112(10):1406–1413.

289. Pai JK, Mukamal KJ, Rimm EB. Long-term alcohol consumption in relation to all-cause and cardiovascular

mortality among survivors of myocardial infarction: the Health Professionals Follow-up Study. *Eur Heart J* 2012;33(13):1598–1605.

290. Bagnardi V, Zatonski W, Scotti L, et al. Does drinking pattern modify the effect of alcohol on the risk of coronary heart disease? Evidence from a meta-analysis. *J Epidemiol Commun Health*, 2008;62:615–619.

291. Chen Y, Tseng SH. Review. Pro- and anti-angiogenesis effects of resveratrol. *In Vivo* 2007;21:365–370.

292. Agewall S, Wright S, Doughty R, et al. Does a glass of red wine improve endothelial function? *Eur Heart J* 2000;21:74–78.

293. Chiva-Blanch G, Urpi-Sarda M, Ros E, et al. Dealcoholized red wine decreases systolic and diastolic blood pressure and increases plasma nitric oxide: short communication. *Circ Res* 2012;111(8):1065–1068.

294. Criqui M. Alcohol and coronary heart disease: consistent relationship and public health implications. *Clin Chim Acta* 1996;246:51–57.

295. Kannell W, Ellison R. Alcohol and coronary heart disease: the evidence for a protective effect. *Clin Chim Acta* 1996;246:59–76.

296. Brooks PJ, Zakhari S. Moderate alcohol consumption and breast cancer in women: from epidemiology to mechanisms and interventions. *Alcohol Clin Exp Res* 2013;37(1):23–30.

297. Seitz HK, Becker P. Alcohol metabolism and cancer risk. *Alcohol Res Health* 2007;30(1):38–47.

298. Boffetta P, Hashibe M. Alcohol and cancer. *Lancet Oncol* 2006;7:149–156.

299. Beulens JW, Rimm EB, Ascherio A, et al. Alcohol consumption and risk for coronary heart disease among men with hypertension. *Ann Intern Med* 2007;146:10–19.

300. Mukamal KJ, Chiuve SE, Rimm EB. Alcohol consumption and risk for coronary heart disease in men with healthy lifestyles. *Arch Intern Med* 2006;166:2145–2150.

301. Koppes LL, Dekker JM, Hendriks HF, et al. Meta-analysis of the relationship between alcohol consumption and coronary heart disease and mortality in type 2 diabetic patients. *Diabetologia* 2006;49:648–652.

302. Mukamal KJ, Chung H, Jenny NS, et al. Alcohol consumption and risk of coronary heart disease in older adults: the Cardiovascular Health Study. *J Am Geriatr Soc* 2006;54:30–37.

303. Ebrahim S, Lawlor DA, Shlomo YB, et al. Alcohol dehydrogenase type 1C (ADH1C) variants, alcohol consumption traits, HDL-cholesterol and risk of coronary heart disease in women and men: British Women's Heart and Health Study and Caerphilly cohorts. *Atherosclerosis* 2008;196:871–878.

304. Solomon CG, Hu FB, Stampfer MJ, et al. Moderate alcohol consumption and risk of coronary heart disease among women with type 2 diabetes mellitus. *Circulation* 2000;102:494–499.

305. Krenz M, Korthuis RJ. Moderate ethanol ingestion and cardiovascular protection: from epidemiologic associations to cellular mechanisms. *J Mol Cell Cardiol* 2010;52(1):93–104.

306. Franco OH, Bonneux L, de Laet C, et al. The Polymeal: a more natural, safer, and probably tastier (than the Polypill) strategy to reduce cardiovascular disease by more than 75%. *BMJ* 2004;329:1447–1450.

307. Valk BD, Marx J. Iron, atherosclerosis, and ischemic heart disease. *Arch Intern Med* 1999;159:1542–1548.

308. Depalma RG, Hayes VW, Chow BK, et al. Ferritin levels, inflammatory biomarkers, and mortality in peripheral arterial disease: a substudy of the Iron (Fe) and Atherosclerosis Study (FeAST) Trial. *J Vasc Surg* 2010;51(6):1498–1503.

309. Zacharski LR, Chow BK, Howes PS, et al. Reduction of iron stores and cardiovascular outcomes in patients with peripheral arterial disease: a randomized controlled trial. *JAMA* 2007;297(6):603–610.

310. Wood RJ. The iron-heart disease connection: is it dead or just hiding? *Ageing Res Rev* 2004;3:355–367.

311. Ma J, Stampfer MJ. Body iron stores and coronary heart disease. *Clin Chem* 2002;48:601–603.

312. Lee DH, Jacobs DR Jr. Serum markers of stored body iron are not appropriate markers of health effects of iron: a focus on serum ferritin. *Med Hypotheses* 2004;62:442–445.

313. Sun Q, Ma J, Rifai N, et al. Excessive body iron stores are not associated with risk of coronary heart disease in women. *J Nutr* 2008;138(12):2436–2441.

314. Ford E. Serum magnesium and ischaemic heart disease: findings from a national sample of US adults. *Int J Epidemiol* 1999;28:645–651.

315. Ueshima K. Magnesium and ischemic heart disease: a review of epidemiological, experimental, and clinical evidences. *Magnes Res* 2005;18:275–284.

316. Delva P. Magnesium and coronary heart disease. *Mol Aspects Med* 2003;24:63–78.

317. Touyz RM. Role of magnesium in the pathogenesis of hypertension. *Mol Aspects Med* 2003;24:107–136.

318. Chakraborti S, Chakraborti T, Mandal M, et al. Protective role of magnesium in cardiovascular diseases: a review. *Mol Cell Biochem* 2002;238:163–179.

319. Gums JG. Magnesium in cardiovascular and other disorders. *Am J Health Syst Pharm* 2004;61:1569–1576.

320. Song Y, Manson JE, Cook NR, et al. Dietary magnesium intake and risk of cardiovascular disease among women. *Am J Cardiol* 2005;96:1135–1141.

321. Al-Delaimy WK, Rimm EB, Willett WC, et al. Magnesium intake and risk of coronary heart disease among men. *J Am Coll Nutr* 2004;23:63–70.

322. Houston M. The role of magnesium in hypertension and cardiovascular disease. *J Clin Hypertens* (Greenwich) 2011;13(11):843–847.

323. Kupetsky-Rincon EA, Uitto J. Magnesium: novel applications in cardiovascular disease—a review of the literature. *Ann Nutr Metab* 2012;61:102–110.

324. Grundy SM. Stanol esters as a component of maximal dietary therapy in the National Cholesterol Education Program Adult Treatment Panel III report. *Am J Cardiol* 2005;96:47d–50d.

325. Cater NB, Garcia-Garcia AB, Vega GL, et al. Responsiveness of plasma lipids and lipoproteins to plant stanol esters. *Am J Cardiol* 2005;96:23d–28d.

326. Scholle JM, Baker WL, Talati R, et al. The effect of adding plant sterols or stanols to statin therapy in hypercholesterolemic patients: systematic review and meta-analysis. *J Am Coll Nutr* 2009;28(5):517–524.

327. Talati R, Sobieraj DM, Makanji SS, et al. The comparative efficacy of plant sterols and stanols on serum lipids: a systematic review and meta-analysis. *J Am Diet Assoc* 2010;110(5):719–726.

328. Gardner CD, Lawson LD, Block E, et al. Effect of raw garlic vs commercial garlic supplements on plasma lipid concentrations in adults with moderate

hypercholesterolemia: a randomized clinical trial. *Arch Intern Med* 2007;167:346–353.

329. Stabler SN, Tejani AM, Huynh F, et al. Garlic for the prevention of cardiovascular morbidity and mortality in hypertensive patients. *Cochrane Database Syst Rev* 2012;8:CD007653.

330. Feldman EB. The scientific evidence for a beneficial health relationship between walnuts and coronary heart disease. *J Nutr* 2002;132:1062s–1101s.

331. Hu FB, Stampfer MJ. Nut consumption and risk of coronary heart disease: a review of epidemiologic evidence. *Curr Atheroscler Rep* 1999;1:204–209.

332. Ros E, Mataix J. Fatty acid composition of nuts—implications for cardiovascular health. *Br J Nutr* 2006;96:s29–s35.

333. Ros E. Nuts and novel biomarkers of cardiovascular disease. *Am J Clin Nutr* 2009;89(5):1649S–1656S.

334. Sabaté J, Ang Y. Nuts and health outcomes: new epidemiologic evidence. *Am J Clin Nutr* 2009;89(5):1643S–1648S.

335. O'Neil CE, Keast DR, Nicklas TA, et al. Nut consumption is associated with decreased health risk factors for cardiovascular disease and metabolic syndrome in U.S. adults: NHANES 1999-2004. *J Am Coll Nutr* 2011;30(6):502–510.

336. Sabate J. Nut consumption and body weight. *Am J Clin Nutr* 2003;78:647s–650s.

337. Vadivel V, Kunyanga CN, Biesalski HK. Health benefits of nut consumption with special reference to body weight control. *Nutrition* 2012;28(11–12):1089–1097.

338. Sabaté J, Ang Y. Nuts and health outcomes: new epidemiologic evidence. *Am J Clin Nutr* 2009;89(5):1643S–1648S.

339. Bes-Rastrollo M, Sabaté J, Gómez-Gracia E, et al. Nut consumption and weight gain in a Mediterranean cohort: the SUN study. *Obesity* (Silver Spring) 2007;15(1):107–116.

340. Tey SL, Brown R, Gray A, et al. Nuts improve diet quality compared to other energy-dense snacks while maintaining body weight. *J Nutr Metab* 2011;2011:357–350.

341. Guasch-Ferre M, Bullo M, Martinez-Gonzalez MA, et al. Frequency of nut consumption and mortality risk in the PREDIMED nutrition intervention trial. *BMC medicine* 2013;11:164.

342. Wien M, Bleich D, Raghuwanshi M, et al. Almond consumption and cardiovascular risk factors in adults with prediabetes. *J Am Coll Nutr* 2010;29(3):189–97.

343. Griel AE, Kris-Etherton PM. Tree nuts and the lipid profile: a review of clinical studies. *Br J Nutr* 2006;96 (suppl 2):S68–S78.

344. Phung OJ, Makanji SS, White CM, et al. Almonds have a neutral effect on serum lipid profiles: a meta-analysis. *J Am Diet Assoc* 2009;109(5):865–873.

345. Jaceldo-Siegl K, Sabaté J, Batech M, et al. Influence of body mass index and serum lipids on the cholesterol-lowering effects of almonds in free-living individuals. *Nutr Metab Cardiovasc Dis* 2011;21(suppl 1):S7–S13.

346. Sundram K, Karupaiah T, Hayes K. Stearic acid-rich interesterified fat and trans-rich fat raise the LDL/HDL ratio and plasma glucose relative to palm olein in humans. *Nutr Metab* (Lond) 2007;4:3.

347. Berry SE. Triacylglycerol structure and interesterification of palmitic and stearic acid rich fats: an overview and implications for cardiovascular disease. *Nutr Res Rev* 2009;22(1):3–17.

348. US Department of Health and Human Services. *Dietary guidelines for Americans, 2010*. Available at www.cnpp.usda.gov/dietaryguidelines.htm.

349. Lapinleimu H, Viikari J, Jokinen J, et al. Prospective randomized trial in 1062 infants of diet low in saturated fat and cholesterol. *Lancet* 1995;345:471–476.

350. Writing Group for the DISC collaborative research group. Efficacy and safety of lowering dietary intake of fat and cholesterol in children with elevated low-density lipoprotein cholesterol. The Dietary Intervention Study in Children (DISC). *JAMA* 1995;273:1429–1435.

SUGGESTED READING

Aviram M, Kaplan M, Rosenblat M, et al. Dietary antioxidants and paraoxonases against LDL oxidation and atherosclerosis development. *Handb Exp Pharmacol* 2005;170:263–300.

Binkoski AE, Kris-Etherton PM, Wilson TA, et al. Balance of unsaturated fatty acids is important to a cholesterol-lowering diet: comparison of mid-oleic sunflower oil and olive oil on cardiovascular disease risk factors. *J Am Diet Assoc* 2005;105:1080–1086.

Chahoud G, Aude YW, Mehta JL. Dietary recommendations in the prevention and treatment of coronary heart disease: do we have the ideal diet yet? *Am J Cardiol* 2004;94:1260–1267.

Denke MA. Cholesterol-lowering diets. *Arch Intern Med* 1995;155:17–26.

Denke MA. Diet, lifestyle, and nonstatin trials: review of time to benefit. *Am J Cardiol* 2005;96:3f–10f.

Denke MA. Dietary fats, fatty acids, and their effects on lipoproteins. *Curr Atheroscler Rep* 2006;8:466–471.

Diaz M, Frei B, Vita J, et al. Antioxidants and atherosclerotic heart disease. *N Engl J Med* 1997;337:408–416.

Dwyer J. Overview: dietary approaches for reducing cardiovascular disease risks. *J Nutr* 1995;125:656s–665s.

Erkkila AT, Herrington DM, Mozaffarian D, et al. Cereal fiber and whole-grain intake are associated with reduced progression of coronary-artery atherosclerosis in postmenopausal women with coronary artery disease. *Am Heart J* 2005;150:94–101.

Esrey KL, Joseph L, Grover SA. Relationship between dietary intake and coronary heart disease mortality: lipid research clinics prevalence follow-up study. *J Clin Epidemiol* 1996;49:211–216.

Ferguson LR. Nutrigenomics: integrating genomic approaches into nutrition research. *Mol Diagn Ther* 2006;10:101–108.

Fitzpatrick D, Bing B, Rohdewald P. Endothelium-dependent vascular effects of Pycnogenol. *J Cardiovasc Pharmacol* 1998;32:509–515.

Fraser G. Associations between diet and cancer, ischemic heart disease, and all-cause mortality in non-Hispanic white California Seventh-day Adventists. *Am J Clin Nutr* 1999;70:532s–538s.

Gaziano J. Antioxidants in cardiovascular disease: randomized trials. *Nutrition* 1996;12:583–588.

Gaziano JM, Manson JE. Diet and heart disease. The role of fat, alcohol, and antioxidants. *Cardiol Clin* 1996;14:69–83.

Giugliano D, Ceriello A, Esposito K. The effects of diet on inflammation: emphasis on the metabolic syndrome. *J Am Coll Cardiol* 2006;48:677–685.

Goldman L, Cook EF. The decline in ischemic heart disease mortality rates. *Ann Intern Med* 1984;101:825–836.

Heber D, Yip I, Ashley J, et al. Cholesterol-lowering effects of a proprietary Chinese red-yeast-rice dietary supplement. *Am J Clin Nutr* 1999;69:231–236.

Hensrud DD, Heimburger DC. Antioxidant status, fatty acids, and cardiovascular disease. *Nutrition* 1994;10:170–175.

Hodis H, Mack W, LaBree L, et al. Serial coronary angiographic evidence that antioxidant vitamin intake reduces progression of coronary artery atherosclerosis. *JAMA* 1995;273:1849–1854.

Hollman PC, Katan MB. Bioavailability and health effects of dietary flavonols in man. *Arch Toxicol* 1998;20:237–248.

Howard BV, Van Horn L, Hsia J, et al. Low-fat dietary pattern and risk of cardiovascular disease: the Women's Health Initiative Randomized Controlled Dietary Modification Trial. *JAMA* 2006;295:655–666.

Jenkins DJA. Optimal diet for reducing the risk of arteriosclerosis. *Can J Cardiol* 1995;11:118g–122g.

Jha P, Flather M, Lonn E, et al. The antioxidant vitamins and cardiovascular disease. A critical review of epidemiologic and clinical trial data. *Ann Intern Med* 1995;123:860–872.

Jiang R, Jacobs DR Jr, Mayer-Davis E, et al. Nut and seed consumption and inflammatory markers in the multi-ethnic study of atherosclerosis. *Am J Epidemiol* 2006;163:222–231.

Katz DL. Lifestyle and dietary modification for prevention of heart failure. *Med Clin North Am* 2004;88:1295–1320, xii.

Knoops KT, de Groot LC, Kromhout D, et al. Mediterranean diet, lifestyle factors, and 10-year mortality in elderly European men and women: the HALE project. *JAMA* 2004;292:1433–1439.

Koop C. *The Surgeon General's report on nutrition and health.* Washington, DC: Department of Health and Human Services, 1988.

Kromhout D, Bosschieter EB, Coulander C. The inverse relation between fish consumption and 20-year mortality from coronary heart disease. *N Engl J Med* 1985;312:1205–1209.

Libby P. Inflammation and cardiovascular disease mechanisms. *Am J Clin Nutr* 2006;83:456s–460s.

Marchioli R, Levantesi G, Macchia A, et al. Antiarrhythmic mechanisms of n-3 PUFA and the results of the GISSI–Prevenzione Trial. *J Membr Biol* 2005;206:117–128.

McNamara DJ. Dietary cholesterol and the optimal diet for reducing risk of atherosclerosis. *Clin J Cardiol* 1995;11:123g–126g.

Mendis S, Abegunde D, Yusuf S, et al. WHO study on Prevention of REcurrences of Myocardial Infarction and StrokE (WHO-PREMISE). *Bull World Health Organ* 2005;83: 820–829.

Menotti A. Diet, cholesterol and coronary heart disease. A perspective. *Acta Cardiol* 1999;54:169–172.

Meydani M. Vitamin E. *Lancet* 1995;345:170–175.

Nalsen C, Vessby B, Berglund L, et al. Dietary (n-3) fatty acids reduce plasma F2-isoprostanes but not prostaglandin F2alpha in healthy humans. *J Nutr* 2006;136:1222–1228.

Ordovas JM. Genetic interactions with diet influence the risk of cardiovascular disease. *Am J Clin Nutr* 2006;83:443s–446s.

Reiffel JA, McDonald A. Antiarrhythmic effects of omega-3 fatty acids. *Am J Cardiol* 2006;98:50i–60i.

Rexrode K, Manson J. Antioxidants and coronary heart disease: observational studies. *J Cardiovasc Risk* 1996;3:363–367.

Rimm E, Stampfer M. The role of antioxidants in preventive cardiology. *Curr Opin Cardiol* 1997;12:188–194.

Sanders TA, Lewis F, Slaughter S, et al. Effect of varying the ratio of n-6 to n-3 fatty acids by increasing the dietary intake of alpha-linolenic acid, eicosapentaenoic and docosahexaenoic acid, or both on fibrinogen and clotting factors VII and XII in persons aged 45–70 y: the OPTILIP study. *Am J Clin Nutr* 2006;84:513–522.

Serra-Majem L, Roman B, Estruch R. Scientific evidence of interventions using the Mediterranean diet: a systematic review. *Nutr Rev* 2006;64:s27–s47.

Song Y, Manson JE, Cook NR, et al. Dietary magnesium intake and risk of cardiovascular disease among women. *Am J Cardiol* 2005;96:1135–1141.

Stone NJ, Nicolosi RJ, Kris-Etherton P, et al. Summary of the scientific conference on the efficacy of hypocholesterolemic dietary interventions. *Circulation* 1996:94:3388–3391.

Sumner MD, Elliott-Eller M, Weidner G, et al. Effects of pomegranate juice consumption on myocardial perfusion in patients with coronary heart disease. *Am J Cardiol* 2005;96:810–814.

Suter PM. Carbohydrates and dietary fiber. *Handb Exp Pharmacol* 2005;170:231–261.

Tribble DL. AHA Science Advisory. Antioxidant consumption and risk of coronary artery disease: emphasis on vitamin C, vitamin E, and beta-carotene: a statement for healthcare professionals from the American Heart Association. *Circulation* 1999;99:591–595.

Trichopoulou A, Bamia C, Trichopoulos D. Mediterranean diet and survival among patients with coronary heart disease in Greece. *Arch Intern Med* 2005;165:929–935.

Trichopoulou A, Orfanos P, Norat T, et al. Modified Mediterranean diet and survival: EPIC–elderly prospective cohort study. *BMJ* 2005;330:991.

Virtamo J, Rapola J, Rippatti S, et al. Effect of vitamin E and beta carotene on the incidence of primary nonfatal myocardial infarction and fatal coronary heart disease. *Arch Intern Med* 1998;158:668–675.

CHAPTER 8

Diet and Hypertension

T here has long been epidemiologic evidence of variations in mean blood pressure among diverse populations. Although attribution is complicated by the multitude of potentially confounding variables that hamper transcultural comparisons, some of the observed variation is clearly engendered by variations in dietary pattern. Epidemiologic data suggest and recent clinical trial data affirm an effect of sodium chloride intake on blood pressure. Population data suggest that sodium may influence blood pressure levels in 50% or more of hypertensives and a smaller but still substantial proportion of normotensives. Data from multiple sources, including the INTERSALT trial, suggest that high intakes of sodium may shift mean population blood pressure upward (1). This is important because the influence of blood pressure on cardiovascular risk is continuous over a range both above and below the somewhat arbitrary cutpoints that define normotension and hypertension. There is decisive evidence that modification of the overall dietary pattern can be effective in modulating blood pressure. With good patient compliance, diet at times may even substitute for pharmacotherapy. In addition, there is decisive evidence that weight management is often effective in reducing blood pressure in overweight patients, an issue of increasing public health importance as the prevalence of obesity steadily rises. There is suggestive evidence that a variety of micronutrients, in addition to sodium, may modify blood pressure somewhat independently of the overall dietary pattern.

OVERVIEW

Diet

Hypertension is unusually prevalent in the United States, with nearly 60 million cases in a population of approximately 300 million. Trends had been favorable over recent decades, with data from the National Health Examination Surveys demonstrating both a decline in the prevalence of hypertension—defined as a systolic blood pressure ≥140 mm Hg and/or a diastolic blood pressure ≥90 mm Hg (see Table 8-1)—and a downward shift in the mean population blood pressure between 1971 and 1991. Since 1991, however, the prevalence of hypertension has risen by roughly 4%, apparently due to the rising prevalence of obesity.

Evidence linking hypertension to diet has been derived in part from transcultural comparisons, demonstrating higher rates of hypertension in industrialized countries. To compensate for the

---

TABLE 8.1

Classification of Blood Pressure Levels

Category	Systolic BP[a]		Diastolic BP[a]
Normal	<120	and	<80
Prehypertension	120 to 139	or	80 to 89
Stage 1 hypertension	140 to 159	or	90 to 99
Stage 2 hypertension	≥160	or	≥100

[a]BP = blood pressure. All measures are in mm Hg.

Source: Reproduced with permission from National Heart, Lung, and Blood Institute. Reference card from the seventh report of the Joint National Committee on Prevention, Detection, Evaluation, and Treatment of High Blood Pressure (JNC 7). Bethesda, MD: National Institutes of Health, 2003. Available at http://www.nhlbi.nih.gov/guidelines/hypertension/phycard.pdf; accessed 6/29/07.

plethora of confounding variables intrinsic to such transcultural comparisons, migration studies have been conducted. Hypertension, like hyperlipidemia, is more prevalent in Asians living in the United States than in their non-emigrating counterparts (2). Similar effects of migration have been reported in other populations (3).

Whereas African Americans have particularly high rates of hypertension, the rate is low among native Africans living in rural settings and intermediate in Africans exposed to some aspects of the Western lifestyle (4). Among populations in the United States, hypertension is less common among the lean than the overweight and among vegetarians than the general population (5). Isolating the direct effects of diet on blood pressure is difficult due to the prevalence of obesity in the United States and the strong association between obesity and hypertension (see Chapters 5 and 6). Epidemic obesity is almost certainly the explanation for rising prevalence of hypertension in the United States in recent years, after a steady decline over preceding decades. The association between higher body mass index (BMI) and hypertension may be especially strong for black Americans (6). A number of mechanisms have been proposed to account for obesity's causative role in the development of hypertension: increased sodium retention, activation of renin-angiotensin system, intrarenal compression by adipose tissue, and sleep disturbance (7,8).

From a practical perspective, patients benefit comparably from dietary interventions that lower blood pressure directly, or indirectly as a result of weight loss (see Table 8-2). There is decisive evidence that weight loss among obese hypertensives frequently results in blood pressure reduction. Even modest weight loss may lower blood pressure in patients who do not reach or even approximate their ideal body weight (9).

Secular trends in the epidemiology of hypertension suggest an important influence of obesity (10). In particular, central adiposity is associated with insulin resistance and the metabolic syndrome, of which hypertension is a key feature. In addition, up to 50% of nonobese hypertensives may be insulin resistant; a recent trial in Spain found impairments in glucose metabolism in a majority of patients presenting to a specialty clinic with essential hypertension (11). Obesity, insulin resistance, and central adiposity are independent predictors of risk for hypertension (12). Insulin resistance and compensatory hyperinsulinemia are thought to promote hypertension by increasing renal sodium reabsorption, stimulating sympathetic nervous system overactivity, and inducing a proinflammatory state (13). Hypertensive patients with the metabolic syndrome may be at higher cardiovascular risk than those without it (14,15). Weight loss and dietary pattern may exert both interdependent and independent effects on blood pressure (16). The topics of obesity and insulin

---

TABLE 8.2

Lifestyle Interventions for Blood Pressure Control Recommended by the National Heart, Lung, and Blood Institute

Intervention	Specific Guidance	Average Systolic Blood Pressure Reduction[a]
Weight reduction	Maintain a normal body weight (BMI 18.5 to 24.9 kg/m²).	5 to 20 mm Hg/10 kg
DASH eating plan	Adopt a diet rich in fruits, vegetables, and low-fat dairy products with reduced content of saturated and total fat.	8 to 14 mm Hg
Dietary sodium reduction	Reduce dietary sodium to ≤100 mmol per day (2.4 g sodium or 6 g sodium chloride).	2 to 8 mm Hg
Aerobic physical activity	Regular aerobic physical activity (e.g., brisk walking) at least 30 minutes per day, most days of the week.	4 to 9 mm Hg
Moderation of alcohol consumption	Men: limit to ≤2 drinks[b] per day. Women and lighter-weight men: limit to ≤1 drink[a] per day.	2 to 4 mm Hg

[a]Effects are dose and time dependent.

[b]One drink equals 0.5 oz of 15 ml ethanol (e.g., 12 oz. beer, 5 oz. wine, 1.5 oz. 80-proof whiskey).

Source: Reproduced with permission from National Heart, Lung, and Blood Institute. Reference card from the seventh report of the Joint National Committee on Prevention, Detection, Evaluation, and Treatment of High Blood Pressure (JNC 7). Bethesda, MD: National Institutes of Health, 2003. Available at http://www.nhlbi.nih.gov/guidelines/hypertension/phycard.pdf; accessed 6/29/07.

resistance are addressed fully in Chapters 5 and 6, respectively.

In general, diets associated with optimal blood pressure control are similar to diets associated with a variety of other salutary health effects (see Chapter 45). Vegetarianism is associated with lower average blood pressure (see Chapter 43), as are the Mediterranean diet and the low-fat diet typical of the nonindustrialized Far East (5). The association between dietary pattern and blood pressure was confirmed by the results of the DASH (Dietary Approaches to Stop Hypertension) study (17), which demonstrated that adherence to a diet high in fruit, vegetables, and low-fat dairy and restricted in total fat effectively lowered blood pressure among randomized, hypertensive subjects. The DASH diet is apparently particularly beneficial in African Americans (18). The DASH dietary pattern in combination with sodium restriction to 1,200 mg per day reduced systolic blood pressure on average by more than 10 mm Hg among hypertensive subjects (19). The DASH sodium trial demonstrated independent effects on blood pressure reduction of modifying the overall dietary pattern and restricting sodium, and additive benefits by combining the two approaches.

The PREMIER trial tested the value of established lifestyle approaches to blood pressure reduction—weight loss, sodium reduction, increased physical activity, and limited alcohol intake—alone and in combination with the dietary pattern tested in DASH. Significant reductions in systolic blood pressure were seen in both groups; reductions were greater in the combined treatment group (20,21). These effects were somewhat greater in African Americans than in whites and in those with stage 1 hypertension as compared with prehypertension, but they were generally robust across population subgroups (22).

The DISC study suggests that the relationship between diet and blood pressure in children is similar to that in adults (23) and that growing children can safely adopt and maintain a cardioprotective diet (24,25).

Several recent studies have examined the effects on blood pressure of reducing intake of dietary carbohydrate and substituting a higher intake of protein (26). Reduction in blood pressure has been seen, with a shift toward higher protein derived from either plant sources or lean meat (27,28) and with substitution of unsaturated fat for carbohydrate (29). In general, though, such comparisons have relied on the carbohydrate sources that prevail in the typical American diet rather than the sources deemed most healthful: vegetables, fruits, whole grains, beans, and legumes. Thus, the diets tend to differ substantially in glycemic load. A low glycemic load (see Chapter 6) may be achieved with a diet high in carbohydrate as well by emphasizing natural rather than processed foods. When tested, such a diet shows very favorable effects across an array of cardiovascular risk factors, including blood pressure (30,31). Meat intake, when less selective, has been associated with elevations rather than reductions in blood pressure (32). For instance, red meat intake has been associated with hypertension and other components of the metabolic syndrome, as well as increased risk for cardiovascular disease and premature death (33,34). In the aggregate, this literature suggests that glycemic load and the specific foods chosen rather than the percentage of calories derived from carbohydrate, per se, is of importance to dietary management of blood pressure. Of note, the DASH diet has a relatively high-carbohydrate, low-glycemic-load pattern. Blood pressure reduction has been observed with several patterns of macronutrient intake (35); combining these benefits may be achievable with a diet based predominantly on natural carbohydrate sources, low-fat dairy, lean protein sources, and unsaturated fats.

As is the case with the prevention and modification of other cardiovascular risk factors, the optimal diet for management of incipient and established hypertension is not known with certainty. Some avenues of research suggest that restricting total fat may be less beneficial than selectively restricting saturated and trans fat, while liberalizing the intake of monounsaturated and polyunsaturated fat (particularly n-3 polyunsaturates) (36,37); this is advisable for health promotion as well (see Chapters 7 and 45). Recommendations for calorie control, abundant intake of fruits and vegetables, and restriction of saturated and trans fat intake may be made with confidence. Of note, such a diet is naturally rich in the micronutrients associated with blood pressure lowering, relatively rich in fiber, and relatively low in sodium. Which of these modifications in dietary behavior is responsible for blood pressure control is important to advance our understanding but unnecessary to make recommendations likely to benefit patients.

Although stage 1 hypertension has been effectively treated with diet in studies, two caveats should be noted. First, the compliance in a controlled trial is generally greater than is achieved in practice (38). Second, more advanced hypertension has not been shown to respond to dietary management in the absence of pharmacotherapy. One suitable approach in efforts at managing more significant hypertension with lifestyle modification is to initiate pharmacotherapy as indicated and then taper medications when the blood pressure is well controlled, and evidence accrues that the patient is engaged in recommended dietary and lifestyle modifications.

Nutrigenomics, the study of the effects of diet on gene expression, is increasingly recognized as an important contributor to understanding the etiology and treatment of hypertension. The DASH study found that those individuals with the AA genotype of the angiotensin gene had higher risk for hypertension but also were more responsive to the diet. A recent study found further evidence of gene–diet interplay for blood pressure modification (39). The results indicated that the DASH diet was particularly effective at lowering blood pressure in individuals carrying the G46A polymorphism of the β-2-androgen receptor, suggesting that this receptor may be a modifier of DASH-diet responsiveness (40). As nutrigenomic technologies continue to develop, they will provide additional avenues to illuminate genetic predispositions and identify specific, tailored treatments.

There are also a several diet–drug interactions that clinicians should be aware of when treating patients with hypertension. Grapefruit juice should not be consumed by patients taking calcium-channel blockers, commonly prescribed antihypertensives, as it interferes with the breakdown of this class of drugs (41). Grapefruit juice may also increase the absorption of these drugs. Similarly, patients taking angiotensin-converting enzyme inhibitors such as lisinopril should avoid drinking alcoholic beverages (42).

NUTRIENTS, NUTRICEUTICALS, AND FUNCTIONAL FOODS

Sodium

Sodium is the most extensively studied nutrient influencing blood pressure. Evidence from a variety of sources, including epidemiologic studies

as well as intervention trials, indicates rather conclusively that sodium contributes to blood pressure elevations on a population and individual basis (43,44). This conclusion is supported by results of the INTERSALT study, which examined the association between sodium intake and blood pressure in multiple cohorts around the globe (1). Generally, each 100 mEq per day incremental increase in sodium intake increases mean systolic blood pressure in a population by 3 to 6 mm Hg. But recent Cochrane Reviews and a report from the IOM have cast some doubt on the extent of blood pressure reduction seen with sodium restriction, and whether salt reduction decreases risk of cardiovascular disease and death (45,46). These reviews have, however, been criticized by some for methodological flaws (47). While there may indeed be the possibility of consuming too little sodium, this concern becomes less relevant given our population's prevailing sodium intake levels. The preponderance of evidence suggests that, given the vast majority of Americans consume far more than the recommended amount of daily sodium, reduction of sodium intake is an important tool for reducing blood pressure and improving health outcomes.

Although there is substantial evidence that sodium contributes to blood pressure elevation, the causal role of sodium in hypertension is less well established. Studies suggest that roughly 50% of hypertensives in the United States are responsive to sodium, demonstrating blood pressure variation with change in sodium intake; this figure was previously set at about 10% (48). A substantial but smaller percentage of normotensives are salt sensitive. Salt sensitivity is more prevalent among African Americans than among others; up to 75% of hypertensive African Americans are responsive to dietary sodium.

The efficacy of sodium restriction in the management of hypertension has been demonstrated in the context of clinical trials, but establishing real-world effectiveness is a greater challenge. Adherence to a low-sodium diet is difficult for most patients (49), and such diets inevitably introduce other changes that may account in part for blood pressure reduction. Cook et al. (50) asserted that the effect of salt restriction on blood pressure has generally been underestimated. In 2005, the Center for Science in the Public Interest (CPSI) filed suite against the U.S. Food and Drug Administration for according sodium the designation "generally recognized as safe" (GRAS). CSPI alleges that excess dietary salt is responsible for as many as 150,000 premature deaths each year in the United States (51). Kumanyika has suggested that achieving recommended sodium intake levels in the United States with any consistency will require appreciable changes to the food supply (49). Currently, over 99% of adults in the United States consume more sodium daily than recommended by the American Heart Association (<1,500 mg), and 90% consume more than the Institute of Medicine's Tolerable Upper Intake Level (2,300 mg) (52).

Despite the uncertainties, recommendations for sodium restriction below prevailing levels in the United States can be made with considerable confidence. Intake in the United States generally exceeds the recommended limit of 2,400 mg per day. Ancestral intake, which may indicate optimal levels, was approximately 700 to 800 mg per day, less than one-fourth the average intake today (53). Advocacy of a health-promoting diet will result in sodium restriction by reducing the intake of fast foods and other highly processed foods. It is estimated that even modest reductions in salt intake may have significant beneficial health effects and result in major healthcare cost savings (54).

Patients should be advised of the importance of reading food labels. The sodium content of many commercial breakfast cereals is comparable to that of potato chips and pretzels, although the taste of salt in such products is masked by the sugar (see Chapter 38). In attempting to limit sodium intake, many patients will report not using a salt shaker. However, the salt added to food during preparation is less readily tasted than the salt shaken on just as the food is eaten. Therefore, selection and preparation of relatively low-salt foods and continued, albeit controlled, use of a salt shaker may be a preferred approach. As with other dietary changes, salt restriction becomes less objectionable as it becomes familiar. Whereas the salt content of many processed foods goes unnoticed by most consumers, those acclimated to a lower-sodium diet begin to taste salt more readily and to prefer lower intake levels (55,56). Acclimation to a high-salt diet has the opposite effect (57) (see Chapter 38).

Salt Substitutes

So-called salt substitutes, which replace some of the sodium with potassium or calcium, may serve as a useful aid to patients struggling to acclimate to a salt-restricted diet. There is some evidence suggesting that the preference for dietary salt may vary with factors other than taste perception (58,59), so acceptance of salt substitutes is variable. Clinical trial outcomes suggest a favorable influence on blood pressure of salt substitution (60–62).

Potassium

Diets rich in potassium tend to be relatively low in sodium, and vice versa, making the study of isolated dietary potassium difficult. Nonetheless, there is convincing evidence that potassium supplementation has a blood pressure–lowering effect (63). The evidence is decisive that total dietary modification that results in increased potassium intake, and particularly a potassium intake that exceeds sodium intake, lowers blood pressure (17,64). Blacks may demonstrate larger reductions in blood pressure than do Caucasians with equal potassium intake (65). The average intake of sodium in the United States is up to 4,000 mg per day, while average daily intake of potassium is approximately 2,500 to 3,400 mg (53). Our prehistoric ancestors are estimated to have consumed approximately 750 to 800 mg per day of sodium and nearly 10,500 mg of potassium (53). As potassium is abundant in a variety of fruits and vegetables, high intake of potassium generally is associated with other dietary changes that may independently lower blood pressure. In the INTERSALT study, blood pressure rose with age in all populations consuming more sodium than potassium, but not in those consuming more potassium than sodium (1).

Calcium

There is suggestive evidence that high dietary calcium intake contributes to lowering of blood pressure. In the DASH trial, calcium is considered a potentially important mediator of the hypotensive effects of nonfat dairy products (17). Meta-analysis suggests that calcium, either in the diet or as a supplement, has a modest antihypertensive effect (66,67). However, on the basis of an extensive literature review, the Canadian Hypertension Society has advised against calcium supplementation as a means of either treating or preventing hypertension (68,69). The isolated effects of calcium supplementation on blood pressure appear to be modest; a dietary pattern providing abundant calcium may be of greater benefit. A particular benefit of calcium in the management and prevention of pregnancy-induced hypertension has been suggested (69) (see Chapter 27). A recent study suggests that higher dairy consumption leads to lower blood pressures in children (70). In the aggregate, evidence supports a hypotensive benefit of calcium intake at levels advisable on other grounds (71) (see Chapter 14).

Magnesium

Diets rich in potassium tend to be rich in magnesium and vice versa (see Chapter 4). Magnesium supplementation may be beneficial in the treatment of hypertension in magnesium-deficient patients (68,72). Meta-analysis of clinical trials suggests a modest hypotensive effect of supplemental magnesium (73,74). While routine supplementation of magnesium is not advocated on the basis of current evidence, a dietary pattern providing abundant magnesium certainly is (75,76).

Fiber

A potential benefit of dietary fiber in the regulation of blood pressure has been reported in both adults (77,78) and children (23). At the population level, the isolated effects of dietary fiber on blood pressure are difficult to establish (44), as dietary patterns associated with high fiber intake tend to exert a favorable influence on blood pressure by other means as well. Clinical trials have suggested a beneficial effect of soluble fiber from oats on blood pressure (79) and indicated that regular intake of oats may reduce the need for medication in hypertensives (80). A recent meta-analysis revealed a modest hypotensive effect of supplemental dietary fiber independent of other factors (81). In the aggregate, the evidence is persuasive that increasing dietary fiber intake is likely to exert a favorable influence on blood pressure. Patients should be encouraged to increase fiber intake on general principles, as both soluble and insoluble fiber offer a potential array of health benefits; average intake levels in the United States are well below the recommended levels, and a healthful dietary pattern is naturally high in fiber. Health effects of fiber and dietary sources are addressed in Chapter 1 and Section VIIE.

Alcohol

Alcohol contributes to blood pressure elevations when intake exceeds 30 to 45 g of ethanol daily and may contribute at lower intakes in patients with hypertension. Moderate alcohol intake below this level may actually lower blood pressure slightly or may have no effect on blood pressure. The cardiovascular benefits of alcohol (see Chapters 7 and 40) may help reduce the risk of myocardial infarction in well-controlled hypertensives. When blood pressure is not well controlled, alcohol intake should be discouraged. Moderation of alcohol intake is among the established interventions for blood pressure control advocated by the National Heart, Lung, and Blood Institute (see Table 8-2).

Garlic

Garlic is reputed to have antihypertensive effects. Garlic stimulates nitric oxide synthase (82), providing a mechanism by which it might lower blood pressure. Meta-analysis supports a modest antihypertensive effect of garlic, but the evidence is limited (83,84). Reliance on garlic to control blood pressure based on available evidence is not advisable (85).

Amino Acids

Arginine and taurine may have antihypertensive properties, but evidence to date is limited (86). Arginine is a precursor in the synthesis of nitric oxide, an endothelium-derived vasodilator; a link between blood pressure and endothelial function is clear, although the direction of causality is not (87,88). Limited data suggest a favorable influence of supplemental sustained-release arginine on both blood pressure and endothelial function (89). Evidence is insufficient at present to justify recommendations of amino acid supplementation in efforts to regulate blood pressure.

Coenzyme Q$_{10}$

An antihypertensive effect of coenzyme Q$_{10}$ is claimed, and practitioners of alternative medicine use coenzyme Q$_{10}$ in the management of hypertension. The evidence for such an effect is limited and not sufficient to justify routine clinical application (90–93). Small clinical trials have been promising, however (94), and further study of the compound for a role in blood pressure control is warranted (95,96). Coenzyme Q_{10} is discussed in more detail in Section VIIE.

Caffeine

Caffeine is a pressor and acutely raises blood pressure, generally to a modest degree. The effects of caffeine on blood pressure are apparently greater in hypertensives than in normotensives (97). Evidence is insufficient to warrant population-wide recommendations for caffeine restriction as a means of improving blood pressure. However, caffeine restriction in hypertensives is both reasonable and prudent, even though additional research is needed to provide definitive evidence of benefit. For further discussion, see Chapter 41.

CLINICAL HIGHLIGHTS

There is decisive evidence that a diet rich in fruits, vegetables, grains, and nonfat dairy products; restricted in saturated and trans fat and their sources; and low in highly processed foods is associated with reductions in blood pressure in hypertensives and preservation of normal blood pressure in normotensives. There is suggestive evidence that such a diet may prevent hypertension on a population basis. Evidence suggests that restriction of dietary sodium to less than 2,400 mg per day will contribute to blood pressure control in many, if not most, individuals. While recent reports have raised concerns about consuming too little sodium, most patients in the United States will be a long way from doing so, and still likely to benefit from reduced intake. Weight control, regular physical activity, and moderation of alcohol intake are of established benefit as well. The combination of these strategies is particularly effective and offers benefits beyond blood pressure regulation (see Chapter 45).

Most individuals can be expected to acclimate to a salt-reduced diet over a period of weeks so that preference for higher salt intake abates. Adherence to the dietary patterns advisable both for blood pressure control and health promotion will lead naturally to a salt intake far closer to the recommended 2.4 g or less per day than the prevailing level in the United States, which can be up to twice that amount. Similarly, although there is

suggestive evidence of hypotensive effects of potassium, calcium, and magnesium, these nutrients are abundant in the dietary pattern advocated for blood pressure control and, therefore, generally need not be singled out (98). A recent Cochrane review indicates that data are as yet insufficient to make the case for routine supplementation of these minerals alone or in combination for the primary purpose of blood pressure control (99).

Hypertensive patients should be advised to read food labels and minimize the intake of processed foods with greater sodium than potassium content. A useful guideline is to limit foods with more milligrams of sodium per serving than calories; to approximate the 2.4 g upper limit for sodium per day in a 2,000 kcal diet requires that foods average 1.2 mg sodium per calorie over the course of a typical day. Supplemental calcium, of potential value in the prevention of osteoporosis in many patients (see Chapter 14), may contribute slightly to blood pressure control. Alcohol should be restricted or avoided until blood pressure is normalized, and it should be kept to moderate levels in normotensives. Although there is little evidence that salt substitutes effectively control blood pressure, use of such products as one means of reducing sodium intake is reasonable. Caffeine should be restricted in poorly controlled hypertensives; moderate intake is acceptable for all others. Patients with blood pressure in the prehypertension range or in the upper range of normal generally develop hypertension over time (100) and should be encouraged to modify diet in an effort to prevent such progression. Adherence to the recommended dietary pattern can be expected to lower systolic blood pressure by approximately 11 and 6 mm Hg in hypertensives and normotensives, respectively, and diastolic blood pressure by approximately 6 and 3 mm Hg in hypertensives and normotensives, respectively (20,101).

REFERENCES

1. Stamler J. The INTERSALT Study: background, methods, findings, and implications. *Am J Clin Nutr* 1997;65: 626s–642s.
2. Imazu M, Sumida K, Yamabe T, et al. A comparison of the prevalence and risk factors of high blood pressure among Japanese living in Japan, Hawaii, and Los Angeles. *Public Health Rep* 1996;111:59.
3. He J, Tell GS, Tang YC, et al. Effect of migration on blood pressure: the Yi People Study. *Epidemiology* 1991;2:88.

4. Grim CE, Robinson M. Blood pressure variation in blacks: genetic factors. *Semin Nephrol* 1996;16:83.

5. Moore TJ, McKnight JA. Dietary factors and blood pressure regulation. *Endocrinol Metab Clin North Am* 1995;24:643.

6. Brown CD, Higgins M, Donato KA, et al. Body mass index and the prevalence of hypertension and dyslipidemia. *Obes Res* 2000;8(9):605–619.

7. Grundy S. Inflammation, hypertension, and the metabolic syndrome. *JAMA* 2003;290(22):3000–3002.

8. Hall JE, Kuo JJ, da Silva AA, de Paula RB, Liu J, Tallam L. Obesity-associated hypertension and kidney disease. Curr Opin Nephrol Hypertens. 2003 Mar;12(2):195–200.

9. Landsberg L. Weight reduction and obesity. *Clin Exp Hypertens* 1999;21:763.

10. Silva DA, Petroski EL, Peres MA. Is high body fat estimated by body mass index and waist circumference a predictor of hypertension in adults? a population-based study. *Nutr J* 2012;11(1):112.

11. Garcia-Puig J, Ruilope LM, Luque M, et al. Glucose metabolism in patients with essential hypertension. *Am J Med* 2006;119:318–326.

12. Sung KC, Kim BJ, Kim BS, et al. In normoglycemic Koreans, insulin resistance and adiposity are independently correlated with high blood pressure. *Circ J* 2004;68:898–902.

13. Expert Panel on Detection, Evaluation, and Treatment of High Blood Cholesterol in Adults. Executive Summary of the Third Report of the National Cholesterol Education Program (NCEP) Expert Panel on detection, evaluation, and treatment of high blood cholesterol in adults (Adult Treatment Panel III). *JAMA* 2001;285:2486–2497.

14. Schillaci G, Pirro M, Vaudo G, et al. Prognostic value of the metabolic syndrome in essential hypertension. *J Am Coll Cardiol* 2004;43(10):1817–1822.

15. Pierdomenico SD, Lapenna D, Di Tommaso R, et al. Prognostic relevance of metabolic syndrome in hypertensive patients at low-to-medium risk. *Am J Hypertens* 2007;20(12):1291–1296.

16. Nowson CA, Worsley A, Margerison C, et al. Blood pressure change with weight loss is affected by diet type in men. *Am J Clin Nutr* 2005;81:983–989.

17. Harsha DW, Lin PH, Obarzanek E, et al. Dietary approaches to stop hypertension: a summary of study results. DASH Collaborative Research Group. *J Am Diet Assoc* 1999;99:s35.

18. Tucker K. Dietary patterns and blood pressure in African Americans. *Nutr Rev* 1999;57:356.

19. Sacks FM, Svetkey LP, Vollmer WM, et al. Effects on blood pressure of reduced dietary sodium and the Dietary Approaches to Stop Hypertension (DASH) diet. DASH–Sodium Collaborative Research Group. *N Engl J Med* 2001;344:3–10.

20. Appel LJ, Champagne CM, Harsha DW, et al. Effects of comprehensive lifestyle modification on blood pressure control: main results of the PREMIER clinical trial. *JAMA* 2003;289:2083–2093.

21. Elmer PJ, Obarzanek E, Vollmer WM, et al. Effects of comprehensive lifestyle modification on diet, weight, physical fitness, and blood pressure control: 18-month results of a randomized trial. *Ann Intern Med* 2006;144:485–495.

22. Svetkey LP, Erlinger TP, Vollmer WM, et al. Effect of lifestyle modifications on blood pressure by race, sex, hypertension status, and age. *J Hum Hypertens* 2005;19:21–31.

23. Simons-Morton DG, Hunsberger SA, Van Horn L, et al. Nutrient intake and blood pressure in the Dietary Intervention Study in Children. *Hypertension* 1997;29:930.

24. Obarzanek E, Kimm SY, Barton BA, et al. Long-term safety and efficacy of a cholesterol-lowering diet in children with elevated low-density lipoprotein cholesterol: seven-year results of the Dietary Intervention Study in Children (DISC). *Pediatrics* 2001;107:256–264.

25. Gopinath B, Flood VM, Rochtchina E, et al. Influence of high glycemic index and glycemic load diets on blood pressure during adolescence. *Hypertension* 2012;59(6):1272–1277.

26. He J, et al. Effect of dietary protein supplementation on blood pressure: a randomized, controlled trial. *Circulation* 2011;124(5):589–595.

27. Hodgson JM, Burke V, Beilin LJ, et al. Partial substitution of carbohydrate intake with protein intake from lean red meat lowers blood pressure in hypertensive persons. *Am J Clin Nutr* 2006;83:780–787.

28. Sargrad KR, Homko C, Mozzoli M, et al. Effect of high protein vs high carbohydrate intake on insulin sensitivity, body weight, hemoglobin A1c, and blood pressure in patients with type 2 diabetes mellitus. *J Am Diet Assoc* 2005;105:573–580.

29. Appel LJ, Sacks FM, Carey VJ, et al. Effects of protein, monounsaturated fat, and carbohydrate intake on blood pressure and serum lipids: results of the OmniHeart randomized trial. *JAMA* 2005;294:2455–2564.

30. McMillan-Price J, Petocz P, Atkinson F, et al. Comparison of 4 diets of varying glycemic load on weight loss and cardiovascular risk reduction in overweight and obese young adults: a randomized controlled trial. *Arch Intern Med* 2006;166:1466–1475.

31. Ebbeling CB, Leidig MM, Sinclair KB, et al. Effects of an ad libitum low-glycemic load diet on cardiovascular disease risk factors in obese young adults. *Am J Clin Nutr* 2005;81:976–982.

32. Steffen LM, Kroenke CH, Yu X, et al. Associations of plant food, dairy product, and meat intakes with 15-y incidence of elevated blood pressure in young black and white adults: the Coronary Artery Risk Development in Young Adults (CARDIA) Study. *Am J Clin Nutr* 2005;82:1169–1177.

33. Azadbakht L, Esmaillzadeh A. Red meat intake is associated with metabolic syndrome and the plasma C-reactive protein concentration in women. *J Nutr* 2009;139(2):335–339.

34. Pan A, Sun Q, Bernstein AM, et al. Red meat consumption and mortality: results from 2 prospective cohort studies. *Arch Intern Med* 2012;172(7):555–563.

35. Miller ER III, Erlinger TP, Appel LJ. The effects of macronutrients on blood pressure and lipids: an overview of the DASH and OmniHeart trials. *Curr Atheroscler Rep* 2006;8:460–465.

36. Horrocks LA, Yeo YK. Health benefits of docosahexaenoic acid. *Pharmacol Res* 1999;40:211.

37. Grimsgaard S, Bonaa KH, Jacobsen BK, et al. Plasma saturated and linoleic fatty acids are independently associated with blood pressure. *Hypertension* 1999;34:478.

38. Windhauser MM, Ernst DB, Karanja NM, et al. Translating the Dietary Approaches to Stop Hypertension diet from research to practice: dietary and behavior change techniques. DASH Collaborative Research Group. *J Am Diet Assoc* 1999;99:s90.

39. Simopoulos AP. Genetic variation and dietary response: nutrigenetics/nutrigenomics. *Asia Pac J Clin Nutr* 2002; 11(S6):S117–S128.

40. Sun B, Williams JS, Svetkey LP, et al. Beta2-adrenergic receptor genotype affects the renin-angiotensin-aldosterone system response to the Dietary Approaches to Stop Hypertension (DASH) dietary pattern. *Am J Clin Nutr* 2010; 92(2):444–449.

41. Cuciureanu M, Vlase L, Muntean D, et al. Grapefruit juice—drug interactions: importance for pharmacotherapy. *Rev Med Chir Soc Med Nat Iasi* 2010;114(3):885–891.

42. Odou P, Ferrari N, Barthélémy C, et al. Grapefruit juice-nifedipine interaction: possible involvement of several mechanisms. *J Clin Pharm Ther* 2005;30(2):153–158.

43. Cutler JA. The effects of reducing sodium and increasing potassium intake for control of hypertension and improving health. *Clin Exp Hypertens* 1999;21:769.

44. He J, Whelton PK. Role of sodium reduction in the treatment and prevention of hypertension. *Curr Opin Cardiol* 1997;12:202.

45. Graudal NA, Hubeck-Graudal T, Jurgens G. Effects of low sodium diet versus high sodium diet on blood pressure, renin, aldosterone, catecholamines, cholesterol, and triglyceride. *Cochrane Database Syst Rev* 2011;(11):CD004022.

46. Taylor RS, Ashton KE, Moxham T, et al. Reduced dietary salt for the prevention of cardiovascular disease. *Cochrane Database Syst Rev* 2011;(7):CD009217.

47. He FJ, MacGregor GA. Salt reduction lowers cardiovascular risk: meta-analysis of outcome trials. *Lancet.* 2011;378: 380–382.

48. Chrysant GS, Bakir S, Oparil S. Dietary salt reduction in hypertension–what is the evidence and why is it still controversial? *Prog Cardiovasc Dis* 1999;42:23.

49. Kumanyika S. Behavioral aspects of intervention strategies to reduce dietary sodium. *Hypertension* 1991;17:i190.

50. Cook NR, Kumanyika SK, Cutler JA. Effect of change in sodium excretion on change in blood pressure corrected for measurement error. The Trials of Hypertension Prevention, phase I. *Am J Epidemiol* 1998;148:431.

51. Center for Science in the Public Interest. *In re Center for Science in the Public Interest.* United States Court of Appeals for the District of Columbia Circuit. Petition for a Writ of Mandamus Compelling Respondent Food and Drug Administration to Take Agency Action Unreasonably Delayed. February 24, 2005. Available at http://www.cspinet.org/new/pdf/salt_lawsuit.pdf; accessed 10/11/07.

52. Cogswell ME, et al. Sodium and potassium intakes among US adults: NHANES 2003–2008. *Am J Clin Nutr* 2012;96(3):647–657.

53. Eaton SB, Eaton SB III, Konner MJ. Paleolithic nutrition revisited: a twelve-year retrospective on its nature and implications. *Eur J Clin Nutr* 1997;51:207.

54. He FJ, Macgregor GA. Salt intake, plasma sodium, and worldwide salt reduction. *Ann Med* 2012;44(suppl 1): S127–S137.

55. Bertino M, Beauchamp GK, Engelman K. Long-term reduction in dietary sodium alters the taste of salt. *Am J Clin Nutr* 1982;36:1134.

56. Rogers PJ. Eating habits and appetite control: a psychobiological perspective. *Proc Nutr Soc* 1999;58:59.

57. Bertino M, Beauchamp GK, Engelman K. Increasing dietary salt alters salt taste preference. *Physiol Behav* 1986;38:203.

58. Drewnowski A, Henderson SA, Driscoll A, et al. Salt taste perceptions and preferences are unrelated to sodium consumption in healthy older adults. *J Am Diet Assoc* 1996;96:471.

59. Mattes RD. The taste for salt in humans. *Am J Clin Nutr* 1997;65:692s.

60. Gilleran G, O'Leary M, Bartlett WA, et al. Effects of dietary sodium substitution with potassium and magnesium in hypertensive type II diabetics: a randomised blind controlled parallel study. *J Hum Hypertens* 1996;10:517–521.

61. Geleijnse JM, Witteman JC, Bak AA, et al. Reduction in blood pressure with a low sodium, high potassium, high magnesium salt in older subjects with mild to moderate hypertension. *BMJ* 1994;309:436–440.

62. Zhou B, Wang HL, Wang WL, et al. Long-term effects of salt substitution on blood pressure in a rural North Chinese population. *J Hum Hypertens* 2013;27(7):427–433. doi: 10.1038/jhh.2012.63.

63. Whelton PK, He J. Potassium in preventing and treating high blood pressure. *Semin Nephrol* 1999;19:494.

64. van Bommel E, Cleophas T. Potassium treatment for hypertension in patients with high salt intake: a meta-analysis. *Int J Clin Pharmacol Ther* 2012;50(7):478–482.

65. Houston MC. The importance of potassium in managing hypertension. *Curr Hypertens Rep* 2011;13(4):309–317.

66. Griffith LE, Guyatt GH, Cook RJ, et al. The influence of dietary and nondietary calcium supplementation on blood pressure: an updated metaanalysis of randomized controlled trials. *Am J Hypertens* 1999;12:84.

67. van Mierlo LA, Arends LR, Streppel MT, et al. Blood pressure response to calcium supplementation: a meta-analysis of randomized controlled trials. *J Hum Hypertens* 2006;20:571–580.

68. Burgess E, Lewanczuk R, Bolli P, et al. Lifestyle modifications to prevent and control hypertension. 6. Recommendations on potassium, magnesium and calcium. Canadian Hypertension Society, Canadian Coalition for High Blood Pressure Prevention and Control, Laboratory Centre for Disease Control at Health Canada, Heart and Stroke Foundation of Canada. *CMAJ* 1999;160:s35.

69. Yabes-Almirante C. Calcium supplementation in pregnancy to prevent pregnancy induced hypertension (PIH). *J Perinat Med* 1998;26:347.

70. Rangan AM, Flood VI, Denyer G, et al. The effect of dairy consumption on blood pressure in mid-childhood: CAPS cohort study. *Eur J Clin Nutr* 2012;66(6):652–657.

71. McCarron DA, Reusser ME. Finding consensus in the dietary calcium-blood pressure debate. *J Am Coll Nutr* 1999;18:398s.

72. Houston M. The role of magnesium in hypertension and cardiovascular disease. *J Clin Hypertens* (Greenwich). 2011;13(11):843–847.

73. Jee SH, Miller ER III, Guallar E, et al. The effect of magnesium supplementation on blood pressure: a meta-analysis of randomized clinical trials. *Am J Hypertens* 2002;15:691–696.

74. Kass L, Weekes J, Carpenter L. Effect of magnesium supplementation on blood pressure: a meta-analysis. *Eur J Clin Nutr* 2012;66(4):411–418.

75. Appel LJ. Nonpharmacologic therapies that reduce blood pressure: a fresh perspective. *Clin Cardiol* 1999;22:iii1–iii5.

76. Rosanoff A, Weaver CM, Rude RK. Suboptimal magnesium status in the United States: are the health consequences underestimated? *Nutr Rev* 2012;70(3):153–164.

77. Stamler J, Caggiula AW, Grandits GA. Relation of body mass and alcohol, nutrient, fiber, and caffeine intakes to

blood pressure in the special intervention and usual care groups in the Multiple Risk Factor Intervention Trial. *Am J Clin Nutr* 1997;65:338s–365s.

78. Ascherio A, Hennekens C, Willett WC, et al. Prospective study of nutritional factors, blood pressure, and hypertension among US women. *Hypertension* 1996;27:1065.

79. Keenan JM, Pins JJ, Frazel C, et al. Oat ingestion reduces systolic and diastolic blood pressure in patients with mild or borderline hypertension: a pilot trial. *J Fam Pract* 2002;51:369.

80. Pins JJ, Geleva D, Keenan JM, et al. Do whole-grain oat cereals reduce the need for antihypertensive medications and improve blood pressure control? *J Fam Pract* 2002;51: 353–359.

81. Streppel MT, Arends LR, van't Veer P, et al. Dietary fiber and blood pressure: a meta-analysis of randomized placebo-controlled trials. *Arch Intern Med* 2005;165:150–156.

82. Pedraza-Chaverri J, Tapia E, Medina-Campos ON, et al. Garlic prevents hypertension induced by chronic inhibition of nitric oxide synthesis. *Life Sci* 1998;62:pl71–pl77.

83. Silagy CA, Neil HA. A meta-analysis of the effect of garlic on blood pressure. *J Hypertens* 1994;12:463.

84. Ried K, Frank OR, Stocks NP. Aged garlic extract reduces blood pressure in hypertensives: a dose-response trial. *Eur J Clin Nutr* 2013;67:64–70.

85. Capraz M, Dilek M, Akpolat T. Garlic, hypertension and patient education. *Int J Cardiol* 2006;121:130–131.

86. Nittynen L, Nurminen ML, Korpela R, et al. Role of arginine, taurine and homocysteine in cardiovascular diseases. *Ann Med* 1999;31:318–326.

87. Hedner T, Sun X. Measures of endothelial function as an endpoint in hypertension? *Blood Press* 1997;2:58–66.

88. Panza JA. Endothelial dysfunction in essential hypertension. *Clin Cardiol* 1997;20:11–26.

89. Miller AL. The effects of sustained-release-L-arginine formulation on blood pressure and vascular compliance in 29 healthy individuals. *Altern Med Rev* 2006;11:23–29.

90. Langsjoen P, Langsjoen P, Willis R, et al. Treatment of essential hypertension with coenzyme Q_{10}. *Mol Aspects Med* 1994;15:s265–s272.

91. Singh RB, Niaz MA, Rastogi SS, et al. Effect of hydrosoluble coenzyme Q_{10} on blood pressures and insulin resistance in hypertensive patients with coronary artery disease. *J Hum Hypertens* 1999;13:203–208.

92. Digiesi V, Cantini F, Oradei A, et al. Coenzyme Q_{10} in essential hypertension. *Mol Aspects Med* 1994;15:s257–s262.

93. Ho MJ, Bellusci A, Wright JM. Blood pressure lowering efficacy of coenzyme Q10 for primary hypertension. *Cochrane Database Syst Rev* 2009.

94. Hodgson JM, Watts GF, Playford DA, et al. Coenzyme Q_{10} improves blood pressure and glycaemic control: a controlled trial in subjects with type 2 diabetes. *Eur J Clin Nutr* 2002;56:1137–1142.

95. Hodgson JM, Watts GF. Can coenzyme Q_{10} improve vascular function and blood pressure? Potential for effective therapeutic reduction in vascular oxidative stress. *Biofactors* 2003;18:129–136.

96. Young JM, et al. A randomized, double-blind, placebo-controlled crossover study of coenzyme Q10 therapy in hypertensive patients with the metabolic syndrome. *Am J Hypertens* 2012;25(2):261–270.

97. Nurminen ML, Niittynen L, Korpela R, et al. Coffee, caffeine and blood pressure: a critical review. *Eur J Clin Nutr* 1999;53:831.

98. Wexler R, Aukerman G. Nonpharmacologic strategies for managing hypertension. *Am Fam Physician* 2006;73: 1953–1956.

99. Beyer FR, Dickinson HO, Nicolson DJ, et al. Combined calcium, magnesium and potassium supplementation for the management of primary hypertension in adults. *Cochrane Database Syst Rev* 2006;3:CD004805.

100. Sagie A, Larson MG, Levy D. The natural history of borderline isolated systolic hypertension. *N Engl J Med* 1993;329:1912.

101. Kolasa KM. Dietary approaches to stop hypertension (DASH) in clinical practice: a primary care experience. *Clin Cardiol* 1999;22:iii16.

SUGGESTED READING

The sixth report of the Joint National Committee on prevention, detection, evaluation, and treatment of high blood pressure. *Arch Intern Med* 1997;157:2413–2446.

Chobanian AV, Bakris GL, Black HR, et al. Seventh report of the Joint National Committee on Prevention, Detection, Evaluation, and Treatment of High Blood Pressure: The JNC 7 report. *JAMA* 2003;289:2560–2572. Available at http:// www.nhlbi.nih.gov/guidelines/hypertension/phycard.pdf; accessed 10/11/07.

Karanja NM, Obarzanek E, Lin PH, et al. Descriptive characteristics of the dietary patterns used in the Dietary Approaches to Stop Hypertension Trial. DASH Collaborative Research Group. *J Am Diet Assoc* 1999;99:s19.

Kawano Y, Matsuoka H, Takishita S, et al. Effects of magnesium supplementation in hypertensive patients: assessment by office, home, and ambulatory blood pressures. *Hypertension* 1998;32:260–265.

Kotchen TA, Kotchen JM. Nutrition, diet, and hypertension. In: Shils ME, Shike M, Ross AC, et al., eds. *Modern nutrition in health and disease*, 10th ed. Philadelphia, PA: Lippincott Williams & Wilkins, 2006:1095–1107.

Krousel-Wood MA, Muntner P, He J, et al. Primary prevention of essential hypertension. *Med Clin North Am* 2004;88:223–238.

CHAPTER 9

Diet and Hemostasis

Nutrition plays a vital role in both the manufacture of blood products and in the homeostatic mechanisms governing the function of both cellular and noncellular constituents of blood. Hematopoiesis requires an adequate intake of both energy and an array of micronutrients, including minerals such as iron, vitamins such as folate and B_{12}, and specific amino acids. The manufacture of clotting factors II, VII, IX, and X is dependent on adequate intake of vitamin K and normal hepatocyte function. Inflammation is an increasing focus of pathophysiology in cardiovascular disease (CVD), diabetes, and other chronic diseases. In fact, obesity has a strong inflammatory component that can be stimulated by diet-induced increases in arachidonic acid.

Provided that both macronutrient and micronutrient intake meet or exceed recommended levels, diet is unlikely to be a limiting factor in hematopoiesis. However, variations in dietary pattern and in the metabolic responses to such variations appear to play an important and as yet incompletely understood role in modifying hemostasis. Roles for total energy intake, adiposity, alcohol, the quantity and type of dietary fat, and various micronutrients have been tentatively or reliably identified in promoting or inhibiting thrombotic tendencies.

DIET

Excess energy intake leading to obesity appears to be associated with increased thrombotic tendencies. Obesity is associated with increased levels of fibrinogen, factor VII, factor VIII, and plasminogen activator inhibitor (PAI-1) as well as increased blood viscosity (1,2). Adipose tissue is considered a true organ, made up of fat and vascular cells, and capable of producing hormones as well as inflammatory mediators. Adiposity, as measured by the waist circumference, has been positively correlated with fibrinogen levels (1) and may be particularly associated with a prothrombotic tendency (3). Faber et al. explains that adipose

tissue induces thrombocyte activation by the production of adipose tissue-derived hormones, called adipokines, which directly and indirectly (via insulin resistance) affect platelet function (4). Recent evidence suggests that the nonfat cells (5) produce PAI-1 (6,7). The molecule PAI-1 is the major physiologic inhibitor of tissue-type plasminogen activator in plasma, thus preventing thrombolysis in vivo and increasing one's risk of myocardial infarction. Numerous studies have demonstrated significant associations among increased serum concentration of PAI-1, insulin resistance, and central adiposity, suggesting that PAI-1 can be considered part of the metabolic syndrome complex and may contribute to the impaired fibrinolysis in type 2 diabetes (8–10) (see Chapter 6). A recent study found that both weight loss and medication-induced improvement of insulin sensitivity significantly decreased platelet activation in obese women, suggesting that insulin resistance is itself an independent contributor to platelet activation (11). In fact, another study demonstrated that patients with metabolic syndrome who take aspirin have higher levels of serum thromboxane B(2), indicating less effective inhibition of cyclooxygenase-1 (COX-1) and a higher risk of clot formation (12).

Beneficial effects of weight loss on hemostasis have been reported. Short-term studies have shown variable effects on fibrinogen, apparently mediated by fluctuations in the levels of free fatty acids (1). Rapid weight loss may elevate fibrinogen because of free fatty acid mobilization, whereas more measured weight loss, and the maintenance of such loss, appears to be associated with reduced levels of both fibrinogen and other prothrombotic factors (1,13). Even weight reduction in obese children has been associated with decreased levels of fibrinogen, IL-6, C-reactive protein (CRP), and other inflammatory mediators (14). Fibrinogen levels may only decline with fairly significant weight loss. In contrast, both modest and substantial weight loss have been found to significantly reduce PAI-1 levels, especially in type-2 diabetics (15). Weight loss has also been associated with reductions in factor VII coagulant activity (factor VIIc), an effect that may be mediated through reductions in plasma triglycerides (16).

Physical activity appears to influence hemostasis, reducing levels of fibrinogen, factor VII, and PAI-1; however, these effects have been notably found only with regular exercise; acute exercise reduces PAI-1 as well but is associated with increases in fibrinogen and plasma viscosity (17). The benefits of regular activity may be especially robust in diabetics, suggesting that improved insulin sensitivity may reduce thrombotic tendencies. In addition, a recent study demonstrated that exercise, independent of inflammatory mediators, can speed cutaneous wound healing in obese mice (18), which has important implications for diabetic patients at increased risk for lower extremity injuries. In healthy, untrained adults, moderate exercise significantly elevates fibrinolytic activity, while strenuous exercise enhances coagulation as well as fibrinolysis; however, it appears that hemostasis remains in balance after both moderate and strenuous activity (19). Athletes show even higher rates of fibrinolytic activity via increased antithrombin III levels and markedly decreased PAI-1, suggesting greater vascular efficiency in this group (20). In contrast, unfavorable hemostatic changes at the extremes of exercise intensity may predispose to the formation of intravascular thrombus and may contribute to the phenomenon of sudden cardiac death after exercise (21). It has been found that strenuous exercise promotes thrombin generation by shear stress that causes the release of procoagulant microparticles from platelets, and this phenomenon seems to be more important in sedentary people (22). Thus, very strenuous physical activity such as marathon running may not be beneficial to some people, and one of the mechanisms behind this may be an unequal activation of the coagulation and fibrinolytic cascades.

Intensive lifestyle interventions that combine a healthy diet with increased physical activity appear to have the greatest benefit on hemostatic factors. The Finnish Diabetes Prevention Study found a significant beneficial long-term effect of such an intervention on fibrinolysis, measured by reduced levels of PAI-1, in obese subjects with impaired glucose tolerance (23). Likewise, Lindahl et al. (24) showed that intense behavioral intervention producing significant weight loss also produced significant reductions in PAI-1. Although the intervention subjects also showed declines in tissue plasminogen activator (tPA), these effects were smaller than those on PAI-1, suggesting enhanced fibrinolysis. The Diabetes Prevention Program clinical trial, which studied the effect of an intensive lifestyle intervention or metformin on progression to diabetes in adults with impaired glucose tolerance, found modest but significant reductions in fibrinogen levels in the lifestyle group compared to both metformin and placebo (25).

In a randomized trial of physical activity and a low-fat diet with or without daily fish in type 2 diabetics, Dunstan et al. (26) found some prothrombotic and some antithrombotic effects of the interventions. Interestingly, electroacupuncture, which can induce analgesia and thus decrease inflammation, has been shown to reduce PAI-1 and fibrinogen levels in women with polycystic ovarian syndrome (27).

High dietary fat intake is associated with relatively high levels of factors VIIc and X. Levels of PAI-1 and tPA may rise with increasing fat consumption. Reductions in fat intake have been shown to lower PAI-1 levels, but only if substantial. Similarly, changing to a healthy diet with reduced energy density may decrease endogenous thrombin generation (27). Elevated serum lipids associated with high dietary fat intake may promote thrombosis both directly and indirectly (1). These effects likely vary with the composition of dietary fat, as well as with its quantity, and may also be determined by certain genetic factors (28). In addition, a recent study demonstrated that implementation of the low-sodium DASH diet in diabetic patients for 8 weeks, resulted in decreased CRP and plasma fibrinogen levels as compared to a standard diabetic diet (29).

Adherence to the Mediterranean diet, which is high in mono- and polyunsaturated fatty acids, fruits, and vegetables, is associated with lower levels of fibrinogen (30). However, the effects of specific fatty acids on thrombotic tendencies remain somewhat controversial. Olive oil is a major constituent of the Mediterranean diet, and largely composed of the most important monounsaturated fatty acid (MUFA), oleic acid. Replacing saturated fats with MUFA yields a graded reduced aggregation response of platelets to ADP. As reviewed by Delgado-Lista et al., maintaining a basic Mediterranean diet rich in MUFA leads to decreased factor VII, tissue factor, PAI-1, and thromboxane levels (31).

Alterations in the intake of both saturated and MUFAs have yielded inconsistent and conflicting effects on the hemostatic profile, as reviewed by Miller (32). Even the n-3 polyunsaturated fatty acids (PUFAs), well known to inhibit platelet aggregability, have been associated with reductions in tPA, thus suggesting that fibrinolysis might be impaired by excessive intake. Fish oil may lower fibrinogen levels only when supplemented with vitamin E, and the major beneficial effect of n-3 PUFA may be antiarrhythmic (33) rather than antithrombotic (34); however, recent studies have found that fish oil may be pro- or antiarrhythmic and intake should be tailored to the individual patient's cardiac status and type of rhythm disturbance (35). On the other hand, adding 1 g per day of ω-3 PUFAs to dual antiplatelet therapy actually decreases thrombin formation in patients undergoing percutaneous coronary intervention (36). Likewise, giving fish oil to patients in severe CHF leads to a dose-dependent decrease in platelet activation and tissue factor levels, and higher doses result in decreased Il-6 and TNF-α (37).

The association between vegetarianism and reduced cardiac risk would suggest possible salutary effects on hemostasis; however, evidence to date is inconclusive. Four out of five cross-sectional studies examining hemostatic factors associated with vegetarian diet have found reduced levels of prothrombotic factors and enhanced fibrinolytic activity in vegetarians compared to nonvegetarians (38–40). In contrast, vegetarian diets, especially vegan diets, are also associated with increased platelet aggregation, which may be explained by lower consumption of foods rich in n-3 PUFAs, leading to lower platelet levels of LC n-3 PUFA, as well as eicosapentanoic acid and docosahexanoic acid (41,42).

Preliminary investigations have begun to identify the antithrombotic potential of specific fruits, vegetables, and other components of diets shown to have overall hemostatic benefit. Tomatoes (43), certain berries (44,45), and commonly used herbs and spices, such as thyme, rosemary, and cardamom, have shown significant antithrombotic activity in vitro and in vivo (45,46). Further, orange juice fortified with plant sterols reduces biomarkers of inflammation in healthy humans (47).

Vegetarian diets are associated with reduced cardiovascular risk (see Chapters 7 and 43); as is a Mediterranean pattern characterized by a relatively generous intake of poly- and monounsaturated fat (see Chapters 7 and 45). Thus, whether such dietary components yield consistently favorable effects on hemostasis is debatable; however, their net effect on overall cardiovascular risk is clearly beneficial.

In addition to obesity and CVD, the impact of diet on inflammation is also seen in deep venous thrombosis (DVT), further evidenced by the occurrence of holiday thrombolysis. This phenomenon entails acute thrombosis due to an accumulation of holiday-related factors, such as overindulgence, travel, increased alcohol intake, and emotional stress (48). Prophylaxis and treatment of DVT are typically accomplished through pharmacological anticoagulation and less commonly via endovascular or surgical intervention. Without treatment, patients with DVT are at risk of life-threatening pulmonary embolism, stroke, and other end results of embolic phenomena; however, anticoagulation imposes its own risk of fatal hemorrhage. As reviewed by Cundiff et al. (49), epidemiological evidence suggests that a diet made up mostly of fruits and vegetables (i.e., Mediterranean diet) rather than meat may significantly reduce the risk of DVT; however, the DASH diet does not appear to affect risk of DVT (50). In 2012, Varraso et al. investigated the impact of diet on the development of DVT among 129,430 US women and men in the Nurses' Health Study and Health Professionals Follow-up Study (51). They found that adherence to a Western diet, and intake of red meat and trans-fatty acids, were associated with an increased risk of DVT in men but not in women, while vitamins E and B$_6$ and fiber were beneficial in preventing DVT. The reasons for the gender discrepancy are unclear. This study was limited by infrequent follow-up (every 2 to 4 years) and sampling bias as subjects responded using questionnaires, rather than in an interview. Randomized, controlled, prospective noninferiority trials are needed to substantiate these claims.

NUTRIENTS, NUTRICEUTICALS, AND FUNCTIONAL FOODS

Alcohol

Light to moderate alcohol intake (1 to 2 drinks per day for men and 1 drink per day for women) has been shown to lower levels of fibrinogen, activate fibrinolysis through increased tPA, and reduce platelet aggregation over time (52,53). Acutely, alcohol may do just the opposite, thereby inducing a prothrombotic profile in the postprandial state, but this effect seems to depend on the type of alcohol consumed. Tousoulis et al. randomized healthy young individuals to receive equal amounts (30 g) of alcohol as either red wine, white wine, beer, whisky, or water. They found that Von Willebrand factor was only decreased in the beer and red wine groups, suggesting an improvement in endothelial function (54). Moreover, while moderate alcohol consumption is associated with reduced levels of fibrinogen, heavier intake has been shown to elevate levels. Notably, alcoholism, with resultant cirrhosis, is associated with a severe and potentially life-threatening coagulopathy, due to impaired production of vitamin K-dependent clotting factors and other effects.

Overall, at a dose of 10 to 30 g per day, alcohol appears to impart greater antithrombotic than prothrombotic effects, accounting for some portion of its association with reduced risk of cardiovascular events (55). More specifically, red wine has been found to contain resveratrol, a compound naturally found in certain fruits and nuts, which shows particular antiplatelet properties (56). A recent randomized controlled study investigated the anti-inflammatory effects of a resveratrol-rich grape supplement (resveratrol 8 mg) for 6 months followed by a double dose for the next 6 months in patients undergoing primary prevention for CVD. The investigators found that the resveratrol-rich supplement significantly decreased CRP, TNF-α, PAI-1, and Il-6/Il-10 ratio, and increased Il-10 (anti-inflammatory) levels (57). These results have important implications for the prevention of CVD. Further, it is now believed that alcohol and resveratrol may act synergistically to mitigate the process of atherosclerosis as well as coagulation (58).

Soluble Fiber

Current recommended forms of soluble fiber gaining FDA approval are psyllium seed husks (7 g per day), and β-glucan from oats, whole grains, or barley (3 g per day). In both male and female adolescents, dietary fiber is negatively associated with adipose tissue, CRP, and plasma fibrinogen levels (59). Soluble fiber has been shown to lower fibrinogen levels in diabetics. Raising soluble fiber intake also may improve fibrinolytic activity by increasing levels of tPA. Overall, the evidence is suggestive that dietary soluble fiber should correlate inversely

with thrombotic tendency. The mechanism by which fiber decreases inflammation is unknown, but it is possible that a reduction in visceral adiposity, which is known to be associated with inflammatory mediators, may be the link. An indirect effect is also possible, as soluble fiber attenuates postprandial elevations in insulin (see Chapter 6).

n-3 Fatty Acids

The effects of n-3 fatty acid supplementation on the hemostatic profile remain controversial (60,61). A review of randomized controlled trials published through 2005 by Robinson and Stone (62) found no consistent effects of n-3 supplementation on hemostatic parameters; approximately half of 24 trials reviewed demonstrated increased fibrinogen with n-3 supplementation, while the other half showed no effect or reduced levels.

Animal data suggest that long-chain n-3 fatty acids reduce platelet aggregation (63,64), while dietary supplementation with fish oil prolongs bleeding time (65). Across the range of typical fish consumption in the United States, no effect on hemostatic factors was seen among young adults in the CARDIA study (66). Likewise, a recent study measuring the effect of 6 week supplementation with OMACOR fish oil in 150 patients receiving aspirin and statin therapy revealed no change in vWF, fibrinogen binding, platelet aggregation, or CRP levels (67).

It is possible that effects may vary depending on the composition of the fish oil. Supplementation for 3 months with docosahexaenoic acid did not appreciably alter hemostatic factors in a group of healthy young adults (68). The OPTILIP trial of older adults found that decreasing the n-6:n-3 ratio to approximately 3:1 through increased intake of eicosapentaenoic and docosahexaenoic acids lowered triacylglycerol concentrations but had no significant effect on hemostasis markers (69). Another study showed that plasma n-3 and n-6 fatty acids were independently inversely associated with CRP and fibrinogen, but the ratio of n-6/n-3 fatty acids was actually positively correlated with the hemostatic and inflammatory biomarkers studied (70). Further, fibrinogen levels may only be lowered by fish oil if vitamin E supplementation is also provided. As reviewed by Thijssen et al., the most consistent finding is the potential beneficial effect of moderate amounts of fish oil on platelet aggregation (71).

Whereas the serum markers of hemostasis in humans show variable responses, a meta-analysis by Gapinski et al. (72) reported promising clinical effects. These investigators reported a nearly 14% reduction in the risk of restenosis at 6 months after coronary angioplasty and recommended intake of 4 to 5 g per day of n-3 fatty acids. Studies evaluated by Gapinski et al., such as that of Dehmer et al. (73), demonstrated a benefit of n-3 fatty acid supplementation in conjunction with aspirin use. In the context of coronary stenting and use of GpIIb/IIIa inhibitors, these findings are promising, Gajos et al. demonstrated that adding 1 g per day of ω-3 PUFAs to dual antiplatelet therapy actually decreases thrombin formation in patients undergoing percutaneous coronary intervention (36). Likewise, giving fish oil to patients with severe CHF leads to a dose-dependent decrease in platelet activation and tissue factor levels, and higher doses result in decreased Il-6 and TNF-α (37).

Monounsaturated Fatty Acids

The substitution of monounsaturated fat (oleic acid) for saturated fat appears to have a favorable effect on thrombotic tendency. Initial in vitro data suggested an increase in platelet aggregability (74), but recent clinical trials have found that a high-MUFA diet sustains potentially beneficial effects on platelet aggregation (75). MUFA has been inversely correlated with CRP and Il-6 levels (76). Sustained MUFA supplementation has also been associated with reduced postprandial activation of factor VII (77–79). In a randomized crossover study examining effects of diets rich in varying compositions of fatty acids, Pacheco et al. (80) observed increases in postprandial concentrations of TF (prothrombotic effect) and PAI-1 (antifibrinolytic effect) when the ratio of oleic to palmitic acid decreased (i.e., MUFA:SFA). As mentioned above, the replacement of saturated fats with MUFA yields a graded reduction in the aggregation response of platelets to ADP as well as decreased factor VII, tissue factor, PAI-1, and thromboxane levels (81).

Saturated Fatty Acids

Inconsistent effects of saturated fatty acids on thrombotic tendency have been observed. Irrespective of the type of fat consumed, there exists a postprandial procoagulant state, which may be enhanced by increased intake of SFA (82). Tholstrup et al. (83) administered meals rich in either stearic or myristic acid to 10 healthy men and found variable effects on thrombotic factors including PAI-1, factor VIIc, and β-thromboglobuli. Both fatty acids diminished platelet aggregability in the postprandial phase (84). Other studies have reported increased levels of factor VIIc induced by a high saturated fat diet relative to a high monounsaturated fat diet in women (85,86), and Lahoz et al. (87) reported increased thromboxane excretion in association with a high saturated fat test diet. A recent study on palmitate demonstrated increased levels of the procoagulant molecule, tissue factor, via extracellular release of histone H3, further suggesting that the effects of saturated fatty acids may be related to the specific type of fatty acid studied (88). Evidence to date does not strongly support assignation of cardiac risk associated with saturated fat intake to effects on hemostasis, although increased levels of activated factor VII and PAI-1 induced by diets rich in saturated fat may raise the risk of occlusive thrombosis from preexisting unstable atheromatous plaques (55). Notably, ω-6 PUFAs (e.g., arachidonic acid) and ω-3 PUFAs (e.g. eicosapentaenoic acid) are precursors to eicosanoids, which are lipid mediator signaling molecules; however, only those derived from ω-6 PUFA are proinflammatory, while those derived from ω-3 PUFA are anti-inflammatory. In recent decades, our diets have changed to favor intake of ω-6 PUFA over ω-3's in a 15:1 ratio, which may contribute to the rise in chronic inflammatory diseases, including obesity and heart disease (89).

Antioxidant Vitamins

Animal data suggest that both vitamins E and C can inhibit platelet aggregation and delay thrombus formation (90,91). However, investigations into the antithrombotic effects of antioxidant supplementation in humans have had mixed results.

Endothelial dysfunction is a known contributor to diabetes mellitus, and it would thus be expected that vitamin C, a chain-breaking antioxidant, would mitigate this effect; however, it has been shown that 800 mg per day of vitamin C only partially replenishes vitamin C levels in type 2 diabetics and fails to improve endothelial dysfunction or insulin resistance (92).

One study of short-term vitamin E supplementation (400 IU per day) in hypercholesterolemic subjects demonstrated reduced platelet aggregation after 6 weeks (93). It has also been shown that 600 mg of vitamin E daily for 2 weeks leads to normalization of 8-iso-PGF2-α urinary excretion and decreased thromboxane metabolite excretion (94). Further, Cangemi et al. showed that patients with hypercholesterolemia had lower vitamin E levels. Treatment with atorvastatin not only led to decreased isoprostane levels but also to increased vitamin E levels, suggesting that statins may enhance the antioxidant effects of vitamin E (95). Enhanced anticoagulant effect in response to high-dose vitamin E supplementation has been reported in patients taking oral anticoagulants, prompting preliminary investigations into possible antagonistic effects of vitamin E on vitamin K (96). In contrast, a recent trial of vitamin E supplementation in healthy volunteers showed no significant effects on the coagulation profile or platelet aggregation (97).

Studies of antioxidant supplements, including vitamins E and C, for cardiac risk reduction have generally been disappointing (see Chapter 7). Moreover, some studies have found that supplementation with vitamins C or E may even portend a higher mortality risk (98,99). Most of these studies have used α-tocopherols only; further studies of vitamin E supplementation in the form of mixed tocopherols, shown to have greater potency in inhibiting platelet aggregation, may be warranted (100).

Vitamin K

Vitamin K plays a crucial role in hemostasis, as it is required for the formation of clotting factors II, VII, IX, and X, which can be disrupted in fat malabsorption syndromes (such as cystic fibrosis, short gut, celiac sprue, and chronic pancreatitis). In addition, neonates are inherently deficient in vitamin K. The goal of oral anticoagulant therapy is to achieve a balance that results in the production of clotting factors at a reduced rate. It is suggested that adaptive hepatic mechanisms are present to compensate for the variable intake of daily phylloquinone. The highest concentrations of vitamin K (400 to 700 μg per 100 g) are found in green vegetables but other foods such as fruits and grains contain as low as 1 to 10 μg per 100 g (101). Preliminary evidence suggests that

dietary vitamin K may interfere with anticoagulation stability in patients on oral anticoagulants, a phenomenon of clear relevance to the practicing clinician (102). High vitamin K diets lead to decreased warfarin sensitivity indices and thus decreased INR values, leading to higher anticoagulant dosage requirements; however diets low in vitamin K are more likely to cause unstable anticoagulation than diets higher in the vitamin. Patients receiving warfarin should be advised to keep their dietary intake of vitamin K stable and supplementation with 100 to 150 μg per day may even help improve INR stability (101).

Flavonoids

Flavonoids, a family of polyphenol compounds found in a variety of foods, including grapes, nuts, and cocoa, have been shown to inhibit platelet aggregation in vitro. Human studies are not yet conclusive but suggest beneficial effects. One recent randomized, controlled crossover study in 23 patients with coronary artery disease demonstrated 200 mg of Pycnogenol per day for 8 weeks leads to decreased isoprostane levels and improved endothelial function (103). Another study showed that both in vitro incubation and oral supplementation with purple grape juice reduced platelet aggregation in healthy subjects (104). A small trial by Hermann et al. (105) found flavonoid-containing dark chocolate to induce a rapid, significant improvement of platelet function in smokers, a demographic known to have baseline platelet dysfunction. Similarly, a recent study implementing 3-week consumption of 50 g flavonoid-rich dark chocolate found improvement in the lipoprotein profile in healthy individuals, with a greater effect on women than men (106). A placebo-controlled trial found significantly decreased platelet function in healthy subjects after 28 days of cocoa flavonol supplementation (65) (see Chapter 39). Moreover, Pycnogenol may have protective antithrombotic properties for individuals following a thrombotic event and are synergistic with compression stockings for the prevention of post-thrombotic syndrome (107).

There have been some contradictory findings (108), including studies examining isoflavone phytoestrogens found in soy (109), and it is as yet unclear whether the cardioprotective effects of flavonoids can be attributed directly to hemostatic mechanisms (110).

Arginine

Arginine is a precursor in the manufacture of nitric oxide by the vascular endothelium; nitric oxide levels may influence platelet–endothelium interactions. Animal data have been reported suggesting that L-arginine supplementation reduces levels of thromboxane relative to prostacyclin and inhibits platelet aggregation (111). A recent study on New Zealand white rabbits showed that L-arginine was even more effective than aspirin in reducing platelet aggregation (112). Administration of L-arginine has been shown to inhibit platelet aggregation in healthy human subjects (113); Neri et al. (114) found this effect to be reproducible in pregnant women with normal blood pressure and with chronic hypertension, but not in the preeclamptic state. However, an older study of L-arginine supplementation in subjects with hypercholesterolemia showed no favorable effects on levels of endothelin or platelet adhesion molecules (115).

Diet/Drug Interactions

Not only does nutrient intake play a role in disease development and progression, but it also affects pharmacological treatments for CVD.

Aspirin has wide spread applications and while generally safe in low doses, it does put patients at risk of gastrointestinal bleeding and renal damage. Caffeine increases the rate of appearance, the maximum concentration of salicylate in the blood plasma, and its time to excretion; however, the specific mechanism is unclear (116). Drinking alcohol while taking aspirin may enhance platelet dysfunction and dangerously prolong bleeding time, and significantly increase the risk of gastrointestinal or other bleeding (117,118).

Similarly, nutrition affects the functioning of heparin and warfarin, antithrombotic medications used to treat and prevent DVT, stroke, and other thrombotic events. Heparin activates antithrombin III to inactivate thrombin, while warfarin inhibits the production of vitamin K, an essential component of clotting factors II, VII, IX, and X, and proteins C, S, and Z. A diet rich in vitamin K (i.e., lettuce, broccoli, brussels sprouts) can diminish the effects of warfarin and heparin and result in thrombosis (119); however, a reduction in vitamin K intake while taking these drugs will cause an increased risk of bleeding. Likewise, a small study in Brazil demonstrated variation in warfarin drug levels with fluctuations in phylloquinone intake (120), particularly from kidney beans. Herbs also affect vitamin K metabolism, including biliberry, bromelains, coenzyme Q-10, danshen, dong quai, feverfew, garlic, ginger, gingko biloba, ginseng, horse chestnut, meadowsweet, St John's wort, turmeric, and willow. It is thus recommended to maintain a stable diet while on antithrombotic medications, especially if taking warfarin over the long term.

There are no known food interactions with clopidogrel, ticagrelor, and dipyridamole, antiplatelet drugs used in cardiac catheterization procedures (i.e., endovascular stenting); however, in combination with aspirin or antithrombotic drugs, they will increase the risk of bleeding. In addition, a recent study found that despite exclusion or control of various patient factors, including diet, clopidogrel pharmacokinetics and pharmacodynamics varied widely, accounting for the high risk of major adverse cardiovascular events seen with this drug (121).

NUTRIGENOMICS

The presence of endogenous or exogenous antioxidants affects the development of thrombus formation. Therefore there are therapeutic opportunities in the area of nutrigenomics for vascular diseases, for example, the use of nutriceuticals to prevent and manage thrombosis in women with inherited mutations in their thrombophilic genes (122). The methylene tetrahydrofolate reductase (MTHFR) enzyme converts homocysteine to methionine and has been implicated in thrombotic disease and neural tube defects. There are two known single nucleotide polymorphisms (C677T and A1298C) that result in reduced enzyme activity, which can be treated effectively with folic acid supplementation (122).

It is well established that oral contraceptive use and hormone replacement therapy increase the risk of thrombosis in women (123). That risk is increased significantly in women with prothrombotic blood abnormalities, such as factor V Leiden mutation (124,125). Before prescribing hormone therapy, the patient's medical and family history should be considered and if there is a history of thrombosis, the risks and benefits of therapy need to be evaluated. In addition, women may benefit from the herb, guarana (*Paulinia cupana, Saponidaceae*), which is native to the central Amazon Basin, where it is consumed as a high-caffeine stimulant or for medicinal purposes. Old studies have reported that aqueous extracts of guarana seeds demonstrate powerful inhibitory properties toward platelet aggregation and thromboxane synthesis (126,127), and thus may be beneficial to women with thrombophilic gene mutations.

CLINICAL HIGHLIGHTS

Hemostatic factors, such as fibrinogen, PAI-1, and factor VIIc, are strongly associated with the risk of cardiovascular events (128,129). Evidence from a variety of sources indicates that dietary pattern may play an important role in influencing hemostasis. However, due in part to the wide range of circulating factors involved in hemostatic mechanisms and in part to the difficulties of controlled dietary interventions, little is known with certainty about the effects of specific foods or nutrients on overall thrombotic tendency (130). Evidence available to date suggests that dietary recommendations to reduce risk of thromboembolic disease are consistent with recommendations to lower risk of CVD. Protective factors include the avoidance of excess energy intake and obesity; the avoidance of excess fat consumption; physical activity; abundant dietary fiber, especially soluble fiber; moderate alcohol consumption; and possibly dietary supplementation with n-3 fatty acids and vitamin E at moderate doses (130). A shift of calories from saturated fat to unsaturated fats; and increased intake of fruits, vegetables, and concentrated sources of flavonoids such as cocoa and green tea all conform with the weight of evidence, although definitive knowledge of hemostatic effects is lacking in each case. Weight loss in obese patients may be of particular importance. Before definitive dietary recommendations can be offered to modify hemostasis for clinical benefit, observational and ideally interventional studies of diet and clinically important thrombotic events rather than surrogate markers will be needed. Careful monitoring prior to anticoagulation therapy may be indicated for patients on ketogenic diets (131) as well as those with high dietary consumption or supplementation of vitamin K or n-3 fatty acids.

REFERENCES

1. Vorster HH, Cummings JH, Veldman FJ. Diet and haemostasis: time for nutrition science to get more involved. *Br J Nutr* 1997;77:671–684.
2. Yarnell JW, Sweetnam PM, Rumley A, et al. Lifestyle and hemostatic risk factors for ischemic heart disease: the Caerphilly study. *Arterioscler Thromb Vasc Biol* 2000;20:271–279.
3. Anderssen SA, Holme I, Urdal P, et al. Associations between central obesity and indexes of hemostatic, carbohydrate and lipid metabolism. Results of a 1-year intervention from the Oslo Diet and Exercise study. *Scand J Med Sci Sports* 1998;8:109–115.
4. Faber DR, de Groot PG, Visseren FL. Role of adipose tissue in haemostasis, coagulation and fibrinolysis. *Obes Rev* 2009;10(5):554–563.
5. Fain JN. Release of inflammatory mediators by human adipose tissue is enhanced in obesity and primarily by the nonfat cells: a review. *Mediators Inflamm* 2010;513948.
6. Lundgren CH, Brown SL, Nordt TK, et al. Elaboration of type-1 plasminogen activator inhibitor from adipocytes: a potential pathogenetic link between obesity and cardiovascular disease. *Circulation* 1996;93:106–110.
7. Ronti T, Lupattelli G, Mannarino E. The endocrine function of adipose tissue: an update. *Clin Endocrinol* (Oxford) 2006;64:355–365.
8. Trost S, Pratley R, Sobel B. Impaired fibrinolysis and risk for cardiovascular disease in the metabolic syndrome and type 2 diabetes. *Curr Diab Rep* 2006;6:47–54.
9. Aso Y, Okumura KI, Yoshida N, et al. Enhancement of fibrinolysis in poorly controlled, hospitalized type 2 diabetic patients by short-term metabolic control: association with a decrease in plasminogen activator inhibitor 1. *Exp Clin Endocrinol Diabetes* 2004;112:175–180.
10. Godsland IF, Crook D, Proudler AJ, et al. Hemostatic risk factors and insulin sensitivity, regional body fat distribution, and the metabolic syndrome. *J Clin Endocrinol Metab* 2005;90:190–197.
11. Basili S, Pacini G, Guagnano MT, et al. Insulin resistance as a determinant of platelet activation in obese women. *J Am Coll Cardiol* 2006;48:2531–2538.
12. Smith JP, Haddad EV, Oates JA. Suboptimal inhibition of platelet cyclooxygenase-1 by aspirin in metabolic syndrome. *Hypertension* 2012;59(3):719–725.
13. Marckmann P, Toubro S, Astrup A. Sustained improvement in blood lipids, coagulation, and fibrinolysis after major weight loss in obese subjects. *Eur J Clin Nutr* 1998;52:329–333.
14. Garanty-Bogacka B, Syrenicz M, Goral J, et al. Changes in inflammatory biomarkers after successful lifestyle intervention in obese children. *Endokrynol Pol* 2011;62(6):499–505.
15. Belalcazar LM, Ballantyne CM, Lang W, et al. Metabolic factors, adipose tissue, and plasminogen activator inhibitor-1 levels in type 2 diabetes: findings from the look AHEAD study. *Arterioscler Thromb Vasc Biol* 2011; 31(7):1689–1695.
16. Mertens I, Van Gaal LF. Obesity, haemostasis and the fibrinolytic system. *Obes Rev* 2002;3:85–101.
17. Lee KW, Lip GY. Effects of lifestyle on hemostasis, fibrinolysis, and platelet reactivity. *Arch Intern Med* 2003;163:2368–2392.

18. Pence BD, Dipietro LA, Woods JA. Exercise speeds cutaneous wound healing in high-fat diet-induced obese mice. *Med Sci Sports Exerc* 2012;44(10):1846–1854.

19. Menzel K, Hilberg T. Blood coagulation and fibrinolysis in healthy, untrained subjects: effects of different exercise intensities controlled by individual anaerobic threshold. *Eur J Appl Physiol* 2011;111(2):253–260.

20. Cerneca E, Simeone R, Burno G, et al. Coagulation parameters in senior athletes practicing endurance sporting activity. *J Sports Med Phys Fitness* 2005;45(4):576–579.

21. Smith JE. Effects of strenuous exercise on haemostasis. *Br J Sports Med* 2003;37:433–435.

22. Chen YW, Chen JK, Wang JS. Strenuous exercise promotes shear-induced thrombin generation by increasing the shedding of procoagulant microparticles from platelets. *Thromb Haemost* 2010;104(2):293–301.

23. Hämäläinen H, Rönnemaa T, Virtanen A, et al. Improved fibrinolysis by an intensive lifestyle intervention in subjects with impaired glucose tolerance. The Finnish Diabetes Prevention Study. *Diabeteologia* 2005;48:2248–2253.

24. Lindahl B, Nilsson TK, Jansson JH, et al. Improved fibrinolysis by intense lifestyle intervention. A randomized trial in subjects with impaired glucose tolerance. *J Intern Med* 1999;246:105–112.

25. Haffner S, Temprosa M, Crandall J, et al. Intensive lifestyle intervention or metformin on inflammation and coagulation in participants with impaired glucose tolerance. *Diabetes* 2005;54:1566–1572.

26. Dunstan DW, Mori TA, Puddey IB, et al. A randomised, controlled study of the effects of aerobic exercise and dietary fish on coagulation and fibrinolytic factors in type 2 diabetics. *Thromb Haemost* 1999;81:367–372.

27. Stener-Victorin E, Baghaei F, Holm G, et al. Effects of acupuncture and exercise on insulin sensitivity, adipose tissue characteristics, and markers of coagulation and fibrinolysis in women with polycystic ovary syndrome: secondary analyses of a randomized controlled trial. *Fertil Steril* 2012;97(2):501–508.

28. Sanders TA, de Grassi T, Acharya J, et al. Postprandial variations in fibrinolytic activity in middle-aged men are modulated by plasminogen activator inhibitor I 4G-675/5G genotype but not by the fat content of a meal. *Am J Clin Nutr* 2004;79:577–581.

29. Azadbakht L, Surkan PJ, Willett WC, et al. The Dietary Approaches to Stop Hypertension eating plan affects C-reactive protein, coagulation abnormalities, and hepatic function tests among type 2 diabetic patients. *J Nutr* 2011; 141(6):1083–1088.

30. Chrysohoou C, Panagiotakos DB, Pitsavos C, et al. Adherence to the Mediterranean diet attenuates inflammation and coagulation process in healthy adults: The ATTICA study. *J Am Coll Cardiol* 2004;44:152–158.

31. Delgado-Lista J, Garcia-Rios A, Perez-Martinez P, et al. Olive oil and haemostasis: platelet function, thrombogenesis and fibrinolysis. *Curr Pharm Des* 2011;17(8): 778–785.

32. Miller GJ. Dietary fatty acids and the haemostatic system. *Atherosclerosis* 2005;179:213–227.

33. Siscovick DS, Raghunathan T, King I, et al. Dietary intake of long-chain n-3 polyunsaturated fatty acids and the risk of primary cardiac arrest. *Am J Clin Nutr* 2000; 71:208s–212s.

34. Anand RG, Alkadri M, Lavie CJ, et al. The role of fish oil in arrhythmia prevention. *J Cardiopulm Rehabil Prev* 2008;28(2):92–98.

35. Den Ruijter HM, Berecki G, Opthof T, et al. Pro- and anti-arrhythmic properties of a diet rich in fish oil. *Cardiovasc Res* 2007;73(2):316–325.

36. Gajos G, Zalewski J, Rostoff P, et al. Reduced thrombin formation and altered fibrin clot properties induced by polyunsaturated omega-3 fatty acids on top of dual antiplatelet therapy in patients undergoing percutaneous coronary intervention (OMEGA-PCI clot). *Arterioscler Thromb Vasc Biol* 2011;31(7):1696–1702.

37. Moertl D, Berger R, Hammer A, et al. Dose-dependent decrease of platelet activation and tissue factor by omega-3 polyunsaturated fatty acids in patients with advanced chronic heart failure. *Thromb Haemost*; 2011;106(3): 457–465.

38. Mezzano D, Munoz X, Martinez C, et al. Vegetarians and cardiovascular risk factors: hemostasis, inflammatory markers and plasma homocysteine. *Thromb Haemost* 1999; 81:913–917.

39. Famodu AA, Osilesi O, Makinde YO, et al. The influence of a vegetarian diet on haemostatic risk factors for cardiovascular disease in Africans. *Thromb Res* 1999;95:31–36.

40. Li D, Sinclair A, Mann N, et al. The association of diet and thrombotic risk factors in healthy male vegetarians and meat-eaters. *Eur J Clin Nutr* 1999;53:612–619.

41. Rajaram S. The effect of vegetarian diet, plant foods, and phytochemicals on hemostasis and thrombosis. *Am J Clin Nutr* 2003;78:552s–558s.

42. Li D, Sinclair A, Mann N, et al. The association of diet and thrombotic risk factors in healthy male vegetarians and meat-eaters. *Eur J Clin Nutr* 1999;53(8):612–619.

43. O'Kennedy N, Crosbie L, van Lieshout M, et al. Effects of antiplatelet components of tomato extract on platelet function in vitro and ex vivo: a time-course cannulation study in healthy humans. *Am J Clin Nutr* 2006;84:570–579.

44. Naemura A, Mitani T, Ijiri Y, et al. Anti-thrombotic effect of strawberries. *Blood Coagul Fibrinolysis* 2005;16:501–509.

45. Yamamoto J, Naemura A, Ura M, et al. Testing various fruits for anti-thrombotic effect: I. Mulberries. *Platelets* 2006;17:555–564.

46. Verma SK, Jain V, Katewa SS. Blood pressure lowering, fibrinolysis enhancing and antioxidant activities of cardamom (*Elettaria cardamomum*). *Indian J Biochem Biophys* 2009;46(6):503–506.

47. Devaraj S, Jialal I, Rockwood J, et al. Effect of orange juice and beverage with phytosterols on cytokines and PAI-1 activity. *Clin Nutr* 2011;30(5):668–671.

48. Lippi G, Franchini M, Favaloro EJ. Holiday thrombosis. *Semin Thromb Hemost* 2011;37(8):869–874.

49. Cundiff DK, Agutter PS, Malone PC, et al. Diet as prophylaxis and treatment for venous thromboembolism? *Theor Biol Med Model* 2010;7:31.

50. Fitzgerald KC, Chiuve SC, Buring JE, et al. Comparison of associations of adherence to a Dietary Approaches to Stop Hypertension (DASH)-style diet with risks of cardiovascular disease and venous thromboembolism. *J Thromb Haemost* 2012;10(2):189–198.

51. Varraso R, Kabrhel C, Goldhaber SZ, et al. Prospective study of diet and venous thromboembolism in US women and men. *Am J Epidemiol* 2012;175(2):114–126.

52. Mukamal KJ, Jadhav PP, D'Agostino RB, et al. Alcohol consumption and hemostatic factors: analysis of the Framingham Offspring cohort. *Circulation* 2001;104:1367–1373.

53. Salem RO, Laposata M. Effects of alcohol on hemostasis. *Am J Clin Pathol* 2005;123:s96–s105.

54. Tousoulis D, Ntarladimas I, Antoniades C, et al. Acute effects of different alcoholic beverages on vascular endothelium, inflammatory markers and thrombosis fibrinolysis system. *Clin Nutr* 2008;27(4):594–600.

55. Rimm EB, Williams P, Fosher K, et al. Moderate alcohol intake and lower risk of coronary heart disease: meta-analysis of effects on lipids and haemostatic factors. *BMJ* 1999;319:1523–1528.

56. Olas B, Wachowicz B. Resveratrol, a phenolic antioxidant with effects on blood platelet functions. *Platelets* 2005; 16:251–260.

57. Tome-Carneiro J, Gonzalvez M, Larrosa M, et al. One-year consumption of a grape nutraceutical containing resveratrol improves the inflammatory and fibrinolytic status of patients in primary prevention of cardiovascular disease. *Am J Cardiol* 2012;110(3):356–363.

58. Lippi G, Franchini M, Favaloro EJ, et al. Moderate red wine consumption and cardiovascular disease risk: beyond the "French paradox". *Semin Thromb Hemost* 2010;36(1):59–70.

59. Parikh S, Pollock NK, Bhagatwala J, et al. Adolescent fiber consumption is associated with visceral fat and inflammatory markers. *J Clin Endocrinol Metab* 2012; 97(8):E1451–E1457.

60. Allman-Farinelli MA, Hall D, Kingham K, et al. Comparison of the effects of two low fat diets with different alpha-linolenic: linoleic acid ratios on coagulation and fibrinolysis. *Atherosclerosis* 1999;142:159–168.

61. Sanders TA, Oakley FR, Miller GJ, et al. Influence of n-6 versus n-3 polyunsaturated fatty acids in diets low in saturated fatty acids on plasma lipoproteins and hemostatic factors. *Arterioscler Thromb Vasc Biol* 1997;17:3449–3460.

62. Robinson JG, Stone NJ. Antiatherosclerotic and antithrombotic effects of omega-3 fatty acids. *Am J Cardiol* 2006;98:39–49.

63. Adan Y, Shibata K, Sato M, et al. Effects of docosahexaenoic and eicosapentaenoic acid on lipid metabolism, eicosanoid production, platelet aggregation and atherosclerosis in hypercholesterolemic rats. *Biosci Biotechnol Biochem* 1999;63:111–119.

64. Chen LY, Jokela R, Li DY, et al. Effect of stable fish oil on arterial thrombogenesis, platelet aggregation, and superoxide dismutase activity. *J Cardiovasc Pharmacol* 2000;35:502–505.

65. Lefevre M, Kris-Etherton PM, Zhao G, et al. Dietary fatty acids, hemostasis, and cardiovascular disease risk. *J Am Diet Assoc* 2004;104:410–419.

66. Archer SL, Green D, Chamberlain M, et al. Association of dietary fish and n-3 fatty acid intake with hemostatic factors in the Coronary Artery Risk Development in Young Adults (CARDIA) study. *Arterioscler Thromb Biol* 1998;18:1119–1123.

67. Mackay I, Ford I, Thies F, et al. Effect of omega-3 fatty acid supplementation on markers of platelet and endothelial function in patients with peripheral arterial disease. *Atherosclerosis* 2012;221(2):514–520.

68. Nelson GJ, Schmidt PS, Bartolini GL, et al. The effect of dietary docosahexaenoic acid on platelet function, platelet fatty acid composition, and blood coagulation in humans. *Lipids* 1997;32:1129–1136.

69. Sanders TA, Lewis F, Slaughter S, et al. Effect of varying the ratio of n-6 to n-3 fatty acids by increasing the dietary intake of alpha-linolenic acid, eicosapentaenoic and docosahexaenoic acid, or both on fibrinogen and clotting factors VII and XII in persons aged 45–70 y: the OPTILIP study. *Am J Clin Nutr* 2006;84:513–522.

70. Kalogeropoulos N, Panagiotakos DB, Pitsavos C, et al. Unsaturated fatty acids are inversely associated and n-6/n-3 ratios are positively related to inflammation and coagulation markers in plasma of apparently healthy adults. *Clin Chim Acta* 2010;411(7–8):584–591.

71. Thijssen MA, Mensink RP. Fatty acids and atherosclerotic risk. *Handb Exp Pharmacol* 2005;(170):165–194.

72. Gapinski JP, VanRuiswyk JV, Heudebert GR, et al. Preventing restenosis with fish oils following coronary angioplasty. A meta-analysis. *Arch Intern Med* 1993;153: 1595–1601.

73. Dehmer GJ, Popma JJ, Van den Berg EK, et al. Reduction in the rate of early restenosis after coronary angioplasty by a diet supplemented with n-3 fatty acids. *N Engl J Med* 1988;319:733–740.

74. Turpeinen AM, Pajari AM, Freese R, et al. Replacement of dietary saturated by unsaturated fatty acids: effects of platelet protein kinase C activity, urinary content of 2,3-dinor-TXB2 and *in vitro* platelet aggregation in healthy man. *Thromb Haemost* 1998;80:649–655.

75. Smith RD, Kelly CN, Fielding BA, et al. Long-term monounsaturated fatty acid diets reduce platelet aggregation in healthy young subjects. *Br J Nutr* 2003;90:597–606.

76. Kalogeropoulos N, et al. Unsaturated fatty acids are inversely associated and n-6/n-3 ratios are positively related to inflammation and coagulation markers in plasma of apparently healthy adults. *Clin Chim Acta* 2010;411(7–8):584–591.

77. Roche HM, Zampelas A, Knapper JM, et al. Effect of long-term olive oil dietary intervention on postprandial triacylglycerol and factor VII metabolism. *Am J Clin Nutr* 1998;68:552–560.

78. Silva KD, Kelly CN, Jones AE, et al. Chylomicron particle size and number, factor VII activation and dietary monounsaturated fatty acids. *Atherosclerosis* 2003;166: 73–84.

79. Allman-Farinelli MA, Gomes K, Favaloro EJ, et al. A diet rich in high-oleic-acid sunflower oil favorably alters low-density lipoprotein cholesterol, triglycerides, and factor VII coagulant activity. *Am Diet Assoc* 2005; 105:1071–1079.

80. Pacheco YM, Bermudez B, Lopez S, et al. Ratio of oleic to palmitic acid is a dietary determinant of thrombogenic and fibrinolytic factors during the postprandial state in men. *Am J Clin Nutr* 2006;84:342–349.

81. Lopez-Miranda J, Delgado-Lista J, Perez-Martinez P, et al. Olive oil and the haemostatic system. *Mol Nutr Food Res* 2007;51(10):1249–1259.

82. Delgado-Lista J, Lopez-Miranda J, Cortes B, et al. Chronic dietary fat intake modifies the postprandial response of hemostatic markers to a single fatty test meal. *Am J Clin Nutr* 2008;87(2):317–322.

83. Tholstrup T, Andreasen K, Sandstrom B. Acute effect of high-fat meals rich in either stearic or myristic acid on hemostatic factors in healthy young men. *Am J Clin Nutr* 1996;64:168–176.

84. Tholstrup T, Miller GJ, Bysted A, et al. Effect of individual dietary fatty acids on postprandial activation of blood coagulation factor VII and fibrinolysis in healthy young men. *Am J Clin Nutr* 2003;77:1125–1132.

85. Temme EH, Mensink RP, Hornstra G. Effects of diets enriched in lauric, palmitic or oleic acids on blood coagulation and fibrinolysis. *Thromb Haemost* 1999;81:259–263.

86. Lindman AS, Muller H, Seljeflot I, et al. Effects of a dietary fat quantity and composition on fasting and postprandial levels of coagulation factor VII and serum choline-containing phospholipids. *Br J Nutr* 2003;90:329–336.

87. Lahoz C, Alonso R, Ordovas JM, et al. Effects of dietary fat saturation on eicosanoid production, platelet aggregation and blood pressure. *Eur J Clin Invest* 1997; 27:780–789.

88. Shrestha C, Ito T, Kawahara K, et al. Saturated fatty acid palmitate induces extracellular release of histone H3: a possible mechanistic basis for high-fat diet-induced inflammation and thrombosis. *Biochem Biophys Res Commun* 2013;437:573–578.

89. Patterson E, Wall R, Fitzgerald GF, et al. Health implications of high dietary omega-6 polyunsaturated Fatty acids. *J Nutr Metab* 2012;2012:539426.

90. Mehta J, Li D, Mehta JL. Vitamins C and E prolong time to arterial thrombosis in rats. *J Nutr* 1999;129:109–112.

91. Harris A, Devaraj S, Jialal I. Oxidative stress, alpha-tocopherol therapy, and atherosclerosis. *Curr Atheroscler Rep* 2002;4:373–380.

92. Chen H, Karne RJ, Hall G, et al. High-dose oral vitamin C partially replenishes vitamin C levels in patients with Type 2 diabetes and low vitamin C levels but does not improve endothelial dysfunction or insulin resistance. *Am J Physiol Heart Circ Physiol* 2006;290(1):H137–H145.

93. Williams JC, Forster LA, Tull SP, et al. Dietary vitamin E supplementation inhibits thrombin-induced platelet aggregation, but not monocyte adhesiveness, in patients with hypercholesterolaemia. *Int J Exp Pathol* 1997;78:259–266.

94. Davi G, Ciabattoni G, Consoli A, et al. In vivo formation of 8-iso-prostaglandin $f_{2\alpha}$ and platelet activation in diabetes mellitus: effects of improved metabolic control and vitamin E supplementation. *Circulation* 1999;99(2): 224–229.

95. Cangemi R, Loffredo L, Carnevale R, et al. Early decrease of oxidative stress by atorvastatin in hypercholesterolaemic patients: effect on circulating vitamin E. *Eur Heart J* 2008;29(1):54–62.

96. Booth SL, Golly I, Sacheck JM, et al. Effect of vitamin E supplementation on vitamin K status in adults with normal coagulation status. *Am J Clin Nutr* 2004;80:143–148.

97. Dereska NH, McLemore EC, Tessier DJ, et al. Short-term, moderate dosage vitamin E supplementation may have no effect on platelet aggregation, coagulation profile, and bleeding time in healthy individuals. *J Surg Res* 2006;132:121–129.

98. Miller ER 3rd, Pastor-Burriuso R, Dalal D, et al. Meta-analysis: high-dosage vitamin E supplementation may increase all-cause mortality. *Ann Intern Med* 2005;142(1): 37–46.

99. Bjelakovic G, Nikolova D, Gluud LL, et al. Mortality in randomized trials of antioxidant supplements for primary and secondary prevention: systematic review and meta-analysis. *JAMA* 2007;297(8):842–857.

100. Liu M, Wallmon A, Olsson-Mortlock C, et al. Mixed tocopherols inhibit platelet aggregation in humans: potential mechanisms. *Am J Clin Nutr* 2003;77:700–706.

101. Holmes MV, Hunt BJ, Shearer MJ. The role of dietary vitamin K in the management of oral vitamin K antagonists. *Blood Rev* 2012;26(1):1–14.

102. Franco V, Polanczyk CA, Clausell N, et al. Role of dietary vitamin K intake in chronic oral anticoagulation: prospective evidence from observational and randomized protocols. *Am J Med* 2004;116:651–656.

103. Enseleit F, Sudano I, Periat D, et al. Effects of pycnogenol on endothelial function in patients with stable coronary artery disease: a double-blind, randomized, placebo-controlled, cross-over study. *Eur Heart J* 2012; 33(13):1589–1597.

104. Freedman JE, Parker C 3rd, Li L, et al. Select flavonoids and whole juice from purple grapes inhibit platelet function and enhance nitric oxide release. *Circulation* 2001;103:2792–2798.

105. Hermann F, Spieker LE, Ruschitzka F, et al. Dark chocolate improves endothelial and platelet function. *Heart* 2006;92:119–120.

106. Nanetti L, Raffaelli F, Tranquilli AL, et al. Effect of consumption of dark chocolate on oxidative stress in lipoproteins and platelets in women and in men. *Appetite* 2012;58(1):400–405.

107. Errichi BM, Belcaro G, Hosoi M, et al. Prevention of post thrombotic syndrome with Pycnogenol® in a twelve month study. *Panminerva Med* 2011;53(3 suppl 1):21–27.

108. Janssen K, Mensink RP, Cox FJ, et al. Effects of the flavonoids quercetin and apigenin on hemostasis in healthy volunteers: results from an *in vitro* and a dietary supplement study. *Am J Clin Nutr* 1998;67:255–262.

109. Teede HJ, Dalais FS, Kotsopoulos D, et al. Dietary soy containing phytoestrogens does not activate the hemostatic system in postmenopausal women. *J Clin Endocrinol Metab* 2005;90:1936–1941.

110. Vita JA. Polyphenols and cardiovascular disease: effects on endothelial and platelet function. *Am J Clin Nutr* 2005;81:292s–297s.

111. Bode-Boger SM, Boger RH, Kienke S, et al. Chronic dietary supplementation with L-arginine inhibits platelet aggregation and thromboxane A2 synthesis in hypercholesterolaemic rabbits *in vivo*. *Cardiovasc Res* 1998;37:756–764.

112. Saleh AI, Abdel Maksoud SM, El-Maraghy SA, et al. Protective effect of L-arginine in experimentally induced myocardial ischemia: comparison with aspirin. *J Cardiovasc Pharmacol Ther* 2011;16(1):53–62.

113. Adams MR, Forsyth CJ, Jessup W, et al. Oral L-arginine inhibits platelet aggregation but does not enhance endothelium-dependent dilation in healthy young men. *J Am Coll Cardiol* 1995;26:1054–1061.

114. Neri I, Piccinini F, Marietta M, et al. Platelet responsiveness to L-arginine in hypertensive disorders of pregnancy. *Hypertens Pregnancy* 2000;19:323–330.

115. Abdelhamed AI, Reis SE, Sane DC, et al. No effect of an L-arginine-enriched medical food (HeartBars) on endothelial function and platelet aggregation in subjects with hypercholesterolemia. *Am Heart J* 2003;145:E15.

116. Miners JO. Drug interactions involving aspirin (acetylsalicylic acid) and salicylic acid. *Clin Pharmacokinet* 1989;17(5):327–344.

117. Tsuda T, Okamoto Y, Sakaguchi R, et al. Purpura due to aspirin-induced platelet dysfunction aggravated by drinking alcohol. *J Int Med Res* 2001;29(4):374–380.

118. Kaufman DW, Kelly JP, Wiholm BE, et al. The risk of acute major upper gastrointestinal bleeding among users of aspirin and ibuprofen at various levels of alcohol consumption. *Am J Gastroenterol* 1999;94(11):3189–3196.

119. Walker FBT. Myocardial infarction after diet-induced warfarin resistance. *Arch Intern Med* 1984;144(10): 2089–2090.

120. Custodio das Dores SM, Booth SL, Martini LA, et al. Relationship between diet and anticoagulant response to warfarin: a factor analysis. *Eur J Nutr* 2007;46(3):147–154.

121. Frelinger AL 3rd, Bhatt DL, Lee RD, et al. Clopidogrel pharmacokinetics and pharmacodynamics vary widely despite exclusion or control of polymorphisms (cyp2c19, abcb1, pon1), noncompliance, diet, smoking, co-medications (including proton pump inhibitors), and pre-existent variability in platelet function. *J Am Coll Cardiol* 2013;61(8):872–879.

122. Subbiah MT. Nutrigenetics and nutraceuticals: the next wave riding on personalized medicine. *Transl Res* 2007;149(2):55–61.

123. Tanis BC, Rosendaal FR. Venous and arterial thrombosis during oral contraceptive use: risks and risk factors. *Semin Vasc Med* 2003;3(1):69–84.

124. Douketis JD, Julian JA, Crowther MA, et al. The effect of prothrombotic blood abnormalities on risk of deep vein thrombosis in users of hormone replacement therapy: a prospective case-control study. *Clin Appl Thromb Hemost* 2011;17(6):E106–E113.

125. Mohllajee AP, Curtis KM, Martins SL, et al. Does use of hormonal contraceptives among women with thrombogenic mutations increase their risk of venous thromboembolism? A systematic review. *Contraception* 2006;73(2):166–178.

126. Bydlowski SP, Yunker RL, Subbiah MT. A novel property of an aqueous guarana extract (*Paullinia cupana*): inhibition of platelet aggregation in vitro and in vivo. *Braz J Med Biol Res* 1988;21(3):535–538.

127. Bydlowski SP, D'amico EA, Chamone DA. An aqueous extract of guarana (*Paullinia cupana*) decreases platelet thromboxane synthesis. *Braz J Med Biol Res* 1991;24(4):421–424.

128. Smith A, Patterson C, Yarnell J, et al. Which hemostatic markers add to the predictive value of conventional risk factors for coronary heart disease and ischemic stroke? The Caerphilly study. *Circulation* 2005;112:3080–3087.

129. Montalescot G, Collet JP, Choussat R, et al. Fibrinogen as a risk factor for coronary heart disease. *Eur Heart J* 1998;19:h11–h17.

130. Hamer M, Steptoe A. Influence of specific nutrients on progression of atherosclerosis, vascular function, haemostasis and inflammation in coronary heart patients: a systematic review. *Br J Nutr* 2006;95:849–859.

131. Berry-Kravis E, Booth G, Taylor A, et al. Bruising and the ketogenic diet: evidence for diet-induced changes in platelet function. *Ann Neurol* 2001;49:98–103.

CHAPTER 10

Diet and Cerebrovascular and Peripheral Vascular Disease

S troke is the fourth leading cause of death in the United States, just behind heart disease, cancer, and chronic lower respiratory diseases, and accounts for approximately 130,000 deaths annually (1). Most strokes are the result of thromboembolic events and are associated with atherosclerotic vascular disease. Peripheral vascular disease is the result of systemic atherogenesis and is associated with the same predisposing factors as coronary atherosclerosis. Therefore, dietary recommendations for the prevention and modification of cardiovascular risk generally are pertinent for peripheral vascular disease and stroke risk reduction as well. However, some observational evidence that dietary fat restriction may be associated with increased stroke risk suggests a possible disparity in the optimal dietary interventions for the two conditions. The weight of evidence would still favor fat restriction, and particularly saturated/trans fat restriction, below levels currently prevailing in the United States. The leading modifiable risk factor for stroke is hypertension, which is amenable to dietary prevention and management, as described in Chapter 8. Approximately 25% of all strokes are cardioembolic, and the prevention of ischemic heart disease might most effectively eliminate events in this category. Fewer than 10% of all strokes are hemorrhagic. The incidence of hemorrhagic stroke is elevated in Inuit populations with extremely high intake of marine oils rich in n-3 fatty acids, suggesting that the risk of intracranial hemorrhage may be elevated by excessive intake of platelet-inhibiting nutrients. However, thromboembolic stroke risk is reduced by the same practices. The overall evidence that stroke can be prevented by dietary means is convincing, but definitive intervention studies are still limited.

OVERVIEW

Diet

The risk of stroke is strongly correlated with both systolic and diastolic blood pressure, and advances in the pharmacologic management of hypertension are thought to be the principal explanation for declining stroke incidence and mortality over recent decades. Nonetheless, stroke remains the fourth leading cause of death and a leading cause of long-term disability among adults in the United States (2).

Elevated levels of total cholesterol, low-density lipoprotein (LDL), triglycerides, and very low-density lipoprotein, as well as depressed levels of high-density lipoprotein (HDL), are linked with atherosclerotic heart disease. Atherosclerosis is known to be a systemic disease, and the same lipid patterns are inferentially linked to cerebrovascular disease. Observational and retrospective studies have been inconclusive. A case-controlled study by Hachinski et al. (3) showed total cholesterol, LDL, and triglyceride levels to be significantly higher and HDL to be significantly lower among subjects with thromboembolic stroke compared to matched controls. Nagaraj et al. recently reported no difference in the serum lipid profiles between controls and thrombotic stroke patients (4). Recent prospective population-based studies have demonstrated significantly increased rates of ischemic stroke among men and women with low HDL levels (5–10).

Reduction of cholesterol levels in high-risk patients has been shown to reduce significantly the incidence of stroke (11,12). Whereas most trials have used pharmacotherapy, namely statin drugs, for lipid reduction, the achievement of lipid reduction by dietary means is thought to confer similar benefit. The possibility that statin-related stroke risk reduction is due to effects other than lipid lowering complicates inferences about diet, serum lipids, and stroke risk (13,14). Lifestyle intervention to reduce cholesterol would also induce diverse effects, however (see Chapter 45), and thus might lower stroke by other means as well. Additionally, although statins are commonly used and well-tolerated medications, a recent meta-analysis reviewed 13 statin trials with a total of 91,140 participants and determined that statin therapy is associated with a 9% increased risk of incident diabetes (15). However, other meta-analyses have shown a reduction in all-cause mortality with statin use (16–19).

Dietary patterns associated with optimal lipid profiles are described in detail in Chapters 7 and 45. In general, restriction of atherogenic fat (i.e., saturated and trans fat) to below 10% of total calories (and preferably below 5%); a substitution of healthful unsaturated oils from nuts, seeds, olives, and avocado; an abundant intake of fruits, vegetables, and whole grains; regular consumption of fish, beans, and lentils; and moderate intake of lean meats would be indicated. Plant-based diets have been shown to confer a large reduction in lipid levels when compared with diets that include animal products. Randomized controlled trials have shown that ovo-lacto vegetarian diets were associated with a 10% to 15% decrease in total cholesterol and LDL levels, a vegan diets were associated with 15% to 25% decreases, and combining a vegetarian diet with additional fiber, soy, and nuts was associated with a 20% to 35% decline in those lipid levels (20). Cholesterol is exclusively found in animal-based products; however, it is possible that the benefit from a plant-based diet is due to a mechanism other than purely a reduction in dietary cholesterol. Recent prospective observational studies and randomized trials have shown that the consumption of dietary cholesterol is not significantly associated with serum lipid profiles (21–23).

The Mediterranean diet, along with high-quality dietary patterns and consumption of vegetables and nuts, has been shown to be significantly associated with coronary heart disease in cohort studies and randomized controlled trials (24) and has recently been shown to be associated with decreased stroke risk. The Mediterranean diet consists of abundant intake of fresh vegetables, fruits, legumes, olive oil, and nuts, a moderate amount

of fish, poultry, dairy products, and red wine with meals, and low amounts of red meat and processed foods (25). A recent multicenter randomized trial compared cardiovascular endpoints in participants on two versions of the Mediterranean diet (one with olive oil supplementation and one with nuts) with a control low-fat diet (26). There was a significant risk reduction for stroke in Mediterranean diet groups relative to the control group (HR, 0.61; 95% CI, 0.44–0.86).

Traditional recommendations for cardiovascular disease include restriction of saturated fat and trans fat, combined, to less than 5% of total calories, with 15% of calories from monounsaturates and 10% to 15% from polyunsaturates. The ratio of n-3 to n-6 polyunsaturated should be between 1:1 and 1:4 (see Chapters 2, 7, 44, and 45), achieved by including fish, seafood, and flaxseed in the diet routinely and/or taking a fish oil supplement. However, the diet recommendations regarding saturated fat have been challenged. Saturated fats are often lumped together as one group, but should be considered as a class of compounds (27). Stearic acid, found in dark chocolate, and lauric acid, found in coconut oil, have not been proven to have detrimental effects (28). However, other saturated fatty acids, such as palmitic and myristic acid, have been shown to be associated with inflammation and atherogenesis (29,30). One observational study by Gillman et al. (31) followed 832 men in the Framingham cohort over 20 years for incident strokes. Dietary intake was assessed using a single 24-hour recall at baseline. Total intake of fat, saturated fat, and monounsaturated fat was negatively associated with stroke risk. The reliability of dietary intake assessment in this study is suspect, as is the control of confounders. Nevertheless, these results have been reproduced by subsequent epidemiological investigations (32–34), which have found inverse associations between intake of animal fat and risk of stroke. Recent diet intervention studies have also found no difference or higher adjusted stroke mortality in subjects advised to eat lower-fat diets (35–37). A recent meta-analysis of prospective cohort studies demonstrated that there is no significant evidence for concluding that dietary saturated fat is associated with an increased risk of stroke (RR, 0.81; 95% CI, 0.62 to 1.05) or cardiovascular disease (RR, 1.00; 95% CI, 0.89 to 1.11) (38). These findings are certainly provocative and suggest a need for more research but should not, on their own, refute the weight of evidence favoring restriction of potentially atherogenic fat for health promotion.

Cigarette smoking, a sedentary lifestyle, and obesity (39,40) have all been shown to contribute to stroke risk. A case-control study completed in England suggests that 80% of strokes might potentially be preventable by avoidance of these risk factors (41). A recent cohort study of nearly 40,000 women found that a healthy lifestyle— consisting of smoking abstinence, moderate alcohol consumption, regular exercise, healthy diet, and lowering of body mass index—was associated with a more than 50% reduction in risk of ischemic stroke (42).

Hypertension is the single most important modifiable risk factor for stroke, and improved detection and treatment of hypertension is thought to be the principal explanation for declining rates of cerebrovascular disease (43,44). The primary prevention of hypertension is often feasible, with diet playing a major role (see Chapter 8). The consistent prevention of hypertension by dietary means would almost certainly result in the prevention of cerebrovascular events as well (45,46).

Recent reports have demonstrated that stroke incidence in younger adults has been increasing (47), possibly secondary to increasing obesity in children and adolescents. A recent retrospective population-based study also demonstrated rising rates of acute ischemic stroke in adolescents and young adults (aged 15 to 44) along with a concurrent increase in the prevalence of hypertension, diabetes, obesity, and tobacco use in that age group. A meta-analysis of prospective studies demonstrated that overweight (RR, 1.22; 95% CI, 1.05 to 1.41) and obesity (RR, 1.64; 95% CI, 1.36 to 1.99) were independently associated with increased risk of ischemic stroke (48).

Type 2 diabetes mellitus is a strong predictor of cardiovascular disease and appears to be an independent risk factor for stroke (49). HbA1c levels and smoking appear to be associated with increased risk for first stroke among diabetics (50). As with nondiabetics, tight blood pressure control significantly reduces stroke incidence (51,52).

Consumption of dietary fiber via whole grains has been shown to predict lower risk of total and ischemic stroke (53–55); influence of glycemic load on serum lipids, glucose levels, and insulin sensitivity may play a role in this association. There is some evidence that oat consumption

lowers blood pressure (56–58), although this evidence has been challenged (59); the evidence for a cardioprotective effect of grains was deemed suggestive but not definitive in a recent Cochrane review (60).

The hypothesis that antioxidant nutrients may prevent stroke was tested in the Chicago Western Electric Study. A total of 1,843 men contributed to 46,102 person-years of observation, during which 222 incident strokes occurred (61). Although reported intakes of β-carotene and vitamin C were inversely associated with stroke risk, the relationships did not achieve statistical significance. Subsequent studies of antioxidant supplementation have been inconclusive to date, although diets rich in foods containing such micronutrients have shown strong evidence of benefit (62,63). Data from the Honolulu Heart Program were used to assess the association between milk consumption and stroke risk, given an association between dietary calcium and reduced blood pressure (64). A significant inverse association between milk consumption and stroke risk, but not between calcium intake and stroke risk, was reported. The authors suggest that milk consumption might reduce stroke risk or might be associated with other dietary and lifestyle factors contributing to risk reduction.

The importance of adequate micronutrient intake to stroke prevention is supported by data from the Linxian Nutrition Intervention Trial. Subjects from a rural Chinese population with a micronutrient-poor diet had reduced rates of hypertension and stroke when given a multivitamin/multimineral supplement rather than placebo; the effect was more pronounced in men than in women (65).

Population data have shown consistently that fruit and vegetable consumption is associated with reduced stroke risk (55,66,67). A recent review by He et al. (68) used subgroup analysis to demonstrate that this strong association holds for both hemorrhagic and ischemic stroke. For each additional serving of fruits and vegetables, the risk of stroke was reduced by 6% (95% CI, 1% to 10%) (69). Data from the Zutphen study were used to determine the role of specific micronutrients in this association (70). A total of 42 strokes occurred among 552 men followed for 15 years. Dietary histories were obtained at three times, after 5-year intervals. A strong and statistically significant relationship between flavonoid intake, particularly quercetin from black tea, and reduced stroke risk was reported (relative risk = 0.27 by quartile; 95% CI, 0.11 to 0.7). A weaker, inverse association with stroke risk was observed for carotenoids. Data extracted from vital statistics in Spain suggest a marked decline in the incidence of cerebrovascular disease over recent years related to increased fruit and decreased wine consumption (71).

Partial substitution of protein for carbohydrates in a balanced diet has been shown to improve blood pressure and lipid profiles and decrease cardiovascular risk (72). However, the source of the protein may have a strong influence on stroke risk. With respect to coronary heart disease, red meat and high-fat dairy products have been associated with increased risk, while nuts, fish, and poultry protein sources were associated with a lower risk (73). A recent prospective study of men and women observed that both unprocessed and processed red meat was linked to a higher risk of stroke (74). In comparison to a serving of red meat, a serving per day of poultry, nuts, fish, low-fat dairy, and whole-fat dairy were associated with 27%, 17%, 11%, and 10% lower risk of stroke, respectively.

Fish consumption is associated with reduced risk of cardiovascular disease. The association between stroke and fish consumption was assessed in the Chicago Western Electric Study. Among 1,847 men followed for 30 years, stroke incidence was highest among subjects in the highest quartile of fish intake (75), thus failing to suggest any benefit. Results of retrospective case-control studies of fish intake and stroke risk have likewise been conflicting (76). However, the accumulating prospective studies investigating associations between fish intake and risk of stroke have generally found significant inverse associations (77). A recent meta-analysis fish intake 3 times a week was associated with a 6% decrease in total stroke and a subanalysis of studies with stroke subtypes demonstrated a 10% reduction in ischemic and hemorrhagic strokes (78). Of note, this level of consumption was not linked to an increased risk of hemorrhagic stroke, which has been seen in association with very high intake of marine oils in the Inuit population (79,80).

In addition to its role in stroke prevention, diet may play a role in recovery. Evidence suggests that a large proportion of acute stroke patients either have preexisting malnutrition or develop malnutrition within 1 week after the event (81). Protein-energy malnutrition in this group significantly predicts poor outcome, including death (81,82). Dietary interventions to build and maintain lean body mass may offer benefit; dietary consultation is generally warranted.

Although stroke can be prevented by the pharmacologic treatment of hypertension, projections from Framingham and National Health and Nutrition Examination Survey (NHANES) data suggest that a population-based approach would confer additional benefits. Modeling by Cook et al. (83) suggests that a reduction of 2 mm Hg in the mean population diastolic blood pressure achieved through lifestyle modification could prevent 67,000 cardiovascular events and 34,000 strokes annually in the 35- to 64-year-old age group. Adherence to the so-called Mediterranean diet, rich in fruits and vegetables, fatty fish, and whole grains, has been associated with reduced risk of total and ischemic stroke (84).

Alcohol taken in low doses may protect against cerebrovascular disease, whereas higher intakes appear to increase risk (85,86). Wine may offer increased protection over other alcohol types (86,87). Modest alcohol intake—approximately 15 to 30 g per day of ethanol, or the equivalent of two drinks—may independently of other behaviors reduce the risk of atherosclerosis in the carotid arteries (88) (see Chapter 40). Alcohol consumption increases the risk of hemorrhagic stroke in a dose-dependent manner (89).

Moderate coffee and tea consumption has been shown to be correlated with a lower risk of stroke (90,91). A recent large prospective study in Japan observed that coffee and green tea consumption was associated with an inverse risk of cerebrovascular disease and stroke (92). Other smaller prospective studies have demonstrated that consumption of coffee and tea may reduce the risk of ischemic stroke in men (93) and both ischemic stroke and subarachnoid hemorrhage in women (94).

Physical activity appears to protect against both incident stroke and the degree of functional disability resulting from stroke (95–97). Moderate and high levels of activity are associated with reduced risk of total, ischemic, and hemorrhagic strokes (98). Exercise contributes directly to blood pressure control, produces favorable influences on both serum lipids and glucose, and helps control body weight, all of which may influence stroke risk.

Elevated homocysteine levels have been associated with cardiovascular disease and, to a lesser extent, cerebrovascular disease (99–105). There has been some evidence linking reduction of homocysteine with reduced carotid intimal thickness (106). A diet rich in B vitamins and folate, or a supplement containing these nutrients, may confer some protection against stroke in vulnerable individuals (107). Recent prospective trials have demonstrated, however, that while B vitamin supplementation lowers homocysteine, there is no clear evidence of protection against cardiovascular or cerebrovascular events; an adverse influence is even a possibility (108–110). Despite these data, the relatively high prevalence of vitamin B_{12} deficiency in the population at risk for ischemic stroke suggests that additional supplement trials may be warranted (111).

Magnesium supplementation, particularly in magnesium-deficient individuals, may mitigate stroke risk by inhibiting spasm of intracranial vessels. A recent prospective study evaluating the relationship between dietary magnesium intake (comparing highest and lowest quintiles of magnesium intake) and cardiovascular disease demonstrated an inverse relationship between dietary magnesium intake and mortality from hemorrhagic strokes in men (HR, 0.68; 95% CI, 0.48 to 0.96) and from total (HR, 0.47; 95% CI, 0.29 to 0.77) and ischemic strokes in women (HR, 0.50; 95% CI, 0.30 to 0.84) (112).

Higher sodium intake is associated with hypertension and increased cardiovascular morbidity and mortality (see Chapter 8). The American Public Health Association has called for a 50% reduction in sodium in processed food. If fully implemented, this measure is estimated to significantly reduce deaths due to heart disease and stroke, saving as many as 150,000 lives annually (113). A meta-analysis reported that higher salt intake was associated with a greater risk of stroke (RR, 1.23; 95% CI, 1.06 to 1.43) (114). Studies have shown that a reduction in salt intake is a cost-effective public health measure, with a significant impact on morbidity and mortality (115–117). However, several studies have suggested that there are potential harms associated with too little sodium intake (118,119). An observational study of over 28,880 patients used salt excretion as a proxy for salt intake and determined that there was J-shaped association between sodium excretion and cardiovascular events. Sodium excretion of >7 g per day was associated with an increased risk of all cardiovascular events and excretion of <3 g per day associated with increased risk of cardiovascular mortality (120).

PERIPHERAL VASCULAR DISEASE

Peripheral vascular disease is the result of systemic atherosclerosis and shares risk factors with coronary and cerebrovascular disease. Dietary interventions to modify coronary artery disease risk, described in Chapter 7, should be applied in peripheral arterial disease as well. There is evidence that clinicians tend to modify risk factors less aggressively in peripheral than in coronary arterial disease (121–123). As in patients with stroke, malnutrition is common in people with peripheral vascular disease and may lead to poorer outcomes (124). Peripheral vascular disease is associated with elevated plasma homocysteine and, therefore, may be amenable to intervention with B vitamin and folate supplementation in certain patients (125,126), although as noted, vascular benefit of homocysteine lowering is increasingly uncertain. As is the case for atherosclerotic disease in general, dietary modification of risk factors should be coupled to other lifestyle interventions, such as smoking cessation and increased physical activity, as well as all indicated pharmacologic interventions (127). A recent trial found that 1 year of daily supplementation with n-3 fatty acids, oleic acid, and vitamins B_6 and E significantly ameliorated peripheral vascular disease (128).

Plasma levels of n-3 fatty acids have been reported to correlate inversely with risk of peripheral vascular disease (129), and evidence from prospective trials to date is promising but inconclusive (130). A strong positive association between smoking and peripheral vascular disease has been consistently reported (131,132). Elevated postprandial insulin levels appear to be an independent risk factor as well, suggesting that dietary intervention to improve glycemic control (see Chapter 6) may play a role in the prevention and control of peripheral vascular disease (133,134).

NUTRIENTS, NUTRICEUTICALS, AND FUNCTIONAL FOODS

Nutrients and nutriceuticals pertinent to the prevention or management of atherosclerosis and dyslipidemias are discussed in Chapter 7; those related to the control of hypertension in Chapter 8; and those related to control of insulin levels in Chapter 6. Evidence is generally insufficient to characterize the role of single nutrients in the prevention or amelioration of cerebrovascular or peripheral vascular disease independent of these effects. The literature offers strongest support for fish oil supplementation (135–138). Intravenous magnesium as a therapy in acute stroke is a topic of ongoing investigation (139) but is not yet referable to standard care. An association between low levels of vitamin D in circulation and increased stroke risk has been observed, but implications for risk reduction are as yet speculative (140). Studies of vitamin E supplementation have demonstrated no significant clinical benefit to using vitamin E for stroke prevention (141).

An evolving area of discussion is how the interaction between genetic variation and dietary intake impacts the development of cerebrovascular disease. The gene coding for apolipoprotein A-I (apo A-I), a component of HDL, is highly variable and a particular single nucleotide polymorphism in its promoter region ($-75G>A$) results in a rare A allele that has been associated with increased apo A-I concentrations (142). A study of 755 men and 822 women demonstrated that higher dietary intake of polyunsaturated fatty acids was associated with higher HDL concentration in women who had the A allele, but the inverse effect was seen in women who had the G allele. This effect was not seen in men with either allele (143). Polyunsaturated fatty acids are also thought to interact with genetic polymorphisms in the peroxisome proliferator-activated receptor α-family (Leu162Val). For both men and women, those with the V162 allele experienced decreased fasting triglyceride concentrations with increased polyunsaturated fatty acid intake, while those with the L162 allele did not experience any association between polyunsaturated fatty acid intake and fasting triglyceride levels (144). Nutrigenomic considerations in cerebrovascular disease is an evolving field, and further research is needed in order to be able to provide dietary recommendations based on genotype.

Dietary compounds can also interact with pharmacotherapy. Statins, other than pravastatin, are metabolized via cytochrome P-450, so the consumption of grapefruit juice may inhibit cytochrome P-450 and reduce the metabolism of many statins. Additionally, preliminary research suggests that oils rich in polyunsaturated fats could interact with statins and lead to greater protective effects than either alone. A small study demonstrated that patients on statins who consumed olive oil rather than sunflower oil had improved lipid profiles (145).

■ CLINICAL HIGHLIGHTS

The predominant risk factor for stroke is hypertension, which can be prevented and modified by dietary interventions (see Chapter 8). Additional risk may be conferred by low dietary intake of n-3 fatty acids, obesity, hyperinsulinemia, hyperlipidemia, micronutrient deficiencies, and elevated plasma homocysteine. The possibility exists that excessive fat restriction may increase stroke risk, although the data are not definitive. Certain factors that reduce the risk of thromboembolic stroke, such as platelet-inhibiting nutrients—notably fish oil—may increase the risk of hemorrhagic stroke in a dose-dependent manner.

Dietary recommendations for prevention of stroke and peripheral vascular disease parallel recommendations for general health promotion. Dietary cholesterol is not associated with serum lipid profiles, but a plant-based diet has been shown to confer a reduction in lipid levels. Total dietary fat intake should be moderate (approximately 25% to 30% of total calories), with a preponderance of monounsaturated and polyunsaturated fatty acids. The possibility exists that saturated fat consumption may not be associated with increased stroke risk.

Consumption of fish and the use of flaxseed oil to increase the proportion of n-3 fatty acids in the diet appear safe and reasonable in efforts to prevent stroke and peripheral vascular disease, although risk of hemorrhage is raised if consumption is extreme. Fish oil, which provides eicosapentaenoic acid and docosahexaenoic acid, is of more certain benefit than flaxseed, which provides α-linolenic acid. Supplemental fish oil at a dose of 1 to 2 g per day is reasonable for most patients, barring intolerance or contraindications (e.g., hypersensitivity; coagulopathy).

A variety of fruits and vegetables may provide all needed micronutrients, but a multivitamin/multimineral supplement is a reasonable precaution against isolated, subclinical deficiencies, the most pertinent of which are apt to be B vitamins and folate. Definitive evidence of benefit is

lacking. Dietary sodium restriction and generous intake of potassium, magnesium, and calcium may lower blood pressure. Regular physical
activity and smoking cessation are essential elements in lifestyle management of risk for both
stroke and peripheral vascular disease. Alcohol
intake should not exceed the range consistent
with health promotion (i.e., 15 to 30 g per day
of ethanol) and at this dose may confer benefit
(see Chapter 40). The value of micronutrient
supplements in megadoses for the prevention
or modification of either stroke or peripheral
vascular disease is unsubstantiated at present,
although investigation of various nutrients (e.g.,
magnesium, vitamin D, vitamin E, flavonoids,
L-arginine) is ongoing, and thus recommendations in this area will evolve.

REFERENCES

1. Centers for Disease Control and Prevention. *Leading causes of death.* 2010. Available at http://www.cdc.gov/nchs/fastats/lcod.htm; accessed 11/21/13.
2. Miniño AM, Murphy SL, Xu J, et al. Deaths: final data for 2008. *National Vital Statistics Reports*; vol 59 no 10. Hyattsville, MD: National Center for Health Statistics, 2011.
3. Hachinski V, Graffagnino C, Beaudry M, et al. Lipids and stroke: a paradox resolved. *Arch Neurol* 1996;53:303.
4. Nagaraj S, Pai P, Bhat G, et al. Lipoprotein (a) and other lipid profile in patients with thrombotic stroke: is it a reliable marker? *J Lab Physicians* 2011;3(1):28.
5. Wannamethee SG, Shaper AG, Ebrahim S. HDL-cholesterol, total cholesterol, and the risk of stroke in middle-aged British men. *Stroke* 2000;31:1882–1888.
6. Soyama Y, Miura K, Morikawa Y, et al. Oyabe Study. High-density lipoprotein cholesterol and risk of stroke in Japanese men and women: the Oyabe Study. *Stroke* 2003;34:863–868.
7. Shahar E, Chambless LE, Rosamond WD, et al. Atherosclerosis risk in communities study. Plasma lipid profile and incident ischemic stroke: the Atherosclerosis Risk in Communities (ARIC) Study. *Stroke* 2003;34:623–631.
8. Amarenco P, Labreuche J, Touboul P-J. High-density lipoprotein-cholesterol and risk of stroke and carotid atherosclerosis: a systematic review. *Atherosclerosis* 2008;196(2):489–496. doi:10.1016/j.atherosclerosis.2007.07.033.
9. Tirschwell DL, Smith NL, Heckbert SR, et al. Association of cholesterol with stroke risk varies in stroke subtypes and patient subgroups. *Neurology* 2004;63(10):1868–1875.
10. Zhang Y, Tuomilehto J, Jousilahti P, et al. Total and high-density lipoprotein cholesterol and stroke risk. *Stroke* 2012;43(7):1768–1774.
11. Sever PS, Dahlof B, Poulter NR, et al. Prevention of coronary and stroke events with atorvastatin in hypertensive patients who have average or lower-than-average cholesterol concentrations, in the Anglo-Scandinavian Cardiac Outcomes Trial–Lipid Lowering Arm (ASCOT-LLA): a multicentre randomised controlled trial. *Lancet* 2003;361:1149–1158.
12. Waters D, Schwart GG, Olsson AG, et al. Effects of atorvastatin on stroke in patients with unstable angina on non-Q-wave myocardial infarction: a Myocardial Ischemia Reduction with Aggressive Cholesterol Lowering (MIRACL) substudy. *Circulation* 2002;106:1690–1695.
13. Endres M, Laufs U, Huang Z, et al. Stroke protection by 3-hydroxy-3-methylglutaryl (HMG)-CoA reductase inhibitors mediated by endothelial nitric oxide synthase. *Proc Natl Acad Sci USA* 1998;95:8880.
14. Vaughan CJ. Prevention of stroke and dementia with statins: effects beyond lipid lowering. *Am J Cardiol* 2003;91:23–29.
15. Sattar N, Preiss D, Murray HM, et al. Statins and risk of incident diabetes: a collaborative meta-analysis of randomised statin trials. *Lancet* 2010;375(9716):735–742. doi:10.1016/S0140-6736(09)61965-6.
16. Taylor F, Huffman MD, Macedo AF, et al. Statins for the primary prevention of cardiovascular disease. *Cochrane Database Syst Rev* 2013;1:CD004816.
17. de Vries FM, de Denig P, Pouwels KB, et al. Primary prevention of major cardiovascular and cerebrovascular events with statins in diabetic patients. *Drugs* 2012;72(18):2365–2373.
18. Kostis WJ, Cheng JQ, Dobrzynski JM, et al. Meta-analysis of statin effects in women versus men. *J Am Coll Cardiol* 2012;59(6):572–582.
19. Cholesterol Treatment Trialists' (CTT) Collaborators. The effects of lowering LDL cholesterol with statin therapy in people at low risk of vascular disease: meta-analysis of individual data from 27 randomised trials. *Lancet* 2012;380(9841):581–590.
20. Ferdowsian HR, Barnard ND. Effects of plant-based diets on plasma lipids. *Am J Cardiol* 2009;104(7):947–956.
21. Hu FB, Stampfer MJ, Rimm EB, et al. A prospective study of egg consumption and risk of cardiovascular disease in men and women. *JAMA* 1999;281(15):1387–1394.
22. Njike V, Faridi Z, Dutta S, et al. Daily egg consumption in hyperlipidemic adults—effects on endothelial function and cardiovascular risk. *Nutr J* 2010;9:28. doi:10.1186/1475-2891-9-28.
23. Lindeberg S, Jönsson T, Granfeldt Y, et al. A Palaeolithic diet improves glucose tolerance more than a Mediterranean-like diet in individuals with ischaemic heart disease. *Diabetologia* 2007;50(9):1795–1807.
24. Mente A, de Koning L, Shannon HS, et al. A systematic review of the evidence supporting a causal link between dietary factors and coronary heart disease. *Arch Intern Med.* 2009;169(7):659–669.
25. Willett WC, Sacks F, Trichopoulou A, et al. Mediterranean diet pyramid: a cultural model for healthy eating. *Am J Clin Nutr* 1995;61(6 suppl):1402S–1406S.
26. Estruch R, Ros E, Salas-Salvadó J, et al. Primary prevention of cardiovascular disease with a Mediterranean diet. *N Engl J Med* 2013;368(14):1279–1290.
27. Katz DL. Scapegoats, saints and saturated fats: old mistakes in new directions. *Huffington Post.* 2013. Available at: http://www.huffingtonpost.com/david-katz-md/saturated-fat_b_4156320.html.
28. Hunter JE, Zhang J, Kris-Etherton PM. Cardiovascular disease risk of dietary stearic acid compared with trans, other saturated, and unsaturated fatty acids: a systematic review. *Am J Clin Nutr* 2010;91(1):46–63.

29. Katz DL. Is all saturated fat the same? *Huffington Post.* 2011. Available at: http://www.huffingtonpost.com/david-katz-md/saturated-fat_b_875401.html.

30. Shrestha C, Ito T, Kawahara K, et al. Saturated fatty acid palmitate induces extracellular release of histone H3: a possible mechanistic basis for high-fat diet-induced inflammation and thrombosis. *Biochem Biophys Res Commun* 2013;437(4):573–578. doi:10.1016/j.bbrc.2013.06.117.

31. Gillman MW, Cupples LA, Millen BE, et al. Inverse association of dietary fat with development of ischemic stroke in men. *JAMA* 1997;278:2145.

32. Sauvaget C, Nagano J, Hayashi M, et al. Animal protein, animal fat, and cholesterol intakes and risk of cerebral infarction mortality in the adult health study. *Stroke* 2004;35:1531–1537.

33. Iso H, Sato S, Kitamura A, et al. Fat and protein intakes and risk of intraparenchymal hemorrhage among middle-aged Japanese. *Am J Epidemiol* 2003;157:32–39.

34. Yamagishi K, Folsom AR, Steffen LM, ARIC Study Investigators. Plasma fatty acid composition and incident ischemic stroke in middle-aged adults: the Atherosclerosis Risk in Communities (ARIC) Study. *Cerebrovasc Dis* 2013;36(1):38–46.

35. Ness AR, Hughes J, Elwood PC, et al. The long-term effect of dietary advice in men with coronary disease: follow-up of the Diet and Reinfarction Trial (DART). *Eur J Clin Nutr* 2002;56:512–518.

36. Howard BV, van Horn L, Hsia J, et al. Low-fat dietary pattern and risk of cardiovascular disease: the Women's Health Initiative Randomized Controlled Dietary Modification Trial. *JAMA* 2006;295:655–666.

37. Malhotra A. Saturated fat is not the major issue. *BMJ* 2013;347:f6340–f6340.

38. Siri-Tarino PW, Sun Q, Hu FB, et al. Meta-analysis of prospective cohort studies evaluating the association of saturated fat with cardiovascular disease. *Am J Clin Nutr* 2010;91(3):535–546.

39. Kurth T, Gaziano JM, Berger K, et al. Body mass index and the risk of stroke in men. *Arch Intern Med* 2002;162:2557–2562.

40. Kurth T, Gaziano JM, Rexrode KM, et al. Prospective study of body mass index and risk of stroke in apparently healthy women. *Circulation* 2005;111:1992–1998.

41. Shinton R. Lifelong exposures and the potential for stroke prevention: the contribution of cigarette smoking, exercise, and body fat. *J Epidemiol Community Health* 1997;51:138.

42. Kurth T, Moore SC, Gaziano M, et al. Healthy lifestyle and the risk of stroke in women. *Arch Intern Med* 2006;166:1403–1409.

43. He J, Whelton PK. Epidemiology and prevention of hypertension. *Med Clin North Am* 1997;81:1077.

44. Chobanian AV, Bakris GL, Black HR, et al. The Seventh Report of the Joint National Committee on prevention, detection, evaluation, and treatment of high blood pressure: the JNC 7 report. *JAMA* 2003;289:2560–2572.

45. Lewington S, Clarke R, Qizilbash N, et al. Age-specific relevance of usual blood pressure to vascular mortality: a meta-analysis of individual data for one million adults in 61 prospective studies. *Lancet* 2002;360:1903–1913.

46. Whelton PK, He J, Appel LJ, et al. Primary prevention of hypertension: clinical and public health advisory from the National High Blood Pressure Education Program. *JAMA* 2002;288:1882–1888.

47. Kissela BM, Khoury JC, Alwell K, et al. Age at stroke: temporal trends in stroke incidence in a large, biracial population. *Neurology* 2012;79(17):1781–1787.

48. Strazzullo P, D'Elia L, Cairella G, et al. Excess body weight and incidence of stroke: meta-analysis of prospective studies with 2 million participants. *Stroke* 2010;41(5):e418–e426.

49. Burchfiel CM, Curb JD, Rodriguez BL, et al. Glucose intolerance and 22-year stroke incidence: the Honolulu Heart Program. *Stroke* 1994;25:951–957.

50. Giorda CB, Avogaro A, Maggini M, et al. Incidence and risk factors for stroke in type 2 diabetic patients: the DAI study. *Stroke* 2007;38:1154.

51. Heart Outcomes Prevention Evaluation Study Investigators. Effects of ramipril on cardiovascular and microvascular outcomes in people with diabetes mellitus: results of the HOPE study and MICRO-HOPE substudy. *Lancet* 2000;355:253–259.

52. Lindholm LH, Ibsen H, Dahlof B, et al. Cardiovascular morbidity and mortality in patients with diabetes in the Losartan Intervention for Endpoint reduction in hypertension study (LIFE): a randomised trial against atenolol. *Lancet* 2002;359:1004–1010.

53. Oh K, Hu FB, Cho E. Carbohydrate intake, glycemic index, glycemic load, and dietary fiber in relation to risk of stroke in women. *Am J Epidemiol* 2005;161:161–169.

54. Liu S, Manson JE, Stampfer MJ. Whole grain consumption and risk of ischemic stroke in women: a prospective study. *JAMA* 2000;284:1534–1540.

55. Steffen LM, Jacobs DR, Stevens J, et al. Associations of whole-grain, refined-grain, and fruit and vegetable consumption with risks of all-cause mortality and incident coronary artery disease and ischemic stroke: the Atherosclerosis Risk in Communities (ARIC) Study. *Am J Clin Nutr* 2003;78:383–390.

56. Maki KC, Galant R, Samuel P, et al. Effects of consuming foods containing oat beta-glucan on blood pressure, carbohydrate metabolism and biomarkers of oxidative stress in men and women with elevated blood pressure. *Eur J Clin Nutr* 2006;61:786–795.

57. Keenan JM, Pins JJ, Frazel C, et al. Oat ingestion reduces systolic and diastolic blood pressure in patients with mild or borderline hypertension: a pilot trial. *J Fam Pract* 2002;51:369.

58. Pins JJ, Geleva D, Keenan JM, et al. Do whole-grain oat cereals reduce the need for antihypertensive medications and improve blood pressure control? *J Fam Pract* 2002;51:353–359.

59. Davy BM, Melby CL, Beske SD, et al. Oat consumption does not affect resting casual and ambulatory 24-h arterial blood pressure in men with high-normal blood pressure to stage I hypertension. *J Nutr* 2002;132:394–398.

60. Kelly S, Summerbell C, Brynes A, et al. Wholegrain cereals for coronary heart disease. *Cochrane Database Syst Rev* 2007;2:CD005051.

61. Daviglus ML, Orencia AJ, Dyer AR, et al. Dietary vitamin C, beta-carotene and 30-year risk of stroke: results from the Western Electric Study. *Neuroepidemiology* 1997;16:69.

62. Leppala JM, Virtamo J, Fogelholm R. Controlled trial of alpha-tocopherol and beta-carotene supplements on stroke incidence and mortality in male smokers. *Arterioscler Thromb Vasc Biol* 2000;20:230–235.

63. Hirvonen T, Virtamo J, Korhonen P, et al. Intake of flavonoids, carotenoids, vitamins C and E, and risk of stroke in male smokers. *Stroke* 2000;31:2301–2306.

64. Abbott RD, Curb JD, Rodriguez BL, et al. Effect of dietary calcium and milk consumption on risk of thromboembolic stroke in older middle-aged men. The Honolulu Heart Program. *Stroke* 1996;27:813.

65. Mark SD, Wang W, Fraumeni JF, et al. Lowered risks of hypertension and cerebrovascular disease after vitamin/mineral supplementation: the Linxian Nutrition Intervention Trial. *Am J Epidemiol* 1996;143:658.

66. Johnsen SP, Overvad K, Stripp C, et al. Intake of fruit and vegetables and the risk of ischemic stroke in a cohort of Danish men and women. *Am J Clin Nutr* 2003;78:57–64.

67. Sauvaget C, Nagano J, Allen N, et al. Vegetable and fruit intake and stroke mortality in the Hiroshima/Nagasaki Life Span Study. *Stroke* 2003;34:2355–2360.

68. He FJ, Nowson CA, MacGregor GA. Fruit and vegetable consumption and stroke: meta-analysis of cohort studies. *Lancet* 2006;367:320–326.

69. Joshipura KJ, Ascherio A, Manson JE, et al. Fruit and vegetable intake in relation to risk of ischemic stroke. *JAMA* 1999;282(13):1233–1239.

70. Keli SO, Hertog MG, Feskens EJ, et al. Dietary flavonoids, antioxidant vitamins, and incidence of stroke: the Zutphen study. *Arch Intern Med* 1996;156:637.

71. Rodriguez Artalejo F, Guallar-Castillon P, Banegas JR, et al. Consumption of fruit and wine and the decline in cerebrovascular disease mortality in Spain (1975–1993). *Stroke* 1998;8:1556.

72. Appel LJ, Sacks FM, Carey VJ, et al. Effects of protein, monounsaturated fat, and carbohydrate intake on blood pressure and serum lipids: results of the OmniHeart randomized trial. *JAMA* 2005;294(19):2455–2464.

73. Bernstein AM, Sun Q, Hu FB, et al. Major dietary protein sources and risk of coronary heart disease in women. *Circulation* 2010;122(9):876–883.

74. Micha R, Wallace SK, Mozaffarian D. Red and processed meat consumption and risk of incident coronary heart disease, stroke, and diabetes mellitus. A systematic review and meta-analysis. *Circulation* 2010;121(21):2271–2283.

75. Orencia AJ, Daviglus ML, Dyer AR, et al. Fish consumption and stroke in men. 30-year findings of the Chicago Western Electric Study. *Stroke* 1996;27:204.

76. Caicoya M. Fish consumption and stroke: a community case-control study in Asturias, Spain. *Neuroepidemiology* 2002;21:107–114.

77. Ding EL, Mozaffarian D. Optimal dietary habits for the prevention of stroke. *Semin Neurol* 2006;26:11–23.

78. Larsson SC, Orsini N. Fish consumption and the risk of stroke: a dose-response meta-analysis. *Stroke* 2011;42(12):3621–3623.

79. Bjerregaard P, Dyerberg J. Mortality from ischaemic heart disease and cerebrovascular disease in Greenland. *Int J Epidemiol* 1988;17:514–519.

80. Kromann N, Green A. Epidemiological studies in the Upernavik district, Greenland. Incidence of some chronic diseases 1950–1974. *Acta Med Scan* 1980;208:401–406.

81. Davalos A, Ricart W, Gonzalez-Huix F, et al. Effect of malnutrition after acute stroke on clinical outcome. *Stroke* 1996;27:1028.

82. FOOD Trial Collaboration. Poor nutritional status on admission predicts poor outcome after stroke: observational data from the FOOD trial. *Stroke* 2003;34:1450–1455.

83. Cook NR, Cohen J, Hebert PR, et al. Implications of small reductions in diastolic blood pressure for primary prevention. *Arch Intern Med* 1995;155:701.

84. Fung TT, Stampfer MJ, Manson JE, et al. Prospective study of major dietary patterns and stroke risk in women. *Stroke* 2004;35:2014–2019.

85. Reynolds K, Lewis LB, Nolen JD, et al. Alcohol consumption and risk of stroke: a meta-analysis. *JAMA* 2003;289:579–588.

86. Mukamal KJ, Ascherio A, Mittelman MA, et al. Alcohol and risk for ischemic stroke in men: the role of drinking patterns and usual beverage. *Ann Intern Med* 2005;142:11–19.

87. Malarcher AM, Giles WH, Croft JB, et al. Alcohol intake, type of beverage, and the risk of cerebral infarction in young women. *Stroke* 2001;32:77.

88. Kiechl S, Willeit J, Egger G, et al. Alcohol consumption and carotid atherosclerosis: evidence of dose-dependent atherogenic and antiatherogenic effects. Results from the Bruneck study. *Stroke* 1994;25:1593.

89. Klatsky AL, Armstrong MA, Sidney S, et al. Alcohol drinking and risk of hemorrhagic stroke. *Neuroepidemiology* 2002;21:115–122.

90. Hankey GJ. Nutrition and the risk of stroke. *Lancet Neurol* 2012;11(1):66–81.

91. Larsson SC, Orsini N. Coffee consumption and risk of stroke: a dose-response meta-analysis of prospective studies. *Am. J. Epidemiol* 2011;174(9):993–1001.

92. Kokubo Y, Iso H, Saito I, et al. The impact of green tea and coffee consumption on the reduced risk of stroke incidence in Japanese population: the Japan public health center-based study cohort. *Stroke.* 2013, May;44(5):1369-74.

93. Larsson SC, Männistö S, Virtanen MJ, et al. Coffee and tea consumption and risk of stroke subtypes in male smokers. *Stroke* 2008;39(6):1681–1687.

94. Larsson SC, Virtamo J, Wolk A. Coffee consumption and risk of stroke in women. *Stroke* 2011;42(4):908–912.

95. Fletcher GF. Exercise in the prevention of stroke. *Health Rep* 1994;6:106.

96. Hu FB, Stampfer MJ, Colditz GA, et al. Physical activity and risk of stroke in women. *JAMA* 2000;283:2961–2967.

97. Wendel-Vos GCW, Schuit AJ, Feskens EJM, et al. Physical activity and stroke. A meta-analysis of observational data. *Int J Epidemiol* 2004;33:787–798.

98. Lee CD, Folsom AR, Blair SN. Physical activity and stroke risk: a meta-analysis. *Stroke* 2003;34:2475.

99. Furie KL, Kelly PJ. Homocyst(e)ine and stroke. *Semin Neurol* 2006;26:24–32.

100. Clarke R, Lewington S. Homocysteine and coronary heart disease. *Semin Vasc Med* 2002;2:391–399.

101. Clarke R. Homocysteine-lowering trials for prevention of heart disease and stroke. *Semin Vasc Med* 2005;5:215–222.

102. Clarke R, Armitage J. Vitamin supplements and cardiovascular risk: review of the randomized trials of homocysteine-lowering vitamin supplements. *Semin Thromb Hemost* 2000;26:341–348.

103. B-Vitamin Treatment Trialists' Collaboration. Homocysteine-lowering trials for prevention of cardiovascular events: a

review of the design and power of the large randomized trials. *Am Heart J* 2006;151(2):282–287.

104. Stanger O, Herrmann W, Pietrzik K, et al. Clinical use and rational management of homocysteine, folic acid, and B vitamins in cardiovascular and thrombotic diseases. *Z Kardiol* 2004;93:439–453.

105. Schwammenthal Y, Tanne D. Homocysteine, B-vitamin supplementation, and stroke prevention: from observational to interventional trials. *Lancet Neurol* 2004;3: 493–495.

106. Tungkasereerak P, Ong-ajyooth L, Chaiyasoot W, et al. Effect of short-term folate and vitamin B supplementation on blood homocysteine level and carotid artery wall thickness in chronic hemodialysis patients. *J Med Assoc Thai* 2006;89:1187–1193.

107. van Guelpen B, Hultdin J, Johansson I, et al. Folate, vitamin B_{12}, and risk of ischemic and hemorrhagic stroke: a prospective, nested case-referent study of plasma concentrations and dietary intake. *Stroke* 2005;36(7): 1426–1431.

108. Toole JF, Malinow MR, Chambless LE, et al. Lowering homocysteine in patients with ischemic stroke to prevent recurrent stroke, myocardial infarction, and death: the Vitamin Intervention for Stroke Prevention (VISP) randomized controlled trial. *JAMA* 2004;291:565–574.

109. Lonn E, Yusuf S, Arnold MJ, et al. Homocysteine lowering with folic acid and B vitamins in vascular disease. *N Engl J Med* 2006;354:1567–1577.

110. Bonaa KH, Njolstad I, Ueland PM, et al. Homocysteine lowering and cardiovascular events after acute myocardial infarction. *N Engl J Med* 2006;354:1578–1588.

111. Fisher M, Lees K, Spence JD. Nutrition and stroke prevention. *Stroke* 2006;37:2430.

112. Zhang W, Iso H, Ohira T, et al. Associations of dietary magnesium intake with mortality from cardiovascular disease: the JACC study. *Atherosclerosis* 2012;221(2): 587–595.

113. Havas S, Roccella EJ, Lenfant C. Reducing the public health burden from elevated blood pressure levels in the United States by lowering intake of dietary sodium. *Am J Public Health* 2004;94(1):19–22.

114. Strazzullo P, D'Elia L, Kandala N-B, et al. Salt intake, stroke, and cardiovascular disease: meta-analysis of prospective studies. *BMJ* 2009;339(1):b4567–b4567.

115. Selmer RM, Kristiansen IS, Haglerod A, et al. Cost and health consequences of reducing the population intake of salt. *J Epidemiol Commun Health* 2000;54: 697–702.

116. Murray CJ, Lauer JA, Hutubessy RC, et al. Effectiveness and costs of interventions to lower systolic blood pressure and cholesterol: a global and regional analysis on reduction of cardiovascular-disease risk. *Lancet* 2003; 361:717–725.

117. Asaria P, Chisholm D, Mathers C, et al. Chronic disease prevention: health effects and financial costs of strategies to reduce salt intake and control tobacco use. *Lancet* 2007;370:2044–2053.

118. Paterna S, Parrinello G, Cannizzaro S, et al. Medium term effects of different dosage of diuretic, sodium, and fluid administration on neurohormonal and clinical outcome in patients with recently compensated heart failure. *Am J Cardiol* 2009;103(1):93–102.

119. Ekinci EI, Clarke S, Thomas MC, et al. Dietary salt intake and mortality in patients with type 2 diabetes. *Diabetes Care* 2011;34(3):703–709. doi:10.2337/dc10-1723.

120. O'Donnell MJ, Yusuf S, Mente A, et al. Urinary sodium and potassium excretion and risk of cardiovascular events. *JAMA* 2011;306(20):2229–2238.

121. McDermott MM, Mehta S, Ahn H, et al. Atherosclerotic risk factors are less intensively treated in patients with peripheral arterial disease than in patients with coronary artery disease. *J Gen Intern Med* 1997;12:209.

122. Tornwall ME, Virtamo J, Haukka JK, et al. Prospective study of diet, lifestyle, and intermittent claudication in male smokers. *Am J Epidemiol* 2000;151:892–901.

123. Mukherjee D, Lingam P, Chetcuti S, et al. Missed opportunities to treat atherosclerosis in patients undergoing peripheral vascular interventions: insights from the University of Michigan Peripheral Vascular Disease Quality Improvement Initiative, (PVD-QI2). *Circulation* 2002; 106:1909–1912.

124. Spark JI, Robinson JM, Gallavin L, et al. Patients with chronic critical limb ischemia have reduced total antioxidant capacity and impaired nutrition status. *Eur J Vasc Endovasc Surg* 2002;24:535–539.

125. Cheng SW, Ting AC, Wong J. Fasting total plasma homocysteine and atherosclerotic peripheral vascular disease. *Ann Vasc Surg* 1997;11:217.

126. Merchant AT, Hu FB, Spiegelman D, et al. The use of B vitamin supplements and peripheral arterial disease risk in men are inversely related. *J Nutr* 2003;133: 2863–2867.

127. Cooke JP, Ma AO. Medical therapy of peripheral arterial occlusive disease. *Surg Clin North Am* 1995;75:569.

128. Carrero JJ, Lopez-Huertas E, Salmeron LM, et al. Daily supplementation with (n-3) PUFAs, oleic acid, folic acid, and vitamins B-6 and E increases pain-free walking distance and improves risk factors in men with peripheral vascular disease. *J Nutr* 2005;135:1393–1399.

129. Leng GC, Horrobin DF, Fowkes FG, et al. Plasma essential fatty acids, cigarette smoking, and dietary antioxidants in peripheral arterial disease. A population-based case-control study. *Arterioscler Thromb* 1994;14:471.

130. Sommerfield T, Hiatt WR. Omega-3 fatty acids for intermittent claudication. *Cochrane Database Syst Rev* 2004;3:CD003833.

131. Fowkes FG, Housley E, Riemersma RA, et al. Smoking, lipids, glucose intolerance, and blood pressure as risk factors for peripheral atherosclerosis compared with ischemic heart disease in the Edinburgh Artery Study. *Am J Epidemiol* 1992;135:331.

132. Powell JT, Edwards RJ, Worrell PC, et al. Risk factors associated with the development of peripheral arterial disease in smokers: a case-control study. *Atherosclerosis* 1997;129:41.

133. Price JF, Lee AJ, Fowkes FG. Hyperinsulinemia: a risk factor for peripheral arterial disease in the non-diabetic general population. *J Cardiovasc Risk* 1996;3:501.

134. Carrero JJ, Grimble. Does nutrition have a role in peripheral vascular disease? *Br J Nutr* 2006;95:217–229.

135. Riccioni G, Bucciarelli T, Mancini B, et al. The role of the antioxidant vitamin supplementation in the prevention of cardiovascular diseases. *Expert Opin Investig Drugs* 2007;16:25–32.

136. Psota TL, Gebauer SK, Kris-Etherton P. Dietary omega-3 fatty acid intake and cardiovascular risk. *Am J Cardiol* 2006;98:3i–18i.

137. Huang HY, Caballero B, Chang S, et al. The efficacy and safety of multivitamin and mineral supplement use to prevent cancer and chronic disease in adults: a systematic review for a National Institutes of Health state-of-the-science conference. *Ann Intern Med* 2006;145:372–385.

138. Wang C, Harris WS, Chung M, et al. n-3 Fatty acids from fish or fish-oil supplements, but not alpha-linolenic acid, benefit cardiovascular disease outcomes in primary- and secondary-prevention studies: a systematic review. *Am J Clin Nutr* 2006;84:5–17.

139. Aslanyan S, Weir CJ, Muir KW, et al. Magnesium for treatment of acute lacunar stroke syndromes: further analysis of the IMAGES trial. *Stroke* 2007;38:1269–1273.

140. Poole KE, Loveridge N, Barker PJ, et al. Reduced vitamin D in acute stroke. *Stroke* 2006;37:243–245.

141. Bin Q, Hu X, Cao Y, et al. The role of vitamin E (tocopherol) supplementation in the prevention of stroke. A meta-analysis of 13 randomised controlled trials. *Thromb Haemost* 2011;105(4):579–585.

142. Juo S-HH, Wyszynski DF, Beaty TH, et al. Mild association between the A/G polymorphism in the promoter of the apolipoprotein A-I gene and apolipoprotein A-I levels: a meta-analysis. *Am J Med Genet* 1999;82(3):235–241.

143. Ordovas JM, Corella D, Cupples LA, et al. Polyunsaturated fatty acids modulate the effects of the APOA1 G-A polymorphism on HDL-cholesterol concentrations in a sex-specific manner: the Framingham study. *Am J Clin Nutr* 2002;75(1):38–46.

144. Tai ES, Corella D, Demissie S, et al. Polyunsaturated fatty acids interact with the PPARA-L162V polymorphism to affect plasma triglyceride and apolipoprotein C-III concentrations in the Framingham Heart Study. *J Nutr* 2005;135(3):397–403.

145. Sánchez-Muniz FJ, Bastida S, Gutiérrez-García O, et al. Olive oil-diet improves the simvastatin effects with respect to sunflower oil-diet in men with increased cardiovascular risk: a preliminary study. *Nutr Hosp* 2009;24(3):333–339.

CHAPTER 11

Diet and Immunity

I mmune function refers broadly to the various means by which the body distinguishes and defends self from nonself. Because not all moieties identified as "nonself" are pathogenic, and because mistakes in such differentiation are made, not all immune responses are salutary. Atopy and autoimmune disease represent aspects of immune function, albeit undesirable ones (see Chapters 20 and 24).

Physical barriers—the skin and mucous membranes—serve the purpose of delimiting exposure to foreign materials and thus comprise important constituents of immunity. To the extent that nutrition influences the integrity of such barriers (see Chapters 18, 22, and 23 for GI; skin; and wound healing respectively), it influences both the structures and function of the immune system.

When immunity is discussed, however, it is most often the actions of both the humoral and cell-mediated systems in defense of the body against microbial and toxic invasions that are implied. The humoral immune system comprises the five immunoglobulin classes IgA, D, E, G, and M produced by B lymphocytes, along with other noncellular elements such as the complement cascade. Immunoglobulins are glycoproteins and therefore are dependent on adequate protein nutriture, as well as on the enzymes and cofactors essential to protein metabolism. The cell-mediated system includes T lymphocytes and various granulocytes, both phagocytic and nonphagocytic. Increasingly, the immune system is discussed in terms of innate and adaptive components, the former referring to monocyte and macrophage cell lines that do not require antigenic priming and the latter referring to antigen-specific responses for which such priming is required (1). After immune cell activation, the metabolic needs are met by increased utilization of glucose, amino acids, and fatty acids.

Along with the cellular elements, normal immune function is dependent on cytokines and complement, chemical messengers orchestrating the response of immune cells. Included in an immune response are hematopoietic mitotic divisions, cell–cell interactions, and the expression of reactive cell-surface proteins. The entire immune system is subject to neuroendocrine regulation, which in turn is influenced in various ways by nutritional status. For instance, Leptin regulates both appetite, T-cell activity, and promotion of innate immune cells (2).

The bone marrow is one of the largest and most metabolically active tissues in the body, producing billions of blood cells daily. Hematopoiesis is dependent on the availability of adequate substrate for cell formation. Intake of nutrients likely to be rate limiting in the production of immune system components offers the possibility of modifying immunocompetence through dietary manipulation. Also relevant are dietary components that influence everything from oxidation to the rate of apoptosis.

OVERVIEW

Diet

Antibody formation is impaired by deficiencies in total protein and/or B-complex vitamins. Natural conditions make the study of single-nutrient deficiencies on immune function difficult, as nutrient deficiency is typically the result of generalized malnutrition. Environmental circumstances conducive to malnutrition tend to favor the transmission of infectious disease as well (e.g., poverty, poor sanitation, displacement), further complicating interpretation of naturally occurring states of nutritional immunosuppression in humans. Therefore, the effects of isolated nutrient deficiencies on immune function have been investigated predominantly by use of animal models.

Data on the effects of dietary patterns on the immune system are limited. The anti-inflammatory effects of the Mediterranean diet are well known, and are mostly related to its antioxidative effects. Additional studies have also shown decreased immune cell activation associated with the Mediterranean diet (3). There is some evidence relating gluten intake and an increase in IgA immune complexes, which may be related to the geographic prevalence of IgA nephropathy (4). A study on the immune status of vegans compared to nonvegetarians demonstrated that vegans had a significantly lower level of platelets, leukocytes, lymphocytes, and complement factor 3, yet there was no difference in functional immunocompetence as measured by mitogen stimulation or natural killer cell cytotoxic assay (5). There have also been several reports demonstrating the clinical benefit of a vegetarian diet for patients with rheumatoid arthritis (RA). A study examining laboratory variables in RA patients treated with a vegetarian diet noticed a decrease in several inflammatory markers, notably leukocyte count, IgM rheumatoid factor, and complement components C3 and C4 (6). Additionally, a systemic review analyzing the effect of a vegetarian diet on patients with RA showed a statistically and clinically significant long-term disease improvement with the dietary intervention (7).

Protein-energy malnutrition in humans is associated with impairment of both humoral and cell-mediated immunity; T-helper cells are suppressed, whereas T-suppressor cells are spared or even generated at an increased rate. Production of, and response to, interleukin 1 appears to be diminished by protein malnutrition. Globally, protein-energy malnutrition, vitamin A deficiency, and iron deficiency constitute important and prevalent adverse influences on immune function (8).

Of the B complex, pyridoxine, pantothenic acid, riboflavin, folate, and B_{12} have the greatest impact on immune function. B_{12} repletion in patients with pernicious anemia has been shown to reverse anergy on skin testing.

Malnutrition during gestation apparently can result in prolonged immunocompromise even if the diet is adequate during the neonatal period. Low birth weight is associated with impaired development of the spleen and thymus and possibly impaired placental transfer of maternal immunoglobulin G (see Chapter 26).

Overnutrition may interfere with immunity, although the data are limited. Specifically, obesity has been shown to impair immune function through alteration of inflammatory mediators and the subsequent derangement of leukocyte counts and the cell-mediated immune response (9). Chronic low-grade inflammation associated with obesity can increase the risk of developing multiple diseases, including type 2 diabetes, atherosclerosis, hypertension, liver disease, asthma, cancer, chronic kidney disease, and infection (1,10). Calorie restriction, studied for effects on longevity, may enhance immune function, although variable results have been generated, and human data are scant. Animal studies may indicate a benefit of caloric restriction on the immune system; however, these studies are confounded by the energy requirements necessary to mount a response to infections, and similar studies in humans are limited (11). Excess intake of dietary fat may interfere with reticuloendothelial system function. Phagocyte function is impaired by hyperglycemia in diabetes; the role of dietary sugar in nondiabetics is less clear. In general, the rate of infection in states of extreme malnutrition is lower than the immune system disruption would suggest. Some authorities have speculated that malnutrition might result in some enhancement of immune function or merely render the body less accommodating to microbial pathogens.

Epidemiologic data reveal the total leukocyte count to be a potent predictor of various morbidities and all-cause mortality. Leukocyte activity generates reactive oxygen moieties, a possible mechanism for adverse effects. Reactive oxidant species such as H_2O_2 and HOCl exert an inhibitory influence on both T and B lymphocytes and natural killer cells. Dietary intake levels and serum levels of several antioxidant nutrients, including vitamin C, vitamin E, and β-carotene, are inversely correlated with neutrophil and total leukocyte counts. Thus, the white blood cell count may emerge as a convenient gauge of the adequacy of antioxidant intake (12). These findings are preliminary and require further study before any clinical application ensues. Studies of isolated antioxidants in humans convey a generally precautionary message, with little evidence of benefit and some of potential harm (13–16).

The health benefits of a diet with relatively high fruit and vegetable intake are thought to include enhanced immunity. Although the nutrient complexity of whole foods makes nutrient-specific causality difficult to establish, potential benefits have been proposed for vitamins, minerals, sterols, fiber, and antioxidant phytochemicals.

Gradual attenuation of immune function with aging is well established and may be an important contributor to functional deterioration with age. Reduced T-cell function may be the earliest harbinger of age-related immunocompromise and may be related to thymic involution (17). Although a decline in immune function with age has been deemed normal, epidemiologic evidence suggests that age-related immune dysfunction may be due, at least in part, to nutritional deficiencies. The regulation of T-cell function tends to deteriorate with age, whereas immunoglobulin levels tend to rise. Specific antibody responses diminish. Protein and zinc deficiencies appear to be particularly prevalent and important contributors to dysregulation of immune function in elderly individuals. Limited evidence suggests that supplementation can confer clinical benefit (18). There is some evidence, reviewed by Bogden and Louria (17), that a daily multivitamin/multimineral supplement for 6 to 12 months in older adults improves measures of cell-mediated immunity. Data on the benefits of multivitamin supplementation much beyond 1 year are lacking. Given that deficiencies of one or more micronutrients are found in up to one-third of all free-living elderly, a multivitamin/multimineral supplement for all individuals over age 50 is likely to be both appropriate and cost-effective, and it conforms to recommendations for general health promotion while offering a potential, if uncertain, boost to immune system function (19). That said, the evidence of health benefit is uncertain at present (20).

NUTRIENTS, NUTRICEUTICALS, AND FUNCTIONAL FOODS

Zinc

Zinc deficiency is considered one of the most prevalent nutritional deficiencies worldwide, due both to limited dietary intake and the presence in the food supply of phytic acid (found in wheat bran, whole grain cereals, and many raw vegetables), a zinc chelator. Zinc is an essential cofactor in more than 90 metalloenzyme systems; its deficiency interferes with cellular replication. Zinc deficiency in particular appears to arrest T-cell maturation. Studies in mice have shown that moderate-to-severe zinc deficiency leads to bone marrow depletion of B lymphocytes and to peripheral lymphopenia. Further, observational studies in humans have demonstrated that inadequate zinc stores were a risk factor for pneumonia in the elderly (21).

These studies suggest that zinc deficiency leads to chronic elevation of glucocorticoid levels, which in turn suppress immunity. The combination of zinc deficiency and elevated cortisol is thought to augment apoptosis of prelymphocytes in the bone marrow. The same conditions that lead to lymphopenia apparently spare, at least relatively, granulocyte precursors. The possibility exists that granulocytosis and lymphopenia in response to zinc deficiency represent a form of homeostatic prioritization in the face of resource shortages, although this is unverified. Phagocytic cells, representing a first line of defense, may be favored over lymphocytes during periods of malnutrition. Zinc repletion appears to restore normal immunity in zinc-deficient organisms within as little as 2 weeks. Studies have shown that younger adults have higher plasma zinc, lower oxidative markers, and decreased inflammatory markers when compared to elderly subjects. Following zinc supplementation, elderly subjects developed increased plasma zinc levels, and subsequently decreased oxidative stress markers and inflammatory markers (22). However, excessive zinc supplementation may adversely affect immune function (17).

Iron

Iron deficiency is associated with impaired cell-mediated immunity. If iron deficiency occurs in the context of general malnutrition, protein deficiency will suppress levels of anti-inflammation. Under such circumstances, repleted iron is more readily available to microorganisms than to a human host; therefore, iron repletion before protein repletion might be harmful, promoting bacterial replication. Iron excess is also associated with impaired immunity, along with susceptibility to tumorigenesis.

Essential Amino Acids/Arginine

Deficiency of any of the essential amino acids appears to suppress humoral immunity, whereas intake of nonessential amino acids appears not to be limiting given adequate total protein intake. Animal studies suggest that imbalances of protein intake can impair immunity even in the absence of overt deficiency; excessive dietary leucine, for example, has been shown to reduce antibody responses in animals. Sulfur-containing amino acids involved in the synthesis of glutathione may be in particular demand during infection/inflammation due to the increased oxidative stresses, suggesting that supplementation might be beneficial (23).

Arginine is a conditionally essential amino acid (see Chapter 3). Studies in animals and in vitro suggest that supplemental L-arginine may be immunostimulatory (24). The use of L-arginine in states of human immunodeficiency has been proposed. Reduced hospital stay following surgery has been observed in supplemented patients. Arginine is an essential nitrogen donor in nitric oxide synthesis. Macrophages produce nitric oxide after Toll-like receptor activation, which is consequently toxic to several pathogens and thus plays an important role in the innate arm of the immune response. Of note, certain pathogens have inherent arginase activity, which blocks arginine availability for nitric oxide synthase (25). The effects of nitric oxide on the vasculature are potentially an important component of the response to severe infection (26); enhancement of endothelial function with arginine supplementation has been reported (27–29). Immune enhancement has been ascribed to both glutamine (30) and taurine (31) as well.

Uracil

The ribonucleotide uracil is manufactured from ingested amino acids and is not considered an essential nutrient. There is some evidence that dietary supplementation is beneficial to immune function during states of high metabolic stress (32).

Vitamin C

Whereas overt vitamin C deficiency interferes with normal immune function, studies of high-dose supplementation as a means of enhancing immunity have not produced convincing results. Normal vitamin C nutriture is vital to skin integrity, with skin representing a vital immune system barrier (see Chapters 22 and 23). The importance of at least adequate vitamin C intake to immune function is well established (33). Megadoses of vitamin C cannot be recommended, however, as a means of enhancing resistance to viral infection on the basis of available data. A recent study reviewed the benefits of using vitamin C

as a prophylactic or therapeutic measure against pneumonia. They found weak evidence supporting its use prophylactically. However, vitamin C may be beneficial for treating community acquired pneumonia if the patient was found to have low vitamin C levels (34). The current recommended dietary allowance (RDA) for vitamin C is 90 mg for men and 75 mg for women (35).

Vitamin A and Carotenoids

Vitamin A deficiency is associated with disruption of mucosal and epithelial barriers, as well as impaired antibody responses. Vitamin A metabolites are also known to enhance cytotoxicity, T-cell proliferation via upregulation of IL-2 secretion and T-cell signaling, dendritic cell maturation and antigen presenting capabilities, and gut IgA production (36). High-dose supplementation of vitamin A may cause immunosuppression. Carotenoid supplementation, particularly β-carotene, has been studied as a means of reducing cancer risk (see Chapter 12). Randomized trial data do not support a beneficial effect to date. The relationship between vitamin A and infection appears to be bidirectional; for example, infection with *Schistosoma mansoni* has been reported to deplete vitamin A (37). Malaria has been reported to induce acute-phase reactants that deplete carrier proteins and thereby lower levels of serum carotenoids and retinol. Thus, the reliability of serum measures of these micronutrients during acute infection is highly suspect (38). Vitamin A supplementation of children in the developing world has been established as a means of preventing infectious disease and death, specifically decreasing diarrhea and mortality in malnourished or HIV-infected children, and is a priority for the World Health Organization (39).

Vitamin E

Vitamin E, a term that actually refers to a group of related compounds of both the tocopherol and tocotrienol chemical classes, is important to immune function both in its role as antioxidant and as a cell membrane constituent. A relatively high amount of vitamin E is found in the membranes of immune cells since they are highly susceptible to oxidative damage (40). There is suggestive evidence that vitamin E supplementation can enhance both cellular and humoral immunity.

Vitamin E may be of particular importance in combination with n-3 fatty acids (see Essential Fatty Acids). The RDA for vitamin E intake may not be optimal with regard to immune function, particularly in the elderly (41). A randomized trial of vitamin E supplementation for 4 months in healthy elderly subjects demonstrated enhancement of clinically relevant measures of T-cell function (42); a dose of 200 mg per day was superior to both higher and lower doses. The possibility of adverse effects of high doses of vitamin E on immune function and other aspects of health is noteworthy (13–15). Optimal dosing, nutrient context, and formulation remain uncertain. Vitamin E is found in foods in the company of polyunsaturated fat, and it mitigates the effects of n-3 polyunsaturated fatty acid (PUFA) on various aspects of immune function (43). Thus, some combination of vitamin E and fish oil supplementation may offer benefits as yet to be clarified. A total daily intake of vitamin E from both food sources and supplements up to but not exceeding 200 mg per day seems prudent while awaiting further research. The RDA for adults is 15 mg of α-tocopherol or equivalent (35).

Vitamin D

The active form of vitamin D, 1,25-dihydroxyvitamin D (3), regulates bone formation and additionally modulates multiple immune cells, including monocytes, macrophages, dendritic cells, and lymphocytes. Additionally, immune cells contain vitamin D–activating enzymes, which allow local activation within the immune system. Multiple epidemiologic reports have associated vitamin D deficiency with increased risk of chronic infections, specifically from *Mycobacterium tuberculosis*, and autoimmune disorders. Recent studies have shown that active vitamin D has multiple effects on the immune system, including increase in chemotaxis, phagocytosis, and T-cell activation. Supplementation has been associated with a decreased overall mortality in a recent randomized control trial (44), and has been reported to increase sputum clearance of acid fast bacilli and promote radiologic improvement of patients with tuberculosis (45). Vitamin D supplementation has also shown benefits in chronic obstructive pulmonary disease patients with a baseline deficiency by reducing the incidence of exacerbations (46). Further, supplementation has been associated with a lower risk of developing autoimmune disorders (47). However, a recent study showed that vitamin D_3 supplementation did not reduce the incidence or severity of upper respiratory tract infections in healthy adults (48).

Essential Fatty Acids

Diets high in n-6 PUFAs appear to promote tumorigenesis. Dietary n-3 PUFAs inhibit the generation of arachidonic acid and inflammatory eicosanoids. This effect may be beneficial in states of chronic inflammation, as discussed in Chapter 20. A randomized trial involving 40 healthy adults over age 65 showed that 2 months of supplementation with black currant seed oil, a source of both n-6 and n-3 essential fatty acids, enhanced delayed-type hypersensitivity skin responses, and reduced production of prostaglandin E_2 (49). The clinical significance of these results and the effects of n-3 PUFA supplementation on susceptibility to infection are as yet uncertain. However, a new study demonstrates that fish oil supplementation may be beneficial in reducing neutropenia secondary to chemotherapy (50). There has long been speculation that increasing n-3 fatty acid intake may serve to reduce the risk of chronic, inflammatory diseases such as atherosclerosis but at the cost of increased vulnerability to certain infectious pathogens (51). Benefits of fish oil supplementation in chronic inflammatory states, such as RA, have been reported (52) (see Chapter 20).

In general, high intake of long-chain n-3 PUFA inhibits a wide range of immune functions, including antigen presentation, adhesion molecule expression, proinflammatory cytokine, and eicosanoid production, while inducing lymphocyte apoptosis. Although n-3 fatty acids have an anti-inflammatory effect deemed beneficial, they also tend to suppress T-cell function; the latter effect apparently is mitigated by vitamin E supplementation (53). At present, arguments that total dietary n-3 PUFA, the ratio of n-3 to n-6 PUFA, or the total amount of each of these fat classes in the diet is most germane to health outcomes (43).

Selenium

Selenium is an essential trace element shown to enhance immune function and mitigate cancer risk when supplemented in selenium-deficient individuals. Some of the most convincing evidence has been derived from study in the Linxian province in China, an area of selenium-deficient soil and hyperendemic rates of upper GI tumors (54). The utility of selenium supplementation in selenium-replete individuals is a matter of conjecture. The topic has been extensively reviewed (55–59), and the consensus at present is that much will depend on the results of ongoing clinical trials.

CLA

Conjugated linolenic acid (CLA) refers to a mix of 18-carbon n-6 PUFAs of both cis and trans configuration. CLA has of late generated interest for a potential role in weight control (see Chapter 5), although evidence for such an effect is inconclusive if not contrary (60). Potential effects of CLA on immune function are of increasing interest, as evidenced by coverage in the popular press. A current study suggested oral CLA supplementation may decrease disease activity and improve quality of life in patients with Crohn's disease (61). Certain reviews, however, suggest that evidence for salutary effects is as yet unconvincing and that studies to date have been hampered by inconsistency in the selection of CLA isomers (62,63).

SPECIAL TOPICS

Physical Activity

Whereas moderate, regular physical activity facilitates weight control, improves vascular health, and generally supports optimal immune function, intense exertion is consistently associated with immunosuppression in the short term. This effect, which lasts from 3 to 72 hours, is apparently exacerbated by relative carbohydrate depletion and mitigated by carbohydrate ingestion before or during exercise (64,65). Potential attenuation of the immunosuppressive effect of intense exercise by various nutrient supplements is of considerable interest and the subject of ongoing research, but available evidence is as yet unconvincing. Saliva IgA secretion has been shown to increase in military personnel receiving nutritional supplementation during an 8-week intense training program. Additionally, there was a prevention in training induced decrease in total leucocyte, lymphocyte, and monocyte counts (66).

Breast Milk

Breast-feeding is addressed in Chapter 27. Breast milk imparts to the neonate preformed antibodies that supplement innate immunity. Increasing evidence suggests that breast milk also functions in priming the acquired immune system of the newborn. There is speculation that the substitution of formula for breast milk may be a contributing factor to increases in the prevalence of atopy, asthma, and autoimmune disease (67).

Probiotics

The potential health benefits of commensal bacteria known as probiotics are of considerable interest at present; the literature on the topic and the gut microbiota is rapidly expanding (68–73). There is a strong link between the gut microbiota and the development of the gut-associated lymphoid tissue, immune system, and mucosal barrier. Alterations to the microbiota, whether through antibiotics or sanitation efforts, may predispose patients to a variety of diseases, including allergies, asthma, autoimmune diseases, diabetes, heart disease, and cancer (73–75). Whether the ingestion of bacteria, including lactobacilli and bifidobacteria, is correctly considered a nutrition topic may itself be debatable. The topic, however, is generally included in discussions of functional food development (76). There is evidence that probiotics can enhance specific aspects of immune function as measured in vitro. Further, in vivo studies in mice demonstrated that probiotic mixtures can reduce T-cell and B-cell responsiveness and downregulate certain cytokine production, which may be beneficial in certain autoimmune disease (77). A review of studies examining probiotic effect on immune function has shown that probiotic use improves phagocytosis, natural killer cell activity, and mucosal immunoglobulin A production (78). Interestingly, gut microbiota play a vital role in nutrient processing, specifically short chain fatty acids (SCFAs), which is an end product of microbial fermentation of micronutrients such as plant polysaccharides, and micronutrient synthesis and absorption, including B vitamins, folate, and vitamin K. SCFAs provide both an energy source and influence on immune cell response (2). Studies in infants have shown that probiotic use may decrease episodes of diarrhea and prevent necrotizing enterocolitis (79,80).

However, a clear mechanism for the influence of probiotics on infection or immune disorders over time remains to be established. Studies show that these effects are closely related to specific bacterial strain supplementation and individual responsiveness (1,81). The use of probiotics specifically for gastrointestinal disorders is addressed in Chapter 18.

Human Immunodeficiency Virus Infection

Energy expenditure rises with human immunodeficiency virus (HIV) infection, and depletion of vitamin B_{12}, vitamin D, folate, zinc, and selenium have been reported as the CD4 count falls below 500 (82). The acquired immunodeficiency syndrome (AIDS) is associated with wasting; the wasting syndrome seen in HIV infection is an AIDS-defining condition (83). Loss of 10% or more of baseline body weight generally is associated with diminished functional capacity.

In addition to appropriate antiretroviral therapy, nutritional supplementation and appetite stimulation are important adjuvants in this syndrome (84). There is some evidence for improving CD4 counts in HIV patients on antiretroviral therapy with micronutrient supplementation (85). However, the evidence for high-dose supplementation is not as clear. High-dose supplementation did not confer added benefits and may increase alanine transaminase levels in a recent randomized control trial (86), yet another review reports improved CD4 cell counts and survival in five out of six trials using high-dose micronutrient interventions; vitamin A supplementation was not beneficial (87). Of note, vitamin B, C, and E supplementation did not reduce mortality in HIV-exposed infants in another recent randomized control trial (88), yet there has been evidence supporting zinc supplementation and prevention of immune failure and diarrhea in HIV patients (89). Decreased bone mineral density (BMD) is seen in HIV patients; however, vitamin D did not increase bone mass despite elevating serum vitamin D concentrations in HIV affected youth (90). Although, there have been studies in adults which may show improvement of BMD with vitamin D supplementation. Of note, HIV medication may be involved in vitamin D metabolism and could make these results difficult to interpret (91). Vitamin D deficiency is common in both pediatric and adult HIV patients and may be related

to various comorbidities in pediatric HIV patients, including infections, growth failure, wasting, and coronary artery disease (91,92). An imbalance between caloric intake and the metabolic demands imposed by the primary HIV infection as well as any secondary opportunistic infections is thought to be the principal antecedent of wasting, but effects of specific inflammatory cytokines have been suggested (83). Reviews conducted in the past two decades address the role of pharmacologic support with megestrol acetate, dronabinol, and/or testosterone analogues, as well as growth hormone (83,93–95). Clinical trials suggest that resistance training may offer the benefits of anabolic steroids without the attendant adverse metabolic effects (96,97); the inclusion of exercise in the treatment of AIDS-related wasting should be routine (94). Benefits suggested for recombinant human growth hormone (rHGH) administration may be achievable with a combination of resistance and aerobic training, both of which augment endogenous growth hormone production (94). Nutritional supplementation should focus on adequate total energy to prevent ongoing weight loss, as well as balanced intake of macronutrients and micronutrients. Nutrition counseling apparently is more effective when combined with an appropriate oral supplement than when given alone (98). Glutamine supplementation has been studied with limited evidence of benefit. The role, if any, of potentially immune-enhancing nutrients, such as zinc, arginine, or n-3 fatty acids, in HIV in general, and the AIDS wasting syndrome specifically, is unknown. There has been recent evidence suggesting a relationship between selenium deficiency in HIV patients and worse outcomes. Certain randomized trials suggest that selenium supplementation in HIV patients may reduce morbidity and CD4 cell counts (99).

CLINICAL HIGHLIGHTS

An association between nutritional status and immune function is of clear clinical importance. Less clear is the means for optimizing immune responses when overt nutritional deficiency is not a threat. Although the evidence supporting immune enhancement by specific nutrients in humans is preliminary, the confluence of lines of evidence from animal, in vitro, in vivo, and epidemiologic studies allows for some general recommendations. The maintenance of macronutrient balance, including adequate protein intake with regard to both quantity and quality, is essential for immunocompetence across the lifespan. Dietary intake of arginine, taurine, and glutamine, along with the essential amino acids, may be of some importance. Abundant intake of fruits and vegetables is advisable on the basis of epidemiologic evidence, even as the potential mediators of immune effects (e.g., vitamins, minerals, sterols, flavonoids) are investigated. Multivitamin/multimineral supplementation for all individuals over age 50 offers potential benefit and virtually no known toxicity. Additional supplementation with zinc (up to 30 mg per day) and vitamin E (200 IU per day) may confer additional benefit. Excessive dosing of single nutrients may have adverse effects and should be discouraged; zinc is a notable example. Inclusion in the diet of n-3 fatty acids from plant or marine food sources may be beneficial, particularly if vitamin E is supplemented; a ratio of n-3 to n-6 fatty acids of not less than 1:4 is supported by available evidence. Recommendations for probiotic use are still difficult to provide due to variations in strains and individual responses. Regular, moderate physical activity and avoidance of obesity may confer benefit to immune function and are advisable on other grounds.

Optimizing the maternal diet during gestation should be a high priority in all populations at risk for nutritional deficiencies (see Chapter 27); such deficiencies during fetal development appear to produce long-lasting immunologic impairment, regardless of the quality of the perinatal diet. Megadosing of micronutrients may be hazardous; even nutrients of clear benefit to immune function, such as zinc, iron, and vitamin E, are immunoinhibitory at high doses.

Although adequate iron in conjunction with adequate levels of transport proteins is of clear importance to immune function, iron repletion during acute infection, particularly if globulin levels are low, should be avoided, as the iron under such conditions is preferentially available for bacterial metabolism. There is some preliminary evidence of benefit from the administration of immunomodulating nutrients in the setting of acute illness. The combination of uracil, arginine, and n-3 fatty acid supplementation has shown particular promise. (A proprietary product, Impact [Sandoz], offers this combination in an enteral formula.) Even though conclusive evidence

from outcome studies of infectious disease in humans to support a role for dietary manipulations in the enhancement of immunity is lacking, the available evidence supports a diet consistent with recommendations supported by other lines of evidence. New trends are supporting a new paradigm to nutrient supplementation to treat disease. The new paradigm, labeled pharmaconutrition, tailors nutrient supplementation directly with the underlying disease process (100). Similar evidence supports daily supplementation with a multivitamin/multimineral. Recommendations for a diet that may enhance immune function may be made to patients with confidence in the probability of health benefits and the improbability of toxicity; a more cautious approach to supplements is advised.

REFERENCES

1. Calder PC, Kew S. The immune system: a target for functional foods? *Br J Nutr* 2002;88(suppl 2):S165–S177. doi:10.1079/bjn2002682.
2. Kau AL, Ahern PP, Griffin NW, et al. Human nutrition, the gut microbiome and the immune system. *Nature* 2011; 474(7351):327–336. doi: http://www.nature.com/nature/journal/v474/n7351/abs/10.1038-nature10213-unlocked.html#supplementary-information.
3. Mena M-P, Sacanella E, Vazquez-Agell M, et al. Inhibition of circulating immune cell activation: a molecular anti-inflammatory effect of the Mediterranean diet. *Am J Clin Nutr* 2009;89(1):248–256. doi: 10.3945/ajcn.2008.26094.
4. Coppo R, Basolo B, Rollino C, et al. Mediterranean diet and primary IgA nephropathy. *Clin Nephrol* 1986;26(2):72–82.
5. Haddad EH, Berk LS, Kettering JD, et al. Dietary intake and biochemical, hematologic, and immune status of vegans compared with nonvegetarians. *Am J Clin Nutr* 1999;70(3):586s–593s.
6. Kjeldsen-Kragh J, Mellbye O, Haugen M, et al. Changes in laboratory variables in rheumatoid arthritis patients during a trial of fasting and one-year vegetarian diet. *Scand J Rheumatol* 1995;24(2):85–93.
7. Müller H, de Toledo FW, Resch KL. Fasting followed by vegetarian diet in patients with rheumatoid arthritis: a systematic review. *Scand J Rheumatol* 2001;30(1):1–10. doi:10.1080/030097401750065256.
8. Field CJ, Johnson IR, Schley PD. Nutrients and their role in host resistance to infection. *J Leukocyte Biol* 2002;71(1): 16–32.
9. de Heredia FP, Gomez-Martinez S, Marcos A. Obesity, inflammation and the immune system. *Proc Nutr Soc* 2012;71(2):332–338. doi:10.1017/S0029665112000092.
10. Tilg H, Moschen AR. Adipocytokines: mediators linking adipose tissue, inflammation and immunity. *Nature Rev Immunol* 2006;6(10):772–783. doi:10.1038/nri1937.
11. Falagas ME, Kompoti M. Obesity and infection. *Lancet Infect Dis* 2006;6(7):438–446. doi:10.1016/s1473-3099 (06)70523-0.

12. Anderson R. Antioxidant nutrients and prevention of oxidant-mediated, smoking-related diseases. In: Bendich A, Deckelbaum RJ, eds. *Preventive nutrition: the comprehensive guide for health professionals*. Totowa, NJ: Humana Press, 1997:303–316.

13. Lonn E, Bosch J, Yusuf S, et al. Effects of long-term vitamin E supplementation on cardiovascular events and cancer: a randomized controlled trial. *JAMA* 2005;293(11):1338–1347. doi:10.1001/jama.293.11.1338.

14. Dietary supplementation with n-3 polyunsaturated fatty acids and vitamin E after myocardial infarction: results of the GISSI-Prevenzione trial. Gruppo Italiano per lo Studio della Sopravvivenza nell'Infarto miocardico. *Lancet* 1999;354(9177):447–455.

15. The Alpha-Tocopherol Beta Carotene Cancer Prevention Study Group. The effect of vitamin E and beta carotene on the incidence of lung cancer and other cancers in male smokers. *N Engl J Med* 1994;330(15):1029–1035. doi:10.1056/NEJM199404143301501.

16. Omenn GS, Goodman GE, Thornquist MD, et al. Risk factors for lung cancer and for intervention effects in CARET, the Beta-Carotene and Retinol Efficacy Trial. *J Natl Cancer Inst* 1996;88(21):1550–1559.

17. Bogden J, Louria D. Micronutrients and immunity in older people. In: Bendich A, Deckelbaum RJ, eds. *Preventive nutrition: the comprehensive guide for health professionals*. Totowa, NJ: Humana Press, 1997:317–336.

18. Lesourd BM. Nutrition and immunity in the elderly: modification of immune responses with nutritional treatments. *Am J Clin Nutr* 1997;66(2):478S–484S.

19. Chandra RK. Graying of the immune system. Can nutrient supplements improve immunity in the elderly? *JAMA* 1997;277(17):1398–1399.

20. Huang HY, Caballero B, Chang S, et al. The efficacy and safety of multivitamin and mineral supplement use to prevent cancer and chronic disease in adults: a systematic review for a National Institutes of Health state-of-the-science conference. *Ann Intern Med* 2006;145(5):372–385.

21. Barnett JB, Hamer DH, Meydani SN. Low zinc status: a new risk factor for pneumonia in the elderly? *Nutr Rev* 2010;68(1):30–37.doi:10.1111/j.1753-4887.2009.00253.x.

22. Prasad AS, Beck FW, Bao B, et al. Zinc supplementation decreases incidence of infections in the elderly: effect of zinc on generation of cytokines and oxidative stress. *Am J Clin Nutr* 2007;85(3):837–844.

23. Grimble RF, Grimble GK. Immunonutrition: role of sulfur amino acids, related amino acids, and polyamines. *Nutrition* (Burbank, Los Angeles County, Calif) 1998;14(7–8):605–610.

24. Evoy D, Lieberman MD, Fahey TJ 3rd, et al. Immunonutrition: the role of arginine. *Nutrition* (Burbank, Los Angeles County, Calif) 1998;14(7–8):611–617.

25. Morris SM Jr. Arginine: master and commander in innate immune responses. *Sci Signal* 2010;3(135):e27. doi:10.1126/scisignal.3135pe27.

26. Kelly E, Morris SM Jr, Billiar TR. Nitric oxide, sepsis, and arginine metabolism. *JPEN* 1995;19(3):234–238.

27. Jiang J, Valen G, Tokuno S, et al. Endothelial dysfunction in atherosclerotic mice: improved relaxation by combined supplementation with L-arginine-tetrahydrobiopterin and enhanced vasoconstriction by endothelin. *Br J Pharmacol* 2000;131(7):1255–1261. doi:10.1038/sj.bjp.0703705.

28. Schulze F, Lenzen H, Hanefeld C, et al. Asymmetric dimethylarginine is an independent risk factor for coronary heart disease: results from the multicenter Coronary Artery Risk Determination (CARDIAC) study. *Am Heart J* 2006;152(3):493e1–8. doi:10.1016/j.ahj.2006.06.005.

29. Jiang DJ, Jia SJ, Yan J, et al. Involvement of DDAH/ADMA/NOS pathway in nicotine-induced endothelial dysfunction. *Biochem Biophys Res Commun* 2006;349(2):683–693. doi:10.1016/j.bbrc.2006.08.115.

30. Wilmore DW, Shabert JK. Role of glutamine in immunologic responses. *Nutrition* (Burbank, Los Angeles County, Calif) 1998;14(7–8):618–626.

31. Redmond HP, Stapleton PP, Neary P, et al. Immunonutrition: the role of taurine. *Nutrition* (Burbank, Los Angeles County, Calif) 1998;14(7–8):599–604.

32. Hess JR, Greenberg NA. The role of nucleotides in the immune and gastrointestinal systems: potential clinical applications. *Nutr Clin Prac* 2012;27(2):281–294. doi:10.1177/0884533611434933.

33. Wintergerst ES, Maggini S, Hornig DH. Immune-enhancing role of vitamin C and zinc and effect on clinical conditions. *Ann Nutr Metab* 2006;50(2):85–94. doi:10.1159/000090495.

34. Hemila H, Louhiala P. Vitamin C for preventing and treating pneumonia. *Cochrane Database Syst Rev* (Online) 2013;8:CD005532. doi:10.1002/14651858.CD005532.pub3.

35. Institute of Medicine. *Dietary reference intakes: vitamins*. 2009. http://www.iom.edu/~/media/Files/Activity%20Files/Nutrition/DRIs/DRI_Vitamins.pdf

36. Mora JR, Iwata M, von Andrian UH. Vitamin effects on the immune system: vitamins A and D take centre stage. *Nature Rev Immunol* 2008;8(9):685–698. doi:10.1038/nri2378.

37. Friis H, Ndhlovu P, Kaondera K, et al. Serum concentration of micronutrients in relation to schistosomiasis and indicators of infection: a cross-sectional study among rural Zimbabwean schoolchildren. *Eur J Clin Nutr* 1996;50(6):386–391.

38. Das BS, Thurnham DI, Das DB. Plasma alpha-tocopherol, retinol, and carotenoids in children with falciparum malaria. *Am J Clin Nutr* 1996;64(1):94–100.

39. Semba RD. Impact of vitamin A on immunity and infection in developing countries. In: Bendich A, Deckelbaum RJ, eds. *Preventive nutrition: the comprehensive guide for health professionals*, 2nd ed. Totowa, NJ: Humana Press, 1997:329–346.

40. Meydani SN, Beharka AA. Recent developments in vitamin E and immune response. *Nutr Rev* 1998;56(1 Pt 2):S49–S58.

41. Beharka A, Redican S, Leka L, et al. Vitamin E status and immune function. *Methods Enzymol* 1997;282:247–263.

42. Meydani SN, Meydani M, Blumberg JB, et al. Vitamin E supplementation and in vivo immune response in healthy elderly subjects. A randomized controlled trial. *JAMA* 1997;277(17):1380–1386.

43. Harbige LS. Fatty acids, the immune response, and autoimmunity: a question of n-6 essentiality and the balance between n-6 and n-3. *Lipids* 2003;38(4):323–341.

44. Autier P, Gandini S. Vitamin D supplementation and total mortality: a meta-analysis of randomized controlled trials. *Arch Intern Med* 2007;167(16):1730–1737. doi:10.1001/archinte.167.16.1730.

45. Nursyam EW, Amin Z, Rumende CM. The effect of vitamin D as supplementary treatment in patients with moderately advanced pulmonary tuberculous lesion. *Acta Medica Indonesiana* 2006;38(1):3–5.

46. Lehouck A, Mathieu C, Carremans C, et al. High doses of vitamin D to reduce exacerbations in chronic obstructive pulmonary disease: a randomized trial. *Ann Intern Med* 2012;156(2): 105–114. doi:10.1059/0003-4819-156-2-201201170-00004.

47. Baeke F, Takiishi T, Korf H, et al. Vitamin D: modulator of the immune system. *Curr Opin Pharmacol* 2010;10(4):482–496. doi:10.1016/j.coph.2010.04.001.

48. Murdoch DR, Slow S, Chambers ST, et al. Effect of vitamin D_3 supplementation on upper respiratory tract infections in healthy adults: the VIDARIS randomized controlled trial. *JAMA* 2012;308(13):1333–1339. doi:10.1001/jama.2012 .12505.

49. Wu D, Meydani M, Leka LS, et al. Effect of dietary supplementation with black currant seed oil on the immune response of healthy elderly subjects. *Am J Clin Nutr* 1999;70(4):536–543.

50. Bonatto SJ, Oliveira HH, Nunes EA, et al. Fish oil supplementation improves neutrophil function during cancer chemotherapy. *Lipids* 2012;47(4):383–389. doi:10.1007/ s11745-011-3643-0.

51. Meydani SN, Lichtenstein AH, Cornwall S, et al. Immunologic effects of national cholesterol education panel step-2 diets with and without fish-derived N-3 fatty acid enrichment. *J Clin Invest* 1993;92(1):105–113. doi:10.1172/ jci116537.

52. Calder PC. N-3 polyunsaturated fatty acids and inflammation: from molecular biology to the clinic. *Lipids* 2003;38(4):343–352.

53. Wu D, Meydani SN. n-3 Polyunsaturated fatty acids and immune function. *Proc Nutr Soc* 1998;57(4):503–509.

54. Taylor PR, Li B, Dawsey SM, et al. Prevention of esophageal cancer: the nutrition intervention trials in Linxian, China. Linxian Nutrition Intervention Trials Study Group. *Cancer Res* 1994;54(7 suppl):2029s–2031s.

55. Ryan-Harshman M, Aldoori W. The relevance of selenium to immunity, cancer, and infectious/inflammatory diseases. *Can J Diet Pract Res* 2005;66(2):98–102.

56. Rayman MP, Rayman MP. The argument for increasing selenium intake. *Proc Nutr Soc* 2002;61(2):203–215.

57. Rayman MP. Selenium in cancer prevention: a review of the evidence and mechanism of action. *Proc Nutr Soc* 2005;64(4):527–542.

58. Neve J. Selenium as a 'nutraceutical': how to conciliate physiological and supra-nutritional effects for an essential trace element. *Curr Opin Clin Nutr Metab Care* 2002;5(6):659–663. doi:10.1097/01.mco.0000038809.16540.36.

59. Brenneisen P, Steinbrenner H, Sies H. Selenium, oxidative stress, and health aspects. *Mol Aspects Med* 2005;26(4–5): 256–267.

60. Rainer L, Heiss CJ. Conjugated linoleic acid: health implications and effects on body composition. *J Am Diet Assoc* 2004;104(6):963–968, quiz 1032. doi:10.1016/j.jada.2004 .03.016.

61. Bassaganya-Riera J, Hontecillas R, Horne WT, et al. Conjugated linoleic acid modulates immune responses in patients with mild to moderately active Crohn's disease. *Clin Nutr* (Edinburgh, Scotland) 2012;31(5):721–727. doi:10.1016/j.clnu.2012.03.002.

62. Bhattacharya A, Banu J, Rahman M, et al. Biological effects of conjugated linoleic acids in health and disease. *J Nutr Biochem* 2006;17(12):789–810. doi:10.1016/j. jnutbio.2006.02.009.

63. Tricon S, Yaqoob P. Conjugated linoleic acid and human health: a critical evaluation of the evidence. *Curr Opin Clin Nutr Metab Care* 2006;9(2):105–110. doi:10.1097/01. mco.0000214567.44568.fb.

64. Gleeson M, Nieman DC, Pedersen BK. Exercise, nutrition and immune function. *J Sports Sci* 2004;22(1):115–125. doi:10.1080/0264041031000140590.

65. Nieman DC. Nutrition, exercise, and immune system function. *Clin Sports Med* 1999;18(3):537–548.

66. Diment BC, Fortes MB, Greeves JP, et al. Effect of daily mixed nutritional supplementation on immune indices in soldiers undertaking an 8-week arduous training programme. *Eur J Appl Physiol* 2012;112(4):1411–1418. doi:10.1007/s00421-011-2096-8.

67. Kelly D, Coutts AG. Early nutrition and the development of immune function in the neonate. *Proc Nutr Soc* 2000;59(2):177–185.

68. Williams HC. Two "positive" studies of probiotics for atopic dermatitis: or are they? *Arch Dermatol* 2006;142(9): 1201–1203. doi:10.1001/archderm.142.9.1201.

69. Geier MS, Butler RN, Howarth GS. Probiotics, prebiotics and synbiotics: a role in chemoprevention for colorectal cancer? *Cancer Biol Ther* 2006;5(10):1265–1269.

70. Gassull MA. Review article: the intestinal lumen as a therapeutic target in inflammatory bowel disease. *Aliment Pharmacol Ther* 2006;24(suppl 3):90–95. doi:10.1111/j. 1365-2036.2006.03067.x.

71. Haghighi HR, Gong J, Gyles CL, et al. Probiotics stimulate production of natural antibodies in chickens. *Clin Vacc Immunol* 2006;13(9):975–980. doi:10.1128/cvi.00161-06.

72. Gill HS, Prasad J, Donkor O. Probiotics and human immune function. In: Salminen S, Wright AV, Ouwehand A, eds. *Lactic acid bacteria: microbiological and functional aspects*. Boca Raton, FL: CRC Press, 2011:439.

73. Velasquez-Manoff M. *An epidemic of absence: a new way of understanding allergies and autoimmune diseases*. New York, NY: Scribner, 2012.

74. Fujimura KE, Slusher NA, Cabana MD, et al. Role of the gut microbiota in defining human health. *Expert Rev Anti Infect Ther* 2010;8(4):435–454.

75. Round JL, Mazmanian SK. The gut microbiota shapes intestinal immune responses during health and disease. *Nature Rev Immunol* 2009;9(5):313–323.

76. Bidlack W, Wang W. Designing functional foods. In: Shils ME, Shike M, eds. *Modern nutrition in health and disease*. Philadelphia, PA: Lippincott Williams & Wilkins, 2006: 1789–1808.

77. Kwon H-K, Lee C-G, So J-S, et al. Generation of regulatory dendritic cells and CD4+Foxp3+ T cells by probiotics administration suppresses immune disorders. *Proc Nat Acad Sci* 2010;107(5):2159–2164. doi:10.1073/ pnas.0904055107.

78. Lomax AR, Calder PC. Probiotics, immune function, infection and inflammation: a review of the evidence

from studies conducted in humans. *Curr Pharm Des* 15(13):1428–1518. doi:10.2174/138161209788168155.

79. Weizman Z, Asli G, Alsheikh A. Effect of a probiotic infant formula on infections in child care centers: comparison of two probiotic agents. *Pediatrics* 2005;115(1):5–9. doi:10.1542/peds.2004-1815.

80. Alfaleh K, Anabrees J, Bassler D, et al. Probiotics for prevention of necrotizing enterocolitis in preterm infants. *Cochrane Database Syst Rev* (Online) 2011(3):CD005496. doi:10.1002/14651858.

81. Klaenhammer TR, Kleerebezem M, Kopp MV, et al. The impact of probiotics and prebiotics on the immune system. *Nature Rev Immunol* 2012;12(10):728–734.

82. Walsek C, Zafonte M, Bowers JM. Nutritional issues and HIV/AIDS: assessment and treatment strategies. *J Assoc Nurses AIDS Care*: JANAC. 1997;8(6):71–80.

83. Corcoran C, Grinspoon S. Treatments for wasting in patients with the acquired immunodeficiency syndrome. *N Engl J Med* 1999;340(22):1740–50. doi:10.1056/nejm199906033402207.

84. Siegfried N, Irlam JH, Visser ME, et al. Micronutrient supplementation in pregnant women with HIV infection. *Cochrane Database Syst Rev* (Online) 2012;3:CD009755. doi:10.1002/14651858.cd009755.

85. Kaiser JD, Campa AM, Ondercin JP, et al. Micronutrient supplementation increases CD4 count in HIV-infected individuals on highly active antiretroviral therapy: a prospective, double-blinded, placebo-controlled trial. *J Acquir Immune Defic Syndr* (1999)2006;42(5):523–528. doi:10.1097/01.qai.0000230529.25083.42.

86. Isanaka S, Mugusi F, Hawkins C, et al. Effect of high-dose vs standard-dose multivitamin supplementation at the initiation of HAART on HIV disease progression and mortality in Tanzania: a randomized controlled trial. *JAMA* 2012;308(15):1535–1544. doi:10.1001/jama.2012.13083.

87. Forrester JE, Sztam KA. Micronutrients in HIV/AIDS: is there evidence to change the WHO 2003 recommendations? *Am J Clin Nut* 2011;94(6):1683S–1689S. doi:10.3945/ajcn.111.011999.

88. Duggan C, Manji KP, Kupka R, et al. Multiple micronutrient supplementation in Tanzanian infants born to HIV-infected mothers: a randomized, double-blind, placebo-controlled clinical trial. *Am J Clin Nutr* 2012;96(6):1437–1446. doi:10.3945/ajcn.112.044263.

89. Baum MK, Lai S, Sales S, et al. Randomized, controlled clinical trial of zinc supplementation to prevent immunological failure in HIV-infected adults. *Clin Infect Dis* 2010;50(12):1653–1660.

90. Arpadi SM, McMahon DJ, Abrams EJ, et al. Effect of supplementation with cholecalciferol and calcium on 2-y bone mass accrual in HIV-infected children and adolescents: a randomized clinical trial. *Am J Clin Nutr* 2012;95(3):678–685. doi:10.3945/ajcn.111.024786.

91. Overton E, Yin M. The rapidly evolving research on vitamin D among HIV-infected populations. *Curr Infect Dis Rep* 2011;13(1):83–93. doi:10.1007/s11908-010-0144-x.

92. Finkelstein JL. Maternal vitamin D status and child morbidity, anemia, and growth in human immunodeficiency virus-exposed children in Tanzania. *Pediatr Infect Dis J* 2012;31(2):171.

93. Abrams DI. Potential interventions for HIV/AIDS wasting: an overview. *J Acquir Immune Defic Syndr* 2000;25(suppl 1): S74–S80.

94. Roubenoff R. Acquired immunodeficiency syndrome wasting, functional performance, and quality of life. *Am J Manag Care* 2000;6(9):1003–1016.

95. Steinhart CR. HIV-associated wasting in the era of HAART: a practice-based approach to diagnosis and treatment. *The AIDS Reader* 2001;11(11):557–560, 66–69.

96. Fairfield WP, Treat M, Rosenthal DI, et al. Effects of testosterone and exercise on muscle leanness in eugonadal men with AIDS wasting. *J Appl Physiol* (Bethesda, MD: 1985) 2001;90(6):2166–2171.

97. Grinspoon S, Corcoran C, Parlman K, et al. Effects of testosterone and progressive resistance training in eugonadal men with AIDS wasting. A randomized, controlled trial. *Ann Intern Med* 2000;133(5):348–355.

98. Rabeneck L, Palmer A, Knowles JB, et al. A randomized controlled trial evaluating nutrition counseling with or without oral supplementation in malnourished HIV-infected patients. *J Am Diet Assoc* 1998;98(4):434–438. doi:10.1016/s0002-8223(98)00099-6.

99. Stone CA, Kawai K, Kupka R, et al. Role of selenium in HIV infection. *Nutr Rev* 2010;68(11):671–681. doi:10.1111/j.1753-4887.2010.00337.x.

100. Dupertuis YM, Meguid MM, Pichard C. Advancing from immunonutrition to a pharmaconutrition: a gigantic challenge. *Curr Opin Clin Nutr Metab Care* 2009;12(4):398–403. doi:10.1097/MCO.0b013e32832c4ce1.

SUGGESTED READING

Ahluwalia N. Aging, nutrition and immune function. *J Nutr Health Aging* 2004;8:2–6.

Beaumier L, Castillo L, Yu YM, et al. Arginine: new and exciting developments for an "old" amino acid. *Biomed Environ Sci* 1996;9:296.

Beisel WR, Edelman R, Nauss K, et al. Single-nutrient effects on immunologic functions. Report of a workshop sponsored by the department of Food and Nutrition and its Nutrition Advisory Group of the American Medical Association. *JAMA* 1981;245:53–58.

Calder PC. n-3 polyunsaturated fatty acids and cytokine production in health and disease. *Ann Nutr Metab* 1997; 41:203.

Calder PC. Immunoregulatory and anti-inflammatory effects of n-3 polyunsaturated fatty acids. *Braz J Med Biol Res* 1998;31:467–490.

Cummings JH, Antoine JM, Azpiroz F, et al. PASSCLAIM—gut health and immunity. *Eur J Nutr* 2004;43:ii118–ii173.

Ergas D, Eilat E, Mendlovic S, et al. n-3 fatty acids and the immune system in autoimmunity. *Isr Med Assoc J* 2002; 4:34–38.

Fernandes G, Jolly CA, Lawrence RA. Nutrition and the immune system. In: Shils ME, Shike M, Ross AC, et al., eds. *Modern nutrition in health and disease*, 10th ed. Philadelphia, PA: Lippincott Williams & Wilkins, 2006:670–684.

Levy J. Immunonutrition: the pediatric experience. *Nutrition* 1998;14:641.

Lopez-Varela S, Gonzalez-Gross M, Marcos A. Functional foods and the immune system: a review. *Eur J Clin Nutr* 2002;56:s29–s33.

Mainous MR, Deitch EA. Nutrition and infection. *Surg Clin North Am* 1994;74:659.

Marcos A, Nova E, Montero A. Changes in the immune system are conditioned by nutrition. *Eur J Clin Nutr* 2003;57: S66–S69.

Scrimshaw NS, SanGiovanni JP. Synergism of nutrition, infection, and immunity: an overview. *Am J Clin Nutr* 1997;66:464s.

Thies F, Miles EA, Nebe-von-Caron G, et al. Influence of dietary supplementation with long-chain n-3 or n-6 polyunsaturated fatty acids on blood inflammatory cell populations and functions and on plasma soluble adhesion molecules in healthy adults. *Lipids* 2001;36:1183–1193.

Thies F, Nebe-von-Caron G, Powell JR, et al. Dietary supplementation with eicosapentaenoic acid, but not with other long-chain n-3 or n-6 polyunsaturated fatty acids, decreases natural killer cell activity in healthy subjects aged >55 y. *Am J Clin Nutr* 2001;73:539–548.

Thomas JA. Oxidant defense in oxidative and nitrosative stress. In: Shils ME, Shike M, Ross AC, et al., eds. *Modern nutrition in health and disease*, 10th ed. Philadelphia, PA: Lippincott Williams & Wilkins, 2006:685–694.

Wintergerst ES, Maggini S, Hornig DH. Immune-enhancing role of vitamin C and zinc and effect on clinical conditions. *Ann Nutr Metab* 2006;50:85–94.

CHAPTER 12

Diet and Cancer

T he link between diet and cancer, supported by in vitro, animal, and epidemiologic studies, is convincing. Decisive intervention trials are for the most part lacking, however, because of the protracted time course of carcinogenesis and a lack of reliable surrogate markers in most cases. An exception is studies in populations with well-defined nutrient deficiencies that increase the risk of specific cancers, where supplementation may dramatically reduce risk; the Linxian study in rural China is noteworthy in this regard (1,2). Most reviews of diet and cancer cite the work of Doll and Peto (3) and suggest that one-third or more of all cancer is related to nutritional factors and potentially preventable by nutritional means. Dietary factors may influence cancer initiation, promotion, and progression via direct effects on DNA, indirect effects on immune function (see Chapter 11), and overall vitality (see Chapter 45).

As is the case for atherogenesis, the process of carcinogenesis may be affected both favorably and unfavorably by micronutrients and macronutrients. Initiation is fostered by mutagenic exposures, including nutrient compounds, and forestalled by immunosurveillance (the detection and destruction of neoplastic cells by the immune system), the robustness of which is influenced by dietary pattern. Cancer promotion and progression appear to be more meaningfully associated with macronutrient intake and overall health than with specific nutrient compounds, although the aggregate influence of certain nutrient groups, such as antioxidants and essential fatty acids, may be considerable. Procarcinogens in the diet include heterocyclic amines (HCAs) and polycyclic aromatic hydrocarbons (PAHs) that result from pyrolysis (i.e., charring); acrylamide formed when starchy foods are cooked at high temperature (4); nitrosamines used or produced in the curing of meats; naturally occurring contaminants, such as aflatoxin B-1; naturally occurring

chemicals in plants; and chemicals added to the food supply as a result of agricultural practices and food handling. While all of potential importance, the net effect of carcinogenic compounds in foods is generally thought to be small relative to the effects of dietary pattern on general health, and its profound influence on cancer risk. This contention is highlighted by the presence of naturally occurring mutagens in many plant foods, yet a consistent and strong inverse association between the consumption of such foods and cancer risk. Also germane is the issue of chemical contamination of food; there is widespread concern that pesticide residues on produce, for example, may at times be carcinogenic (5). If so, voluminous data largely from observational trials suggest that the benefits of a generally nutritious diet clearly outweigh any harmful effects of such residues on otherwise healthful foods. Nonetheless, a potential benefit from choosing organic alternatives—particularly in certain food groups (6)—is worthy of both consideration and study.

Whereas mutagenicity has been demonstrated for most of the compounds noted above, there are, of course, no intervention trials demonstrating carcinogenicity directly in humans. Epidemiologic studies support an association between excess saturated fat intake and cancer incidence at a variety of sites; a relative excess of n-6 polyunsaturated fats has been implicated as well. The literature linking trans fat to cancer risk is limited, but suggests the association may be especially strong (7,8). Overall, balance in dietary fat intake may be an important determinant of cancer risk (see Chapters 2, 7, and 45) as may the balance of dietary fat to other macronutrients. Carbohydrate content may be of particular concern with high-glycemic-load carbohydrates potentially increasing risk of cancer (9–16), possibly through insulin and insulin-like growth factors (17–22). Also, diet may lead indirectly to cancer by contributing to obesity, which is consistently and strongly associated with the risk of almost all cancers and of particular importance in breast and prostate cancer (23). Associations with cancer incidence have been suggested for both excess dietary protein of animal origin and excessive intake of simple sugars.

The most convincing evidence for the cancer-fighting potential of diet supports a high total intake of fruits and vegetables. Increasing public interest in organic foods, apparently motivated by concerns for both personal and planetary health, while a welcome trend, has the potential to exaggerate the dangers of chemical residues on produce. A net benefit of higher intake of fruits and vegetables is not limited to organic produce only. Thus, any harms attached to chemical residues on plant foods appear to be overwhelmed by the benefits of produce intake, as noted previously. Recent data reaffirm that prevailing intake of fruits and vegetables in the United States falls well short of recommended levels (24).

Less extensive evidence suggests that energy restriction may reduce cancer risk, either directly or indirectly through effects on body fat. Conversely, overweight and obesity are convincingly associated with increased cancer risks (25). Dietary fiber and a variety of micronutrients to be discussed are thought to reduce cancer risk. Nutrients with antioxidant properties are thought to be particularly important in cancer prevention by neutralizing the carcinogenic potential of free radicals ingested or generated by metabolism and radiation exposure. Efforts to isolate the "active ingredients" from cancer-fighting foods and diets, however, have been largely disappointing to date. Whether this is due to errors in dosing and/or choice of compound or to the differential effects of nutrients in the native context of foods versus isolation in supplements is at present unknown.

In clinical practice, dietary recommendations may be made based on available evidence to reduce both aggregate cancer risk and the risk of certain specific cancers. Similar recommendations are indicated for secondary prevention. In general, dietary recommendations for cancer prevention are entirely consistent with recommendations for health promotion (see Chapter 45) and substantially confluent with those for cancer recovery (26). In areas where dietary recommendations for cancer prevention rest on slight or inconclusive evidence, alternative, stronger sources of evidence consistently support very comparable recommendations.

As clinically overt cancer is invariably a catabolic process, nutritional support is important in the management and tertiary prevention of cancer. Malnutrition is a frequent concomitant of cancer and its treatment, with the potential to forestall recovery and impair functional ability. Strategies to promote and preserve lean body mass during cancer treatment likely warrant greater attention than they have received to date (27–29). Limited study of branched-chain amino acids suggests that certain combinations provided as a dietary supplement may meaningfully enhance lean body mass reserves and cancer recovery (30–33).

OVERVIEW

Diet

Cancer as a pathologic category is diverse and complex, as is the literature associating carcinogenesis, and its suppression, with diet. Numerous attempts have been made to review and summarize the pertinent literature (3,34–51), but none is truly conclusive. The lack of readily measurable and modifiable risk factors for cancer renders the study of human carcinogenesis extremely difficult. Surrogate markers of cancer risk are improving but do not compare to those relied on routinely to assess the cardioprotective effects of lifestyle interventions (see Chapter 7). Prospective interventions still must rely on actual cancer or precancerous dysplasia/neoplasms as endpoints. Of necessity, such interventions are lengthy and large and often prohibitively expensive. In addition, the study of cancer prevention by dietary means may be obviated by assessing individuals in whom signs of increased risk or damage done are already evident, if the benefit of diet pertains to initiation and the earliest stages of promotion. Further complicating the relationship between diet and cancer is the prevailing view that cancer is a nonthreshold risk. Establishing a dose–response relationship between any isolated dietary factor and cancer may prove daunting.

Despite the complexity of both cancer and nutritional epidemiology, there is considerable uniformity in published recommendations for prevention of cancer by dietary means. As summarized by the American Cancer Society, current guidelines for the dietary prevention of cancer include achievement and maintenance of healthy weight, a generous intake of vegetables and fruits, and a relative abundance of other plant-based foods such as cereals and grains; regular physical activity; and limitation of alcohol intake (52). These recommendations are generally consistent with those for the prevention of both heart disease and diabetes, inspiring a joint effort by the American Cancer Society, American Heart Association, and American Diabetes Association to promote the same basic pattern of healthful lifestyle change (53).

Evidence in support of these recommendations derives principally from observational and retrospective studies and is of varying strength with regard to specific cancers and specific aspects of diet (34). A mechanistic understanding of nutrients in the prevention of cancer is developing and should guide future studies and recommendations.

Diet and Specific Neoplasms

Colon Cancer

Colon cancer is the leading cause of cancer death in the United States, and diet is thought to be one of the most potent determinants of colon cancer risk (54). A link between diet and colon cancer risk would seem virtually intuitive, and indeed diet is thought to be one of the, if not the, most important modifiable risk factors (54,55). Diet and nutrition are estimated to explain as much as 30% to 50% of the worldwide incidence of colorectal cancer, according to a recent report (56). Evidence of an inverse association between dietary fiber intake and the risk of colorectal cancer has been consistent overall and convincing (41,57,58). High intake of fruits and vegetables is associated with reduced risk, but the extent to which this is due to fiber or other nutrients is uncertain. A positive association has been reported for high intake of dietary fat and red meat, although these, too, tend to covary. Physical inactivity and obesity may increase risk, while physical activity is associated with a reduced risk of both proximal colon and distal colon cancers (59).

High fiber intake is thought to lower risk by any of several possible mechanisms, including dilution of mutagens, reduction of gastrointestinal transit time, alteration of pH, and alteration of the gut flora and microbiome (60,61). The source of fiber may also be important for influencing cancer risk. The prospective Scandinavian HELGA cohort study, which examined 108,081 subjects, found that fiber from cereal foods may play a particularly strong role in the prevention of colon cancer (62). Another recent study found that high compliance with a low-fat, high-fiber diet is in fact associated with reduced risk of adenoma recurrence (63). Furthermore, data from the Iowa Women's Health Study, obtained prospectively over a five-year period, demonstrated an inverse association between vegetable and fiber intake and colon cancer risk, although the associations were not statistically significant. A protective effect of garlic was also reported in this study but has not since been convincingly replicated (64).

Negative studies of fiber and colonic polyp recurrence, however, have raised doubts about the potential for dietary fiber to reduce colon cancer risk. In one such study (65), subjects with a prior history of colonic polyps were randomly assigned to receive counseling conducive to high dietary fiber intake or a control condition. The rate of recurrent polyp development did not differ between groups. In the second (66), more than 1,000 subjects with colonic polyps were randomly assigned to high (13.5 g) or low (2 g) daily supplements of wheat-bran fiber. Again, no difference was seen in the rate of polyp recurrence between groups. An accompanying editorial by Byers (67) appropriately concludes that these studies, while suggesting lack of short-term benefit of fiber in the prevention of polyp recurrence, provide little information about the potential role of fiber in colon cancer prevention. In particular, the long latency of cancer and the segregation of its pathogenesis into initiation, promotion, and expression raise the possibility that preventive measures may need to occur years before clinical features might otherwise develop to exert a meaningful influence. Injury to colonic epithelial cells is apt to have occurred years earlier in these study participants (i.e., long before polyps first appeared). Thus, these studies cannot be inferred to offer meaningful information about the impact of varying lifelong fiber intake on colon cancer risk (67). While provocative, these short-term studies do not refute the weight of evidence suggesting a benefit of high fiber intake over the course of a lifetime. The European Prospective Investigation of Cancer and Nutrition (EPIC) suggests an approximate 9% reduction in the risk of colorectal cancer for each quintile increase in total dietary fiber intake (68).

A recent examination of seven cohort studies suggests that methodological differences may account for inconsistencies in previous studies evaluating the inverse association between fiber intake and colorectal cancer risk (69). The studies do, however, raise important questions about both the reliability and magnitude of any benefit fiber offers and the role of timing over the lifespan. The negative evidence generated by such trials should neither be exaggerated nor dismissed. Perhaps dietary fiber offers protection against colon cancer only by preserving the health of an uninjured colon but provides no safeguard against polyps or cancer once injury related to diet and luminal pressures has accrued. Future study will be needed to make such determinations.

In an innovative application of factor analysis, Slattery et al. (70) studied nearly 2,000 cases of colon cancer in comparison to 2,400 controls. They found that a "Western"-style diet (with high intake of fat, cholesterol, and protein and a high body mass index [BMI]) was associated with significantly increased risk compared to other dietary patterns. These data are consistent with those of most other studies but are novel in providing an assessment of associations with overall dietary patterns (71). In the dietary arm of the Women's Health Initiative, nearly 50,000 postmenopausal women were randomly assigned to a fat-reduced diet with abundant intake of fruits and vegetables or to a control group given information about the current dietary guidelines. After 8 years of follow-up, colon cancer rates did not differ between groups (72). However, the dietary patterns achieved differed minimally between groups, and the advice to restrict all varieties of dietary fat indiscriminately is at odds with current thinking. Thus, the study has been criticized for methodologic failings and is not generally seen as refuting other evidence regarding the protective effects of fruits and vegetables or of restricting dietary fats selectively.

Recommendations supported by the weight of available evidence include a diet rich in vegetables and other plant-based foods and still support a high intake of insoluble fiber from whole grains, beans, and lentils, along with vegetables and fruits. Consumption of red meat (at least conventionally raised, factory-farmed red meat) and particularly processed meat should be moderate. Alcohol intake should be kept at moderate levels. There may be a particular benefit from

including dairy foods in the diet. To date, no definitive evidence supports micronutrient supplements as a specific strategy for preventing colon cancer, although arguments may be made for calcium, vitamin D, folate, probiotics, and glutamine (see Chapters 4 and 18).

Prospective data from the Nurses' Health Study demonstrate an association between animal fat consumption and colon cancer risk (73). Recent meta-analyses show that high consumers of cured meats and red meat are at increased risk of colorectal cancer (74). The same study revealed no association between low-fat meats, specifically fish and skinless poultry, and colon cancer risk. A case-control study conducted by Neugut et al. (75) using patients with colorectal adenomatous polyps as cases demonstrated an increased risk of colon cancer among those in the highest quartile of saturated fat intake, red meat consumption, and total dietary fat. Other recent studies further support an association between high red meat consumption and colon cancer risk (76,77). High dietary fat intake is thought to influence colon cancer development through effects on bile acid production and bacterial flora (54). High consumption of fiber showed a strong protective effect. Fiber has been shown to prevent the induction of colon cancer in rats fed a "high-risk" diet (78,79). Results of the Health Professionals Follow-up Study suggest an inverse association between physical activity and colon cancer risk and an independent association between BMI and colon cancer risk. The association was even stronger for the waist-to-hip ratio than for BMI, suggesting that adiposity and fat distribution may influence colon cancer development (80). Data from Calle et al. (23) reveal a relative risk increase of 50% or more for cancer death in those with a BMI above 40 as compared to those of normal weight.

Recent studies have linked red meat consumption to colorectal and other types of cancers. Evidence suggests that processed red meats have the strongest association with cancer, potentially because meat cooked at high temperatures may form carcinogenic compounds such as PAHs and HCAs. A recent observational study of more than 120,000 individuals found that a daily increase of 3 oz of red meat was associated with a 10% greater risk of cancer mortality (81). Pastured or "grass-fed" beef has a different fat composition than "conventional" factory-farmed beef, and this difference could matter for cancer risk in general and for colon cancer specifically (82). Grass-fed beef is higher in ω-3 polyunsaturated fatty acids (PUFAs), which may be protective, and lower in ω-6 PUFA, which may be harmful (83). Moreover, the beef fat from cows raised on grass (cow's natural diet) is very different than beef fat from factory-farmed cows raised on grain, offal, and various industrial chemicals. There is interest in how fat-stored pesticides, antibiotics, and other growth promoters from factory farming might impact on human disease, but evidence at this time (notwithstanding health effects through environmental damage) is mostly speculative.

The hypothesis that calcium, vitamin D, and/or dairy products rich in both reduce colon cancer risk is currently among the most provocative topics in the field (84). Some observational data support a protective effect, but such an association was not supported by data from either the Health Professionals Follow-up Study or the Nurses' Health Study (85). A recent intervention trial suggested significant reduction in colon cancer risk with vitamin D supplementation (86), but these findings are contradicted by a longer, larger trial (87). Meta-analyses have shown reduced colon cancer risk with consumption of dairy products (88,89), however, there are also other rationales for recommending both dairy intake (see Chapter 8) and calcium/vitamin D supplements (see Chapters 4 and 14) (90,91). Data from the Iowa Women's Health Study, obtained prospectively over a five-year period, demonstrated an inverse association between vegetable and fiber intake and colon cancer risk, although the associations were not statistically significant. A protective effect of garlic was reported in this study but has not since been convincingly replicated (64).

Diet is thought to be one of the most potent determinants of colon cancer risk (54). High dietary fat intake is thought to influence colon cancer development through effects on bile acid production and bacterial flora (54). High fiber intake is thought to lower risk by any of several possible mechanisms, including dilution of mutagens, reduction of gastrointestinal transit time, and alteration of pH.

Breast Cancer

Evidence linking dietary factors to breast cancer risk is based on a combination of animal studies, ecologic studies between and among populations,

retrospective studies within populations, observational cohort studies, and, to a lesser extent, intervention studies.

The American Cancer Society recommends avoidance or limitation of alcohol intake, avoidance of obesity, maintenance of physical activity, and abundant intake of vegetables and fruits as means to lower breast cancer risk (52). The evidence is stronger for alcohol and obesity than for other aspects of diet. Most reviews over recent years offer similar advice, albeit with variable degrees of enthusiasm for the quality of evidence gathered to date (92–94).

In an effort to quantify the relationship between micronutrient intake and breast cancer risk, Kushi et al. (95) assessed the association between breast cancer incidence and intake of vitamins A, C, and E, retinol, and carotenoids among more than 34,000 women in the Iowa Women's Health Study. No protective effect was found for women with high intake of any of these nutrients. Some protective effect was noted for megadose supplements of vitamins C and A, but the associations did not reach significance. Similar results were reported from the Nurses' Health Study, where intake of vitamins C and E showed no association with breast cancer risk; vitamin A intake was inversely associated with risk in this study (96). A recent meta-analysis supports the role of vitamin A intake to reduce breast cancer risk (97). This inverse relationship may be mediated by the effect of vitamin A on reducing oxidative stress (98).

Hebert and Rosen (99), comparing breast cancer incidence among 66 countries, used food intake and socioeconomic status (SES) data to develop predictive multivariable models. The strongest predictors of breast cancer risk in their study were total calories, total dietary fat, red meat, dairy, and alcohol. Fish and cereal products showed protective effects. The strength of association for dietary factors was commensurate with that for fertility; SES factors dropped out in multivariable models due to covariance with dietary and fertility factors. The biologic plausibility for a relationship between dietary fat intake and breast cancer is supported by prior literature (100–104).

Dorgan et al. (105) compared serum levels of carotenoids, retinol, selenium, and α-tocopherol between 105 breast cancer cases and matched controls. Only lycopene emerged as significantly protective, whereas the trend for β-cryptoxanthin was favorable but did not reach statistical significance. Lycopene is found principally in tomatoes, and β-cryptoxanthin is found in tangerines, nectarines, oranges, peaches, papaya, and mango.

Evidence linking alcohol consumption to breast cancer risk has been fairly consistent, as recently reported in a meta-analysis by Smith-Warner et al. (106), Schatzkin et al. (107), and van den Brandt et al. (108). The pooled data suggest a relative risk of approximately 1.4 among moderate to moderately heavy drinkers (30 to 60 g of ethanol per day; 2 to 5 drinks) compared with nondrinkers.

In a recent analysis of data from a large case-control study in Italy, Mezzetti et al. (109) suggest that modification of dietary antioxidant intake, body weight, alcohol consumption, and physical activity level could eliminate up to one-third of breast cancers in the population studied.

The association between dietary fat intake and breast cancer risk is both controversial and complex. Animal studies and cross-cultural comparisons in humans suggest that total fat, saturated fatty acids, and n-6 PUFAs may increase breast cancer risk (110), whereas n-3 PUFAs and possibly monounsaturates decrease risk (92,111–113). Dietary fat may have disparate effects on pre- and postmenopausal women, possibly conferring a protective effect on premenopausal women, while elevating cancer risk in postmenopausal women (114).

Data from recent case-control and observational cohort studies, however, have largely failed to corroborate such associations (115–118). Similar doubts have been cast on the relationship between adiposity and breast cancer risk (119). A case-control study found no significant effect of dietary fat intake during adolescence on subsequent risk of breast cancer (120).

A case-control study in Italy found an inverse association between intake of unsaturated fat and breast cancer and a positive association for starch, although fat and vegetable intake were highly correlated (112). Thus, the dietary contributors to breast cancer risk may vary with population characteristics and prevailing dietary patterns. Complications in establishing a definitive link between dietary fat and breast cancer have been described elsewhere (94). Factor analysis has been used to demonstrate an association between a Western dietary pattern and increased risk of breast cancer (121).

Among the most controversial of dietary trials for cancer prevention, the dietary arm of the Women's Health Initiative randomly assigned roughly 40,000 subjects to intervention and control groups. The intervention group received guidance for a fat-reduced diet with increased intake of fruits and vegetables; the control group received information about the current dietary guidelines. After approximately 8 years of follow-up, differences in breast cancer were not significant between the groups, although trends favored the intervention group (122). The between-group differences in dietary pattern achieved were very modest, and the guidance to restrict dietary fat indiscriminately was questionable. The study has generated a great deal of criticism and certainly does not provide evidence to refute the apparent benefits of increasing fruit and vegetable intake or moderating intake of certain fats like n-6 PUFAs.

A diet rich in fruits, vegetables, and grains, with modest to no alcohol intake, and without excess meat, fat, calories, and obesity are consistent with recommendations for health promotion. The aggregated evidence suggests that such recommendations may serve to reduce breast cancer risk as well (93,123,124). A recent study suggests better breast cancer survival among women who are physically active and eat an abundance of vegetables and fruits (125). An online database is now available that provides summary evidence for a wide array of potential carcinogens that might contribute to breast cancer risk (5).

Lung Cancer

As is widely known, tobacco is by far the most important modifiable risk factor for lung cancer. However, as only a minority of smokers develop cancer, there are likely to be other important exposures, as well as variability in genetic susceptibility (126). There has long been evidence of a protective effect of fruit and vegetable intake. American Cancer Society data indicate that obesity is a risk factor for lung cancer (23).

The association of reduced risk of lung cancer with consumption of green and yellow vegetables suggested a protective effect of β-carotene (126). The results of randomized clinical trials have largely refuted a role for supplemental β-carotene in cancer prevention. Specifically with regard to lung cancer, two negative trials are noteworthy. In the CARET (beta-carotene and retinol efficacy trial) trial, current smokers and asbestos-exposed workers had a statistically significant increase in risk of both incident lung cancer and lung cancer mortality when taking supplemental β-carotene as opposed to placebo (127). Similarly, β-carotene supplementation was associated with a higher incidence of lung cancer than placebo in the Alpha-Tocopherol, Beta-Carotene (ATBC) Cancer Prevention Study (128–130).

In a case-control study of lung cancer among nonsmoking women, Alavanja et al. (131) reported increased risk in association with red meat and dairy intake and particularly total and saturated fat intake; a protective effect of vegetables was not seen. A subsequent meta-analysis did not support an important relationship between fat or cholesterol intakes and lung cancer risk (132). A case-control study among men in Sweden identified low vegetable intake and high milk consumption as lung cancer risk factors in a mixed group of smokers and nonsmokers (133). A subsequent meta-analysis in the United Kingdom suggested an overall survival advantage with dairy consumption, limited not just to cancer (134). In a review of studies of lung cancer risk factors among nonsmoking women in China, the dietary factors reported to be most consistently associated with increased risk were low intake of vegetables and fruits, particularly vegetables and fruits rich in carotene and vitamin C (135).

A separate case-control study in Chinese women identified frequent consumption of fried food as a risk factor and frequent carrot consumption as protective (136). At least one case-control study in China demonstrated a decreased risk of lung cancer with increasing intake of meat as well as vegetables among men in a mining town (137). The discrepant findings with regard to red meat are likely due to variable population characteristics; red meat may be protective when diet is marginal and harmful when diet tends to be excessive. Alternatively, as yet unspecified confounders may account for the observed associations between meat consumption and lung cancer.

The results of a large cohort study conducted in Finland suggest that flavonoids, particularly quercetin, confer protection against cancer in general and lung cancer in particular (138). The primary source of flavonoids in the study population was apples (139). The results of this study were relatively unaffected by adjusting for intake of vitamins C and E and β-carotene. A recent study found little evidence of a link between B vitamins or methionine and lung cancer risk (140). Overall, there are suggestions in the literature of protective effects against lung cancer of several antioxidant nutrients (141). Definitive

evidence is lacking, however, and further study will be required to reach secure conclusions.

The sum of available evidence supports recommendations to consume an abundance of fruits and vegetables and dairy products. Recommendations to limit meat are reasonable. Recommendations to consume any particular micronutrient cannot be made with confidence (41).

Prostate Cancer

There is considerable interest in dietary and lifestyle risk factors for prostate cancer, but there is little definitive evidence to date. Ecologic and migrant studies suggest that the dietary patterns of industrialized countries, associated with high saturated fat and protein intake and relatively low intake of fruits and vegetables, contribute to increased risk (142). There is evidence of an increased risk in association with high intake of saturated fat from animal and dairy sources (143–145). However, fat intake was not predictive of risk in a case-control study in England, thought to be due in part to a high mean fat intake and a relatively narrow range (146). Based on the results of a case-control study in Sweden, Andersson et al. (147) suggest that the association between prostate cancer risk and dietary fat is eliminated by controlling for total energy intake. The discrepancies in the available literature may be interpreted as suggesting that intake of saturated fat or total energy, or both, are among the factors contributing to population risk for prostate cancer, but that other important factors remain to be identified to further stratify the risk among members of a population with high or low mean fat and energy intake.

As with virtually all other cancers, there is an association between prostate cancer risk and obesity. American Cancer Society data suggest a marked increase in prostate cancer risk with rising BMI (23).

Fish intake may not protect against prostate cancer incidence but may have a decided benefit for prostate cancer mortality (148). Although a recent trial showed higher prostate cancer risk with higher plasma level of long-chain ω-3 PUFAs (like those derived from fish intake) (149), commentators have been critical of the plasma measure used in the study, which does not accurately reflect long-term intake, and of the conclusion, which may erroneously attribute disordered ω-3 partitioning to high consumption (150). Still, meta-analyses of a shorter-chain ω-3 PUFA (specifically α-linolenic acid) show inconsistent findings; there may be increased risk of prostate cancer overall with higher intakes, blood levels, or adipose concentrations, but prospective studies do not show a clear association (151,152).

A variety of micronutrients have been suggested to protect against prostate cancer, although for most, the evidence is limited. However, as virtually all of the putatively protective nutrients are found in fruits and vegetables, the evidence is more convincing that fruit and vegetable intake may be protective (145). The evidence in support of a specific protective effect of tomatoes and/or their lycopene content raises the possibility that high fruit and vegetable intake is a marker of high tomato intake (142). Of note, whereas the incidence of clinically apparent prostate cancer varies markedly among populations, the incidence of latent cancer appears to be fairly consistent among diverse populations (153,154). This observation suggests that the role of dietary factors may be to inhibit or stimulate the promotion of microscopic tumor foci. Such inhibitory effects have been observed for fat-restricted and soy-supplemented diets in animals (153).

Preliminary evidence has suggested protective effects of vitamins D and E, but further study is required before a basis for recommendations is established (143,155). Recent data from the ATBC trial suggest that α-tocopherol may inhibit the transformation of clinically latent to clinically active prostate cancer. The same study showed a decrease in prostate cancer risk in non-alcohol drinkers receiving β-carotene but an increased risk in drinkers (156,157). Like lycopene, β-carotene is concentrated in the prostate (158).

An inverse association between intake of retinoid (which regulates epithelial cell growth and is chemically related to vitamin A) and prostate cancer risk has been reported fairly consistently. In contrast, intake of retinol—a first generation retinoid—has been positively associated with risk in several studies (143). Data from the Health Professionals Follow-up Study suggested an inverse association between prostate cancer risk and intake of lycopene but not other carotenoids, the organic pigments found in carrots and apricots (159). A positive association between retinol and cancer risk was not seen. Studies suggesting a protective effect of lycopene generated considerable interest (158), but an association with lycopene was not seen in recent case-control studies (146,160). The largest cohort study to date, involving nearly 30,000 participants, does not support a protective effect of lycopene against prostate cancer (161,162). As tomatoes are the highly predominant source of dietary lycopene, associations observed between lycopene intake and prostate cancer risk may pertain to some other nutrient in tomatoes (159). At this point, data from ongoing randomized controlled trials will be required to establish a role for lycopene in defense against prostate cancer. Uncertainties about dietary factors in the etiology of prostate cancer are highlighted by a case-control study conducted in the United Kingdom, which revealed essentially no association with either fat or carotenoid intake (146).

Other Cancers

The principal risk factor for cancer of the esophagus appears to be tobacco exposure, but the effect is apparently promoted by alcohol (163). Fruit and vegetable intake is inversely associated with risk for esophageal cancer. An association with obesity has been suggested and derives support from the American Cancer Society's large observational cohort study (23).

The link between alcohol consumption and gastric cancer risk is less clear. Epidemiologic studies suggest that risk is increased by high intake of salted, cured, smoked, and pickled foods (114), with salt apparently the dominant factor (164). High fruit and vegetable intake has been consistently associated with reduced risk of gastric cancer (163).

An ecologic study of populations in 24 European countries suggests that when total fat intake is high, fish and fish oil confer protection against both colorectal and breast cancers (165). The etiology of childhood cancers is poorly understood at present. An association between maternal consumption of cured meats containing N-nitroso compounds and brain tumor risk has been suggested (166). Recommendations to avoid such products are consistent with general dietary guidelines. Other specific recommendations to reduce the risk of childhood cancer cannot be made on the basis of available evidence.

Data from the Iowa Women's Health Study suggest that fat from animal sources and a diet high in meat may increase risk of non-Hodgkin's lymphoma (167); fruit consumption appeared to be protective.

A case-control study in Japan, where the incidence of pancreatic cancer is rising concurrently with lifestyle changes, suggests that a predominantly plant-based diet is protective, whereas meat consumption increases risk (168). The prevailing consensus is that fruits and vegetables are protective, whereas high intake of meat, saturated fat, or both increases risk (169). Obesity is associated with increased risk (170). Obesity and adiposity have been associated with several tumors of hormonal tissues, including ovary, uterus, breast, and prostate. Obesity is thought to promote tumorigenesis by raising estrogen levels, as well as by promoting insulin resistance and insulin-like growth factor, as noted above (41,170). Obesity also has been linked to renal cell cancer, particularly in women (171). A large, ongoing American Cancer Society observational cohort study suggests an association between obesity and virtually all varieties of cancer (23). In a case-control study, Davies et al. (172) found an association between the risk of testicular cancer and milk consumption, compatible with prior work suggesting an association with fat intake. A case-control study in Washington State suggested that fried food consumption may increase bladder cancer risk, whereas fruit, vitamin C from both diet and supplements, and multivitamin use may decrease risk (173).

Animal and in vitro studies implicate nitrates, nitrites, and N-nitroso compounds, but no definitive evidence is available in humans (174). In a concise summary, Willett (34) made the following observations: Cancer of the oral cavity is inversely associated with fruit and possibly vegetable intake and positively associated with alcohol intake; esophageal cancer is inversely associated with fruit and vegetable intake and positively associated with alcohol and hot drink consumption; gastric cancer is inversely associated with fruit and vegetable intake, is positively associated with salt intake, and may be positively associated with egg and total carbohydrate intake; pancreatic cancer risk may be reduced by fruit, vegetable, and fiber intake and increased by intake of alcohol, meat, protein, and carbohydrate; both endometrial and renal cancers are convincingly associated with obesity; and fruit and vegetable consumption appears to be at least weakly protective against most cancers studied. Summary recommendations of most agencies attempting to prevent cancer are consistent with these associations and include reduced fat intake; increased fruit, vegetable, and fiber intake; maintenance of body weight near ideal; and minimal consumption of salt-cured, pickled, and smoked foods, and alcohol (35). It should be noted that with our evolving understanding, total dietary fat may be less important for cancer prevention than the distribution of fats in the diet.

NUTRIENTS, NUTRICEUTICALS, AND FUNCTIONAL FOODS

The natural reductionist tendencies of Western science are perhaps nowhere more evident, for good or for bad, than in efforts to elucidate the relationships between dietary constituents and cancer risk. As stated earlier, the weight of evidence clearly favors a diet rich in fruits and vegetables. Whether or not isolated nutrients found in plant foods can provide the benefits of a prudent dietary pattern is far from established. Most studies to date in pursuit of such evidence have proved disappointing. Nonetheless, a variety of nutrients and nutrient categories have received considerable attention in both the professional literature and lay press, and they are addressed briefly here.

Vitamin C

Despite long-standing interest in the potential for vitamin C to prevent cancer by virtue of its antioxidant properties, to date there is no convincing evidence that supplementation effectively prevents or treats cancer. High dietary intake of vitamin C is consistently associated with reduced cancer risk, but such intake invariably is associated with high fruit and vegetable consumption (175). The evidence regarding vitamin C supplementation is summarized in Section VIIE.

Carotenoids

There are more than 600 carotenoids in nature, most of which are widespread in plants, lending pigment that functions in photoprotection and photosynthesis (176). Approximately 50 carotenoids are retinoids, moieties with varying vitamin A activity (177). The hypothesis that carotenoids in general may prevent cancer is based on associations between cancer risk and dietary intake patterns (178) and on a mechanistic rationale (179). However, no definitive evidence of benefit from isolated supplements has been produced to date.

β–Carotene

Abundant in dark green, yellow, and orange fruits and vegetables, β-carotene is the most extensively studied of the carotenoids. Interest in the cancer-fighting properties of the nutrient derived from observational and ecologic studies. Intervention trials to date report consistently negative results, however, with β-carotene in supplement form increasing cancer risk in smokers in both CARET (127) and the ATBC trial (129). β-carotene failed to reduce the development of colorectal adenomas in an intervention trial (180) and showed no benefit in a prospective study of prostate cancer (181). Results from these and other studies resulted in recommendations to avoid supplemental β-carotene, particularly in smokers, and have shifted interest to other carotenoids, alone or in combination with each other and unrelated antioxidants. The evidence regarding β-carotene supplementation is summarized in Section VIIE.

Lycopene

Lycopene is the carotenoid responsible for the bright red color of tomatoes. It differs from other carotenoids in several respects. Lycopene lacks a ring structure; therefore, it cannot be converted to vitamin A. Because of its 11-carbon chain of conjugated double bonds, lycopene has exceptional antioxidant capacity. Recent data from a large, prospective cohort study mitigate against a protective effect (161,162). Clinical trial data should be available in the near future. The evidence regarding lycopene supplementation is summarized in Section VIIE.

Vitamin E

Vitamin E, inevitably provided as α-tocopherol, is a lipid-soluble antioxidant. Like β-carotene, it has been studied in cancer prevention with largely disappointing results. The ATBC and CARET studies both included vitamin E and showed no significant benefit (127,128). In contrast to β- carotene, vitamin E appeared relatively innocuous in these studies, although there have been hints of potential cardiovascular harms at high doses in other studies (see Chapter 7). Some interest persists in the potential role of vitamin E in combination with water-soluble antioxidants such as vitamin C in cancer prevention. Evidence supporting a role for supplemental vitamin E in cancer prevention is in the aggregate unconvincing at present (182). The evidence regarding vitamin E supplementation is summarized in Section VIIE.

Selenium

Selenium is an essential mineral with antioxidant properties. Studies in China, where soil is generally selenium poor, provide definitive evidence for selenium in cancer prevention (183–186). In the United States, where selenium deficiency is rare, a role for supplemental selenium in cancer prevention is much less certain (187), although some trials have been suggestive (188). A recent study in the United States found that dietary selenium intake was associated with reduced risk of pancreatic cancer (189). The evidence regarding selenium supplementation is summarized in Section VIIE.

Fiber

Dietary fiber, a diverse group of indigestible components of plant cell walls, is thought to mediate cancer risk by several mechanisms (190). By increasing fecal bulk and reducing intestinal transit time, insoluble fibers may reduce the risk of colon cancer. Dietary fiber has shown inverse associations with colon cancer risk in both retrospective (191,192) and prospective studies (193). Wheat-bran fiber has been shown to reduce bile acid excretion in patients with resected colon adenomas, suggesting an additional mechanism by which colon cancer risk may be reduced (194). The effect of fiber on the microbiome is also an emerging area of interest. Fiber may exert its protective influence on colon cancer risk and irritable bowel disease partially through fermentation of butyrate, which may decrease the inflammatory response in the colon (195). However, data from the Health Professionals Follow-up Study failed to demonstrate an association between fiber intake and colon cancer risk (196), as have intervention trials of polyp recurrence, as noted previously (65,66). As the overall evidence on the effects of fiber supplementation rather than fiber from dietary sources is mixed at best, use of supplemental fiber to reduce colon cancer risk has been discouraged (197). A protective effect of soluble fibers and cellulose in breast cancer has been reported from a large case-control study

(198). The weight of evidence favors a diet rich in both soluble and insoluble fibers found in fruits, vegetables, beans, lentils, and whole grains. Evidence is insufficient to support supplementation as a means of reducing cancer risk (190). Soluble and insoluble fibers are discussed in Section VIIE.

Green Tea

There is considerable interest in a potential role for green tea, and a particular constituent, epigallocatechin gallate (EGCG), in cancer prevention. Evidence to date derives from epidemiologic studies, animal research, and early-phase intervention trials (199–203). Evidence of benefit is as yet far from definitive, but such benefit is biologically plausible. The inclusion of green, black, white (the most concentrated in bioflavonoids), or oolong in the diet may be recommended as a strategy with some potential to confer health benefit and negligible, if any, potential to confer harm.

Olive Oil

Olive oil is among the salient components of the health-promoting Mediterranean diet, which has been associated with reduced rates of cancer as well as heart disease. There is conjecture that olive oil may offer specific protection against cancer (204). Such effects are attributed to high levels of monounsaturated fatty acids, squalene, tocopherols, and phenolic compounds (205). Whether or not definitive evidence ensues that olive oil protects against cancer, its inclusion in the diet as a health-promoting cooking oil is certainly advisable.

Ethanol

Ethanol is well established as a promoter of head and neck cancers, and its consumption is consistently associated with increased risk of cancers of the gastrointestinal tract, respiratory tract, and breast (206–208). These associations and their implications for advice to patients about alcohol intake are addressed in Chapter 40.

Artificial Sweeteners

The potential carcinogenicity of artificial sweeteners, particularly aspartame, but also sucralose and saccharin, is frequent fodder for the media (209). Such associations from animal research as have been seen are not coupled to any direct evidence in humans. Given the enormous population level exposure to aspartame and other artificial sweeteners, even a very small but meaningful effect on cancer risk would likely have long since been discernible. While the topic is deserving of ongoing scrutiny, there does not appear to be cause for particular concern at present (see Chapter 42). Current guidelines from the U.S. National Cancer Institute report that there is no clear evidence that artificial sweeteners available in the United States are associated with cancer risk in humans (210).

Soy

The evidence linking soy intake and cancer risk is mixed for breast cancer as well as prostate cancer. Population studies generally show lower breast (and other) cancer rates in populations that eat more soy. However, studies that have intervened with soy supplements and examined effects on cancer cells in vitro have actually suggested that the plant estrogens in soy can cause breast cancer to grow faster (211–216).

The explanations for such discordant findings are as yet uncertain. It may be that the effects of soy in vitro and in vivo differ. It may be that soy has some favorable and some unfavorable influences on cancer cell proliferation and cancer biology. It may be that populations eating soy are actually benefiting from something else altogether, such as not eating the foods soy often replaces, meat salient among them. Soy is widely used as a meat substitute, and red meat has been linked to higher cancer risk. It may also be that the soy products the Japanese eat, such as edamame (boiled soybeans in their pods) and miso, a fermented soybean product, have different effects than popular soy foods in the United States, such as soy-based energy bars and soy milk. A recent National Cancer Institute workshop on soy and breast cancer risk concluded that the evidence is inconclusive to date (217). Soy may be recommended as a healthful component of the diet, but reliance on soy as a targeted strategy for cancer prevention is not supported by the available data (218).

While soy has been shown to have mixed effects on cancer in some lab studies, studies in humans have shown no consistent detrimental effect of soy intake on cancer risk. Indeed, the 2012 American Cancer Society Guidelines on Nutrition and Physical Activity for Cancer Survivors concluded that current research suggests no harmful effects of eating soy for breast cancer survivors. A recent study of breast cancer patients in China found that soy consumption was linked to reduced risk of cancer recurrence and mortality (219). Another recent study found similar results among a mixed cohort of women in the United States and China (220). At this point, soy foods appear to be safe for both cancer survivors and the general population. However, the effect of soy on cancer risk may vary considerably by fermentation, cancer type, and patient population. For example, the Shanghai Women's Health Study found that soy consumption may reduce lung cancer risk in nonsmoking women, especially for aggressive tumors (221), while a recent meta-analysis found that soy food consumption may lower lung cancer risk overall, but that more standardized studies were necessary to fully understand the effect of soy (222). Another study found that soy intake may be associated with better survival for breast cancer patients, especially ER negative, ER+/PR+, and postmenopausal patients (223). Kim et al. (224) found that fermented soy foods did not reduce gastric cancer risk, but that high consumption of nonfermented soy foods did. Other studies have found potential associations between soy food consumption and reduced stomach, gynaecological, and colorectal cancer risk, but emphasize the need for further research to confirm these effects (225–227).

Organic versus Conventional Food

Currently, there is no clear evidence that organic meat and produce lower cancer risk as compared to conventionally grown foods. A recent meta-analysis found that organic foods are no more nutritious than conventional foods (228). The study did find that organic produce had less pesticide residue than conventional foods, though both organic and conventional foods had pesticide levels under the safety limits set by the Environmental Protection Agency. Organic produce also contained more phenols, which may prevent cancer,

but authors of the study indicate these results should be interpreted with caution.

Conjugated Linoleic Acid

There is some preliminary evidence of an anticancer effect of conjugated linoleic acid (CLA) (229–231) (see Chapter 2). Such early reports are consistent with the expansive literature suggesting that the quantity and distribution of dietary fats may influence overall cancer risk substantially. The clinical implications for CLA in efforts to attenuate cancer risk remain to be elucidated (232).

Folate

Low folate intake has been associated with increased risk of colorectal and cervical cancers (233). While these associations remain investigational (234), there are other compelling reasons to ensure that all patients (especially female patients) consume at least 400 μg of folate daily (see Chapters 4, 7, and 27), which may offer the added benefit of reduced risk of prostate cancer and potentially melanoma (235,236). However, there is cause for concern with folic acid supplementation as trials have shown increased cancer incidence in the supplementation arms (237).

Other Nutrients

To date, no other micronutrients have been studied adequately to permit definitive recommendations regarding a role in cancer prevention in humans. However, numerous substances are biologically plausible inhibitors of cancer and are supported in this role by preliminary evidence.

Allyl compounds, found in garlic, onion, chives, and leeks, demonstrate inhibition of tumor induction in vitro and are associated with reduced rates of cancer, particularly gastric cancer, in epidemiologic studies. Isothiocyanates, organic compounds distributed widely in plants and particularly abundant in cruciferous vegetables, appear to suppress carcinogen activation by the cytochrome P-450 system. Indole compounds, also abundant in cruciferous vegetables, demonstrate inhibition of carcinogenesis in mammary cell lines, possibly mediated by effects on estrogen. Flavonoids, organic antioxidants widely distributed in plants, may have cancer-fighting properties. This class of compounds includes flavones, flavonols, and iso-flavones. Flavones found in citrus fruit have been shown to inhibit growth of malignant cells in tissue culture. Of the flavonols, quercetin has been most extensively studied and has been shown to inhibit growth of neoplastic cells.

Tea leaves used to prepare green, black, white, and oolong tea contain polyphenols, including catechins and flavonols. Quinones are produced when the tea is oxidized. The constituents of such tea have been shown to inhibit nitrosamine formation in vitro. Tea consumption has been associated with reduced cancer risk in observational studies (238,239).

Soybeans are a rich source of isoflavones, which are converted by intestinal bacteria to substances with weak estrogen activity and the capacity to function as estrogen antagonists in certain tissues. These substances appear to inhibit the growth of mammary cell tumors as well as tumor-induced angiogenesis.

Terpenes, lipid-soluble compounds found in a variety of herbs, have demonstrated a variety of anticancer properties, including suppression of cellular proliferation and induction of apoptosis (240,241).

The list of nutrients with the potential to influence cancer risk by diverse mechanisms is long and continuously growing. The clinician is obligated to remain alert for significant trial results with potential clinical implications.

OTHER TOPICS OF INTEREST

Acrylamide

Acrylamide, a carcinogenic compound formed when starchy foods are cooked at high temperature, has been identified in products as diverse as breakfast cereals and french fries (242). Whether acrylamide poses a meaningful risk to humans at typical exposure levels and what implications this may have for food manufacturing and preparation are as yet uncertain. A recent meta-analysis evaluating 25 relevant studies concluded there was no increased risk of most types of cancer from exposure to acrylamide (243). Nonetheless, the U.S. National Toxicology Program states acrylamide is "reasonable anticipated to be a human carcinogen" and the U.S. Environmental Protection Agency reports it is "likely to be carcinogenic to humans" (244).

Pesticide Residues

Many environmental contaminants, including pesticide residues on foods, are potential carcinogens (5). Concern about such associations contributes to widespread enthusiasm for organic foods. There is, however, no direct evidence in humans of differential cancer rates attributable to chemical residues on food, and as yet, there is no conclusive evidence of benefit from choosing organic foods to avoid such exposures. For example, arsenic—found in agricultural products such as insecticides—was recently found in rice and rice products in the United States at levels high enough to cause of concern for some experts. While arsenic in insecticides is limited to organic arsenic, which is likely nontoxic, arsenic in ground water and rice is inorganic, and may be concerning for increased cancer risk. However, it is not clear that the levels of arsenic found in rice increases risk of cancer, and indeed, the benefits of eating rice—especially whole grain brown rice, which has more arsenic than white rice—may outweigh the risks. Of course, alternative arguments may readily be made to support the preferential production and selection of organically grown foods.

Calorie Restriction

Energy restriction has been shown to have tumor-inhibiting properties in animal studies (245,246) A recent study conducted in mice found that a high-fat, low-carbohydrate ketogenic diet may reduce glucose availability and inhibit tumor growth of malignant brain cancers (247). No long-term studies of calorie restriction have been conducted in humans, nor do such studies seem probable. Most cancers, including breast, prostate, ovarian, endometrial, and renal, may be promoted by either high calorie intake or the resultant high BMI (248). Energy restriction and decreased adiposity may be especially important for breast cancer prevention (249,250). Further study of calorie restriction in cancer prevention is warranted and may be most effectively approached in the context of secondary prevention studies (i.e., prevention of cancer recurrence following successful treatment). In that setting, however, restriction of calories would need to be judiciously balanced against the quality of the diet and nutritional support to preserve lean body mass.

Calorie restriction has recently been studied in the context of SIRT1 gene expression. SIRT1 is an enzyme with a range of cellular functions related to calorie restriction, insulin sensitivity, and cancer development. It acts as an important sensor of nutrient availability in cells and may protect adipose tissue from inflammation under normal feeding conditions. SIRT1 seems to be downregulated in cells with high insulin resistance, and inducing its expression may increase insulin sensitivity (251). Recent evidence suggests SIRT1 enhances skeletal muscle insulin sensitivity during caloric restriction (252). Furthermore, a high-fat diet may act to cleave the SIRT1 protein, and promote inflammation and metabolic dysfunction (253).

SIRT1 also plays a role in cancer metabolism. It has been suggested to have both oncogenic and tumor-suppressor effects, depending on the p53 gene status (254). A recent study found that SIRT1 expression in mice may be a key mediator of the influence of caloric restriction on improved longevity, as SIRT1 may serve to protect colonic mucosa from excessive cell growth (255).

Diet and Cancer Management

By a variety of mechanisms, cancer tends to induce malnutrition (256). Although there is theoretical concern that nutritional support might stimulate tumor growth, there is no evidence of such an effect in humans (257). While in part the result of cancer and treatment factors that may reduce nutrient intake, cancer cachexia differs from starvation in that basal energy expenditure, lipolysis, and protein turnover are increased rather than decreased (256). Optimizing dietary quality to preserve lean body mass and support immune system activity may have important implications for recovery (258–260).

Patients with cancer are at particularly high nutritional risk and often content with continuous loss of lean body mass. The American Society for Parenteral and Enteral Nutrition (ASPEN) has issued guidelines stating that at risk patients should undergo nutrition screening and development of a nutrition care plan, if necessary. Recent studies suggest that oral nutritional interventions may help maintain lean body mass in cancer patients and elderly individuals.

A 2012 systematic review and meta-analysis of 13 studies and 1,414 individuals conducted by Baldwin and colleagues found that oral nutritional interventions increase nutrition intake and improve some quality of life measures in patients with cancer, but do not seem to improve mortality (261). Similarly, Baier et al. (262) found that a simple amino-acid cocktail was effective for increasing lean tissue and protein turnover in elderly individuals.

Learned Food Aversions

Foods associated circumstantially with the unpleasant effects of cancer treatments may result in aversions. Nearly 50% of untreated cancer patients have such aversions, and new ones develop with treatment in more than 50% of all patients. Although several approaches have been tried to prevent learned food aversions from developing, the most promising approach to date is the administration of nutritionally unimportant foods near treatment times so that learned food aversions are directed toward such foods rather than those with important nutritional value (263).

CLINICAL HIGHLIGHTS

Inconsistent and conflicting literature on the relative effectiveness of specific nutrients in preventing cancer of various tissues may be seen as a challenging quagmire of evidence from which no meaningful message can be extracted. If one looks at dietary pattern rather than nutrient consumption, however, the literature is remarkably consistent. The risk for virtually all cancers influenced by diet can likely be reduced with a diet rich in whole plant-based foods like fruits and vegetables. Avoidance of conventionally produced red meat and processed foods has strong support. Dairy foods may be of benefit. Both obesity and high total energy intake, which are correlated with one another, appear to increase risk of most cancers. When fat intake is relatively high, the greater the proportion of fat that is n-3 polyunsaturated, such as that found in fish, the lower the cancer risk; such benefit appears to be absent when fat intake is low. Similarly, a variety of micronutrients that show benefit in populations with marginal diets show no such benefits in populations with abundant diets.

Genetic polymorphisms induce variable susceptibility to diet-related diseases of all kinds but may be especially important in carcinogenesis. Numerous trials highlight the potential importance of genetic polymorphisms and gene/nutrient interactions in cancer development and prevention. Advances in the field of nutrigenomics will undoubtedly foster tailored advice to patients about dietary strategies for minimizing personal cancer risk, but the field remains inchoate at present.

Patients wishing to minimize cancer risk using the knowledge presently at hand should be encouraged to eat a diet rich in fruits and vegetables. Meat should be predominantly poultry and fish. Alcohol consumption should be limited. Ideal body weight should be maintained by prudent energy intake and regular physical activity. Regular consumption of green, black, white, or oolong (oolong is a partially oxidized tea, between green and black tea) tea might confer some benefit. Inclusion of soy in the diet might also confer some benefit, particularly if used as a substitute for red meat. The avoidance of charred food, deep-fried food, and smoke-cured food may be reasonably advised. High doses of any single micronutrient cannot be recommended based on currently available evidence.

REFERENCES

1. Greenwald P, Anderson D, Nelson SA, et al. Clinical trials of vitamin and mineral supplements for cancer prevention. *Am J Clin Nutr* 2007;85:314s–317s.

2. Tran GD, Sun XD, Abnet CC, et al. Prospective study of risk factors for esophageal and gastric cancers in the Linxian general population trial cohort in China. *Int J Cancer* 2005;113:456–463.

3. Doll R, Peto R. The causes of cancer: quantitative estimates of avoidable risks of cancer in the United States today. *J Natl Cancer Inst* 1981;66:1191–1308.

4. Zhang Y, Zhang Y. Formation and reduction of acrylamide in Maillard reaction: a review based on the current state of knowledge. *Crit Rev Food Sci Nutr* 2007;47:521–542.

5. Silent Spring Institute. *Environment and breast cancer: science review.* Available at http://sciencereview.silentspring.org/index.cfm; accessed 10/12/07.

6. Consumer Reports. *When it pays to buy organic.* February 2006. Available at http://www.consumerreports.org/cro/food/organic-products-206/overview/index.htm; accessed 10/12/07.

7. Lopez-Garcia E, Schulze MB, Meigs JB, et al. Consumption of trans fatty acids is related to plasma biomarkers of inflammation and endothelial dysfunction. *J Nutr* 2005;135:562–566.

8. Theodoratou E, McNeill G, Cetnarskyj R, et al. Dietary fatty acids and colorectal cancer: a case-control study. *Am J Epidemiol* 2007;166:181–195.

9. Choi Y, Giovannucci E, Lee JE. Glycaemic index and glycaemic load in relation to risk of diabetes-related cancers: a meta-analysis. *Br J Nutr* 2012;108(11):1934–1947.

10. Gnagnarella P, Gandini S, La Vecchia C, et al. Glycemic index, glycemic load, and cancer risk: a meta-analysis. *Am J Clin Nutr* 2008;87(6):1793–1801.

11. Nagle CM, Olsen CM, Ibiebele TI, et al. Glycemic index, glycemic load and endometrial cancer risk: results from the Australian National Endometrial Cancer study and an updated systematic review and meta-analysis. *Eur J Nutr* 2013;52(2):705–715.

12. Mulholland HG, Murray LJ, Cardwell CR, et al. Dietary glycaemic index, glycaemic load and endometrial and ovarian cancer risk: a systematic review and meta-analysis. *Br J Cancer* 2008;99(3):434–441.

13. Aune D, Chan DS, Vieira AR, et al. Dietary fructose, carbohydrates, glycemic indices and pancreatic cancer risk: a systematic review and meta-analysis of cohort studies. *Ann Oncol* 2012;23(10):2536–2546.

14. Aune D, Chan DS, Lau R, et al. Carbohydrates, glycemic index, glycemic load, and colorectal cancer risk: a systematic review and meta-analysis of cohort studies. *Cancer Causes Control* 2012;23(4):521–535.

15. Mulholland HG, Murray LJ, Cardwell CR, et al. Glycemic index, glycemic load, and risk of digestive tract neoplasms: a systematic review and meta-analysis. *Am J Clin Nutr* 2009;89(2):568–576.

16. Mulholland HG, Murray LJ, Cardwell CR, et al. Dietary glycaemic index, glycaemic load and breast cancer risk: a systematic review and meta-analysis. *Br J Cancer* 2008;99(7):1170–1175.

17. Aleksandrova K, Nimptsch K, Pischon T. Obesity and colorectal cancer. *Front Biosci* (Elite Ed). 2013;5:61–77.

18. Chi F, Wu R, Zeng YC, et al. Circulation insulin-like growth factor peptides and colorectal cancer risk: an updated systematic review and meta-analysis. *Mol Biol Rep* 2013;40(5):3583–3590.

19. Rowlands MA, Gunnell D, Harris R, et al. Circulating insulin-like growth factor peptides and prostate cancer risk: a systematic review and meta-analysis. *Int J Cancer* 2009;124(10):2416–2429.

20. Roddam AW, Allen NE, Appleby P, et al. Insulin-like growth factors, their binding proteins, and prostate cancer risk: analysis of individual patient data from 12 prospective studies. *Ann Intern Med* 2008;149(7):461–471, W83–8.

21. Shi R, Yu H, McLarty J, et al. IGF-I and breast cancer: a meta-analysis. *Int J Cancer* 2004;111(3):418–423.

22. Giovannucci E. Insulin, insulin-like growth factors and colon cancer: a review of the evidence. *J Nutr* 2001;131(11):3109S–3120S.

23. Calle EE, Rodriguez C, Walker-Thurmond K, et al. Overweight, obesity, and mortality from cancer in a prospectively studied cohort of US adults. *N Engl J Med* 2003;348:1625–1638.

24. Centers for Disease Control and Prevention. Fruit and vegetable consumption among adults—United States, 2005. *MMWR* 2007;56:213–217. Available at http://www.cdc.gov/mmwr/preview/mmwrhtml/mm5610a2.htm; accessed 10/12/07.

25. Key TJ, Schatzkin A, Willett WC, et al. Diet, nutrition and the prevention of cancer. *Public Health Nutr* 2004;7: 187–200.

26. Nixon WD. *The cancer recovery eating plan.* New York, NY: Three Rivers Press, 1996.

27. Hyltander A, Bosaeus I, Svedlund J, et al. Supportive nutrition on recovery of metabolism, nutritional state, health-related quality of life, and exercise capacity after major surgery: a randomized study. *Clin Gastroenterol Hepatol* 2005;3:466–474.

28. Ng K, Leung SF, Johnson PJ, et al. Nutritional consequences of radiotherapy in nasopharynx cancer patients. *Nutr Cancer* 2004;49:156–161.

29. Bozzetti F. Nutritional issues in the care of the elderly patient. *Crit Rev Oncol Hematol* 2003;48:113–121.

30. Baracos VE, Mackenzie ML. Investigations of branched-chain amino acids and their metabolites in animal models of cancer. *J Nutr* 2006;136:237s–242s.

31. Laviano A, Muscaritoli M, Cascino A, et al. Branched-chain amino acids: the best compromise to achieve anabolism? *Curr Opin Clin Nutr Metab Care* 2005;8:408–414.

32. Mantovani G, Maccio A, Madeddu C, et al. Cancer-related cachexia and oxidative stress: beyond current therapeutic options. *Expert Rev Anticancer Ther* 2003;3:381–392.

33. Gomes-Marcondes MC, Ventrucci G, Toledo MT, et al. A leucine-supplemented diet improved protein content of skeletal muscle in young tumor-bearing rats. *Braz J Med Biol Res* 2003;36:1589–1594.

34. Willett WC. Nutrition and cancer: a summary of the evidence. *Cancer Causes Control* 1996;7:178–180.

35. Greenwald P. The potential of dietary modification to prevent cancer. *Prev Med* 1996;25:41.

36. Fraser D. Nutrition and cancer: epidemiological aspects. *Public Health Rev* 1996;24:113.

37. Prasad KN, Cole W, Hovland P. Cancer prevention studies: past, present, and future directions. *Nutrition* 1998;14: 197–210.

38. Laviano A, Meguid MM. Nutritional issues in cancer management. *Nutrition* 1996;12:358–371.

39. Butrum RR, Clifford CK, Lanza E. NCI dietary guidelines: rationale. *Am J Clin Nutr* 1988;48:888.

40. Lindsay DG. Dietary contribution to genotoxic risk and its control. *Food Chem Toxicol* 1996;34:423.

41. The American Cancer Society 1996 Advisory Committee on Diet, Nutrition, and Cancer Prevention. Guidelines on diet, nutrition, and cancer prevention: reducing the risk of cancer with healthy food choices and physical activity. *CA Cancer J Clin* 1996;46:325.

42. Divisi D, Di Tommaso S, Salvemini S, et al. Diet and cancer. *Acta Biomed* 2006;77:118–123.

43. de Lorgeril M, Salen P. Modified cretan Mediterranean diet in the prevention of coronary heart disease and cancer: An update. *World Rev Nutr Diet* 2007;97:1–32.

44. Linos E, Holmes MD, Willett WC. Diet and breast cancer. *Curr Oncol Rep* 2007;9:31–41.

45. Jones LW, Demark-Wahnefried W. Diet, exercise, and complementary therapies after primary treatment for cancer. *Lancet Oncol* 2006;7:1017–1026.

46. Kapiszewska M. A vegetable to meat consumption ratio as a relevant factor determining cancer preventive diet. The Mediterranean versus other European countries. *Forum Nutr* 2006;59:130–153.

47. Tercyak KP, Tyc VL. Opportunities and challenges in the prevention and control of cancer and other chronic diseases: children's diet and nutrition and weight and physical activity. *J Pediatr Psychol* 2006;31:750–763.

48. Colomer R, Menendez JA. Mediterranean diet, olive oil and cancer. *Clin Transl Oncol* 2006;8:15–21.

49. Bougnoux P, Giraudeau B, Couet C. Diet, cancer, and the lipidome. *Cancer Epidemiol Biomarkers Prev* 2006;15:416–421.

50. Uauy R, Solomons N. Diet, nutrition, and the life-course approach to cancer prevention. *J Nutr* 2005;135:2934s–2945s.

51. Jolly CA. Diet manipulation and prevention of aging, cancer and autoimmune disease. *Curr Opin Clin Nutr Metab Care* 2005;8:382–387.

52. Kushi LH, Byers T, Doyle C, et al. Reducing the risk of cancer with healthy food choices and physical activity. *CA Cancer J Clin* 2006;56:254–281.

53. American Diabetes Association. *Everyday choices for a healthier life.* Available at http://www.diabetes.org/everydaychoices/default.jsp; accessed 10/12/07.

54. Peipins LA, Sandler RS. Epidemiology of colorectal adenomas. *Epidemiol Rev* 1994;16:273.

55. Tantamango YM, Knutsen SF, Beeson L, et al. Association between dietary fiber and incident cases of colon polyps: the adventist health study. *Gastrointest Cancer Res* 2011;4(5–6):161–167.

56. Vargas AJ, Thompson PA. Diet and nutrient factors in colorectal cancer risk. *Nutr Clin Pract* 2012;27(5):613–623.

57. Kushi LH, Doyle C, McCullough M, et al; American Cancer Society 2010 Nutrition and Physical Activity Guidelines Advisory Committee. American Cancer Society Guidelines on nutrition and physical activity for cancer prevention: reducing the risk of cancer with healthy food choices and physical activity. *CA Cancer J Clin* 2012;62(1):30–67.

58. Aune D, Chan DS, Lau R, et al. Dietary fibre, whole grains, and risk of colorectal cancer: systematic review and dose-response meta-analysis of prospective studies. *BMJ* 2011;343:d6617.

59. Boyle T, Keegel T, Bull F, et al. Physical activity and risks of proximal and distal colon cancers: a systematic review and meta-analysis. *J Natl Cancer Inst* 2012;104(20):1548–1561.

60. McCullougha JS, Ratcliffeb B, Mandirc N, et al. Dietary fibre and intestinal microflora: effects on intestinal morphometry and crypt branching. *Gut* 1998;42:799–806.

61. Tilg H, Kaser A. Gut microbiome, obesity, and metabolic dysfunction. *J Clin Invest* 2011;121(6):2126–2132.

62. Hansen L, Skeie G, Landberg R, et al. Intake of dietary fiber, especially from cereal foods, is associated with lower incidence of colon cancer in the HELGA cohort. *Int J Cancer* 2012;131(2):469–478.

63. Sansbury LB, Wanke K, Albert PS, et al; Polyp Prevention Trial Study Group. The effect of strict adherence to a high-fiber, high-fruit and -vegetable, and low-fat eating pattern on adenoma recurrence. *Am J Epidemiol* 2009;170(5):576–584.

64. Steinmetz KA, Kushi LH, Bostik RM, et al. Vegetables, fruit, and colon cancer in Iowa Women's Health Study. *Am J Epidemiol* 1994;139:1.

65. Schatzkin A, Lanza E, Corle D, et al. Lack of effect of a low-fat, high-fiber diet on the recurrence of colorectal adenomas. *N Engl J Med* 2000;342:1149–1155.

66. Alberts DS, Martinez ME, Roe DJ, et al. Lack of effect of a high-fiber cereal supplement on the recurrence of colorectal adenomas. *N Engl J Med* 2000;342:1156–1162.

67. Byers T. Diet, colorectal adenomas, and colorectal cancer. *N Engl J Med* 2000;342:1206–1207.

68. Bingham S. The fibre–folate debate in colo-rectal cancer. *Proc Nutr Soc* 2006;65:19–23.

69. Dahm CC et al. Dietary fiber and colorectal cancer risk: a nested case-control study using food diaries. *J Natl Cancer Inst* 2010;102(9):614–626.

70. Slattery ML, Boucher KM, Caan BJ, et al. Eating patterns and risk of colon cancer. *Am J Epidemiol* 1998;148:4.

71. Erdelyi I, Levenkova N, Lin EY, et al. Western-style diets induce oxidative stress and dysregulate immune responses in the colon in a mouse model of sporadic colon cancer. *J Nutr* 2009;139(11):2072–2078.

72. Beresford SA, Johnson KC, Ritenbaugh C, et al. Low-fat dietary pattern and risk of colorectal cancer: the Women's Health Initiative Randomized Controlled Dietary Modification Trial. *JAMA* 2006;295:643–654.

73. Willett WC, Stampfer MJ, Colditz GA, et al. Relation of meat, fat, and fiber intake to the risk of colon cancer in a prospective study among women. *N Engl J Med* 1990;323:1664.

74. Corpet DE. Red meat and colon cancer: should we become vegetarians, or can we make meat safer? *Meat Sci* 2011;89(3):310–316.

75. Neugut AI, Garbowski GC, Lee WC, et al. Dietary risk factors for the incidence and recurrence of colorectal adenomatous polyps. A case-control study. *Ann Intern Med* 1993;118:91.

76. Miller PE, Lazarus P, Lesko SM, Meat-related compounds and colorectal cancer risk by anatomical subsite. *Nutr Cancer* 2013;65(2):202–226.

77. Aune D, Chan DS, Vieira AR, et al. Red and processed meat intake and risk of colorectal adenomas: a systematic review and meta-analysis of epidemiological studies. *Cancer Causes Control* 2013;24(4):611–627.

78. Alabaster O, Tang Z, Shivapurkar N. Dietary fiber and the chemopreventive modulation of colon carcinogenesis. *Mutat Res* 1996;350:185.

79. Park H, Kim M, Kwon GT, et al. A high-fat diet increases angiogenesis, solid tumor growth, and lung metastasis of CT26 colon cancer cells in obesity-resistant BALB/c mice. *Mol Carcinog* 2012;51(11):869–880.

80. Giovannucci E, Ascherio A, Rimm EB, et al. Physical activity, obesity, and risk for colon cancer and adenoma in men. *Ann Intern Med* 1995;122:327.

81. Pan A, Sun Q, Bernstein AM, et al. Red meat consumption and mortality: results from 2 prospective cohort studies. *Arch Intern Med* 2012;172(7):555–563.

82. Daley CA, Abbott A, Doyle PS, et al. A review of fatty acid profiles and antioxidant content in grass-fed and grain-fed beef. *Nutr J* 2010;9:10.

83. Bartsch H, Nair J, Owen RW. Dietary polyunsaturated fatty acids and cancers of the breast and colorectum: emerging evidence for their role as risk modifiers. *Carcinogenesis* 1999;20(12):2209–2218.

84. Huth PJ, DiRienzo DB, Miller GD. Major scientific advances with dairy foods in nutrition and health. *J Dairy Sci* 2006;89:1207–1221.

85. Kampman E, Giovannucci E, van't Veer P, et al. Calcium, vitamin D, dairy foods, and the occurrence of colorectal adenomas among men and women in two prospective studies. *Am J Epidemiol* 1994;139:16.

86. Lappe JM, Travers-Gustafson D, Davies KM, et al. Vitamin D and calcium supplementation reduces cancer risk: results of a randomized trial. *Am J Clin Nutr* 2007;85:1586–1591.

87. Wactawski-Wende J, Kotchen JM, Anderson GL, et al. Women's Health Initiative Investigators. Calcium plus vitamin D supplementation and the risk of colorectal cancer. *N Engl J Med* 2006;354:684–696.

88. Aune D, Lau R, Chan DS, et al. Dairy products and colorectal cancer risk: a systematic review and meta-analysis of cohort studies. *Ann Oncol* 2012;23(1):37–45.

89. Huncharek M, Muscat J, Kupelnick B. Colorectal cancer risk and dietary intake of calcium, vitamin D, and dairy products: a meta-analysis of 26,335 cases from 60 observational studies. *Nutr Cancer* 2009;61(1):47–69.

90. Jenab M, Bas Bueno-de-Mesquita H, Ferrari P, et al. Association between pre-diagnostic circulating vitamin D concentration and risk of colorectal cancer in European populations: a nested case-control study. *BMJ* 2010;340:b5500.

91. Carroll C, Cooper K, Papaioannou D, et al. Supplemental calcium in the chemoprevention of colorectal cancer: a systematic review and meta-analysis. *Clin Ther* 2010;32(5):789–803.

92. Hulka BS, Stark AT. Breast cancer: cause and prevention. *Lancet* 1995;346:883–887.

93. Hunter DJ, Willet WC. Nutrition and breast cancer. *Cancer Causes Control* 1996;7:56.

94. Greenwald P, Sherwood K, McDonald SS. Fat, caloric intake, and obesity: lifestyle risk factors for breast cancer. *J Am Diet Assoc* 1997;97:s24.

95. Kushi LH, Fee RM, Sellers TA, et al. Intake of vitamins A, C, E and postmenopausal breast cancer. *Am J Epidemiol* 1996;144:165.

96. Hunter DJ, Manson JE, Olditz GA, et al. A prospective study of the intake of vitamins C, E, and A and the risk of breast cancer. *N Engl J Med* 1993;329:234.

97. Fulan H, Changxing J, Baina WY, et al. Retinol, vitamins A, C, and E and breast cancer risk: a meta-analysis and meta-regression. *Cancer Causes Control* 2011;22(10):1383–1396.

98. Yeon JY, Suh YJ, Kim SW, et al. Evaluation of dietary factors in relation to the biomarkers of oxidative stress and inflammation in breast cancer risk. *Nutrition* 2011;27(9):912–918.

99. Hebert JR, Rosen A. Nutritional, socioeconomic, and reproductive factors in relation to female breast cancer mortality: findings from a cross-national study. *Cancer Detect Prev* 1996;20:234.

100. Hershcoppf RJ, Bradlow HL. Obesity, diet, endogenous estrogens and the risk of hormone-sensitive cancer. *Am J Clin Nutr* 1987;45:283.

101. Gregario DI, Emrich LJ, Graham S, et al. Dietary fat consumption and survival among women with breast cancer. *J Natl Cancer Inst* 1985;75:37.

102. Zumoff B. Hormonal profiles in women with breast cancer. *Anticancer Res* 1988;8:627.

103. Johnston PV. Dietary fat, eicosanoids, and immunity. *Adv Lipid Res* 1985;21:103.

104. Hebert JR, Augustine A, Barone J, et al. Weight, height and body mass in the prognosis of breast cancer: early results of a prospective study. *Int J Cancer* 1988;42:315.

105. Dorgan JF, Sowell A, Swanson CA, et al. Relationships of serum carotenoids, retinol, α-tocopherol, and selenium with breast cancer risk: results from a prospective study in Columbia, Missouri (United States). *Cancer Causes Control* 1998;9:89.

106. Smith-Warner SA, Spiegelman D, Yaun SS, et al. Alcohol and breast cancer in women: a pooled analysis of cohort studies. *JAMA* 1998;279:535.

107. Schatzkin A, Jones Y, Hoover RN, et al. Alcohol consumption and breast cancer in the epidemiologic follow-up study of the first National Health and Nutrition Examination Survey. *N Engl J Med* 1987;316:1169.

108. van den Brandt PA, Goldbohm A, van't Veer P. Alcohol and breast cancer: results from the Netherlands cohort study. *Am J Epidemiol* 1995;141:907.

109. Mezzetti M, La Vecchia C, Decarli A, et al. Population attributable risk for breast cancer: diet, nutrition, and physical exercise. *J Natl Cancer Inst* 1998;90:389.

110. Turner LB. A meta-analysis of fat intake, reproduction, and breast cancer risk: an evolutionary perspective. *Am J Hum Biol* 2011;23(5):601–608.

111. Schatzkin A, Greenwald P, Byar DP, et al. The dietary fat–breast cancer hypothesis is alive. *JAMA* 1989;261:3284.

112. Franceschi S, Favero A, Decarli A, et al. Intake of macronutrients and risk of breast cancer. *Lancet* 1996;347:1351.

113. Zheng JS, Hu XJ, Zhao YM, et al. Intake of fish and marine n-3 polyunsaturated fatty acids and risk of breast cancer: meta-analysis of data from 21 independent prospective cohort studies. *BMJ* 2013;346:f3706.

114. Boyd NF, Stone J, Vogt KN, et al. Dietary fat and breast cancer risk revisited: a meta-analysis of the published literature. *Br J Cancer* 2003;89(9):1672–1685.

115. Willett WC, Hunter DJ, Stampfer MJ, et al. Dietary fat and fiber in relation to risk of breast cancer. An 8-year follow-up. *JAMA* 1992;268:2037.

116. Willett WC, Stampfer MJ, Colditz GA, et al. Dietary fat and the risk of breast cancer. *N Engl J Med* 1987;316:22.

117. Holmberg L, Ohlander EM, Byers T, et al. Diet and breast cancer risk. Results from a population-based, case-control study in Sweden. *Arch Intern Med* 1994;154:1805.

118. Hunter DJ, Spiegelman D, Adami H-O, et al. Cohort studies of fat intake and the risk of breast cancer—a pooled analysis. *N Engl J Med* 1996;334:356.

119. Petrek JA, Peters M, Cirrincione C, et al. Is body fat topography a risk factor for breast cancer? *Ann Intern Med* 1993;118:356.

120. Potischman N, Weiss HA, Swanson CA, et al. Diet during adolescence and risk of breast cancer among young women. *J Natl Cancer Inst* 1998;90:226.

121. Ronco AL, De Stefani E, Boffetta P, et al. Food patterns and risk of breast cancer: a factor analysis study in Uruguay. *Int J Cancer* 2006;119:1672–1678.

122. Prentice RL, Caan B, Chlebowski RT, et al. Low-fat dietary pattern and risk of invasive breast cancer: the Women's Health Initiative Randomized Controlled Dietary Modification Trial. *JAMA* 2006;295:629–642.

123. Howe GR. Nutrition and breast cancer. In: Bendich A, Deckelbaum RJ, eds. *Preventive nutrition. The comprehensive guide for health professionals.* Totowa, NJ: Humana Press, 1997:97–108.

124. Linos E, Holmes MD, Willett WC. Diet and breast cancer. *Curr Oncol Rep* 2007;9:31–41.

125. Pierce JP, Stefanick ML, Flatt SW, et al. Greater survival after breast cancer in physically active women with high vegetable fruit intake regardless of obesity. *J Clin Oncol* 2007;25:2345–2351.

126. Colditz GA, Stampfer MJ, Willett WC. Diet and lung cancer. A review of the epidemiologic evidence in humans. *Arch Intern Med* 1987;147:157.

127. Omenn GS, Goodman GE, Thornquist MD, et al. Risk factors for lung cancer and for intervention effects in CARET, the Beta-Carotene and Retinol Efficacy Trial. *J Natl Cancer Inst* 1996;88:1550.

128. The Alpha-Tocopherol, Beta-Carotene Cancer Prevention Study Group. The effect of vitamin E and beta carotene on the incidence of lung cancer and other cancers in male smokers. *N Engl J Med* 1994;330:1029.

129. Albanes D, Heinonen OP, Taylor PR, et al. α-Tocopherol and β-carotene supplements and lung cancer incidence in the Alpha-Tocopherol, Beta-Carotene Cancer Prevention Study: effects of base-line characteristics and study compliance. *J Natl Cancer Inst* 1996;88:1560.

130. Challem JJ. Re: Risk factors for lung cancer and for intervention effects in CARET, the Beta-Carotene and Retinol Efficacy Trial [Letter]. *J Natl Cancer Inst* 1997;89:326.

131. Alavanja MCR, Brownson RC, Benichou J. Estimating the effect of dietary fat on the risk of lung cancer in nonsmoking women. *Lung Cancer* 1996;14:s63.

132. Smith-Warner SA, Ritz J, Hunter DJ, et al. Dietary fat and risk of lung cancer in a pooled analysis of prospective studies. *Cancer Epidemiol Biomarkers Prev* 2002;11(10 Pt 1):987–992.

133. Rylander R, Axelsson G, Andersson L, et al. Lung cancer, smoking and diet among Swedish men. *Lung Cancer* 1996;14:s75.

134. Elwood PC, Givens DI, Beswick AD, et al. The survival advantage of milk and dairy consumption: an overview of evidence from cohort studies of vascular diseases, diabetes and cancer. *J Am Coll Nutr* 2008;27(6):723S–734S.

135. Gao Y. Risk factors for lung cancer among nonsmokers with emphasis on lifestyle factors. *Lung Cancer* 1996;14:s39.

136. Dai X, Lin C, Sun X, et al. The etiology of lung cancer in nonsmoking females in Harbin, China. *Lung Cancer* 1996;14:s85.

137. Sanson CA, Mao BL, Li JY, et al. Dietary determinants of lung cancer risk: results from a case-control study in Hunan Province. *Int J Cancer* 1992;50:876.

138. Christensen KY, Naidu A, Parent MÉ, et al. The risk of lung cancer related to dietary intake of flavonoids. *Nutr Cancer* 2012;64(7):964–974.

139. Knekt P, Jarvinen R, Seppanen R, et al. Dietary flavonoids and the risk of lung cancer and other malignant neoplasms. *Am J Epidemiol* 1997;146:223–230.

140. Bassett JK, Hodge AM, English DR, et al. Dietary intake of B vitamins and methionine and risk of lung cancer. *Eur J Clin Nutr* 2012;66(2):182–187.

141. Ruano-Ravina A, Figueiras A, Freire-Garabal M, et al. Antioxidant vitamins and risk of lung cancer. *Curr Pharm Des* 2006;12:599–613.

142. Giovannucci E, Clinton SK. Tomatoes, lycopene, and prostate cancer. *Proc Soc Exp Biol Med* 1998;218:129–139.

143. Giovannucci E. How is individual risk for prostate cancer assessed? *Hematol Oncol Clin North Am* 1996;10:537.

144. Kolonel LN. Nutrition and prostate cancer. *Cancer Causes Control* 1996;7:83–94.

145. Pienta KJ, Esper PS. Risk factors for prostate cancer. *Ann Intern Med* 1993;118:793–803.

146. Key TJA, Silcocks PB, Davey GK, et al. A case-control study of diet and prostate cancer. *Br J Cancer* 1997;76:678.

147. Andersson S, Wolk A, Bergstrom R, et al. Energy, nutrient intake and prostate cancer risk: a population-based case-control study in Sweden. *Int J Cancer* 1996;68:716.

148. Szymanski KM, Wheeler DC, Mucci LA. Fish consumption and prostate cancer risk: a review and meta-analysis. *Am J Clin Nutr* 2010;92(5):1223–1233.

149. Brasky TM, Darke AK, Song X, et al. Plasma phospholipid fatty acids and prostate cancer risk in the SELECT trial. *J Natl Cancer Inst* 2013;105(15):1132–1141.

150. DiNicolantonio JJ, McCarty MF, Lavie CJ, et al. Do omega-3 fatty acids cause prostate cancer? *Mo Med* 2013;110(4):293–295.

151. Simon JA, Chen YH, Bent S. The relation of alpha-linolenic acid to the risk of prostate cancer: a systematic review and meta-analysis. *Am J Clin Nutr* 2009;89(5):1558S–1564S.

152. Brouwer IA. Omega-3 PUFA: good or bad for prostate cancer? *Prostaglandins Leukot Essent Fatty Acids* 2008;79(3–5):97–99.

153. Fair WR, Fleshner NE, Heston W. Cancer of the prostate: a nutritional disease? *Urology* 1997;50:840.

154. Giles G, Ireland P. Diet, nutrition, and prostate cancer. *Int J Cancer* 1997;10:s13.

155. Kristal AR, Arnold KB, Neuhouser ML, et al. Diet, supplement use, and prostate cancer risk: results from the prostate cancer prevention trial. *Am J Epidemiol* 2010;172(5):566–577.

156. Heinonen OP, Albanes D, Virtamo J, et al. Prostate cancer and supplementation with α-tocopherol and β-carotene: incidence and mortality in a controlled trial. *J Natl Cancer Inst* 1998;90:440.

157. Olson KB, Pienta KJ. Vitamins A and E: further clues for prostate cancer prevention. *J Natl Cancer Inst* 1998;90:414.

158. Clinton SK, Emenhiser C, Schwartz SJ, et al. Cis-trans Lycopene isomers, carotenoids, and retinol in the human prostate. *Cancer Epidemiol Biomarkers Prev* 1996;5:823.

159. Giovannucci E, Ascherio A, Rimm EB, et al. Intake of carotenoids and retinol in relation to risk of prostate cancer. *J Natl Cancer Inst* 1995;87:1767.

160. Nomura AM, Stemmermann GN, Lee J, et al. Serum micronutrients and prostate cancer in Japanese Americans in Hawaii. *Cancer Epidemiol Biomarkers Prev* 1997;6:487.

161. Peters U, Leitzmann MF, Chatterjee N, et al. Serum lycopene, other carotenoids, and prostate cancer risk: a nested case-control study in the prostate, lung, colorectal, and ovarian cancer screening trial. *Cancer Epidemiol Biomarkers Prev* 2007;16:962–968.

162. Kirsh VA, Mayne ST, Peters U, et al. A prospective study of lycopene and tomato product intake and risk of prostate cancer. *Cancer Epidemiol Biomarkers Prev* 2006;15:92–98.

163. Fontham ETH. Prevention of upper gastrointestinal tract cancers. In: Bendich A, Deckelbaum RJ, eds. *Preventive nutrition. The comprehensive guide for health professionals.* Totowa, NJ: Humana Press, 1997:33–56.

164. Joosens JV, Hill MJ, Elliott P, et al. Dietary salt, nitrate and stomach cancer mortality in 24 countries. *Int J Epidemiol* 1996;25:494.

165. Caygill CPJ, Charlett A, Hill MJ. Fat, fish, fish oil, and cancer. *Br J Cancer* 1996;74:159.

166. Bunin GR, Cary JM. Diet and childhood cancer. In: Bendich A, Deckelbaum RJ, eds. *Preventive nutrition. The comprehensive guide for health professionals.* Totowa, NJ: Humana Press, 1997:17–32.

167. Chiu BC-H, Cerhan JR, Folsom AR, et al. Diet and risk of non-Hodgkin lymphoma in older women. *JAMA* 1996;275:1315.

168. Ohba S, Nishi M, Miyake H. Eating habits and pancreas cancer. *Int J Pancreatol* 1996;20:37.

169. Warshaw AL, Fernandez-Del Castillo C. Pancreatic carcinoma. *N Engl J Med* 1992;326:455.

170. Rao GN. Influence of diet on tumors of hormonal tissues. In: Huff J, Boyd J, Barrett JC, eds. *Cellular and molecular mechanisms of hormonal carcinogenesis: environmental influences.* New York, NY: Wiley-Liss, 1996.

171. Chow W-H, McLaughlin JK, Mandel JS, et al. Obesity and risk of renal cell cancer. *Cancer Epidemiol Biomarkers Prev* 1996;5:17.

172. Davies TW, Palmer CR, Ruja E, et al. Adolescent milk, dairy product and fruit consumption and testicular cancer. *Br J Cancer* 1996;74:657.

173. Bruemmer B, White E, Vaughan TL, et al. Nutrient intake in relation to bladder cancer among middle-aged men and women. *Am J Epidemiol* 1996;144:485.

174. Eichholzer M, Gutzwiller F. Dietary nitrates, nitrites, and N-nitroso compounds and cancer risk: a review of the epidemiologic evidence. *Nutr Rev* 1998;56:95.

175. Weber P, Bendich A, Schalch W. Vitamin C and human health–a review of recent data relevant to human requirements. *Int J Vit Nutr Res* 1996;66:19.

176. Mayne ST. Beta-carotene, carotenoids, and disease prevention in humans. *FASEB J* 1996;10:690.

177. Lotan R. Retinoids in cancer chemoprevention. *FASEB J* 1996;10:1031.

178. Ziegler RG. A review of epidemiologic evidence that carotenoids reduce the risk of cancer. *J Nutr* 1989;119:116.

179. Edge R, McGarvey DJ, Truscott TG. The carotenoids as antioxidants—a review. *J Photochem Photobiol B* 1997;41:189.

180. Greenberg ER, Baron JA, Tosteson TD, et al. A clinical trial of antioxidant vitamins to prevent colorectal adenoma. *N Engl J Med* 1994;331:141.

181. Daviglus ML, Dyer AR, Persky V, et al. Dietary beta-carotene, vitamin C, and the risk of prostate cancer: results from the Western Electric Study. *Epidemiology* 1996;7:472.

182. Meydani M. Vitamin E. *Lancet* 1995;345:170.

183. Greenwald P, Anderson D, Nelson SA, et al. Clinical trials of vitamin and mineral supplements for cancer prevention. *Am J Clin Nutr* 2007;85:314s–317s.

184. Wei WQ, Abnet CC, Qiao YL, et al. Prospective study of serum selenium concentrations and esophageal and gastric cardia cancer, heart disease, stroke, and total death. *Am J Clin Nutr* 2004;79:80–85.

185. Blot WJ, Li JY, Taylor PR, et al. The Linxian trials: mortality rates by vitamin-mineral intervention group. *Am J Clin Nutr* 1995;62:1424s–1426s.

186. Taylor PR, Li B, Dawsey SM, et al. Prevention of esophageal cancer: the nutrition intervention trials in

Linxian, China. Linxian Nutrition Intervention Trials Study Group. *Cancer Res* 1994;54:2029s–2031s.

187. Blot WJ. Vitamin/mineral supplementation and cancer risk: international chemoprevention trials. *Proc Soc Exp Biol Med* 1997;216:291.

188. Clark LC, Dalkin B, Krongrad A, et al. Decreased incidence of prostate cancer with selenium supplementation: results of a double-blind cancer prevention trial. *Br J Urol* 1998;81:730–734.

189. Han X, Li J, Brasky TM, et al. Antioxidant intake and pancreatic cancer risk: The Vitamins and Lifestyle (VITAL) Study. *Cancer* 2013;119(7):1314–1320.

190. Gallaher DD, Schneeman BO. Dietary fiber. In: Ziegler EE, Filer LJ Jr, eds. *Present knowledge in nutrition*, 7th ed. Washington, DC: ILSI Press, 1996.

191. Martinez ME, McPherson RS, Annegers JF, et al. Association of diet and colorectal adenomatous polyps: dietary fiber, calcium, and total fat. *Epidemiology* 1996;7:264.

192. Le Marchand L, Hankin JH, Wilkens LR, et al. Dietary fiber and colorectal cancer risk. *Epidemiology* 1997;8:658.

193. Giovannucci E, Stampfer MJ, Colditz G, et al. Relationship of diet to risk of colorectal adenoma in men. *J Natl Cancer Inst* 1992;84:91.

194. Alberts DS, Ritenbaugh C, Story JA, et al. Randomized, double-blind, placebo-controlled study of effect of wheat bran fiber and calcium on fecal bile acids in patients with resected adenomatous colon polyps. *J Natl Cancer Inst* 1996;88:81.

195. Rose DJ, DeMeo MT, Keshavarzian Ali, et al. Influence of dietary fiber on inflammatory bowel disease and colon cancer: importance of fermentation pattern. *Nutr Rev* 2007;65(2):51–62.

196. Giovannucci E, Rimm EB, Stampfer MJ, et al. Intake of fat, meat, and fiber in relation to risk of colon cancer in men. *Cancer Res* 1994;54:2390.

197. Wasan HS, Goodlad RA. Fibre-supplemented foods may damage your health. *Lancet* 1996;348:319.

198. LaVecchia C, Ferraroni M, Franceschi S, et al. Fibers and breast cancer risk. *Nutr Cancer* 1997;28:264.

199. Tsugane S, Sasazuki S. Diet and the risk of gastric cancer: review of epidemiological evidence. *Gastric Cancer* 2007;10:75–83.

200. Shankar S, Ganapathy S, Srivastava RK. Green tea polyphenols: biology and therapeutic implications in cancer. *Front Biosci* 2007;12:4881–4899.

201. Berletch JB, Liu C, Love WK, et al. Epigenetic and genetic mechanisms contribute to telomerase inhibition by EGCG. *J Cell Biochem* 2008;103(2):509–519.

202. Carlson JR, Bauer BA, Vincent A, et al. Reading the tea leaves: anticarcinogenic properties of (-)-epigallocatechin-3-gallate. *Mayo Clin Proc* 2007;82:725–732.

203. Landis-Piwowar KR, Huo C, Chen D, et al. A novel prodrug of the green tea polyphenol (-)-epigallocatechin-3-gallate as a potential anticancer agent. *Cancer Res* 2007;67:4303–4310.

204. Colomer R, Menendez JA. Mediterranean diet, olive oil and cancer. *Clin Transl Oncol* 2006;8:15–21.

205. Hashim YZ, Eng M, Gill CI, et al. Components of olive oil and chemoprevention of colorectal cancer. *Nutr Rev* 2005;63:374–386.

206. Brooks PJ, Zakhari S. Moderate alcohol consumption and breast cancer in women: from epidemiology to mechanisms and interventions. *Alcohol Clin Exp Res* 2013;37(1):23–30.

207. Seitz HK, Becker P. Alcohol metabolism and cancer risk. *Alcohol Res Health* 2007;30(1):38–41, 44–47.

208. Boffetta P, Hashibe M. Alcohol and cancer. *Lancet Oncol* 2006;7(2):149–156.

209. Center for Science in the Public Interest. *FDA should reconsider Aspartame cancer risk, say experts: New rat study links artificial sweetener with lymphomas, breast cancer.* June 25, 2007. Available at http://www.cspinet.org/new/200706251.html; accessed 10/12/07.

210. Gallus S, Scotti L, Negri E, et al. Artificial sweeteners and cancer risk in a network of case-control studies. *Ann Oncol* 2007;18(1):40–44.

211. Hu SA. Risks and benefits of soy isoflavones for breast cancer survivors. *Oncol Nurs Forum* 2004;31:249–263.

212. Yamamoto S, Sobue T, Kobayashi M, et al. Soy, isoflavones, and breast cancer risk in Japan. *J Natl Cancer Inst* 2003;95:906–913.

213. Brown BD, Thomas W, Hutchins A, et al. Types of dietary fat and soy minimally affect hormones and biomarkers associated with breast cancer risk in premenopausal women. *Nutr Cancer* 2002;43:22–30.

214. Messina MJ, Loprinzi CL. Soy for breast cancer survivors: a critical review of the literature. *J Nutr* 2001;131:3095S–3108S.

215. Wu AH, Ziegler RG, Nomura AM, et al. Soy intake and risk of breast cancer in Asians and Asian Americans. *Am J Clin Nutr* 1998;68:1437s–1443s.

216. Stoll BA. Eating to beat breast cancer: potential role for soy supplements. *Ann Oncol* 1997;8:223–225.

217. Messina M, McCaskill-Stevens W, Lampe JW. Addressing the soy and breast cancer relationship: review, commentary, and workshop proceedings. *J Natl Cancer Inst* 2006;98:1275–1284.

218. Trock BJ, Hilakivi-Clarke L, Clarke R. Meta-analysis of soy intake and breast cancer risk. *J Natl Cancer Inst* 2006;98:459–471.

219. Shu XO, Zheng Y, Cai H, et al. Soy food intake and breast cancer survival. *JAMA* 2009;302(22):2437–2443.

220. Nechuta SJ, Caan BJ, Chen WY, et al. Soy food intake after diagnosis of breast cancer and survival: an in-depth analysis of combined evidence from cohort studies of US and Chinese women. *Am J Clin Nutr* 2012;96(1):123–132.

221. Yang G, Shu XO, Chow W, et al. Soy food intake and risk of lung cancer: evidence from the Shanghai Women's Health Study and a meta-analysis. *Am J Epidemiol* 2012;176(10):846–55.

222. Yang WS, Va P, Wong MY, et al. Soy intake is associated with lower lung cancer risk: results from a meta-analysis of epidemiologic studies. *Am J Clin Nutr* 2011;94(6):1575–1583.

223. Chi F, Wu R, Zeng Y-C, et al. Post-diagnosis soy food intake and breast cancer survival: a meta-analysis of cohort studies. *Asian Pac J Cancer Prev* 2013;14(4):2407–2412.

224. Kim J, Kang M, Lee JS, et al. Fermented and nonfermented soy food consumption and gastric cancer in Japanese and Korean populations: a meta-analysis of observational studies. *Cancer Sci* 2011;102(1):231–244.

225. Yan L, Spitznagel EL, Bosland MC. Soy consumption and colorectal cancer risk in humans: a meta-analysis. *Cancer Epidemiol Biomarkers Prev* 2010;19(1):148–158.

226. Myung SK, Ju W, Choi HJ, et al. Korean Meta-Analysis (KORMA) Study Group. Soy intake and risk of endocrine-related gynaecological cancer: a meta-analysis. *BJOG* 2009;116(13):1697–1705.

227. Wu AH, Yang D, Pike MC. A meta-analysis of soyfoods and risk of stomach cancer: the problem of potential confounders. *Cancer Epidemiol Biomarkers Prev* 2000;9(10): 1051–1058.

228. Smith-Spangler C, Brandeau ML, Hunter GE, et al. Are organic foods safer or healthier than conventional alternatives?: a systematic review. *Ann Intern Med* 2012;157(5): 348–66.

229. Ou L, Ip C, Lisafeld B, et al. Conjugated linoleic acid induces apoptosis of murine mammary tumor cells via Bcl-2 loss. *Biochem Biophys Res Commun* 2007;356:1044–1049.

230. Sauer LA, Blask DE, Dauchy RT. Dietary factors and growth and metabolism in experimental tumors. *J Nutr Biochem* 2007;18:637–649.

231. Soel SM, Choi OS, Bang MH, et al. Influence of conjugated linoleic acid isomers on the metastasis of colon cancer cells in vitro and in vivo. *J Nutr Biochem* 2007;18: 650–657.

232. Heinze VM, Actis AB. Dietary conjugated linoleic acid and long-chain n-3 fatty acids in mammary and prostate cancer protection: a review. *Int J Food Sci Nutr* 2012;63(1):66–78.

233. Powers HJ. Interaction among folate, riboflavin, genotype, and cancer, with reference to colorectal and cervical cancer. *J Nutr* 2005;135:2960S–2966S.

234. Strohle A, Wolters M, Hahn A. Folic acid and colorectal cancer prevention: molecular mechanisms and epidemiological evidence [Review]. *Int J Oncol* 2005;26: 1449–1464.

235. Lin HL, An QZ, Wang QZ, et al. Folate intake and pancreatic cancer risk: an overall and dose-response meta-analysis. *Public Health* 2013;127(7):607–613.

236. Qin X, Cui Y, Shen L, et al. Folic acid supplementation and cancer risk: a meta-analysis of randomized controlled trials. *Int J Cancer* 2013;133(5):1033–1041.

237. Baggott JE, Oster RA, Tamura T. Meta-analysis of cancer risk in folic acid supplementation trials. *Cancer Epidemiol* 2012;36(1):78–81.

238. Zheng W, Doyle TJ, Kushi LH, et al. Tea consumption and cancer incidence in a prospective cohort study of postmenopausal women. *Am J Epidemiol* 1996;144:175.

239. Gao YT, McLaughlin JK, Blot WJ, et al. Reduced risk of esophageal cancer associated with green tea consumption. *J Natl Cancer Inst* 1994;86:855.

240. Milner JA. Nonnutritive components in foods as modifiers of the cancer process. In: Bendich A, Deckelbaum RJ, eds. *Preventive nutrition. The comprehensive guide for health professionals.* Totowa, NJ: Humana Press, 1997: 135–152.

241. Murray MT. *Encyclopedia of nutritional supplements.* Rocklin, CA: Prima Publishing, 1996.

242. Jagerstad M, Skog K. Genotoxicity of heat-processed foods. *Mutat Res* 2005;574:156–172.

243. Pelucchi C, La Vecchia C, Bosetti C, et al. Exposure to acrylamide and human cancer—a review and meta-analysis of epidemiologic studies. *Ann Oncol* 2011;22(7):1487–1499.

244. Lineback DR, Coughlin JR, Stadler RH. Acrylamide in foods: a review of the science and future considerations. *Annu Rev Food Sci Technol* 2012;3:15–35.

245. Kolaja KL, Bunting KA, Klauning JE. Inhibition of tumor promotion and heptocellular growth by dietary restriction in mice. *Carcinogenesis* 1996;17:1657.

246. Dirx MJ, Zeegers MP, Dagnelie PC, et al. Energy restriction and the risk of spontaneous mammary tumors in mice: a meta-analysis. *Int J Cancer* 2003;106(5): 766–770.

247. Seyfried TN, Marsh J, Shelton LM, et al. Is the restricted ketogenic diet a viable alternative to the standard of care for managing malignant brain cancer? *Epilepsy Res* 2012;100(3):310–326.

248. Longo VD, Fontana L. Calorie restriction and cancer prevention: metabolic and molecular mechanisms. *Trends Pharmacol Sci* 2010;31(2):89–98.

249. Howell A, Chapman M, Harvie M. Energy restriction for breast cancer prevention. *Recent Results Cancer Res* 2009;181:97–111.

250. Harvie M, Howell A. Energy restriction and the prevention of breast cancer. *Proc Nutr Soc* 2012;71(2):263–275.

251. Sun C, Zhang F, Ge X, et al. SIRT1 improves insulin sensitivity under insulin-resistant conditions by repressing PTP1B. *Cell Metab* 2007;6(4):307–319.

252. Schenk S, McCurdy CE, Philp A, et al. Sirt1 enhances skeletal muscle insulin sensitivity in mice during caloric restriction. *J Clin Invest* 2011;121(11):4281–4288.

253. Chalkiadaki A, Guarente L. High-fat diet triggers inflammation-induced cleavage of SIRT1 in adipose tissue to promote metabolic dysfunction. *Cell Metab* 2012;16(2):180–188.

254. Brooks CL, Gu W. How does SIRT1 affect metabolism, senescence and cancer? *Nat Rev Cancer* 2009;9(2):123–128.

255. Tomita M. Caloric restriction reduced 1, 2-dimethylhydrazine-induced aberrant crypt foci and induces the expression of Sirtuins in colonic mucosa of F344 rats. *J Carcinog* 2012;11:10.

256. Rivadeneira DE, Evoy D, Fahey TJ 3rd, et al. Nutritional support of the cancer patient. *CA Cancer J Clin* 1998;48:69.

257. Copeland EM 3rd. Historical perspective on nutritional support of cancer patients. *CA Cancer J Clin* 1998;48:67.

258. Hyltander A, Bosaeus I, Svedlund J, et al. Supportive nutrition on recovery of metabolism, nutritional state, health-related quality of life, and exercise capacity after major surgery: a randomized study. *Clin Gastroenterol Hepatol* 2005;3:466–474.

259. Ng K, Leung SF, Johnson PJ, et al. Nutritional consequences of radiotherapy in nasopharynx cancer patients. *Nutr Cancer* 2004;49:156–161.

260. Bozzetti F. Nutritional issues in the care of the elderly patient. *Crit Rev Oncol Hematol* 2003;48:113–121.

261. Baldwin C, Spiro A, Ahern R, et al. Oral nutritional interventions in malnourished patients with cancer: a systematic review and meta-analysis. *J Natl Cancer Inst* 2012;104(5):371–385.

262. Baier S, Johannsen D, Abumrad N, et al. Year-long changes in protein metabolism in elderly men and women supplemented with a nutrition cocktail of

beta-hydroxy-beta-methylbutyrate (HMB), L-arginine, and L-lysine. *JPEN* 2009;33(1):71–82.

263. Mattes RD, Kare MR. Nutrition and the chemical senses. In: Shils ME, Olson JA, Shike M, eds. *Modern nutrition in health and disease,* 8th ed. Philadelphia, PA: Lea & Febiger, 1994.

SUGGESTED READING

Ahmed FE. Effect of diet, life style, and other environmental/ chemopreventive factors on colorectal cancer development, and assessment of the risks. *J Environ Sci Health C Environ Carcinog Ecotoxicol Rev* 2004;22:91–147.

Banning M. The carcinogenic and protective effects of food. *Br J Nurs* 2005;14:1070–1074.

Bendich A, Deckelbaum RJ, eds. *Preventive nutrition. The comprehensive guide for health professionals.* Totowa, NJ: Humana Press, 1997.

Birt DF, Pelling JC, Nair S, et al. Diet intervention for modifying cancer risk. In: *Genetics and cancer susceptibility: implications for risk assessment.* New York, NY: Wiley-Liss, 1994:223–234.

Bostik RM. Diet and nutrition in the etiology and primary prevention of colon cancer. In: Bendich A, Deckelbaum RJ, eds. *Preventive nutrition. The comprehensive guide for health professionals.* Totowa, NJ: Humana Press, 1997;57–96.

Bougnoux P, Giraudeau B, Couet C. Diet, cancer, and the lipidome. *Cancer Epidemiol Biomarkers Prev* 2006;15: 416–421.

Brenner DE, Gescher AJ. Cancer chemoprevention: lessons learned and future directions. *Br J Cancer* 2005;93:735–739.

Chan JM, Gann PH, Giovannucci EL. Role of diet in prostate cancer development and progression. *J Clin Oncol* 2005;23:8152–8160.

Cheng TY, Vassy J, Prokopowicz G, et al. The efficacy and safety of multivitamin and mineral supplement use to prevent cancer and chronic disease in adults: a systematic review for a National Institutes of Health state-of-the-science conference. *Ann Intern Med* 2006;145:372–385.

Clinton SK. Diet, anthropometry and breast cancer: integration of experimental and epidemiologic approaches. *J Nutr* 1997;127:916s.

Clinton SK. Lycopene: chemistry, biology, and implications for human health and disease. *Nutr Rev* 1998;56:35.

Committee on Diet and Health, Food and Nutrition Board, Commission on Life Sciences, National Research Council. *Diet and health. Implications for reducing chronic disease burden.* Washington, DC: National Academy Press, 1989.

de Lorgeril M, Salen P. Modified cretan Mediterranean diet in the prevention of coronary heart disease and cancer: An update. *World Rev Nutr Diet* 2007;97:1–32.

Divisi D, Di Tommaso S, Salvemini S, et al. Diet and cancer. *Acta Biomed* 2006;77:118–123.

Ensminger AH, Ensminger ME, Konlande JE, et al. *The concise encyclopedia of foods and nutrition.* Boca Raton, FL: CRC Press, 1995.

Finley JW. Bioavailability of selenium from foods. *Nutr Rev* 2006;64:146–151.

Fresco P, Borges F, Diniz C, et al. New insights on the anticancer properties of dietary polyphenols. *Med Res Rev* 2006;26:747–766.

Garcia-Closas R, Castellsague X, Bosch X, et al. The role of diet and nutrition in cervical carcinogenesis: a review of recent evidence. *Int J Cancer* 2005;117:629–637.

Greenwald P, Anderson D, Nelson SA, et al. Clinical trials of vitamin and mineral supplements for cancer prevention. *Am J Clin Nutr* 2007;85:314s–317s.

Goldin-Lang P, Kreuser ED, Zunft HJF. Basis and consequences of primary and secondary prevention of gastrointestinal tumors. *Recent Results Cancer Res* 1996;142:163.

Gonzalez CA, Riboli E. Diet and cancer prevention: where we are, where we are going. *Nutr Cancer* 2006;56:225–231.

Hanf V, Gonder U. Nutrition and primary prevention of breast cancer: foods, nutrients and breast cancer risk. *Eur J Obstet Gynecol Reprod Biol* 2005;123:139–149.

Jolly CA. Diet manipulation and prevention of aging, cancer and autoimmune disease. *Curr Opin Clin Nutr Metab Care* 2005;8:382–387.

Jones LW, Demark-Wahnefried W. Diet, exercise, and complementary therapies after primary treatment for cancer. *Lancet Oncol* 2006;7:1017–1026.

Kanadaswami C, Lee LT, Lee PP, et al. The antitumor activities of flavonoids. *In Vivo* 2005;19:895–909.

Kapiszewska M. A vegetable to meat consumption ratio as a relevant factor determining cancer preventive diet. The Mediterranean versus other European countries. *Forum Nutr* 2006;59:130–153.

Key TJ, Appleby PN, Rosell MS. Health effects of vegetarian and vegan diets. *Proc Nutr Soc* 2006;65:35–41.

Kohlmeier L, Mendez M. Controversies surrounding diet and breast cancer. *Proc Nutr Soc* 1997;56:369.

Kotsopoulos J, Narod SA. Towards a dietary prevention of hereditary breast cancer. *Cancer Causes Control* 2005;16: 125–138.

Lamb DJ, Zhang L. Challenges in prostate cancer research: animal models for nutritional studies of chemoprevention and disease progression. *J Nutr* 2005;135:3009s–3015s.

Lowenfels AB, Maisonneuve P. Risk factors for pancreatic cancer. *J Cell Biochem* 2005;95:649–656.

Margen S. *The wellness nutrition counter.* New York, NY: Health Letter Associates, 1997.

Martin KR. Targeting apoptosis with dietary bioactive agents. *Exp Biol Med (Maywood)* 2006;231:117–129.

McCarty MF, Block KI. Toward a core nutraceutical program for cancer management. *Integr Cancer Ther* 2006;5:150–171.

McNaughton SA, Marks GC, Green AC. Role of dietary factors in the development of basal cell cancer and squamous cell cancer of the skin. *Cancer Epidemiol Biomarkers Prev* 2005;14:1596–1607.

McTiernan A. Obesity and cancer: the risks, science, and potential management strategies. *Oncology (Williston Park)* 2005;19:871–881.

Murray MT. *Encyclopedia of nutritional supplements.* Rocklin, CA: Prima Publishing, 1996.

Nahleh Z, Tabbara IA. Complementary and alternative medicine in breast cancer patients. *Palliat Support Care* 2003;1:267–273.

National Research Council. *Recommended dietary allowances,* 10th ed. Washington, DC: National Academy Press, 1989.

National Research Council. *Carcinogens and anticarcinogens in the human diet.* Washington, DC: National Academy Press, 1996.

Noguchi M, Rose DP, Miyazaki I. Breast cancer chemoprevention: clinical trials and research. *Oncology* 1996;53:175.

Rathkopf D, Schwartz GK. Molecular basis of carcinogenesis. In: Shils ME, Shike M, Ross AC, et al., eds. *Modern nutrition in health and disease*, 10th ed. Philadelphia, PA: Lippincott Williams & Wilkins, 2006:1260–1266.

Rose DP. The mechanistic rationale in support of dietary cancer prevention. *Prev Med* 1996;25:34.

Scalbert A, Manach C, Morand C, et al. Dietary polyphenols and the prevention of diseases. *Crit Rev Food Sci Nutr* 2005;45:287–306.

Schattner M, Shike M. Nutrition support of the patient with cancer. In: Shils ME, Shike M, Ross AC, et al., eds. *Modern nutrition in health and disease*, 10th ed. Philadelphia, PA: Lippincott Williams & Wilkins, 2006:1290–1313.

Schottenfeld D, Fraumeni JF, eds. *Cancer epidemiology and prevention*, 2nd ed. New York, NY: Oxford University Press, 1996.

Serra-Majem L, Roman B, Estruch R. Scientific evidence of interventions using the Mediterranean diet: a systematic review. *Nutr Rev* 2006;64:s27–s47.

Shils ME, Olson JA, Shike M, eds. *Modern nutrition in health and disease*, 8th ed. Philadelphia, PA: Lea & Febiger, 1994.

Sonn GA, Aronson W, Litwin MS. Impact of diet on prostate cancer: a review. *Prostate Cancer Prostatic Dis* 2005;8:304–310.

Sporn MB. Chemoprevention of cancer. In: Shils ME, Shike M, Ross AC, et al., eds. *Modern nutrition in health and disease*, 10th ed. Philadelphia, PA: Lippincott Williams & Wilkins, 2006:1280–1289.

Tercyak KP, Tyc VL. Opportunities and challenges in the prevention and control of cancer and other chronic diseases: children's diet and nutrition and weight and physical activity. *J Pediatr Psychol* 2006;31:750–763.

Thomas B. *Nutrition in primary care*. Oxford, UK: Blackwell Science, 1996.

Thomas PR, ed. *Improving America's diet and health: from recommendations to action*. Washington, DC: National Academy Press, 1991.

Tsubura A, Uehara N, Kiyozuka Y, et al. Dietary factors modifying breast cancer risk and relation to time of intake. *J Mammary Gland Biol Neoplasia* 2005;10:87–100.

Uauy R, Solomons N. Diet, nutrition, and the life-course approach to cancer prevention. *J Nutr* 2005;135:2934s–2945s.

United States Department of Agriculture. *USDA nutrient database for standard reference*. Release 11–1, 1997.

Whiting SJ, Calvo MS. Dietary recommendations to meet both endocrine and autocrine needs of Vitamin D. *J Steroid Biochem Mol Biol* 2005;97:7–12.

Willett WC, Giovannucci E. Epidemiology of diet and cancer risk. In: Shils ME, Shike M, Ross AC, et al., eds. *Modern nutrition in health and disease*, 10th ed. Philadelphia, PA: Lippincott Williams & Wilkins, 2006:1267–1279.

Wolk A. Diet, lifestyle and risk of prostate cancer. *Acta Oncol* 2005;44:277–281.

Woodside JV, McCall D, McGartland C, et al. Micronutrients: dietary intake v. supplement use. *Proc Nutr Soc* 2005;64:543–553.

World Cancer Research Fund in Association with American Institute for Cancer Research. *Food, nutrition and the prevention of cancer: a global perspective*. Washington, DC: American Institute for Cancer Research, 1997.

Ziegler EE, Filer LJ Jr, eds. *Present knowledge in nutrition*, 7th ed. Washington, DC: ILSI Press, 1996.

CHAPTER 13

Diet and Hematopoiesis: Nutritional Anemias

N utritional status is, of course, a vital determinant of all aspects of health. The influence of nutriture is more readily apparent in some aspects of physiology than others, however. In particular, tissues with a high rate of turnover and metabolic processes with high energy requirements are more likely to manifest impairments due to even nominal nutrient deficiencies than are more sedate aspects of physiology. One of the tissues with the highest rate of cellular turnover is the bone marrow, and thus, as would be expected, nutrient deficiencies are readily manifest as abnormalities in hematopoiesis.

Significant chronic disease of almost any variety, energy malnutrition, protein malnutrition, and/or specific nutrient deficiencies account for a significant percentage of all clinically relevant anemias (1). Anemia can be defined by an insufficient mass of red blood cells and screening tests include an evaluation of the major red blood cell indices, including hemoglobin, hematocrit, or red blood cell count. According to the World Health Organization, a cost-effective approach to defining anemia is by measuring when hemoglobin concentrations are 2 standard deviations below the distribution mean when controlled for age, gender, and altitude (2). Deficiencies of iron, folate, and vitamin B_{12} (cobalamin) will all eventually contribute to decreasing hemoglobin levels and are the most important epidemiological markers nutritionally affecting hematopoiesis. In addition, each deficiency is associated with a particular set of demographic characteristics and risk factors. Nutritional supplementation may be therapeutic in a significant percentage of all anemias seen in primary care. Thus, awareness of and attention to nutritional anemias is incumbent upon all health care providers.

OVERVIEW

Diet

The production of blood cells is an energy-intensive process, and thus overall dietary adequacy is a critical determinant of the vitality of hematopoiesis. The manufacture of red and white cells consumes the building blocks of cells and cell components and thus depends on the availability of proteins and fatty acids in particular. Hematopoiesis is maintained at optimal levels only when an adequate amount of high-quality protein and, more specifically, essential amino acids are consumed. Similarly, the composition of blood cell membranes requires the provision of essential fatty acids (3).

Micronutrients directly involved in hematopoiesis also may influence the rate of blood cell manufacture. These include iron, which is required in the construction of hemoglobin, as well as vitamin B_{12} and folate, cofactors required for erythrocyte DNA synthesis. Deficiencies of several other nutrients—including vitamin A, vitamin B_6, riboflavin, vitamin C, vitamin E, and copper—may be associated with the development or exacerbation of anemia (4).

Approximately one-quarter (1.62 billion) of the world's population has been estimated to have anemia, most commonly in preschool-aged children and nonpregnant women (5). Prevalence is highest in developing countries, but children and pregnant women everywhere are vulnerable; up to 20% of children in the United States and 80% of children in developing countries are estimated to develop anemia at some point before age 18, mostly due to iron deficiency (6). Anemia is also a relatively common condition in the elderly; approximately 1 in 10 men and women over

65 years of age and nearly 1 in 3 non-Hispanic black elderly persons in the US population are estimated to be anemic. The National Health and Nutrition Examination Survey (NHANES III) evaluated causes of anemia in men and women over 65 and found that one-third of cases were nutritional anemias (7). Of these, more than half involved iron deficiency. The other two-thirds of the cases were split between those related to chronic disorders (e.g., renal disease, arthritis, diabetes) and those that were unexplained or myelodysplastic in nature. Although hemoglobin and hematocrit levels for older adults tend to decrease with increasing age, the exact parameters for anemia continue to be strongly debated. However, it is clear that there is a marked increase in morbidity and mortality with worsening degrees of anemia in this population (8).

Iron-deficiency anemia (IDA) is the most common nutritional deficiency worldwide, and it is the main etiology of anemia in infancy, childhood, and pregnancy (9). In the United States, 2% of adult men, 9% to 12% of white women, and up to 20% of black and Mexican American women are estimated to have IDA. The racial differences are pronounced especially in the African American population, most likely due to genetic variation; in fact many researchers recommend using lower parameters for red blood cell indices in this population (10,11). Due to the prolonged life span, 120 days, of the mature RBC it is important to consider the stages necessary to reach IDA. The process of reaching IDA must first occur with a negative iron balance, followed by iron depletion (iron storage is low but the body is still able to maintain normal physiology), followed by iron-deficient erythropoiesis, and finally IDA (12,13). Iron deficiency is the result of an imbalance between the iron demand by the body and iron absorption from the diet. Typical causes include inadequate dietary intake in infants and children, absorption hindrances in older adults, and physiologic losses in menstruating women. Iron deficiency in adults may also be a sign of chronic blood loss and may stem from malignancy, so simply prescribing iron supplements is not appropriate until the exact cause has been determined.

Risk factors for IDA are present across the life cycle. Prenatal vitamins with iron are prescribed to all pregnant women, and compliance has been shown to reduce the number of low-birth-weight infants (14) (see Chapter 27). Infants may be at high risk if they are living in poverty, were preterm or low birth weight, or are fed primarily unfortified cow's milk, which has been demonstrated to increase blood loss and infections in infants (see Chapter 29). Child and adolescent obesity is now known to be a risk factor for IDA (body mass index [BMI] $\geq$ 95th percentile; odds ratio [OR] 2.3; 95% CI, 1.4 to 3.9). Using NHANES III data, researchers evaluated a group of children age 2 to 16 years at varying BMIs and found children who were overweight/obese were twice as likely as normal weight children to be iron deficient, showing a linear trend as BMI increased (15). Many theories have been proposed to describe this correlation between increased weight and iron deficiency including increased energy-density consumption with nutrient-poor foods, increased iron requirements, dilutional hypoferremia by increased plasma volumes, and the chronic inflammatory state associated with increased adiposity. The increased inflammatory state is further elucidated in a theory proposed through proinflammatory cytokines causing a greater release of hepcidin (an important peptide hormone produced by the liver that binds and limits iron's gut absorption and inhibits irons release from macrophages, thereby causing systemic regulation of iron). Additional research is required before a definite association between obesity and IDA can be made (16,17). Lastly, the type of iron in the diet greatly influences the absorption in the gut. Heme iron, mostly found in meats, is more efficiently absorbed (15% to 40%) and less influenced by modifiers, while nonheme iron, the predominant form in iron-containing plant foods and meats, is less well absorbed(1% to 15%) and very influenced by enhancers and inhibitors in the diet (18,19). In Western societies vegetarians and nonvegetarians have a similar prevalence of true IDA. Although vegetarian woman in particular do tend to have lower iron stores (i.e. low serum ferritin levels), and lower but normal hemoglobin and hematocrit levels, there is no resulting associated morbidity or mortality described in the literature (18,20).

Anemia of chronic disease is the second most prevalent anemia worldwide and is often coexistent with IDA. Its diagnosis is usually associated with acute/chronic inflammation, cancer, or chronic infection. Treatment of underlying disease is the mainstay of therapy; however, when this is not feasible, there are alternate strategies that may be assisted with the use of micronutrient therapy (21).

In a state of iron deficiency, oral iron supplementation has been considered but continues to be very controversial because of iron's importance in the proliferation of bacteria as well as its contribution to the formation of free radicals that may lead to tissue damage (22). It is important to remember that the use of iron is never a mainstay in therapy but can be used as an adjuvant treatment in some triggers for anemia of chronic disease (23).

The most recent dietary reference intake for iron is 8 mg per day for healthy, nonmenstruating adults, 18 mg per day for menstruating women, and 16 mg per day for vegetarians (24). As previously mentioned, dietary iron consists of meat-derived heme iron, and nonheme iron, occurring in meats, plants, and supplemented in foods. Nonheme iron constitutes the majority of the daily iron intake, and its absorption is dependent on other dietary factors. It requires acid digestion, and bioavailability may be enhanced by vitamin C (Ascorbic Acid) or meat, while it is inhibited by calcium (and therefore dairy products), fiber, tea, coffee, wine, and any medicine that reduces stomach acidity (H_2 blockers, proton pump inhibitors, and antacids).

In adults, dietary sources of iron provide only 5% of total daily iron needs; in infants and children, this proportion is approximately 30%, due to increased needs for growth and development. Children and adolescents are therefore at increased risk for iron deficiency due to inadequate dietary iron intake. A study of 800 Bolivian children less than 5 years old and their mothers found a highly significant correlation between body iron stores of the mothers and children, highlighting the importance of household dietary patterns on the nutritional status of individual family members (25). Clinical consequences of iron deficiency in infants and children include impairment of psychomotor development (26), cognitive function, and reduced leukocyte and lymphocyte function (27). One cross-sectional study of school-aged children and adolescents found lower standardized math scores among those who were iron deficient, even after controlling for possible confounders (28). Pica or pagophagia may be observed in severe cases (29). Rapid growth during adolescence predisposes this demographic to iron deficiency; even higher risk is seen in menstruating or pregnant adolescent girls (30). Strenuous athletic training among both girls and boys may lead to "sports anemia" due to increased iron demands (31).

While iron deficiency is the major cause of nutritional anemia, several vitamins appear to play an important role in determining its development and severity. For example, riboflavin and vitamin A have been shown to enhance the response of supplemental iron and folic acid (32). Vitamin C and copper enhances the absorption of iron, while copper also assists with its utilization.

Vitamin B_{12} (cobalamin) deficiency is another common cause of nutritional anemia, especially in the elderly. Approximately 20% of older adults have some form of cobalamin deficiency (33,34), most commonly caused by absorption difficulties due to either pernicious anemia or the food-cobalamin malabsorption syndrome, characterized by an inability to release B_{12} from food (35). Food-cobalamin malabsorption is thought to stem from atrophic gastritis and long-term use of antacids or biguanides (36). However, it is important to note that in all of these cases, B_{12} deficiency may not always become full-blown anemia. Other groups at risk for vitamin B_{12} deficiency are strict vegetarians and vegans, individuals with gastrointestinal surgery limiting absorption, and pregnant and lactating women following strict vegetarian diets along with their infants. Vitamin B_{12} naturally exists in animal products, including meat, eggs, fish, and milk. In addition, it is fortified in many cereals and other foods with good bioavailability. Infants are at greatest risk for deficiency when their mother's do not consume enough vitamin B_{12}, because during periods of pregnancy and lactation the maternal intake through gastric absorption have a more potent influence in transmission than the maternal stores. These children become symptomatic within months of birth (2 to 10 months), with symptoms including failure to thrive, anorexia, and developmental regression (37,38). Pregnant or lactating women who are vegans or lacto-ovo vegetarians are recommended to start vitamin B_{12} supplementation for the adequate intake of their child (39).

The USDA recommended dietary intake of vitamin B_{12} for most adults around 2.4 μg per day with slight increases required for pregnancy and lactating women. The average US diet consumes approximately 5 μg per day (40). Body stores of vitamin B_{12} are 2 to 5 mg, enough to support a person for up to 5 years after dietary B_{12} is no longer present. Insufficiency due to diet alone is therefore unusual, though it is possible in cases of severe dietary restriction.

In contrast, the most common cause of folate deficiency is nutritional, due to poor diet, increased requirements, as in pregnancy, and alcoholism (see Chapter 40). Pregnancy and lactation increase daily folate requirements from 400 to 800 μg; prophylactic supplementation is therefore recommended for all pregnant and lactating women and may be advisable in all women of reproductive age who might become pregnant (see Chapter 27).

Whereas limiting or avoiding red meat intake might be considered advisable for overall purposes of health promotion, some intake of lean red meat offers clear advantages for iron nutriture and hematopoiesis. Veganism, which excludes all animal foods, dairy, and eggs, poses some risk of iron and vitamin B_{12} deficiency, particularly in adolescents who are likely to adopt unbalanced vegetarian practices. However, a diverse and balanced vegan diet that meets all nutrient needs is readily achievable; many soy products are now fortified with vitamin B_{12}, and attention to the dietary practices that optimize iron absorption can ensure adequate intake of both micronutrients. Useful guides have been published (41), and this issue is addressed in more detail in Chapter 43.

When the cause of anemia has been established as being a nutritional deficiency, most cases can be easily treated with oral supplementation. Iron deficiency is easily treated with oral iron supplements if dietary modification is unattainable. The initiation of folic acid food supplementation has led to a documented decline in the prevalence of folate deficiency as well as a significant reduction in the number of babies born with neural tube defects (42). A dose of 1 to 5 mg per day is usually sufficient to treat folate deficiency.

Although vitamin B_{12} deficiency has conventionally been treated with monthly intramuscular cobalamin injections, increasing evidence suggests that as long as pernicious anemia is not the cause, high-dose oral supplementation is equally effective (43), better tolerated, feasible in a community setting (44), and more cost-efficient (45).

NUTRIENTS, NUTRICEUTICALS, AND FUNCTIONAL FOODS

Folate

Natural dietary sources of folate include citrus and other fruits, dark green leafy vegetables, and legumes. Since 1996, all flour and uncooked cereal grains have been supplemented with 140 μg of folate per 100 g of flour or grain, making fortified breakfast cereals and other grain products an important dietary source of folate in the United States (see Chapter 4). As discussed in Chapter 27, this practice has reduced the prevalence of pregnancy-induced folate deficiency and megaloblastic anemia, as well as occurrence and recurrence of neural tube defects associated with folate deficiency (46). In addition, it is important to mention that certain individuals have a higher predilection for folic acid deficiency due to gene mutations, specifically polymorphisms in the methylene tetrahydrofolate reductase (MTHFR) gene. Functional folate deficiency occurs due to the multiple variations in genetic mutations, causing poor folate utilization and thereby increased likelihood for neural tube defects (47).

Iron

The best dietary sources of iron include beef and other meats, beans, lentils, iron-fortified cereals, dark green leafy vegetables, dried fruits, nuts, and seeds (see Chapter 4). Iron is best absorbed as the ferrous (Fe^{2+}) salt in a mildly acidic medium; taking 250 mg vitamin C or eating citrus fruits along with iron supplements or iron-rich foods is therefore recommended to optimize absorption. Calcium is a potent inhibitor of iron absorption, so patients should be told not to take iron supplements with milk and to take them 2 hours before or 4 hours after ingestion of antacids. Other dietary factors that can inhibit absorption of iron salts include certain antibiotics as well as simultaneous consumption of coffee, tea, eggs, dietary fiber, or cereals. Enteric coated or sustained-release capsules are largely unnecessary as iron is best absorbed from the duodenum and proximal jejunum. Iron supplements come in two forms: Ferrous (Fe^{2+}) and ferric (Fe^{3+}). Ferrous is better absorbed, whereas the ferric forms tend to be better tolerated with less GI complaints (nausea, constipation, abdominal pain, diarrhea). These side effects can also be limited by slowly titrating the dose and temporarily dose with food (12,48). The recommended daily dose for treatment of iron deficiency in adults is approximately 150 to 200 mg per day of elemental iron; this would correlate to one 325 mg ferrous sulfate tablet (each providing 65 mg elemental iron) taken orally three times daily between meals. Patients who are unable to tolerate oral supplementation, dialysis patients, or patients with increased need of iron supplementation may be given parenteral forms of iron. Intramuscular iron has often been encouraged due to concerns of anaphylactoid-like reactions from intravenous iron. However, these concerns have been challenged due to more recent and safer formulations of intravenous iron, as well as a better understanding of the adverse reactions. Intramuscular iron supplementation has been described as very painful, poorly absorbed, and linked to an increase in gluteal sarcomas. High molecular weight intravenous iron dextran has been rarely but most commonly associated with myalgias and arthralgias which self-resolve and are not associated with hypotension, tachycardia, wheezing, or periorbital edema. These symptoms are often worsened by giving epinephrine or diphenhydramine. Newer intravenous formulations including low-molecular-weight iron dextran and iron salt formations (Ferric Gluconate and Iron Sucrose) have shown an improved safety profile and are encouraged more readily over IM treatments and when oral supplements are suboptimal for patient care (49–51).

Vitamin B_{12}

Vitamin B_{12} is found primarily in meat and dairy products, as well as fortified soy products. A recent Cochrane review concluded that daily oral therapy may be equivalent in efficacy to intramuscular administration for short-term therapy (52). However, a review of vitamin B_{12} disorders by Solomon notes that the available intervention trials have used immediate-release tablets or liquid suspensions, while most over-the-counter supplements are formulated for timed release and may not have the same efficacy (53). Two newer formulations include intranasal and sublingual; however, they also have not been thoroughly studied and tend to be rather expensive. Sublingual forms are considered to be just as efficacious as oral forms and intranasal formulations (54,55). As previously described, the intramuscular therapy is most frequently used for treatment of vitamin B_{12} deficiency. It is available in three forms, cyanocobalamin, hydroxycobalamin, and methylcobalamin. In the United States, cyanocobalamin is the most commonly used form; however, it does require conversion into meythlcobalamin before use in the body.

Methylcobalamin is the form most commonly used in Japan. Proponents of methylcobalamin claim that it is more potent and effective; however, this light sensitive form has no clear increased superiority in the literature (56,57).

RELEVANT NUTRIGENOMIC CONSIDERATIONS

As previously described, the utilization of folic acid is greatly influenced by polymorphisms on the MTHFR gene. These changes result in changes in gene expression and ultimately lead to folate deficiency. One example occurs with the single nucleotide polymorphism occurring on the MTHFR gene at allele position 222, resulting in a simple change of an alanine to valine. Although clinically these changes may result in increased neural tube defects and cardiovascular disease, it also seems to be protective against some cancers such as colon cancer. More broadly, this polymorphism does not change the recommended dietary allowance for folate in the different variants, but if micronutrient recommendations are not followed, the results could greatly affect infant birth and maturation (58). Similar studies have evaluated the HFE gene Cys282Tyr polymorphisms surrounding iron storage disease and iron fortification policies as well as polymorphisms affecting B_{12} metabolism (59,60). Although in its early stages, the opportunity to explore the nutritional genomics surrounding these micronutrients will greatly improve healthcare to be tailored and personalized to individuals globally.

CLINICAL HIGHLIGHTS

Nutritional anemias constitute one of the most common preventable conditions in both the developing world and industrialized countries. Iron deficiency is a public health problem in all countries but particularly among children in developing countries. Most cases of IDA and other nutritional anemias can be avoided by consuming a healthful, varied diet rich in dietary sources of iron, folate, and vitamin B_{12}. Heme iron is best absorbed, but adequate iron may be obtained from a vegetarian diet under most conditions. A diet rich in iron-containing foods should be particularly encouraged for those with high iron requirements, such as infants, children, and pregnant and menstruating women; when lean meat is not a part of the diet in these populations, supplementation may be warranted. In addition, during times where oral supplementation may not suffice, it is perfectly appropriate to consider the newer and safer intravenous iron formulations for better treatment of severe IDA. Attention to adequate iron intake is recommended for all strict vegetarians and long-distance athletes. Pregnant women should be counseled to take prenatal vitamins containing extra folic acid, B_{12}, and iron.

REFERENCES

1. World Health Organization. *The world health report 2002—reducing risks, promoting healthy life.* 2002. Available at http://www.who.int/whr/2002/en/; accessed 10/16/13.
2. WHO, UNICEF, UNU. Iron deficiency anaemia: assessment, prevention, and control. A guide for programme managers. Geneva, World Health Organization, 2001. WHO/NHD/01.3.
3. Okpala I. Leukocyte adhesion and the pathophysiology of sickle cell disease. *Curr Opin Hematol* 2006;13:40–44.
4. Fishman SM, Christian P, West KP. The role of vitamins in the prevention and control of anaemia. *Public Health Nutr* 2000;3:125–150.
5. World Health Organization. *Worldwide Prevalence of Anaemia 1993–2005,* Geneva, Switzerland, 2008. Available at http://whqlibdoc.who.int/publications/2008/9789241596657_eng.pdf; accessed 10/16/13.
6. Irwin JJ, Kirchner JT. Anemia in children. *Am Fam Physician* 2001;64:1379–1386.
7. Guralnik JM, Eisenstaedt RS, Ferrucci L, et al. Prevalence of anemia in persons 65 years and older in the United States: evidence for a high rate of unexplained anemia. *Blood* 2004;104:2263–2268
8. Mindell J, Moody A, Ali A, et al. Using longitudinal data from the Health Survey for England to resolve discrepancies in thresholds for haemoglobin in older adults. *Br J Haematol* 2013;160:368–376.
9. Dugdale M. Anemia. *Obstet Gynecol Clin North Am* 2001;28:363–381.
10. Beutler E, West C. Hematologic differences between African-Americans and whites: the roles of iron deficiency and alpha thalassemia on hemoglobin levels and mean corpuscular volume. *Blood* 2005;106:740–745.
11. Beutler E, Waalen J. The definition of anemia: what is the lower limit of normal of the blood hemoglobin concentration? *Blood* 2006;107:1747–1750.
12. Clark SF. Iron Deficiency Anemia. *Nutr Clin Pract* 2008;23:128–141.
13. WHO. Nutrition for Health and Development, Centers for Disease Control and Prevention(U.S.), et. al. *Assessing the iron status of populations: report of a joint World Health Organization/ Centers for Disease Control and Prevention technical consultation on the assessment of iron status at the population level,* 2nd ed., Geneva, Switzerland, 2004. Available at http://www.who.int/nutrition/publications/micronutrients/anaemia_iron_deficiency/9789241596107.pdf; accessed 10/16/13.
14. Cogswell ME, Parvanta I, Ickes L, et al. Iron supplementation during pregnancy, anemia, and birth weight: a randomized controlled trial. *Am J Clin Nutr* 2003;78:773–781.
15. Nead KG, Halterman JS, Kaczorowski JM, et al. Overweight children and adolescents: a risk group for iron deficiency. *Pediatrics* 2004;114:104–108.
16. McClung JP, Karl JP. Iron deficiency and obesity: the contribution of inflammation and diminished iron absorption. *Nutr Rev* 2009;67:100–104.
17. Cepeda-Lopez AC, Aeberli I, Zimmermann MB. Does obesity increase risk for iron deficiency? A review of the literature and the potential mechanisms. *Int J Vitam Nutr Res* 2010;80:263–270.
18. Hunt JR. Bioavailability of iron, zinc, and other trace minerals from vegetarian diets. *Am J Clin Nutr* 2003;78:633S–639S.
19. Monson ER. Iron and absorption: dietary factors which impact iron bioavailability. *J Am Diet Assoc* 1988;88:786–790.
20. Haas JD, Brownlie T. Iron deficiency and reduced work capacity: a critical review of the research to determine a causal relationship. *J Nutr* 2001;131:676–688.
21. Weis G, Goodnough LT. Anemia of chronic disease. *N England J Med* 2005;352:1011–1023.
22. Sullivan JL. Iron therapy and cardiovascular disease. *Kidney Int Suppl* 1999;69:135–137.
23. Auerbach M, Ballard H, Trout JR, et al. Intravenous iron optimizes the response to recombinant human erythropoietin in cancer patients with chemotherapy-related anemia: a multicenter, open-label, randomized trial. *J Clin Oncol* 2004;22:1301–1307.
24. Food and Nutrition Board, Institute of Medicine. Iron. In: *Dietary reference intakes for vitamin A, vitamin K, arsenic, boron, chromium, copper, iodine, iron, manganese, molybdenum, nickel, silicon, vanadium, and zinc.* Washington, DC: National Academy Press, 2001:290–393.
25. Cook JD, Boy E, Flowers C, et al. The influence of high-altitude living on body iron. *Blood* 2005;106:1441–1446.
26. Sherriff A, Emond A, Bell JC, et al. Should infants be screened for anaemia? A prospective study investigating the relation between haemoglobin at 8, 12, and 18 months and development at 18 months. *Arch Dis Child* 2001;84:480–485.
27. Ekiz C, Agaoglu L, Karakas Z, et al. The effect of iron deficiency anemia on the function of the immune system. *Hematol J* 2005;5:579–583.
28. Halterman JS, Kaczorowski JM, Aligne CA, et al. Iron deficiency and cognitive achievement among school-aged children and adolescents in the United States. *Pediatrics* 2001;107:1381–1386.
29. Osman YM, Wali YA, Osman OM. Craving for ice and iron-deficiency anemia: a case series from Oman. *Pediatr Hematol Oncol* 2005;22:127–131.
30. Beard JL. Iron requirements in adolescent females. *J Nutr* 2000;130:440s–442s.
31. Merkel D, Huerta M, Grotto I, et al. Prevalence of iron deficiency and anemia among strenuously trained adolescents. *J Adolesc Health* 2005;37:220–223.
32. Ahmed F, Kahn MR, Jackson AA. Concomitant supplemental vitamin A enhances the response to weekly supplemental iron and folic acid in anemic teenagers in urban Bangladesh. *Am J Clin Nutr* 2001;74:108–115.
33. Clarke R, Girmley Evans J, Schneede J, et al. Vitamin B_{12} and folate deficiency in later life. *Age Ageing* 2004;33:34–41.

34. Figlin E, Chetrit A, Shahar A, et al. High prevalences of vitamin B_{12} and folic acid deficiency in elderly subjects in Israel. *Br J Haematol* 2003;123:696–701.

35. Andres E, Loukili NH, Noel E, et al. Vitamin B_{12} (cobalamin) deficiency in elderly patients. *CMAJ* 2004;171:251–259.

36. Andres E, Federici L, Affenberger S, et al. Food-cobalamin malabsorption in elderly patients. *Agro Food Ind Hi Tec* 2006;17:v–viii.

37. Rosenblatt DS, Whitehead VM. Cobalamin and folate definceincy: acquired and hereditarydisorders in children. *Semin Hematol* 1999;36:19–34.

38. von Schenck U, Bender-Götze C, Koletzko B. Persistence of neurological damage induced by dietary vitamin B12 deficiency in infancy. *Arch Dis Child* 1997;77:137–139.

39. Kaiser L, Allen LH. Position of the American Dietetic Association: nutrition and lifestyle for ahealthy pregnancy outcome. *J Am Diet Assoc* 2008;108:553–561.

40. Bailey LB. Folate and vitamin B_{12} recommended intakes and status in the United States. *Nutr Rev* 2004;62:s14–s20.

41. Davis B, Melina V. *Becoming vegan*. Summertown, TN: Book Publishing Company, 2000.

42. Ray JG, Vermeulen MJ, Boss SC, et al. Declining rate of folate insufficiency among adults following increased folic acid food fortification in Canada. *Can J Public Health* 2002;93:249–253.

43. Bolamen Z, Kadikoylu G, Yukselen V, et al. Oral versus intramuscular cobalamin treatment in megaloblastic anemia: a single-center, prospective, randomized open-label study. *Clin Ther* 2003;25:3124–3134.

44. Nyholm E, Turpin P, Swain D, et al. Oral vitamin B_{12} can change our practice. *Postgrad Med J* 2003;79:218–220.

45. van Walraven C, Austin P, Naylor C. Vitamin B_{12} injections versus oral supplements. How much money could be saved by switching to pills? *Can Fam Physician* 2001;57:79–86.

46. Tamura T, Picciano MF. Folate and human reproduction. *Am J Clin Nutr* 2006;83:993–1016.

47. National Library of Medicine (US). Genetics Home Reference (Internet). Bethesda (MD): The Library. January 22, 2014. MTHFR; (reviewed July 2011; cited January 24, 2014. Available at http://ghr.nlm.nih.gov/gene/MTHFR.

48. Cancelo-Hidalgo MJ, Castelo-Branco C, Palacios S, et al. Tolerability of different oral iron supplements: a systematic review. *Curr Med Res Opin* 2013;29:291–303.

49. Auerbach M, Ballard H, Glaspy J. Clinical update: intravenous iron for anaemia. *Lancet* 2007;369:1502–1504.

50. Auerbach M, Rodgers GM. Intravenous iron. *N Engl J Med* 2007;357:93–94.

51. Auerbach M, Ballard H. Clinical use of intravenous iron: administration, efficacy, and safety. *Hematol Am Soc Hematol Educ Program* 2010;2010:338–347.

52. Vidal-AIaball J, Butler CC, Cannings-John R, et al. Oral vitamin B_{12} versus intramuscular B_{12} for vitamin B_{12} deficiency. *Cochrane Database Syst Rev* 2005;3:1–21.

53. Solomon LR. Oral vitamin B_{12} therapy: a cautionary note. *Blood* 2004;103:2863.

54. Slot WB, Merkus FW, Van Deventer SJ, et al. Normalization of plasma vitamin B12 concentration by intranasal hydroxocobalamin in vitamin B12-deficient patients. *Gastroenterology* 1997;113:430.

55. Delpre G, Stark P, Niv Y. Sublingual therapy for cobalamin deficiency as an alternative to oral and parenteral cobalamin supplementation. *Lancet* 1999;354:740–741.

56. Hvas AM, Nexo E. Diagnosis and treatment of vitamin B12 deficiency—an update. *Haematologica* 2006;91:1506–1512.

57. Carmel R. How I treat cobalamin (vitamin B12) deficiency. *Blood* 2008;112:2214–2221.

58. Stover PJ. Influence of human genetic variation on nutritional requirements. *Am J Clin Nutr* 2006;83:436s–442s.

59. Beutler E, Gelbart T, West C, et al. Mutation analysis in hereditary hemochromatosis. *Blood Cells Mol Dis* 1996;22:187–194.

60. Wilson A, Platt R, Wu Q, et al. A common variant in methionine synthase reductase combined with low cobalamin(vitamin B12) increases risk for spina bifida. *Mol Genet Metab* 1999;67:317–323.

CHAPTER 14

Diet, Bone Metabolism, and Osteoporosis

T he hydroxyapatite crystals of bone are made up predominantly of calcium and phosphorus. Osteoporosis is the demineralization of bone due to a net movement of calcium from bone to serum, mediated by a predominance of osteoclast over osteoblast activity. Osteoporosis is to be distinguished from osteomalacia, a different pattern of demineralization resulting from vitamin D deficiency.

Osteoporosis likely affects more than 20 million adults in the United States. Risk factors include gender (female), early menopause, ethnicity (white or Asian), thin bone structure, low body mass index, smoking, heavy consumption of alcohol, sedentary lifestyle, and family history.

Dietary pattern, use of supplements, physical activity, and sunlight exposure at various periods of life have the potential to affect peak bone density, the rate of bone mineral losses, and the propensity to bone injuries such as traumatic and pathologic/fragility fractures. The principal dietary consideration in the prevention and management of osteoporosis has long been lifetime calcium intake, although understanding of this association continues to evolve. In addition to lifestyle interventions, various pharmacologic interventions may be indicated in efforts to prevent disability from skeletal demineralization.

OVERVIEW

Bone metabolism is influenced by a variety of hormone actions. The serum calcium level is a stimulus to both parathyroid hormone (PTH) and calcitonin. PTH varies inversely, and calcitonin directly, with circulating calcium; PTH mobilizes calcium from bone, whereas calcitonin enhances skeletal deposition of calcium. PTH also increases activation of vitamin D, enhancing intestinal calcium absorption, and reduces urinary calcium excretion.

Peak bone mass is reached in the third to fourth decade of life, with gradual demineralization thereafter. Relatively rapid bone loss occurs in women during the 5 years following cessation of menses, and spine density diminishes by 3% to 6% annually. Bone loss in men apparently occurs at a fairly constant rate of 0.5% to 2% annually, depending on site, after peak bone mass is achieved. The clinical sequelae of osteoporosis result from fracture, most commonly at the wrist, hip, and spine. More than 50% of women past the age of 80 have experienced compression fracture of the spine.

Diet

Definitive evidence that increasing dietary intake of calcium increases peak bone density is lacking. However, suggestive evidence is available. A National Institutes of Health (NIH) consensus panel convened in 1994 concluded that average calcium intake in the United States is too low to support optimal bone health, and it revised recommended intake ranges upward (1). The NIH currently recommends a daily calcium intake of 1,000 mg in men aged 51 to 70 and 1,200 mg in men over 70 and women over 50 (2). The basis for the NIH-recommended intake levels is the evidence of threshold doses above which further incorporation of calcium into bone does not occur. Optimal calcium intake over time is the level that allows bone density to reach the maximum genetically "encoded" for a given individual. Paleolithic intake of calcium is estimated in the range of 2 g per day for adults (3) (see Section VIIE). Relative inefficiency in the absorption of ingested calcium is protection against calcium excess under the conditions prevailing during our evolutionary history.

Although supplements may be useful in achieving the recommended intake of calcium, food sources offer the benefits of other nutrients known or thought to confer benefits on the skeleton, including vitamin D and trace minerals. A diet rich in dairy products and a variety of vegetables and grains will provide all of the nutrients thought to optimize bone health and may be recommended on other grounds as well. Calcium intake up to 2,500 mg per day is generally safe, although extreme intake may contribute to the formation of renal calculi (see Chapter 16) and interfere with the absorption of iron, zinc, and other minerals. Physical activity, particularly repetitive weight-bearing activities and resistance training, confer benefit to bone mass and strength in addition to that attainable by nutritional means (4). In addition, fitness reduces the risk of injurious falls (5,6).

Calcium requirements are lower when sodium and protein intake is low, as both of these increase urinary losses of calcium (7). The reduced calcium requirements associated with non-Western diets may partly explain the inability to demonstrate a transcultural dietary calcium gradient that corresponds with osteoporosis or fracture risk. A comparison of the characteristics of matched samples of elderly vegetarians and nonvegetarians demonstrated similar calcium profiles (8). Vegetarianism (see Chapter 43) need not, therefore, have adverse effects on calcium nutriture, unless the diet followed is one that is low in calcium and high in sodium. There is longitudinal evidence from the Framingham cohort that diets high in alkaline-producing components, specifically fruits, vegetables, potassium, and magnesium, are associated with preservation of bone mass in both men and women (9,10). A study of participants following the Dietary Approaches to Stop Hypertension (DASH) diet, which emphasizes fruits, vegetables, and whole foods, along with varying levels of sodium intake, found significantly reduced bone turnover in subjects who consumed the lowest-sodium DASH diet (11).

Controversy persists regarding the significance to bone mass of protein intake (12). Protein, and therefore nitrogen, intake results in increased urinary calcium losses. The mobilization of mineral from bone induced by protein intake is thought to be due to the buffering of acid generated during protein metabolism. Most dietary sources of protein are also sources of phosphorus, which, as noted, reduces urinary calcium. To the extent that protein ingestion contributes to calcium loss in urine, it is the result of the sulfur load imposed

and consequent acidification of serum and urine. As vegetable protein imposes less of a sulfur load than animal protein, protein from vegetable sources may be less likely to contribute to urinary loss of calcium.

Thus, there appears to be little net effect of moderate protein intake (approximately 100% to 150% of the recommended dietary allowance [RDA], or 1.0 to 1.5 g protein per kg) on bone density (13); however, only approximately 30% to 50% of US adults have been estimated to consume moderate levels of daily protein (14). Recent evidence suggests that low protein intake, as often occurs among older adults, reduces intestinal calcium absorption and stimulates PTH, which may lead to increased bone loss (15,16). Postmenopausal women with hip fractures have been shown to have low protein intake (<0.8 g/kg body weight/day), and protein supplementation was associated with decreased postfracture bone loss, medical complications, and length of rehabilitation hospital stays (17). Protein may therefore be beneficial to bone when habitual intake is low or in the context of malnutrition (18–20).

In contrast, high protein intake from omnivorous sources, as is characteristic of the typical Western diet, has been shown to produce sustained hypercalciuria (13), though long-term sequelae of this are not fully understood. A recent review by Calvez et al. (21) demonstrated that the increased calcium excretion in high-protein diets was not associated with bone loss, and data suggest that the hypercalciuria may be due to increased intestinal calcium absorption induced by the high-protein diet.

Evidence from the National Health and Nutrition Examination Survey II suggests that a diet high in saturated fat may have deleterious effects on the mineral content of cancellous bone (22,23). A recent review of 40 women with high bone mineral density demonstrated that lower fat intake, body fat levels, and LDL were strongly correlated with higher bone mineral density (adjusted $R^2 = 0.347$; $p < 0.001$) (24). It is hypothesized that a high-fat diet may decrease absorption of calcium, negatively affect osteoclastogenesis, and increase overall oxidative stress.

Dietary factors thought to influence the incorporation of calcium into bone include vitamin D, copper, zinc, manganese, fluorine, silicon, and boron. The predominant effects of protein and phosphorus on bone metabolism are mediated by the fractional reabsorption of calcium in the renal tubule. Protein decreases and phosphorus increases calcium reabsorption. The concomitant ingestion of protein and phosphorus in meat and dairy products has little net effect on calcium loss.

The recommended intakes of calcium at different stages of life (see Section VIIE) are based on what is known about obligate daily calcium losses in stool and urine (200 to 250 mg per day in adults), an absorption rate of 30% to 40%, and the rate of calcium incorporation into bone during the growth phase (140 to 500 mg per day during various stages). Finally, recent recommendations have been revised up to account for the rate of bone loss in older adults, as well as reduced intestinal absorption.

Calcium needs in adolescence have been studied by examining variation in dietary intake and associated variation in bone density in populations, by calcium balance studies, and by the provision of supplements in controlled trials. Bone density in adolescence is consistently influenced by age, weight, height, and pubertal status (25). Recent studies suggest that regular exercise is an important determinant of bone strength in young women (26,27), although excessive exercising in girls may lead to the female athlete triad, characterized by disordered eating, amenorrhea, and osteoporosis (28) (see Chapter 25). Evidence indicating a role for dietary calcium supplementation is less consistent, though observational studies have found that high intake of carbonated soft drinks among adolescents is associated with lower bone mineral density, particularly in girls (29,30); whether due to direct effects of the soft drinks or displacement of milk from the diet (31), this is a concerning finding as soft drink consumption continues to rise among this age group. To some degree, inconsistency in the results with dietary supplementation may be due to limited sample sizes, variation in the calcium preparations used, habitual calcium intake, or the predominant effects of physical activity, weight, and hormonal status. Despite the inconsistency in research findings to date, the possible benefits and lack of potential harm in raising calcium intake during adolescence have resulted in recommendations from the NIH to increase the recommended calcium intake for adolescents to 1,200 to 1,300 mg per day (2).

Pregnancy (see Chapter 27) is associated with the diversion of approximately 30 g of calcium

from the maternal circulation to the fetal skeleton. The effects of this process on the maternal skeleton remain uncertain. Were maternal calcium absorption or ingestion not to increase or excretion not to decrease, the formation of the fetal skeleton would consume 3% of maternal bone calcium. However, the increased levels of estrogen in pregnancy, resulting from placental estradiol production, favor osteoblast action and calcium deposition in bone. Exercise may help reduce the physiologic decrease in bone mineral density that occurs in pregnancy. In comparison to nonexercising low-risk women, very active women who performed over 10 hours of weight-bearing exercises per week experienced less of reduction in bone density during pregnancy (32).

Despite this so-called transient osteoporosis of pregnancy, most women undergo complete recovery of bone marrow density, and the risk of postmenopausal bone fractures appears to be inversely associated with parity (33,34). If multiparity contributes to increased bone mass, the extent to which it is due to pregnancy versus increased weight is uncertain. Pregnancy is associated with increased levels of circulating active vitamin D (1,25-dihydroxy vitamin D) and consequently with enhanced intestinal absorption of calcium. The effects of adolescent pregnancy on bone mass are uncertain. There is concern that the need for both fetal and maternal bone mineralization might exceed compensatory mechanisms. Without compensatory mechanisms, each pregnancy might reduce maternal bone mass by 3%.

Lactation (see Chapter 27) is associated with an initial loss of bone mineral, with subsequent compensation when menses is restored. Approximately 150 to 200 mg per day of calcium is diverted to breast milk at 3 months postpartum, and nearly 300 mg is diverted at 6 months. A total of 6 months of breast-feeding would require 4% to 6% of the maternal skeletal calcium without compensation. A recent study reported that after at least 6 months of lactation, approximately 5% of the bone mineral density is lost in the lumbar spine and femoral neck (35).

High levels of prolactin and reduced levels of estrogen are associated with reductions in bone mass. Net loss of maternal bone apparently does not occur at detectable levels if breast-feeding is sustained for less than 6 months. Loss of calcium from bone apparently occurs with breast-feeding beyond 6 months, even with optimal dietary intake (36). With restoration of menses, bone density is restored provided that dietary intake is adequate; neither pregnancy nor lactation has been found to be associated with increased risk of osteoporotic fracture (37). Case reports have shown that pregnancy and lactation-associated vertebral fractures treated with active vitamin D supplementation resulted in long-term improvement in bone mineral density and bone turnover markers (38). As with pregnancy, the effects of lactation on bone density in adolescents are less certain and of potentially greater concern. The net effect of lactation on the skeleton when vitamin D or calcium intake is deficient has not been adequately addressed.

Celiac disease has significant effects on skeletal health and low bone mineral density is commonly found in patients with celiac disease. Initially, it was thought that the low bone mineral density was directly related to intestinal malabsorption (39). Patients with active celiac disease undergo significant histological changes that alter their ability to absorb nutrients. One such change is the loss of villi from the proximal gut, where calcium is actively absorbed. Additionally, unabsorbed fatty acids can bind up calcium in the intestinal lumen and further contribute to the malabsorption. A gluten-free diet has been shown to reverse both the histological changes and calcium malabsorption, but often bone mineral density does not normalize. This may be due to the fact that celiac patients are in a state of chronic inflammation, and inflammatory cytokines are thought to be one possible mechanism for osteoporosis. Studies have shown that a gluten-free diet is often nutritionally deficient in calcium and vitamin D and has a higher percentage of fat relative to carbohydrates than a typical diet (40,41). Some studies have shown improvement in bone mineral density after calcium and vitamin D supplementation (42), while others did not show any improvement with supplementation (43,44). Senescence (see Chapter 31) in both men and women is associated with progressive demineralization of bone and increasing fracture risk. In women, the rapid phase of bone demineralization following menopause results in the loss of approximately 15% of skeletal calcium before a new steady state is reached. This loss is approximately equal to one standard deviation of bone density; thus, greater-than-average bone density during premenopause can result in ostensibly

"normal" bone density even after rapid postmenopausal bone loss. Conversely, failure to optimize bone density before menopause renders a woman much more susceptible to clinical sequelae of the bone loss induced by menopause. Based on currently available evidence, a total daily intake of 1,500 mg of calcium is appropriate for both elderly men and women, with supplementation indicated to compensate for lesser dietary intake. Vitamin D supplementation also is reasonable; the 400 IU contained in a typical multivitamin is likely sufficient, although more may be needed for fracture prevention among those without adequate sun exposure or dietary intake.

There is some evidence that calcium supplementation may retard bone loss in postmenopausal women with habitually low calcium intake (less than 400 mg per day). The efficacy of calcium supplementation when dietary intake is greater than 400 mg daily is unclear (36), although there is some evidence of slowed bone loss even in women with high to normal habitual intake (750 mg per day). Particular benefits have been demonstrated when calcium supplementation has been combined with vitamin D supplementation; increased bone density and reduced fracture rate in elderly women have been reported.

Whereas the rapid phase of postmenopausal bone loss is highly dependent on estrogen, and therefore relatively unaffected by supplemental calcium, more than 5 years after menopause, when the rate of bone loss slows, responsiveness to supplementation increases, particularly in women with relatively low dietary intake. Although evidence has been gathered demonstrating a reduction in the fracture rate with calcium supplementation, particularly when combined with vitamin D, the benefit would likely be much greater were calcium intake to be adequate throughout life. Thus, it is probable that the fracture rates in the treatment groups of even the most successful trials are higher than they would have to be if lifelong calcium intake were optimized.

A recent randomized trial found that men over 50 years of age with baseline calcium intake at or only slightly below recommended levels, who drank 400 mL per day of reduced-fat milk supplemented with 1,000 mg of calcium and 800 IU of vitamin D_3, demonstrated reduced bone loss at clinically relevant skeletal sites (i.e., femoral neck, total hip, ultradistal radius) after 2 years of supplementation (45). This suggests potential benefit of additional calcium and vitamin D supplementation in elderly men, even those with near-adequate calcium intake. Epidemiological data suggest that hip fracture rates are lower in populations with high habitual intake of dietary calcium, and preliminary evidence from randomized trials suggests that supplementation can be effective (46), but poor compliance may limit its viability as a broad preventive measure (47).

Although the focus in the elderly was until recently on calcium intake, interest has shifted somewhat to stores of vitamin D. Vitamin D intake among adults in the United States is generally about 100 IU per day; the most recent RDA is 400 IU per day for people 51 to 70 years old and at least 700 to 800 IU per day for people older than 70. Circulating levels of vitamin D tend to be lower during the winter in higher latitudes; effects on bone metabolism have not been established with certainty. Epidemiological data support an association between osteoporosis and low serum vitamin D and reduced rates of intestinal calcium absorption. A positive association has been found between circulating serum 25-hydroxy vitamin D levels and bone mineral density in both younger and older adults (48). Vitamin D levels in the elderly are generally lower than in younger adults, with actual deficiency not uncommon in institutionalized elderly not exposed to natural light (49). Because of reduced sunlight exposure among the elderly in general, dietary intake of vitamin D appears to be an important determinant of circulating levels. The principal source of dietary vitamin D is fortified milk.

Vitamin D supplementation as an isolated intervention has not shown consistent utility in preventing fractures in osteoporotic or healthy postmenopausal women, though recent evidence suggests that high-dose oral vitamin D supplementation (700 to 800 IU) given to elderly men and women can increase bone density and decrease the fracture rate, especially in those with documented vitamin D deficiency (50,51). A recent randomized trial of the effect of vitamin D supplementation on calcium absorption in postmenopausal women observed that vitamin D supplementation did not significantly improve calcium absorption except when serum 25-hydroxyvitamin D levels were below 10 ng per ml (52). The potential benefits of vitamin D supplementation are most likely to be realized in subjects with low habitual vitamin D intake or limited sun exposure, and if coadministered with supplemental calcium (53).

Phosphorus, the other main mineral in bone, is abundantly available in the diet. Excess intake of phosphorus suppresses activation of vitamin D, with resultant reduction in intestinal absorption of calcium. PTH levels rise when phosphorus intake is high. However, high dietary phosphorus is associated with reduced urinary calcium losses, so no net effect on bone has been demonstrated. Sodas contain phosphorus. Diets high in processed foods with phosphate additives, meat, and soda may contain an excess of phosphorus that is detrimental to bone. If calcium and phosphorus in the diet remain proportional, high phosphorus intake does not appear to be harmful.

Once osteoporosis has developed, dietary manipulations are relatively, if not completely, ineffective at restoring bone density. Pharmacotherapy is required for this effect; a recent review of treatment options is available (54). Estrogen directly stimulates osteoblasts and enhances production of active vitamin D, and estrogen supplementation effectively prevents the rapid bone loss that occurs at menopause, but use of hormone replacement has not been considered first-line treatment since the publication of the results of the Women's Health Initiative (55). The selective estrogen receptor modulators (SERMs), such as raloxifene, appear to have comparable effects on bone, decreasing risk of vertebral fracture by up to 30% (56). Bisphosphonates, such as alendronate, etidronate, and risedronate, inhibit osteoclast activity. Marketed as Fosamax, alendronate has been shown to increase bone density in osteoporosis and to reduce the fracture rate (57,58). Similar results have been reported for other bisphosphonates (59,60). Calcitonin reduces osteoclast activity and bone resorption. Salmon calcitonin, which is available as a nasal spray, offers analgesic action helpful for patients with acute osteoporotic fracture (61). It reduces osteoclast activity and bone resorption. Teriparatide, a recombinant form of PTH, can help stimulate new bone formation. Phytoestrogens (see Chapter 33) have estrogen-like properties, and limited evidence suggests that high intake of foods or supplements containing isoflavone phytoestrogens may help reduce bone turnover rates and increase bone mineral density (62,63).

The role of pharmacotherapeutics warrants mention in defining the limitations of dietary management of osteoporosis. Malnutrition contributes importantly to adverse outcomes following hospitalization of elderly patients for hip fracture. Sequelae are partly preventable with a vigorous program of nutritional support, which should be a part of the management plan for every such patient (see Chapter 26).

NUTRIENTS, NUTRICEUTICALS, AND FUNCTIONAL FOODS

Calcium

Calcium intake is essential to bone health and the prevention of osteoporosis, as discussed earlier. More detail regarding calcium intake is provided in the Nutrient Reference Data Table in Section VIIE. Good sources include dairy products, mustard greens, almonds, tofu, and sardines. Other seafood is a moderately good source. High-oxalate vegetables, such as spinach, provide little calcium that is bioavailable. Recent data suggest that dietary calcium may have more favorable effects than calcium supplements on estrogen metabolism and bone mineral density in postmenopausal women (64).

The association between calcium supplements and cardiovascular events is unclear. A recent meta-analysis by Bolland et al. (65) reviewed over 12,000 participants from 15 placebo-controlled double-blind randomized trials and demonstrated that a 31% increase in the relative risk of myocardial infarction in the individuals taking ≥500 mg of daily calcium supplementation (HR, 1.31; 95% CI, 1.02 to 1.67). It is thought that perhaps calcium supplements result in an acute increase in calcium levels that may result in vascular calcification. However, the meta-analysis did not observe any increase in any vascular-associated endpoints, such as the incidence of stroke or death. Other studies have shown that overall increased calcium intake may be protective against cardiovascular events. The Iowa Women's Health Study of 34,486 postmenopausal women aged 55 to 69 years demonstrated that women who had the highest quartile of calcium intake had a 33% reduction in ischemic heart disease deaths (RR, 0.67; 95% CI, 0.47 to 0.94) (66). There is also continued debate regarding the association between calcium and cancer risk. A Cochran review of two RCTs demonstrated that calcium supplementation may help

prevent the development of adenomatous polyps in the colon, but there is not enough evidence to recommend the use of calcium supplementation to prevent colorectal cancer (67).

A variety of calcium preparations are available, and most are well absorbed. Calcium carbonate predominates in the United States. Its absorption is enhanced if the tablet is chewed or disintegrates readily. Calcium citrate and phosphate are widely available, and evidence suggests that calcium citrate is better absorbed than calcium carbonate (68). Split dosing enhances absorption, as only a portion of calcium ingested at any time is absorbed. Although some controversy exists regarding the optimal dose of calcium for prevention of osteoporosis, a teleologic view would favor fairly high intake. Our paleolithic ancestors apparently consumed considerably more calcium than we do (3,69).

Magnesium

Although magnesium is essential for the secretion and action of PTH, supplementation of magnesium has not been shown to benefit bone metabolism, even though the average intake in the United States is below the RDA (70,71); however, fruit and vegetable consumption has been linked to bone health, and one mechanism for this association is thought to be their high magnesium content (72). Magnesium supplementation concurrent with calcium may limit calcium absorption.

Approximately half of the body's magnesium stores are in bone: one-third on the bone surface and two-thirds incorporated into hydroxyapatite. Under conditions of calcium deficiency, magnesium may displace calcium in bone mineral. The exact influences of magnesium nutriture on osteoporosis or fracture risk are uncertain (71,73).

Vitamin K

Vitamin K functions in the γ-carboxylation of glutamic acid, contributing to the production of a variety of physiologically important proteins. The most prominent products of vitamin K metabolism participate in coagulation (see Chapters 4 and 9). Several protein products that are dependent on vitamin K are incorporated in bone. One such product, osteocalcin, can be measured in serum as a marker of bone turnover. Circulating osteo-calcin is low in low vitamin K states, such as use of warfarin (Coumadin). In vitro, vitamin K has been shown to inhibit osteoclastogenesis and promote osteoblastogenesis (74). Further, signs of impaired vitamin K metabolism are common in patients with osteoporosis (75).

Several studies have demonstrated that vitamin K supplementation decreases fracture risk (76,77). A recent randomized trial reported that vitamin K supplementation did not prevent age-related declines in bone mineral density, but did reduce fracture risk (76). In transplant patients, postoperative vitamin K supplementation was demonstrated to have a positive effect on lumbar spine bone mineral density (78). A meta-analysis of observational and experimental trials concluded that supplementation with oral vitamin K (phytonadione and menaquinone) reduces bone loss and prevent fractures; the investigators found an odds ratio favoring menaquinone of 0.40 (95% CI, 0.25 to 0.65) for vertebral fractures, 0.23 (95% CI, 0.12 to 0.47) for hip fractures, and 0.19 (95% CI, 0.11 to 0.35) for all nonvertebral fractures (79).

Iron

Calcium in a meal or supplement ingested with iron will interfere with iron absorption.

Phosphorus

Phosphorus is stored in bone at a ratio of 1:2 with calcium, based on mass. Although 85% of body phosphorus is stored in the skeleton, it contributes to a wide range of physiologic functions, including the storage and generation of energy in the phosphate bonds of ATP. Phosphorus is widely distributed in the diet; a typical American diet provides approximately 1 g per day for adult women and 1.5 g for adult men. The major sources are dairy, meat, poultry, and fish; cereals contribute approximately 12% of the total. Phosphorus is abundant in food additives; a highly processed diet may provide as much as 30% of intake in the form of additives. Of note, the ratio of calcium to phosphorus in human milk is nearly twice as high as that in bovine milk.

Phosphorus deficiency does not occur under normal dietary conditions. It may be induced by protracted use of aluminum bases, which bind phosphorus. Recent evidence suggests that intake of carbonated soft drinks, containing both caffeine and phosphoric acid, are associated with reduced bone mineral density in women (80). Bone loss results when phosphorus deficiency occurs, though the ratio of phosphorus to calcium appears to be more important than the absolute intake (81). Recommended intake of phosphorus is based on the maintenance of a 1:1 ratio with calcium.

Vitamin D

Vitamin D is essential in the intestinal absorption of calcium and may be derived from food sources or synthesized in skin with exposure to sunlight. The RDA for vitamin D is based on age, as follows: for those 1 to 70 years of age, the RDA is 600 IU daily, 15 mg of cholecalciferol activity; for those 71 years and older, 800 IU daily; and for pregnant and lactating women, 600 IU daily (82). Although the evidence base is limited, an intake of 400 IU per day is recommended for children 0 to 12 months. These RDAs are based on minimal sun exposure. The principal dietary source of vitamin D in the United States is fortified milk, which contains 400 IU per quart. The vitamin is stable with regard to processing, storage, and cooking.

Vitamin E

Vitamin E is an antioxidant that has been shown to decrease cartilage resorption (83) and improve bone structure in animal models (84). It is hypothesized that vitamin E counteracts the increased bone resorption resulting from oxidative stress. In several human studies, vitamin E supplementation was associated with a decreased risk of hip fracture in smokers only (85,86).

Phytoestrogens

Although there is considerable interest in the potential of phytoestrogens to ameliorate the impact of ovarian endocrine failure at menopause on bone density, to date there are only limited data to suggest that phytoestrogens may help protect postmenopausal bone loss (87,88). Isoflavones, a group of phytoestrogens, are particularly abundant in soy; diets rich in soy products have been associated with low rates of osteoporotic fracture (89) (see Chapter 33).

Boron

Boron appears to influence calcium balance, reducing urinary losses. The mechanisms of boron's action on calcium metabolism are uncertain. Postulated effects include hydroxylation of vitamin D and stimulation of increased estradiol production. Boron may enhance the effects of estrogen on bone. Excess from diet is unlikely, and doses up to 10 mg per day are nontoxic. Doses exceeding 50 mg per day in the form of supplements have induced gastrointestinal discomfort and possibly seizures. Estimated intake in the United States ranges from 0.5 to just over 3 mg per day; 1 mg per day is believed to be sufficient. Boron is found in beans, beer, nuts, legumes, wine, and green leafy vegetables (see Section VIIE).

Fluoride

Fluoride is nearly ubiquitous in soil and water, but in small and variable amounts. The incorporation of fluoride into bone is proportional to intake. Food sources of fluoride in the United States contribute an estimated 0.3 to 0.6 mg per day, with the distribution of foods obscuring differences in the regional fluoride contents of soil.

The principal determinant of variation in fluoride intake is water and beverages. An intake of 1.5 to 4.0 mg per day is recommended for adults; average intake is in this range. Intake of 0.1 to 1 mg daily during the first year of life, and up to 1.5 mg for the next 2 years, is recommended. Mottling of teeth occurs in children with a fluoride intake above 2 mg per day. Chronic intake of more than 20 mg per day induces toxicity in adults, leading to disruption of bone architecture and adverse effects on kidney, muscle, and nerve.

Fluoride is incorporated into hydroxyapatite and stimulates the action of osteoblasts. Fluoride increases bone density and strength, but, because of reduced elasticity, the resistance of bone to fracture is not necessarily enhanced by fluoride supplementation. High-dose fluoride (50 mg per day) has been shown to increase bone density in osteoporosis and to reduce the rate of vertebral fracture (90,91). For benefit to occur with fluoride supplementation, sufficient calcium must be provided concomitantly; fluoride induces osteogenesis and especially consequent "bone hunger" in the spine. If calcium is unavailable from the diet, it may be leached from other skeletal sites (92).

Variation in doses and regimens used in clinical trials has perpetuated controversy regarding the role of fluoride in the treatment and prevention of osteoporosis (92–96). Evidence from recent randomized trials suggests that a low-dose fluoride regimen (approximately 11.2 mg per day) may be more effective at preventing fractures, even though higher doses (20 mg per day) have been associated with greater increases in bone density (97,98).

Caffeine

Caffeine apparently reduces active transport of calcium in the intestine, thereby reducing absorption and inducing a slight negative shift in calcium balance. The effect is modest and completely compensated by the addition of milk to coffee (see Chapter 41).

Sodium

Sodium and calcium share a transport system in the kidney, and filtered sodium is accompanied by calcium. For every 2.3 g of sodium excreted in urine, 20 to 60 mg of calcium is lost (70,99). High-sodium diets therefore increase calcium requirements (100).

Omega-3 Fatty Acids

Since increased expression of inflammatory cytokines with aging is thought to be one mechanism contributing to osteoporosis, anti-inflammatory nutrients such as ω-3 fatty acids are hypothesized to be beneficial for bone health. A recent review of 10 randomized trails investigating skeletal outcomes in individuals with ω-3 fatty acid supplementation versus placebo demonstrated that 4 of the 10 studies reported improvements in bone mineral density or bone turnover markers (101). However, given that three of these studies combined high calcium supplementation with ω-3 fatty acid supplementation and the limited number of trials, there is insufficient evidence to draw conclusions regarding the effect of ω-3 supplementation on skeletal health.

Other Nutrient Effects

Phytate and oxalate in food complex with calcium. They are abundant in cruciferous vegetables and limit the bioavailability of calcium from such sources. Although phytate and oxalate levels are high in beans, calcium from beans is relatively bioavailable. Fiber can interfere with calcium absorption, and wheat bran seems to have a particularly strong influence.

Unlike with phytate and oxalate, the effects of concomitantly ingested fiber generalize to calcium from other foods. In the average US diet, the effects of fiber intake on calcium absorption are negligible (70,102).

A role for zinc, manganese, and copper as cofactors in enzymatic processes germane to bone metabolism has stimulated interest in the influence that dietary levels of these trace minerals may have on bone. To date, there is no more than preliminary evidence in humans that these trace minerals exacerbate osteoporosis when intake is low or ameliorate it when intake is raised (103).

Elevated serum homocysteine levels have been associated with osteoporosis, as well as vascular disease, raising the possibility that vitamins B_{12}, B_6, and folate may affect bone metabolism (104,105). In particular, these nutrients tend to be deficient in the diets of elderly people. Recent evidence indicates an association between vitamin B_{12} status and bone mineral density, particularly in frail older women (106,107); however, evidence that B vitamin supplementation may play a role in the prevention of osteoporosis is not yet available.

Evidence suggests that antioxidant intake may protect against osteoporotic hip fracture; however, this effect may be significantly reduced in patients who smoke (85). Conversely, high intake of vitamin C, E, or both, may protect against the adverse effects of smoking on bone, presumably because oxidation plays a role in the acceleration of osteoporosis in smokers (108).

There is increasing evidence that chronic proton-pump inhibitor (PPI) use or high-dose PPI treatment is associated with increased risk of bone fractures. A meta-analysis demonstrated that PPI use was associated with increased risk of hip (RR, 1.30; 95% CI, 1.19 to 1.43), spine (RR, 1.56; 95% CI, 1.31 to 1.85), and any-site fractures (RR, 1.16; 95% CI, 1.04 to 1.30) (109). This was corroborated by a recently published meta-analysis of 12 studies covering 1,521,062 patients (110). The mechanism underlying this relationship between PPI and bone fractures is unclear. One hypothesis is that the hypochlorhydria induced by the PPI results in decreased absorption

of important vitamins and nutrients, including calcium, magnesium, and vitamin B_{12} (111). PPIs have been shown to increase gastric pH to 5.5, and in vitro studies have reported that calcium dissociation decreases from 96% at pH 1 to 23% at pH 6.1 (112). PPIs have also been shown to induce hypomagnesemia (113) and cause malabsorption of vitamin B_{12} (114).

CLINICAL HIGHLIGHTS

Dietary management is fundamental to the primary and secondary prevention of osteoporosis, and it plays an important role in tertiary prevention. The origins of osteoporosis are in childhood and adolescence, during which time adequate physical activity, vitamin D, and dietary calcium are particularly important. Peak bone density is reached by around the end of the third decade. Calcium intake of about 1,300 mg per day is advisable during adolescence, along with moderate sun exposure and/or at least 600 IU of vitamin D. To achieve these thresholds and to optimize bone metabolism, the diet should be rich in nonfat dairy products and a variety of vegetables, fruits, and grains. Moderation in protein and sodium intake is advisable.

These recommendations are compatible with the dietary pattern advisable on other grounds (see Chapter 45). Hormone replacement therapy is no longer recommended as first-line treatment for postmenopausal women; instead, the use of SERMs, calcium and fluoride supplementation, calcitonin, or alendronate might be considered. These options have not been studied for primary prevention, but evidence supports consideration of their use for secondary prevention.

In older adults, vitamin D supplementation to achieve an intake of at least 800 IU per day is indicated; such an intake can be achieved with use of a multivitamin. As calorie intake declines, the need to supplement calcium to achieve recommended intake levels is more probable. Calcium carbonate is readily available and inexpensive. Any calcium preparation should be given in divided doses to optimize absorption.

A diet in compliance with overall recommendations for fruit, vegetable, grain, meat, and dairy intake will provide various nutrients—including magnesium, zinc, boron, and vitamin K—in amounts adequate to contribute to the health of bone. Brief recommendations in office practice should focus on consuming a diverse diet, consuming nonfat dairy products, avoiding or quitting smoking, limiting alcohol intake, and engaging in consistent weight-bearing physical activity, at least some of which should be outdoors in sunlight.

REFERENCES

1. NIH Consensus Conference. Optimal calcium intake. NIH Consensus Development Panel on optimal calcium intake. *JAMA* 1994;272:1942–1948.
2. Dietary Supplement Fact Sheet. *Calcium—health professional fact sheet.* Available at: http://ods.od.nih.gov/factsheets/Calcium-HealthProfessional/; accessed 5/12/13.
3. Eaton SB, Eaton SB 3rd, Konner MJ. Paleolithic nutrition revisited: a twelve-year retrospective on its nature and implications. *Eur J Clin Nutr* 1997;51:207–216.
4. Todd JA, Robinson RJ. Osteoporosis and exercise. *Postgrad Med J* 2003;79:320–323.
5. Lewis RD, Modlesky CM. Nutrition, physical activity, and bone health in women. *Int J Sport Nutr Exerc Metab* 1998;8:250–284.
6. Tinetti ME. Preventing falls in elderly persons. *N Engl J Med* 2003;348:42–49.
7. Heaney RP. Role of dietary sodium in osteoporosis. *J Am Coll Nutr* 2006;25:271s–276s.
8. Deriemaeker P, Aerenhouts D, De Ridder D, et al. Health aspects, nutrition and physical characteristics in matched samples of institutionalized vegetarian and non-vegetarian elderly (>65yrs). *Nutr Metab (Lond)*. 2011;8(1):37.
9. Tucker KL, Hannan MT, Chen H, et al. Potassium, magnesium, and fruit and vegetable intakes are associated with greater bone mineral density in elderly men and women. *Am J Clin Nutr* 1999;69:727–736.
10. Buclin T, Cosma M, Appenzeller M, et al. Diet acids and alkalis influence calcium retention in bone. *Osteoporos Int* 2001;12:493–499.
11. Lin P-H, Ginty F, Appel LJ, et al. The DASH diet and sodium reduction improve markers of bone turnover and calcium metabolism in adults. *J Nutr* 2003;133:3130–3136.
12. Bonjour J-P. Dietary protein: an essential nutrient for bone health. *J Am Coll Nutr* 2005;24:526s–536s.
13. Kerstetter JE, O'Brien KO, Insogna KL. Dietary protein, calcium metabolism, and skeletal homeostasis revisited. *Am J Clin Nutr* 2003;78:584s–592s.
14. US Department of Agriculture. *Supplementary data tables, USDA's 1994–1996 continuing survey of food intakes by individuals.* Riverdale, MD: Food Surveys Research Group BHNRC, Agricultural Research Service, 1999.
15. Munger RG, Cerhan JR, Chiu BC. Prospective study of dietary protein intake and risk of hip fracture in postmenopausal women. *Am J Clin Nutr* 1999;69:147–152.
16. Kerstetter JE, Svastisalee CM, Caseria DM, et al. A threshold for low-protein-diet-induced elevations in parathyroid hormone. *Am J Clin Nutr* 2000;72:168–173.
17. Bonjour J-P. Protein intake and bone health. *Int J Vitam Nutr Res* 2011;81(2–3):134–142.
18. Bonjour JP, Schurch MA, Rizzoli R. Nutritional aspects of hip fractures. *Bone* 1996;18:139s–144s.
19. Promislow JHE, Goodman-Gruen D, Slymen DJ, et al. Protein consumption and bone mineral density in the elderly: the Rancho Bernardo Study. *Am J Epidemiol* 2002;155:636–644.
20. Devine A, Dick IM, Islam AFM, et al. Protein consumption is an important predictor of lower limb bone mass in elderly women. *Am J Clin Nutr* 2005;81:1423–1428.
21. Calvez J, Poupin N, Chesneau C, et al. Protein intake, calcium balance and health consequences. *Eur J Clin Nutr* 2012;66(3):281–295.
22. Wohl GR, Loehrke L, Watkins BA, et al. Effects of high-fat diet on mature bone mineral content, structure, and mechanical properties. *Calcif Tissue Int* 1998;63:74–79.
23. Corwin RL, Hartman TJ, Maczuga SA, et al. Dietary saturated fat intake is inversely associated with bone density in humans: analysis of NHANES III. *J Nutr* 2006;136:159–165.
24. Sarkis KS, Martini LA, Szejnfeld VL, et al. Low fatness, reduced fat intake and adequate plasmatic concentrations of LDL-cholesterol are associated with high bone mineral density in women: a cross-sectional study with control group. *Lipids Health Dis* 2012;11:37. doi:10.1186/1476-511X-11-37.
25. Vatanparast H, Bailey DA, Baxter-Jones ADG, et al. Calcium requirements for bone growth in Canadian boys and girls during adolescence. *Br J Nutr* 2010;103(4):575–580.
26. Lloyd T, Petit MA, Lin HM, et al. Lifestyle factors and the development of bone mass and bone strength in young women. *J Pediatr* 2004;144:776–782.
27. Lloyd T, Beck TJ, Lin HM, et al. Modifiable determinants of bone status in young women. *Bone* 2002;30:416–421.
28. Golden NH. A review if the female athlete triad (amenorrhea, osteoporosis and disordered eating). *Int J Adolesc Med Health* 2002;14:9–17.
29. Whiting SJ, Vatanparast H, Baxter-Jones A, et al. Factors that affect bone mineral accrual in the adolescent growth spurt. *J Nutr* 2004;134:696s–700s.
30. Libuda L, Alexy U, Remer T, et al. Association between long-term consumption of soft drinks and variables of bone modeling and remodeling in a sample of healthy German children and adolescents. *Am J Clin Nutr* 2008;88(6):1670–1677.
31. McGartland C, Robson PJ, Murray L, et al. Carbonated soft drink consumption and bone mineral density in adolescence: the Northern Ireland Young Hearts project. *J Bone Miner Res* 2003;18:1563–1569.
32. To WWK, Wong MWN. Bone mineral density changes during pregnancy in actively exercising women as measured by quantitative ultrasound. *Arch Gynecol Obstet* 2012;286(2):357–363.
33. Cure-Cure C, Cure-Ramirez P, Teran E, et al. Bone-mass peak in multiparity and reduced risk of bone-fractures in menopause. *Int J Gynaecol Obstet* 2002;76:285–291.
34. Michaelsson K, Baron JA, Farahmand BY, et al. Influence of parity and lactation on hip fracture risk. *Am J Epidemiol* 2001;153:1166–1172.
35. Sowers MF, Hollis BW, Shapiro B, et al. Elevated parathyroid hormone-related peptide associated with lactation and bone density loss. *JAMA* 1996;276(7):549–554.
36. Ziegler EE, Filer LJ Jr, eds. *Present knowledge in nutrition,* 7th ed. Washington, DC: ILSI Press, 1996.
37. Kalkwarf HJ, Specker BL. Bone mineral changes during pregnancy and lactation. *Endocrine* 2002;17:49–53.
38. Iwamoto J, Sato Y, Uzawa M, et al. Five-year follow-up of a woman with pregnancy and lactation-associated osteoporosis and vertebral fractures. *Ther Clin Risk Manag* 2012;8:195–199.

39. Larussa T, Suraci E, Nazionale I, et al. Bone mineralization in celiac disease. *Gastroenterol Res Prac* 2012;1–19.

40. Bardella MT, Fredella C, Prampolini L, et al. Body composition and dietary intakes in adult celiac disease patients consuming a strict gluten-free diet. *Am J Clin Nutr* 2000;72(4):937–939.

41. Kinsey L, Burden ST, Bannerman E. A dietary survey to determine if patients with coeliac disease are meeting current healthy eating guidelines and how their diet compares to that of the British general population. *Eur J Clin Nutr* 2008;62(11):1333–1342.

42. Bai JC, Gonzalez D, Mautalen C, et al. Long-term effect of gluten restriction on bone mineral density of patients with coeliac disease. *Aliment Pharmacol Ther* 1997;11(1):157–164.

43. Ciacci C, Maurelli L, Klain M, et al. Effects of dietary treatment on bone mineral density in adults with celiac disease: factors predicting response. *Am J Gastroenterol* 1997;92(6):992–996.

44. Caraceni MP, Molteni N, Bardella MT, et al. Bone and mineral metabolism in adult celiac disease. *Am J Gastroenterol* 1988;83(3):274–277.

45. Daly RM, Brown M, Bass S, et al. Calcium- and vitamin D₃-fortified milk reduces bone loss at clinically relevant skeletal sites in older men: a 2-year randomized controlled trial. *J Bone Miner Res* 2006;21:397–405.

46. Jackson RD, LaCroix AZ, Gass M, et al. Calcium plus vitamin D supplementation and the risk of fractures. *N Engl J Med* 2006;354:669–683.

47. Prince RL, Devine A, Dhaliwal SS, et al. Effects of calcium supplementation on clinical fracture and bone structure: results of a 5-year, double-blind, placebo-controlled trial in elderly women. *Arch Intern Med* 2006;166:869–875.

48. Bischoff-Ferrari HA, Dietrich T, Orav EJ, et al. Positive association between 25-hydroxy vitamin D levels and bone mineral density: a population-based study of younger and older adults. *Am J Med* 2004;116:634–639.

49. Gennari C. Calcium and vitamin D nutrition and bone disease of the elderly. *Public Health Nutr* 2001;4:547–559.

50. Bischoff-Ferrari HA, Willett EC, Wong JB, et al. Fracture prevention with vitamin D supplementation: a meta-analysis of randomized controlled trials. *JAMA* 2005;293:2257–2264.

51. Trivedi DP, Doll R, Khaw KT. Effect of four monthly oral vitamin D₂ (cholecalciferol) supplementation on fractures and mortality in men and women living in the community: randomized double blind controlled trial. *BMJ* 2003;326:469.

52. Gallagher JC, Yalamanchili V, Smith LM. The effect of vitamin D on calcium absorption in older women. *JCEM* 2012;97(10):3550–3556.

53. Katz D. Is the IOM right to recommend we get less? Vitamin D and calcium? *The Huffington Post*. Available at: http://www.huffingtonpost.com/david-katz-md/vitamind--andcalcium-shouldwe--becautious_b_789842.html; accessed 5/5/13.

54. Simon LS. Osteoporosis. *Rheum Dis Clin North Am* 2007;33:149–176.

55. Rossouw JE, Anderson GL, Prentice RL, et al. Risks and benefits of estrogen plus progestin in healthy postmenopausal women: principal results from the Women's Health Initiative Randomized Controlled Trial. *JAMA* 2002;288:321–333.

56. Srivastava M, Deal C. Osteoporosis in elderly: prevention and treatment. *Clin Geriatr Med* 2002;3:529–555.

57. Liberman UA, Weiss SR, Broll J, et al. Effect of oral alendronate on bone mineral density and the incidence of fractures in postmenopausal osteoporosis. *N Engl J Med* 1995;333:1437–1443.

58. Cranney A, Wells G, Willan A, et al. Meta-analyses of therapies for postmenopausal osteoporosis. II. Meta-analysis of alendronate for the treatment of postmenopausal women. *Endocr Rev* 2002;23:508–516.

59. Watts NB, Harris ST, Genant HK, et al. Intermittent cyclical etidronate treatment of postmenopausal osteoporosis. *N Engl J Med* 1990;323:73–79.

60. Cohen SB. An update on bisphosphonates. *Curr Rheumatol Rep* 2004;6:59–65.

61. Munoz-Torres M, Alonso G, Raya MP. Calcitonin therapy in osteoporosis. *Treat Endocrinol* 2004;3:117–132.

62. Nikander E, Metsa-Heikkila M, Klikorkala O, et al. Effects of phytoestrogens on bone turnover in postmenopausal women with a history of breast cancer. *J Clin Endocrinol Metab* 2004;89:1207–1212.

63. Mei J, Yeung SS, Kung AW. High dietary phytoestrogen intake is associated with higher bone mineral density in postmenopausal but not premenopausal women. *J Clin Endocrinol Metab* 2001;86:5217–5221.

64. Napoli N, Thompson J, Civitelli R, et al. Effects of dietary calcium compared with calcium supplements on estrogen metabolism and bone mineral density. *Am J Clin Nutr* 2007;85:1428–1433.

65. Bolland MJ, Barber PA, Doughty RN, et al. Vascular events in healthy older women receiving calcium supplementation: randomised controlled trial. *BMJ* 2008;336(7638):262–266.

66. Bostick RM, Kushi LH, Wu Y, et al. Relation of calcium, vitamin D, and dairy food intake to ischemic heart disease mortality among postmenopausal women. *Am J Epidemiol* 1999;149(2):151–161.

67. Weingarten MA, Zalmanovici A, Yaphe J. Dietary calcium supplementation for preventing colorectal cancer and adenomatous polyps. *Cochrane Database Syst Rev.* 2008;(1):CD003548.

68. Heller HJ, Greer LG, Haynes SD, et al. Pharmacokinetic and pharmacodynamic comparison of two calcium supplements in postmenopausal women. *J Clin Pharmacol* 2000;40:1237–1244.

69. Patrick L. Comparative absorption of calcium sources and calcium citrate malate for the prevention of osteoporosis. *Altern Med Rev* 1999;4:74–85.

70. Heaney HP. Osteoporosis: vitamins, minerals, and other micronutrients. In: Bendich A, Deckelbaum RJ, eds. *Preventive nutrition. The comprehensive guide for health professionals.* Totowa, NJ: Humana Press, 1997:285–302.

71. Rude RK, Gruber HE. Magnesium deficiency and osteoporosis: animal and human observations. *J Nutr Biochem* 2004;15:710–716.

72. New SA, Robins SP, Campbell MK, et al. Dietary influences on bone mass and bone metabolism: further evidence of a positive link between fruit and vegetable consumption and bone health? *Am J Clin Nutr* 2000;71:142–151.

73. Shils ME. Magnesium. In: Shils ME, Olson JA, Shike M, eds. *Modern nutrition in health and disease*, 8th ed. Philadelphia, PA: Lea & Febiger, 1994:164–184.

74. Koshihara Y, Hoshi K, Okawara R, et al. Vitamin K stimulates osteoblastogenesis and inhibits osteoclastogenesis in human bone marrow cell culture. *J Endocrinol* 2003;176(3):339–348.

75. Booth SL, Broe KE, Gagnon DR, et al. Vitamin K intake and bone mineral density in women and men. *Am J Clin Nutr* 2003;77:512–516.

76. Cheung AM, Tile L, Lee Y, et al. Vitamin K supplementation in postmenopausal women with osteopenia (ECKO Trial): a randomized controlled trial. *PLoS Med.* 2008;5(10):e196.

77. Feskanich D et al. Vitamin K intake and hip fractures in women: a prospective study. *Am J Clin Nutr* 1999; 69(1):74–79.

78. Forli L, Bollerslev J, Simonsen S, et al. Dietary vitamin K2 supplement improves bone status after lung and heart transplantation. *Transplantation* 2010;89(4):458–464.

79. Cockayne S, Adamson J, Lanham-New S, et al. Vitamin K and the prevention of fractures: systematic review and meta-analysis of randomized controlled trials. *Arch Intern Med* 2006;166:1256–1261.

80. Tucker KL, Morita K, Qiao N, et al. Colas, but not other carbonated beverages, are associated with low bone mineral density in older women: the Framingham osteoporosis study. *Am J Clin Nutr* 2006;84:936–942.

81. Heaney RP. Dietary protein and phosphorus do not affect calcium absorption. *Am J Clin Nutr* 2000;72:758–761.

82. Institute of Medicine, Food and Nutrition Board. *Dietary reference intakes for calcium and vitamin D.* Washington, DC: National Academy Press, 2010.

83. Garett IR, Boyce BF, Oreffo RO, et al. Oxygen-derived free radicals stimulate osteoclastic bone resorption in rodent bone in vitro and in vivo. *J Clin Invest* 1990;85:632–639.

84. Xu H, Watkins BA, Seifert MF. Vitamin E stimulates trabecular bone formation and alters epiphyseal cartilage morphometry. *Calcif Tissue Int* 1995;57:293–300.

85. Zhang J, Munger R, West NA, et al. Antioxidant intake and risk of osteoporotic hip fracture in Utah: an effect modified by smoking status. *Am J Epidemiol* 2006;163:9–17.

86. Pasco J, Henry M, Wilkinson L, et al. Antioxidant vitamin supplements and markers of bone turnover in a community sample of nonsmoking women. *J Womens Health (Larchmt).* 2006;15:295–300.

87. Strauss L, Santti R, Saarinen N, et al. Dietary phytoestrogens and their role in hormonally dependent disease. *Toxicol Lett* 1998;102–103:349–354.

88. Weaver CM, Cheong MK. Soy isoflavones and bone health: the relationship is still unclear. *J Nutr* 2005;135:1243–1247.

89. Tham DM, Gardner CD, Haskell WL. Clinical review 97: potential health benefits of dietary phytoestrogens: a review of the clinical, epidemiological, and mechanistic evidence. *J Clin Endocrinol Metab* 1998;83:2223–2235.

90. Pak CY, Sakhaee K, Piziak V, et al. Slow-release sodium fluoride in the management of postmenopausal osteoporosis. A randomized, controlled trial. *Ann Intern Med* 1994;120:625–632.

91. Haguenauer D, Welch V, Shea B, et al. Fluoride for the treatment of postmenopausal osteoporotic fractures: a meta-analysis. *Osteoporos Int* 2000;11:727–738.

92. Heaney RP. Fluoride and osteoporosis. *Ann Intern Med* 1994;120:689–690.

93. Meunier PJ. Evidence-based medicine and osteoporosis: a comparison of fracture risk reduction data from osteoporosis randomised clinical trials. *Int J Clin Pract* 1999;53:122–129.

94. Fluoride and bone: a second look. No use in osteoporosis. *Prescrire Int* 1998;7:110–111.

95. Meunier PJ, Sebert JL, Reginster JY, et al. Fluoride salts are no better at preventing new vertebral fractures than calcium-vitamin D in postmenopausal osteoporosis: the FAVOStudy. *Osteoporos Int* 1998;8:4–12.

96. Kleerekoper M. The role of fluoride in the prevention of osteoporosis. *Endocrinol Metab Clin North Am* 1998;27:441–452.

97. Meunier PJ. Evidence-based medicine and osteoporosis: a comparison of fracture risk reduction data from osteoporosis randomised clinical trials. *Int J Clin Pract* 1999;53:122–129.

98. Reid IR, Cundy T, Grey AB, et al. Addition of monofluorophosphate to estrogen therapy in postmenopausal osteoporosis: a randomized controlled trial. *J Clin Endocrinol Metab* 2007;92:2446–2452.

99. Devine A, Criddle RA, Dick IM, et al. A longitudinal study of the effect of sodium and calcium intakes on regional bone density in postmenopausal women. *Am J Clin Nutr* 1995;62:740–745.

100. Heaney RP. Role of dietary sodium in osteoporosis. *J Am Coll Nutr* 2006;25:271s–276s.

101. Orchard TS, Pan X, Cheek F, et al. A systematic review of omega-3 fatty acids and osteoporosis. *Br J Nutr* 2012;107(suppl 2):S253–S260.

102. Chen ZC, Stini WA, Marshall JR, et al. Wheat bran fiber supplementation and bone loss among older people. *Nutrition* 2004;20:747–751.

103. Palacios C. The role of nutrients in bone health, from A to Z. *Crit Rev Food Sci Nutr* 2006;46:621–628.

104. Bunker VW. The role of nutrition in osteoporosis. *Br J Biomed Sci* 1994;51:228–240.

105. Sasaki S, Yanagibori R. Association between current nutrient intakes and bone mineral density at calcaneus in pre- and postmenopausal Japanese women. *J Nutr Sci Vitaminol (Tokyo).* 2001;47:289–294

106. Dhonukshe-Rutten RA, Lips M, de Jong N, et al. Vitamin B-12 status is associated with bone mineral content and bone mineral density in frail elderly women but not in men. *J Nutr* 2003;133:801–807.

107. Tucker KL, Hannan MT, Qiao N, et al. Low plasma vitamin B_{12} is associated with lower BMD: the Framingham osteoporosis study. *J Bone Miner Res* 2005;20:152–158.

108. Nawaz H, Katz DL. American College of Preventive Medicine position statement on post-menopausal hormone replacement therapy. *Am J Prev Med* 1999;17:250–254.

109. Yu EW, Bauer SR, Bain PA, et al. Proton pump inhibitors and risk of fractures: a meta-analysis of 11 international studies. *Am J Med* 2011;124(6):519–526.

110. Kwok CS, Yeong JK-Y, Loke YK. Meta-analysis: risk of fractures with acid-suppressing medication. *Bone* 2011;48(4):768–776.

111. Maggio M, Lauretani F, Ceda GP, et al. Use of proton pump inhibitors is associated with lower trabecular bone density in older individuals. *Bone* doi:10.1016/j.bone.2013.09.014.

112. Verdu EF, Fraser R, Armstrong D, et al. Effects of omeprazole and lansoprazole on 24-hour intragastric pH in Helicobacter pylori-positive volunteers. *Scand J Gastroenterol* 1994;29(12):1065–1069.

113. Hoorn EJ, van der Hoek J, de Man RA, et al. A case series of proton pump inhibitor–induced hypomagnesemia. *Am J Kidney Dis* 2010;56:112–6.

114. Marcuard SP, Albernaz L, Khazanie PG. Omeprazole therapy causes malabsorption of cyanocobalamin (vitamin B_{12}). *Ann Intern Med* 1994;120:211–5.

SUGGESTED READING

Feskanich D, Weber P, Willett WC, et al. Vitamin K intake and hip fractures in women: a prospective study. *Am J Clin Nutr* 1999;69:74–79.

Heaney HP. Osteoporosis: vitamins, minerals, and other micronutrients. In: Bendich A, Deckelbaum RJ, eds. *Preventive nutrition. The comprehensive guide for health professionals.* Totowa, NJ: Humana Press, 1997:285–302.

Krall EA, Dawson-Hughes B. Osteoporosis. In: Shils ME, Olson JA, Shike M, eds. *Modern nutrition in health and disease,* 8th ed. Philadelphia, PA: Lea & Febiger, 1994:1559–1568.

Lau EM, Woo J. Nutrition and osteoporosis. *Curr Opin Rheumatol* 1998;10:368.

Nawaz H, Katz DL. American College of Preventive Medicine position statement on post-menopausal hormone replacement therapy. *Am J Prev Med* 1999;17:250–254.

Nordin BE. Calcium and osteoporosis. *Nutrition* 1997;13:664.

Nordin BE, Need AG, Steurer T, et al. Nutrition, osteoporosis, and aging. *Ann N Y Acad Sci* 1998;20:336–351.

Sowers MF. Nutritional advances in osteoporosis and osteomalacia. In: Ziegler EE, Filer LJ Jr, eds. *Present knowledge in nutrition,* 7th ed. Washington, DC: ILSI Press, 1996:456–463.

Standing Committee on the Scientific Evaluation of Dietary Reference Intakes, Food and Nutrition Board, Institute of Medicine. *Dietary reference intakes for calcium, phosphorus, magnesium, vitamin D, and fluoride.* Washington, DC: National Academy Press, 1997.

CHAPTER 15

Diet and Respiratory Disease

N utritional and respiratory status are related in a variety of ways. Malnutrition, either in isolation or as the result of acute or chronic illness, impairs respiratory function directly by weakening diaphragmatic contractions and overall diaphragmatic strength, making it more difficult to expel mucous (see Chapter 26). Malnutrition impacts the respiratory system indirectly by causing relative immunosuppression (see Chapter 11). As pneumonia is a leading cause of hospitalization due to infectious disease and is a leading nosocomial infection, the relationship among nutritional status, immune function, and the respiratory system is of particular importance.

The link between diet and the pulmonary system is especially clear in patients with limited respiratory reserve and CO_2 retention. The respiratory quotient of carbohydrate is higher than that of either fat or protein, justifying the restriction of carbohydrate in certain patients. A recent meta-analysis supported the manipulation of diet to reduce the respiratory quotient for modification of long-term outcomes in patients with chronic obstructive pulmonary disease (COPD) (1).

Dietary triggers of asthma and exacerbations of COPD are under investigation. Dietary intake may influence the production of surfactant. Whereas conclusive evidence supports a role for adequate nutritional status in obstructive pulmonary disease, evidence for a protective or provocative role of specific micronutrients is mostly preliminary to date. Generally, obesity and asthma have been closely linked, and a diet high in fiber and low in fat has been linked with improved respiratory function in asthmatics. The anti-inflammatory properties of n-3 fatty acids described in other chapters pertain to airway inflammation as well and may prove to be of benefit in obstructive disease such as asthma and chronic bronchitis.

OVERVIEW

Diet

Malnutrition has been shown to be common among patients with clinically significant obstructive airway disease, ranging from 20% to 70% (2–4). Mortality rates among patients with COPD rise substantially with the advent of malnutrition. Airway obstruction increases the metabolic costs of breathing, as does the need for higher respiratory rates to compensate for a reduction in the proportion of tidal volume effective in gas exchange. In addition, malnourished COPD patients have decreased diffusion capacity and increased CO_2 retention.

Macronutrient intake patterns may directly influence the adequacy of gas exchange by leading to variable CO_2 production. Every molecule of carbohydrate ingested results in a molecule of CO_2 produced; therefore, the respiratory quotient of carbohydrate has a value of 1. The respiratory quotient of protein is 0.8, whereas that of fat is 0.7. Protein supplementation may increase oxygen consumption due to its relatively high thermic effect. Protein consumption also tends to increase ventilation, potentially leading to dyspnea in patients with limited reserve. Thus, on the basis of metabolic effects, a relatively high-fat, carbohydrate-restricted diet is indicated for patients with CO_2 retention. Although the capacity of such diets to reduce CO_2 production has been shown, the capacity of such diets to modify clinical outcomes has not been demonstrated conclusively to date.

Weight loss in chronic pulmonary disease, such as COPD and cystic fibrosis, has been attributed to increased resting energy expenditure, although evidence in support of this is inconsistent. An increased work of breathing may contribute to an elevation of resting energy expenditure, but inefficiency in oxygen metabolism with exertion may contribute more. Cytokines associated with the disease state may contribute to catabolism and attenuate appetite. Negative energy balance during acute exacerbations of COPD apparently is due to both reduced energy intake relative to baseline and an increase in resting energy expenditure (5,6). Elevated levels of tumor necrosis factor α (TNF-α), and other acute-phase-reactant proteins, have been reported in patients with COPD and weight loss, although causality has not been adequately studied to date (5,7).

A review of nutritional support for severe pulmonary disease of diverse etiologies suggests that weight loss, particularly loss of fat-free mass, is a poor prognostic sign and an independent risk factor for mortality. Preliminary evidence suggests there is some benefit to nutritional support combined with an anabolic stimulus such as exercise in order to avoid adipose weight gain from supplemental calories (8–10). A recent meta-analysis examining the clinical outcomes in COPD patients who received nutritional support showed that oral nutritional supplements improved anthropometric measures and grip strength in patients with COPD (1). Further investigation of effective means of suppressing inflammatory mediator activity and preferentially restoring lean body mass is indicated. The use of nutrients to help preserve or increase lean body mass is addressed more thoroughly in Chapter 32.

In COPD, energy intake of 1.4 to 1.6 times the resting energy expenditure is indicated during periods when lean body mass is being recovered; energy then should be maintained at 1 to 1.2 times the resting energy expenditure to avoid increased CO_2 generation (11). Protein supplementation at approximately 1.5 g/kg/day is advocated by some in the aftermath of COPD exacerbation to facilitate the reconstitution of lean body mass (5). Ingestion and postprandial gastric distension may impair gas exchange slightly, leading to reduced calorie consumption as a means to avoid dyspnea.

The energy requirements of patients with COPD and malnutrition are estimated at 45 kcal/kg/day, approximately 80% to 90% higher than predicted resting energy expenditure (see Nutrition Formulas in Section VIIA). In such patients, expert opinion favors a diet relatively high in total fat (45% to 55% of total calories), with low intake of saturated fat to avoid cardiovascular sequelae (12). Population-based survey data suggest an inverse association between dietary fish intake and the development of smoking-related COPD (13).

Although nutritional support with high-fat rather than high-carbohydrate preparations offers the theoretical advantage of a lower respiratory quotient, in most cases, the actual clinical significance appears to be small (11). Nevertheless, Cai et al. (14) demonstrated improvement in lung function measurements and other clinical parameters with this approach as compared to the traditional high-carbohydrate diet.

Reduction in the mass and contractility of the diaphragm has been observed in both animals and humans subject to malnutrition. Muscle wasting of the diaphragm results in decreased ability to expel mucous as well as the patient's ability to exercise. Nutritional support may reverse this effect (15,16). Growth hormone and anabolic steroids have been used with some success, but their roles in clinical management are uncertain (17,18). Muscle wasting is characteristic during exacerbations of COPD and is compounded by the administration of corticosteroids. Dietary supplementation has been shown to attenuate, but not reverse, this tendency (19).

One small study showed long-term smokers with respiratory symptoms (dyspnea on exertion, cough, and sputum production) and without a diagnosis of COPD had a similar level of malnutrition as patients with COPD. The study found that body mass index, body weight, body fat, serum albumin, pre-albumin, and transferrin levels were similar to COPD patients compared to long-term smokers (20).

Difficulty in achieving measurable improvements in anthropometry or pulmonary function with energy-supplemented diets has been reported (20–22). Therefore, current interest has largely shifted from isolated dietary intervention to diet combined with exercise and/or anabolic agents.

Oxidative injury by free radicals is thought to be a key factor in acute lung injury. Preliminary evidence suggests that antioxidant supplementation in the form of vitamin E and C, retinol, and β-carotene may have protective effects. Dietary addition of n-3 fatty acids may also be beneficial in patients with acute lung injury (23).

An area of active investigation is the potential associations between both dietary antioxidants and n-3 fatty acids and the rising incidence of asthma. Although epidemiological and observational studies suggest benefits from higher intake of these nutrients, clinical intervention trials have, for the most part, been less encouraging (24).

Data from the Nurses' Health Study suggest that vitamin E intake may be inversely associated with the risk of asthma development, although the association was relatively weak; other antioxidants did not reveal significant effects (25). Evidence that a variety of dietary antioxidants may protect against COPD is preliminary but provocative (26). The evidence and biologic plausibility of antioxidant benefits in asthma are less robust, although vitamins E and C and selenium appear to be protective, based on available evidence.

There is increasing work focusing on pregnancy and early childhood periods as potentially crucial times for dietary intervention to influence respiratory health (27). Early breast-feeding has been shown to reduce the risk of asthma (28). An observational study of antioxidant intake in pregnancy found that infants born to mothers who had consumed the highest amounts of vitamin E and zinc during pregnancy were less likely to develop a recurrent wheeze by age 2 (29).

The generation of lactic acid, and resultant cellular acidosis, is thought to contribute to muscle fatigue by a variety of mechanisms, including interference with calcium release, glycolytic enzyme activity, and neural impulse propagation (30). The retention of CO_2 and the resultant systemic acidosis impose a respiratory workload on patients with COPD, limiting exercise capacity. Sodium bicarbonate has been studied as an ergogenic aid in healthy subjects with mixed results; approximately half of the published trials show benefit (see Chapter 32). In a small study, Coppoolse et al. (30) demonstrated no increase in exercise capacity in COPD subjects given an acute oral bicarbonate load. Potential benefits of chronic bicarbonate supplementation remain speculative.

Folklore has long suggested that dairy product consumption increases the production of respiratory tract mucus and exacerbates asthma. A double-blind, placebo-controlled crossover trial in 20 subjects showed no effect of acute milk consumption on symptoms or pulmonary function (31). A recent review article further solidified this point; even in patients with upper respiratory infections, milk consumption did not change the amount of mucus production (32).

In a survey of readers of a peer-reviewed journal of alternative and complementary medical practices, nutritional therapy for asthma was the most frequently cited practice among MD and non-MD providers, testifying to widespread interest in the topic (33,34). Use of nutrition and other alternative medical practices has been reported by approximately 50% of patients with asthma in both the adult and pediatric populations (35,36).

A link between asthma and obesity has been widely postulated in the medical literature. Most cross-sectional and prospective studies have demonstrated obesity as a risk factor for developing asthma. Hypothesized mechanisms for this association include change in lung physiology, increase in inflammatory mediators, and modification of hormonal factors. Changes in lung physiology of obese patients involve decreased pulmonary compliance secondary to increased blood volume and fatty infiltration of the lung (37). Inflammatory mediators, such as IL-6, have been shown to be increased in obesity and correlate with the severity of asthma (38). Furthermore, the link between obesity and asthma has been found to be greater in women. This is thought to be secondary to elevated estrogen levels linked to increased adipose tissue (39). The mechanism is still unclear, but may be related to estrogen-mediated effects on mast cells and eosinophils (40). A Cochrane review evaluated weight loss interventions on asthma severity. Four randomized controlled trials with a total of 197 adults were evaluated in this review. The study showed that there may be improvement in FEV1 and FEV1/FVC ratio in patients who were successful with weight loss, but because of the poor quality of studies no definitive conclusion could be made (41). In children, weight gain has also been linked to an increased risk of developing asthma. Infants with an increase in body mass index during the first 2 years of life have been shown to be at increased risk of asthma until age 6 (42).

Dietary intake can modify the severity of asthma in patients. One study showed through food questionnaires and spirometry that patients who consumed a low-fiber and high-fat diet were more likely to have severe persistent asthma and lower FEV1 (43). In addition, patients who consume a high-antioxidant diet (as measured by 5 servings of vegetables and 2 servings of fruits per day) have been shown to have better FEV1 than patients who consume less (44).

Respiratory Infections

Respiratory infections pose a great burden on the healthcare system. Pulmonary infections from *Streptococcus pneumoniae* are still a major source of morbidity and mortality in children of developing countries. The World Health Organization defines probiotic as "a live micro-organism which confers a health benefit to the host and are generally regarded as safe in humans" (45). Recent literature suggests probiotics may not only be helpful in intestinal flora, but also in respiratory pathogenesis. Probiotics have shown to change the micro flora in the nasopharynx and to help maintain the integrity of the epithelial layer in the nasopharynx. As a result, probiotics containing *Lactobacillus* and *Bifidobacterium* can be helpful even in the pediatric population in decreasing the infection rate of respiratory pathogens like *S. pneumoniae* (45).

NUTRIENTS, NUTRICEUTICALS, AND FUNCTIONAL FOODS

Phosphorus

Hypophosphatemia is known to impair diaphragmatic contractility and exacerbate CO_2 retention. Phosphorus depletion commonly occurs due to intracellular shifts following the correction of respiratory acidosis (2,46).

Impaired skeletal muscle function, attributable to loss of lean body mass, is associated with functional deterioration in COPD (17). Weight loss generally correlates with loss of respiratory muscle strength, which in turn is predictive of CO_2 retention. Nonetheless, patients not demonstrably underweight may be impaired due to losses of fat-free mass.

Monosodium Glutamate

The perception among asthma sufferers that the condition is exacerbated by food additives is widespread (see Chapter 15). A Cochrane review included two randomized controlled trials with a total of 24 subjects comparing monosodium glutamate challenge to placebo. There were no statistically significant differences between the monosodium glutamate and placebo groups when evaluating FEV1 fall of 15% or 200 mL (47).

Antioxidants

Inverse associations between dietary antioxidants and both asthma and COPD have been reported in epidemiological and observational studies. A case-control study noted inverse associations with zinc, magnesium, and manganese, as well as vitamin C (48). Theoretical support is strongest for vitamin C, which is found abundantly in pulmonary secretions (49); however, interventional studies have not shown significant clinical benefit (50–52). One recent randomized trial found that supplementation with vitamin C or magnesium over a period of 16 weeks, as compared to placebo, led to significant reduction in required corticosteroid dosage in adult asthmatics (53). In addition, a cross-sectional study including 452 Japanese children who were 3 to 6 years old evaluated the diet of asthmatic and nonasthmatic subjects. The study supported an inverse relationship between asthma and vitamins E and C intake. They found no relationship between asthma and fatty acid intake (54).

Magnesium

Magnesium relaxes bronchial and vascular smooth muscle through its calcium antagonist properties. It has been studied for the treatment of acute, reversible bronchoconstriction, and early studies have shown mixed results in mild to moderate asthma. Randomized controlled trials have demonstrated safety and efficacy of both intravenous (55) and nebulized (56) magnesium sulphate as adjuvant treatment of severe asthma exacerbations. One prospective study evaluated emergency room visits for acute asthma exacerbations in children and found that patients who received intravenous magnesium sulphate had fewer intubations (33% vs. 5% $p < 0.001$) (57).

n-3 Fatty Acids

There is considerable interest in the potential benefits of n-3 fatty acid supplementation on inflammatory conditions in general and pulmonary diseases in particular. n-3 fatty acids are found in abundance in mucosal tissue. They are thought to undergo enzymatic transformation into substances than assist in resolution of inflammation (58). Evidence in support of this interest is limited to date, and interventional trials thus far have yielded conflicting results (59). Several small randomized controlled trials have found beneficial effects such as acute reductions in (TNF-α) (60) and suppression of exercise-induced bronchoconstriction (61). Further research in this area is warranted.

Vitamin D

A positive association between serum vitamin D levels and pulmonary function indices, such as FEV1, has been observed (62). A recent cross-sectional study of children 6 to 18 years of age showed low levels of 25-hydroxy vitamin D was associated with increased odds of having asthma. In addition, levels of 25-hydroxy vitamin D correlated with FEV1 and FEV1/FVC ratio (63). Further prospective trials are needed in order to further elucidate the role vitamin D may play in treatment or prevention of respiratory diseases.

Other Nutrients

Indirect benefits of nutrients on lung function may derive from ergogenic effects (see Chapter 32), vascular effects (see Chapters 7 and 10), or influences on immune function (see Chapter 11).

Nutrigenomic Considerations

As discussed previously, there is an association between asthma and obesity. Questions of whether genetic variations play a role in this association have arisen. One study found various single-nucleotide polymorphisms (SNPs) for both obesity and asthma, but concluded that none of these associations were statistically significant (64). Further research is required to further elucidate the genetic possibility between asthma and obesity.

Gene variations involved in developing cachexia in COPD patients have been evaluated. Particularly, gene polymorphisms for interleukin-1beta (IL-1β), interleukin-6 (IL-6), TNF-α, and lymphotoxin-α have been researched for patients with COPD and cachexia. IL-6 polymorphisms are significantly different in patients with COPD cachexia compared with healthy controls further strengthening the potential role of genetics in developing malnutrition in COPD (65).

Diet/Drug Interactions

Montelukast, a leukotriene inhibitor, often used as a second or third line asthma therapy is metabolized by the cytochrome P450 CYP3A4 enzyme in the liver. A potential dietary interaction of this medication is a potent P450 CYP3A4 inhibitor, grapefruit juice. Therefore the metabolism of montelukast would be decreased if one were to consume a large amount of grapefruit juice.

Hypokalemia after use of inhaled albuterol has been seen on rare occasion. The hypokalemia can require treatment and even cause EKG changes with usual dosages of inhaled albuterol (66).

▌ CLINICAL HIGHLIGHTS

Inflammation is important in the pathogenesis of chronic airway diseases. The inflammatory process leads to oxidative cell injury, implicating oxidation in chronic airway disease as well. Therefore, a theoretical basis exists for optimizing intake of anti-inflammatory and antioxidant nutrients and possibly vitamin D. Although definitive evidence of benefit in airway disease has been reported for neither, both are supported by other lines of evidence and may be recommended on general principles (see Chapter 45). Minimally, a diet rich in fruits, vegetables, whole grains, and fish is advisable. Literature supports a link between obesity and asthma. A diet high in fiber and low in fat can be beneficial in improving FEV1 reading for asthmatic patients.

Supplementation with vitamin C 500 mg per day, vitamin E up to 200 IU per day, and fish oil or flaxseed oil (roughly 2 g per day of the former or 1 tablespoon per day of the latter) would appear to be reasonable components of an overall plan to ameliorate the course of chronic airway disease, despite the lack of conclusive outcome data. Vitamin C and E supplementation may also be an appropriate recommendation for asthmatic children. On general principles, a daily multivitamin/multimineral supplement is appropriate for all patients with chronic airway disease. A daily probiotic supplement may help to decrease respiratory infection and could be considered in patients with frequent infections.

Patients with more advanced airway disease are at risk of malnutrition and should be monitored closely for signs thereof. Nutritional consultation is indicated at the earliest emergence of such signs and, not unreasonably, even before. Increased energy expenditure and decreased intake may both contribute to catabolism, and the diet should be tailored to compensate. Relative restriction of carbohydrate may be indicated to limit CO_2 production in retainers, but conclusive evidence of benefit for this practice is lacking. More convincing is evidence of benefit of maintaining nutritional adequacy, with relatively high protein intake, in combination with a program of conditioning exercise.

REFERENCES

1. Collins PF, Stratton RJ, Elia M. Nutritional support in chronic obstructive pulmonary disease: a systematic review and meta-analysis. *Am J Clin Nutr* 2012;95:1385–1395.
2. Chin R Jr, Haponik EF. Nutrition, respiratory function, and disease. In: Shils ME, Olson JA, Shike M, eds. *Modern nutrition in health and disease*, 8th ed. Philadelphia, PA: Lea & Febiger, 1994.
3. Cano NJ, Roth H, Court-Ortune I, et al. Nutritional depletion in patients on long-term oxygen therapy and/or home mechanical ventilation. *Eur Respir J* 2002;20:30–37.
4. Cote CG. Surrogates of mortality in chronic obstructive pulmonary disease. *Am J Med* 2006;119:54–62.
5. Vermeeren MA, Schols AM, Wouters EF. Effects of an acute exacerbation on nutritional and metabolic profile of patients with COPD. *Eur Respir J* 1997;10:2264.
6. Morley JE, Thomas DR, Wilson MG. Cachexia: pathophysiology and clinical relevance. *Am J Clin Nutr* 2006;83:735–743.
7. Agusti A, Morla M, Sauleda J, et al. NF-kappa β activation and iNOS upregulation in skeletal muscle of patients with COPD and low body weight. *Thorax* 2004;59:483–487.
8. Donahoe MP. Nutrition in end-stage pulmonary disease. *Monaldi Arch Chest Dis* 1995;50:47.
9. Creutzberg EC, Wouters EFM, Mostert R, et al. Efficacy of nutritional supplementation therapy in depleted patients with chronic obstructive pulmonary disease. *Nutrition* 2003;19:120–127.
10. Wouters EFM. Management of severe COPD. *Lancet* 2004;9437:883–895.
11. Pezza M, Iermano C, Tufano R. Nutritional support for the patient with chronic obstructive pulmonary disease. *Monaldi Arch Chest Dis* 1994;49:33.
12. Goldstein-Shapses SA. Nutritional treatment in chronic respiratory failure: the effect of macronutrients on metabolism and ventilation. *Monaldi Arch Chest Dis* 1993; 48:535.
13. Silverman EK, Speizer FE. Risk factors for the development of chronic obstructive pulmonary disease. *Med Clin North Am* 1996;80:501.
14. Cai B, Zhu Y, Ma Y, et al. Effect of supplementing a high-fat, low-carbohydrate enteral formula in COPD patients. *Nutrition* 2003;19:229–232.
15. Dureuil B, Matuszczak Y. Alteration in nutritional status and diaphragm muscle function. *Reprod Nutr Dev* 1998;38:175.
16. Murciano D, Rigaud D, Pingleton S, et al. Diaphragmatic function in severely malnourished patients with anorexia nervosa: effects of renutrition. *Am J Respir Crit Care Med* 1994;150:1569–1574.
17. Schols AM. Nutrition and outcome in chronic respiratory disease. *Nutrition* 1997;13:161.
18. Yeh SS. DeGuzman B, Kramer T. Reversal of COPD-associated weight loss using the anabolic agent oxandrolone. *Chest* 2002;122:421–428.
19. Saudny-Unterberger H, Martin JG, Gray-Donald K. Impact of nutritional support on functional status during an acute exacerbation of chronic obstructive pulmonary disease. *Am J Respir Crit Care Med* 1997;156:794.
20. Obase Y, Mouri K, Shimizu H, et al. Nutritional deficits in elderly smokers with respiratory symptoms that do not fulfill the criteria for COPD. *Int J COPD* 2011;6:679–683.
21. Sridhar MK, Galloway A, Lean MEJ, et al. An out-patient nutritional supplementation programme in COPD patients. *Eur Respir J* 1994;7:720.
22. Ferreira IM, Brooks D, Lacasse Y, et al. Nutritional supplementation for stable chronic obstructive pulmonary disease. *Cochrane Database Syst Rev* 2005;2:CD000998.
23. Nathens AB, Neff MJ, Jurkovich GJ, et al. Randomized, prospective trial of antioxidant supplementation in critically ill surgical patients. *Ann Surg* 2002;236:814–822
24. McKeever TM, Britton J. Diet and asthma. *Am J Respir Crit Care Med.* 2004;170:725–729
25. Troisi RJ, Willett WC, Weiss ST, et al. A prospective study of diet and adult-onset asthma. *Am J Respir Crit Care Med* 1995;151:1401.
26. Burney P. The origins of obstructive airways disease. A role for diet? *Am J Respir Crit Care Med* 1995;151:1292.
27. Devereux G, Seaton A. Diet as a risk factor for atopy and asthma. *J Allergy Clin Immunol* 2005;115:1109–1117.
28. Oddy WH. A review of the effects of breastfeeding on respiratory infections, atopy, and childhood asthma. *J Asthma* 2004;41:605–621.
29. Litonjua AA, Rifas-Shiman SL, Ly NP, et al. Maternal antioxidant intake in pregnancy and wheezing illnesses in children at 2 years of age. *Am J Clin Nutr* 2006;84:903–911.
30. Coppoolse R, Barstow TJ, Stringer WW, et al. Effect of acute bicarbonate administration on exercise responses of COPD patients. *Med Sci Sports Exerc* 1997;29:725.
31. Woods RK, Weiner JM, Abramson M, et al. Do dairy products induce bronchoconstriction in adults with asthma? *J Allergy Clin Immunol* 1998;101:45.
32. Wüthrich B, Schmid A, Walther B, et al. Milk consumption does not lead to mucus production or occurrence of asthma. *J Am Coll Nutr* 2005;24(6 suppl):547S–555S.
33. Davis PA, Gold EB, Hackman RM, et al. The use of complementary/alternative medicine for the treatment of asthma in the United States. *J Investig Allergol Clin Immunol* 1998;8:73.
34. Hassed C. An integrative approach to asthma. *Aust Fam Physician* 2005;34:573–576.
35. Blanc PD, Trupin I, Earnest G, et al. Alternative therapies among adults with a reported diagnosis of asthma or rhinosinusitis: data from a population based survey. *Chest* 2001;120:1461–1467.
36. Shenfield G, Lim E, Allen H. Survey of the use of complementary medicines and therapies in children with asthma. *J Paediatr Child Health* 2002;38:252–257.
37. Delgado J, Barranco P, Quirce S. Obesity and asthma. *J Investig Allergol Clin Immunol* 2008;18(6):420–425.
38. Shore SA. Obesity and asthma: cause for concern. *Curr Opin Pharmacol* 2006;6(3):230–236.
39. Camargo CA Jr, Weiss ST, Zhang S, et al. Prospective study of body mass index, weight change, and risk

of adult-onset asthma in women. *Arch Intern Med* 1999; 159(21):2582–2588.

40. Farah CS, Salome CM. Asthma and obesity: a known association but unknown mechanism. *Respirology* 2012;17(3): 412–421.

41. Adeniyi FB, Young T. Weight loss interventions for chronic asthma. *Cochrane Database Syst Rev* 2012;7:CD009339.

42. Rzehak P, Wijga AH, Keil T, et al. Birth cohorts. Body mass index trajectory classes and incident asthma in childhood: results from 8 European birth cohorts—a Global Allergy and Asthma European Network initiative. *J Allergy Clin Immunol* 2013;131(6):1528–1536.

43. Berthon BS, Macdonald-Wicks LK, Gibson PG, et al. An investigation of the association between dietary intake, disease severity and airway inflammation in asthma. *Respirology* 2013;18(3):447–454. doi:10.1111/resp.12015.

44. Wood LG, Garg ML, Smart JM, et al. Manipulating antioxidant intake in asthma: a randomized controlled trial. *Am J Clin Nutr* 2012;96(3):534–543. doi:10.3945/ajcn.111.032623.

45. Licciardi PV, Toh ZQ, Dunne E, et al. Protecting against pneumococcal disease: critical interactions between probiotics and the airway microbiome. *PLoS Pathog.* 2012;8(6):e1002652. doi:10.1371/journal.ppat.1002652.

46. Fiaccadori E, Coffrini E, Fracchia C, et al. Hypophosphatemia and phosphorus depletion in respiratory and peripheral muscles of patients with respiratory failure due to COPD. *Chest* 1994;105:1392–1398.

47. Zhou Y, Yang M, Dong BR. Monosodium glutamate avoidance for chronic asthma in adults and children. *Cochrane Database Syst Rev* 2012;6:CD004357.

48. Soutar A, Seaton A, Brown K. Bronchial reactivity and dietary antioxidants. *Thorax* 1997;52:166.

49. Hatch GE. Asthma, inhaled oxidants, and dietary antioxidants. *Am J Clin Nutr* 1995;61:625s.

50. Fogarty A, Lewis SA, Scrivener SL, et al. Oral magnesium and vitamin C supplements in asthma: a parallel group randomized placebo-controlled trial. *Clin Exp Allergy* 2003;33:1355–1359.

51. Ram FS, Rowe BH, Kaur B. Vitamin C supplementation for asthma. *Cochrane Database Syst Rev* 2004;3:CD000993.

52. Kaur B, Rowe BH, Arnold E. Vitamin C supplementation for asthma. *Cochrane Database Syst Rev* 2009;(1):CD000993.

53. Fogarty A, Lewis SA, Scrivener SL, et al. Corticosteroid sparing effects of vitamin C and magnesium in asthma: a randomized trial. *Respir Med* 2006;100:174–179.

54. Nakamura K, Wada K, Sahashi Y, et al. Associations of intake of antioxidant vitamins and fatty acids with asthma in preschool children. *Public Health Nutr* 2013;16(11):2040–2045. Available at CJO. doi:10.1017/S1368980012004363

55. Silverman RA, Osborn H, Runge J, et al. IV magnesium sulfate in the treatment of acute severe asthma: a multicenter, randomized controlled trial. *Chest* 2002;122:1870.

56. Hughes R, Goldkorn A, Masoli M, et al. Use of isotonic nebulised magnesium sulphate as an adjuvant to salbutamol in treatment of severe asthma in adults: randomized placebo-controlled trial. *Lancet* 2003;361:2114–2117.

57. Torres S, Sticco N, Bosch JJ, et al. Effectiveness of magnesium sulfate as initial treatment of acute severe asthma in children, conducted in a tertiary-level university hospital: a randomized, controlled trial. *Arch Argent Pediatr* 2012;110(4):291–296.

58. Levy BD, Vachier I, Serhan CN. Resolution of inflammation in asthma. *Clin Chest Med* 2012;33(3):559–570.

59. Woods RK, Thien FC, Abramson MJ. Dietary marine fatty acids (fish oil) for asthma in adults and children. *Cochrane Database Syst Rev* 2002;3:CD001283.

60. Hodge L, Salome CM, Hughes JM, et al. Effect of dietary intake of omega-3 and omega-6 fatty acids on severity of asthma in children. *Eur Respir J* 1998;11:361.

61. Mickleborough TD, Murray RL, Ionesu AA, et al. Fish oil supplementation reduces severity of exercise-induced bronchoconstriction in elite athletes. *Am J Respir Crit Care Med* 2003;168:1181–1189.

62. Black PN, Scragg R. Relationship between serum 25-hydroxyvitamin D and pulmonary function in the third National Health and Nutrition Examination Survey. *Chest* 2005;128:3792–3798.

63. Alyasin S, Momen T, Kashef S, et al. The relationship between serum 25 hydroxy vitamin D levels and asthma in children. *Allergy Asthma Immunol Res* 2011;3(4):251–255.

64. Melén E, Himes BE, Brehm JM, et al. Analyses of shared genetic factors between asthma and obesity in children. *J Allergy Clin Immunol* 2010;126(3):631–637.

65. Broekhuizen R, Grimble RF, Howell WM, et al. Pulmonary cachexia, systemic inflammatory profile, and the interleukin 1b -511 single nucleotide polymorphism. *Am J Clin Nutr* 2005;82(5):1059–1064.

66. Udezue E, D'Souza L, Mahajan M. Hypokalemia after normal doses of neubulized albuterol (salbutamol). *Am J Emerg Med* 1995;13(2):168–171.

SUGGESTED READING

Andrews L, Lokuge S, Sawyer M, et al. The use of alternative therapies by children with asthma: a brief report. *J Paediatr Child Health* 1998;34:131.

Feldman EB. Nutrition and diet in the management of hyperlipidemia and atherosclerosis. In: Shils ME, Olson JA, Shike M, eds. *Modern nutrition in health and disease*, 8th ed. Philadelphia, PA: Lea & Febiger, 1994.

Hill J, Micklewright A, Lewis S, et al. Investigation of the effect of short-term change in dietary magnesium intake in asthma. *Eur Respir J* 1997;10:2225.

Margen S, ed. *The wellness nutrition counter*. New York, NY: Rebus, 1997.

McKeever TM, Lewis SA, Smit H, et al. Serum nutrient markers and skin prick testing using data from the third National Health and Nutrition Examination Survey. *J Allergy Clin Immunol* 2004;114:1398–1402.

McNamar DJ. Cardiovascular disease. In: Shils ME, Olson JA, Shike M, eds. *Modern nutrition in health and disease*, 8th ed. Philadelphia, PA: Lea & Febiger, 1994.

Vincent D. Relationship of dietary fish intake to level of pulmonary function. *Eur J Respir* 1995;8:507.

Weiss ST. Diet as a risk factor for asthma. In: Chadwick DJ, Cardew G, eds. *The rising trends in asthma. Ciba Foundation Symposium 206.* Chichester, UK: Wiley, 1997:244.

Wong KW. Clinical efficacy of n-3 fatty acid supplementation in patients with asthma. *J Am Diet Assoc* 2005;105:98–105.

CHAPTER 16

Diet and Renal Disease

T he development of chronic kidney disease (CKD) often occurs in the context of other chronic conditions, such as hypertension, diabetes, or atherosclerosis, for which dietary management is both essential and of proved benefit. Thus, there is a clear, albeit indirect, role for diet in the prevention of CKD. With the advent of CKD of varying severity, diet is of fundamental importance, both in efforts to delay progression of renal insufficiency and to maintain lean body mass. Despite an extensive literature on the role of dietary protein in the development and progression of renal disease, clear support for a single management strategy is lacking. However, evidence that a range of dietary interventions may contribute to the preservation of renal function at varying levels of compromise is increasingly abundant and compelling. The clinician managing patients with, or at risk for, CKD is obligated to attend to nutrition as well as pharmacotherapy.

Approximately 12% of Americans form renal calculi at some time during their lives. The incidence of stone formation in the urinary tract, and particularly in the upper urinary tract, has been rising over recent decades in Westernized countries. The epidemiology of renal calculi is strongly suggestive of an important role for diet. Most stones contain calcium, and evidence of a link between diet and calcium oxalate stones is convincing.

OVERVIEW

Diet

The two leading causes of renal insufficiency in the United States are diabetes mellitus and hypertension (1–4). There is decisive evidence that diet influences the course of diabetes (see Chapter 6) and accruing evidence that diet may enhance, and at times substitute for, pharmacotherapy in the management of hypertension (see Chapter 8). Both diabetes and hypertension may be preventable with appropriate dietary interventions (see Chapters 6 and 8). Blood pressure reduction appears to retard the progression of CKD in a dose-responsive manner (i.e., the lower the blood pressure, the slower disease progression) (5). However, aggressive blood pressure reduction increases risk for side effects of therapy, and is primarily supported by subgroup and secondary analyses of clinical trials (6). A reasonable target may be <130/80 mm Hg in diabetic CKD and <140/90 mm Hg in nondiabetic CKD without albuminuria (6). Atherosclerosis contributes to the development of renal dysfunction and may be retarded or prevented by dietary management (see Chapter 7). Renal failure is a potential consequence of systemic atherosclerosis and of low cardiac output and thus may often compound the challenges of nutritional therapy in congestive heart failure (7). Dietary intervention to mitigate cardiovascular risk is often warranted in patients with CKD due to the common origins of the two conditions and the tendency of each to propagate the other (8) (see Chapters 7 and 8).

The prevention of risk factors for renal disease may prevent CKD, although evidence for this specific effect is not conclusive. In the absence of evidence, intuition would suggest that if the course and natural history of the leading causes of CKD are substantially modifiable by dietary means (see Chapters 6 and 8), then so, too, is the development of CKD. Consequently, the primary care practitioner may play a role in the prevention of CKD by optimal dietary management of the principal risk factors.

Evidence for the direct influence of diet, particularly dietary protein, on renal function is less clear. With advanced CKD, dietary protein restriction is common practice (9) and generally slows progressive deterioration of renal function (10–13). However, protein restriction may contribute to nutritional deficiencies, with net adverse effects (13,14). CKD in childhood in particular is associated with impairment of growth

TABLE 16.1

Stages of CKD

Stage	GFR (ml/min/1.73 m^2)	Implications
1	≥90	Kidney damage with normal or increased GFR
2	60–89	Kidney damage with mild decrease in GFR
3	30–59	Moderate decrease in GFR
		Moderate protein restriction in nondialyzed patients
		Phosphorus restriction
4	15–29	Severe decrease in GFR
		Moderate protein restriction in nondialyzed patients
		Phosphorus restriction
5	15 (or dialysis)	Kidney failure
		Moderate protein restriction in nondialyzed patients
		Increased protein requirements in dialyzed patients
		Phosphorus restriction

CKD is defined as either kidney damage or GFR <60 mL/min/1.73 m^2 for ≥3 months.

Source: Adapted from K/DOQI Clinical Practice Guidelines For Chronic Kidney Disease: Evaluation, Classification and Stratification.

that can adversely affect quality of life and bone metabolism (15,16). A limited number of studies to date have not found a significant impact of protein restriction on delaying progression to end-stage disease in children (17). Minimum protein intake equivalent to the DRI for ideal body weight has therefore been recommended in pediatric CKD to prevent uremia and reduce dietary phosphorus intake (18). Reconciling the priorities of nutrition for renal protection and for ensuring adequate overall nutritional status is a challenge best met through the application of general principles modified to suit each individual (19–21). Whereas protein restriction is a mainstay in the dietary management of renal disease, declining protein intake as glomerular filtration rate (GFR) declines may independently predict incipient malnutrition (22). The importance of optimizing nutritional status to facilitate wound healing and recovery following renal transplant has received increasing attention as the number of annual transplants has risen (23).

Overall, the evidence supporting protein restriction in established CKD to slow disease progression is convincing (11,24). Evidence for the value of protein restriction in the primary prevention of renal insufficiency and the age-related decline in GFR is inconclusive (25,26). There is evidence that restriction of phosphorus is beneficial in CKD, particularly in the prevention of secondary hyperparathyroidism (24,27,28).

Malnutrition of multifactorial origin often develops in patients with advanced CKD (29–31), and the primary care provider should play a role in ensuring nutritional adequacy. Just as CKD may contribute to malnutrition, malnutrition, particularly protein deficiency, tends to lower GFR and impair the concentrating ability of the kidney. These effects are reversible in healthy individuals with the restitution of adequate protein intake. Creative dietary strategies to maximize dietary choices within the context of a protein-restricted diet may enhance compliance and nutritional status (32).

The complexity of dietary management in advanced renal disease generally requires the input of the primary care provider, a specialized dietitian, and a nephrologist (33). Nutritional management in the setting of acute renal failure may influence prognosis; a potential benefit of essential amino acid supplementation is suggested in particular (34,35). The diet plan in such a setting should result from a collaborative effort involving, minimally, the nephrologist and specialized dietitian.

Once symptomatic or clinically overt CKD has developed, the generalist almost invariably will, and should, be guided by a nephrologist in tailoring both dietary therapy and pharmacotherapy. Such patients are obviously at risk of azotemia (i.e., the accumulation of nitrogenous waste) as well as specific micronutrient abnormalities, including phosphorus retention; impaired absorption of calcium and iron; and deficiencies of thiamin, riboflavin, vitamin B_6, folate, vitamin C, and active vitamin D (37).

The benefits of protein restriction have been convincingly demonstrated for nondialyzed patients with stages 3 to 5 CKD. The standard diet for such patients restricts total protein to approximately 0.6 to 0.8 g/kg/day, with not less than half being of high biologic value (i.e., rich in essential amino acids; see Chapters 3 and 4). For patients with severe CKD (i.e., GFR below 25), commercial supplements of amino acids, keto acids, and hydroxy acids may be indicated. Patients in this group apparently benefit from protein restriction down to 0.3 g/kg/day. The putative benefit of keto or hydroxy acid supplements is that the amino group, which contributes to the body's nitrogen load, is eliminated. Keto and hydroxy acids can be converted into their respective amino acids endogenously. Although such diets help preserve renal function, they are unpalatable, which makes compliance difficult and increases the risk of nutritional deficiencies (38,39). Whether a delay in the need for dialysis is sufficient cause to implement such dietary therapy will depend on an individual patient's preference.

Although a variety of endocrine abnormalities are associated with renal insufficiency and uremia, most are beyond the scope of this discussion. Most relevant to dietary management is the development of both insulin resistance and elevations of glucagon, which contribute to impaired glucose metabolism. The dietary approach to impaired glucose metabolism and insulin resistance is discussed in Chapter 6. The basic approaches are unchanged in the setting of renal failure, although medication doses may need adjustment.

Most patients with end-stage renal disease experience some catabolism while on dialysis. Malnutrition, or at least the risk of it, is considered common in this population. Wasting is due both to increased metabolic demand, perhaps due to dialysis, and poor intake due to malaise, anorexia, and the unpalatability of a therapeutic diet. Poor nutritional status in dialysis patients appears, not surprisingly, to be a poor prognostic sign. In a study of 93 subjects, Young et al. (40) found significant elevations in serum leptin levels in malnourished patients with renal failure, suggesting a role for leptin in the malnutrition seen in CKD. Serum albumin, previously viewed as a reliable marker of protein nutriture, is now recognized as a better indicator of inflammation and disease prognosis than malnutrition (41).

Patients with CKD, particularly stages 3 to 5, generally require a diet restricted in protein, sodium, and phosphorus and supplemented with water-soluble vitamins. Patients undergoing hemodialysis or peritoneal dialysis generally require increased protein intakes to replace losses. The fat intake of uremic patients should be similar to that of nonuremic patients and modified as required to manage comorbid conditions. Carbohydrate intake should represent the majority of calories in these as in other patient groups, with a preponderance of complex carbohydrates rich in fiber.

Nephrolithiasis

The incidence of nephrolithiasis has been increasing sharply over recent decades in affluent populations, and the risk correlates strongly with per capita expenditure on food. Consumption of animal products in particular seems to confer increased susceptibility (42,43). Observational studies reveal a strong protective effect of vegetarianism, despite a high intake of oxalate in vegetables (43). In an analysis of the Health Professionals Follow-up Study and the Nurses' Health Study I and II, dietary patterns consistent with the Dietary Approaches to Stop Hypertension (DASH), as measured by diet scores, were protective. The relative risks of stone formation in the highest compared with the lowest quintile of DASH diet scores were 0.55 for men and 0.58 to 0.60 for older and younger women, respectively (44). Dietary protein, generally of animal origin, has a calciuric effect that correlates well with risk of stone formation, although susceptibility to this effect of protein appears to be highly individualized. High dietary protein intake has an acidifying effect, which diminishes urinary citrate excretion; proximal tubular reuptake of citrate is enhanced by acidosis. In the urine, citrate chelates calcium, inhibiting crystallization. The oncotic properties of protein may result in increased GFR, which in turn increases the filtered load of calcium. Protein also increases urinary urate, which is a risk factor for both calcium and uric acid stones (45). Thus, protein intake is presumed to raise the risk of nephrolithiasis by a variety of mechanisms (46). Observational data suggest the relative risk of stone formation associated with high protein intake to be about 1.3 (45). However, negative results of a randomized trial of protein restriction may indicate that increased fluid intake is of greater importance in the prevention of recurrent stones (47). This finding is supported by a recent meta-analysis showing a benefit for increased fluid intake, as well as reduced soft drink intake in men with high consumption of phosphoric acid–containing beverages at baseline (48).

Mechanisms have been identified by which both dietary fiber and magnesium might protect against stone formation. Insoluble fiber binds calcium in the gastrointestinal tract, potentially reducing urinary calcium. Of greater importance is a positive association between total fiber intake and urinary citrate (49). Magnesium in the urine inhibits the precipitation of calcium oxalate crystals (43). Evidence of clinical benefit specific to fiber or magnesium, except in individuals with demonstrated low magnesium levels, is lacking at present. Data from the Nurses' Health Study suggest a protective effect of dietary phytate intake, as well as benefit from dietary calcium but not calcium supplements (50). Randomized intervention trials for stone recurrence that included dietary fiber have shown mixed results, with no trials testing the independent effect of increasing fiber intake (48). However, meta-analysis of these trials suggested a possible benefit from adequate calcium intake, consistent with earlier epidemiological evidence (48).

Whereas an increase in total fluid intake appears to be protective, the effects of different fluids may be variable (51,52). Beverages containing caffeine and alcohol may lower risk in particular, as both of these substances oppose antidiuretic hormone (ADH) and result in dilute urine (51). Available data have suggested a positive association between soda intake and stones (52). Solute in urine is diluted as urine volume rises, and hydration is protective against stone formation. Ingestion of not less than 2 L of fluid daily, leading to a urine volume not below 2.5 L per day, is protective (48).

Definitive data to support a benefit of dietary modification from controlled trials are lacking to date, and pharmacotherapy is not much better substantiated. Patients with nephrolithiasis; a high dietary intake of protein, oxalate, and/or salt; and less-than-optimal fluid intake are likely to benefit from dietary therapy. Consuming adequate dietary calcium may be particularly useful

to reduce intestinal oxalate absorption in calcium oxalate stone formers (53). Therapeutic goals should include restriction of dietary protein intake to not more than 1 g/kg/day and of sodium to not more than 100 mEq per day; avoidance of foods rich in oxalate; and consumption of not less than 2.5 L per day of fluid (43,48,54).

NUTRIENTS, NUTRICEUTICALS, AND FUNCTIONAL FOODS

Water

In general, thirst is a reliable indicator of appropriate fluid intake. Adequate intake of water is important in the preservation of renal function over time and in the avoidance of nephrolithiasis. An intake of water equal to urine output plus 500 mL is an appropriate guideline as GFR decreases and thirst becomes a less reliable index.

Protein

Studies in humans indicate that protein restriction slows the progression of renal failure once insufficiency has developed (55); efficacy of this approach is limited primarily by poor adherence to what can be an unpalatable dietary pattern (56,57). The ingestion of protein increases renal blood flow and GFR, perhaps through the influence of glucagon. Consequently, the restriction of protein intake reduces glomerular flow and pressures. Protein restriction slows the accumulation of urea, creatinine, and other guanidine compounds in CKD. Studies have examined the benefits of low-protein, low-phosphorus diets with protein intake of approximately 0.6 to 0.8 g/kg/day, as well as very-low-protein diets with protein intake of approximately 0.3 g/kg/day. The very-low-protein diets are supplemented with essential amino acids or keto acids. Essential amino acids can be manufactured in the body from their keto or hydroxy acid analogues, in which the amino group is replaced. The removal of the amino group results in a smaller nitrogen load to the patient. There is preliminary evidence to date that such diets confer greater benefits than standard protein-restricted diets in nondialyzed patients. The addition of keto acids to the diet may allow for the preservation of adequate nutriture with a lower intake of protein than could otherwise be achieved and beneficial effects on renal function

(58–61). Such a diet has been shown to reduce blood pressure as well (61,62), offering another mechanism by which renal function may be preserved. Effective protein restriction appears to reduce the dose of exogenous erythropoietin required to achieve a given target hemoglobin value, apparently by ameliorating secondary hyperparathyroidism (63).

There is less convincing evidence that protein restriction can prevent the onset of CKD in healthy individuals. The average protein intake in the United States exceeds recommendations and may contribute to the age-related decline in GFR. In a review of paleolithic nutrition, Eaton et al. (64) suggest that our ancestors adapted to high protein intake and that such a diet is unlikely to be harmful in the context of healthy activity levels and overall dietary pattern. However, extrapolation from the prehistoric diet may or may not be appropriate in this instance, given a markedly shorter life expectancy until, in evolutionary context, quite recently.

In general, it is difficult to demonstrate the efficacy of preventive measures when disease is not common, does not develop rapidly, or lacks good surrogate markers. Perhaps for these reasons, or perhaps because healthy kidneys do not benefit from protein restriction, the benefits of protein restriction have only been convincingly demonstrated for a GFR below 70 mL/1.73 m^2/min.

Dietary Fat

Atherosclerosis affects the renal arteries and is associated with CKD. The contribution of diabetes and hypertension to atherosclerotic disease of the renal vasculature is one means by which these conditions lead to renal failure. Consequently, dietary interventions to prevent or reverse atherosclerosis may be valuable in preventing or reversing renovascular disease (see Chapter 7). A high intake of dietary fat and cholesterol may contribute to high glomerular pressures. Filtration is impaired by the deposition of foam cells in the glomerular endothelium. Optimal dietary fat intake in the prevention of renal disease is the same as for the prevention of other atherosclerotic conditions. There is evidence that while total, saturated, and trans fat intake should be restricted, intake of polyunsaturated fat, especially n-3 fatty acids, should be liberalized (65,66). Through their effects on eicosanoid and prostaglandin metabolism, polyunsaturated fats may indirectly improve glomerular pressures and function.

Phosphorus

Phosphorus restriction, independent of protein restriction, appears to retard the progression of CKD (27,28,67). Evidence for the isolated effects of phosphorus restriction in humans is limited, however, as diets low in phosphorus tend to be low in protein and vice versa. Calcification of soft tissue is related to the double product (serum levels of phosphorus and calcium, multiplied), and the deposition of calcium in renal tissue is reduced by low phosphorus intake. Serum creatinine rises as the content of calcium in renal tissue rises.

Phosphorus intake should be restricted to 800 to 1,000 mg per day in patients with stages 3 to 5 CKD. Current guidelines recommend restricting dietary phosphorus when hyperphosphatemia develops; however, earlier restriction could help prevent secondary hyperparathyroidism (68). Particular attention should be given to reducing fast food intake. Only a small proportion of all menu items are free of phosphorus-containing additives, according to one study of 15 fast-food chains (69). Fast food intake in patients receiving hemodialysis is associated with higher serum phosphorus levels and greater sodium intakes and interdialytic weight gain (70). As renal function declines, phosphate binders may be necessary to control serum levels. In patients with severe CKD, aluminum toxicity may result from the use of aluminum-containing phosphate binders; this problem can be avoided by using calcium-based binders or newer non-calcium binders, such as lanthanum carbonate or sevelamer. The advantages of phosphorus restriction must be weighed against the risks of malnutrition resulting from an unpalatable diet.

A generous intake of dietary phosphate may inhibit the formation of calcium stones by reducing calcium levels in urine (46); however, data from controlled trials are lacking. Further, dietary sources of phosphate and protein tend to correspond, making dietary phosphate supplementation an impractical recommendation for prevention of nephrolithiasis, given the prevailing view that dietary protein should be restricted.

Calcium

The restriction of protein and phosphorus in CKD often requires avoidance of dairy foods, lowering calcium intake, often down to 300 to 400 mg per day. Calcium absorption generally is impaired due to low levels of active vitamin D. Therefore, nondairy calcium sources and supplemental calcium often are necessary to raise the intake of patients with stage 3 to 5 CKD to the recommended 1,500 to 2,000 mg per day, without exceeding the recommended limit of 2,000 mg per day (71). Patients with CKD are at risk of renal osteodystrophy; chronic ingestion of calcium carbonate may serve to provide needed calcium for skeletal metabolism while compensating for metabolic acidosis. Supplementation of calcium should be deferred if phosphorus levels are elevated, as the double product of calcium and phosphorus correlates with the rate of soft tissue calcification and stone formation. Active vitamin D supplementation is generally indicated as well.

Given that most renal calculi are composed partly or predominantly of calcium, restriction of calcium intake as a means to prevent recurrence has been advocated as an intuitively reasonable precaution. Most of the available evidence now suggests, however, that restriction of dietary calcium results in negative calcium balance, while reducing urinary calcium only slightly and conferring no appreciable protection against stone formation. Calcium in the gastrointestinal tract may complex with oxalate, reducing oxalate absorption and thereby oxalate in the urine. Thus, restriction of dietary calcium may "paradoxically" increase the risk of calcium stone formation and thus is to be discouraged (43). Evidence to date suggests that a high intake of dietary calcium from food sources may protect against stone formation, but this association may not pertain to calcium derived from supplements (45,50).

Oxalate

The precipitation of calcium oxalate from urine is much more sensitive to oxalate than to calcium. Although oxalate levels are influenced by dietary intake, the preponderance of urinary oxalate is derived from metabolism. The metabolism of several amino acids contributes to oxalate levels in blood and urine; therefore, oxaluria correlates

directly with protein intake. Ascorbate can be converted to oxalate. Although this generally contributes minimally to oxalate levels, ingestion of megadoses of vitamin C can lead to hyperoxaluria in susceptible individuals (43). Pyridoxine serves as a cofactor in glycine metabolism, and its deficiency leads to excess oxalate production. Patients with a tendency to produce calcium oxalate stones may benefit from restriction of dietary oxalate and adequate intake of calcium-rich foods in the context of other generally advisable dietary modifications. Among foods known to raise urinary oxalate concentrations are chocolate, rhubarb, beets, wheat bran, nuts, seeds, soy, tea, strawberries, and dark leafy green vegetables (72,72a). Limited data on the bioavailability of oxalate from various dietary sources complicate assessment of the role of dietary oxalate on the risk of nephrolithiasis (45).

Ascorbate

The metabolic conversion of ascorbate to oxalate suggests that high levels of vitamin C intake might increase the risk of stone formation. Urinary oxalate has been shown to increase with high ascorbate intake, but the effects on actual stone formation have not been confirmed. Thus, the risk of nephrolithiasis with an intake of vitamin C above 1.5 g per day may be increased, and this should be considered by those favoring megadosing of this nutrient (73). No change in the risk of nephrolithiasis attributable to vitamin C was seen in the Health Professionals Follow-up Study (74).

Pyridoxine

Vitamin B_6 is a cofactor in the metabolism of glyoxalic acid. High levels of B_6 intake reduce the production of oxalate by shifting the pathway toward the production of glycine. Pyridoxine has been used to treat oxalate stones with anecdotal success. A dose of 100 mg per day has been recommended, increasing up to 300 mg per day if the dose is inadequate, although further study is indicated (75,76). Variation in pyridoxine intake emerged as a predictor of risk of nephrolithiasis in the Nurses' Health Study (RR, 0.66) (77), but not in the Health Professionals Follow-up Study (54,74).

Uric Acid

Uric acid excretion in urine rises with the intake of dietary protein. The solubility of urate is reduced in an acid environment, and ingestion of amino acids acidifies the urine. Thus, purine ingestion both increases urinary urate and reduces its solubility. Hyperuricosuria contributes to the development of calcium oxalate stones by saturating urine and reducing the threshold for solute precipitation. Thus, relative protein restriction may protect against urate and calcium oxalate stone formation by reducing urinary urate.

Magnesium

Magnesium tends to accumulate in renal failure, and intake should generally not exceed 200 mg per day. The restriction of protein and phosphorus generally serves to restrict magnesium intake as well so that it need not be selectively targeted.

Sodium

Sodium filtration and reabsorption are both reduced with CKD; therefore, restriction of sodium intake below levels recommended for the general population in early CKD generally is not necessary. As CKD becomes more severe, sodium restriction to between 1,000 and 2,400 mg per day is appropriate. The role of sodium restriction in the primary prevention of renal disease is unclear, although sodium restriction may play a role in the control of blood pressure (see Chapter 8).

Dietary sodium is related to urinary sodium levels, and calcium excretion in urine tends to parallel that of sodium. High salt intake is associated with calciuria and an increased risk for stone formation (43,78). Stone formation may result in part from enhanced susceptibility to a calciuric effect of dietary sodium (45).

Potassium

Tubular secretion of potassium tends to rise as GFR falls, preserving the ability to excrete potassium in the urine. In stages 3 to 5 of CKD, potassium accumulation becomes a threat. In such patients, the restriction of potassium intake to less than 2.4 g per day is recommended.

Potassium intake appears to be protective against stone formation. Foods rich in potassium, specifically fruits and vegetables, tend to be alkaline and naturally low in sodium. Alkalinity increases urinary citrate, reducing the risk of stone formation. The degree to which potassium provides specific protection versus the degree to which it is simply a marker of a low-protein, low-sodium diet is uncertain (45).

Iron

Iron deficiency is relatively common in chronic CKD and is generally multifactorial. Iron supplementation is appropriate. A multivitamin designed for use in CKD is often adequate. In some patients undergoing hemodialysis, intravenous iron may be required in the setting of elevated hepcidin levels that impair intestinal absorption (79). Provision of adequate iron is necessary for exogenous erythropoietin to be effective.

Zinc

There is increasing evidence of widespread zinc deficiency in the US population. In CKD, zinc absorption may be impaired and zinc may be leached into the dialysate (80). Thus, deficiency is likely to be more significant. Zinc supplementation in CKD is appropriate. A multivitamin designed for use in CKD that contains zinc is generally adequate.

Aluminum

Patients with CKD are at risk of aluminum toxicity if aluminum-based products are used to bind phosphate. Calcium-based phosphate binders are recommended for this reason.

Vitamin D

CKD is associated with decreased activation of 25-hydroxycholecalciferol to 1,25-dihydroxycholecalciferol in the kidney. Vitamin D supplementation is generally indicated; a preparation that does not depend on activation by renal hydroxylation is essential. These preparations include 1,25-dihydroxyvitamin D3 (calcitriol) and its analogs.

Water-Soluble Vitamins

Dietary restrictions and anorexia place patients with chronic CKD at risk for deficiencies of

B vitamins, folate, and vitamin C. Ascorbate can be metabolized to oxalate, and this conversion is accelerated by CKD. Therefore, excessive ascorbate ingestion in renal failure can lead to stone formation; an intake of 60 mg per day should generally not be exceeded. A multivitamin providing the recommended dietary allowance/adequate intake (RDA/AI) of other water-soluble vitamins is appropriate.

Carnitine

Carnitine is a nitrogenous compound abundant in meat and dairy products. Carnitine serves as a cofactor in the mitochondrial oxidation of long-chain fatty acids and buffers the pool of coenzyme A by accepting an acyl group in transfer. Carnitine requirements are met by carnitine ingestion and by carnitine biosynthesis, which occurs in the liver and kidneys. CKD may lead to carnitine deficiency by several mechanisms, including reductions in both intake and manufacture. Hypertriglyceridemia is common in renal failure and may be due in part to impairments in fatty acid oxidation resulting from carnitine deficiency. There is suggestive evidence that carnitine supplementation may be effective in the treatment of hypertriglyceridemia associated with CKD. To date, reliable data characterizing carnitine balance in uremic and dialysis patients are lacking. Carnitine has been used in attempts to lower triglycerides; ameliorate muscle cramps and other symptoms associated with dialysis; improve exercise tolerance; enhance responsiveness to erythropoietin; and improve cardiac function. The current evidence is inconclusive for any of the outcomes. Doses and routes of administration have varied in studies; IV administration of 20 mg per kg following dialysis is typically used (81,81a). Use of carnitine should be considered experimental until additional evidence becomes available.

Fiber

Dietary fiber confers comparable benefits in renal failure patients as in other patients (see Chapter 1). In addition, insoluble fiber may lower serum nitrogen by enhancing fecal nitrogen excretion. High-fiber foods often contain protein of low biologic value, as well as potassium and phosphorus, which may be poorly tolerated by patients with advanced CKD.

Sucrose

Sucrose and other simple sugars in the diet impede tubular reabsorption of calcium and thereby increase calciuria. Although this provides a mechanism for a contribution of dietary sugar to stone formation, this association has not been demonstrated in studies controlling for other aspects of diet (45).

L-Arginine

There is animal evidence that dietary supplementation with L-arginine prevents age-related decline in renal function and protects against acute renal injury (82,83). The mechanism for this effect is unclear and may be independent of nitric oxide (82). Implications for humans are as yet uncertain.

TOPICS OF SPECIAL INTEREST

Nephrotic Syndrome

Evidence suggests that the combination of dietary protein restriction and angiotensin-converting enzyme inhibitor or angiotensin receptor blocker therapy reduces protein loss in urine without contributing to declines in serum albumin levels. Evidence for protein restriction or supplementation in nephrotic syndrome is inconclusive, and modification of protein intake is not routinely recommended (84). Moderate sodium restriction may help to manage edema (84). Nephrotic patients generally require vitamin and mineral supplementation, as they are subject to vitamin D and trace element deficiencies. Hypoalbuminemia results from albumin losses in urine in the nephrotic syndrome, increased albumin catabolism in chronic ambulatory peritoneal dialysis, and reduced synthetic capacity in hemodialysis (82).

Acute Renal Failure

The dietary management of acute renal failure is not well delineated in the literature and depends in part on the etiology. When acute renal failure occurs in the context of shock, parenteral nutrition may be necessary. The composition of parenteral nutrition formulas should be developed with the input of a nephrologist and hospital-based dietitian. Excellent references on total parenteral nutrition in general and renal failure in particular are available (see Chapter 26). Enteral feeding should be maintained whenever possible (see Chapter 26).

Acute renal failure is characterized by a state of accelerated protein breakdown that is not suppressed by provision of exogenous protein. The causes of excessive protein catabolism are diverse, including uremic toxins, insulin resistance, metabolic acidosis, inflammatory mediators, and dialysis-related losses of nutrients, as well as declines in the multiple metabolic and endocrine functions of the kidney. Patient requirements for dietary protein vary and are influenced more by the illness causing renal failure and by the extent of hypercatabolism, as well as by the type and frequency of renal replacement therapy, than by the renal function (83). Patients undergoing continuous renal replacement therapy may need up to 1.8 to 2.5 g/kg protein/day; in hemodialysis, 1.5 g/kg/day is typically required (36). A dietitian should be involved in the management of all patients with acute renal failure that persists for more than several days.

Dialysis

Patients on dialysis tend to lose protein and would benefit from minimum protein intake in the range of 1.0 to 1.2 g/kg/day. In peritoneal dialysis, protein losses are particularly high, and intakes of 1.2 to 1.3 g/kg/day are encouraged. In all dialysis patients, 50% of ingested protein should be of high biologic value (see Chapter 3). To maintain lean body mass, nonobese patients with CKD, whether or not on dialysis, generally should receive an energy intake of approximately 35 kcal/kg/day.

Peritoneal dialysis is conducive to weight gain and obesity in patients receiving adequate nutrition, due to the delivery of 400 to 700 kcal per day in dialysate glucose with most dialysis solutions. Obesity may contribute to the development and progression of CKD and should be avoided due to its other associated hazards (see Chapter 5). Obesity in renal failure is managed as for other patients.

Hyperlipidemia

Elevations of both low-density lipoprotein and very-low-density lipoprotein occur commonly in renal disease. Management is as described in Chapter 7.

Nutrigenomics and Drug–Nutrient Interactions

To date, no specific alleles or drug–nutrient interactions with clear implications for the nutritional management of CKD have been identified.

CLINICAL HIGHLIGHTS

There is no conclusive evidence that diet can prevent CKD. However, the established role of diet in the prevention and management of hypertension, diabetes, atherosclerosis, and obesity suggests that successful primary prevention of renal disease may be achieved by limiting the size of the at-risk population. In CKD, judicious and tailored restriction of protein and phosphorus is indicated, along with supplementation of vitamins and trace elements. Other aspects of the optimal renal diet are similar to the diet recommended for general health promotion (see Chapter 45). The dietary management of patients with severe CKD should be a collaborative effort involving the patient and the patient's family, the primary care provider, the nephrologist, and a dietitian with expertise in renal disease. An effort to delay dialysis in a patient with advanced CKD may involve complex dietary management, including the use of keto or hydroxy acids to minimize nitrogen load while preserving adequate nutriture.

The contribution of dietary pattern to the risk of renal stone formation is uncertain, but it appears to be considerable. The difference in rates of stone formation between developed and developing countries suggests that nephrolithiasis may be largely preventable through dietary modification. A diet rich in fruits and vegetables and restricted in animal protein and sodium is indicated. Fluid intake leading to a urine output of not less than 2.5 L per day is likely protective. Relative restriction of dietary oxalate and purines is a prudent precaution in patients with a history of stone formation. A generous intake of magnesium, potassium, and fiber may be beneficial and is indicated for purposes of health promotion (see Chapter 45). Dietary calcium should not be restricted and actually may be protective. Dietary measures to prevent renal calculi are largely consistent with recommendations for health promotion and may be advocated to patients both with and without a history of nephrolithiasis. Grapefruit juice should be avoided on the basis of available evidence.

Patients with recurrent stone disease despite prudent dietary interventions are candidates for pharmacotherapy and/or more tailored nutritional therapies. Potassium citrate has shown promise in the management of recurrent calcium stones. Thiazide diuretics are indicated for hypercalciuria and allopurinol for hyperuricosuria (52) associated with stone formation. The use of high-dose pyridoxine for oxalate stones may be effective and apparently is safe. Tailored interventions to prevent recurrent nephrolithiasis should be predicated on chemical analysis of a 24-hour urine collection.

REFERENCES

1. Kopple JD. Nutrition, diet, and the kidney. In: Shils ME, Shike M, Ross AC, et al., eds. *Modern nutrition in health and disease*, 10th ed. Philadelphia, PA: Lippincott Williams & Wilkins, 2006:1475–1511.
2. Brazy PC. Epidemiology and prevention of renal disease. *Curr Opin Nephrol Hypertens* 1993;2:211.
3. Mogensen CE. Preventing end-stage renal disease. *Diabet Med* 1998;15:s51–s56.
4. Valderrabano F, Gomez-Campdera F, Jones EH. Hypertension as cause of end-stage renal disease: lessons from international registries. *Kidney Int Suppl* 1998;68:s60.
5. Sarnak MJ, Greene T, Wang X, et al. The effect of a lower target blood pressure on the progression of kidney disease: long-term follow-up of the modification of diet in renal disease study. *Ann Intern Med* 2005;142:342–351.
6. Faqah A, Jafar TH. Control of blood pressure in chronic kidney disease: how low to go? *Nephron Clin Pract* 2011;119:c324–c331.
7. Bennett SJ, Welch JL, Eckert GJ, et al. Nutrition in chronic heart failure with coexisting chronic kidney disease. *J Cardiovasc Nurs* 2006;21:56–62.
8. Beto JA, Bansal VK. Nutrition interventions to address cardiovascular outcomes in chronic kidney disease. *Adv Chronic Kidney Dis* 2004;11:391–397.
9. Maroni BJ, Mitch WE. Role of nutrition in prevention of the progression of renal disease. *Annu Rev Nutr* 1997;17:435.
10. Mandayam S, Mitch WE. Dietary protein restriction benefits patients with chronic kidney disease. *Nephrology (Carlton)* 2006;11:53–57.
11. Levey AS, Adler S, Caggiula AW, et al. Effects of dietary protein restriction on the progression of advanced renal disease in the Modification of Diet in Renal Disease Study. *Am J Kidney Dis* 1996;27:652.
12. Holm EA, Solling K. Dietary protein restriction and the progression of chronic renal insufficiency: a review of the literature. *J Intern Med* 1996;239:99.
13. Burgess E. Conservative treatment to slow deterioration of renal function: evidence-based recommendations. *Kidney Int Suppl* 1999;70:s17–s25.
14. Johnson DW. Dietary protein restriction as a treatment for slowing chronic kidney disease progression: the case against. *Nephrology (Carlton)* 2006;11:58–62.
15. Furth SL. Growth and nutrition in children with chronic kidney disease. *Adv Chronic Kidney Dis* 2005;12:366–371.
16. Bacchetta J, Harambat J, Cochat P, et al. The consequences of chronic kidney disease on bone metabolism and growth in children. *Nephrol Dial Transplant* 2012;27:3063–3071.
17. Chaturvedi S, Jones C. Protein restriction for children with chronic renal failure. *Cochrane Database Syst Rev* 2007;17(4):CD006863.
18. National Kidney Foundation. KDOQI clinical practice guideline for nutrition in children with CKD: 2008 update. *Am J Kidney Dis* 2009;53(suppl 2):S1–S124.
19. Wolfson M. Effectiveness of nutrition interventions in the pre-ESRD and the ESRD population. *Am J Kidney Dis* 1998;32:s126–s130.
20. Wolfson M. Nutrition in elderly dialysis patients. *Semin Dial* 2002;15:113–115.
21. Cupisti A, D'Alessandro C, Morelli E, et al. Nutritional status and dietary manipulation in predialysis chronic renal failure patients. *J Ren Nutr* 2004;14:127–133.
22. Kopple JD, Greene T, Chumlea WC, et al. Relationship between nutritional status and the glomerular filtration rate: results from the MDRD study. *Kidney Int* 2000;57:1688–1703.
23. Tritt L. Nutritional assessment and support of kidney transplant recipients. *J Infus Nurs* 2004;27:45–51.
24. Kent PS. Integrating clinical nutrition practice guidelines in chronic kidney disease. *Nutr Clin Pract* 2005;20:213–217.
25. Brandle E, Sieberth HG, Hautmann RE. Effect of chronic dietary protein intake on the renal function in healthy subjects. *Eur J Clin Nutr* 1996;50:734.
26. Kimmel PL, Lew SQ, Bosch JP. Nutrition, ageing and GFR: is age-associated decline inevitable? *Nephrol Dial Transplant* 1996;11:85–88.
27. Martinez I, Saracho R, Montenegro J, et al. The importance of dietary calcium and phosphorus in the secondary hyperparathyroidism of patients with early renal failure. *Am J Kidney Dis* 1997;29:496–502.
28. Hsu CH. Are we mismanaging calcium and phosphate metabolism in renal failure? *Am J Kidney Dis* 1997;29:641–649.
29. Lusvarghi E, Fantuzzi AL, Medici G, et al. Natural history of nutrition in chronic renal failure. *Nephrol Dial Transplant* 1996;11:75.
30. Dobell E, Chan M, Williams P, et al. Food preferences and food habits of patients with chronic renal failure undergoing dialysis. *J Am Diet Assoc* 1993;93:1129.
31. Oldrizzi L, Rugiu C, Maschio G. Nutrition and the kidney: how to manage patients with renal failure. *Nutr Clin Pract* 1994;9:3–10.
32. Cupisti A, Morelli E, Meola M, et al. Vegetarian diet alternated with conventional low-protein diet for patients with chronic renal failure. *J Ren Nutr* 2002;12:32–37.
33. Beto JA. Which diet for which renal failure: making sense of the options. *J Am Diet Assoc* 1995;95:898–903.
34. Alvestrand A. Nutritional aspects in patients with acute renal failure/multiorgan failure. *Blood Purif* 1996;14:109.

35. Kopple JD. The nutrition management of the patient with acute renal failure. *JPEN* 1996;20:3–12.

36. Brown RO, Compher C; American Society for Parenteral and Enteral Nutrition (A.S.P.E.N.) Board of Directors. A.S.P.E.N. clinical guidelines: nutrition support in adult acute and chronic renal failure. *JPEN* 2010;34:366–377.

37. Steiber AL, Kopple JD. Vitamin status and needs for people with stages 3–5 chronic kidney disease. *J Ren Nutr* 2011;21:355–368.

38. Mitch WE. Dietary protein restriction in chronic renal failure: nutritional efficacy, compliance, and progression of renal insufficiency. *J Am Soc Nephrol* 1991;2:823–831.

39. Kopple JD, Levey AS, Greene T, et al. Effect of dietary protein restriction on nutritional status in the Modification of Diet in Renal Disease Study. *Kidney Int* 1997;52:778.

40. Young GA, Woodrow G, Kendall S, et al. Increased plasma leptin/fat ratio in patients with chronic renal failure: a cause of malnutrition? *Nephrol Dial Transplant* 1997;12:2318–2323.

41. Friedman AN, Fadem SZ. Reassessment of albumin as a nutritional marker in kidney disease. *J Am Soc Nephrol* 2010;21:223–230.

42. Borghi L, Meschi T, Maggiore U, et al. Dietary therapy in idiopathic nephrolithiasis. *Nutr Rev* 2006;64:301–312.

43. Goldfarb S. Diet and nephrolithiasis. *Annu Rev Med* 1994;45:235.

44. Taylor EN, Fung TT, Curhan GC. DASH-style diet associates with reduced risk for kidney stones. *J Am Soc Nephrol* 2009;20:2253–2259.

45. Curhan GC, Curhan SG. Dietary factors and kidney stone formation. *Compr Ther* 1994;20:485–489.

46. Parivar F, Low RK, Stoller ML. The influence of diet on urinary stone disease. *J Urol* 1996;155:432.

47. Hiatt RA, Ettinger B, Caan B, et al. Randomized controlled trial of a low animal protein, high fiber diet in the prevention of recurrent calcium oxalate kidney stones. *Am J Epidemiol* 1996;144:25.

48. Fink HA, Akornor JW, Garimella PS, et al. Diet, fluid, or supplements for secondary prevention of nephrolithiasis: a systematic review and meta-analysis of randomized trials. *Eur Urol* 2009;56:72–80.

49. Jaeger P. Prevention of recurrent calcium stones: diet versus drugs. *Miner Electrolyte Metab* 1994;20:410.

50. Curhan GC, Willett WC, Knight EL, et al. Dietary factors and the risk of incident kidney stones in younger women: Nurses' Health Study II. *Arch Intern Med* 2004;164:885–891.

51. Curhan GC, Willett WC, Rimm EB, et al. Prospective study of beverage use and the risk of kidney stones. *Am J Epidemiol* 1996;143:240.

52. Curhan GC, Willett WC, Speizer FE, et al. Beverage use and risk for kidney stones in women. *Ann Intern Med* 1998;128:534.

53. Finkielstein VA, Goldfarb DS. Strategies for preventing calcium oxalate stones. *CMAJ* 2006;174:1407–1409.

54. Taylor EN, Stampfer MJ, Curhan GC. Dietary factors and the risk of incident kidney stones in men: new insights after 14 years of follow-up. *J Am Soc Nephrol* 2004;15:3225–3232.

55. Ideura T, Shimazui M, Higuchi K, et al. Effect of nonsupplemented low-protein diet on very late stage CRF. *Am J Kidney Dis* 2003;41:s31–s34.

56. Aparicio M, Chauveau P, Combe C. Low protein diets and outcome of renal patients. *J Nephrol* 2001;14:433–439.

57. Kanazawa Y, Nakao T, Ohya Y, et al. Association of sociopsychological factors with the effects of low protein diet for the prevention of the progression of chronic renal failure. *Intern Med* 2006;45:199–206.

58. Feiten SF, Draibe SA, Watanabe R, et al. Short-term effects of a very-low-protein diet supplemented with ketoacids in nondialyzed chronic kidney disease patients. *Eur J Clin Nutr* 2005;59:129–136.

59. Prakash S, Pande DP, Sharma S, et al. Randomized, double-blind, placebo-controlled trial to evaluate efficacy of ketodiet in predialytic chronic renal failure. *J Ren Nutr* 2004;14:89–96.

60. Teplan V, Schuck O, Knotek A, et al. Effects of low-protein diet supplemented with ketoacids and erythropoietin in chronic renal failure: a long-term metabolic study. *Ann Transplant* 2001;6:47–53.

61. Aparicio M, Bellizzi V, Chauveau P, et al. Keto acid therapy in predialysis chronic kidney disease patients: final consensus. *J Ren Nutr* 2012;22(2 suppl):S22–S24.

62. Bellizzi V, Di Iorio BR, De Nicola L, et al. Very low protein diet supplemented with ketoanalogs improves blood pressure control in chronic kidney disease. *Kidney Int* 2007;71:245–251.

63. Di Iorio BR, Minutolo R, De Nicola L, et al. Supplemented very low protein diet ameliorates responsiveness to erythropoietin in chronic renal failure. *Kidney Int* 2003;64:1822–1828.

64. Eaton SB, Eaton SB 3rd, Konner MJ. Paleolithic nutrition revisited. A twelve-year retrospective on its nature and implications. *Eur J Clin Nutr* 1997;51:207.

65. Axelsson TG, Irving GF, Axelsson J. To eat or not to eat: dietary fat in uremia is the question. *Semin Dial* 2010;23:383–388.

66. Lauretani F, Semba RD, Bandinelli S, et al. Plasma polyunsaturated fatty acids and the decline of renal function. *Clin Chem* 2008;54:475–481.

67. Barsotti G, Cupisti A. The role of dietary phosphorus restriction in the conservative management of chronic renal disease. *J Ren Nutr* 2005;15:189–192.

68. Martin KJ, Gonzalez EA. Prevention and control of phosphate retention/hyperphosphatemia in CKD-MBD: what is normal, when to start, and how to treat? *Clin J Am Soc Nephrol* 2011;6:440–446.

69. Sarathy S, Sullivan C, Leon JB, et al. Fast food, phosphorus-containing additives, and the renal diet. *J Ren Nutr* 2008;18:466–470.

70. Butt S, Leon JB, David CL, et al. The prevalence and nutritional implications of fast food consumption among patients receiving hemodialysis. *J Ren Nutr* 2007;17:264–268.

71. National Kidney Foundation. *KDOQI clinical practice guideline for bone metabolism and disease in chronic kidney disease.* Retrieved from http://www.kidney.org/professionals/kdoqi/guidelines_bone/index.htm.

72. Finkielstein VA, Goldfarb DS. Strategies for preventing calcium oxalate stones. *CMAJ.* 2006;174:1407–1409.

72a. Davis M, Wolff M. Patient education: tips for preventing calcium oxalate kidney stones. *J Ren Nutr* 2011;21:e31–e32.

73. Nouvenne A, Meschi T, Guerra A, et al. Dietary treatment of nephrolithiasis. *Clin Cases Miner Bone Metab* 2008;5:135–141.

74. Curhan GC, Willett WC, Rimm EB, et al. A prospective study of the intake of vitamins C and B₆, and the risk of kidney stones in men. *J Urol* 1996;155:1847.

75. Goldenberg RM, Girone JA. Oral pyridoxine in the prevention of oxalate kidney stones [Letter]. *Am J Nephrol* 1996;16:552–553.

76. Reynolds TM. ACP Best Practice No 181: Chemical pathology clinical investigation and management of nephrolithiasis. *J Clin Pathol* 2005;58:134–140.

77. Curhan GC, Willett WC, Speizer FE, et al. Intake of vitamins B₆ and C and the risk of kidney stones in women. *J Am Soc Nephrol* 1999;10:840–845.

78. Sorensen MD, Kahn AJ, Reiner AP. Impact of nutritional factors on incident kidney stone formation: a report from the WHI OS. *J Urol* 2012;187:1645–1649.

79. Besarab A, Coyne DW. Iron supplementation to treat anemia in patients with chronic kidney disease. *Nat Rev Nephrol* 2010;6:699–710.

80. Rucker D, Thadhani R, Tonelli M. Trace element status in hemodialysis patients. *Semin Dial* 2010;23:389–395.

81. Savica V, Santoro D, Mazzaglia G, et al. L-Carnitine infusions may suppress serum C-reactive protein and improve nutritional status in maintenance hemodialysis patients. *J Ren Nutr* 2005;15:225–230.

81a. Duranay M, Akay H, Yilmaz FM, et al. Effects of L-carnitine infusions on inflammatory and nutritional markers in haemodialysis patients. *Nephrol Dial Transplant* 2006;21:3211–3214.

82. Kaysen GA. Albumin turnover in renal disease. *Miner Electrolyte Metab* 1998;24:55.

83. Druml W. Protein metabolism in acute renal failure. *Miner Electrolyte Metab* 1998;24:47.

84. Seigneux SD, Martin P. Management of patients with nephrotic syndrome. *Swiss Med Wkly* 2009;139:416–422.

SUGGESTED READINGS

Beto JA, Bansal VK. Medical nutrition therapy in chronic kidney failure: integrating clinical practice guidelines. *J Am Diet Assoc* 2004;104:404–409.

Broquist HP. Carnitine. In: Shils ME, Olson JA, Shike M, eds. *Modern nutrition in health and disease*, 8th ed. Philadelphia, PA: Lea & Febiger, 1994.

Byham-Gray LD. Outcomes research in nutrition and chronic kidney disease: perspectives, issues in practice, and processes for improvement. *Adv Chronic Kidney Dis* 2005;12:96–106.

Klahr S. Renal disease. In: Ziegler EE, Filer LJ, eds. *Present knowledge in nutrition*, 7th ed. Washington, DC: ILSI Press, 1996.

Kopple JD. Nutrition, diet, and the kidney. In: Shils ME, Shike M, Ross AC, et al., eds. *Modern nutrition in health and disease*, 10th ed. Philadelphia, PA: Lippincott Williams & Wilkins, 2006:1475–1511.

Kopple JD, Massry AG, eds. *Nutritional management of renal disease*. Baltimore, MD: Williams & Wilkins, 1997.

Pietrow PK, Karellas ME. Medical management of common urinary calculi. *Am Fam Physician* 2006;74:86–94.

Pupim LB, Cuppari L, Ikizler TA. Nutrition and metabolism in kidney disease. *Semin Nephrol* 2006;26:134–157.

Reckelhoff JF, Kellum JA Jr, Racusen LC, et al. Long-term dietary supplementation with L-arginine prevents age-related reduction in renal function. *Am J Physiol* 1997;272:R1768.

Sheng H-P. Body fluids and water balance. In: Stipanuk MH, ed. *Biochemical and physiological aspects of human nutrition*. Philadelphia, PA: Saunders, 2000:843–865.

Taylor EN, Curhan GC. Diet and fluid prescription in stone disease. *Kidney Int* 2006;70:835–839.

Wiggins KL, Harvey KS. A review of guidelines for nutrition care of renal patients. *J Ren Nutr* 2002;12:190–196.

CHAPTER 17

Diet and Hepatobiliary Disease

The importance of the liver in the metabolism of ingested nutrients and drugs suggests that hepatic function can be influenced by dietary manipulations. Less obvious is the potential role of specific nutrients in ameliorating the natural history of various chronic liver diseases or toxic exposures. Preliminary evidence supports the use of several nutriceutical agents in the treatment of liver diseases for which conventional therapies are limited.

OVERVIEW

Diet in compensated chronic liver disease need not differ from that recommended for general health promotion (1,2). In uncompensated liver disease, malnutrition is a common sequela (3,4). The increased energy demands in chronic liver disease are at least comparable to those in dialysis patients (5). Malnutrition in patients with chronic liver disease may develop despite near-normal dietary intake, even in mild disease, due to increased muscle protein breakdown and decreased synthesis (6–8).

Liver disease directly influences the biomarkers of nutrient energy deficiency, such as albumin, prealbumin, transferrin, and retinol-binding protein, rendering nutritional assessment difficult (9–11). Upper body anthropometry, such as triceps skin-fold thickness, may be necessary to assess body fat reserves in a patient with ascites. Bioelectrical impedance analysis may also be useful, but it has limitations in patients with ascites (12,13). For bedside assessment, clinical parameters such as weight change, functional status, and visible muscle wasting are reliable indices of nutritional status, particularly when used in combination (9). Where available, indirect calorimetry should be used to determine energy needs in ICU patients with liver disease,

particularly those who do not have the expected response to nutritional therapies (11).

A cross-sectional study compared bedside measurements of handgrip strength, subjective global assessment, and prognostic nutrition index in 50 patients with cirrhosis; the authors found that handgrip strength was the only method that reliably predicted poorer clinical outcome (14). A complete nutritional assessment should include evaluation of micronutrients at high risk of deficiency, including vitamins A, D, and E, folate, zinc, and iron, as well as thiamin in alcoholic liver disease (15). Given the frequency of protein-energy malnutrition in patients with advanced liver disease and the complexity of evaluating the nutritional status of such patients, a dietary consultation is generally indicated for inpatients and outpatients alike.

Maintenance of adequate nutritional status should be a priority in patients with chronic liver disease and hepatic insufficiency, as malnutrition in this population is significantly correlated with poorer clinical outcome (13,16) (see Chapter 26). Ascites is associated with anorexia and has been shown to increase energy expenditure (9). Nausea, which frequently accompanies liver disease, further reduces dietary intake. Malabsorption and poor dietary intake associated with alcoholism are other common reasons for malnutrition in chronic liver disease. A systematic review found a positive effect of nutrition support on clinical outcome of nutritionally at-risk patients with cirrhosis (17). Reduction in the frequency of infectious complications, reduction in hospitalization, and improvement in hepatic function have also been seen in patients with liver disease in response to nutritional support (18).

Protein restriction is no longer recommended for patients with mild to moderate hepatic encephalopathy, as recent evidence suggests that this is not necessary for patients with inadequate dietary intake unless the condition is severe (19). A randomized trial by Córdoba (20) found a higher rate of protein catabolism in patients initially given a low-protein diet compared to those started immediately on a normal protein diet (1.2 g/kg/day). A goal of managing the cirrhotic patient over time should be to provide the maximal level of protein tolerated without inducing encephalopathy (9). Lactulose followed by a nonabsorbable antibiotic, such as rifaximin, is now considered the standard therapy for hepatic encephalopathy; this strategy facilitates clearance of nitrogenous waste while permitting protein intake adequate for metabolic needs (21).

The recommended energy intake for cirrhotic patients is approximately 30 to 35 kcal/kg/day, with 50% to 60% of calories from carbohydrate, 10% to 20% from fat, and 20% to 30% of calories from protein (21). Malnourished patients may need up to 40 kcal/kg/day (22). To prevent negative nitrogen balance in patients with hepatic insufficiency, a protein intake in the range of 1.0 to 1.5 g/kg/day generally is indicated (1,23). Higher protein intake may be indicated during periods of physical stress or in the recovery phase from malnutrition. For maximal effect of caloric consumption, the evidence suggests greatest benefit from frequent feeding, with four to six smaller meals throughout the day and a late-night snack (24). Late-night, carbohydrate-rich snack interventions improve nitrogen balance and quality of life, and potentially reverse sarcopenia, by reducing time spent in the fasting state (25). Snacks include fruit and yogurt, blended smoothies or liquid nutritional supplements, and whole-grain crackers or cereal with milk. There is consensus in the literature that when enteral tube feeding is required to maintain nutritional adequacy in liver disease, esophageal varices are not a contraindication (13).

Dietary fat should be restricted in patients with steatorrhea but otherwise should be unmodified. A reduction in dietary fat may be indicated on general principles if fat intake exceeds recommendations. In a malnourished patient, any reduction in dietary fat should be balanced by an increase in calories from other sources, preferably carbohydrate. Protein malnutrition is exacerbated whenever energy intake is insufficient, as amino acids are extracted from skeletal muscle to support gluconeogenesis (9).

In patients with portal hypertension and ascites, restriction of fluid and sodium intake is generally indicated. An unpalatable diet may exacerbate the tendency toward malnutrition common to patients with advanced liver disease and, therefore, may be harmful even if the dietary restriction imposed would otherwise be judicious. In such situations, there is a trade-off between controlling specific nutrients and ensuring the adequacy of energy intake.

The prevalence of nonalcoholic fatty liver disease (NAFLD) and nonalcoholic steatohepatitis (NASH) has risen along with obesity rates in adults and children (26,27). Because NASH and its precursor, NAFLD, are hepatic manifestations of the metabolic syndrome, nonpharmacologic treatment centers on diet and exercise to promote gradual weight loss and improve insulin resistance (see Chapters 5 and 6). Although a variety of approaches to low-calorie diets may be effective for weight loss, reducing consumption of sugar-sweetened beverages and excess fructose, which stimulates de novo lipogenesis, is of particular importance. Emerging evidence from primarily animal models suggests that fructose also contributes to translocation of gut-derived bacterial endotoxins to promote insulin resistance (26). The role of intestinal microbiota in the pathogenesis of NAFLD suggests potential utility of probiotics in the prevention and treatment of fatty liver disease; however, randomized clinical trials are lacking (28).

Nutritional management of liver disease in the pediatric patient varies with etiology. Given the importance of adequate nutrition in proper neurodevelopment and growth, nutritional assessment is a critical part of the management of children with chronic liver disease (29), and malnutrition is correlated with increased morbidity and mortality in this patient population (30). When liver disease is due to inborn errors of metabolism, such as galactosemia and Wilson's disease, specific dietary interventions are indicated. The management of such children generally should be overseen by a specialist.

NUTRIENTS, NUTRICEUTICALS, AND FUNCTIONAL FOODS

Silymarin

Silymarin is derived from the seeds of *Silybum marianum* (milk thistle). The extract contains a group of chemical compounds in the flavonoid family. There is a long history of its use in traditional medical systems for treatment of liver disease and manifestations of portal hypertension (31).

The hepatoprotective effects of silymarin have been demonstrated in animal studies and in cell culture, the principal mechanism of which appears to be the prevention of lipid peroxidation. In addition, it plays a role in hepatocyte regeneration, and reduces inflammation and fibrogenesis (32). Clinical trials have produced conflicting results. A meta-analysis of placebo-controlled clinical trials found that silymarin significantly reduced liver-related mortality in all trials, but this effect became nonsignificant when analysis was limited to higher-quality trials. The authors concluded that silymarin does not seem to influence the course of patients with alcoholic and/or hepatitis B or C liver disease, but it could potentially affect liver injury, and it is not associated with increased adverse effects (33). Likewise, a recent multicenter randomized trial found that silymarin did not significantly reduce serum ALT more than a placebo in chronic hepatitis C patients previously treated unsuccessfully with interferon (34). True comparison of these studies is difficult, given the heterogeneity of both the study populations and the silymarin doses administered.

In diabetic patients with cirrhosis, insulin resistance results from decreased hepatic uptake of glucose and decreased hepatic degradation of insulin. There is evidence from human trials that silymarin reduces insulin resistance (35), and silymarin supplementation may help lower insulin requirements in patients with cirrhosis-related diabetes mellitus (36). In another insulin-resistant state, NAFLD, a recent randomized controlled pilot study compared the effect of silymarin, metformin, and pioglitazone treatment in 66 patients. Patients in the silymarin group had the largest decrease in average AST and ALT levels. These levels were significantly reduced from baseline in all three groups, and the average change with silymarin was significantly different from the metformin group (37).

Cell culture study suggests that silymarin acts independently of the cytochrome P-450 enzyme system, with free-radical scavenging the dominant action accounting for hepatoprotection (38,39).

Antifibrotic effects of silymarin have been shown in a rat model, suggesting a role in cirrhosis (40). Evidence supporting a role for silymarin in viral hepatitis, drug-induced and toxin-induced hepatitis, and alcoholic liver disease has been summarized (41,42). To date, there is no evidence of toxicity in humans. The possibility of toxic effects on the hepatocyte membrane and cytoskeleton is suggested (38) and requires further investigation. Well-controlled studies of silymarin are small, and the populations studied are heterogeneous; the historical experience and promising results from studies to date indicate a need for additional well-controlled trials.

Picroliv

Extracts of the rhizome *Picrorhiza kurrooa* have been used in traditional Indian medicine for treatment of liver diseases. A variety of mechanisms have been elaborated, including free-radical quenching (31). In animal models, *Picrorhiza*, and its purified derivative Picroliv, have been shown to stimulate liver regeneration, enhance detoxification from malaria-induced damage, and exert potent anti-inflammatory and anticholestatic properties (43). However, evidence of benefit in liver disease remains limited to animal studies.

Vegetable Protein

Benefits from a diet deriving protein from plant sources have been reported to reduce the incidence of hepatic encephalopathy in patients with cirrhosis. Such diets often are poorly tolerated, however, because of their high fiber and high total food volume. To the extent that protein derived from plant sources is tolerated by individual patients, its use is reasonable (9). In addition to vegetable protein, dairy-based proteins may also be better tolerated than meats in patients with cirrhosis (21).

Branched-Chain Amino Acids

Impairment in amino acid metabolism in cirrhosis results in accumulation of aromatic-ring amino acids and depletion of branched-chain amino acids (BCAAs). An imbalance in the amino acid distribution has been implicated in the development of hepatic encephalopathy (18), and it has been thought that the competitive action of BCAAs on amino acid transport across the blood–brain barrier may help alleviate this condition (44). Unfortunately, studies have shown that BCAAs reduce plasma concentrations of aromatic amino acids but fail to consistently improve hepatic encephalopathy (22). However, BCAA supplementation has been shown to improve serum albumin, prevent muscle catabolism, and improve quality of life (22). Randomized studies in outpatient settings suggest that supplementation with BCAAs for 1 to 2 years may slow the progression of liver disease or failure (11). Recent studies suggest that BCAAs may also be helpful in reducing morbidity in patients with hepatocellular carcinoma (45).

Branched-Chain Keto Acids

The keto acid analogues of BCAAs offer the putative advantage of providing a substrate for protein synthesis devoid of the amine group. Metabolic advantages of such preparations have been well described, but the evidence of clinical benefit in advanced liver disease is limited (9). Use of branched-chain keto acids in patients intolerant of standard protein may be appropriate; however, recent research in this area is limited.

S-Adenosyl-L-Methionine

S-adenosyl-L-methionine (SAMe), a precursor in the formation of the essential amino acid methionine, is known to be deficient in many forms of liver disease. Preliminary evidence from both animal studies and clinical trials suggests that SAMe supplementation may improve biochemical parameters of liver disease (46,47). Limited evidence suggests SAMe is not an effective treatment for alcoholic liver disease (48,49), but may improve early response to treatment for hepatitis C (50,51). There is also preclinical evidence for roles in preventing hepatocellular carcinoma in chronic liver disease and treating inflammation in NASH (52).

Amino Acids

Cysteine and tyrosine are nonessential amino acids (see Chapter 3), whose synthesis by hepatocytes is impaired in chronic liver disease (9). Inclusion of these amino acids in the diet may be essential when liver disease is advanced.

Glutamine

Glutamine is a nonessential amino acid (see Chapter 3). Because of abnormal intestinal permeability, endotoxemia in cirrhosis accelerates turnover of skeletal muscle. Glutamine is the predominant amino acid in muscle, and its consumption in cirrhosis might suggest a need for dietary replacement. However, glutamine is metabolized into ammonia and may increase plasma ammonia levels. Clinicians should therefore advise patients with cirrhosis to avoid glutamine supplements (22).

Medium-Chain Triglycerides

Medium-chain triglycerides (MCTs), generally containing 8- to 10-carbon fatty acids, can be absorbed in the intestine without incorporation into chylomicrons and require minimal hepatic metabolism. MCTs are particularly useful in malnourished patients with steatorrhea, which may improve with their administration (9). Preliminary evidence suggests survival benefit from enteral nutrition, with MCTs as therapy for acute alcoholic hepatitis (53). Supplementation with essential fatty acids (see Chapter 2) is required if MCT supplementation is sustained and intake of fat from other sources is negligible.

In patients with cirrhosis, the ability of the liver to extract MCTs from circulation and metabolize them is impaired. Because MCTs cross the blood–brain barrier and have been known to cause encephalopathy and coma, their use generally should be avoided in cirrhotic patients.

Trace Elements

Reduction in the serum levels of zinc and selenium attributable to chronic liver disease has been reported in patients with chronic hepatitis C, with or without cirrhosis (54). Zinc supplementation has been shown to improve both glucose tolerance in patients with cirrhosis (55) and hepatic encephalopathy in alcoholic patients (56). In a recent randomized trial of standard therapy with and without oral zinc supplementation in 79 cirrhotic patients, supplementation significantly decreased hepatic encephalopathy grade and blood ammonia levels (57). Magnesium depletion is also common in end-stage liver disease (58) and may play a role in the development of the insulin resistance commonly seen in conjunction with liver disease (59). Because copper and manganese are excreted in bile, doses of these minerals should be decreased or eliminated from parenteral nutrition in patients with cirrhosis or cholestasis (22).

Vitamins

Use of a multivitamin supplement is advocated for all patients with chronic liver disease (56). Thiamine supplementation is indicated in all alcoholic patients. Vitamin E supplementation of 800 IU daily in adults with NASH reduced liver inflammation and steatosis, but not fibrosis, in a recent randomized controlled trial (60). However, long-term intake of high-dose vitamin E supplements may increase risk for hemorrhagic stroke and all-cause mortality (61).

CLINICAL HIGHLIGHTS

Liver disease, whether cholestatic or noncholestatic, of alcoholic, viral, or other origin imposes significant nutritional demands. Once severe, liver disease increases energy demands considerably. The sequelae of liver disease make malnutrition common.

Nutritional management should be directed toward preventing protein-energy malnutrition. Where available, indirect calorimetry should be used to determine energy needs in ICU patients with liver disease. Protein intake should be unrestricted unless severe encephalopathy is present in a patient without underlying malnutrition. In contrast to previously held clinical belief, recent studies suggest that restricting protein in patients with mild to moderate encephalopathy and malnutrition may actually impair recovery; lactulose and a nonabsorbable antibiotic, such as rifaximin, with adequate protein intake is now recommended in this situation. In patients intolerant of standard protein, BCAAs or keto acids should be considered, although their benefit and particularly their cost-effectiveness are as yet uncertain. All patients should receive vitamin and mineral supplements.

In the case of NAFLD and NASH, nonpharmacologic treatment centers on diet—in particular, avoidance of sugar-sweetened beverages—and exercise to promote gradual weight loss and improve insulin resistance.

Patients with ascites should consume a salt-restricted and, if necessary, water-restricted diet. In the setting of malabsorption, MCTs may be advantageous. The possible benefits of silymarin and other nutriceuticals in the amelioration of hepatocyte function once cirrhosis has developed are intriguing, but such benefits are as yet inadequately demonstrated.

REFERENCES

1. Corish C. Nutrition and liver disease. *Nutr Rev* 1997;55:17.
2. Lieber CS. Nutrition in liver disorders and the role of alcohol. In: Shils ME, Shike M, Ross AC, et al., eds. *Modern nutrition in health and disease*, 10th ed. Philadelphia, PA: Lippincott Williams & Wilkins, 2006:1235–1259.
3. Cabre E, Gassull MA. Nutritional therapy in liver disease. *Acta Gastroenterol Belg* 1994;57:1.
4. Caregaro L, Alberino F, Amodio P, et al. Malnutrition in alcoholic and virus-related cirrhosis. *Am J Clin Nutr* 1996;63:602–609.
5. Cano N, Leverve XM. Influence of chronic liver disease and chronic renal failure on nutrient metabolism and undernutrition. *Nutrition* 1997;13:381.
6. Levine JA, Morgan MY. Weighed dietary intakes in patients with chronic liver disease. *Nutrition* 1996;12:430.
7. Ferreira-Figueiredo FA, De Mello Perez R, Kondo M. Effect of liver cirrhosis on body composition: evidence of significant depletion even in mild disease. *J Gastroenterol Hepatol* 2005;20:209–216.
8. Periyalwar P, Dasarathy S. Malnutrition in cirrhosis: contribution and consequences of sarcopenia on metabolic and clinical responses. *Clin Liver Dis* 2012;16:95–131.
9. Munoz SJ. Nutritional therapies in liver disease. *Semin Liver Dis* 1991;11:278.
10. Crawford DHG, Cuneo RC, Shepherd RW. Pathogenesis and assessment of malnutrition in liver disease. *J Gastroenterol Hepatol* 1993;8:89.
11. McClave SA, Martindale RG, Vanek VW, et al. Guidelines for the provision and assessment of nutrition support therapy in the adult critically ill patient: Society of Critical Care Medicine (SCCM) and American Society for Parenteral and Enteral Nutrition (A.S.P.E.N.). *JPEN* 2009;33:277–316.
12. Pirlich M, Schütz T, Spachos T, et al. Bioelectrical impedance analysis is a useful bedside technique to assess malnutrition in cirrhotic patients with and without ascites. *Hepatology* 2000;32:1208–1215.
13. Plauth M, Cabre E, Riggio O, et al. ESPEN guidelines on enteral nutrition: liver disease. *Clin Nutr* 2006;25:285–294.
14. Alvares-da-Silva MR, Reverbel da Silveira T. Comparison between handgrip strength, subjective global assessment, and prognostic nutritional index in assessing malnutrition and predicting clinical outcome in cirrhotic outpatients. *Nutr* 2005;21:113–117.
15. Figueiredo FA, Dickson ER, Pasha TM, et al. Utility of standard nutritional parameters in detecting body cell mass depletion in patients with end-stage liver disease. *Liver Transpl* 2000;6:575–581.

16. Kondrup J. Nutrition in end stage liver disease. *Best Pract Res Clin Gastroenterol* 2006;20:547–560.

17. Kondrup J, Rasmussen HH, Hamberg O, et al. Nutritional risk screening (NRS2002): a new method based on an analysis of controlled clinical trials. *Clin Nutr* 2003;22:321–336.

18. Siriboonkoom W, Gramlich L. Nutrition and chronic liver disease. *Can J Gastroenterol* 1998;12:201.

19. Mullen KD, Dasarathy S. Protein restriction in hepatic encephalopathy: necessary evil or illogical dogma? *J Hepatol* 2004;41:147–148.

20. Córdoba J, López-Hellín J, Planas M, et al. Normal protein diet for episodic hepatic encephalopathy: results of a randomized study. *J Hepatol* 2004;41:38–43.

21. Chadalavada R, Sappati Biyyani RS, Maxwell J, et al. Nutrition in hepatic encephalopathy. *Nutr Clin Pract* 2010;25:257–264.

22. Johnson TM, Overgard EB, Cohen AE, et al. Nutrition assessment and management in advanced liver disease. *Nutr Clin Pract* 2013;28:15–29.

23. Lochs H, Plauth M. Liver cirrhosis: rationale and modalities for nutritional support: the European Society of Parenteral and Enteral Nutrition consensus and beyond. *Curr Opin Clin Nutr Metab Care* 1999;2:345–349.

24. Swart GR, Zillikens MC, van Vuure JK, et al. Effect of late evening meal on nitrogen balance in patients with cirrhosis of the liver. *BMJ* 1989;200:1202–1203.

25. Tsien CD, McCullough AJ, Dasarathy S. Late evening snack: exploiting a period of anabolic opportunity in cirrhosis. *J Gastroenterol Hepatol* 2012;27:430–441.

26. Rahimi RS, Landaverde C. Nonalcoholic fatty liver disease and the metabolic syndrome: clinical implications and treatment. *Nutr Clin Pract* 2013;28:40–51.

27. Alisi A, Nobili V. Non-alcoholic fatty liver disease in children now: lifestyle changes and pharmacologic treatments. *Nutrition* 2012;28:722–726.

28. Kirpich IA, McClain CJ. Probiotics in the treatment of the liver diseases. *J Am Coll Nutr* 2012;31:14–23.

29. Nobili V. Nutritional considerations in children with chronic liver disease. *J Gastroenterol Hepatol* 2005;20:1805.

30. Ramaccioni V, Soriano HE, Arumugam R, et al. Nutritional aspects of chronic liver disease and liver transplantation in children. *J Pediatr Gastroenterol Nutr* 2000;30:361–367.

31. Utrilla MP. Natural products with hepatoprotective action. *Methods Find Exp Clin Pharmacol* 1996;18:11.

32. Feher J, Lengyel G. Silymarin in the prevention and treatment of liver diseases and primary liver cancer. *Curr Pharm Biotechnol* 2012;13:210–217.

33. Rambaldi A, Jacobs BP, Iaquinto G, et al. Milk thistle for alcoholic and/or hepatitis B or C liver diseases: a systematic Cochrane hepato-biliary group review with meta-analyses of randomized clinical trials. *Am J Gastroenterol* 2005;100:2583–2591.

34. Fried MW, Navarro VJ, Afdhal N, et al. Effect of silymarin (milk thistle) on liver disease in patients with chronic hepatitis C unsuccessfully treated with interferon therapy: a randomized controlled trial. *JAMA* 2012;308:274–282.

35. Velussi M, Cernigoli AM, De Monte A, et al. Long-term (12 months) treatment with an anti-oxidant drug (silymarin) is effective on hyperinsulinemia, exogenous insulin need and malondialdehyde levels in cirrhotic diabetic patients. *J Hepatol* 1997;26:871.

36. Saller R, Meier R, Brignoli R. The use of silymarin in the treatment of liver diseases. *Drugs* 2001;61:2035–2063.

37. Hajiaghamohammadi AA, Ziaee A, Oveisi S, Masroor H. Effects of metformin, pioglitazone, and silymarin treatment on non-alcoholic fatty liver disease: a randomized controlled pilot study. *Hepat Mon* 2012;12:e6099.

38. Miguez M, Anundi I, Sainz-Pardo LA, et al. Hepatoprotective mechanism of silymarin: no evidence for involvement of cytochrome P450 2EI. *Chem Biol Interact* 1994;91:51.

39. Zuber R, Modriansky M, Dvorak Z, et al. Effect of silybin and its congeners on human liver microsomal cytochrome P450 activities. *Phytother Res* 2002;16:632–638.

40. Boigk G, Stroedter L, Herbst H, et al. Silymarin retards collagen accumulation in early and advanced biliary fibrosis secondary to complete bile duct obliteration in rats. *Hepatology* 1997;26:643.

41. Flora K, Hahn M, Rosen H, et al. Milk thistle (Silybum marianum) for the therapy of liver disease. *Am J Gastroenterol* 1998;93:139.

42. Rainone F. Milk thistle. *Am Fam Physician* 2005;72:1285–1288.

43. Picrorhiza kurroa. Monograph. *Altern Med Rev* 2001;6:319–321.

44. Bianchi G, Marzocchi R, Agostini F, et al. Update on branched-chain amino acid supplementation in liver diseases. *Curr Opin Gastroenterol* 2005;21:197–200.

45. Poon RT, Yu WC, Fan ST, et al. Long-term oral branched chain amino acids in patients undergoing chemoembolization for hepatocellular carcinoma: a randomized trial. *Aliment Pharmacol Ther* 2004;19:779–788.

46. Hanje AJ, Fortune B, Song M, et al. The use of selected nutritional supplements and complementary and alternative medicine in liver disease. *Nutr Clin Pract* 2006;21:255–272.

47. Mato JM, Camara J, Fernandez de Paz J, et al. S-adenosylmethionine in alcoholic liver cirrhosis: a randomized, placebo-controlled, double-blind, multicentre clinical trial. *J Hepatol* 1999;30:1081–1089.

48. Medici V, Virata MC, Peerson JM, et al. S-adenosyl-L-methionine treatment for alcoholic liver disease: a double-blinded, randomized, placebo-controlled trial. *Alcohol Clin Exp Res* 2011;35:1960–1965.

49. Rambaldi A, Gluud C. S-adenosyl-L-methionine for alcoholic liver diseases. *Cochrane Database Syst Rev* 2006;19:CD002235.

50. Flipowicz M, Bernsmeier C, Terracciano L, et al. S-adenosylmethionine and betaine improve early virological response in chronic hepatitis C patients with previous nonresponse. *PloS One* 2010;5:e15492.

51. Feld JJ, Modi AA, El-Diwany R. S-adenosyl methionine improves early viral responses and interferon-stimulated gene induction in hepatitis C nonresponders. *Gastroenterology* 2011;140:830–839.

52. Anstee QM, Day CP. S-adenosylmethionine (SAMe) therapy in liver disease: a review of current evidence and clinical utility. *J Hepatol* 2012;57:1097–1109.

53. Cabré E, Rodríguez-Iglesias P, Caballería J, et al. Short- and long-term outcome of severe alcohol-induced hepatitis treated with steroids or enteral nutrition: a multicenter randomized trial. *Hepatology* 2000;32:36–42.

54. Loguercio C, De Girolamo V, Federico A, et al. Trace elements and chronic liver diseases. *J Trace Elem Med Biol* 1997;11:158.

55. Samman S. Zinc supplementation improves glucose disposal in patients with cirrhosis. *Metabolism* 1999;48:1069–1070.

56. Levinson MJ. A practical approach to nutritional support in liver disease. *Gastroenterologist* 1995;3:234.

57. Takuma Y, Nouso K, Makino Y, et al. Clinical trial: oral zinc in hepatic encephalopathy. *Aliment Pharmacol Ther* 2010;32:1080–1090.

58. Koivisto M, Valta P, Hockerstedt K, et al. Magnesium depletion in chronic terminal liver cirrhosis. *Clin Transplant* 2002;16:325–328.

59. Patrick L. Nonalcoholic fatty liver disease: relationship to insulin sensitivity and oxidative stress: treatment approaches using vitamin E, magnesium and betaine. *Altern Med Rev* 2002;7:276–291.

60. Sanyal AJ, Chalasani N, Kowdley KV, et al. Pioglitazone, vitamin E, or placebo for nonalcoholic steatohepatitis. *N Engl J Med* 2010;362:1675–1685.

61. Mullin G. The use of complementary and alternative medicine for liver disease part I. *Nutr Clin Pract* 2013;28:138–139.

SUGGESTED READINGS

Novy MA, Schwarz KB. Nutritional consideration and management of the child with liver disease. *Nutrition* 1997;13:177.

Pares A, Planas R, Torres M, et al. Effects of silymarin in alcoholic patients with cirrhosis of the liver: results of a controlled, double-blind, randomized and multicenter trial. *J Hepatol* 1998;28:615.

CHAPTER 18

Diet and Common Gastrointestinal Disorders

Normal functioning of the gastrointestinal (GI) tract is essential to normal digestion, nutrient absorption, and egestion. GI pathology can impair nutritional status in a variety of ways, depending on the site, nature, and extent of disease or injury. Conversely, nutritional status and specific exposures to ingested substances can significantly affect the health of the GI tract via both direct and systemic influences. GI diseases often can be prevented or managed, in whole or in part, by dietary means.

OVERVIEW

Constipation

Constipation refers to infrequent bowel movements associated with abdominal discomfort and straining. The frequency of bowel movement is quite variable, and there is an insufficient basis for defining a pathologic state. Constipation is associated with hemorrhoids, diverticulosis, and appendicitis. Prolonged GI transit time is thought to increase the risk of colon cancer, and constipation and colon cancer share some risk factors (see Chapter 12). Constipation should be managed with diet whenever possible, as laxatives generally fail to address the problem at its source and may cause worsening of bowel function over time.

Dietary management consists principally of increasing fiber intake, with an emphasis on cereal fibers, and on maintaining good hydration. Whole grain foods and cereals are excellent sources of insoluble fiber, and patients should be encouraged to eat them. Fruits and vegetables provide soluble and insoluble fiber in combination, and their consumption should be encouraged both for the prevention or management of constipation and on general principles. Use of bran supplements such as psyllium may be injudicious, as it poses a threat of esophageal obstruction and may interfere with micronutrient absorption. Prunes (dried plums) are safer and generally more effective than psyllium in treating constipation (1). Used appropriately and in conjunction with adequate fluid intake, wheat bran added to food (as two tablespoons of wheat bran contains 3 g of fiber) can help prevent constipation. Dried fruits are an excellent source of fiber and should be incorporated into the diet in efforts to prevent constipation and on general principles, as they are nutrient dense. Although other dried fruits provide more fiber, prunes also provide phenolphthalein, which is used in commercial laxatives. Therefore, regular consumption of prunes may be particularly helpful.

Constipation in children is likely to be related to dietary fiber intake (2). A case-control study of more than 100 Brazilian children found low intake of fiber, particularly insoluble fiber, to be a risk factor for constipation (2). Similar results were obtained from a larger case-control study in Greece (3). A double-blind crossover study examining the effects of soluble fiber in constipated children demonstrated more frequent, softer stools (4). Goat milk yogurt, with and without *Bifidobacterium longum* probiotics, demonstrated improvement in stool frequency and abdominal pain in a randomized trial in children with constipation, with greater effects seen in the probiotic-containing yogurt (5). Although it is commonly believed that increased juice intake can relieve constipation (because of its association with "toddler's diarrhea"), there is no evidence to support this practice (6).

Even with adequate fiber intake (30 g per day is recommended), hard stools and constipation are likely if hydration status is poor. Fiber increases stool bulk by absorbing water. A glass of water with every meal (and in between) should be encouraged. Anti et al. (7) reported results of a randomized trial in adults that demonstrated a significant benefit in the treatment of constipation of fiber intake and 1.5 to 2.0 L of fluid per day. Physical activity may stimulate GI peristalsis and contribute to the prevention of constipation; it is advisable on general principles as well. Preliminary evidence suggests that products containing probiotics may help improve bowel transit time and reduce symptoms of constipation (8) and constipation-associated irritable bowel syndrome (see Irritable Bowel Syndrome discussed later).

Pediatric Colic

Colic refers to periods of nearly inconsolable crying in infants between the ages of 2 weeks and 4 months, apparently induced by abdominal distention and pain. The etiology of the condition and its pathophysiology are uncertain. Colic occurs more commonly in bottle-fed than in breast-fed infants. Breast-fed infants with colic may benefit from modification of maternal diet, with avoidance of bovine milk, peanuts, eggs, seafood, or wheat, or several of these items. Temporary elimination of bovine milk protein from the diet of a colicky infant with appropriate substitution of soy protein is reasonable, although not certain to alleviate the condition. Bovine milk may be reintroduced after resolution of symptoms; it is then generally well tolerated. A randomized controlled trial demonstrated marked reduction in infants' duration of crying when fed a whey hydrolysate formula compared to conventional formula (9). Probiotics are emerging as a potential treatment for colic (10,11).

Nucleotides, such as nucleic acids and nucleosides, are present in human milk in much greater quantities than in cow's milk or infant formula. There is increasing evidence that dietary nucleotides enhance both immune and GI function in the infant and may account for some of the functional benefit associated with breast-feeding (12,13).

Diarrhea

Diarrhea generally is due to a specific perturbation of GI homeostasis, often infectious, and treatment should be directed at the underlying cause, as indicated. Viral gastroenteritis is among the most common conditions affecting healthy children. The mainstay of management is repletion of lost fluid and electrolytes. Most children do not need intravenous hydration; oral rehydration therapy has been proven just as effective and is the preferred treatment for moderate dehydration (14). Children under age 2 should be given a commercially prepared solution with balanced electrolytes (see Chapter 29). Older children may replenish fluid and electrolyte loss with clear liquids, broth, or commercial drinks. Highly sweetened drinks of any kind may worsen diarrhea and should be avoided.

Gastroenteritis in children may result in a state of temporary lactose intolerance. During and immediately after (up to 1 week) an acute diarrheal illness, milk and milk products should be avoided if there is evidence of lactose intolerance; lactose-free or lactose-reduced products may be substituted. A meta-analysis suggests that most children continue to tolerate nonhuman milk during the period of acute diarrheal illness (15). In a population of Indian children with persistent diarrhea, Bhatnagar et al. (16) demonstrated that moderate milk consumption was well tolerated, producing no meaningful outcome differences as compared to a milk-free diet. The consensus supporting oral rehydration and continuous feeding of staples, including lactose, is well established.

Lactose intolerance may be problematic in children with significant dehydration. There is evidence of some benefit of lactose-free or lactose-reduced refeeding after rehydration in underweight infants (17). Lactose-free formula may also be beneficial in children of Asian descent who may have genetically determined lactase deficiency. Simakachorn et al. (18) found that compared to lactose-containing formula, lactose-free formula was well tolerated and led to reduced duration of diarrhea and better weight gain in Thai infants with acute viral gastroenteritis following oral rehydration therapy.

Breast-fed infants should continue to be breast-fed, and older children generally should continue to receive their normal diet whenever possible (19). The so-called BRAT diet (bananas, rice, apples, toast) is no longer recommended, although these foods may be included as part of a more balanced diet during the illness. The CRAM diet (cereal, rice, applesauce, and milk) is an alternative to the BRAT diet and has a more complete protein and fat profile compared to the

BRAT diet. Other foods rich in soluble fiber, such as oatmeal, have a binding effect and can be helpful. Foods high in insoluble fiber, such as wheat bran, should be avoided during the illness. Excessive fruit juice consumption in toddlers can induce an osmotic diarrhea; fruit juice intake is best limited to 2 to 3 oz per day until after age 2.

Appendicitis

Specific dietary precipitants of appendicitis are generally unknown. Population studies link the disease to relatively low intake of dietary fiber. A diet rich in cereal grains, fruits, and vegetables is thought to be protective. Epidemiological data suggest that improved sanitation and reduced exposure to food-borne pathogens in early life may increase the incidence of childhood appendicitis by fostering a more extreme hyperplasia of appendiceal lymphoid tissue when viral exposure occurs. Uncertainties about the etiology of appendicitis limit the security with which targeted dietary recommendations can be made. A lower-than-average risk of appendicitis has been associated with vegetarianism (20). Low water intake may be associated with appendicitis (21).

Conventional clinical wisdom holds that particulate matter in the diet, such as small seeds, may contribute to episodes of acute appendicitis or diverticulitis by luminal occlusion; however, evidence in support of this perception is lacking in the peer-reviewed literature.

Diverticulosis/Diverticulitis

Diverticula develop as a direct consequence of high intraluminal pressure in the bowel. Outpouchings typically occur in the sigmoid colon, as pressures increase with solidification of the stool. Long GI transit time and increased pressure are associated with low dietary fiber, thought to be a strong determinant of diverticulosis in both populations and individuals (22,23). Diverticulitis occurs when bacteria are trapped within a diverticulum, leading to infection. Dietary interventions to prevent diverticulosis are aimed at preventing constipation and the attendant elevations of intraluminal pressure (see "Constipation," discussed earlier). Historically, low residue diets minimizing food remnants in the intestinal tract (i.e., foods such as nuts, seeds, corn, and popcorn) were recommended to

prevent diverticulosis, though no evidence supports this approach (24). The principal strategy is to achieve and maintain a high intake of dietary fiber, indicated on general principles of health promotion as well. Vegetarianism is associated with reduced risk for diverticulosis (20,25). Data suggest that physical activity, particularly vigorous activity, may be protective against diverticular disease (26,27).

Pancreatitis

The only aspect of diet reliably known to cause pancreatitis is excessive alcohol intake. Diet may contribute indirectly to the development of pancreatitis by leading to cholelithiasis (discussed later; see "Cholestasis/Cholelithiasis"). Bowel rest is standard care in acute pancreatitis, with the goal of eliminating stimulation of pancreatic enzyme release. Resumption of oral intake, preferably of low-fat foods, can generally take place within 5 days of the onset of symptoms.

When pancreatitis is more severe and protracted, enteral nutritional support should be considered. Total parenteral nutrition is one option; enteral nutrition with tube placement in the jejunum is another. The more distally a tube is placed in the small bowel, the less pancreatic stimulation occurs. Placement of a jejunostomy tube beyond the ligament of Treitz, coupled with slow continuous infusion of an enteral formula, results in almost no pancreatic stimulation and offers considerable advantages over total parenteral nutrition (see Chapter 26).

Among the symptoms of chronic pancreatitis associated with exocrine failure of the pancreas is fat malabsorption. Treatment strategies include moderate restriction of dietary fat (advisable on general principles, but potentially ill-advised in a malnourished patient), use of commercial pancreatic enzyme supplements, and supplementation with medium-chain triglycerides. The dietary management of a patient with chronic loss of exocrine pancreatic function should involve both a gastroenterologist and a dietitian.

Cholestasis/Cholelithiasis

Definitive associations between diet and cholelithiasis have not been established. Epidemiological data suggest associations with high intake of dietary fat, excess body weight, rapid weight loss, and low dietary fiber (28). A case-control study in southern Italy found physical inactivity and consumption of animal fats and refined sugars to increase risk, whereas physical activity, monounsaturated fats, and dietary fiber appeared to be protective (29). A comparable study in France had similar findings and suggested that moderate alcohol consumption (20 to 40 g per day of ethanol) is protective (30). Cohort studies have reported associations between caffeinated coffee consumption and reduced risk of cholecystectomy (31,32). Epidemiological data suggest a protective effect of vitamin C (33).

Rapid weight loss seems to lead to cholelithiasis over a range of dietary fat content (34), but risk may vary when the manipulation of dietary fat content is more extreme (35). The level of calorie restriction achievable with over-the-counter meal replacements may be sufficient to raise substantially the risk of gallstone formation (36). There is evidence, however, that energy restriction to 1,200 kcal per day by use of regular food rather than liquid diet does not increase the risk of cholelithiasis (37).

Recommendations for reducing the risk of cholelithiasis consistent with general dietary guidelines include consuming a diet rich in fiber, particularly soluble fiber; restricting dietary fat to 30% or less of total calories; avoiding excess body weight; avoiding "crash" diets with less than 1,000 to 1,200 kcal daily; avoiding rapid swings in weight; avoiding extended fasts followed by binges; and, possibly, increasing n-3 fatty acid intake by consuming fish or plant sources (flaxseed, linseed) regularly (38). The n-3 fatty acids may decrease bile acid synthesis (39). Vegetarianism and high consumption of fruit and vegetables is associated with a reduced risk of gallstone formation (20,40).

Gastroesophageal Reflux Disease

Gastroesophageal reflux disease (GERD) is the preferred term for acid reflux into the esophagus associated with pain typically referred to as heartburn. Symptoms of GERD typically occur postprandially. Dietary precipitants are thought to include large meals, fatty meals, coffee, alcohol, and meat (41). Dietary interventions to control GERD include eating small, regularly spaced meals and/or snacks; avoiding food within several hours of sleep; avoiding meals with high fat content; avoiding carbonated beverages and excess caffeine; and controlling weight (see Chapters 5 and 25). Dietary interventions are complementary to pharmacotherapy with histamine (H_2) receptor antagonists or proton pump inhibitors.

Gastrectomy

Dietary interventions in the advent of surgical gastrectomy are aimed at mitigating the symptoms of the dumping syndrome. The syndrome, as a result of rapid entry of a nutrient load into the jejunum, is characterized by tachycardia, nausea, and even hypotension. Rapid insulin release can result in hypoglycemia. Dietary interventions include small, evenly spaced meals; avoidance of meals with a high content of sugar or processed carbohydrate; use of nutrient-dense foods or supplements to prevent malnutrition due to early satiety; iron supplementation as indicated; and parenteral B_{12} due to loss of intrinsic factor.

Short Bowel Syndrome

Short bowel syndrome, in which resection or loss of major lengths of the small bowel for any reason leads to impaired nutrient absorption, is associated with diarrhea, weight loss, and malnutrition. Resection of the small bowel impairs absorption of salt, water, various nutrients, and bile salts. Loss of bile salts in stool in the short bowel syndrome is associated with impaired fat absorption. Delivery of salt, water, and bile salts to the large bowel induces an osmotic diarrhea. Malabsorption tends to occur when more than 75% of the total small bowel length is lost; parenteral nutrition support generally is required. With lesser degrees of resection, oral intake can be maintained. Vitamin B_{12} generally needs to be supplemented parenterally, and oral calcium supplementation is indicated.

Short bowel syndrome generally is consequent to severe Crohn's disease, radiation enteritis, neoplastic disease, infarction, or trauma. The condition occurs in infants due to congenital malformations or necrotizing enterocolitis. When bowel resections occur at specific sites, there is some adaptation over remaining lengths of bowel to develop compensatory absorptive capacity. Nonetheless, some degree of site specificity persists, so that nutrient deficiencies are characteristic to sites of resection.

The colon principally resorbs water and electrolytes. The duodenum absorbs iron, folate, and calcium preferentially. Water-soluble vitamins, proteins, electrolytes, and minerals (particularly trace elements) are well absorbed in the jejunum and ileum. Glucose uptake is coupled to active sodium absorption in the jejunum. Reduced secretion of cholecystokinin-pancreozymin after jejunal resection is associated with cholestasis and cholelithiasis, whereas loss of various hormones from the jejunum can lead to gastric hypersecretion as a result of unregulated release of gastrin. The distal ileum absorbs fat-soluble vitamins and vitamin B_{12}. Loss of the ileum results in bile salt malabsorption, bile acid delivery to the colon, and diarrhea accompanied by loss of fat-soluble nutrients. Loss of the ileocecal valve can allow colonic bacteria to migrate into the small bowel.

Bacterial metabolism in the small bowel can generate nonmetabolizable D-lactic acid, resulting in acidosis. The condition may manifest with slurred speech and ataxia, mimicking intoxication with ethanol. Treatment of acidosis may require supplemental base, such as bicarbonate or citrate, and reduced carbohydrate to limit the generation of acid. Bile salt malabsorption results in binding of calcium to fatty acids in the gut, which in turn leads to absorption of free oxalate, normally bound by calcium. Oxalate excretion in urine can lead to formation of oxalate stones. Reduction of dietary oxalate may be indicated when significant portions of the ileum are missing. Also of use in preventing formation of renal oxalate stones is the binding of bile salts with cholestyramine, increased calcium intake, increased fluid intake, and alkalinization of urine with citrate to prevent crystallization.

Villous height and crypt depth both increase in response to small bowel resections, facilitating nutritional support with enteral preparations. Adaptation apparently can be expected to continue as long as 2 years after surgery. Enteral feeding stimulates continued adaptation, whereas exclusive parenteral nutrition induces atrophy. Immediately after small bowel resection, total parenteral nutrition is required; careful monitoring of electrolytes is necessary during this period. Enteral feeding should be initiated as soon as feasible (see Chapter 26). Pharmacotherapy likely will be needed to slow motility and reduce gastric acid secretion. Cholestyramine may help control diarrhea induced by malabsorption of bile acids. A period of overlapping enteral and parenteral nutrition is commonly indicated.

Energy requirements are increased by malabsorption, and in the short bowel syndrome it may be twice normal. Supplements of folate, iron, and fat-soluble vitamins generally are indicated; B_{12} injection is indicated after loss of the terminal ileum. Preliminary evidence and data from animal studies suggest that glutamine and pectin may stimulate enhanced intestinal adaptation.

Specific nutritional strategies may be tailored to the site and extent of small bowel resection. When only the jejunum has been resected, a near-normal diet can be maintained. When less than 100 cm of ileum is resected, cholestyramine and parenteral B_{12} are generally indicated. When more than 100 cm of ileum is resected, parenteral B_{12} is required, cholestyramine is not indicated (due to depletion of bile salts), and fat restriction is necessary to limit steatorrhea. Massive bowel resection (less than 60 cm of intact small bowel) requires home parenteral nutrition, although even in this group, gut adaptation may permit restoration of at least partial enteral nutrition in time. Nutritional management of the short bowel syndrome has been reviewed (42–44).

Studies of enteral solutions in malabsorption and the short bowel syndrome have largely failed to demonstrate the superiority of hydrolyzed protein or free amino acids, apparently because of the absorptive capacity of the intestine even when impaired. The higher costs of solutions containing free amino acids or peptides suggest that they be used only when absorption is severely impaired and other solutions are not tolerated.

Celiac Disease (Gluten Enteropathy)

Celiac disease (see Chapter 24) is a cell-mediated hypersensitivity reaction to gluten and other environmental factors. After removing the starch, gluten is the leftover protein found predominantly in wheat, but also in barley, rye, and to a limited extent in oats (45). When severe, celiac disease can lead to nearly complete villous atrophy and thus malabsorption.

Although clearly familial and highly correlated with gluten sensitivity, celiac disease often requires environmental triggers. Adenovirus infection, interferon alfa treatment, and intestinal infections have all been shown to increase risk of celiac disease development in genetically predisposed individuals. Breast-fed babies and those with delayed exposure to wheat have reduced risk of the condition (45).

Celiac Disease is associated with various systemic diseases and particularly autoimmune conditions, such as type 1 diabetes (45). Diagnosis is made definitively by small bowel biopsy; IgA antigliadin, antiendomysial, and antibodies to tissue transglutaminase (anti-tTG) are strongly suggestive of celiac disease. Treatment requires the elimination of all sources of gluten, which is therapeutic but difficult to follow. Gluten can be found in many products that do not even seem related to wheat, barley, or rye (like bread or pasta) and thus great care must be taken when making dietary changes. Patients can be encouraged to join celiac disease support groups as support group members are generally better at managing their diet than those not participating in support groups (45). Print and online information is available to assist a patient in efforts to adhere to a gluten-free diet (see Section VIIJ). Consultation with a dietitian is always indicated.

Irritable Bowel Syndrome

Irritable bowel syndrome affects up to 25% of the population and is responsible for up to 50% of referrals to gastroenterologists. Of unknown etiology, the syndrome is characterized by crampy, abdominal pain and diarrhea, constipation, or cycles of both. The Rome III diagnostic criteria define irritable bowel syndrome as recurrent abdominal pain or discomfort at least 3 days per month in the past 3 months, associated with at least two of the following: change in form or frequency of stool or improvement with defecation (46). Gradual increases in dietary fiber are generally recommended, helping most when constipation predominates. Stress and anxiety are linked with exacerbations (see Chapter 32).

Irritable bowel syndrome and other functional GI disturbances may be associated with dieting practices in young women (47). The role of intolerance of specific foods in irritable bowel syndrome remains unclear (48), but a randomized study of dietary elimination in patients with irritable bowel syndrome found significant improvement in symptoms; further investigation into food elimination based on individual sensitivities is warranted (49). Non-celiac wheat sensitivity resulting in irritable bowel syndrome-like symptoms has been recently characterized (50). Individualization of therapy within a range of general guidelines is most appropriate (51,52). Randomized trials of peppermint oil have been conducted and summarized by meta-analysis (53,54). The data are promising, but further investigation is needed. Fecal microflora have been shown to be altered in irritable bowel syndrome, suggesting a potential therapeutic role for probiotics (55), in particular *Bifidobacterium infants* 35624 and VSL#3 (a high-dose combination of eight different strains of bacteria) (56).

Emerging research suggests that irritable bowel syndrome symptoms may be related to visceral hypersensitivity and alterations in the neuroendocrine system, with similarity to other chronic pain conditions that often occur together, such as fibromyalgia, temporomandibular joint disorder, and chronic regional pain disorder (57). Thus, similar clinical approaches may be relevant to all of these conditions.

Non-Celiac Gluten Intolerance

There is growing interest in the concept of non-celiac gluten intolerance, a general dietary concept attributing a myriad of nonspecific symptoms to gluten consumption, and alleviation of these symptoms after ceasing gluten consumption. Indeed, the rapid growth of the gluten-free food industry is reflective of this concept that has a basis in the peer-reviewed literature, the popular media, and anecdotal reports.

In clinical practice, many patients attribute amelioration of irritable bowel syndrome symptoms after a trial of a gluten-free diet (58). Biesiekierski et al. (59) published a randomized controlled trial of a gluten-free diet in 34 adults with irritable bowel syndrome (without celiac disease) and assessed GI symptoms, as well as markers of intestinal inflammation, injury, and immune activation for 6 weeks. Participants randomized to the gluten-free diet reported less GI pain, bloating, dissatisfaction with stool consistency, fatigue, and overall symptoms compared to those on a gluten-containing diet over the course of the study. Minimal differences were seen between groups in nausea and wind symptoms. Of note, there were no differences seen in celiac disease serology (tissue transglutaminase IgA or whole gliadin IgA/IgG antibodies, intestinal permeability, and high-sensitivity C-reactive protein). In a follow-up study, the same investigators found that in persons considered to have non-celiac gluten intolerance, the reintroduction of gluten to the diet did not change irritable bowel syndrome symptomology after following a diet excluding fermentable, poorly absorbed, short-chain carbohydrates ("FODMAPs"—fermentable, oligo-, di-, monosaccharides, and polyols) (60). Emerging research has demonstrated a low-FODMAPs diet an effective therapeutic approach in persons with irritable bowel syndrome (61). Nevertheless, the low-FODMAPs diet is considerably more restrictive than a gluten-free diet and thus may be challenges in dietary counseling and patient adherence. It may be prudent to try a gluten-free diet initially, and if symptoms are not adequately controlled, to follow-up with a low-FODMAPs diet.

Beyond irritable bowel syndrome, where the emerging literature is most robust, a short (2–4 weeks) trial of a gluten-free diet for functional GI symptoms may be warranted. Rechallenging with gluten-continuing foods (i.e., reintroducing gluten-containing foods after a period of abstinence) will provide stronger evidence regarding causality, but may be undesirable by patients reporting improvements after avoiding gluten. In most instances, a gluten-free diet that is well tolerated by the patient should be supported by the clinician.

Lactose Intolerance

Lactose intolerance is discussed in Chapter 24. The symptom complex of lactose intolerance is very similar to that of irritable bowel syndrome, with the important difference that the etiology and optimal management of the latter are ill-defined (62). Definitive diagnosis of lactose intolerance requires dietary challenge and elimination.

Inflammatory Bowel Disease

Both ulcerative colitis and Crohn's disease can lead to malabsorption and malnutrition. In adults, weight loss is common; in children, growth failure occurs. The adequacy of the diet is threatened not only by malabsorption due to mucosal injury or surgery but also by anorexia, diarrhea, increased metabolic demand, and medication effects. Inflammatory bowel disease (IBD) is more common in industrialized than developing nations, and dietary factors are thought to influence the natural history of the disease. Nutritional management principles of the two variants overlap but are in some ways distinct. Highlights of nutritional management have been summarized (63–65).

Nutritional therapy can be used to influence the course of IBD. Parenteral nutrition and bowel rest are indicated during acute flares and can contribute to induction of remission while preventing malnutrition. However, as enteral feeding can often accomplish the same end with lower cost and risk, it is preferred unless clearly contraindicated (see Chapter 26). Elemental diets have been shown to induce remission in up to two-thirds of patients, but they are costly and generally unpalatable. Meta-analysis indicates that polymeric enteral feeds are as effective as elemental diets at lower cost and with improved palatability (66). Steroids are more effective at inducing remission than enteral formulae of either variety (67). The nutritional risk index, based on serum albumin and weight loss, can be used to gauge the need for and urgency of nutritional support (68).

Dietary fats and their metabolites are involved in inflammation in the intestine as well as immune responses in IBD. A higher ratio of n-6/n-3 polyunsaturated fatty acids is associated with an increased incidence of IBD, while diets low in n-3 PUFAs (as well as fish, fruit, and dietary fiber) are associated with developing inflammatory bowel disease (65). Higher amounts of protein and carbohydrate intake were associated with IBD patients compared to healthy controls in a case-control study (69).

Nutritional deficiencies common in IBD, including both Crohn's and ulcerative colitis, include protein/energy; zinc, magnesium, and selenium; iron (due to GI blood losses); vitamins A, E, and B_6; and thiamine, riboflavin, and niacin (70,71). Zinc deficiency impairs wound healing (see Chapter 23) as well as taste sensation, potentially compounding anorexia. The most reliable measure of zinc status is 24-hour urinary zinc excretion. Magnesium deficiency can similarly impair wound healing and is best gauged via 24-hour urine collection. Serum levels of magnesium and zinc may be altered by globulin status and, therefore, are potentially unreliable in states of generalized malnutrition. Selenium deficiency can be assessed by measurement of serum level, erythrocyte level, or erythrocyte glutathione peroxidase. Routine selenium supplementation in IBD is apparently warranted.

Patients treated with corticosteroids for periods longer than 2 months should be supplemented with vitamin D and calcium (65). There is interest in supplementing with glutamine, believed to reduce intestinal damage in IBD patients (65). The related compound n-acetyl glucosamine was shown to provide benefit in 8 of 12 children with treatment-resistant IBD (72).

Guidelines for the use of enteral formula feeding in the management of Crohn's disease have been published (73,74).

Ulcerative Colitis

Two probiotic preparations (*Escherichia coli* Nissle and VSL#3) have been shown to induce remission and support maintenance in patients with ulcerative colitis (56). Because ulcerative colitis involves only the large bowel, it is potentially curable with total colectomy. After colectomy, dietary interventions pertain to the avoidance of dehydration and electrolyte imbalance and the management of an ileostomy (see Ostomies discussed later). A probiotic formula (VSL#3) can prevent pouchitis in patients post-colectomy (56). Other than the dietary interventions indicated with colectomy, to date there is little to suggest that diet influences the course of ulcerative colitis. A randomized controlled trial found improvement in clinical response of patients given an oral supplement enriched with fish oil, soluble fiber, and antioxidants (75). Dietary consultation is indicated to support efforts to maintain a diet adequate in energy and all essential nutrients.

Crohn's Disease

In general, a balanced diet should be maintained during periods of remission in Crohn's disease. Dietary consultation is indicated to help ensure the adequacy of energy and nutrient intake. Avoidance of excessive fiber is generally indicated to prevent the dilution of nutrient energy and to reduce the risk of obstruction. Restriction of lactose or use of supplemental lactase is often indicated. Restriction of dietary fat intake is useful in the prevention of steatorrhea. Supplementation with n-3 fatty acids may be useful in maintaining remission (76).

Evidence derived from studies subject to methodologic limitations suggests a possible role for corn, wheat, eggs, potatoes, tea, coffee, apples, mushrooms, oats, chocolate, dairy products, and yeast in the induction of flares of Crohn's disease.

Evidence is stronger that elemental diets based on oligopeptides or amino acids are of potential benefit. A semi-vegetarian diet was shown to prevent relapse in Crohn's patients in remission (77). A randomized trial in 40 patients with Crohn's disease demonstrated symptomatic improvement and reductions in ESR when selected foods were eliminated based on IgG4 antibody reactivity (78). Another pilot study found changes in stool frequency in patients given dietary recommendations based on IgG antibody responses (79). There is concern that elimination or restricted diets pose the threat of worsening nutrient deficiencies if they are found to be unpalatable by patients often already experiencing anorexia.

Ostomies

Ileostomies are associated with the passage of rather liquid stool, raising the risk of dehydration and electrolyte imbalance. Patients should be advised to remain well hydrated at all times and to keep handy oral rehydration formula. Diarrhea may be associated with consumption of raw fruit and vegetables, beer, and spicy foods. These reactions are somewhat idiosyncratic, and diet should be adjusted individually, as indicated. Fiber intake should be moderate, as very high fiber intake may lead to stomal blockage.

Colostomies are associated with a risk of constipation, and thus good hydration is important in conjunction with adequate fiber consumption. Flatus may be a problem and is associated particularly with onions, leeks, and garlic; cruciferous vegetables; beans; resistant starches; cucumbers; and yeast. Again, dietary adjustment should be guided by general principles but individualized.

General recommendations in stomal management include chewing food well and maintaining good hydration status at all times. Stomal blockage is associated with very fibrous vegetables such as celery and asparagus; citrus fruits; nuts; cabbage; and the skins of apples, tomatoes, and potatoes. Individual, empirical dietary adjustments are indicated rather than blanket dietary exclusions. Foods particularly associated with stool odor include fish, eggs, cabbage, onion, garlic, and leeks. Stool odor may be reduced in some individuals by consumption of parsley or yogurt. Diarrhea may be induced by raw fruit, highly fibrous vegetables, and beer.

Intestinal Barrier Function, Permeability, and "Leaky Gut Syndrome"

The GI tract houses $1 \times 10^{13-14}$ resident bacteria ("the microbiome") that modulates the normal function and development of the GI tract. The intestinal epithelial barrier is responsible for the equilibrium between tolerance and immunity to nonself antigens. Emerging translational research is determining the roles of the microbiome (and other antigens present in the GI tract) in autoimmune diseases, especially in the context of compromised intestinal permeability (80). This concept, colloquially referred to as "leaky gut syndrome," attributes the development of a variety of chronic conditions to the displacement of antigens into the body and the subsequent immunologic activation (81–88,88a).

A common therapeutic approach follows; that is, to "treat the gut" by restoring compromised intestinal permeably through oral administration of nutrients and probiotics. A number of health claims exist purporting to treat intestinal hyperpermeability with various nutrients and natural products, including L-glutamine, n-acetyl glucosamine, digestive enzymes, and probiotics. The strongest evidence exists for glutamine supplementation, with mixed results with various probiotic formulations.

NUTRIENTS, NUTRICEUTICALS, AND FUNCTIONAL FOODS

Probiotics and Intestinal Microflora

There is rapidly proliferating evidence that manipulation of the intestinal microflora can influence health and alter outcomes of clinical importance (89–91). Probiotics refer generically to commensal organisms (live bacteria) associated with putative health benefits (92). Among the most commonly used species of probiotics are *Lactobacillus, Bifidobacterium, and Saccharomyces* fungi. The intestines are predominantly populated by *Bacteroides, Porphyromonas, Bifidobacterium, Lactobacillus,* and *Clostridium* species (93).

Both *Lactobacillus acidophilus* and *Bifidobacterium bifidum* colonize the intestinal tract after birth; *L. acidophilus* is introduced from foods, whereas *B. bifidum* is introduced through breastfeeding. The concentration of *Lactobacilli* in the GI tract can be increased by ingestion of fermented dairy products, such as yogurt, or certain nondigestible substances, such as oligofructose or other short-chain polysaccharides (94). *Bifidobacteria* growth can be stimulated by introduction of fructo-oligosaccharides, which are prebiotics (nondigestable food ingredients that stimulate the growth of bacteria). Many probiotic strains have been studied in rigorous clinical trials to assess effects on alimentary tract health.

Yogurt may be made with other bacteria, such as *Lactobacillus bulgaricus* and *Streptococcus thermophilus*; therefore, commonly consumed yogurts cannot be assumed to be a source of acidophilus. Yogurts made with acidophilus strains generally are explicit on their labels. Commercial preparations of variable quality are available. Prebiotics preferentially nourish probiotic bacteria and are widely marketed in other countries, especially Japan. Fructo-oligosaccharides are found naturally in onions, garlic, asparagus, and artichokes.

The intestinal flora are involved in nutrient metabolism, immune function, and cholesterol metabolism. They influence the susceptibility of colonic epithelial cells to mutations. Claims made for probiotics include defense against pathogenic bacteria in the GI tract by a variety of mechanisms, including elaboration of lactic acid, hydrogen peroxide, and bacteriocidal proteins known as bacteriocins. Thus, probiotics were initially investigated for their potential to reduce the risk of gastroenteritis (95), though recent research has found a variety of connections between the gut microbiome and human health. The term dysbiosis refers to the alteration of the normal bacterial flora, often secondary to the administration of broad-spectrum antibiotics.

Diarrhea of various etiologies can be either treated or prevented with different strains of probiotics. Infectious diarrhea in children can be treated using *Saccharomyces boulardii, Lactobacillus rhamnosus GG*, or *Lactobacillus reuteri* strains (56), as an adjunct to oral rehydration (96–98). Preliminary evidence also points to the safety and efficacy of oral probiotics in breast milk to reduce the incidence and severity of necrotizing enterocolitis in premature infants (99,100), specifically *Lactobacillus acidophilus* and *Bifidobacterium bifidium* strains (56).

Probiotic supplementation has been advocated after, or during, use of broad-spectrum antibiotics for reconstitution of flora (101,102). A cocktail of *Lactobacillus casei, Lactobacillus bulgaricus,* and *Streptococcus thermophilus* as well as *Lactobacillus reuteri* have been shown to be effective in treating antibiotic-associated diarrhea (56,93) as monotherapy. *Saccharomyces boulardii* is the strain that has shown greatest effectiveness for *Clostridium difficile* infection, a significant cause of nosocomial antibiotic-associated diarrhea (103), though a recent review states that there is not enough evidence to support using *Saccharomyces boulardii* as the primary treatment for *C. difficile* infection (93). The combination of *L. casei, L. bulgaricus, and S. thermophilus* as well as *Lactobacillus acidophilus and L. casei* combined and on their own have also been shown to prevent *C. difficile* infection as well as treat *C. difficile*-associated diarrhea in specific populations, and thus evidence is limited to support this combination as monotherapy (93).

There is promising data regarding clinical benefits of probiotics in IBD and irritable bowel syndrome (104,105). Probiotics may have benefit equivalent to that of standard therapy in preventing relapses of ulcerative colitis (106). *E. coli* Nissle and VSL#3 have been shown to prevent relapses of ulcerative colitis as well as induce remission (56). There is mixed evidence in using probiotic preparations for Crohn's disease (56). *Bifidobacterium infantis, Bifidobacterium bifidum*, and VSL#3 are all supported as having some curative effect on irritable bowel syndrome. There is some evidence that VSL#3 could also be used to treat pouchitis as well as prevent remission, though there is not enough evidence to currently recommend as monotherapy to induce remission (56).

Vaginal douching as well as oral *Lactobacillus acidophilus, Lactobacillus rhamnosus GR-1, and Lactobacillus reuteri* may help prevent recurrences of *Candida* vaginitis and gram-negative urinary tract infection, as well as reduce the risk of developing bacterial vaginosis (56,107). There is early evidence that vaginal colonization with lactobacilli may offer some protection against sexually transmitted disease, including human immunodeficiency virus (108).

Preliminary data suggest reduced cancer risk (109,110), particularly but not necessarily limited to cancers of the GI tract, with high habitual intake or supplementation of *Lactobacillus acidophilus*. A variety of mechanisms by which probiotics and prebiotics may serve as anticarcinogens are under investigation (111,112).

There may be beneficial effects on GI function after radiation therapy; a double-blind controlled trial found probiotics to be effective over placebo in preventing radiation-induced diarrhea (113). Intestinal flora influence lipid metabolism, and salutary effects of probiotics and prebiotics on serum lipids have been reported (114–116).

In the past, Lactobacilli in foods and commercial supplements were generally categorized as GRAS ("generally recognized as safe") by the Food and Drug Administration (FDA) (117,118), though recent considerations may result in probiotics being categorized as biologic products, with more rigorous safety requirements (119). The incorporation of nutrients such as oligosaccharides in the diet may alter more sustainably intestinal flora than the ingestion of probiotic organisms per se; such substances have been characterized as prebiotics, as noted (120–122). As with all supplements, quality control varies by manufacturer; the website www.consumerlab.com is a very useful resource for assessment and verification of product quality.

Probiotic supplements, in particular, have demonstrated poor quality control with some over-the-counter products even containing pathogenic bacteria (123). Thus, products made consistent with FDA Current Good Manufacturing Practices (cGMPs) are recommended (124). The website www.consumerlab.com also provides data about over-the-counter natural products regarding purity and constancy. A number of specialty laboratories offer assays of intestinal microbiota, often with concurrent therapeutic recommendations. Though the potential benefits of this type of testing are rational and reasonable, to date, none of the commercial tests have been independently studied for validity and clinical utility.

In summary, probiotic recommendations are strain specific and include (93):

Clostridium difficile infection
   Saccharomyces boulardii
Irritable bowel syndrome
   Bifidobacterium bifidum MIMBb75
   Bifidobacterium infantis 35624
   Lactobacillus rhamnosus GG
   VSL#3
   Saccharomyces boulardii
IBD
   E. coli Nissle 1917
   Saccharomyces boulardii
   VSL#3
Acute gastroenteritis/Acute diarrheal illness
   Lactobacillus rhamnosus GG

Dosing varies by condition and population. In general, it is difficult to overdose probiotic supplements, as the amount available in commercial preparations (millions to hundreds of billions) is still orders of magnitude less than the total amount of organisms in the human GI tract. Clinical benefit is often seen at daily doses of 5 billion colony-forming units (CFU) or greater; combination products may confer greater benefit than single products.

Glutamine

The amino acid glutamine is utilized preferentially as a fuel source by intestinal epithelial cells (125). There have long been hints in the basic science literature of potential applications in the treatment and prevention of GI and systemic disorders (126–128). At present, therefore, a role for supplemental glutamine in clinical practice is a matter of informed speculation. Most authorities agree that further research is warranted (128,129).

Glutamine is tolerated both orally and intravenously (130) and has been used in critically ill patients to improve nutrition and immune system function (131), reducing protein degradation (132). In persons with HIV/AIDS, administration of 40 g per day was shown to increase weight gain through better intestinal absorption and reduced intestinal permeability (133). Some patients with chemotherapy-induced mucositis (taking 4 g every 4 hours) experienced reduced duration, time, and occurrence of pain (134). There is some evidence that recovery from bone marrow transplants as well as abdominal surgery is improved with high doses, mediated by immune function, nitrogen balance, hepatic function, and shorter hospital stays (135). There are no known significant side effects with oral glutamine. There is, however, concern for negative interactions with anticonvulsants, chemotherapy, and lactulose as well as contraindications in seizure disorders, mania/hypomania, hepatic encephalopathy, and MSG hypersensitivity (135).

Other Natural Products

A variety of herbal (plant-based) remedies, digestive enzymes, and other natural products are widely used in GI conditions. Safety and evidence levels vary based on the intervention and condition. A detailed discussion of these products is beyond the scope of this chapter. High-quality information on natural products can be found on the Natural Standard (www.naturalstandard.com) and Natural Medicines Comprehensive Database (www.naturaldatabase.com) websites.

■ CLINICAL HIGHLIGHTS

That impaired GI function would adversely affect nutritional status and that nutrition would influence GI function and health are rather self-evident. Thus, nutritional management and dietary pattern are of considerable importance in GI disorders. The details of management vary with the specific effort to prevent or ameliorate a particular disorder.

Breast-feeding may offer some protection against infantile colic, which in any event is a self-limited disorder. Diarrhea is best managed with vigorous oral hydration and, generally, maintenance of a varied diet. Constipation is best managed by increasing dietary fiber in combination with adequate hydration and physical activity; the folklore regarding prunes is valid. Abrupt and extreme weight loss increase the risk of cholelithiasis, which is possibly compounded when dietary fat intake is severely restricted. The best preventive measure is to avoid excessive weight gain in the first place. Diverticular disease and appendicitis may be related in part to deficient dietary fiber.

States of malabsorption related to resection or inflammation of the small or large bowel require meticulous attention to nutritional status; collaboration with a dietitian or another nutritionist in all such cases is indicated. Supplements of vitamins and minerals generally are warranted. A growing body of evidence emphasizes the preferability of enteral to parenteral nutrition support unless truly precluded by obstruction or intolerance. Advances in understanding of the immunomodulation of GI tract function by altering the composition of dietary fat or using probiotics or prebiotics offer promise for health promotion and disease prevention.

On general principles, an effort to include n-3 fatty acids in the diet appears to be warranted. In the aggregate, GI health can be promoted, and gastrointestinal disorders prevented, by adherence to a dietary pattern indicated on general principles. These principles include moderate intake of total calories with maintenance of nearly ideal weight; intake of dietary fat at roughly

30% of total calories, distributed appropriately among polyunsaturated (n-6, n-3, and nonessential), monounsaturated, and saturated fats with avoidance of animal fat in particular; abundant and consistent consumption of cereal grains, vegetables, and fruits, with approximately 30 g (or more) of fiber intake per day; moderate intake of refined carbohydrate; moderate alcohol intake; adequate hydration; and regular physical activity.

Daily diets incorporating fermented foods (yogurt, sauerkraut, kefir, etc.) containing a variety of probiotic organisms are associated with decreased all-cause mortality and reduced risk for a variety of chronic diseases (136). Individual probiotic supplements are indicated for specific conditions. Thus, a daily diet containing a variety of fermented foods is preferable for general health and chronic disease prevention.

ACKNOWLEDGMENT

We thank Nicholas Scoulios and Theresa Weiss for their support and technical assistance.

REFERENCES

1. Attaluri A, Donahoe R, Valestin J, et al. Randomised clinical trial: dried plums (prunes) vs. psyllium for constipation. *Alimen Pharmacol Ther* 2011;33(7):822–828.
2. Corkins MR. Are diet and constipation related in children? *Nutr Clin Prac* 2005;20(5):536–539.
3. Roma E, Adamidis D, Nikolara R, et al. Diet and chronic constipation in children: the role of fiber. *J Pediatr Gastroenterol Nutr* 1999;28(2):169–174.
4. Loening-Baucke V, Miele E, Staiano A. Fiber (glucomannan) is beneficial in the treatment of childhood constipation. *Pediatrics* 2004;113(3 pt 1):e259–e264.
5. Guerra PV, Lima LN, Souza TC, et al. Pediatric functional constipation treatment with Bifidobacterium-containing yogurt: a crossover, double-blind, controlled trial. *WJG* 2011;17(34):3916–3921.
6. Committee on Nutrition. American Academy of Pediatrics. The use and misuse of fruit juice in pediatrics. *Pediatrics* 2001;107(5):1210–1213.
7. Anti M, Pignataro G, Armuzzi A, et al. Water supplementation enhances the effect of high-fiber diet on stool frequency and laxative consumption in adult patients with functional constipation. *Hepato-gastroenterology* 1998;45(21):727–732.
8. Bekkali NL, Bongers ME, Van den Berg MM, et al. The role of a probiotics mixture in the treatment of childhood constipation: a pilot study. *Nutr J* 2007;6:17.
9. Lucassen PL, Assendelft WJ, Gubbels JW, et al. Infantile colic: crying time reduction with a whey hydrolysate: a double-blind, randomized, placebo-controlled trial. *Pediatrics* 2000;106(6):1349–1354.
10. Savino F, Pelle E, Palumeri E, et al. *Lactobacillus reuteri* (American Type Culture Collection Strain 55730) versus simethicone in the treatment of infantile colic: a prospective randomized study. *Pediatrics* 2007;119(1):e124–130.
11. Thomas DW, Greer FR; American Academy of Pediatrics Committee on Nutrition, American Academy of Pediatrics Section on Gastroenterology, Hepatology, and Nutrition. Probiotics and prebiotics in pediatrics. *Pediatrics* 2010;126(6):1217–1231.
12. Carver JD. Dietary nucleotides: effects on the immune and gastrointestinal systems. *Acta paediatr* 1999;88(430):83–88.
13. Yu VY. Scientific rationale and benefits of nucleotide supplementation of infant formula. *J Paediatr Child Health* 2002;38(6):543–549.
14. Spandorfer PR, Alessandrini EA, Joffe MD, et al. Oral versus intravenous rehydration of moderately dehydrated children: a randomized, controlled trial. *Pediatrics* 2005;115(2):295–301.
15. Brown KH, Peerson JM, Fontaine O. Use of nonhuman milks in the dietary management of young children with acute diarrhea: a meta-analysis of clinical trials. *Pediatrics* 1994;93(1):17–27.
16. Bhatnagar S, Bhan MK, Singh KD, et al. Efficacy of milk-based diets in persistent diarrhea: a randomized, controlled trial. *Pediatrics* 1996;98(6 pt 1):1122–1126.
17. Wall CR, Webster J, Quirk P, et al. The nutritional management of acute diarrhea in young infants: effect of carbohydrate ingested. *J Pediatr Gastroenterol Nutr* 1994;19(2):170–174.
18. Simakachorn N, Tongpenyai Y, Tongtan O, et al. Randomized, double-blind clinical trial of a lactose-free and a lactose-containing formula in dietary management of acute childhood diarrhea. *J Med Assoc Thai* 2004;87(6):641–649.
19. Brown KH. Dietary management of acute diarrheal disease: contemporary scientific issues. *J Nutr* 1994;124 (8 suppl):1455S–1460S.
20. Key TJ, Davey GK, Appleby PN. Health benefits of a vegetarian diet. *Proc Nutr Soc* 1999;58(2):271–275.
21. Nelson M, Morris J, Barker DJ, et al. A case-control study of acute appendicitis and diet in children. *J Epidemiol Community Health* 1986;40(4):316–318.
22. Aldoori WH, Giovannucci EL, Rimm EB, et al. A prospective study of diet and the risk of symptomatic diverticular disease in men. *Am J Clin Nutr* 1994;60(5):757–764.
23. Unlu C, Daniels L, Vrouenraets BC, et al. A systematic review of high-fibre dietary therapy in diverticular disease. *Int J Colorectal Dis* 2012;27(4):419–427.
24. Tarleton S, DiBaise JK. Low-residue diet in diverticular disease: putting an end to a myth. *Nutr Clin Prac* 2011;26(2):137–142.
25. Leitzmann C. Vegetarian diets: what are the advantages? *Forum Nutr* 2005(57):147–156.
26. Aldoori WH, Giovannucci EL, Rimm EB, et al. Prospective study of physical activity and the risk of symptomatic diverticular disease in men. *Gut* 1995;36(2):276–282.
27. Aldoori W, Ryan-Harshman M. Preventing diverticular disease. Review of recent evidence on high-fibre diets. *Can Fam Physician* 2002;48:1632–1637.
28. Cuevas A, Miquel JF, Reyes MS, et al. Diet as a risk factor for cholesterol gallstone disease. *J Am Coll Nutr* 2004;23(3):187–196.

29. Misciagna G, Centonze S, Leoci C, et al. Diet, physical activity, and gallstones—a population-based, case-control study in southern Italy. *Am J clin nutr* 1999;69(1): 120–126.

30. Caroli-Bosc FX, Deveau C, Peten EP, et al. Cholelithiasis and dietary risk factors: an epidemiologic investigation in Vidauban, Southeast France. General Practitioner's Group of Vidauban. *Dig Dis Sci* 1998;43(9):2131–2137.

31. Leitzmann MF, Stampfer MJ, Willett WC, et al. Coffee intake is associated with lower risk of symptomatic gallstone disease in women. *Gastroenterology* 2002;123(6):1823–1830.

32. Leitzmann MF, Willett WC, Rimm EB, et al. A prospective study of coffee consumption and the risk of symptomatic gallstone disease in men. *JAMA* 1999;281(22):2106–2112.

33. Simon JA, Hudes ES. Serum ascorbic acid and gallbladder disease prevalence among US adults: the Third National Health and Nutrition Examination Survey (NHANES III). *Arch Intern Med* 2000;160(7):931–936.

34. Vezina WC, Grace DM, Hutton LC, et al. Similarity in gallstone formation from 900 kcal/day diets containing 16 g vs 30 g of daily fat: evidence that fat restriction is not the main culprit of cholelithiasis during rapid weight reduction. *Dig Dis Sci* 1998;43(3):554–561.

35. Gebhard RL, Prigge WF, Ansel HJ, et al. The role of gallbladder emptying in gallstone formation during diet-induced rapid weight loss. *Hepatology* 1996;24(3): 544–548.

36. Spirt BA, Graves LW, Weinstock R, et al. Gallstone formation in obese women treated by a low-calorie diet. *Int J Obes Relat Metab Disord* 1995;19(8):593–595.

37. Heshka S, Spitz A, Nunez C, et al. Obesity and risk of gallstone development on a 1200 kcal/d (5025 Kj/d) regular food diet. *Int J Obes Relat Metab Disord* 1996;20(5):450–454.

38. Tseng M, Everhart JE, Sandler RS. Dietary intake and gallbladder disease: a review. *Public Health Nutr* 1999;2(2):161–172.

39. Jonkers IJ, Smelt AH, Princen HM, et al. Fish oil increases bile acid synthesis in male patients with hypertriglyceridemia. *J Nutr* 2006;136(4):987–991.

40. Tsai CJ, Leitzmann MF, Willett WC, et al. Fruit and vegetable consumption and risk of cholecystectomy in women. *Am J Med* 2006;119(9):760–767.

41. Bhatia SJ, Reddy DN, Ghoshal UC, et al. Epidemiology and symptom profile of gastroesophageal reflux in the Indian population: report of the Indian Society of Gastroenterology Task Force. *Indian J Gastroenterol* 2011;30(3):118–127.

42. Nightingale JM. Management of patients with a short bowel. *Nutrition* 1999;15(7–8):633–637.

43. Matarese LE, Steiger E. Dietary and medical management of short bowel syndrome in adult patients. *J Clin Gastroenterol* 2006;40(suppl 2):S85–S93.

44. Jeejeebhoy KN. Short bowel syndrome: a nutritional and medical approach. *CMAJ* 2002;166(10):1297–1302.

45. Di Sabatino A, Corazza GR. Coeliac disease. *Lancet* 2009;373(9673):1480–1493.

46. Longstreth GF, Thompson WG, Chey WD, et al. Functional bowel disorders. *Gastroenterology* 2006; 130(5):1480–1491.

47. Krahn D, Kurth C, Nairn K, et al. Dieting severity and gastrointestinal symptoms in college women. *J Am Coll Health* 1996;45(2):67–71.

48. Niec AM, Frankum B, Talley NJ. Are adverse food reactions linked to irritable bowel syndrome? *Am J Gastroenterol* 1998;93(11):2184–2190.

49. Atkinson W, Sheldon TA, Shaath N, et al. Food elimination based on IgG antibodies in irritable bowel syndrome: a randomised controlled trial. *Gut* 2004;53(10): 1459–1464.

50. Carroccio A, Mansueto P, Iacono G, et al. Non-celiac wheat sensitivity diagnosed by double-blind placebo-controlled challenge: exploring a new clinical entity. *Am J Gastroenterol* 2012;107(12):1898–1906; quiz 1907.

51. Bonis PA, Norton RA. The challenge of irritable bowel syndrome. *Am Fam Physician* 1996;53(4):1229–1236.

52. Paterson WG, Thompson WG, Vanner SJ, et al. Recommendations for the management of irritable bowel syndrome in family practice. IBS Consensus Conference Participants. *CMAJ* 1999;161(2):154–160.

53. Pittler MH, Ernst E. Peppermint oil for irritable bowel syndrome: a critical review and meta-analysis. *Am J Gastroenterol* 1998;93(7):1131–1135.

54. Grigoleit HG, Grigoleit P. Peppermint oil in irritable bowel syndrome. *Phytomedicine* 2005;12(8):601–606.

55. Madden JA, Hunter JO. A review of the role of the gut microflora in irritable bowel syndrome and the effects of probiotics. *Br J Nutr* 2002;88(suppl 1):S67–S72.

56. Floch MH, Walker WA, Madsen K, et al. Recommendations for probiotic use-2011 update. *J Clin Gastroenterol* 2011;45(suppl):S168–S171.

57. Zhou Q, Verne GN. New insights into visceral hypersensitivity—clinical implications in IBS. *Nat Rev Gastroenterol Hepatol* 2011;8(6):349–355.

58. Vazquez-Roque MI, Camilleri M, Smyrk T, et al. A controlled trial of gluten-free diet in patients with irritable bowel syndrome-diarrhea: effects on bowel frequency and intestinal function. *Gastroenterology* 2013;144(5):903–911 e903.

59. Biesiekierski JR, Newnham ED, Irving PM, et al. Gluten causes gastrointestinal symptoms in subjects without celiac disease: a double-blind randomized placebo-controlled trial. *Am J Gastroenterol* 2011;106(3):508–514; quiz 515.

60. Biesiekierski JR, Peters SL, Newnham ED, et al. No effects of gluten in patients with self-reported non-celiac gluten sensitivity after dietary reduction of fermentable, poorly absorbed, short-chain carbohydrates. *Gastroenterol* 2013;145(2):320–328 e321–e323.

61. Halmos EP, Power VA, Shepherd SJ, et al. A diet low in fodmaps reduces symptoms of irritable bowel syndrome. *Gastroenterol* 2014;146(1):67–75 e65.

62. Shaw AD, Davies GJ. Lactose intolerance: problems in diagnosis and treatment. *J Clin Gastroenterol* 1999;28(3):208–216.

63. Dieleman LA, Heizer WD. Nutritional issues in inflammatory bowel disease. *Gastroenterol Clin North Am* 1998;27(2):435–451.

64. Cabre E, Gassull MA. Nutritional and metabolic issues in inflammatory bowel disease. *Curr Opin Clin Nutr Metab Care* 2003;6(5):569–576.

65. Neuman MG, Nanau RM. Inflammatory bowel disease: role of diet, microbiota, life style. *Transl Res* 2012;160(1):29–44.

66. Griffiths AM. Inflammatory bowel disease. *Nutr* 1998; 14(10):788–791.

67. Zachos M, Tondeur M, Griffiths AM. Enteral nutritional therapy for induction of remission in Crohn's disease. *Cochrane Database Syst Rev* 2007(1):CD000542.

68. Duerksen DR, Nehra V, Bistrian BR, et al. Appropriate nutritional support in acute and complicated Crohn's disease. *Nutr* 1998;14(5):462–465.

69. Ueda Y, Kawakami Y, Kunii D, et al. Elevated concentrations of linoleic acid in erythrocyte membrane phospholipids in patients with inflammatory bowel disease. *Nutr Res* 2008;28(4):239–244.

70. Geerling BJ, Badart-Smook A, Stockbrugger RW, et al. Comprehensive nutritional status in patients with long-standing Crohn disease currently in remission. *Am J Clin Nutr* 1998;67(5):919–926.

71. Kim SC, Ferry GD. Inflammatory bowel diseases in pediatric and adolescent patients: clinical, therapeutic, and psychosocial considerations. *Gastroenterology* 2004;126(6):1550–1560.

72. Salvatore S, Heuschkel R, Tomlin S, et al. A pilot study of N-acetyl glucosamine, a nutritional substrate for glycosaminoglycan synthesis, in paediatric chronic inflammatory bowel disease. *Aliment Pharmacol Ther* 2000;14(12):1567–1579.

73. Ferguson A, Glen M, Ghosh S. Crohn's disease: nutrition and nutritional therapy. *Bailliere's Clin Gastroenterol* 1998;12(1):93–114.

74. Lochs H, Dejong C, Hammarqvist F, et al. ESPEN guidelines on enteral nutrition: gastroenterology. *Clin Nutr* 2006;25(2):260–274.

75. Seidner DL, Lashner BA, Brzezinski A, et al. An oral supplement enriched with fish oil, soluble fiber, and antioxidants for corticosteroid sparing in ulcerative colitis: a randomized, controlled trial. *Clin Gastroenterol Hepatol* 2005;3(4):358–369.

76. Romano C, Cucchiara S, Barabino A, et al. Usefulness of omega-3 fatty acid supplementation in addition to mesalazine in maintaining remission in pediatric Crohn's disease: a double-blind, randomized, placebo-controlled study. *World J Gastroenterol* 2005;11(45):7118–7121.

77. Chiba M, Abe T, Tsuda H, et al. Lifestyle-related disease in Crohn's disease: relapse prevention by a semi-vegetarian diet. *World J Gastroenterol* 2010;16(20):2484–2495.

78. Rajendran N, Kumar D. Food-specific IgG4-guided exclusion diets improve symptoms in Crohn's disease: a pilot study. *Colorectal Dis* 2011;13(9):1009–1013.

79. Bentz S, Hausmann M, Piberger H, et al. Clinical relevance of IgG antibodies against food antigens in Crohn's disease: a double-blind cross-over diet intervention study. *Digestion* 2010;81(4):252–264.

80. Ochoa-Reparaz J, Mielcarz DW, Begum-Haque S, et al. Gut, bugs, and brain: role of commensal bacteria in the control of central nervous system disease. *Ann Neurol* 2011;69(2):240–247.

81. Rogler G, Rosano G. The heart and the gut. *Eur Heart J* 2014;35(7):429–430.

82. Schnabl B. Linking intestinal homeostasis and liver disease. *Curr Opin Gastroenterol* 2013;29(3):264–270.

83. Anders HJ, Andersen K, Stecher B. The intestinal microbiota, a leaky gut, and abnormal immunity in kidney disease. *Kidney Int* 2013;83(6):1010–1016.

84. Seo YS, Shah VH. The role of gut-liver axis in the pathogenesis of liver cirrhosis and portal hypertension. *Clin Mol Hepatol* 2012;18(4):337–346.

85. Chassaing B, Aitken JD, Gewirtz AT, et al. Gut microbiota drives metabolic disease in immunologically altered mice. *Adv Immunol* 2012;116:93–112.

86. Ilan Y. Leaky gut and the liver: a role for bacterial translocation in nonalcoholic steatohepatitis. *World J Gastroenterol* 2012;18(21):2609–2618.

87. Maes M, Kubera M, Leunis JC, et al. Increased IgA and IgM responses against gut commensals in chronic depression: further evidence for increased bacterial translocation or leaky gut. *J Affect Disord* 2012;141(1):55–62.

88. Klein GL, Petschow BW, Shaw AL, et al. Gut barrier dysfunction and microbial translocation in cancer cachexia: a new therapeutic target. *Curr Opin Support Palliat Care* 2013;7(4):361–367.

88a. Fasano A. Leaky gut and autoimmune diseases. *Clin Rev Allergy Immunol*. 2012. Feb;42(1):71-8.

89. Salminen S, Bouley C, Boutron-Ruault MC, et al. Functional food science and gastrointestinal physiology and function. *Br J Nutr* 1998;80(suppl 1):S147–S171.

90. Goldin BR. Health benefits of probiotics. *Br J Nutr* 1998;80(4):S203–S207.

91. Guarner F, Malagelada JR. Gut flora in health and disease. *Lancet* 2003;361(9356):512–519.

92. von Wright A, Salminen S. Probiotics: established effects and open questions. *Eur J Gastroenterol Hepatol* 1999;11(11):1195–1198.

93. Balakrishnan M, Floch MH. Prebiotics, probiotics and digestive health. *Curr Opin Clin Nutr Metab Care* 2012;15(6):580–585.

94. Kasper H. Protection against gastrointestinal diseases—present facts and future developments. *Int J Food Microbiol* 1998;41(2):127–131.

95. Salminen S, Isolauri E, Onnela T. Gut flora in normal and disordered states. *Chemotherapy* 1995;41(suppl 1): 5–15.

96. Van Niel CW, Feudtner C, Garrison MM, et al. *Lactobacillus* therapy for acute infectious diarrhea in children: a meta-analysis. *Pediatrics* 2002;109(4):678–684.

97. Allen SJ, Okoko B, Martinez E, et al. Probiotics for treating infectious diarrhoea. *Cochrane Database Syst Rev* 2004(2):CD003048.

98. Parker MW, Schaffzin JK, Lo Vecchio A, et al. Rapid adoption of *Lactobacillus rhamnosus* GG for acute gastroenteritis. *Pediatrics* 2013;131(suppl 1):S96–S102.

99. Lin HC, Su BH, Chen AC, et al. Oral probiotics reduce the incidence and severity of necrotizing enterocolitis in very low birth weight infants. *Pediatrics* 2005;115(1):1–4.

100. Bin-Nun A, Bromiker R, Wilschanski M, et al. Oral probiotics prevent necrotizing enterocolitis in very low birth weight neonates. *J Pediatr* 2005;147(2):192–196.

101. Gismondo MR, Drago L, Lombardi A. Review of probiotics available to modify gastrointestinal flora. *Int J Antimicrob Agents* 1999;12(4):287–292.

102. D'Souza AL, Rajkumar C, Cooke J, et al. Probiotics in prevention of antibiotic associated diarrhoea: meta-analysis. *BMJ* 2002;324(7350):1361.

103. McFarland LV. Meta-analysis of probiotics for the prevention of antibiotic associated diarrhea and the treatment of *Clostridium difficile* disease. *Am J Gastroenterol* 2006;101(4):812–822.

104. Saggioro A. Probiotics in the treatment of irritable bowel syndrome. *J Clin Gastroenterol* 2004;38(6 suppl): S104–S106.

105. Rolfe VE, Fortun PJ, Hawkey CJ, et al. Probiotics for maintenance of remission in Crohn's disease. *Cochrane Database Syst Rev* 2006(4):CD004826.

106. Kruis W, Fric P, Pokrotnieks J, et al. Maintaining remission of ulcerative colitis with the probiotic *Escherichia coli* Nissle 1917 is as effective as with standard mesalazine. *Gut* 2004;53(11):1617–1623.

107. Reid G. Probiotics for urogenital health. *Nutr Clin Care* 2002;5(1):3–8.

108. Martin HL, Richardson BA, Nyange PM, et al. Vaginal lactobacilli, microbial flora, and risk of human immunodeficiency virus type 1 and sexually transmitted disease acquisition. *J Infect Dis* 1999;180(6):1863–1868.

109. Hirayama K, Rafter J. The role of lactic acid bacteria in colon cancer prevention: mechanistic considerations. *Antonie van Leeuwenhoek* 1999;76(1–4):391–394.

110. Rafter J. Probiotics and colon cancer. *Best Prac Res Clin Gastroenterol* 2003;17(5):849–859.

111. Reddy BS. Possible mechanisms by which pro- and prebiotics influence colon carcinogenesis and tumor growth. *J Nutr* 1999;129(7 suppl):1478S–1482S.

112. Commane D, Hughes R, Shortt C, et al. The potential mechanisms involved in the anti-carcinogenic action of probiotics. *Mut Res* 2005;591(1–2):276–289.

113. Delia P, Sansotta G, Donato V, et al. Use of probiotics for prevention of radiation-induced diarrhea. *Tumori* 2007;93(2):suppl 1–6.

114. Taylor GR, Williams CM. Effects of probiotics and prebiotics on blood lipids. *Br J Nutr* 1998;80(4):S225–230.

115. Kiessling G, Schneider J, Jahreis G. Long-term consumption of fermented dairy products over 6 months increases HDL cholesterol. *Eur J Clin Nutr* 2002; 56(9):843–849.

116. Fabian E, Elmadfa I. Influence of daily consumption of probiotic and conventional yoghurt on the plasma lipid profile in young healthy women. *Ann Nutr Metab* 2006;50(4):387–393.

117. Salminen S, von Wright A, Morelli L, et al. Demonstration of safety of probiotics—a review. *Int J Food Microbiol* 1998;44(1–2):93–106.

118. Hammerman C, Bin-Nun A, Kaplan M. Safety of probiotics: comparison of two popular strains. *BMJ* 2006; 333(7576):1006–1008.

119. Degnan FH. The US Food and Drug Administration and probiotics: regulatory categorization. *Clin Infect Dis* 2008;46(suppl 2):S133–S136; discussion S144–S151.

120. Gibson GR, Roberfroid MB. Dietary modulation of the human colonic microbiota: introducing the concept of prebiotics. *J Nutr* 1995;125(6):1401–1412.

121. Sartor RB. Therapeutic manipulation of the enteric microflora in inflammatory bowel diseases: antibiotics, probiotics, and prebiotics. *Gastroenterology* 2004;126(6):1620–1633.

122. Van Loo JA. Prebiotics promote good health: the basis, the potential, and the emerging evidence. *J Clin Gastroenterol* 2004;38(6 suppl):S70–S75.

123. Berman S, Spicer D. Safety and reliability of *Lactobacillus* supplements in Seattle, Washington (a pilot study). *The Internet Journal of Alternative Medicine*. 2003;1(2).

124. http://www.fda.gov/Food/GuidanceRegulation/Guidance DocumentsRegulatoryInformation/DietarySupplements/ ucm238182.htm.

125. Buchman AL. Glutamine: is it a conditionally required nutrient for the human gastrointestinal system? *J Am Coll Nut* 1996;15(3):199–205.

126. Ziegler TR, Bazargan N, Leader LM, et al. Glutamine and the gastrointestinal tract. *Curr Opin Clin Nutr Metab Care* 2000;3(5):355–362.

127. Elia M, Lunn PG. The use of glutamine in the treatment of gastrointestinal disorders in man. *Nutrition* 1997; 13(7–8):743–747.

128. Alpers DH. Glutamine: do the data support the cause for glutamine supplementation in humans? *Gastroenterology* 2006;130(2 suppl 1):S106–S116.

129. Tubman TR, Thompson SW. Glutamine supplementation for prevention of morbidity in preterm infants. *Cochrane Database Syst Rev* 2001(4):CD001457.

130. Garlick PJ. Assessment of the safety of glutamine and other amino acids. *J Nutr* 2001;131(9 suppl):2556S–2561S.

131. Jones C, Palmer TE, Griffiths RD. Randomized clinical outcome study of critically ill patients given glutamine-supplemented enteral nutrition. *Nutr* 1999;15(2):108–115.

132. Holecek M. Relation between glutamine, branched-chain amino acids, and protein metabolism. *Nutr* 2002;18(2): 130–133.

133. Shabert JK, Winslow C, Lacey JM, et al. Glutamine-antioxidant supplementation increases body cell mass in AIDS patients with weight loss: a randomized, double-blind controlled trial. *Nutr* 1999;15(11–12):860–864.

134. Cockerham MB, Weinberger BB, Lerchie SB. Oral glutamine for the prevention of oral mucositis associated with high-dose paclitaxel and melphalan for autologous bone marrow transplantation. *Ann Pharmacotherapy* 2000;34(3):300–303.

135. Therapeutic Research Faculty. Glutamine. *Natural Medicines Comprehensive Database*, 2013.

136. Soedamah-Muthu SS, Masset G, Verberne L, et al. Consumption of dairy products and associations with incident diabetes, CHD and mortality in the Whitehall II study. *Br J Nutr* 2012:1–9.

SUGGESTED READINGS

Fasano A, Shea-Donohue T. Mechanisms of disease: the role of intestinal barrier function in the pathogenesis of gastrointestinal autoimmune diseases. *Nat Clin Pract Gastroenterol Hepatol* 2005;2(9):416–422.

McKenzie YA, Alder A, Anderson W, et al. British Dietetic Association evidence-based guidelines for the dietary management of irritable bowel syndrome in adults. *J Human Nutr Diet* 2012;25(3):260–274.

Velasquez-Manoff M. *An epidemic of absence.* New York, NY: Scribner, 2012.

CHAPTER 19

Diet, Dyspepsia, and Peptic Ulcer Disease

P athologies of the upper gastrointestinal (GI) tract, including peptic ulcer disease, dyspepsia, and gastroesophageal reflux disease (GERD), are very common. Proton pump inhibitors such as omeprazole and esomeprazole are among the most commonly prescribed drugs worldwide.

That diet should play a role in the course of symptoms related to irritation of the upper GI tract seems intuitive. Adjustments in diet, including restrictions of spicy food, acidic food (e.g., citrus, tomatoes), alcohol, and caffeine, are common practices, by both clinicians and patients, in efforts to control symptoms of ulcer disease, reflux disease, and dyspepsia. Evidence in support of these intuitive practices is notably scant. However, emerging evidence supports a role for probiotics in peptic ulcer disease, as well as avoidance of food allergens in eosinophilic esophagitis.

OVERVIEW

Diet

There is widespread belief that diet influences the development of upper GI tract pathology, including peptic ulcer disease, functional (non-ulcer) dyspepsia, GERD, and gastric carcinoma. This impression derives largely from variations in population incidence and observational epidemiological studies. Data substantiating associations between ulcer disease and dietary patterns, alcohol, caffeine, and salt have been inconsistent, of limited quality, and overall relatively sparse.

Results from the Health Professionals Follow-up Study, based on observations of more than 47,000 male health professionals in the United States, indicated that dietary fiber reduces the risk of duodenal ulcer (DU)—perhaps by half—comparing the highest to the lowest quintile of intake (1). The protective effect of soluble fiber appeared particularly strong (relative risk [RR] 0.4 for the highest quintile). Observational studies in India and Africa have found that DU is much more common in regions where refined rice or wheat is the predominant grain and much less common in unrefined rice- or wheat-eating regions; these differences persist even when other potential confounders are addressed, suggesting a true effect of dietary fiber (2,3).

A positive association has been reported between DU and both a low intake of dietary fiber and a high intake of refined sugar. In a case-control study of 78 patients with DU and using a food frequency questionnaire, Katschinski et al. (4) observed an association with refined sugar intake but no independent association with fiber (4). They also noted a modest protective effect of vegetable intake, specifically of vegetable fiber.

Intake of vitamin A appears to be protective as well, with an RR below 0.5 for those in the highest compared to the lowest quintile in the Health Professionals Follow-up Study (1).

A positive association between cigarette smoking and the risk of both gastric ulcer (GU) and DU was noted in an earlier prospective cohort study with more than twice as many total cases (5); a linear dose-response relationship was observed. A cross-sectional study using data from the National Health Interview Survey (NHIS) also found that a history of self-reported GI ulcer was associated with current (OR, 1.99) and former (OR, 1.55) tobacco use (6). Smoking is known to stimulate gastric acid secretion via histamine receptors, potentiate ulceration and increase production of potential ulcerogens, and impair wound healing; these are just a few of the many mechanisms likely to be responsible for an effect of cigarettes on the pathogenesis of ulcers (7).

Alcohol is also known to promote acid secretion, but there is little direct evidence to support an association between alcohol consumption and risk of either GU or DU (5). A population-based cohort study in Denmark found that alcohol did increase the risk of peptic ulcer disease in those with increased antibodies to *Helicobacter pylori*, but this effect was much smaller than the corresponding risk associated with smoking (8). In the NHIS study, increased odds of ulceration were associated with former alcohol use (OR, 1.29) (6). GU recurrence rates may be increased in patients who consume alcohol (9), and alcohol may be a risk factor for bleeding peptic ulcers (10).

Dietary intake in a cohort of Japanese men residing in Hawaii was assessed using both a food frequency questionnaire and 24-hour recall, with a corroborating 7-day food record in a subsample. A Western dietary pattern, particularly regular intake of two or more servings of bread per day, appeared to be protective against DU, whereas high intake of salt and soy sauce appeared to increase risk of GU slightly (5).

Ingestion of linoleic acid, an n-6 essential fatty acid, has been shown to increase the production of gastric prostaglandin. A case-control study in 70 male subjects based on this observation demonstrated significantly less linoleic acid in the adipose tissue of the cases of DU than in matched controls (11). It has been hypothesized that deficiency of dietary n-3 fatty acids might contribute to ulcer disease, but to date, limited clinical evidence exists to support this theory (12).

Associations between higher intake of fermented milk products (e.g., yogurt, cheese) and reduced risk of peptic ulcer have been observed in population studies, whereas consumption of unfermented milk is associated with increased risk. This effect may be attributed to the antimicrobial properties of fermented dairy products; *Lactobacillus* and casein inhibit the replication of *H. pylori* (13). Pretreatment with *Lactobacillus*- and *Bifidobacterium*-containing yogurt has been found prospectively to improve the efficacy of quadruple therapy in eradicating residual *H. pylori* after failed triple therapy (14). In addition, pretreatment with *Lactobacillus*-containing yogurt twice daily for 4 weeks has recently been shown to improve the efficacy of first-line *H. pylori* triple therapy (15). Various *Lactobacillus, Saccharomyces,* and *Bifidobacterium* spp. reduce nausea, taste changes, diarrhea, and epigastric pain with standard *H. pylori* therapy (16).

The positive association between milk and ulcer disease is hypothesized to relate to stimulation of gastric acid secretion and masking of symptoms. An association between milk consumption and risk of peptic ulcer disease (both gastric and duodenal) has been reported in a large, prospective, population-based study in Norway (17). In this study, adjustment for the presence of symptoms likely to have led to increased milk consumption failed to eliminate the association.

There has been inconsistency in the definition of nonulcer, or functional, dyspepsia; an international committee revised the definition and diagnostic criteria, which now include all cases of bothersome postprandial fullness, early satiation, epigastric pain, and epigastric burning, in which there is no evidence of structural disease to explain symptoms (18). There is evidence that eradicating *H. pylori* may still have a small benefit in functional dyspepsia (19). A recent study has linked the prevalence and degree of microscopic duodenitis in *H. pylori* infection to the severity of functional dyspepsia symptoms (20).

Applying such a definition, no specific foods or nutrients have been causally implicated, even though symptoms are often induced by meal consumption (21,22). Study of suspected dietary factors, including alcohol and coffee, has failed to support an association (23,24). Foods implicated anecdotally in dyspepsia include onions, peppers, spices, fatty and fried foods, and citrus (25); however, one study did not find any such association to be significant (26).

Many dyspeptic patients appear to practice avoidance of specific foods in an effort to reduce symptoms. Some differences noted between cases and controls in dietary pattern have varied by gender (27). A few small studies have found that women with functional dyspepsia appear to be especially sensitive to dietary fat and have greater fasting and postprandial cholecystokinin (CCK) levels than healthy subjects (28–30). Assessing the impact of dyspepsia on eating patterns, rather than the other way around, Cuperus et al. (25), in a case-control study involving 100 subjects, found no evidence that diet is systematically altered in an effort to relieve dyspeptic symptoms. In one recent study, patients with unexplained dysmotility-like dyspepsia symptoms, such as fullness, nausea, belching, and vomiting, were offered a gluten-free diet if they exhibited signs of mild upper GI enteropathy and had IgA tissue transglutaminase antibodies or HLA DQ2 or DQ8 genotyping consistent with susceptibility to celiac disease. The gluten-free diet in these patients resulted in symptom improvement in 91.9% of cases and serological or histological response in 87.5%, suggesting a potential role for gluten intolerance in a subset of individuals with functional dyspepsia but not overt villous atrophy (31). The evidence for managing a gluten-free diet in individuals diagnosed with celiac disease is addressed in Chapter 18.

Specific food allergies often play a role in eosinophilic esophagitis, a T-helper 2-type (Th2) inflammatory disease refractory to GERD treatment that presents with symptoms of heartburn, food impaction, and dysphagia. Treatment modalities include corticosteroids, immune-suppressing therapies, dietary management, and esophageal dilation. Food antigens such as milk, egg, and wheat are the most common trigger for the disease in children, who frequently respond to dietary elimination (32). Adults are more likely to have evidence of aeroallergen sensitization (e.g., tree and grass pollen) (32). Treatment of adults with an elemental diet, empiric elimination of six major food allergens, and elimination diets directed by skin testing results have been the subject of recent studies, with varying levels of efficacy reported (33–35). A trial of dietary therapy is recommended for all children and motivated adults with a diagnosis of eosinophilic esophagitis (36).

The evidence of association between diet and gastric carcinoma is addressed in Chapter 12. Some prospective and case-control data suggest that consumption of vegetables and, to a lesser extent, fruits is protective against gastric cancer (37–39).

NUTRIENTS, NUTRICEUTICALS, AND FUNCTIONAL FOODS

Capsaicin

Capsaicin, which mediates burning and pain through the gut transient-receptor potential villanoid-1 (TRPV$_1$) (40), is responsible for evoking the sensation of heat associated with spicy food. The belief that capsaicin contributes to dyspepsia or symptoms of heartburn associated with GERD is widespread. Evidence in the medical literature for an effect of capsaicin-containing foods, however, is limited. A small blinded, controlled trial demonstrated a reduction in time to peak symptoms of heartburn when capsaicin was provided along with a test meal (41). It is noteworthy that acute exposure to a capsaicin solution promotes heartburn (42), but chronic consumption has been shown to protect against development of symptoms in GERD and dyspepsia, possibly due to desensitization of TRPV$_1$ receptors (40).

Ginger

Ginger has anti-inflammatory and analgesic properties and has therefore been used in complementary and alternative medicine for treating a variety of GI ailments (43). In a study of rats with GUs induced by acetic acid, ginger extract significantly reduced the ulcer area (44). Gingerol, a component of ginger extract, has been shown to inhibit the growth of *H. pylori* in vitro (45). However, no human studies have investigated the efficacy of ginger for ameliorating peptic ulcer disease.

◼ CLINICAL HIGHLIGHTS

Despite the prevailing and intuitive view that certain foods irritate the GI tract directly or indirectly by effects on motility, gastroesophageal sphincter tone, or acid production, evidence linking diet or nutrients with peptic ulcer disease, GERD, or dyspepsia is very limited. What evidence there is suggests that a diet high in fiber is likely to be of benefit. There is also increasing evidence for benefit for probiotics in fermented milk products enhancing *H. pylori* eradication therapy and reducing GI side effects of treatment. A trial of dietary therapy is recommended for all children and motivated adults with a diagnosis of eosinophilic esophagitis. On the basis of available evidence, no strong argument can be made for significant adjustment of dietary pattern, including alterations in intake of alcohol or caffeine, specifically to address symptoms of dyspepsia.

Dietary practices consistent with health promotion (see Chapter 45) appear to be appropriate for purposes of preventing or managing dyspepsia or peptic ulcer disease. Because weight loss has been prospectively associated with a dose-dependent reduction in GERD symptoms (46), dietary and physical activity recommendations for weight management in overweight and obese individuals are indicated. A diet rich in fiber should receive emphasis, as is true on general principles. Despite the lack of compelling evidence in the literature, interventions supported by judgment and physiologic mechanism, such as restriction in alcohol, dietary fat, or caffeine intake, are reasonable on a trial basis in individual patients. Advances in the pharmacotherapy of dyspeptic syndromes, including treatment of *H. pylori* and the use of proton pump inhibitors, are such that most patients need not impose dietary restrictions. However, in the setting of emerging evidence for increased risks of bone fractures, B_{12} and magnesium deficiencies, and *Clostridium difficile* infection in elderly and hospitalized patients with long-term proton pump inhibitor use (47), a trial of dietary and lifestyle management is prudent. Avoidance of large meals in close proximity to bedtime is a standard and sensible practice in the treatment of GERD, as are positional adjustments that may diminish reflux.

■ REFERENCES

1. Aldoori WH, Giovannucci EL, Stampfer MJ, et al. Prospective study of diet and the risk of duodenal ulcer in men. *Am J Epidemiol* 1997;145:42.
2. Tovey FI, Hobsley M, Kaushik SP, et al. Duodenal gastric metaplasia and *Helicobacter pylori* infection in high and low duodenal ulcer-prevalent areas in India. *J Gastroenterol Hepatol* 2004;19:497–505.
3. Tovey FI, Hobsley M, Segal I, et al. Duodenal ulcer in South Africa: home-pounded versus milled maize. *J Gastroenterol Hepatol* 2005;20:1008–1111.
4. Katschinski BD, Logan RFA, Edmond M, et al. Duodenal ulcer and refined carbohydrate intake: a case-control study assessing dietary fiber and refined sugar intake. *Gut* 1990;31:993.
5. Kato K, Nomura AM, Stemmerman GN, et al. A prospective study of gastric and duodenal ulcer and its relation to smoking, alcohol, and diet. *Am J Epidemiol* 1992;135:521.
6. Garrow D, Delegge MH. Risk factors for gastrointestinal ulcer disease in the US population. *Dig Dis Sci* 2010;55:66–72.
7. Maity P, Kaushik B, Somenath R, et al. Smoking and the pathogenesis of gastroduodenal ulcer—recent mechanistic update. *Mol Cell Biochem* 2003;253:329–338.
8. Rosenstock S, Jorgensen T, Bennevie O, et al. Risk factors for peptic ulcer disease: a population based prospective cohort study comprising 2416 Danish adults. *Gut* 2003;52:186–193.
9. Miwa H, Sakaki N, Sugano K, et al. Recurrent peptic ulcers in patients following successful *Helicobacter pylori* eradication: a multicenter study of 4940 patients. *Helicobacter* 2004;9:9–16.
10. Kang JM, Kim N, Lee BH, et al. Risk factors for peptic ulcer bleeding in terms of *Helicobacter pylori*, NSAIDs, and antiplatelet agents. *Scand J Gastroenterol* 2011;46:1295–1301.
11. Grant HW, Palmer KR, Riermesma RR, et al. Duodenal ulcer is associated with low dietary linoleic acid intake. *Gut* 1990;31:997.
12. Duggan AE, Atherton JC, Cocaye JC, et al. Clarification of the link between polyunsaturate fats and *Helicobacter pylori*-associated duodenal ulcer disease: a dietary intervention study. *Br J Nutr* 1997;78:515–522.
13. Elmstahl S, Svensson U, Berglund G. Fermented milk products are associated to ulcer disease. Results from a cross-sectional population study. *Eur J Clin Nutr* 1998;52:668.
14. Sheu B, Cheng H, Kao A, et al. Pretreatment with *Lactobacillus-* and *Bifidobacterium*-containing yogurt can improve the efficacy of quadruple therapy in eradicating residual *Helicobacter pylori* infection after failed triple therapy. *Am J Clin Nutr* 2006;83:864–869.
15. Deguchi R, Nakaminami H, Rimbara E, et al. Effect of pretreatment with *Lactobacillus gasseri* OLL2716 on first-line *Helicobacter pylori* eradication therapy. *J Gastroenterol Hepatol* 2012;27:888–892.
16. Malfertheiner P, Selgrad M, Bornschein J. *Helicobacter pylori*: clinical management. *Curr Opin Gastroenterol* 2012;28:608–614.
17. Johnsen R, Forde OH, Straume B, et al. Aetiology of peptic ulcer: a prospective population study in Norway. *J Epidemiol Community Health* 1994;48:156.
18. Tack J, Talley NJ, Camilleri M, et al. Functional gastroduodenal disorders. *Gastroenterology* 2006;130:466.
19. Moayyedi P, Deeks J, Talley NJ, et al. An update of the Cochrane systematic review of *Helicobacter pylori* eradication therapy in nonulcer dyspepsia: resolving the discrepancy between systematic reviews. *Am J Gastroenterol* 2003;98:2621–2626.
20. Mirbagheri SA, Khajavirad N, Rakhshani N, et al. Impact of *Helicobacter pylori* infection and microscopic duodenal histopathological changes on clinical symptoms of patients with functional dyspepsia. *Dig Dis Sci* 2012;57:967–972.
21. Scolapio JS, Camilleri M. Nonulcer dyspepsia. *Gastroenterologist* 1996;4:13.
22. Talley NJ, Phillips SF. Non-ulcer dyspepsia: potential causes and pathophysiology. *Ann Intern Med* 1988;108:865.
23. Talley NJ, McNeil D, Piper DW. Environmental factors and chronic unexplained dyspepsia: association with acetaminophen but no other analgesics, alcohol, coffee, tea or smoking. *Dig Dis Sci* 1988;33:641.
24. Feinle-Bisset C, Horowitz M. Dietary factors in functional dyspepsia. *Neurogastroenterol Motil* 2006;18:608–618.
25. Cuperus P, Keeling PWN, Gibney MJ. Eating patterns in functional dyspepsia: a case control study. *Eur J Clin Nutr* 1996;50:520.
26. Saito YA, Locke GR 3rd, Weaver AL, et al. Diet and functional gastrointestinal disorders: a population-based case-control study. *Am J Gastroenterol* 2005;100:2743–2748.
27. Mullan A, Kavanagh P, O'Mahony P, et al. Food and nutrient intakes and eating patterns in functional and organic dyspepsia. *Eur J Clin Nutr* 1994;48:97.
28. Bjornsson E, Sjoberg J, Ringstrom G, et al. Effects of duodenal lipids on gastric sensitivity and relaxation in patients with ulcer-like and dysmotility-like dyspepsia. *Digestion* 2003;67:209–217.

29. Pilichiewicz AN, Horowitz M, Holtmann GJ, et al. Relationship between symptoms and dietary patterns in patients with functional dyspepsia. *Clin Gastroenterol Hepatol* 2009;7:317–322.

30. Pilichiewicz AN, Feltrin KL, Horowitz M, et al. Functional dyspepsia is associated with a greater symptomatic response to fat but not carbohydrate, increased fasting, and postprandial CCK, and diminished PYY. *Am J Gastroenterol* 2008;103:2613–2623.

31. Santolaria S, Alcedo J, Cuartero B, et al. Spectrum of gluten-sensitive enteropathy in patients with dysmotility-like dyspepsia. *Gastroenterol Hepatol* 2013;36:11–20.

32. Straumann A, Aceves SS, Blanchard C, et al. Pediatric and adult eosinophilic esophagitis: similarities and differences. *Allergy* 2012;67:477–490.

33. Peterson KA, Byrne KR, Vinson LA, et al. Elemental diet induces histologic response in adult eosinophilic esophagitis. *Am J Gastroenterol* 2013;108:759–766.

34. Lucendo AJ, Arias Á, González-Cervera J, et al. Empiric 6-food elimination diet induced and maintained prolonged remission in patients with adult eosinophilic esophagitis: a prospective study on the food cause of the disease. *J Allergy Clin Immunol* 2013;131:797–804.

35. Molina-Infante J, Martin-Noguerol E, Alvarado-Arenas M, et al. Selective elimination diet based on skin testing has suboptimal efficacy for adult eosinophilic esophagitis. *J Allergy Clin Immunol* 2012;130:1200–1202.

36. Liacouras CA, Furuta GT, Hirano I, et al. Eosinophilic esophagitis: updated consensus recommendations for children and adults. *J Allergy Clin Immunol* 2011;128:3–20.e6.

37. Chyou P-H, Nomura AM, Hankin JH, et al. A case-control study of diet and stomach cancer. *Cancer Res* 1990;50:7501.

38. van den Brandt PA, Goldbohm RA. Nutrition in the prevention of gastrointestinal cancer. *Best Pract Res Clin Gastroenterol* 2006;20:589–603.

39. Steevens J, Schouten LJ, Goldbohm RA, et al. Vegetables and fruits consumption and risk of esophageal and gastric cancer subtypes in the Netherlands Cohort Study. *Int J Cancer* 2011;129:2681–2693.

40. Gonlachanvit S. Are rice and spicy diet good for functional gastrointestinal disorders? *J Neurogastroenterol Motil* 2010;16:131–138.

41. Rodriguez-Stanley S, Collings KL, Robinson M, et al. The effects of capsaicin on reflux, gastric emptying and dyspepsia. *Aliment Pharmacol Ther* 2000;14:129.

42. Kindt S, Vos R, Blondeau K, et al. Influence of intra-oesophageal capsaicin instillation on heartburn induction and oesophageal sensitivity in man. *Neurogastroenterol Motil* 2009;21:1032–e82.

43. Ojewole JA. Analgesic, anti-inflammatory and hypoglycaemic effects of ethanol extract of *Zingiber officinale* (Roscoe) rhizomes (Zingiberaceae) in mice and rats. *Phytother Res* 2006;20:764–772.

44. Ko JK, Leung CC. Ginger extract and polaprezinc exert gastroprotective actions by anti-oxidant and growth factor modulating effects in rats. *J Gastroenterol Hepatol* 2010;25:1861–1868.

45. Mahady GB, Pendland SL, Yun GS, et al. Ginger (*Zingiber officinale* Roscoe) and the gingerols inhibit the growth of Cag A+ strains of *Helicobacter pylori*. *Anticancer Res* 2003;23:3699–3702.

46. Ness-Jensen E, Lindam A, Lagergren J, et al. Weight loss and reduction in gastroesophageal reflux. A prospective population-based cohort study: the HUNT study. *Am J Gastroenterol* 2013;108:376–382.

47. Abraham NS. Proton pump inhibitors: potential adverse effects. *Curr Opin Gastroenterol* 2012;28:615–620.

■ SUGGESTED READING

Aldoori WH, Giovannucci EL, Stampfer MJ, et al. A prospective study of alcohol, smoking, caffeine, and the risk of duodenal ulcer in men. *Epidemiology* 1997;8:420.

Barbara L, Camilleri M, Corinaldesi R, et al. Definitions and investigation of dyspepsia, consensus of an international ad hoc working party. *Dig Dis Sci* 1989;34:1272.

Colin-Jones DG, Bloom B, Bodemar G, et al. Management of dyspepsia: report of a working party. *Lancet* 1988;1:576.

Heading RC. Definitions of dyspepsia. *Scand J Gastroenterol* 1991;26:1.

CHAPTER 20

Diet and Rheumatologic Disease

I nterest among patients in dietary management of various inflammatory diseases of soft tissue and joints generally exceeds the availability of rigorously obtained scientific evidence. Much of the evidence in support of nutritional therapies for rheumatologic conditions is preliminary or anecdotal. There are, however, clear links between diet and the natural history of certain arthritides. Further, there is a biologically plausible link between dietary patterns and inflammatory activity in general.

Preliminary evidence of the beneficial effects of n-3 fatty acids in rheumatoid arthritis (RA) is fortified by the clearly established role of polyunsaturated fats in the manufacture of inflammatory and anti-inflammatory cytokines. The impact of diet on weight may indirectly have important effects on the degree to which arthritis of any etiology translates into functional limitations and on its rate of progression. Rheumatologic diseases arising from errors in intermediate metabolism, such as gout, are decisively influenced by diet. There is sufficient evidence of possible benefit, and sufficiently limited evidence of likely toxicity, to support consideration of nutritional interventions for osteoarthritis (OA), RA, and gout.

Evidence for nutritional therapies in other conditions is less interpretable. In general, the magnitude of benefit from nutritional interventions appears insufficient to replace conventional treatments; nutritional and pharmacologic interventions should be considered potentially complementary. Several drugs commonly used to treat rheumatologic diseases may put patients at risk of certain nutritional deficiencies; supplementation may therefore be warranted. The dissemination of unsubstantiated claims for nutrients with healing properties in diverse rheumatologic conditions does a disservice to patients by cultivating misapprehensions and perhaps even more so

to physicians, among whom this trend may cultivate inattention to the actual potential benefits of nutritional therapies. However, in situations in which conventional treatments are undesirable, ineffective, or inadequately effective, dietary therapy may be appropriate even in the absence of robust evidence; absence of evidence is not necessarily evidence of absence.

OVERVIEW

Diet

Overall dietary pattern may influence the risk of rheumatologic disease as well as the risk of functional limitations in the advent of such disease. Mechanisms for these associations are both direct and indirect. Directly, there is a link between dietary pattern and immune function, mediated by a variety of micronutrients, including antioxidant substances and zinc (Chapter 4), as well as the pattern of fatty acid intake (1). Indirectly, diet influences the impact of arthritic conditions on function by contributing to overall health status and the extent of comorbidities, including vascular disease.

Most of the claims for an effect of general dietary pattern on the development and progression of rheumatologic conditions are consistent with dietary recommendations for general health maintenance. Excess body weight secondary to caloric excess increases joint stress and particularly may exacerbate and accelerate OA. In other forms of arthritis, the spondyloarthropathies, and related conditions, obesity may contribute to functional limitations.

General recommendations for abundant fruit and vegetable intake are mostly consistent with the literature on diet and rheumatologic conditions, with some exceptions. Although there is little solid evidence to support the contention, lay literature consistently raises concerns about a link between the nightshade vegetables and "arthritis" in general.

One of the limitations of the abundant, unreviewed literature on nutrition and arthritis is the tendency to refer to arthritis as a collective entity and a failure to distinguish among the many types, etiologies, and pathophysiologies the category includes. Claims for the effects of a particular nutrient or class of nutrients on the whole spectrum of arthritic diseases seem inherently implausible, although some argument may be made for the generalized anti-inflammatory properties of certain aspects of diet. In particular, the anti-inflammatory properties of n-3 fatty acids may confer benefit in a variety of inflammatory conditions, although the effect on RA is most studied (2,3).

Diet and Specific Rheumatologic Disorders

Osteoarthritis

Degenerative arthritis of the weight-bearing joints is convincingly accelerated by obesity; therefore, weight management is an important element in both the prevention and management of OA of the knees and hips (4–7). Rapid, substantial weight loss through dietary restriction may have significant benefits on symptoms and functionality in overweight patients (6,8). Physical activity is beneficial in OA directly by maintaining mobility and indirectly by contributing to weight maintenance (9,10). Messier et al. (11) demonstrated in a large randomized trial that the combination of dietary weight loss plus exercise (compared to either alone, or a control group receiving educational materials) resulted in significant long-term symptomatic improvement in obese sedentary people with OA. If OA is advanced, exercise may need to be selected to minimize stress to joints; swimming is often appropriate.

The relationship between obesity and OA in non–weight-bearing joints such as the hands is poorly understood (12,13), though adipokines (14) may play a role, and systemic inflammation (15) may affect muscle strength.

Observational data suggested an association between low vitamin K levels and increased OA of the hand and knee (16), though clinical trial data suggest no relationship (17). A limited number of cohort and randomized trials suggest that antioxidant supplements may confer some benefit in OA, though evidence from clinical trials has been conflicting (18). In particular, benefit has been seen in observational studies with high dietary intake or supplementation of vitamin E, carotenoids, and vitamin C (12), as well as in clinical trials of various antioxidant supplements of botanical origin (19,20). Data from the Framingham OA Cohort Study suggest that low dietary intake and low serum levels of vitamin D may contribute to the progression of OA; high intake may offer some protection (12,21), although this remains uncertain (22) and under active investigation (23). Methylsulfonylmethane (MSM), an organosulfur compound marketed as a dietary supplement, has shown some promise for the treatment of OA symptoms in two small clinical trials (24,25).

Gout

Gout, the result of a defect in intermediate metabolism leading to uric acid accumulation, is decisively influenced by diet. Foods rich in purines facilitate uric acid production and should be avoided; such foods include beer, organ meats, yeast, shellfish, sardines, herring, and bacon (4,26,27). Alcohol, long implicated in gouty flares, leads to increased purine production and decreases renal urate clearance (4,28). Choi et al. (29) demonstrated definitively that there is an increased risk of gout with increasing daily alcohol intake, particularly from beer. Fructose intake may adversely affect uric acid levels (30), though data supporting this association is conflicting (31). Low-fat dairy products and wine may offer protective benefit (31,32). Obesity is associated with hyperuricemia and flares of gout. Epidemiological studies have confirmed a clear dose-response relationship between BMI and the risk of gout (33,34); increasing obesity levels may in part explain the rapid rise in prevalence of gout among Americans over the past two decades (35). Preliminary evidence suggests beneficial effects of low-carbohydrate, calorie-restricted diets generous in monounsaturated fats and higher in total daily protein than has previously been recommended for patients with gout (36). Coffee consumption (caffeinated or decaffeinated) appears to decrease the risk of gout, possibly related to antioxidant effects and reduction of insulin (37). Based on these recent findings, dietary strategies for gout therapy and prevention are now shifting toward an emphasis on weight loss and reduction of insulin resistance (38).

Rheumatoid Arthritis

The major principal dietary approaches to RA are the addition to the diet of foods with anti-inflammatory properties and the elimination of foods with apparent proinflammatory properties (4). Clinical benefits arising from dietary modification may be attributed to a variety of mechanisms, including the modification of gut flora and reducing intestinal permeability (37,39).

A recent systematic review has confirmed consistent evidence that the addition of n-3 fatty acids to the diet may be beneficial in RA (40–42). Studies have largely demonstrated reduction in number of tender joints, duration of morning stiffness (42). Some patients receiving fish oil supplements may be able to reduce or even stop their usage of nonsteroidal anti-inflammatory drugs (NSAIDs) (43,42). As this practice is of apparent benefit for several other conditions (see Section VIIE) and consistent with recommendations for general health promotion, there is little reason not to include it among routine interventions for RA.

Specific recommendations in the literature include intake of up to 12 g per day of linoleic acid and 4 g per day of α-linolenic acid, while restricting arachidonic acid intake to less than 50 mg per day (44). Therapeutic benefit is often seen with 2 to 3 g per day of eicosapentaenoic acid (EPA) and docosahexaenoic acid (DHA) found in fish oil. Higher doses (>3 g per day) of n-3 fatty acids are associated with reduced production of reactive oxygen species (42). Arachidonic acid, found only in animal foods, is eliminated from the diet in strict vegetarians; vegetarianism has been associated with symptomatic relief in RA (44–46). Fasting appears to confer benefits in RA, perhaps by restricting arachidonic acid; however, the benefits are lost when an omnivorous diet is resumed.

A vegetarian diet may sustain the benefits of a fast; clinically significant benefit has been measured in RA patients who undergo fasting followed by vegetarian diets for at least 3 months (47). Other studies report symptomatic relief of RA symptoms with gluten-free vegan diets (48). One randomized trial found that a gluten-free vegan diet significantly decreased oxidized low-density lipoprotein levels and slightly elevated anti-phosphorylcholine IgM and IgA levels (49). In another study, a gluten-free vegan diet was shown to significantly reduce the number of IgG antigliadin and IgG anti-β-lactoglobulin antibodies (45). In a survey

of RA patients, 27% reported intolerances to cow's milk, wheat, and gluten, though no relationship was seen between patients reporting food intolerances and food challenges in rectal mucosa. A low-arachidonic acid ("anti-inflammatory") vegetarian diet supplemented with fish oil was found to improve clinical signs of inflammation in patients with RA, in a double-blind crossover trial (50).

Oxidation apparently contributes to joint inflammation and destruction in RA, suggesting a therapeutic role for antioxidant nutrients. There is some evidence that a combination of antioxidant nutrients, including vitamins E and C and selenium, confers benefit in RA (44,51), while other evidence demonstrates no effect of combination antioxidants (52). Current dietary recommendations for the management of RA therefore include a diet rich in antioxidants, avoidance of animal fat, regular ingestion of fish or soybeans (or both), and avoidance of alcohol (44). There is inconclusive evidence to date linking coffee consumption and risk of RA; further research may be warranted (53–55). In light of conflicting evidence for specific antioxidant supplements, foods containing high amounts of antioxidant nutrients should be emphasized.

Evidence regarding the role of food allergy in RA is preliminary and inconsistent, with some positive and some negative studies in the literature. As many as one-third of RA cases may be influenced by food (4). Foods commonly implicated include cereals, corn, and dairy products. A 2004 epidemiological study found a significant association between inflammatory polyarthritis and high intake of red meat, animal protein, and total protein (OR = 1.9, 2.3, 2.9, respectively) (56), though a 2007 follow-up prospective cohort study found no clear relationship between meat and protein intake and the incidence of RA using Nurse's Health Study data (n = 82,603 women). Assessment for dietary precipitants of arthritis flares, generally by use of a food and symptom diary, is reasonable if not prudent in most cases, with trial elimination of implicated food items (see Chapter 24).

The variability in food allergy requires that such hypotheses be tested on an individual basis, using elimination diets, as some patients can achieve symptomatic relief with restricted diets (46). Suspected foods are eliminated from the diet, and clinical status is monitored. If there is improvement, the same food is reintroduced into the diet. If symptoms recur in convincing association with reexposure to the implicated food, it should be permanently removed from the patient's diet (57).

Although there is considerable interest in the role food sensitivity might play in RA, the evidence to date is still very limited (46,58). A study of elimination diets in 63 children with chronic arthritis revealed in only one case a fairly clear association between dietary intolerance and disease state (59). The authors conclude that food intolerance is likely to be pertinent to only occasional patients with inflammatory arthritis and is clearly not the principal etiologic factor. A controlled study measuring antibodies to dietary antigens found significantly increased production of cross-reactive antibodies in the intestinal fluid of RA patients compared to healthy control, however. The authors suggest that the combination of multiple minor hypersensitivity reactions may have had adverse additive effects in RA patients, resulting in production of autoimmune reactions in their joints (60).

RA is thought to influence dietary intake as a result of both the course of disease and its treatment. Symptoms of RA may cause discomfort during eating or limit access to food; pharmacotherapy may cause anorexia or nausea. There is some evidence that micronutrient deficiencies may be relatively common among patients with RA (41,61). Several trials have shown reduced gastrointestinal (GI) side effects in patients receiving folate supplementation in addition to methotrexate, a drug commonly used in RA and a known folate antagonist (62). Although the role of some of the nutrients in question on the course of RA is speculative, intake meeting the DRI is advisable on other grounds. Therefore, given the available evidence, multivitamin/multimineral supplementation for all patients with RA seems a prudent recourse.

Ankylosing Spondylitis

The association between the seronegative spondyloarthropathies and the HLA-B27 histocompatibility sequence is well established. Efforts to explain this association led to the identification of molecules on *Klebsiella* organisms in the gut with similar sequencing and generated speculation that the bacteria are causally involved in the diseases (63). Small studies suggest that starch restriction reduces serum immunoglobulin A and

symptoms in patients with ankylosing spondylitis, apparently by inhibiting the growth of enteric *Klebsiella* (64), while other studies found no relationship between diet and ankylosing spondylitis disease activity (65).

Other Rheumatologic Conditions

Subsumed under the rubric of rheumatologic conditions is a wide array of pathologies involving joints and soft tissue by mechanisms of pathology known in some cases and unknown in others. The autoimmune basis for inflammatory conditions of blood vessels, neurons, skin, and so on is clear in many cases, even if the specific antigens are not. In conditions ranging from vasculitis to dermatitis, polymyositis to polyarteritis to systemic lupus, dietary interventions directed toward reduced inflammatory response (see above, and Chapters 11 and 21) are appropriate, if often not of proven therapeutic value. As such dietary adjustments—reduced intake of saturated fat and trans fat as well as increased intake of fruits, vegetables, and unsaturated oils, with particular emphasis on n-3 fatty acids—conform to the features of a health-promoting diet, they are advisable even in the absence of confirmed, condition-specific utility. As Mediterranean-style diets tend to be health-promoting and can reduce risk of a variety of chronic disease, as well as possibly provide symptomatic relief (66), they are prudent recommendations in a variety of inflammatory conditions. As obesity itself is a proinflammatory condition (67,68) and can exacerbate disease activity, targeted weight-loss programs can also be beneficial in obese patients with inflammatory rheumatologic conditions.

In some cases, the etiology and pathogenesis of rheumatologic conditions are entirely unclear. Salient examples include fibromyalgia and chronic fatigue syndrome. Autoimmune mechanisms have been suggested for both but are unconfirmed theories that compete with others (69–77). Dietary management has been espoused for both conditions, although in neither case is there definitive evidence of efficacy for any specific treatment (76,78–83). There is, however, general support for what may be considered "dietary hygiene" (i.e., an effort to improve the overall dietary pattern for health promotion, along with n-3 fatty acid supplementation and consideration of food sensitivities and intolerances).

The use of an intravenous nutrient infusion known as the "Myers' cocktail" (84), containing B vitamins, vitamin C, magnesium, and calcium, is a popular treatment modality for both fibromyalgia and chronic fatigue syndromes (as well as other conditions) in complementary/alternative medicine (CAM) practice. Until recently, reports of therapeutic efficacy were anecdotal, if widespread. The first clinical trial of the Myers' cocktail for fibromyalgia was completed in the author's lab, with equivocal results (84).

NUTRIENTS, NUTRICEUTICALS, AND FUNCTIONAL FOODS

Fatty Acids

As discussed in Chapters 6, 7, 11, 12, 44, and 45, the prevailing diet in the United States provides a preponderance of n-6 over n-3 polyunsaturated fatty acids. Modern diets provide n-6 to n-3 fatty acids in an approximate 11:1 ratio. Paleolithic intake apparently ranged from 4:1 to 1:1 (85). The metabolism of n-3 fatty acids leads to generation of anti-inflammatory cytokines (see Figure xx). Eicosapentaenoic acid and docosahexaenoic acid, ingested as marine oils or manufactured endogenously from α-linolenic acid, inhibit the production of arachidonic acid–derived proinflammatory eicosanoids (86).

Dietary n-3 fatty acids have been shown to ameliorate symptoms in RA (40–42). A systematic review of 23 studies found a consistent, modest improvement in joint swelling and pain with n-3 fatty acids (42). See Chapter 45 for other lines of argument supporting increased n-3 fatty acid intake.

Vitamin D

In addition to effects on bone and calcium metabolism, vitamin D can have immunosuppressive effects. 1,25-dihydroxyvitamin [OH]$_2$ D$_3$, the biologically active form, interacts with vitamin D receptors that are expressed on osteoblasts, T cells, dendritic cells (DCs), macrophages, and B cells (87).

Adequate vitamin D may be a protective factor for various autoimmune diseases (88); vitamin D supplementation may be beneficial for B cell–mediated autoimmune diseases such as RA and systemic lupus erythematosus (87). Thus, clinicians should routinely assess vitamin D status and supplement as warranted in persons with rheumatologic conditions.

Probiotics

Some probiotics have anti-inflammatory properties that are strain- and species-specific (87,89). These anti-inflammatory effects may be modulated through interactions with intestinal epithelial cells. Gut immune function can be modified by the composition of intestinal flora and can affect intestinal barrier function (87). There are shared inflammatory pathways in the GI system and joints; arthralgia and spondyloarthropathy of axial and peripheral joints are often found in patients with inflammatory bowel diseases (90). Thus, targeted probiotic supplementation may be a reasonable intervention in a multimodal approach to inflammatory conditions. There is emerging evidence that alterations in immune stimulation in early childhood (the "hygiene hypothesis") promotes inflammation and autoimmunity (91). Consequently, reduced exposure to parasites and microorganisms may contribute to the increased incidence of a variety of immune-mediated conditions (92). This is an area of active research and interest in treatments such as fecal microbiota transplantation (93).

Glucosamine Sulfate

Glucosamine is found in the body as a precursor of glycosaminoglycans, which are used by chondrocytes in the manufacture of proteoglycans incorporated into articular cartilage. The body's manufacture of glucosamine declines with age at variable rates, apparently leaving some people vulnerable to deficiency. The use of supplemental glucosamine is promoted as a means of compensating for a decline in endogenous production, thereby reconstituting worn articular surfaces.

Although glucosamine is available in various forms, its use as a sulfate salt is most convincingly supported by available evidence, perhaps because sulfur is another integral component of cartilage. Glucosamine available as a nutriceutical agent is derived from the exoskeletons of shrimp, lobsters, and crabs.

Data from a number of methodologically rigorous studies, including double-blind, randomized trials, have suggested the efficacy of glucosamine in OA of the lower limbs (61,94–96). Glucosamine works slowly by reconstituting cartilage and has no known direct analgesic properties, although anti-inflammatory effects have been reported (97); therefore, pain relief is faster with NSAIDs. One recent controlled trial found that glucosamine significantly reduced arthritic joint space narrowing over a period of 3 years (98).

One double-blind trial demonstrated superior pain relief with ibuprofen at 2 weeks but a superior effect of glucosamine at 4 weeks (99). There is evidence that NSAIDs, while alleviating symptoms, may actually accelerate the degeneration of articular cartilage (100,101). There is no known toxicity of glucosamine sulfate. Doses up to 1,500 mg daily are generally recommended (96); higher doses may be required in obese patients or those on diuretics.

A 2009 Cochrane review assessing randomized controlled trials of glucosamine for OA concluded that glucosamine was superior to placebo for treating pain and improving functionality in osteoarthritis, with a safety profile comparable to placebo (94) More recent data demonstrated equivalent effects of glucosamine sulfate, celecoxib (a COX-2 inhibitor), and placebo on pain and function in adults with moderate-to-severe knee OA (102). More recent trials have been negative, however. A 2013 meta-analysis concluded that glucosamine is ineffective for pain control in OA of the knee, but may have functional benefits when used for more than 6 months (103).

Cartilage Extracts and Chondroitin Sulfate

Some alternative medicine publications advocate the use of various cartilage extracts, including shark cartilage, sea cucumber, chondroitin sulfate, and green-lipped mussel for chronic, degenerative arthroses. These products either contain glycosaminoglycans or, in the case of chondroitin, are glycosaminoglycans and putatively function by incorporation into joints (104). However, absorption is very poor, with undetectable levels of dietary chondroitin sulfate in rigorous trials, and may actually reduce absorption of glucosamine in combination (105).

The available evidence and the established pharmacokinetics support the use of glucosamine over these products, although chondroitin does show highly significant efficacy over placebo in

some trials (106,107). The combination of chondroitin sulfate and glucosamine sulfate has become popular, and as noted previously, a recent large multicenter trial found evidence of significant pain reduction in a subgroup of subjects with moderate-to-severe OA of the knee (108), while other studies have found no particular benefits of the combination (107). Thus, as with glucosamine, the therapeutic efficacy of chondroitin deserves further investigation.

S-Adenosyl-L-Methionine (SAMe)

A popular alternative therapy for OA, S-adenosyl-L-methionine (SAMe) is a compound derived from the amino acid L-methionine and ATP. Although evidence is limited, a meta-analysis by Soeken et al. (109) found SAMe to have efficacy equivalent to that of NSAIDs in reducing functional limitation and pain in patients with OA and to have fewer side effects. Most clinical trials have used 600 to 1,200 mg per day.

Nightshade Vegetables

The nightshade family of plants, known scientifically as the *Solanaceae*, has been implicated in the alternative medicine literature as a cause of arthritis. The literature is poorly substantiated and the type of arthritis rarely specified.

The family *Solanaceae* is diverse and includes potatoes, tomatoes, red peppers, eggplant, tobacco, paprika, pimento, cayenne pepper, and chili pepper. There is little evidence to support elimination of one or more of these foods from the diet to manage any particular type of arthritis. Elimination diets, however, are occasionally helpful in RA, and the elimination of nightshades might be considered in that context in an effort to manage refractory disease.

Herbal Products

Several botanicals have shown promise in alleviating symptoms of OA (110). Capsaicin, derived from chili peppers, has shown benefit in improving pain and articular tenderness in patients with OA when applied topically (111) and is conditionally recommended as an initial pharmacologic intervention for OA by the American College of Rheumatology (112). Preliminary evidence is promising for ginger as a treatment for pain in patients with OA (113,114). A systematic review found encouraging evidence for avocado-soybean unsaponifiables, although further research is clearly needed (115). The most clinically effective formulation of avocado-soybean unsaponifiable is considered a prescription drug in some countries (116). Devil's claw (*Harpagophytum procumbens*) may have benefit, but it is thought to be an herbal COX-2 inhibitor, so caution is warranted (117).

Other Nutriceuticals

Genistein, an isoflavone found in a variety of plants (including soybeans) and pycnogenol, an antioxidant derived from pine bark (as well as other sources) has demonstrated some preclinical anti-inflammatory properties. Other nutriceuticals demonstrating anti-inflammatory effects include epigallocatechin-3-gallate (found in green tea), as well as resveratrol (found in red grapes) (116).

Nutrigenomic Considerations

Nutritional factors can affect gene expression through epigenetic modification, and may be an emerging area of focus in autoimmune and inflammatory conditions. Some inflammatory response disease genes have been shown to be affected by epigenetic regulatory mechanisms (118). For example, Rho iso-alpha acids from hops have been shown to have properties that inhibit NF-kappaB-mediated inflammatory markers in some cell models (119). This emerging area of therapeutics has the potential to help tailor nutritional interventions to persons with specific genetic polymorphisms.

Diet/Drug and Nutrient/Drug Interactions of Importance (120)

As RA is a progressive disease, it often requires the successive use of more toxic drugs with serious effects on nutritional status. There is also a risk of developing drug-induced osteoporosis with longer regimens of corticosteroids and cytotoxic drugs.

Many cytotoxic drugs (i.e., methotrexate) are folate antagonists, and will thus decrease folate levels and increase homocysteine levels. Supplemental folate may decrease the efficacy of the drug. Methotrexate can also cause mouth ulcers that can affect food consumption. Cyclosporine can induce hyperglycemia, hypercholesterolemia, electrolyte disturbances, and renal insufficiency.

Other drug–nutrient interactions of significance in rheumatic disease:

- NSAIDs should be taken with food to prevent GI upset.
- Glucocorticoids and corticosteroids can cause stomach upset and should be taken after eating a meal. They may also cause protein wasting.
- Penicillamine is a chelating agent for copper, iron, and zinc, and can cause sodium depletion and vitamin B_6 deficiency.
- Avoid grapefruit juice with cyclosporine
- Sulfasalazine reduces the absorption of folic acid

■ CLINICAL HIGHLIGHTS

There is sufficient evidence to justify offering tailored dietary advice to patients suffering from various forms of arthritis. Avoidance of obesity is a mainstay (see Chapter 5). A Mediterranian-style diet conforming to recommendations for health promotion (see Chapter 45) is advisable on general principles and for its favorable influences on inflammation.

A vegetarian diet may be advantageous in RA and, provided that all nutrient needs are met (see Chapter 43), is conducive to health-promotion goals. Alcohol intake should be restricted or avoided. Regular consumption of fish and regular use of flaxseed oil as a means of increasing n-3 fatty acid intake are advisable both for arthritis management and on general principles (see Chapter 45). Fish oil supplementation containing 1 g of n-3 fatty acids daily is reasonable, and in progressive RA, a trial of higher-dose therapy may be warranted.

The use of glucosamine sulfate shows mixed results regarding efficacy and is safe, but published evidence to date demonstrates greater effects for functionality rather than pain control. A trial of glucosamine sulfate 500 mg three times daily for patients with chronic joint pain seems appropriate, and even more so in patients intolerant of NSAIDs. Fasting and elimination diets may offer at least temporary relief to a minority of patients with RA. The avoidance of nightshade vegetables does not appear to offer any consistent benefit, although the practice is supported by anecdotal reports. Use of food and symptom diaries to identify food sensitivities and intolerances is advisable in virtually all rheumatologic or autoimmune conditions refractory to initial interventions.

ACKNOWLEDGMENT

The technical assistance of Nicholas Scoulios and Theresa Weiss is appreciated.

REFERENCES

1. Alcock J, Franklin ML, Kuzawa CW. Nutrient signaling: evolutionary origins of the immune-modulating effects of dietary fat. *Quart Rev Biol* 2012;87(3):187–223.
2. Sperling RI. Eicosanoids in rheumatoid arthritis. *Rheumatic Dis Clin North Am* 1995;21(3):741–758.
3. Simopoulos AP. Omega-3 fatty acids in inflammation and autoimmune diseases. *J Am Coll Nutr* 2002;21(6):495–505.
4. Cleland LG, Hill CL, James MJ. Diet and arthritis. *Bailliere's Clin Rheumatol* 1995;9(4):771–785.
5. Miller GD, Nicklas BJ, Davis C, et al. Intensive weight loss program improves physical function in older obese adults with knee osteoarthritis. *Obesity* 2006;14(7):1219–1230.
6. Vincent HK, Heywood K, Connelly J, et al. Obesity and weight loss in the treatment and prevention of osteoarthritis. *PM R* 2012;4(5 suppl):S59–S67.
7. Toivanen AT, Heliovaara M, Impivaara O, et al. Obesity, physically demanding work and traumatic knee injury are major risk factors for knee osteoarthritis—a population-based study with a follow-up of 22 years. *Rheumatology* 2010;49(2):308–314.
8. Christensen R, Astrup A, Bliddal H. Weight loss: the treatment of choice for knee osteoarthritis? A randomized trial. *Osteoarthritis Cartilage* 2005;13(1):20–27.
9. Thomas KS, Muir KR, Doherty M, et al. Home based exercise programme for knee pain and knee osteoarthritis: randomised controlled trial. *BMJ* 2002;325(7367):752.
10. Semanik PA, Chang RW, Dunlop DD. Aerobic activity in prevention and symptom control of osteoarthritis. *PM R* 2012;4(5 suppl):S37–S44.
11. Messier SP, Loeser RF, Miller GD, et al. Exercise and dietary weight loss in overweight and obese older adults with knee osteoarthritis: the Arthritis, Diet, and Activity Promotion Trial. *Arthritis Rheum* 2004;50(5):1501–1510.
12. McAlindon T, Felson DT. Nutrition: risk factors for osteoarthritis. *Ann Rheum Dis* 1997;56(7):397–400.
13. Sayer AA, Poole J, Cox V, et al. Weight from birth to 53 years: a longitudinal study of the influence on clinical hand osteoarthritis. *Arthritis Rheum* 2003;48(4):1030–1033.
14. Berenbaum F, Eymard F, Houard X. Osteoarthritis, inflammation and obesity. *Curr opin Rheumatol* 2013;25(1):114–118.
15. Sanchez-Ramirez DC, van der Leeden M, van der Esch M, et al. Association of serum C-reactive protein and erythrocyte sedimentation rate with muscle strength in patients with knee osteoarthritis. *Rheumatology* 2013;52(4):727–732.
16. Neogi T, Booth SL, Zhang YQ, et al. Low vitamin K status is associated with osteoarthritis in the hand and knee. *Arthritis Rheum* 2006;54(4):1255–1261.
17. Neogi T, Felson DT, Sarno R, et al. Vitamin K in hand osteoarthritis: results from a randomised clinical trial. *Ann Rheum Dis* 2008;67(11):1570–1573.
18. Wluka AE, Stuckey S, Brand C, et al. Supplementary vitamin E does not affect the loss of cartilage volume in knee osteoarthritis: a 2 year double blind randomized placebo controlled study. *J Rheumatol* 2002;29(12):2585–2591.
19. Levy R, Khokhlov A, Kopenkin S, et al. Efficacy and safety of flavocoxid compared with naproxen in subjects with osteoarthritis of the knee—a subset analysis. *Adv Ther* 2010;27(12):953–962.
20. Farid R, Rezaieyazdi Z, Mirfeizi Z, et al. Oral intake of purple passion fruit peel extract reduces pain and stiffness and improves physical function in adult patients with knee osteoarthritis. *Nutr Res* 2010;30(9):601–606.
21. Castillo EC, Hernandez-Cueto MA, Vega-Lopez MA, et al. Effects of vitamin D supplementation during the induction and progression of osteoarthritis in a rat model. *Evid Based Complement Alternat Med* 2012;2012:156563.
22. Felson DT, Niu J, Clancy M, et al. Low levels of vitamin D and worsening of knee osteoarthritis: results of two longitudinal studies. *Arthritis Rheu* 2007;56(1):129–136.
23. Cao Y, Jones G, Cicuttini F, et al. Vitamin D supplementation in the management of knee osteoarthritis: study protocol for a randomized controlled trial. *Trials* 2012;13:131.
24. Kim LS, Axelrod LJ, Howard P, et al. Efficacy of methylsulfonylmethane (MSM) in osteoarthritis pain of the knee: a pilot clinical trial. *Osteoarthritis Cartilage* 2006;14(3):286–294.
25. Debbi EM, Agar G, Fichman G, et al. Efficacy of methylsulfonylmethane supplementation on osteoarthritis of the knee: a randomized controlled study. *BMC Complement Alternat Med* 2011;11:50.
26. Dohan JL. Purine-rich foods and the risk of gout in men. *N Engl J Med* 2004;350(24):2520–2521.
27. Choi HK, Liu S, Curhan G. Intake of purine-rich foods, protein, and dairy products and relationship to serum levels of uric acid: the Third National Health and Nutrition Examination Survey. *Arthritis Rheum* 2005;52(1):283–289.
28. Choi HK, Mount DB, Reginato AM; American College of Physicians, American Physiological Society. Pathogenesis of gout. *Ann Intern Med* 2005;143(7):499–516.
29. Choi HK, Atkinson K, Karlson EW, et al. Alcohol intake and risk of incident gout in men: a prospective study. *Lancet* 2004;363(9417):1277–1281.
30. Wang DD, Sievenpiper JL, de Souza RJ, et al. The effects of fructose intake on serum uric acid vary among controlled dietary trials. *J Nutr* 2012;142(5):916–923.
31. Zgaga L, Theodoratou E, Kyle J, et al. The association of dietary intake of purine-rich vegetables, sugar-sweetened beverages and dairy with plasma urate, in a cross-sectional study. *PLoS One* 2012;7(6):e38123.
32. Choi HK, Atkinson K, Karlson EW, et al. Purine-rich foods, dairy and protein intake, and the risk of gout in men. *N Engl J Med* 2004;350(11):1093–1103.
33. Chen JH, Pan WH, Hsu CC, et al. Impact of obesity and hypertriglyceridemia on gout development with or without hyperuricemia: a prospective study. *Arthritis Care Res* 2013;65(1):133–140.

34. Juraschek SP, Miller ER 3rd, Gelber AC. Body mass index, obesity, and prevalent gout in the United States in 1988–1994 and 2007–2010. *Arthritis Care Res* 2013;65(1):127–132.

35. Wallace KL, Riedel AA, Joseph-Ridge N, et al. Increasing prevalence of gout and hyperuricemia over 10 years among older adults in a managed care population. *J Rheumatol* 2004;31(8):1582–1587.

36. Dessein PH, Shipton EA, Stanwix AE, et al. Beneficial effects of weight loss associated with moderate calorie/carbohydrate restriction, and increased proportional intake of protein and unsaturated fat on serum urate and lipoprotein levels in gout: a pilot study. *Ann Rheum Dis* 2000;59(7):539–543.

37. Li S, Micheletti R. Role of diet in rheumatic disease. *Rheum Dis Clin North Am* 2011;37(1):119–133.

38. Lee SJ, Terkeltaub RA, Kavanaugh A. Recent developments in diet and gout. *Curr Opin Rheumatol* 2006;18(2):193–198.

39. Rayman MP, Pattison DJ. Dietary manipulation in musculoskeletal conditions. *Best Pract Res Clin Rheumatol* 2008;22(3):535–561.

40. Calder PC, Zurier RB. Polyunsaturated fatty acids and rheumatoid arthritis. *Curr Opin Clin Nutr Metab Care* 2001;4(2):115–121.

41. Rennie KL, Hughes J, Lang R, et al. Nutritional management of rheumatoid arthritis: a review of the evidence. *J Human Nutr Diet* 2003;16(2):97–109.

42. Miles EA, Calder PC. Influence of marine n-3 polyunsaturated fatty acids on immune function and a systematic review of their effects on clinical outcomes in rheumatoid arthritis. *Br J Nutr* 2012;107(suppl 2):S171–S184.

43. Kremer JM. n-3 Fatty acid supplements in rheumatoid arthritis. *Am J Clin Nutr* 2000;71(1 suppl):349S–351S.

44. Adam O. Anti-inflammatory diet in rheumatic diseases. *Eur J Clin Nutr* 1995;49(10):703–717.

45. Hafstrom I, Ringertz B, Spangberg A, et al. A vegan diet free of gluten improves the signs and symptoms of rheumatoid arthritis: the effects on arthritis correlate with a reduction in antibodies to food antigens. *Rheumatol* 2001;40(10):1175–1179.

46. Smedslund G, Byfuglien MG, Olsen SU, et al. Effectiveness and safety of dietary interventions for rheumatoid arthritis: a systematic review of randomized controlled trials. *J Am Diet Assoc* 2010;110(5):727–735.

47. Muller H, de Toledo FW, Resch KL. Fasting followed by vegetarian diet in patients with rheumatoid arthritis: a systematic review. *Scand J Rheumatol* 2001;30(1):1–10.

48. Liden M, Kristjansson G, Valtysdottir S, et al. Self-reported food intolerance and mucosal reactivity after rectal food protein challenge in patients with rheumatoid arthritis. *Scand J Rheumatol* 2010;39(4):292–298.

49. Elkan AC, Sjoberg B, Kolsrud B, et al. Gluten-free vegan diet induces decreased LDL and oxidized LDL levels and raised atheroprotective natural antibodies against phosphorylcholine in patients with rheumatoid arthritis: a randomized study. *Arthritis Res Ther* 2008;10(2):R34.

50. Adam O, Beringer C, Kless T, et al. Anti-inflammatory effects of a low arachidonic acid diet and fish oil in patients with rheumatoid arthritis. *Rheumatol Int* 2003;23(1):27–36.

51. Darlington LG, Stone TW. Antioxidants and fatty acids in the amelioration of rheumatoid arthritis and related disorders. *Br J Nutr* 2001;85(3):251–269.

52. Bae SC, Jung WJ, Lee EJ, et al. Effects of antioxidant supplements intervention on the level of plasma inflammatory molecules and disease severity of rheumatoid arthritis patients. *J Am Coll Nutr* 2009;28(1):56–62.

53. Karlson EW, Mandl LA, Aweh GN, et al. Coffee consumption and risk of rheumatoid arthritis. *Arthritis Rheum* 2003;48(11):3055–3060.

54. Mikuls TR, Cerhan JR, Criswell LA, et al. Coffee, tea, and caffeine consumption and risk of rheumatoid arthritis: results from the Iowa Women's Health Study. *Arthritis Rheum* 2002;46(1):83–91.

55. Pedersen M, Stripp C, Klarlund M, et al. Diet and risk of rheumatoid arthritis in a prospective cohort. *J Rheumatol* 2005;32(7):1249–1252.

56. Pattison DJ, Symmons DP, Lunt M, et al. Dietary risk factors for the development of inflammatory polyarthritis: evidence for a role of high level of red meat consumption. *Arthritis Rheum* 2004;50(12):3804–3812.

57. Denton C. The elimination/challenge diet. *Minn Med* 2012;95(12):43–44.

58. Martin RH. The role of nutrition and diet in rheumatoid arthritis. *Proc Nutr Soc* 1998;57(2):231–234.

59. Schrander JJ, Marcelis C, de Vries MP, et al. Does food intolerance play a role in juvenile chronic arthritis? *Br J Rheumatol* 1997;36(8):905–908.

60. Hvatum M, Kanerud L, Hallgren R, et al. The gut-joint axis: cross reactive food antibodies in rheumatoid arthritis. *Gut* 2006;55(9):1240–1247.

61. Stone J, Doube A, Dudson D, et al. Inadequate calcium, folic acid, vitamin E, zinc, and selenium intake in rheumatoid arthritis patients: results of a dietary survey. *Sem Arthritis Rheum* 1997;27(3):180–185.

62. Whittle SL, Hughes RA. Folate supplementation and methotrexate treatment in rheumatoid arthritis: a review. *Rheumatology* 2004;43(3):267–271.

63. Ebringer A, Wilson C. The use of a low starch diet in the treatment of patients suffering from ankylosing spondylitis. *Clin Rheumatol* 1996;15(suppl 1):62–66.

64. Ebringer A, Rashid T, Tiwana H, et al. A possible link between Crohn's disease and ankylosing spondylitis via Klebsiella infections. *Clin Rheumatol* 2007;26(3):289–297.

65. Sundstrom B, Wallberg-Jonsson S, Johansson G. Diet, disease activity, and gastrointestinal symptoms in patients with ankylosing spondylitis. *Clin Rheumatol* 2011;30(1):71–76.

66. Skoldstam L, Hagfors L, Johansson G. An experimental study of a Mediterranean diet intervention for patients with rheumatoid arthritis. *Ann Rheum Dis* 2003;62(3):208–214.

67. Tran B, Oliver S, Rosa J, et al. Aspects of inflammation and oxidative stress in pediatric obesity and type 1 diabetes: an overview of ten years of studies. *Exp Diabetes Res* 2012;2012:683680.

68. Hursting SD, Dunlap SM. Obesity, metabolic dysregulation, and cancer: a growing concern and an inflammatory (and microenvironmental) issue. *Ann NY Acad Sci* 2012;1271:82–87.

69. Katz DL, Greene L, Ali A, et al. The pain of fibromyalgia syndrome is due to muscle hypoperfusion induced by regional vasomotor dysregulation. *Med Hypotheses* 2007;69(3):517–525.

70. Van Houdenhove B, Luyten P. Stress, depression and fibromyalgia. *Acta Neurol Belg* 2006;106(4):149–156.

71. Buskila D, Sarzi-Puttini P, Ablin JN. The genetics of fibromyalgia syndrome. *Pharmacogenomics* 2007;8(1):67–74.

72. Shah MA, Feinberg S, Krishnan E. Sleep-disordered breathing among women with fibromyalgia syndrome. *J Clin Rheumatol* 2006;12(6):277–281.

73. Appel S, Chapman J, Shoenfeld Y. Infection and vaccination in chronic fatigue syndrome: myth or reality? *Autoimmunity* 2007;40(1):48–53.

74. Kato K, Sullivan PF, Evengard B, et al. Premorbid predictors of chronic fatigue. *Arch Gen Psychiatry* 2006; 63(11):1267–1272.

75. Heim C, Wagner D, Maloney E, et al. Early adverse experience and risk for chronic fatigue syndrome: results from a population-based study. *Arch Gen Psychiatry* 2006;63(11): 1258–1266.

76. Ozgocmen S, Ozyurt H, Sogut S, et al. Current concepts in the pathophysiology of fibromyalgia: the potential role of oxidative stress and nitric oxide. *Rheumatol Int* 2006;26(7):585–597.

77. van de Putte EM, Uiterwaal CS, Bots ML, et al. Is chronic fatigue syndrome a connective tissue disorder? A cross-sectional study in adolescents. *Pediatrics.* 2005;115(4): e415–422.

78. Brouwers FM, Van Der Werf S, Bleijenberg G, et al. The effect of a polynutrient supplement on fatigue and physical activity of patients with chronic fatigue syndrome: a double-blind randomized controlled trial. *QJM* 2002;95(10):677–683.

79. Lim A, Lubitz L. Chronic fatigue syndrome: successful outcome of an intensive inpatient programme. *J Paediatr Child Health* 2002;38(3):295–299.

80. Tamizi far B, Tamizi B. Treatment of chronic fatigue syndrome by dietary supplementation with omega-3 fatty acids—a good idea? *Med Hypotheses* 2002;58(3):249–250.

81. Craig T, Kakumanu S. Chronic fatigue syndrome: evaluation and treatment. *Am Fam Physician* 2002;65(6):1083–1090.

82. Logan AC, Wong C. Chronic fatigue syndrome: oxidative stress and dietary modifications. *Alternat Med Rev* 2001;6(5):450–459.

83. Gray JB, Martinovic AM. Eicosanoids and essential fatty acid modulation in chronic disease and the chronic fatigue syndrome. *Med Hypotheses* 1994;43(1):31–42.

84. Ali A, Njike VY, Northrup V, et al. Intravenous micronutrient therapy (Myers' Cocktail) for fibromyalgia: a placebo-controlled pilot study. *J Alternat Complement Med* 2009;15(3):247–257.

85. Eaton SB, Eaton SB 3rd, Konner MJ. Paleolithic nutrition revisited: a twelve-year retrospective on its nature and implications. *Eur J Clin Nutr* 1997;51(4):207–216.

86. Calder PC. n-3 polyunsaturated fatty acids and cytokine production in health and disease. *Ann Nutr Metab* 1997;41(4):203–234.

87. Firestein GS, Budd RC, Gabriel SE, et al. *Kelley's textbook of rheumatology,* 9th ed. Philadelphia, PA: Elsevier, 2013.

88. Fletcher JM, Basdeo SA, Allen AC, et al. Therapeutic use of vitamin D and its analogues in autoimmunity. *Recent Pat Inflamm Allergy Drug Discov* 2012;6(1):22–34.

89. Lomax AR, Calder PC. Probiotics, immune function, infection and inflammation: a review of the evidence from studies conducted in humans. *Curr Pharm Des* 2009;15(13):1428–1518.

90. Karimi O, Pena AS. Indications and challenges of probiotics, prebiotics, and synbiotics in the management of arthralgias and spondyloarthropathies in inflammatory bowel disease. *J Clin Gastroenterol* 2008;42(suppl 3 pt 1):S136–S141.

91. Kramer A, Bekeschus S, Broker BM, et al. Maintaining health by balancing microbial exposure and prevention of infection: the hygiene hypothesis versus the hypothesis of early immune challenge. *J Hosp Infect* 2013;83(Suppl 1): S29–S34.

92. Velasquez-Manoff M. *An epidemic of absence: a new way of understanding allergies and autoimmune diseases,* 1st Scribner hardcover ed. New York, NY: Scribner, 2012.

93. Borody TJ, Khoruts A. Fecal microbiota transplantation and emerging applications. *Nature Rev Gastroenterol Hepatol* 2012;9(2):88–96.

94. Towheed TE, Maxwell L, Anastassiades TP, et al. Glucosamine therapy for treating osteoarthritis. *Cochrane Database Syst Rev* 2005(2):CD002946.

95. McAlindon TE, LaValley MP, Gulin JP, et al. Glucosamine and chondroitin for treatment of osteoarthritis: a systematic quality assessment and meta-analysis. *JAMA* 2000;283(11):1469–1475.

96. Reginster JY, Neuprez A, Lecart MP, et al. Role of glucosamine in the treatment for osteoarthritis. *Rheumatol Int* 2012;32(10):2959–2967.

97. Gottlieb MS. Conservative management of spinal osteoarthritis with glucosamine sulfate and chiropractic treatment. *J Manipulative Physiol Ther* 1997;20(6):400–414.

98. Pavelka K, Gatterova J, Olejarova M, et al. Glucosamine sulfate use and delay of progression of knee osteoarthritis: a 3-year, randomized, placebo-controlled, double-blind study. *Arch Intern Med* 2002;162(18):2113–2123.

99. Lopes Vaz A. Double-blind clinical evaluation of the relative efficacy of ibuprofen and glucosamine sulphate in the management of osteoarthrosis of the knee in outpatients. *Curr Med Res Opin* 1982;8(3):145–149.

100. Newman NM, Ling RS. Acetabular bone destruction related to non-steroidal anti-inflammatory drugs. *Lancet* 1985;2(8445):11–14.

101. Brandt KD. Effects of nonsteroidal anti-inflammatory drugs on chondrocyte metabolism in vitro and in vivo. *Am J Med* 1987;83(5A):29–34.

102. Sawitzke AD, Shi H, Finco MF, et al. Clinical efficacy and safety of glucosamine, chondroitin sulphate, their combination, celecoxib or placebo taken to treat osteoarthritis of the knee: 2-year results from GAIT. *Ann Rheum Dis* 2010;69(8):1459–1464.

103. Wu D, Huang Y, Gu Y, et al. Efficacies of different preparations of glucosamine for the treatment of osteoarthritis: a meta-analysis of randomised, double-blind, placebo-controlled trials. *Int J Clin Pract* 2013;67(6):585–594.

104. Pipitone VR. Chondroprotection with chondroitin sulfate. *Drugs Exp Clin Res* 1991;17(1):3–7.

105. Jackson CG, Plaas AH, Sandy JD, et al. The human pharmacokinetics of oral ingestion of glucosamine and chondroitin sulfate taken separately or in combination. *Osteoarthritis And Cartilage* 2010;18(3):297–302.

106. Richy F, Bruyere O, Ethgen O, et al. Structural and symptomatic efficacy of glucosamine and chondroitin in knee osteoarthritis: a comprehensive meta-analysis. *Arch Intern Med* 2003;163(13):1514–1522.

107. Miller KL, Clegg DO. Glucosamine and chondroitin sulfate. *Rheum Dis Clin North Am* 2011;37(1):103–118.

108. Clegg DO, Reda DJ, Harris CL, et al. Glucosamine, chondroitin sulfate, and the two in combination for painful knee osteoarthritis. *N Engl J Med* 2006;354(8):795–808.

109. Soeken KL, Lee WL, Bausell RB, et al. Safety and efficacy of S-adenosylmethionine (SAMe) for osteoarthritis. *J Fam Pract* 2002;51(5):425–430.

110. Ernst E. Complementary or alternative therapies for osteoarthritis. *Nature Clin Pract Rheumatol* 2006;2(2):74–80.

111. Zhang WY, Li Wan Po A. The effectiveness of topically applied capsaicin. A meta-analysis. *Eur J Clin Pharmacol* 1994;46(6):517–522.

112. Hochberg MC, Altman RD, April KT, et al. American College of Rheumatology 2012 recommendations for the use of nonpharmacologic and pharmacologic therapies in osteoarthritis of the hand, hip, and knee. *Arthritis Care Res* 2012;64(4):465–474.

113. Altman RD, Marcussen KC. Effects of a ginger extract on knee pain in patients with osteoarthritis. *Arthritis Rheum* 2001;44(11):2531–2538.

114. Wigler I, Grotto I, Caspi D, et al. The effects of Zintona EC (a ginger extract) on symptomatic gonarthritis. *Osteoarthritis and Cartilage* 2003;11(11):783–789.

115. Ernst E. Avocado-soybean unsaponifiables (ASU) for osteoarthritis - a systematic review. *Clin Rheumatol* 2003;22(4–5):285–288.

116. Henrotin Y, Lambert C, Couchourel D, et al. Nutraceuticals: do they represent a new era in the management of osteoarthritis?—a narrative review from the lessons taken with five products. *Osteoarthritis and Cartilage* 2011;19(1):1–21.

117. Jang MH, Lim S, Han SM, et al. Harpagophytum procumbens suppresses lipopolysaccharide-stimulated expressions of cyclooxygenase-2 and inducible nitric oxide synthase in fibroblast cell line L929. *J Pharmacol Sci* 2003;93(3):367–371.

118. Wilson AG. Epigenetic regulation of gene expression in the inflammatory response and relevance to common diseases. *J Periodontol* 2008;79(8 suppl):1514–1519.

119. Konda VR, Desai A, Darland G, et al. Rho iso-alpha acids from hops inhibit the GSK-3/NF-kappaB pathway and reduce inflammatory markers associated with bone and cartilage degradation. *J Inflamm* 2009;6:26.

120. Boullata JI, Armenti VT. *Handbook of drug-nutrient interactions*, 2nd ed. New York, NY: Humana Press, 2010.

SUGGESTED READINGS

Calder PC. Fatty acids and inflammation: the cutting edge between food and pharma. *Eur J Pharmacol* 2011; 668(suppl 1):S50–S58.

El-Chammas K, Danner E. Gluten-free diet in nonceliac disease. *Nutr Clin Pract* 2011;26(3):294–299.

Yeoh N, Burton JP, Suppiah P, et al. The role of the microbiome in rheumatic diseases. *Curr Rheumatol Rep* 2013; 15(3):314.

CHAPTER 21

Diet and Neurologic Disorders

E vidence in support of a direct role for diet in most neurologic disorders affecting well-nourished populations is limited. Malnutrition, however, which affects more than 800 million people worldwide, is a well-established and important cause of both cognitive impairment and neuropathy (see Chapter 26). The importance of diet in brain development and of folic acid in the prevention of neural tube defects is discussed elsewhere (see Chapters 27 and 29), as is the clear importance of diet and nutrition to cerebrovascular disease (see Chapter 10). The ketogenic diet has been used since at least the 1920s in efforts to control intractable childhood seizures. Overall results have been promising, with published reports indicating efficacy in approximately one-third of treated subjects; in recent years, interest has developed in applying the somewhat less restrictive low-carbohydrate diets popularized for weight loss (see Chapter 5) in addition to medium-chain triglyceride (MCT) diets. Popular belief supports a link between dietary factors and headache; supportive evidence in the medical literature is convincing in certain areas. Individuals with reduced activity of the enzyme diamine oxidase are intolerant of dietary histamine and develop headache with ingestion of histamine-rich foods, such as cheese and wine. The role of chocolate in triggering headache is uncertain, with some evidence refuting the widely held view that chocolate is provocative. Inflammatory conditions of the nervous tissues may be influenced by dietary patterns, as is inflammation in other systems. Certain nutrients directly involved in the metabolism of neurons may be applied therapeutically; pyridoxine in the treatment of neuropathy is an example.

OVERVIEW

Diet

Cognitive Function

A detailed discussion of the myriad effects of nutriture on cognition, via direct and indirect

mechanisms, is beyond the scope of this chapter. Dementia is addressed in Chapter 35, early brain development in Chapter 29, senescence in Chapter 31, and cognition in Chapter 35. The influence of nutrition on the vitality of the various organ systems addressed throughout this text is obviously germane to brain health as well. Healthy brain function is dependent on the steady delivery to the brain of glucose, amino acids, fatty acids, and micronutrients. The brain of an adult constitutes roughly 2% of body mass but requires nearly 20% of calories consumed. In newborns, nearly 60% of caloric intake is directed toward brain function and growth.

As many as 50 million people worldwide have cognitive impairment related to iodine deficiency. This problem has largely been eliminated in the United States by virtue of routine salt iodization, and efforts to make iodized salt available to the global population are a priority for the World Health Organization. Some recent successes have been reported (1). Iron deficiency in childhood also induces cognitive impairment through multiple pathways. Iron deficiency anemia impairs oligodendrocyte growth, resulting in decreased myelination of white matter during critical periods of infant brain development. Neurotransmission is also dependent on adequate iron availability (2). Iron supplementation following an extended period of deficiency may not fully compensate. A recent longitudinal study evaluated Chilean iron-deficient patients diagnosed at 6, 12, or 18 months and followed until 10 years of age. This study found that auditory brainstem responses and visually evoked potentials had decreased speed of transmission in iron deficient patients as compared to those in the control group (2). Iron deficiency–associated cognitive impairment is still a concern in the United States but far more common elsewhere; iron deficiency is considered the most common nutritional disorder in the world (3).

Headache

Survey research suggests a role for chocolate, cheese, red wine, and beer in the precipitation of migraines, but there is no clear association between these foods and tension headache (4). Sensitivity to alcohol in general is described but apparently is unrelated to other food sensitivities. A study of adolescents found a correlation between elevated alcohol intake and migraine headaches (5). The role of chocolate in the precipitation of both migraine and tension headache was examined in a double-blind, crossover trial with 63 women (6). Acute ingestion of chocolate did not induce headache more consistently than carob, which served as the placebo. A recent meta-analysis evaluated use of intravenous magnesium for acute treatment of migraine headaches and found no benefit with an increase in side effects and adverse events (7).

Induction of vascular headache by wine occurs in individuals sensitive to dietary histamine, apparently as a result of reduced diamine oxidase activity (8). Diamine oxidase is involved in the metabolism of histamine. Wine is a particularly potent precipitator of headache in such individuals because it contains histamine, and alcohol competitively inhibits the enzyme. In addition to the avoidance of wine and cheese, such patients may benefit from vitamin B_6 supplementation, as pyridoxine is a cofactor in histamine metabolism, and from the use of histamine receptor (type 1) blocking agents. Recent evidence suggests that some degree of intolerance to dietary histamine may be fairly common and that headache is among the relatively frequent reactions (9). Concentrated food sources of histamine include cheese, sausages, sauerkraut, tuna, and tomatoes in addition to alcoholic beverages.

Epidemiologically, the link between foods and food additives and migraine is convincing, and there are plausible physiologic mechanisms to account for the associations in most cases (10–15). Commonly reported dietary precipitants of migraine include cheese, chocolate, citrus fruits, hot dogs, monosodium glutamate, aspartame, fatty foods, ice cream, caffeine withdrawal, and alcoholic drinks, red wine and beer in particular. Because dietary triggers tend to be idiosyncratic, a standard elimination diet for migraine is not generally recommended. Rather, a food and symptom diary may prove useful in elucidating triggers unique to a given patient. Reduced headache

frequency and/or severity often ensue when exposure to such triggers is eliminated or reduced.

Fasting has been reported as a trigger of headache, although the mechanism is unclear. Fasting apparently is more likely to induce headache in chronic headache sufferers, and the risk rises with the duration of the fast (16). Muslim patients with migraine headaches were studied while fasting during Ramadan. Researchers found length of migraine episodes were three times greater in fasting patients when compared to their nonfasting state (17).

Dehydration is associated with headache, and the effects of dehydration are often invoked to account for many of the symptoms characteristic of hangover, headache prominent among them (18,19). An intervention study in which hypohydration was intentionally induced in a small group of healthy young adults produced headache as a common reaction (20). What this means for recurrent tension headache in general is uncertain, but a trial of increased fluid intake would seem to be a reasonable consideration.

Headache is among the symptoms commonly associated with gluten enteropathy (celiac disease); avoidance of gluten reliably offers relief (21). The prevalence of otherwise occult celiac disease has been found to be higher among migraine sufferers than among matched controls. Removing gluten from the diet in such cases will generally reduce the frequency and severity of migraine attacks (22). The association between headaches of various types and gluten enteropathy suggests that other, and often less overt, food allergies and intolerances may contribute to headache as well. When other explanations for chronic or recurrent headache are not identified, consideration of food allergy is both reasonable and warranted (see Chapter 24). Use of a food and symptom diary to identify potential dietary precipitants of recurrent headache should be routine under such circumstances.

Seizure

Dietary precipitants of seizure have not been described, nor has a role of overall dietary pattern in general susceptibility to epilepsy been characterized. Animal research suggests that iron deficiency may lower the seizure threshold, at least in the context of lead exposure (23). Human case reports suggest that selenium deficiency lowers the seizure threshold and may result in intractable seizures in epileptics (24). Hypoglycemia is an established risk factor for seizure.

The ketogenic diet has been used as primary or adjunctive therapy of childhood seizures since the 1920s (25). The diet originally was developed following observations that seizure activity was suppressed in epileptics during fasting and starvation (26). The utility of high-fat diets in raising the seizure threshold has been demonstrated in animal studies (26). The ketogenic diet is designed to induce ketosis and to shift brain metabolism from glucose to ketone bodies, as occurs during a period of caloric restriction. The diet is initiated with a fast, generally lasting about 38 hours (26,27). The diet, which is started when ketones are detectable in serum, relies on a ratio of fat to protein and carbohydrate combined in the range from 3:1 to 4:1 (27). A mild degree of dehydration is advocated by some to preserve circulating ketone levels (28), but the need for this is not well substantiated (26). Recent modifications of the original diet have been developed in an attempt to facilitate compliance (27). One such modification is the MCT diet. A randomized trial compared the classical ketogenic diet to MCT, showing comparable efficacy in treating epilepsy (29). The mechanism by which ketosis influences seizure activity is uncertain, although progress in this areas is being made (30). Insights gained regarding mechanism of effect may lead to generalized advances in seizure management; Swink et al. (31) have suggested that the efficacy of the ketogenic diet should be exploited in seeking novel approaches to the pharmacologic management of epilepsy.

Observational studies suggest that approximately one-third of treated patients respond favorably to the ketogenic diet. A recent meta-analysis with data from more than 1,000 patients corroborates this (32). Furthermore, patient response to the ketogenic diet was found to be comparable to modern antiepileptic medications in a Cochrane review (33). A systematic review suggests that roughly 15% of patients may experience complete relief of seizure activity with the regimen, and another 15% or so may experience a reduction of seizure frequency of 50% or more (34). Numerous adverse reactions to the diet have been reported, including micronutrient deficiencies, particularly carnitine deficiency; hypoglycemia; hyperlipidemia; osteoporosis; abnormal liver function; optic neuropathy; urolithiasis; and

hemolytic anemia (25,35). The principal limitation of the diet is its unpalatability, which hinders adherence; seizure relief is greatest among those who adhere strictly to the diet, although this association likely goes both ways (34). Furthermore, families reported preparation time and the restrictive nature of the diet as large barriers to compliance. Interestingly, socioeconomic status and family stability were not noted to be factors associated with an inability to maintain the ketogenic diet (36). Given the potential adverse effects and the difficulties in achieving compliance, the ketogenic diet is generally indicated only for those patients resistant to or intolerant of pharmacotherapy (37). However, some advocate more widespread use of the ketogenic diet because it is less expensive, ostensibly safer, and potentially more effective than most available drugs (31).

The low-carbohydrate and ketogenic diet advocated by the late Dr. Robert Atkins for weight loss (38) has been tested for seizure control, as an alternative to the more restrictive ketogenic diet typically used in this context (39). A recent study evaluated pediatric patients with epilepsy in relation to the Atkins diet. The study found that long-term adherence (>6 months) to the Atkins diet resulted in a decrease in seizures similar to that seen in patients who followed the Atkins diet for only a short-term basis (33). Data are as yet limited but suggest that the modified Atkins diet may work at least as well for control of intractable seizures, with easier implementation and better adherence. Further study is clearly warranted.

The ketogenic diet may be of particular benefit in epilepsy syndromes most resistant to pharmacotherapy, such as the West and Lennox-Gastaut syndromes (40). Diet and drug therapy may be used in combination, but interactions are possible. In particular, the ketogenic diet and valproic acid may represent a hazardous combination (35). The limited extent and quality of evidence elucidating the efficacy, toxicity, and mechanism of the ketogenic diet remains cause for both caution and concern (41).

Neurodegenerative Conditions

Chronic, degenerative conditions of the nervous system, such as multiple sclerosis (MS), typically are inflammatory in nature. The putative mechanism of demyelination in MS is autoimmune activity. There is limited evidence to suggest that diet may play a role in the etiology of

MS (42). More plausible on theoretical grounds than an etiologic role is a role for diet in the course of MS. Dietary pattern has an important influence on immune function (see Chapter 11) and susceptibility to inflammatory processes (see Chapter 20). A potentially beneficial role for a diet rich in fruits, vegetables, and fish or other sources of n-3 fatty acids and restricted in total and animal fat, in inflammatory conditions of the central nervous system, is plausible but certainly not established. Popular in alternative medicine practice for the treatment of MS, the Swank diet emphasizes saturated fat restriction and a generous intake of n-3 fatty acids. Further research has found the presence of antigliadin antibodies in some patients with MS. One hypothesis is as a result of a diet rich in refined carbohydrates and saturated fat, there is a change in gut flora. This change in gut flora contributes to disruption of the mucosal barrier in the GI tract and elevated levels of lipopolysaccharide in plasma, promoting a proinflammatory state (43). There does not appear to be any definitive evidence for a therapeutic effect of the Swank diet, but both theoretical justification and trial data have been published and offer some support (44–48).

There is an epidemiological association between MS and relative vitamin D deficiency (49,50). Higher 25-hydroxyvitamin D levels (>75 nmol per L) has been associated with a decreased risk of developing MS (51). The effects of vitamin D on T-cell function offer a plausible mechanism by which vitamin D nutriture could influence the development and course of MS (50). Evidence for a therapeutic effect of vitamin D supplementation in MS is limited to date (52). High-dose vitamin D_2 (6,000 IU) versus low-dose vitamin D_2 (1,000 IU) has not been shown to provide any therapeutic benefit in treating MS (53), and more research in this area is clearly warranted. An argument for increasing vitamin D intake on the basis of diverse health effects is increasingly persuasive (54).

Chronic neurologic conditions resulting in disability, including cerebrovascular disease (see Chapter 10) and Parkinson's disease (55), are associated with a risk of malnutrition. For example, a higher prevalence of neuropathy has been found in patients with Parkinson's disease, likely a result of B_{12} deficiency associated with levodopa exposure (56). Nutritional assessment at regular intervals is indicated in all such patients, with nutritional support as required to maintain muscle mass and metabolic balance (57) (see Chapter 26). In terms of treatment for chronic neurologic conditions, N-acetylcysteine has been shown to increase brain and blood levels of glutathione in neurodegenerative disorders such as Parkinson's and Gaucher's diseases (58).

Amyotrophic lateral sclerosis (ALS) is a disease associated with rapidly progressing weakness with both upper motor neuron and lower motor neuron findings. The disease is marked by inclusions in both upper and lower motor neurons, although the exact pathogenesis is unknown. Hyperlipidemia (elevated total cholesterol or LDL cholesterol) may be protective in patients with ALS. Research shows an increase survival of greater than 12 months for patients with hyperlipidemia and ALS (59).

Coenzyme Q is used by the body as a cofactor in mitochondria as part of the electron transport chain. It has been used as therapy for patients with disorders of mitochondrial dysfunction (60). Recent questions of the use of coenzyme Q in treating ALS have arisen for its antioxidant properties as oxidative stress might be a key pathogenic component of the disease. The superoxide dismutase 1 (SOD1) gene has been implicated in 20% of cases of familial ALS. In sporadic cases of ALS, autopsy analysis has shown oxidative damage to proteins, lipids, or DNA. Studies in transgenic SOD1G93A mice showed that low doses of coenzyme Q increased survival by 4.4% (6 days) (61). However, a phase-II study in patients with ALS taking coenzyme Q for 9 months did not warrant a phase-III trial due to poor efficacy (61). Further research is needed to elucidate the role coenzyme Q may play in treating ALS.

Neuropathy

Vitamin B_6 (pyridoxine) is routinely administered in conjunction with isoniazid for prevention of peripheral neuropathy. It has been studied for the treatment of neuropathy, especially carpal tunnel syndrome, with mixed results (62,63). Some randomized controlled trials have shown a benefit of B_6 at a dose of 50 mg two to three times daily for a period of weeks, whereas others have shown no benefit. In the aggregate, the literature does not provide convincing evidence for the therapeutic efficacy of pyridoxine but does not preclude it either. The result at present is seemingly rather divisive (62,64–66). However, one recent study showed an alleviation in symptoms of diabetic neuropathy when treated with L-methylfolate, methylcobalamin, and pyridoxal-5'-phosphate (67). More study is clearly required to reach an evidence-based conclusion either way; in the interim, the clinician is left to draw upon judgment and interpretation of the limited studies available.

Smith et al. (68) recently tested the effects of the lifestyle intervention of the Diabetes Prevention Program (69) (see Chapter 6) on lower extremity neuropathy in 32 adults with impaired glucose tolerance but not frank diabetes. The same lifestyle intervention that ameliorated glycemic responses to a glucose tolerance test resulted in reduced neuropathic pain and improvement in intraepidermal nerve fiber density, as measured by biopsy.

The potential for nutrient deficiencies to induce a variety of neuropathic syndromes is well established. Thiamine deficiency is associated with polyneuropathy and the Wernicke-Korsakoff syndrome, usually in the context of alcoholism but also reported in the context of impaired dietary intake following bariatric surgery (70). An epidemic of optic, peripheral, and mixed neuropathy in Cuba in the early 1990s has been attributed principally to deficiencies in B complex vitamins (71–74). One area of widespread interest is vitamin B_{12} deficiency and long-term metformin use. Metformin use may result in vitamin B_{12} deficiency, predisposing patients to neuropathy. Routine monitoring of B_{12} in patients taking metformin is underutilized and may be warranted (75). The extent to which nutrients, especially B vitamins, are of potential therapeutic value in neuropathic states unrelated to overt deficiency is less clear but an area of interest.

NUTRIENTS, NUTRICEUTICALS, AND FUNCTIONAL FOODS

Manganese

Manganese is widely distributed in grains, cereals, and nuts and is present in lower levels in fruits and vegetables. As a result, overt deficiency is extremely rare. However, low levels have been associated with epilepsy, and optimal intake is uncertain. Paleolithic intake of manganese has not yet been estimated in a published report, but given the characteristics of our ancestral diet, intake was likely to have been greater than it is today. Any benefit of manganese supplementation

in reducing the severity or frequency of seizures in some patients with epilepsy remains to be shown.

Thiamine

As noted previously, thiamine deficiency in the context of alcoholism may result in Wernicke's encephalopathy or Korsakoff psychosis. The latter may cause unconsciousness or coma; thus, parenteral thiamine supplementation (generally 1 mg) is an established component in the early response to coma of uncertain etiology. It is important in such situations to administer thiamine prior to glucose, as carbohydrate induces thiamine metabolism. Thiamine supplementation has been shown to enhance cognition in epileptic patients on long-term phenytoin (Dilantin) therapy (76).

Pyridoxine (Vitamin B_6)

Seizures resulting from pyridoxine deficiency have been reported in infants, and they respond when pyridoxine is given in doses approximating the recommended dietary allowance. Other infantile seizures of uncertain etiology have been characterized as pyridoxine dependent and occur despite ostensibly adequate pyridoxine intake. These seizures reportedly respond to high-dose supplementation, in the range from 25 to 50 mg per day (77). There is some suggestion that pyridoxine-dependent seizures, thought to be due to an inborn derangement of γ-aminobutyric acid synthesis (78), may represent only the extreme form of a syndrome with various neurocognitive deficits (79). A potential role for pharmacologic dosing of pyridoxine (50 mg b.i.d. to t.i.d.) in the treatment of carpal tunnel syndrome remains controversial, as noted earlier.

Selenium

Brain cells are apparently guarded against oxidative injury, at least in part, by two enzymes that require selenium: glutathione peroxidase and phospholipid hydroperoxide glutathione peroxidase. In other tissues, catalase inactivates hydrogen peroxide, but the central nervous system is catalase deficient. At least one report suggests that selenium deficiency should be considered when intractable seizures develop in children (24). The value of routine selenium supplementation as adjuvant therapy in epilepsy has not been established. Serum selenium levels have been measured in febrile children with and without simple febrile seizures. Children with simple febrile seizures had lower selenium levels than those without seizure activity (80).

n-3 Fatty Acids

A potential role for n-3 fatty acid supplementation, docosahexaenoic acid (DHA) in particular, in the prevention and amelioration of peripheral neuropathy has been suggested (81–83). The well-established importance of this nutrient class to neurologic development and health is addressed in Chapters 27 and 29.

Aspartame

Controversies over the health effects of aspartame have long been debated. It has been linked as a migraine headache trigger for a subset of patients (84). Furthermore, concerns over the possibility that aspartame can increase susceptibility to brain tumors have arisen. A prospective trial found no significant associations between consumption of aspartame and developing either hematopoietic cancers or gliomas after 5 years of follow-up (85).

Aspartame may also have analgesic properties. In rat models, the substance had antinociceptive properties; however, when given with opioid and serotonergic antagonists, the analgesic effect was diminished (86). A more detailed discussion of the chemical nature of aspartame can be found in Chapter 42.

Nutrigenomic Considerations

Researchers have evaluated gene polymorphisms to the vitamin D receptor (VDR) in relationship to an increased risk of developing MS. A recent meta-analysis found no association between VDR polymorphisms and MS (87).

Diet/Drug Interactions

Antiepileptic medications are notorious for drug–drug interactions, but less publicized are their potential drug–food interactions. One study showed butter was found to increase the absorption of phenytoin and carbamazepine in mice (88). In addition, honey has been found in rabbits to increase the extent and rate of absorption of phenytoin, whereas Coca-Cola increases the extent of absorption of phenytoin in rabbits (89,90). Carbamazepine and phenytoin may have increased bioavailability with the mere intake of food, possibly due to increased disintegration of the medication (91).

CLINICAL HIGHLIGHTS

The specific role for nutritional management of neurologic conditions as defined by outcome data is limited but nonetheless important. Malnutrition is a common sequela of chronic, disabling neurologic conditions and can be prevented through continual monitoring and early intervention. Diet may play a role in the precipitation of headaches in some patients, although this appears not to be a predominant factor on a population basis. Diet and symptom diaries are a simple and expedient means of identifying dietary triggers of headaches, in particular migraines. The use of dietary interventions for the management of seizures, alone or in combination with pharmacotherapy, is well established. The therapeutic efficacy of the ketogenic diet is supported by definitive evidence, but the circumstances under which it should be applied remain controversial. Modifications of this dietary approach, such as the Atkins diet and the MCT diet, may offer therapeutic efficacy along with relative ease and palatability. Pyridoxine is of well-defined benefit in certain cases of pediatric seizure disorder; its role in the treatment of peripheral neuropathies remains controversial; however, new data are promising in treatment of diabetic neuropathy with L-methylfolate, methylcobalamin, and pyridoxal-5'-phosphate. Vitamin D supplementation, n-3 fatty acid supplementation, and restricted intake of saturated fats may offer specific benefit in MS and are defensible on the basis of other likely health benefits (see Chapter 45). Coenzyme Q supplementation may be a potential avenue in survival and treatment of ALS.

Although direct evidence of specific neurologic benefit is lacking, a balanced diet rich in the sources of micronutrients and with a judicious distribution of macronutrients (see Chapter 45) could be expected to be supportive of optimal neurologic health on theoretical grounds. The dietary pattern advocated for health promotion offers benefit with regard to immune function (see Chapter 11), susceptibility to inflammation (see Chapter 20), cognitive function (see Chapter 35), brain development (see Chapter 29), and susceptibility to cerebrovascular disease (see Chapter 10). Thus, although largely indirect, the evidence linking dietary practices to the prevention and mitigation of neurologic disorders is substantial in the aggregate.

REFERENCES

1. World Health Organization. *Macronutrient deficiencies: iodine deficiency disorders*. Available at http://www.who.int/nutrition/topics/idd/en/; accessed 1/07.
2. Congdon EL, Westerlund A, Algarin CR, et al. Iron deficiency in infancy is associated with altered neural correlates of recognition memory at 10 years. *J Pediatr* 2012;160(6):1027–1033.
3. World Health Organization. *Macronutrient deficiencies: iron deficiency anaemia*. Available at http://www.who.int/nutrition/topics/ida/en/index.html; accessed 1/07.
4. Peatfield RC. Relationship between food, wine, and beer-precipitated migrainous headaches. *Headache* 1995;35:355.
5. Milde-Busch A, Blaschek A, Borggräfe I, et al. Associations of diet and lifestyle with headache in high-school students: results from a cross-sectional study. *Headache* 2010;50(7):1104–1114.
6. Marcus DA, Scharff L, Turk D, et al. A double-blind provocative study of chocolate as a trigger of headache. *Cephalalgia* 1997;17:855.
7. Choi H, Parmar N. The use of intravenous magnesium sulphate for acute migraine: meta-analysis of randomized controlled trials. *Eur J Emerg Med* 2014;21(1):2–9.
8. Jarisch R, Wantke F. Wine and headache. *Int Arch Allergy Immunol* 1996;110:7.
9. Wohrl S, Hemmer W, Focke M, et al. Histamine intolerance-like symptoms in healthy volunteers after oral provocation with liquid histamine. *Allergy Asthma Proc* 2004;25:305–311.
10. Millichap JG, Yee MM. The diet factor in pediatric and adolescent migraine. *Pediatr Neurol* 2003;28:9–15.
11. Coelho RS, Gomes CM, Teixeira RA. Cerebral vasoreactivity is influenced by the prandial state among migraineurs. *Headache* 2006;46:1191–1194.
12. Damen L, Bruijn J, Koes BW, et al. Prophylactic treatment of migraine in children. Part 1: a systematic review of non-pharmacological trials. *Cephalalgia* 2006;26:373–383.
13. Woolhouse M. Migraine and tension headache—a complementary and alternative medicine approach. *Aust Fam Physician* 2005;34:647–651.
14. Joubert J. Migraine—diagnosis and treatment. *Aust Fam Physician* 2005;34:627–632.
15. Wober C, Holzhammer J, Zeitlhofer J, et al. Trigger factors of migraine and tension-type headache: experience and knowledge of the patients. *J Headache Pain* 2006;7:188–195.
16. Mosek A, Korczyn AD. Yom Kippur headache. *Neurology* 1995;45:1953.
17. Abu-Salameh I, Plakht Y, Ifergane G. Migraine exacerbation during Ramadan fasting. *J Headache Pain.* 2010;11(6):513–517.
18. Rohsenow DJ, Howland J, Minsky SJ, et al. The acute hangover scale: a new measure of immediate hangover symptoms. *Addict Behav* 2006;32:1314–1320.
19. Wiese JG, Shlipak MG, Browner WS. The alcohol hangover. *Ann Intern Med* 2000;132:897–902.
20. Shirreffs SM, Merson SJ, Fraser SM, et al. The effects of fluid restriction on hydration status and subjective feelings in man. *Br J Nutr* 2004;91:951–958.
21. Zarkadas M, Cranney A, Case S, et al. The impact of a gluten-free diet on adults with coeliac disease: results of a national survey. *J Hum Nutr Diet* 2006;19:41–49.
22. Gabrielli M, Cremonini F, Fiore G, et al. Association between migraine and celiac disease: results from a preliminary case-control and therapeutic study. *Am J Gastroenterol* 2003;98:625–629.
23. Barzideh O, Burright RG, Donovick PJ. Dietary iron and exposure to lead influence susceptibility to seizures. *Psychol Rep* 1995;76:971.
24. Ramaekers VT, Calomme M, Vanden Berghe D, et al. Selenium deficiency triggering intractable seizures. *Neuropediatrics* 1994;25:217.
25. Tallian KB, Nahata MC, Tsao CY. Role of the ketogenic diet in children with intractable seizures. *Ann Pharmacother* 1998;32:349.
26. Nordli DR, De Vivo C. The ketogenic diet revisited: back to the future. *Epilepsia* 1997;38:743.
27. Carroll J, Koenigsberger D. The ketogenic diet: a practical guide for caregivers. *J Am Diet Assoc* 1998;98:316.
28. Berryman MS. The ketogenic diet revisited. *J Am Diet Assoc* 1997;97:s192–s194.
29. Neal EG, Chaffe H, Schwartz RH, et al. A randomized trial of classical and medium-chain triglyceride ketogenic diets in the treatment of childhood epilepsy. *Epilepsia* 2009;50(5):1109–1117.
30. Freeman J, Veggiotti P, Lanzi G, et al. The ketogenic diet: from molecular mechanisms to clinical effects. *Epilepsy Res* 2006;68:145–180.
31. Swink TD, Vining EP, Freeman JM. The ketogenic diet: 1997. *Adv Pediatr* 1997;44:297.
32. Henderson CB, Filloux FM, Alder SC, et al. Efficacy of the ketogenic diet as a treatment option for epilepsy: meta-analysis. *J Child Neurol* 2006;21:193–198.
33. Chen W, Kossoff EH. Long-term follow-up of children treated with the modified Atkins diet. *J Child Neurol* 2012;27(6):754–758.
34. Keene DL. A systematic review of the use of the ketogenic diet in childhood epilepsy. *Pediatr Neurol* 2006;35:1–5.
35. Ballaban-Gil K, Callahan C, O'Dell C, et al. Complications of the ketogenic diet. *Epilepsia* 1998;39:744.
36. McNamara NA, Carbone LA, Shellhaas RA. Epilepsy characteristics and psychosocial factors associated with ketogenic diet success. *J Child Neurol* 2013;28(10):1233–1237.
37. Bazil CW, Pedley TA. Advances in the medical treatment of epilepsy. *Annu Rev Med* 1998;49:135.
38. Atkins RC. *Dr. Atkins' new diet revolution*. New York, NY: HarperCollins, 2002.
39. Kossoff EH, McGrogan JR, Bluml RM, et al. A modified Atkins diet is effective for the treatment of intractable pediatric epilepsy. *Epilepsia* 2006;47:421–424.

40. Arnold ST, Dodson WE. Epilepsy in children. *Baillere's Clin Neurol* 1996;5:783.

41. Prasad AN, Stafstrom CF, Holmes GL. Alternative epilepsy therapies: the ketogenic diet, immunoglobulins, and steroids. *Epilepsia* 1996;37:s81.

42. Ghadirian P, Jain M, Ducic S, et al. Nutritional factors in the aetiology of multiple sclerosis: a case-control study in Montreal, Canada. *Int J Epidemiol* 1998;27:845.

43. Riccio P. The molecular basis of nutritional intervention in multiple sclerosis: a narrative review. *Complement Ther Med* 2011;19(4):228–237.

44. Swank RL, Goodwin J. Review of MS patient survival on a Swank low saturated fat diet. *Nutrition* 2003;19:161–162.

45. Das UN. Is there a role for saturated and long-chain fatty acids in multiple sclerosis? *Nutrition* 2003;19:163–166.

46. Schwarz S, Leweling H. Multiple sclerosis and nutrition. *Mult Scler* 2005;11:24–32.

47. Swank RL, Goodwin JW. How saturated fats may be a causative factor in multiple sclerosis and other diseases. *Nutrition* 2003;19:478.

48. Weinstock-Guttman B, Baier M, Park Y, et al. Low fat dietary intervention with omega-3 fatty acid supplementation in multiple sclerosis patients. *Prostaglandins Leukot Essent Fatty Acids* 2005;73:397–404.

49. Munger KL, Levin LI, Hollis BW, et al. Serum 25-hydroxyvitamin D levels and risk of multiple sclerosis. *JAMA* 2006;296:2832–2838.

50. Cantorna MT. Vitamin D and its role in immunology: multiple sclerosis, and inflammatory bowel disease. *Prog Biophys Mol Biol* 2006;92:60–64.

51. Salzer J, Hallmans G, Nyström M, et al. Vitamin D as a protective factor in multiple sclerosis. *Neurology* 2012;79(21):2140–2145.

52. Wingerchuk DM, Lesaux J, Rice GP, et al. A pilot study of oral calcitriol (1,25-dihydroxyvitamin D3) for relapsing-remitting multiple sclerosis. *J Neurol Neurosurg Psychiatry* 2005;76:1294–1296.

53. Stein MS, Liu Y, Gray OM, et al. A randomized trial of high-dose vitamin D_2 in relapsing-remitting multiple sclerosis. *Neurology* 2011;77(17):1611–1618.

54. Vieth R. Why the optimal requirement for vitamin D_3 is probably much higher than what is officially recommended for adults. *J Steroid Biochem Mol Biol* 2004;89–90:575–579.

55. Beyer PL, Palarino MY, Michalek D, et al. Weight change and body composition in patients with Parkinson's disease. *J Am Diet Assoc* 1995;95:979.

56. Rajabally YA, Martey J. Neuropathy in Parkinson disease: prevalence and determinants. *Neurology* 2011;77(22):1947–1950.

57. Britton JER, Lipscomb G, Mohr PD, et al. The use of percutaneous endoscopic gastrostomy (PEG) feeding tubes in patients with neurological disease. *J Neurol* 1997;244:431.

58. Holmay MJ, Terpstra M, Coles LD, et al. N-acetylcysteine boosts brain and blood glutathione in Gaucher and Parkinson diseases. *Clin Neuropharmacol* 2013;36(4):103–106.

59. Dupuis L, Corcia P, Fergani A, et al. Dyslipidemia is a protective factor in amyotrophic lateral sclerosis. *Neurology* 2008;70(13):1004–1009.

60. Orsucci D, Mancuso M, Ienco EC, et al. Targeting mitochondrial dysfunction and neurodegeneration by means of coenzyme Q10 and its analogues. *Curr Med Chem* 2011;18(26):4053–4064.

61. Siciliano G, Carlesi C, Pasquali L, et al. Clinical trials for neuroprotection in ALS. *CNS Neurol Disord Drug Targets* 2010;9(3):305–313.

62. Gerritsen AA, de Krom MC, Struijs MA, et al. Conservative treatment options for carpal tunnel syndrome: a systematic review of randomised controlled trials. *J Neurol* 2002;249:272–280.

63. Bender DA. Non-nutritional uses of vitamin B_6. *Br J Nutr* 1999;81:7.

64. Goodyear-Smith F, Arroll B. What can family physicians offer patients with carpal tunnel syndrome other than surgery? A systematic review of nonsurgical management. *Ann Fam Med* 2004;2:267–273.

65. Aufiero E, Stitik TP, Foye PM, et al. Pyridoxine hydrochloride treatment of carpal tunnel syndrome: a review. *Nutr Rev* 2004;62:96–104.

66. Holm G, Moody LE. Carpal tunnel syndrome: current theory, treatment, and the use of B6. *J Am Acad Nurse Pract* 2003;15:18–22.

67. Fonseca VA, Lavery LA, Thethi TK, et al. Metanx in type 2 diabetes with peripheral neuropathy: a randomized trial. *Am J Med* 2013;126(2):141–149.

68. Smith AG, Russell J, Feldman EL, et al. Lifestyle intervention for pre-diabetic neuropathy. *Diabetes Care* 2006;29:1294–1299.

69. Knowler WC, Barrett-Connor E, Fowler SE, et al. Reduction in the incidence of type 2 diabetes with lifestyle intervention or metformin. *N Engl J Med* 2002;346:393–403.

70. Chaves LC, Faintuch J, Kahwage S, et al. A cluster of polyneuropathy and Wernicke–Korsakoff syndrome in a bariatric unit. *Obes Surg* 2002;12:328–334.

71. Arnaud J, Fleites-Mestre P, Chassagne M, et al. Vitamin B intake and status in healthy Havanan men, 2 years after the Cuban neuropathy epidemic. *Br J Nutr* 2001;85:741–748.

72. Barnouin J, Verdura Barrios T, Chassagne M, et al. Nutritional and food protection against epidemic emerging neuropathy. Epidemiological findings in the unique disease-free urban area of Cuba. *Int J Vitam Nutr Res* 2001;71:274–285.

73. Dominguez YL, Hernandez M, Matos CM, et al. Is B vitamins deficiency associated with prevalence of Alzheimer's disease in Cuban elderly? *Nutr Health* 2006;18:103–118.

74. Rodriguez-Hernandez M, Hirano M, Naini A, et al. Biochemical studies of patients with Cuban epidemic neuropathy. *Ophthalmic Res* 2001;33:310–313.

75. Pierce SA, Chung AH, Black KK. Evaluation of vitamin B_{12} monitoring in a veteran population on long-term, high-dose metformin therapy. *Ann Pharmacother* 2012;46(11):1470–1476.

76. Botez MI, Botez T, Ross-Chouinard A, et al. Thiamine and folate treatment of chronic epileptic patients: a controlled study with the Wechsler IQ scale. *Epilepsy Res* 1993;16:157.

77. Jiao FY, Gao DY, Takuma Y, et al. Randomized, controlled trial of high-dose intravenous pyridoxine in the treatment of recurrent seizures in children. *Pediatr Neurol* 1997;17:54.

78. Gospe SM Jr, Hecht ST. Longitudinal MRI findings in pyridoxine-dependent seizures. *Neurology* 1998;51:74.

79. Baxter P, Griffiths P, Kelly T, et al. Pyridoxine-dependent seizures: demographic, clinical, MRI and psychometric features and effect of dose on intelligence quotient. *Dev Med Child Neurol* 1996;38:998.

80. Mahyar A, Ayazi P, Fallahi M, et al. Correlation between serum selenium level and febrile seizures. *Pediatr Neurol* 2010;43(5):331–334.

81. Coste TC, Gerbi A, Vague P, et al. Neuroprotective effect of docosahexaenoic acid-enriched phospholipids in experimental diabetic neuropathy. *Diabetes* 2003;52: 2578–2585.

82. Gerbi A, Maixent JM, Ansaldi JL, et al. Fish oil supplementation prevents diabetes-induced nerve conduction velocity and neuroanatomical changes in rats. *J Nutr* 1999;129:207–213.

83. Uauy R, Dangour AD. Nutrition in brain development and aging: role of essential fatty acids. *Nutr Rev* 2006;64: s24–s33; discussion s72–s91.

84. Sun-Edelstein C, Mauskop A. Foods and supplements in the management of migraine headaches. *Clin J Pain* 2009;25(5):446–452.

85. Lim U, Subar AF, Mouw T, et al. Consumption of aspartame-containing beverages and incidence of hematopoietic and brain malignancies. *Cancer Epidemiol Biomarkers Prev* 2006;15(9):1654–1659.

86. Rani S, Gupta MC. Evaluation and comparison of antinociceptive activity of aspartame with sucrose. *Pharmacol Rep* 2012;64(2):293–298.

87. Huang J, Zehng FX. Polymorphisms in the vitamin D receptor gene and multiple sclerosis risk: A meta-analysis of case control studies. *J Neurol Sci* 2012;313(1–2):79–85.

88. Sidhu S, Malhotra S, Garg SK. Influence of high fat diet (butter) on pharmacokinetics of phenytoin and carbamazepine. *Methods Find Exp Clin Pharmacol* 2004;26(8):634–638.

89. Sukriti, Garg SK. Influence of honey on the pharmacokinetics of phenytoin in healthy rabbits. *Methods Find Exp Clin Pharmacol* 2003;25(5):367–370.

90. Kondal A, Garg SK. Influence of an acidic beverage (Coca-Cola) on the pharmacokinetics of phenytoin in healthy rabbits. *Methods Find Exp Clin Pharmacol* 2003;25(10):823–825.

91. Melander A. Influence of food on the bioavailability of drugs. *Clin Pharmacokinet* 1978;3(5):337–351.

SUGGESTED READINGS

Roman GC. Nutritional disorders of the nervous system. In: Shils ME, Shike M, Ross AC, et al., eds. *Modern nutrition in health and disease*, 10th ed. Philadelphia, PA: Lippincott Williams & Wilkins, 2006:1362–1380.

CHAPTER 22

Diet and Dermatoses

C ommon ailments of the skin are often related to hypersensitivity and autoimmunity. These states are in turn influenced by diet. Cutaneous manifestations of food allergy and intolerance are common; many of the dermatologic conditions influenced by food are atopic responses to food itself (see Chapter 24). There is an array of dermatopathology associated with excessive intake of alcohol, and there is some evidence that ethanol tends to exacerbate autoimmune dermatoses. Atopic dermatitis (AD) in children is common and may respond to dietary manipulations. Gluten enteropathy often presents with dermatitis that may be evident even in the absence of overt gastrointestinal symptoms. Some studies suggest benefits of probiotic bacteria and ω-3 fatty acids in the treatment of dermatitis. In nickel-sensitive individuals, the nickel used in stainless steel cookware may induce dermatitis. Increasing evidence is suggesting a link between high-glycemic-load foods and acne development and psoriasis. Further, psoriasis symptoms may be improved with low-energy diets rich in fruits, vegetables, and n-3 fatty acids. Highly processed diets, refined sugar, saturated fat, and trans fat may exert adverse influences, whereas vegetables, fruit, and organic foods free of contaminants may reduce the risk of food-induced dermatopathology.

OVERVIEW

Effects of the overall quality of the diet on the health and integrity of the skin are well established. Skin is a complex tissue, or group of tissues, with a high rate of cellular turnover, and is thus dependent on a consistent intake of diverse nutrients. Epidermal regeneration requires approximately 2 weeks, and malnutrition can affect this process, resulting in skin dryness, atrophy, and wrinkling. Acute dermatitis has been observed with mixed nutrient deficiencies in the aftermath of surgery (1). The influence of specific micronutrients on skin health is addressed in Chapter 4, and the importance of diet and nutrients to wound healing (2,3) is covered in Chapter 23. The effects of nutrition on vascular health, immune function, and even weight have important, indirect effects on the health of skin, also addressed in other chapters.

Cutaneous reactions, encompassing pruritus, urticaria, angioedema, AD, and even contact dermatitis of the oral cavity are a common expression of food allergy and intolerance (4,5) (see Chapter 24). Diverse food additives have been implicated in chronic urticaria, although it appears that often combinations of additives are responsible, increasing the challenges in identifying the offending compounds and removing them from the diet (6).

Food allergy has been attributed to abnormal permeability of the bowel wall to food antigens. Chronic urticaria has been associated with increased gastrointestinal permeability in at least a subgroup of affected patients (7). Probiotic bacteria (see Chapter 18) are posited to improve gut barrier function and to consequently offer a defense against and potential treatment for AD, along with other manifestations of food allergy and intolerance (8). A previous clinical trial suggests that a 3-month course of synbiotics (probiotic bacteria in combination with "prebiotic" fructo-oligosaccharides) and prebiotics alone can both significantly ameliorate the course of AD in children age 2 and older (9). A more recent study demonstrated that supplementation with *Lactobacillus rhamnosus* reduced the cumulative risk of eczema by age 2 (10). Multiple reviews examining randomized controlled trials on the effect of probiotic use for reducing AD have shown some evidence for the benefits of probiotics (11,12). Certain probiotic strains may have greater effect on prevention of AD, and the mechanisms behind their effects remain unclear (10). There is currently an inadequate amount of evidence to support probiotic use for management of AD; however, the field is only recently emerging as a treatment option for AD, and still requires further studies.

Atopic eczema is known to flare following the ingestion of allergenic foods. A reduced ability to metabolize histamine in food may contribute to dermatitis in a subgroup of patients (13). Identifying and avoiding culprit foods may ameliorate the course of the condition. Associations between AD and high intake of refined sugar, high intake of saturated fat, low intake of n-3 fatty acids, low intake of fruits, and low intake of vitamin D have been reported, although the clinical importance of these observational data remains uncertain (14).

The clinical manifestations of gluten enteropathy (see Chapters 18 and 24) often involve the skin (15). Well-characterized associations include dermatitis herpetiformis, alopecia, angular stomatitis, and aphthous ulcerations; psoriasis has been associated as well (16). Chronic, intermittent urticaria may be seen as well, in children as well as adults (17). Occasionally, cutaneous manifestations of celiac disease are seen in the absence of any other overt signs or symptoms (18). A high index of suspicion is clearly required in such cases, and diagnosis is facilitated by general awareness of the potential link between food intolerances and otherwise chronic and enigmatic dermatopathology. Removal of gluten from the diet reliably ameliorates the cutaneous as well as the gastrointestinal symptoms resulting from celiac disease.

The association between heavy, chronic alcohol intake and pathology of the skin is long established. Less well known is the potential contribution of lesser alcohol consumption to dermatopathology (19). Alcohol intake may induce, or exacerbate, psoriasis, cutaneous infections, and eczema. Excessive consumption of alcohol—a term that implies variable intake depending on individual vulnerability to adverse effects—is also associated with acne, rosacea, porphyria cutanea tarda, pruritus and urticara, seborrhea, and increased susceptibility to superficial skin infections (20,21). Many of these conditions develop long before the well-characterized cutaneous stigmata of chronic alcohol abuse and liver disease, such as spider angiomata. Familiarity with the diverse dermal manifestations of alcohol may help reveal an otherwise occult alcohol problem (21). Control of alcohol intake may meaningfully improve the course of otherwise refractory dermatoses, particularly psoriasis (22). Studies have shown that serum biotin levels are significantly lower with chronic alcohol abuse, and animal studies suggest decreased intestinal biotin absorption and decreased renal biotin reabsorption with chronic alcohol feeding (23,24). Biotin deficiency is commonly associated with skin inflammation including seborrhoeic dermatitis.

The important influence of essential fatty acid intake on eicosanoid production and inflammation is addressed extensively throughout the text (see, in particular, Chapter 11 and Section VIIE). Essential fatty acids influence inflammatory markers relevant in dermatitis (25,26), and there is evidence that n-3 fatty acid intake may influence the course of several chronic skin conditions. The pattern of fatty acid intake may have some effect on overall atopic tendencies, with n-3 fatty acids exerting a protective influence (27). The evidence in this area is far from conclusive, and debate over the relative importance of total amounts of ingested fat in various classes versus the ratio of one intake level to another (in particular that of n-6 to n-3 polyunsaturated fatty acid) is lively.

A trial of α-linolenic acid, an n-3 fatty acid, for AD in a mouse model was negative (28). In a small sample of adults hospitalized with AD, Mayser et al. (29) saw improvement with infusion of either n-3 or n-6 fatty acid emulsions. Others have seen beneficial effects of both n-3 and n-6 fatty acids (30). Consistent with this finding is a suggestion that atopic eczema may derive, at least in some cases, from a minor defect in essential fatty acid metabolism, specifically the failure to convert linoleic acid to γ-linolenic acid, an n-6 fatty acid, and other long-chain polyenes, for which supplementation may be compensatory (31). Newer studies have demonstrated that γ-linolenic acid supplementation has limited to no effects on reducing AD (32–34). Further, a recent review failed to support that n-3 and n-6 supplementation was beneficial for prevention of allergic disease (35).

There have been studies demonstrating the risk of breast milk high in saturated fats and low in n-3 fatty acids in the development of AD in infants (36). A study showed n-3 supplementation during pregnancy resulted in decreased childhood asthma and food allergy (37). Dunstan et al. (38) tested the influence of fish oil supplementation during pregnancy, beginning at gestational week 20, on atopy in newborns. There was no difference between groups in the rate of AD, but disease severity was less in the supplemented neonates. Cytokine levels and skin prick test responses differed significantly between groups, suggesting a reduction in atopy with fish oil administration. Others have suggested that n-3 fatty acids may show more promise in the prevention than in the treatment of atopic disease and that supplementation in utero or infancy may be of particular benefit (39). A recent randomized control trial observed a decrease in atopic eczema and egg sensitization with n-3 fatty acid supplementation in pregnancy; however, the overall incidence of immunoglobulin E associated allergies were not diminished (40).

Delayed introduction of solid food in infancy is thought to attenuate the risk of atopy, although recent birth cohort data do not lend much support to this notion (41,42). Some benefit of delaying solid food past 4 months of age is suggested, with no appreciable, additional benefit attached to delaying past 6 months. Whether more extended periods of breast-feeding defend against food allergy is uncertain (see Chapter 27). Exclusive breast-feeding for 6 months or longer is advisable on other grounds (see Chapters 27 and 29). Breast-feeding may decrease AD in infants, and hydrolyzed formulas may be preferred over cow's milk formulas if breast-feeding is not an option (43). Antigen avoidance during pregnancy and lactation has also been considered as a possible strategy for minimizing atopy in high-risk patients, yet a recent systemic review failed to demonstrate adequate evidence for antigen avoidance. Of note, it is important to consider the possible nutritional deficiencies that may arise from suggesting such a diet (44).

Nickel can induce contact dermatitis, with secondary generalization (45). Nickel from food, from water, or released from stainless steel cookware has been implicated (45,46). The removal of nickel from stainless steel formulations has been suggested (46). Nickel-sensitive individuals should substitute alternatives for stainless steel cooking utensils.

There has been an association between diet and acne since the 1930s. Bowe et al. (47) provided epidemiologic data suggesting an association between dairy and acne, and high glycemic loads may exacerbate acne. Additional studies have added further support for the influence of high-glycemic-load diet, milk, and hormonal mediators on increasing acne risk (48–51). Preliminary studies have demonstrated a decrease in acne with low-glycemic-load diet interventions. These investigations suggest glycemic load may influence sebaceous lipogenesis, sex hormone activity, and IGF-1 production (52–54). Further studies are necessary to adequately characterize the mechanisms underlying these associations.

Psoriasis, an inflammatory skin disease marked by keratinocyte hyperproliferation and abnormal differentiation, is primarily a genetic disease but has been associated with certain dietary habits. Specifically, low-energy, vegetarian diets, diets rich in n-3 fatty acids, and gluten-free diets have shown to improve psoriasis symptoms (55). Nutrition is not well studied in regards to psoriasis treatment; however, obesity and diets low in fruits and vegetables have been associated with worse symptoms. A current prospective randomized trial found that obese psoriatic patients treated with a low-energy diet had improved dermatologic involvement and significantly better Dermatology Life Quality Index (56). There have been several findings of decreased antioxidant levels in psoriatic patients, which could potentially be remedied by adequate fruit and vegetable intake. Additionally, psoriasis is common in patients with insulin resistance, which is in turn exacerbated with foods containing a high glycemic index (57). Further, oral vitamin D supplementation can decrease keratinocyte proliferation as well as minimize psoriatic arthropathy (58). Nutritional therapies for psoriasis include vitamin D, n-3 fatty acid, retinoid, selenium, and vitamin B_{12} supplementation (59).

The effect of nutritional factors on cancer has been active area of research for several decades. Early epidemiological studies have demonstrated an association with diet and cancer, specifically, a reduced risk of cancer at all sites with increased fruit and vegetable intake (60). There are emerging data suggesting that certain dietary factors may alter the risk for developing skin cancer in particular. It was originally thought that β-carotene supplementation may be protective for patients with prior nonmelanoma skin cancer against tumor recurrence; however, subsequent studies were nonsupportive (61). Further, plasma levels of β-carotene, as well as other micronutrients, including lycopene, retinal, α-carotene, α-tocopherol, carotene, and vitamin E, did not alter risks for malignant melanoma. Although, reduced risk for melanoma was observed with decreased alcohol consumption (62). The effect of a low-fat diet intervention on skin cancer patients demonstrated a significantly lower recurrence of nonmelanoma skin cancer after 8 months of intervention (63). A Danish population based case-control study, however, found no association of diet and alcohol on risk for malignant melanoma (64). Selenium supplementation was also not beneficial in preventing basal cell carcinoma in skin cancer patients, and, interestingly, increased the risk of nonmelanoma skin cancer (65).

CLINICAL HIGHLIGHTS

The overall adequacy and quality of the diet have important implications for the health and integrity of skin. Food intolerance and food allergy commonly manifest with cutaneous reactions, and chronic dermatitis often relates to food intolerance. AD in children and chronic dermatitis or pruritus in adults warrants assessment of diet with a food and symptom diary to probe for dietary triggers. Elimination of such foods or food additives is reliably of therapeutic value. Gluten enteropathy is a noteworthy example of food allergy in which skin manifestation may predominate, at least early, and for which removal of the offending food item, in this case gluten, is effective treatment.

Irritants in both food and cookware may induce dermatitis; nickel in stainless steel is a noteworthy example. Contact dermatitis of the mouth may secondarily generalize, but a careful history that reveals the original site of symptoms will help disclose the source.

Alcohol intake, in some cases at levels that would not otherwise be deemed excessive, can induce and exacerbate a wide array of dermatoses, including eczema, cellulitis, and psoriasis. In patients with chronic dermatitis or pruritus, a therapeutic trial of alcohol avoidance is warranted.

The anti-inflammatory effects of n-3 fatty acids are well established; a role in the treatment of inflammatory skin conditions is less clear. Fish oil supplementation in pregnancy may reduce atopic tendencies in newborns, raising the prospect that n-3 fatty acids are of greater utility in preventing than treating AD. The evidence of treatment effects is equivocal, but there is a strong case for

n-3 fatty acid supplementation on other grounds. Thus, a trial of fish oil for any chronic or refractory dermatitis is reasonable. A standard adult dose of fish oil is roughly 1 g, twice daily.

Abnormal intestinal permeability has been invoked to explain food allergy and associated dermatitis. The literature is suggestive of potential benefits of probiotics, prebiotics, and their combination in synbiotics. A course of probiotic is of potential benefit and unlikely harm in any case of chronic dermatitis or pruritus. Products meeting high quality control standards can be identified at www.consumerlab.com.

There is some suggestion that dermatitis risk increases with intake of refined sugar and saturated fat and declines with intake of several micronutrients, fruits, and unsaturated oils. The link between high-energy foods and worsening acne and psoriasis is becoming increasingly evident. Additionally, current studies are observing new associations between nutritional factors and skin cancer. Overall, these associations indicate that a dietary pattern advisable for purposes of general health promotion (see Chapter 45) may offer some protection against various dermatoses as well.

REFERENCES

1. Kim YJ, Kim MY, Kim HO, et al. Acrodermatitis enteropathica-like eruption associated with combined nutritional deficiency. *J Korean Med Sci* 2005;20(5):908–911.
2. Lansdown AB. Nutrition 2: a vital consideration in the management of skin wounds. *Br J Nurs* (Mark Allen Publishing) 2004;13(20):1199–1210.
3. Lansdown AB. Nutrition 1: a vital consideration in the management of skin wounds. *Br J Nurs* (Mark Allen Publishing) 2004;13(19):S22–S28.
4. Pastar Z, Lipozencic J. Adverse reactions to food and clinical expressions of food allergy. *J Skinmed* 2006;5(3):119–125; quiz 26–27.
5. Heine RG, Laske N, Hill DJ. The diagnosis and management of egg allergy. *Curr Allergy Asthma Rep* 2006;6(2):145–152.
6. Di Lorenzo G, Pacor ML, Mansueto P, et al. Food-additive-induced urticaria: a survey of 838 patients with recurrent chronic idiopathic urticaria. *Int Arch Allergy Immunol* 2005;138(3):235–242.
7. Buhner S, Reese I, Kuehl F, et al. Pseudoallergic reactions in chronic urticaria are associated with altered gastroduodenal permeability. *Allergy* 2004;59(10):1118–1123.
8. Bongaerts GP, Severijnen RS. Preventive and curative effects of probiotics in atopic patients. *Med Hypotheses* 2005;64(6):1089–1092.
9. Passeron T, Lacour JP, Fontas E, et al. Prebiotics and synbiotics: two promising approaches for the treatment of atopic dermatitis in children above 2 years. *Allergy* 2006;61(4):431–437.

10. Wickens K, Black PN, Stanley TV, et al. A differential effect of 2 probiotics in the prevention of eczema and atopy: a double-blind, randomized, placebo-controlled trial. *J Allergy Clin Immunol* 2008;122(4):788–794.

11. van der Aa LB, Heymans HS, van Aalderen WM, et al. Probiotics and prebiotics in atopic dermatitis: review of the theoretical background and clinical evidence. *Pediatr Allergy Immunol* 2010; 21(2 pt 2):e355–e367.

12. Betsi GI, Papadavid E, Falagas ME. Probiotics for the treatment or prevention of atopic dermatitis: a review of the evidence from randomized controlled trials. *Am J Clin Dermatol* 2008;9(2):93–103.

13. Maintz L, Benfadal S, Allam JP, et al. Evidence for a reduced histamine degradation capacity in a subgroup of patients with atopic eczema. *J Allergy Clin Immunol* 2006;117(5):1106–1112.

14. Solvoll K, Soyland E, Sandstad B, et al. Dietary habits among patients with atopic dermatitis. *Eur J Clin Nutr* 2000; 54(2):93–97.

15. Abenavoli L, Proietti I, Leggio L, et al. Cutaneous manifestations in celiac disease. *World J Gastroenterol* 2006;12(6):843–852.

16. Humbert P, Pelletier F, Dreno B, et al. Gluten intolerance and skin diseases. *Eur J Dermatol* 2006; 16(1):4–11.

17. Caminiti L, Passalacqua G, Magazzu G, et al. Chronic urticaria and associated coeliac disease in children: a case-control study. *Pediatr Allergy Immunol* 2005; 16(5):428–432.

18. Haussmann J, Sekar A. Chronic urticaria: a cutaneous manifestation of celiac disease. *Can J Gastroenterol* 2006; 20(4):291–293.

19. Higgins EM, du Vivier AW. Alcohol and the skin. *Alcohol and Alcoholism* (Oxford, Oxfordshire) 1992;27(6):595–602.

20. Higgins EM, du Vivier AW. Cutaneous disease and alcohol misuse. *Br Med Bull* 1994;50(1):85–98.

21. Kostovic K, Lipozencic J. Skin diseases in alcoholics. *Acta Dermatovenerol Croat* 2004;12(3):181–90.

22. Smith KE, Fenske NA. Cutaneous manifestations of alcohol abuse. *J Am Acad Dermatol* 2000; 43(1 pt 1):1–16; quiz 8.

23. Subramanian VS, Subramanya SB, Said HM. Chronic alcohol exposure negatively impacts the physiological and molecular parameters of the renal biotin reabsorption process. *Am J Physiol* 2011;300(3):F611–F617.

24. Subramanya SB, Subramanian VS, Kumar JS, et al. Inhibition of intestinal biotin absorption by chronic alcohol feeding: cellular and molecular mechanisms. *Am J Physiol* 2011;300(3):G494–G501.

25. Sakai K, Okuyama H, Shimazaki H, et al. Fatty acid compositions of plasma lipids in atopic dermatitis/asthma patients. *Arerugi* 1994; 43(1):37–43.

26. Soyland E, Lea T, Sandstad B, et al. Dietary supplementation with very long-chain n-3 fatty acids in man decreases expression of the interleukin-2 receptor (CD25) on mitogen-stimulated lymphocytes from patients with inflammatory skin diseases. *Eur J Clin Investig* 1994;24(4):236–242.

27. Trak-Fellermeier MA, Brasche S, Winkler G, et al. Food and fatty acid intake and atopic disease in adults. *Eur Respir J* 2004; 23(4):575–582.

28. Suzuki R, Shimizu T, Kudo T, et al. Effects of n-3 polyunsaturated fatty acids on dermatitis in NC/Nga mice. *Prostaglandins Leukot Essent Fatty Acids* 2002; 66(4):435–440.

29. Mayser P, Mayer K, Mahloudjian M, et al. A double-blind, randomized, placebo-controlled trial of n-3 versus n-6 fatty acid-based lipid infusion in atopic dermatitis. *JPEN* 2002;26(3):151–158.

30. Soyland E, Funk J, Rajka G, et al. Dietary supplementation with very long-chain n-3 fatty acids in patients with atopic dermatitis. A double-blind, multicentre study. *Br J Dermatol* 1994;130(6):757–764.

31. Horrobin DF. Essential fatty acid metabolism and its modification in atopic eczema. *Am J Clin Nutr* 2000;71(1 suppl): 367S–372S.

32. Das UN. Polyunsaturated fatty acids and atopic dermatitis. *Nutrition* 2010;26(7–8):719–720.

33. Foolad N, Brezinski EA, Chase EP, et al. Effect of nutrient supplementation on atopic dermatitis in children: a systematic review of probiotics, prebiotics, formula, and fatty acids. *Arch Dermatol* 2012;17:1–6.

34. Van Gool CJ, Zeegers MP, Thijs C. Oral essential fatty acid supplementation in atopic dermatitis—a meta-analysis of placebo-controlled trials. *Br J Dermatol* 2004;150(4): 728–740.

35. Anandan C, Nurmatov U, Sheikh A. Omega 3 and 6 oils for primary prevention of allergic disease: systematic review and meta-analysis. *Allergy* 2009;64(6):840–848.

36. Hoppu U, Rinne M, Lampi A-M, et al. Breast milk fatty acid composition is associated with development of atopic dermatitis in the infant. *J Pediatr Gastroenterol Nutr* 2005;41(3):335–338.

37. Klemens CM, Berman DR, Mozurkewich EL. The effect of perinatal omega-3 fatty acid supplementation on inflammatory markers and allergic diseases: a systematic review. *BJOG* 2011;118(8):916–925.

38. Dunstan JA, Mori TA, Barden A, et al. Fish oil supplementation in pregnancy modifies neonatal allergen-specific immune responses and clinical outcomes in infants at high risk of atopy: a randomized, controlled trial. *J Allergy Clin Immunol* 2003;112(6):1178–1184.

39. Prescott SL, Calder PC. N-3 polyunsaturated fatty acids and allergic disease. *Curr Opin Clin Nutr Metab Care* 2004;7(2):123–129.

40. Palmer DJ, Sullivan T, Gold MS, et al. Effect of n-3 long chain polyunsaturated fatty acid supplementation in pregnancy on infants' allergies in first year of life: randomised controlled trial. *BMJ* 2012;344:e184.

41. Zutavern A, Brockow I, Schaaf B, et al. Timing of solid food introduction in relation to atopic dermatitis and atopic sensitization: results from a prospective birth cohort study. *Pediatrics* 2006;117(2):401–411.

42. Tromp II, Kiefte-de Jong JC, Lebon A, et al. The introduction of allergenic foods and the development of reported wheezing and eczema in childhood: the Generation R study. *Arch Pediatr Adolesc Med* 2011; 165(10):933–938.

43. Finch J, Munhutu MN, Whitaker-Worth DL. Atopic dermatitis and nutrition. *Clin Dermatol* 2010;28(6):605–614.

44. Kramer MS, Kakuma R. Maternal dietary antigen avoidance during pregnancy or lactation, or both, for preventing or treating atopic disease in the child. *Cochrane Database Syst Rev* (Online). 2012;9:CD000133.

45. Jensen CS, Menne T, Johansen JD. Systemic contact dermatitis after oral exposure to nickel: a review with a modified meta-analysis. *Contact Dermat* 2006;54(2):79–86.

46. Kuligowski J, Halperin KM. Stainless steel cookware as a significant source of nickel, chromium, and iron. *Arch Environ Contam Toxicol* 1992;23(2):211–215.

47. Bowe WP, Joshi SS, Shalita AR. Diet and acne. *J Am Acad Dermatol* 2010;63(1):124–141.
48. Ferdowsian HR, Levin S. Does diet really affect acne? *Skin Therapy Lett* 2010;15(3):1–2, 5.
49. Ismail NH, Manaf ZA, Azizan NZ. High glycemic load diet, milk and ice cream consumption are related to acne vulgaris in Malaysian young adults: a case control study. *BMC Dermatol* 2012;12:13.
50. Melnik B. Acne vulgaris. Role of diet. *Der Hautarzt*; Zeitschrift fur Dermatologie, Venerologie, und verwandte Gebiete. 2010;61(2):115–125.
51. Adebamowo CA, Spiegelman D, Danby FW, et al. High school dietary dairy intake and teenage acne. *J Am Acad Dermatol* 2005; 52(2):207–214.
52. Smith RN, Mann NJ, Braue A, et al. A low-glycemic-load diet improves symptoms in acne vulgaris patients: a randomized controlled trial. *Am J Clin Nutr* 2007;86(1):107–115.
53. Smith RN, Mann NJ, Braue A, et al. The effect of a high-protein, low glycemic-load diet versus a conventional, high glycemic-load diet on biochemical parameters associated with acne vulgaris: a randomized, investigator-masked, controlled trial. *J Am Acad Dermatol* 2007;57(2):247–256.
54. Smith RN, Braue A, Varigos GA, et al. The effect of a low glycemic load diet on acne vulgaris and the fatty acid composition of skin surface triglycerides. *J Dermatol Sci* 2008; 50(1):41–52.
55. Wolters M. Diet and psoriasis: experimental data and clinical evidence. *Br J Dermatol* 2005;153(4):706–714.
56. Jensen P, Zachariae C, Christensen R, et al. Effect of weight loss on the severity of psoriasis: a randomized clinical study. *JAMA dermatol* 2013;149(7):795–801.
57. Treloar V. Integrative dermatology for psoriasis: facts and controversies. *Clin Dermatol* 2010;28(1):93–99.
58. Kamangar F, Koo J, Heller M, et al. Oral vitamin D, still a viable treatment option for psoriasis. *J Dermatol Treat* 2013;24(4):261–267.
59. Ricketts JR, Rothe MJ, Grant-Kels JM. Nutrition and psoriasis. *Clin Dermatol* 2010;28(6):615–626.
60. Steinmetz K, Potter J. Vegetables, fruit, and cancer. I: epidemiology. *Cancer Causes Control* 1991;2(5):325–357.
61. Greenberg ER, Baron JA, Stukel TA, et al. A clinical trial of beta carotene to prevent basal-cell and squamous-cell cancers of the skin. *N Engl J Med* 1990;323(12):789–795.
62. Stryker WS, Stamper MJ, Stein EA, et al. Diet, plasma levels of beta-carotene and alpha-tocopherol, and risk of malignant melanoma. *Am J Epidemiol* 1990;131(4):597–611.
63. Black HS, Thornby JI, Wolf JE, et al. Evidence that a low-fat diet reduces the occurrence of non-melanoma skin cancer. *Int J Cancer* 1995;62(2):165–169.
64. Østerlind A, Tucker MA, Stone BJ, et al. The Danish case-control study of cutaneous malignant melanoma. IV. No association with nutritional factors, alcohol, smoking or hair dyes. *Int J Cancer* 1988;42(6):825–828.
65. Duffield-Lillico AJ, Slate EH, Reid ME, et al. Selenium supplementation and secondary prevention of nonmelanoma skin cancer in a randomized trial. *J Natl Cancer Inst* 2003;95(19):1477–1481.

SUGGESTED READINGS

Barre DE. Potential of evening primrose, borage, black currant, and fungal oils in human health. *Ann Nutr Metab* 2001;45:47–57.

Barth GA, Weigl L, Boeing H, et al. Food intake of patients with atopic dermatitis. *Eur J Dermatol* 2001;11:199–202.

Ryan AS, Goldsmith LA. Nutrition and the skin. *Clin Dermatol* 1996;14:389–406.

CHAPTER 23

Diet and Wound Healing

O verall nutritional status influences the response of the body to metabolic stress. Wound healing requires sufficient nutritional substrate to support the formation of granulation tissue. Adequate intake of energy, protein, and various micronutrients before, during, and after either surgical or traumatic injury can influence the speed and vitality of tissue repair. Nutritional assessment and management strategies for the promotion of optimal wound healing have been elaborated, although evidence for certain interventions remains preliminary.

OVERVIEW

A patient's nutritional status is of vital importance to tissue repair in the advent of injury. Susceptibility to skin breakdown and the development of pressure ulcers is related in part to nutritional status (1,2), whereas wound development increases metabolic demand (3) (see Table 23-1). The adequacy of various micronutrients, total protein, and total energy influence wound healing. Metabolic demand is increased during wound healing, increasing the likelihood of negative nitrogen balance and catabolism. Energy, protein, and micronutrient deficiencies are among the most common impediments to optimal wound healing (4).

Evaluation of all patients' nutritional status should be performed before elective surgery. In patients with no clinical evidence of compromised nutritional status and who are clearly robust preoperatively, no laboratory testing is indicated. Patients with recent weight loss or who are chronically underweight require a more extensive evaluation (see Chapter 26, Sections VIIA, and VIID). A comprehensive assessment of nutritional status includes measures of dietary intake pattern, anthropometry, and biochemical assays. Dietary consultation in such cases is indicated. Preoperative nutritional support may be important to postoperative healing. Total parenteral nutrition

(TPN; see Chapter 26) is an intervention of last resort; it has been shown to reduce noninfectious complications of surgery in select patients while increasing infectious complications.

In general, preoperative nutrition support is indicated in patients unfed for a period of 7 days or more as well as patients expected not to eat for 10 days or more and patients with loss of more than 10% of lean body mass. Such patients should receive enteral nutrition support; only if contraindicated by intolerance or gastrointestinal tract dysfunction should TPN be used. In patients with evidence of poor nutritional status before elective surgery, enteral supplementation preoperatively may shorten recovery time (5). In patients who are well nourished before surgery, a 5% dextrose infusion for up to 1 week postoperatively has not been shown to impair recovery.

Because elderly patients have reduced appetite possibly compounded by impaired sensorium or functional status, they are highly subject to protein–calorie malnutrition and involuntary weight loss during wound healing. Nutritional status is correlated with the rate of wound healing. If compromised nutritional status results in loss of lean body mass, wound healing is delayed; therefore, nutritional support during wound healing should begin early, even when there is no evidence of nutritional impairment (6). Children, particularly neonates, are susceptible to loss of lean body mass during wound healing because their tissue reserves are limited (7).

The effects of specific nutrient deficiencies and isolated nutrient supplements on wound healing have been studied predominantly in animals. There is some evidence that pantothenic acid (vitamin B_5) supplementation can increase the tensile strength of aponeuroses and dermal scars. Thiamine is essential to normal collagen synthesis and metabolism, and animal studies have demonstrated impaired wound healing with deficiency.

Animal studies have demonstrated enhanced scar-tissue strength with vitamin A or provitamin A carotenoid supplementation and impaired

TABLE 23.1

Relative Increases in Metabolic Demand Associated with Various Physical Stressors[a]

Representative Stress Factors

Condition	Stress Factor
Alcoholism	0.9
Burn (<40%)	2.0–2.5
Cancer	1.10–1.45
Head trauma	1.35
Long-bone fracture	1.25–1.30
Mild starvation	0.85–1.0
Multiple trauma	1.30–1.55
Peritonitis	1.05–1.25
Severe infection	1.30–1.55
Uncomplicated postoperative recovery	1.00–1.05

[a]Uncomplicated surgical recovery increases metabolic demand above baseline levels by roughly 5%, but surgical complications or other forms of trauma, such as burns, can drive metabolic demand to much higher levels.

Source: Adapted from Frankenfield DC, Muth ER, Rowe WA. The Harris-Benedict studies of human basal metabolism: history and limitations. *J Am Diet Assoc* 1998;98:439–445.

healing with deficiency. Vitamin C, which is essential to the metabolism of both collagen and elastin, has been studied in humans to a limited extent. Studies summarized by Werbach (8) suggest that vitamin C supplementation at a dose of 500 mg per day can accelerate the healing of surgical wounds and pressure sores.

Evidence regarding zinc to date suggests that its nutriture is essential to healing, but that supplementation is of importance only when zinc stores are deficient. Animal evidence suggests that zinc is concentrated at the site of wound healing, with impaired tensile strength of skin resulting when zinc is deficient (9). Recent epidemiological data suggest that incipient zinc deficiency may be relatively widespread worldwide, concentrated in developing countries (10).

In a human study of pantothenic acid and ascorbic acid on skin wound healing, no direct benefit of supplementation was seen on the wound healing process, though supplementation seemed to modulate the concentration of trace minerals in the scars (11). In a randomized controlled trial of 32 children with burns, an antioxidant combination containing vitamins E and C and zinc was found to reduce wound healing time and decrease markers of lipid peroxidation (12).

In a randomized trial of 16 inpatients with pressure ulcers, Desneves et al. (13) compared standard care to the addition of two high-protein, high-energy supplements daily, with and without the addition of 9 g of arginine, 500 mg of vitamin C, and 30 mg of zinc daily. Healing was significantly faster, as measured by the Pressure Ulcer Scale for Healing (PUSH), in the group receiving arginine, vitamin C, and zinc than in either of the other two groups. A 2005 systematic review showed that oral nutritional supplements (of various ingredients) were associated with a reduced risk of developing pressure ulcers (14–16). The specific evidence surrounding supplemental arginine for wound healing is inconclusive, however, and there are potential risks (i.e., possibly causing hemodynamic instability in critically ill patients) (17).

Lee et al. (18) demonstrated similar benefits in a larger group using a concentrated, fortified collagen protein hydrolysate supplement. Nearly 90 residents in 23 long-term care facilities with pressure ulcers were randomized to the supplement or placebo three times daily for 8 weeks in conjunction with standard care. Nearly twice the rate of healing was observed in the supplemented group as compared to the controls. Collagen synthesis can also be enhanced with supplementation of a combination of arginine, glutamine, and β-hydroxy-β-methylbutyrate (HMB), a leucine metabolite. This combination has also shown benefit in increasing exercise-related lean muscle mass (19).

In a case-control study of chronic lower-extremity ulcers, Rojas and Phillips (20) found patients to have lower serum levels of vitamin A and carotenes, vitamin E, and zinc. These nutrients are generally thought to influence wound healing capacity (21). Supplements of the amino acids glutamine and arginine, and n-3 fatty acids, have shown promise in accelerating a patient's recovery from burns (17,22). n-3 fatty acids, however, may impair the postoperative healing response by impairing collagen fibril crosslinking or orientation (23).

Of increasing relevance is the adverse influence of obesity on wound healing (24). Surgical wound closure and wound perfusion may be compromised by excess subcutaneous fat. Metabolic derangements associated with obesity (see Chapter 5) may interfere with tissue recovery as well. Obese individuals frequently face wound complications, including skin wound infection, dehiscence, hematoma and seroma formation, pressure ulcers, and venous ulcers (24) (www.cdc.gov/nccdphp/dnpa/obesity). An increased frequency of wound complications has been reported for obese individuals undergoing both bariatric and non-bariatric operations (25–27). In particular, a higher rate of surgical site infection occurs in obese patients. Many of these complications may be a result of a relative hypoperfusion and ischemia that occurs in subcutaneous adipose tissue. This situation may be caused by a decreased delivery of antibiotics as well. In surgical wounds, the increased tension on the wound edges that is frequently seen in obese patients also contributes to wound dehiscence. Wound tension increases tissue pressure, reducing microperfusion and the availability of oxygen to the wound (24–28).

Wound infection has the potential to disrupt the healing process, while placing further metabolic demands on the patient. The adequacy of nutrition during wound healing has systemic effects on immune function (see Chapter 11), thereby influencing susceptibility to wound infection (29).

Among the metabolic derangements associated with trauma is accelerated gluconeogenesis, which contributes to a state of catabolism (30). Protein requirements rise during recovery from trauma, and supplemental protein should be provided during periods of wound healing.

In addition to adequate nutritional support, pain control, conditioning exercises, and anabolic agents may contribute to preservation of lean body mass and to wound healing. In a study of eight patients with nonhealing wounds, Demling and De Santi (30) found that all subjects had lost at least 10% of body weight. Nutritional support alone failed to restore the lost weight or influence wound closure. The addition of oxandrolone, an oral anabolic agent, in combination with nutritional support led to weight gain and wound healing, with complete or partial wound closure in all subjects over 12 weeks. The authors noted a high correlation between restoration of lean body mass and wound healing (31).

Other Dietary Supplements

Bromelain

Bromelain is an extract of proteolytic enzymes derived from pineapple stems. In culinary use, it is used as a meat tenderizer. A number of studies have demonstrated anti-inflammatory, fibrinolytic, and skin debridement properties (32). Oral bromelain supplements may help reduce swelling and improve healing time for surgical wounds and soft tissue injuries. Animal studies have shown improved blood perfusion in firearm wounds when supplemented with bromelain (33). Preliminary studies have found effectiveness in a relatively noninvasive debridement of deep burns with minimal blood loss (34). Caution should be exercised in the use of bromelain as it also inhibits platelet aggregation and thus can cause bleeding (23).

Probiotics

Preclinical (laboratory) studies show that a probiotic may be useful for mucosal injuries as experienced in inflammatory bowel disease. A preparation of E. coli Nissle 1917 was shown to enhance the wound-healing migration of human enterocytes (35).

Nutrigenomic considerations

Topical dexpanthenol (vitamin B_5) is often used in clinical practice to improve wound healing. A clinical trial found that the application of topical dexpanthenol resulted in the upregulation of IL-6, IL-1β, CYP1B1, CXCL1, CCL18, and KAP 4-2 gene expression and downregulation of psoriasin mRNA and protein expression (36).

The probiotic E. coli 1917 induced COX-2 expression and PGE(2) secretion in intestinal epithelial cells (37).

Nutrient–Drug Interactions

Aspirin—Vitamin C

Aspirin increases vitamin C excretion, reducing tissue and leukocyte uptake of vitamin C, leaving more in the plasma to be filtered into the urine. Aspirin may also reduce gut absorption of vitamin C (38).

Antibiotics—Calcium

Calcium can affect the absorption of multiple classes of antibiotics (tetracyclines, quinolones). Dosing should be adjusted such that calcium supplements and antibiotic administration are at least 2 to 6 hours apart. There also exists a potentially fatal precipitation of ceftriaxone-calcium salts in infants (39).

CLINICAL HIGHLIGHTS

Evidence in the aggregate is conclusive that overall nutritional status influences the pace and quality of wound healing. Evidence for specific nutritional manipulations to enhance wound healing capacity is generally less definitive. Patients scheduled for elective surgery should routinely be assessed for the adequacy of their diets, recent weight loss history, and preservation of lean body mass. Preoperative nutrition supplementation in marginally malnourished patients may be of benefit and is of clear benefit when malnutrition is advanced.

Energy and protein needs are increased in patients recovering from surgical trauma as well as during healing of traumatic wounds. Multivitamin/multimineral supplements are advisable in older adults on general principles and may be of particular benefit in wound healing, as trace minerals (magnesium, copper, and zinc) are involved in wound healing (17). Bromelain supplements show promise, but should be used with caution. Supplementation with glutamine and arginine (and combinations) may be of benefit, but this is uncertain. A beneficial role of n-3 fatty acids has been suggested.

Dietary consultation to optimize nutrition is prudent in patients with nonhealing wounds, as case reports of rapid recovery following nutritional adjustments have been published. In general, the nutritional guidelines to promote wound healing are consistent with those that can be advocated on general principles. While the use of various supplements has shown promise, no single regimen has yet emerged as the clearly preferred, evidence-based approach (40,41). Thus, the mainstay of nutritional care in wound healing is individualized assessment and care, with general principles of healthful nutrition underlying.

REFERENCES

1. Raffoul W, Far MS, Cayeux MC, et al. Nutritional status and food intake in nine patients with chronic low-limb ulcers and pressure ulcers: importance of oral supplements. *Nutrition* 2006;22(1):82–88.
2. Todorovic V. Food and wounds: nutritional factors in wound formation and healing. *Br J Commun Nurs* 2002:43–44,46,48 passim.
3. Casey G. Nutritional support in wound healing. *Nurs Stand* 2003;17(23):55–58.
4. Stadelmann WK, Digenis AG, Tobin GR. Impediments to wound healing. *Am J Surg* 1998;176(2A suppl):39S–47S.
5. McClave SA, Snider HL, Spain DA. Preoperative issues in clinical nutrition. *Chest* 1999;115(5 suppl):64S–70S.
6. Himes D. Protein-calorie malnutrition and involuntary weight loss: the role of aggressive nutritional intervention in wound healing. *Ostomy Wound Manag* 1999;45(3):46–51,54–45.
7. Shew SB, Jaksic T. The metabolic needs of critically ill children and neonates. *Semi Pediatr Surg* 1999;8(3):131–139.
8. Werbach MR. *Nutritional Influences on Illness: a sourcebook of clinical research*, 2nd ed. Tarzana, CA: Third Line Press, 1988.
9. Nezu R, Takagi Y, Ito T, et al. The importance of total parenteral nutrition-associated tissue zinc distribution in wound healing. *Surg Today* 1999;29(1):34–41.
10. Wessells KR, Brown KH. Estimating the global prevalence of zinc deficiency: results based on zinc availability in national food supplies and the prevalence of stunting. *PloS One* 2012;7(11):e50568.
11. Vaxman F, Olender S, Lambert A, et al. Effect of pantothenic acid and ascorbic acid supplementation on human skin wound healing process. A double-blind, prospective and randomized trial. *Eur Surg Res* 1995;27(3):158–166.
12. Barbosa E, Faintuch J, Machado Moreira EA, et al. Supplementation of vitamin E, vitamin C, and zinc attenuates oxidative stress in burned children: a randomized, double-blind, placebo-controlled pilot study. *J Burn Care Res* 2009;30(5):859–866.
13. Desneves KJ, Todorovic BE, Cassar A, et al. Treatment with supplementary arginine, vitamin C and zinc in patients with pressure ulcers: a randomised controlled trial. *Clin Nutr* 2005;24(6):979–987.
14. Stratton RJ, Ek AC, Engfer M, et al. Enteral nutritional support in prevention and treatment of pressure ulcers: a systematic review and meta-analysis. *Ageing Res Rev* 2005;4(3):422–450.
15. Biesalski H. Micronutrients, wound healing, and prevention of pressure ulcers. *Nutrition* 2010;26(9):858.
16. van Anholt RD, Sobotka L, Meijer EP, et al. Specific nutritional support accelerates pressure ulcer healing and reduces wound care intensity in non-malnourished patients. *Nutrition* 2010;26(9):867–872.
17. Stechmiller JK. Understanding the role of nutrition and wound healing. *Nutr Clin Pract* 2010;25(1):61–68.
18. Lee SK, Posthauer ME, Dorner B, et al. Pressure ulcer healing with a concentrated, fortified, collagen protein hydrolysate supplement: a randomized controlled trial. *Adv Skin Wound Care* 2006;19(2):92–96.
19. Williams JZ, Abumrad N, Barbul A. Effect of a specialized amino acid mixture on human collagen deposition. *Ann Surg* 2002;236(3):369–374; discussion 374–365.
20. Rojas AI, Phillips TJ. Patients with chronic leg ulcers show diminished levels of vitamins A and E, carotenes, and zinc. *Dermatol Surg* 1999;25(8):601–604.
21. Thomas DR. Specific nutritional factors in wound healing. *Adv Wound Care* 1997;10(4):40–43.
22. De-Souza DA, Greene LJ. Pharmacological nutrition after burn injury. *J Nutr* 1998;128(5):797–803.
23. Kavalukas SL, Barbul A. Nutrition and wound healing: an update. *Plast Reconstr Surg* 2011;127(suppl 1):38S–43S.
24. Wilson JA, Clark JJ. Obesity: impediment to postsurgical wound healing. *Adv Skin Wound Care* 2004;17(8):426–435.
25. Anaya DA, Dellinger EP. The obese surgical patient: a susceptible host for infection. *Surg Infect* 2006;7(5):473–480.

26. Greco JA 3rd, Castaldo ET, Nanney LB, et al. The effect of weight loss surgery and body mass index on wound complications after abdominal contouring operations. *Ann Plast Surg* 2008;61(3):235–242.

27. Momeni A, Heier M, Bannasch H, et al. Complications in abdominoplasty: a risk factor analysis. *Journal Plast, Reconstr Aesthetic Surg* 2009;62(10):1250–1254.

28. Guo S, Dipietro LA. Factors affecting wound healing. *J Dent Res* 2010;89(3):219–229.

29. Thornton FJ, Schaffer MR, Barbul A. Wound healing in sepsis and trauma. *Shock* 1997;8(6):391–401.

30. Demling RH, DeSanti L. Involuntary weight loss and the nonhealing wound: the role of anabolic agents. *Adv Wound Care* 1999;12(1 suppl):1–14; quiz 15–16.

31. Demling R, De Santi L. Closure of the "non-healing wound" corresponds with correction of weight loss using the anabolic agent oxandrolone. *Ostomy Wound Manag* 1998;44(10):58–62,64,66 passim.

32. Therapeutic Research Faculty. Bromelain. *Nat Med Compr Database* 2013.

33. Wu SY, Hu W, Zhang B, et al. Bromelain ameliorates the wound microenvironment and improves the healing of firearm wounds. *J Surg Res* 2012;176(2):503–509.

34. Koller J, Bukovcan P, Orsag M, et al. Enzymatic necrolysis of acute deep burns—report of preliminary results with 22 patients. *Acta Chir Plast* 2008;50(4):109–114.

35. Choi HJ, Ahn JH, Park SH, et al. Enhanced wound healing by recombinant Escherichia coli Nissle 1917 via human epidermal growth factor receptor in human intestinal epithelial cells: therapeutic implication using recombinant probiotics. *Infect Immun* 2012;80(3):1079–1087.

36. Heise R, Skazik C, Marquardt Y, et al. Dexpanthenol modulates gene expression in skin wound healing in vivo. *Skin Pharmacol Physiol* 2012;25(5):241–248.

37. Otte JM, Mahjurian-Namari R, Brand S, et al. Probiotics regulate the expression of COX-2 in intestinal epithelial cells. *Nutr Cancer* 2009;61(1):103–113.

38. Therapeutic Research Faculty. Vitamin C. *Nat Med Compr Database* 2013.

39. Therapeutic Research Faculty. Calcium. *Nat Med Compr Database* 2013.

40. Thompson C, Fuhrman MP. Nutrients and wound healing: still searching for the magic bullet. *Nutr Clin Pract* 2005;20(3):331–347.

41. Arnold M, Barbul A. Nutrition and wound healing. *Plast Reconstr Surg* 2006;117(7 suppl):42S–58S.

SUGGESTED READINGS

DeSanti L. Pathophysiology and current management of burn injury. *Adv Skin Wound Care* 2005;18:323–332.

Kudsk KA, Sacks GS. Nutrition in the care of the patient with surgery, trauma, and sepsis. In: Shils ME, Shike M, Ross AC, et al., eds. *Modern nutrition in health and disease*, 10th ed. Philadelphia, PA: Lippincott Williams & Wilkins, 2006:1414–1435.

Posthauer ME. When is enteral nutrition support an effective strategy? *Adv Skin Wound Care* 2006;19:257–260.

Whitney JD, Heitkemper MM. Modifying perfusion, nutrition, and stress to promote wound healing in patients with acute wounds. *Heart Lung* 1999;28:123.

CHAPTER 24

Food Allergy and Intolerance

A dverse reactions to food include intolerance, a non-immune–mediated abnormal physiologic response, and true food allergy, an immunologic reaction to ingested antigens. Intolerance may be mediated by metabolic processes (e.g., lactose intolerance), contaminants (e.g., bacteria or toxins), or pharmacologic effects of ingested food chemicals (e.g., alcohol, caffeine). True food allergy is typically an antibody-mediated, immediate hypersensitivity response. A cell-mediated, delayed hypersensitivity reaction is well established only for gluten but is posited to occur with other food antigens as well. Other adverse reactions are idiosyncratic. Although there is considerable uncertainty about the epidemiology of food allergy, due to methodological differences and uncertainty in diagnostic testing, the data suggest an increasing prevalence over the last decade with a 2010 meta-analysis displaying a range between 2% to 10% (1). The overall improved public health measures and vaccination systems have lead groups to believe that the "hygiene hypothesis" is to blame for our increase in atopy. The "hygiene hypothesis" indicates that the lack of early childhood exposure to infectious disease, crowded environments, and unhygienic conditions increases susceptibility to allergic diseases, such as eczema, allergic rhinitis, and asthma. Although there are many associations with the change in environment and the increase in atopy globally, there are very limited data to indicate an association with respect to food allergies (2,3).

Generally, the predominant antibody reaction to ingested antigen is mediated by immunoglobulin A (IgA). Systemic hypersensitivity reactions to food are predominantly mediated by immunoglobulin E (IgE), and thus IgE-mediated food allergy is generally deemed most important. True food allergy is broken down into three categories, IgE-mediated (i.e., acute urticaria/angioedema, anaphylaxis, oral allergy syndrome), non-IgE-mediated (i.e., food protein-induced enterocolitis,

Heiner syndrome), and mixed IgE and non-IgE (i.e., atopic dermatitis, Eosinophilic Esophagitis). The majority of our discussion will focus on IgE-mediated reactions; these are unique in that they are associated with mediator release from tissue mast cells and circulating basophils. Therefore, these reactions are very rapid in onset (minutes to 2 hours), mainly affecting the skin, gastrointestinal (GI) tract, respiratory and/or cardiovascular systems. Ingested antigens must traverse the intestinal mucosa and enter the circulation to elicit a hypersensitivity response; thus, food antigens are stable, water-soluble proteins of predictable size. Categorically any food may cause an allergic response and over 170 of them have been reported to be linked to IgE-mediated reactions. The foods most commonly responsible for hypersensitivity reactions include eggs, peanuts, other nuts, milk, soy, wheat, fish, and shellfish. Bovine milk allergy is common in infancy.

OVERVIEW

Diet

The prevalence of true food allergy is estimated at approximately 2% to 10%, although in most self-reported surveys, a much larger majority of the population believe themselves to have food allergy. A meta-analysis comparing self-reported data to clinical testing was done in 2007 comparing food allergies to milk, eggs, peanuts, fish, and shellfish found that 12% to 13% reported food allergy while clinical testing only indicated around a 3% yield. (4). The gold standard for food allergy testing is a double-blind, placebo-controlled oral food challenges; however, due to the increased risk of anaphylaxis, most of the data relies on retrospective case series studies. Intolerance to food additives is quite uncommon, estimated to be 1 per 10,000 population. There is some preliminary evidence associating food allergy in childhood with *Helicobacter pylori* infection;

disruption of the GI barrier by ingested antigens is the presumed mechanism (5). The prevalence of food allergy in children under age 3 is estimated at 5% to 8%; the early identification, management, and prevention of food allergy in infants remain quite challenging (6).

With the exception of hypersensitivity to peanuts, tree nuts, fish, and shellfish, most food allergies occur in infancy and are outgrown by early childhood. Overall, approximately 40% of food allergies in children subside by age 5. Once a food allergen is identified and excluded from the diet, rechallenge after 1 to 2 years is appropriate, as most allergies abate with time. Allergies to tree nuts, peanuts, and seafood are particularly persistent, and rechallenge at 4- to 8-year intervals is more appropriate when these foods are implicated. Recent attention has been drawn to the particular hazards of food allergies in adolescence. Social circumstances frequently appear to increase adolescents risk exposure to known allergens and forgo use of injectable epinephrine, suggesting a need for targeted educational programs. Adolescents frequently have a false sense of security concerning their food allergies, are often inadequately trained, and may find it difficult to manage their emotions surrounding emergencies (7).

Theoretically, exposure to food antigens in early infancy may be particularly likely to lead to hypersensitivity in susceptible individuals because of low levels of secretory IgA. Limited binding of antigen in the GI tract leads to greater absorption and more IgE generation. These theories contributed to the previous recommendations by the American Academy of Pediatrics (AAP) in 2000. These recommendations once advised for the most hyperallergenic foods to be introduced slowly into the atopic infant's diet by adding cow's milk at 1 year old, eggs at 2 years old and peanuts, tree nuts, and fish at 3 years old (8). The goal was to discourage the likelihood of reaction to these foods; however, with the increasing prevalence of food allergies, there have been drastic changes in the recommendations by the AAP. In 2008, the AAP stated that there was no convincing evidence to delay the introduction of these hyperallergenic foods (9). In fact, more recent studies indicate that the delayed introduction of many of these foods actually may increase the risk of allergy and allergic disease. In addition, guidelines published in the American Academy of Allergy, Asthma & Immunology in 2012 have now recommended against restricting highly allergenic foods in nonatopic

infants during lactation, as well as against restricting essential foods like milk and eggs during pregnancy. Inconclusive evidence exists around peanut ingestion during pregnancy, and at this time no recommendation can be made (10). There is some evidence that maternal use of probiotic supplements during lactation may be protective.

There is no evidence that the substitution of soy-based formulas for milk-based formulas attenuates the risk of atopy (11). Hypoallergenic formulas are available (Alimentum, Nutramigen, Pregestimil) (12) and are preferred, at least for high-risk infants weaned before 6 months. Although strict avoidance of these hyperallergenic foods is the primary therapy, it is essential that families have close clinical follow-up with a dietician to ensure proper nutritional adequacy of the diet. The current literature has hypothesized a so-called "window of opportunity," described as a poorly defined period of time in which children develop tolerance to foods requiring direct exposure to these foods (10,13). Not exposing children to these hyperallergenic foods may actually make them more susceptible to reactions in the future. The dual-allergen exposure hypothesis also heavily challenges the current debate that the allergic sensitization to food is best accomplished through elimination diets. This hypothesis has been studied extensively in murine models, evaluated thoroughly in retrospective studies, and is now undergoing two randomized clinical trials. The theory is based on the idea that allergic sensitization is mainly achieved through cutaneous sensitization and the early consumption of food protein leads to oral tolerance. Therefore, the order and balance of exposure to specific antigens will determine the child's development of allergy or tolerance. Children with severe eczema by definition have highly disruptive cutaneous barriers and this hypothesis has linked the presence of early severe eczema with early development of food allergies. One cross-sectional study compared Jewish children in Israel and the United Kingdom. They observed a 10-fold higher prevalence of peanut allergy in the United Kingdom children compared to the Israeli children, noting that peanuts were introduced earlier, eaten more often and in much larger quantities in Israel as compared to the UK families (3,14). These studies offer some fascinating insight into early oral exposure of known allergens to infants, and have the potential for drastically shifting the approach for introduction of complementary foods in the near future.

The most common manifestation of true food allergy is cutaneous, ranging from urticaria and angioedema to atopic dermatitis; the link between food allergy and atopic dermatitis is particularly important. The 2012: ICON Food allergy review describes a 2.4-fold increased likelihood of atopic dermatitis in children with food allergies (13,15). The spectrum of cutaneous manifestations of food allergy has been reviewed (16,17). GI reactions such as nausea, vomiting, and abdominal pain (IgE-mediated) tend to occur acutely within 1 hour of ingestion, while symptoms like blood in stool(non-IgE-mediated or mixed) tend to be more associated with infants and young children and often are delayed/chronic in onset taking >2 hours to present. A condition known as Heiner's syndrome is a form of pulmonary hemosiderosis associated with hypersensitivity to bovine milk protein or, less commonly, egg or pork. Symptoms resolve with avoidance of the implicated food.

Oral allergy syndrome (pollen-food allergy syndrome) is also an IgE-mediated response that is more of a contact hypersensitivity of the oropharynx and typically associated with fresh fruits and raw vegetables. These reactions tend to occur minutes after ingesting the allergen and result in mild swelling of lips and throat, pruritus, and localized irritation. Only 1% to 2% of these cases ever result in full blown anaphylaxis (18). Specifically, the syndrome is induced in individuals with respiratory allergy to birch pollen, potatoes, carrots, celery, hazelnuts, and apples; in individuals with respiratory allergy to ragweed pollen, melons and bananas are implicated. The putative mechanism is antigenic cross-reactivity, although the responsible antigens have, for the most part, not been identified.

Among the varieties of food intolerance distinct from allergy is pseudoallergy, in which symptoms are related to the release of histamine. The histamine release appears to be related to chemical rather than immunologic mechanisms, and it requires a large exposure. Dietary chemicals with pharmacologic properties often produce intolerance. Caffeine may be poorly tolerated, as may vasoactive amines such as histamine in fermented deli meats (sausage) and sauerkraut and tyramine in cheese, chocolate, and red wine. Monosodium glutamate, typically associated with Chinese food, may lead to flushing and palpitations. Sulfites added to wine may be poorly tolerated, as may strong spices and capsaicin.

An association between "colic" in infants and the presence of bovine milk immunoglobulin G in breast milk has been established, suggesting that hypersensitivity may account for some cases of colic (10% to 15%). Chronic constipation in young children may be a manifestation of allergy to bovine milk proteins (19). Although isolated respiratory manifestations of food allergy are relatively less common, rhinitis and exacerbations of asthma have been convincingly associated with foods in blinded challenges.

Food-mediated anaphylaxis does occur, as does a variant, in which both food hypersensitivity and exercise are required in combination to induce the anaphylactic response. Both are IgE-type reactions that result in systemic reactions often involving combinations of systems including the skin, respiratory, and GI tracts or less commonly may involve cardiovascular comprise. As described previously the potent vasoconstrictor, epinephrine, is crucial in individuals experiencing anaphylaxis, and use is usually limited to two pens in the home setting for unrelenting symptoms spaced 5 to 15 minutes apart. Although the epinephrine pen has played a crucial role in preventing many fatalities, there are cases in which the early and repeated administrations of the pen have still resulted in fatality (13). Peanuts and tree nuts are the most common triggers for these reactions, and delayed use of epinephrine is far and away the most common associated factor leading to death. Other common factors include being a teenager/young adult with asthma, absence of skin symptoms, or reliance on oral antihistamines (13,20).

Mixed-IgE- and non-IgE-mediated reactions commonly involve the GI tract. Eosinophilic gastroenteritis may be induced by milk protein hypersensitivity in infants and may require 12 weeks to resolve after removal of the offending antigen from the diet; short-term corticosteroid therapy may be indicated for both eosinophilic gastroenteritis and food-induced enterocolitis.

Food allergy has been implicated in some cases of migraine headache. Although there is interest in the possible role of food allergy in inflammatory arthritis, inflammatory bowel disease, dysmenorrhea, chronic fatigue, and a variety of other constitutional symptoms, there is currently no convincing evidence. The means by which allergens are presented to cells of the GI tract and how these mechanisms might be used in vaccine development are topics of ongoing investigation (21,22), as is a potential role for food allergy in irritable bowel syndrome (23).

The diagnosis of food allergy is facilitated by a history that establishes a temporal link between ingestion and the manifestations of hypersensitivity. Food allergy is much more likely when a family history of atopy is present. A diet diary is useful in identifying potential allergens.

Skin testing is fairly reliable and speedy in excluding IgE-mediated food allergy, as the test is quite sensitive, although skin testing to rule out food allergy has recently been challenged (24). Skin testing is generally not considered reliable for ruling in food allergy because of limited specificity (25). Data suggest that skin prick tests may be of variable utility, depending on the allergen (26); such tests perform poorly for soy allergy in particular (27). A more specific test is serum IgE immunoassay testing. This testing is also very reliable and is more sensitive than the often previously performed serum radioallergosorbent tests (RAST). In combination, these tests with a thorough clinical history and physical examination provide invaluable information to make more complete medical decision-making. However, the most important thing to remember is that the degree of positivity of either test does not correlate with the severity of reactions (13). No laboratory tests are available for the detection of non-IgE-mediated food allergies. Novel testing methods, such as patch testing (28,29) and basophil activation (30), are under investigation. Thus far, however, no testing method fully substitutes for food elimination and blinded challenges (31).

Elimination diets are useful both diagnostically and therapeutically, requiring that the correct food antigen be entirely eliminated from the diet for a period of 1 to 2 weeks. Software to facilitate the detection of food allergens and safe foods in food diaries is available (32). As mentioned previously, the most definitive diagnostic and specific method is double-blind, placebo-controlled oral challenge with the suspected antigen; such testing is potentially hazardous and should be done only when truly necessary, and then only under carefully controlled circumstances. The diagnostic approach to food allergy has been reviewed (26).

There are multiple advances being introduced in the arena of curative medicine for food allergies, including oral immunotherapy, extensively heated egg and milk diets, sublingual immunotherapy, epicutaneous immunotherapy, modified recombinant food protein vaccines, as well as adjuvants such as Chinese herbal formulations, anti-IgE monoclonal antibody therapy, and the use of helminthes (22). In addition, there is great promise shown in the arena of gut microflora and food allergy prevention and treatment. It is evident that gut microflora plays a crucial role in development and maintenance of building tolerance to antigens most likely by a combination of factors including T-cell regulation. Although epidemiological studies yield strong correlations between food allergy and the gut microbiota, thus far the limited clinical data have shown weak correlations (33–35). At present, the treatment of food allergy depends on elimination of the implicated antigen(s) from the diet (36). Whenever possible, the antigenic proteins should be identified, rather than the whole food most likely to contain them, as the proteins may be present in other foods. For example, the milk proteins responsible for hypersensitivity, casein and whey, may be included on ingredient lists independent of milk. Lecithin often is derived from either soy or egg, but the source is frequently not included on ingredient labels.

Because food allergens tend to be widely distributed in the food supply, elimination requires expert dietary advice both to achieve full elimination and to avoid nutrient deficiencies. Importantly, families must continue to be very vigilant concerning their higher risk atopic children and practice the necessary preventive strategies in order to promote wellness while still maintaining a sense of normalcy. Other treatment approaches, such as herbal remedies and oral desensitization, are receiving increasing attention in the research literature but are not yet advisable as standard clinical practice (13,37). The hope for these alternate therapies is that they one day will provide true clinical tolerance, in order for the patient to experience permanent freedom from allergic response even if the allergen is eliminated and later reintroduced. At the present moment, the treatments are mostly showing desensitization, requiring individual to continue daily/frequent maintenance therapy and only protecting individuals to a limited exposure based on the current dose of allergen. These studies are in Phase-I/II trials and hold the key for the first curative therapeutic agents (22).

The most common food allergies in adults are to fish, shellfish, nuts, and peanuts. In children, the most common reactions are to milk, eggs, peanuts, soy, and wheat. Peanuts are in the legume family and, therefore, have antigens that do not generally cross-react with those of other nuts.

NUTRIENTS, NUTRICEUTICALS, AND FUNCTIONAL FOODS

Lactose

Intolerance to lactose, a milk sugar, results from deficiency of the enzyme lactase. Deficiency actually is considered the normal condition for adult mammals, with preservation of enzyme activity into adulthood the result of a genetic mutation. Lactase deficiency is considered the most common enzyme deficiency; more than half of all adults are affected. Deficiency is especially common in individuals of African, Asian, Mediterranean, and Native-American origin. These individuals typically have enough lactase enzyme till around 5 years of age, than will have a precipitous drop in lactase causing a variability in tolerance of lactose loads in the large intestines. Lactose tolerance is highly prevalent in northern Europeans.

Lactose intolerance is distinct from allergy to milk proteins. For individuals allergic to bovine milk protein, alternative milks may be substituted. However, all milks (cow, goat, sheep) contain lactose. Milk products such as cheese and butter contain milk protein, so they cannot be eaten by individuals with true allergy, but they contain trivial amounts of lactose. Most individuals with lactose intolerance of genetic origin can tolerate at least 5 g of lactose contained in 100 mL of milk with no symptoms. In a randomized, double-blind crossover trial, Suarez et al. (38) demonstrated that adults self-reporting severe lactose intolerance could tolerate up to 15 g of lactose in 250 mL of milk.

In a separate study, Suarez et al. (39) demonstrated that lactose intolerance is unlikely to interfere meaningfully with a dietary pattern providing the recommended 1,500 mg of daily calcium in adult women. The GI symptoms attributed by many individuals to lactose intolerance may represent a form of irritable bowel syndrome of as yet uncertain etiology (40–43). To the extent that symptoms are induced by lactose in maldigesters, there is no appreciable difference between whole-fat and fat-free milk; recommendations to such individuals to use whole-fat dairy products to reduce symptoms are unfounded (44). For lactose-intolerant patients consuming more than 15 g per day of lactose, a variety of lactose-free or hydrolyzed-lactose products are available (see Sections VIIH and VIIJ).

Gluten

Gluten is a protein found in many cereal grains, and it is especially abundant in wheat. Other implicated grains include rye and barley. Other products under these categories include products cross-contaminated with wheat, rye, or barley, in addition products containing triticale (cross between wheat and rye), along with wheat products (spelt, kamut, semolina, bulgur, farina, etc.). Intolerance to gluten has a variety of conditions associated including non-celiac gluten sensitivity, wheat allergy, and celiac disease. In 2011, an expert panel came together to discuss new nomenclature for these varied gluten-related disorders (45). Non-celiac gluten sensitivity is by far the most common, with an assumed prevalence of 6% of the US population. These individuals may present with similar GI manifestations common to celiac disease such as bloating and abdominal pain, in addition to a variety of other symptoms including headaches, confusion, and ataxia. However, there is no associated damage to the small intestine, no specific celiac antibodies, and is mainly considered a diagnosis of exclusion. Symptoms usually resolve after onset of a gluten-free diet. Wheat allergy on the other hand is an IgE-mediated reaction and occurs in <1% of children and rarely in adult populations. The most well studied gluten-related disorder is celiac disease, which is autoimmune in nature, with its prevalence at about 1% of the population. Its hallmark is gluten-induced villous atrophy that occurs in the small intestine (45–47). Dermatitis herpetiformis and gluten ataxia are other autoimmune conditions associated with gluten intolerance. Antibody testing to endomysial tissue indicates that gluten sensitivity is more prevalent than the number of clinically overt cases would suggest; thus, mild cases may go clinically undetected (48). The prevalence of gluten intolerance is estimated to be 1 in 300 for individuals of European origin. Gluten intolerance is lifelong, and exclusion of gluten from the diet is the only known treatment to date (49). While gluten enteropathy is immune mediated, and thus a true food allergy, it is cell mediated and manifests as a delayed hypersensitivity reaction rather than an acute, antibody-mediated reaction, and thus it is atypical. Various sources refer to the condition as allergy or intolerance, in part because it is not a typical example of either.

The increased prevalence of gluten intolerance is often challenged and considered difficult to define (50). However, there is a rising amount of literature leading toward a likely increase in prevalence throughout the world correlated with the widened spectrum of disorders associated with gluten sensitivity, along with the empiric evidence of increased purchasing and ingestion of gluten-free products (45,51). The reason for this increased prevalence is unclear but has been speculated to be associated with multiple factors, including the compromised intestinal barrier function (i.e., leaky gut syndrome theory), human genetics, environmental toxins, intestinal infections, autoimmune diseases, increased ingestion of Westernized gluten diets, and also genetically modified foods (46,50). These factors are common in popular science and remain as speculations due to limited data availability. It is clear that Western diets are becoming more common all over the world, and as more gluten rich products are introduced into cultures we are likely to see more cases of gluten intolerance (52). In addition, it is conceivable that as wheat products, starches, and other foods have been modified, there may also be an association with increased prevalence's of gluten intolerance (50,53). The leaky gut syndrome theory concludes that intestinal barrier compromise leads to systemic and intestinal damage and is often associated with gluten intolerance. This compromised intestinal barrier appears to be more associated with celiac disease than non-celiac gluten sensitivity disorders based on recent evidence (46). Although, this theory provides great promise, thus far there is no direct evidence linking effective drug repair of barrier permeability with improved celiac pathophysiology (54).

Lymphoma risk rises with celiac disease but is mitigated by adherence to a gluten-free diet. As gluten is virtually ubiquitous in the diet, expert dietary advice is essential. (registries of gluten-free foods are available online; see Section VIIJ.) Most gluten-free diets traditionally exclude oats, due to cross-contamination, but this may prove to be unnecessary for some patients (55) (see Chapter 18). Facilities that process oats often process wheat as well, and thus contamination of oats with wheat proteins may complicate inclusion of oats in a gluten-free diet. For further discussion of gluten enteropathy, see Chapter 18.

CLINICAL HIGHLIGHTS

Food allergy is sufficiently common that most clinicians are likely to encounter it. The condition often imposes a considerable burden on patient and family alike, particularly when children are affected (56). The manifestations span a wide spectrum, although the most common manifestations are fairly prototypical. The prevalence of true food allergy is higher in children than in adults, and many children can be expected to outgrow their allergies. Diagnosis can be confirmed with non-IgE-mediated reactions by elimination diets and IgE-mediated reactions require food challenges with IgE-specific immunoassays or skin testing. The most common food allergies in adults are to fish, shellfish, nuts and peanuts; in children, the most common reactions are to milk, eggs, peanuts, soy, and wheat. If food allergy is confirmed, a dietitian should be consulted to help the patient (or the patient's parents) develop a nutritionally complete diet completely free of the offending antigen. Allergy to gluten can produce celiac disease or be associated with non-celiac gluten intolerance and both require nearly complete and permanent elimination of gluten from the diet (see Chapter 18).

Food intolerance, as opposed to allergy, is not immune mediated. Lactose intolerance is perhaps the most common and best-known example. Although patients with lactose intolerance may report an inability to tolerate any milk, randomized double-blind trials are consistent in demonstrating that most individuals can tolerate up to 15 g per day of lactose and that adequate calcium intake from dairy sources remains feasible. Breast-feeding up to the age of 4 to 6 months may reduce the risk of cow's milk allergy but not general food allergy before the age of 2 years old. Providers are encouraged to tell families to not delay introduction of highly allergenic foods >4 to 6 months unless child has sibling or first-degree relative with peanut allergy, worsening moderate-severe eczema, or previous reaction to other foods. In these cases, foods may continue to be introduced, but recommendations are to refer to allergy specialist for more structured introduction and allergy testing (10). The role of food allergy in a host of conditions and constitutional symptoms remains speculative at present. Progress is considerable in identifying common food antigens. The modification of food antigenicity through bioengineering to remove offending proteins is an area of intense activity and considerable promise (57). The use of probiotics to adjust intestinal microflora also shows promise for the prevention and management of food allergy.

REFERENCES

1. Chafen JJ, Newberry SJ, Riedl MA, et al. Diagnosing and managing common food allergies: a systematic review. *JAMA* 2010;303:1848–1856.
2. Brooks C, Pearce N, Douwes J. The hygiene hypothesis in allergy and asthma: an update. *Curr Opin Allergy Clin Immunol* 2013;13:70–77.
3. Lack G. Update on risk factors for food allergy. *J Allergy Clin Immunol* 2012;129:1187–1197.
4. Rona RJ, Keil T, Summers C, et al. The prevalence of food allergy: a meta-analysis. *J Allergy Clin Immunol* 2007;120:638–646.
5. Corrado G, Luzzi I, Lucarelli S, et al. Positive association between Helicobacter pylori infection and food allergy in children. *Scand J Gastroenterol* 1998;33:1135–1139.
6. Cox H. Food allergy in infants: practical and clinical considerations (1). *Community Pract* 2006;79:370–371.
7. Sampson MA, Munoz-Furlong A, Sicherer SH. Risk-taking and coping strategies of adolescents and young adults with food allergy. *J Allergy Clin Immunol* 2006;117: 1440–1445.
8. American Academy of Pediatrics Committee on Nutrition. Hypoallergenic infant formulas. *Pediatrics* 2000;106:346–349.
9. Greer FR, Sicherer SH, Burks AW, et al. Effects of early nutritional interventions on the development of atopic disease in infants and children: the role of maternal dietary restriction, breastfeeding, timing of introduction of complementary foods, and hydrolyzed formulas. *Pediatrics* 2008;121:183–191.
10. Fleischer DM, Spergel JM, Assa'ad AH, et al. Primary prevention of allergic disease through nutritional interventions. *J Allergy Clin Immunol* 2013;1:29–36.
11. Osborn DA, Sinn J. Soy formula for prevention of allergy and food intolerance in infants. *Cochrane Database Syst Rev* 2006;4:CD003741.
12. Host A, Koletzko B, Dreborg S, et al. Dietary products used in infants for treatment and prevention of food allergy. Joint statement of the European society for paediatric allergology and clinical immunology (ESPACI) committee on hypoallergenic formulas and the European society for paediatric gastroenterology, hepatology and nutrition (ESPGHAN) committee on nutrition. *Arch Dis Child* 1999;81:80–84.
13. Burks AW, Tang M, Sicherer S, et al. ICON: food allergy. *J Allergy Clin Immunol* 2012;129:906–920.
14. Du Toit G, Katz Y, Sasienei P, et al. Early consumption of peanuts in infancy is associated with alow prevalence of peanut allergy. *J Allergy Clin Immunol* 2008;122: 984–991.
15. Branum AM, Lukacs SL. Food allergy among children in the United States. *Pediatrics* 2009;124:1549–1555.
16. Wuthrich B. Food-induced cutaneous adverse reactions. *Allergy* 1998;53:131–135.
17. Fasano MB. Dermatologic food allergy. *Pediatr Ann* 2006;35:727–731.
18. Ortolani C, Pastorello EA, Farioli L, et al. IgE-mediated allergy from vegetable allergens. *Ann Allergy* 1993;71: 470–476.
19. Iacono G, Cavataio F, Montalto G, et al. Intolerance of cow's milk and chronic constipation in children. *N Engl J Med* 1998;339:1100–1104.
20. Bock SA, Muñoz-Furlong A, Sampson HA. Further fatalities caused by anaphylactic reactions to food, 2001–2006. *J Allergy Clin Immunol* 2007;119:1016–1018.
21. Untersmayr E, Jensen-Jarolim E. Mechanisms of type I food allergy. *Pharmacol Ther* 2006;112:787–798.
22. Virkud YV, Vickery BP. Advances in immunotherapy for food allergy. *Discov Med* 2012;14:159–165.
23. Park MI, Camilleri M. Is there a role of food allergy in irritable bowel syndrome and functional dyspepsia? A systematic review. *Neurogastroenterol Motil* 2006;18: 595–607.
24. Cantani A, Micera M. The prick by prick test is safe and reliable in 58 children with atopic dermatitis and food allergy. *Eur Rev Med Pharmacol Sci* 2006;10:115–120.
25. Majamaa H, Moiso P, Holm K, et al. Wheat allergy: diagnostic accuracy of skin prick and patch test and specific IgE. *Allergy* 1999;54:851–856.
26. Knight AK, Bahna SL. Diagnosis of food allergy. *Pediatr Ann* 2006;35:709–714.
27. Eigenmann PA, Sampson HA. Interpreting skin prick tests in the evaluation of food allergy in children. *Pediatr Allergy Immunol* 1998;9:186–191.
28. Spergel JM, Brown-Whitehorn T. The use of patch testing in the diagnosis of food allergy. *Curr Allergy Asthma Rep* 2005;5:86–90.
29. Hill DJ, Heine RG, Hosking CS. The diagnostic value of skin prick testing in children with food allergy. *Pediatr Allergy Immunol* 2004;15:435–441.
30. Shreffler WG. Evaluation of basophil activation in food allergy: present and future applications. *Curr Opin Allergy Clin Immunol* 2006;6:226–233.
31. Eigenmann PA. Do we have suitable in-vitro diagnostic tests for the diagnosis of food allergy? *Curr Opin Allergy Clin Immunol* 2004;4:211–213.
32. Allergy Advisor. *Allergy and intolerance software.* Available at http://www.allergyadvisor.com/index.html; accessed 12/16/06.
33. Molloy J, Allen K, Collier F, et al. The potential link between gut microbiota and IgE-mediated food allergy in early life. *Int J Environ Res Public Health* 2013;10:7235–7256.
34. Rivas MN, Burton OT, Wise P, et al. A microbiota signature associated with experimental food allergy promotes allergic sensitization and anaphylaxis. *J Allergy Clin Immunol* 2013;131:201–212.

35. Kinross JM, Darzi AW, Nicholson JK. Gut microbiome-host interactions in health and disease. *Genome Med* 2011;3:14.

36. Fiocchi A, Martelli A. Dietary management of food allergy. *Pediatr Ann* 2006;35:755–756, 758–763.

37. Kattan JD, Srivastava KD, Zou ZM, et al. Pharmacological and immunological effects of individual herbs in the Food Allergy Herbal Formula-2 (FAHF-2) on peanut allergy. *Phytother Res* 2008;22:651–659.

38. Suarez FL, Savaiano DA, Levitt MD. A comparison of symptoms after the consumption of milk or lactose-hydrolyzed milk by people with self-reported severe lactose intolerance. *N Engl J Med* 1995;333:1–4.

39. Suarez FL, Adshead J, Furne JK, et al. Lactose maldigestion is not an impediment to the intake of 1500 mg calcium as dairy products. *Am J Clin Nutr* 1998;68:1118–1122.

40. Vesa TH, Korpela RA, Sahi T. Tolerance to small amounts of lactose in lactose maldigesters. *Am J Clin Nutr* 1996;64:197–201.

41. Suarez F, Levitt MD. Abdominal symptoms and lactose: the discrepancy between patients' claims and the results of blinded trials. *Am J Clin Nutr* 1996;64:251–252.

42. Mascolo R, Saltzman JR. Lactose intolerance and irritable bowel syndrome. *Nutr Rev* 1998;56:306–308.

43. Vesa TH, Seppo LM, Marteau PR, et al. Role of irritable bowel syndrome in subjective lactose intolerance. *Am J Clin Nutr* 1998;67:710–715.

44. Vesa TH, Lember M, Korpela R. Milk fat does not affect the symptoms of lactose intolerance. *Eur J Clin Nutr* 1997;51:633–636.

45. Sapone A, Bai JC, Ciacci C, et al. Spectrum of gluten-related disorders: consensus on new nomenclature and classification. *BMC Med* 2012;10:13.

46. Sapone A, Lammers KM, Casolaro V, et al. Divergence of gut permeability and mucosal immune gene expression in two gluten-associated conditions: celiac disease and gluten sensitivity. *BMC Med* 2011;9:23.

47. Verdu EF, Armstrong D, Murray JA. Between celiac disease and irritable bowel syndrome: the "no man's land" of gluten sensitivity. *Am J Gastroenterol* 2009;104:1587–1594.

48. Parnell ND, Ciclitira PJ. Review article: coeliac disease and its management. *Aliment Pharmacol Ther* 1999;13:1–13.

49. Murray JA. The widening spectrum of celiac disease. *Am J Clin Nutr* 1999;69:354–365.

50. Brown AC. Gluten sensitivity: problems of an emerging condition separate from celiac disease. *Expert Rev Gastroenterol Hepatol* 2012;6:43–55.

51. Rubio-Tapia A, Kyle RA, Kaplan EL, et al. Increased prevalence and mortality in undiagnosed celiac disease. *Gastroenterology* 2009;137:88–93.

52. Catassi C, Gobellis G. Coeliac disease epidemiology is alive and kicking, especially in the developing world. *Dig Liver Dis* 2007, 39:908–910.

53. Anjum FM, Khan MR, Din A, et al. Wheat gluten: high molecular weight glutenin subunits—structure, genetics, and relation to dough elasticity. *J Food Sci* 2007;72:R56–R63.

54. Odenwald MA, Turner JR. Intestinal permeability defects: is it time to treat? *ClinGastroenterol Hepatol* 2013;11:1075–1083.

55. Thompson T. Do oats belong in a gluten-free diet? *J Am Diet Assoc* 1997;97:1413–1416.

56. Bollinger ME, Dahlquist LM, Mudd K, et al. The impact of food allergy on the daily activities of children and their families. *Ann Allergy Asthma Immunol* 2006;96:415–421.

57. Perr HA. Novel foods to treat food allergy and gastrointestinal infection. *Curr Allergy Asthma Rep* 2006;6:153–159.

SUGGESTED READINGS

Burks AW, Jones SM, Boyce JA, et al. NIAID-sponsord 2010 guidelines for managing food allergy: applications in the pediatric population. *Pediatrics* 2011;128:955–965.

Dreskin SC. Genetics of food allergy. *Curr Allergy Asthma Rep* 2006;6:58–64.

Freeman HJ, Chopra A, Clandinin MT, et al. Recent advances in celiac disease. *World J Gastroenterol* 2011;17:2259–2272.

Kueper T, Martinelli D, Konetzki W, et al. Identification of problem foods using food and symptom diaries. *Otolaryngol Head Neck Surg* 1995;112:415–420.

Lack G. Food allergy. *N Eng J Med* 2008;359;1252–1260.

Lomer MC, Parkes GC, Sanderson JD. Review article: lactose intolerance in clinical practice—myths and realities. *Aliment Pharmacol Ther* 2008;27:93–103.

NIAID-Sponsored Expert Panel. Guidelines for the diagnosis and management of food allergy in the United States: report of the NIAID-Sponsored Expert Panel. *J Allergy Clin Immunol* 2010;126:S1–S58.

Nowak-Wegrzyn A, Assa'ad AH, Bahna SL, et al. Work group report: oral food challenge testing. *J Allergy Clin Immunol* 2009;123:365–383.

Pirson F. Food allergy: a challenge for the clinician. *Acta Gastroenterol Belg* 2006;69:38–42.

Taylor SL, Baumert JL. Food allergies and intolerances. In: Ross CA, Benjamin C, Cousins RJ, et al., eds. *Modern nutrition in health and disease*, 11th ed. Philadelphia, PA: Lippincott Williams & Wilkins, 2012:1421–1439.

Terho EO, Savolainen J. Diagnosis and food hypersensitivity. *Eur J Clin Nutr* 1996;50:1–5.

van Ree R, Vieths S, Poulsen LK. Allergen-specific IgE testing in the diagnosis of food allergy and the event of a positive match in the bioinformatics search. *Mol Nutr Food Res* 2006;50:645–654.

Zuercher AW, Fritsche R, Corthesy B, et al. Food products and allergy development, prevention and treatment. *Curr Opin Biotechnol* 2006;17:198–203.

CHAPTER 25

Eating Disorders

ating disorders refer to aberrant eating behavior, with or without discernible physical consequences. The prototypical conditions are anorexia nervosa (AN) and bulimia nervosa (BN). A more recent addition is binge-eating disorder (BED).

As obesity is a state of imbalance between energy needs and energy intake, it, too, may be considered a disorder of eating, although it is generally categorized and managed differently, partly because of its prevalence. Disorder or not, obesity and overweight now afflict more than two-thirds of the adult population in the United States, with rates of severe obesity rising even faster than that of moderate obesity (1,2) (see Chapter 5). By virtue of prevalence alone, it cannot be considered "aberrant." Extreme degrees of obesity represent aberrancy and as such share characteristics with the other eating disorders. In these cases, elements of management borrowed from the other disorders may be helpful. Conversely, as social pressures increase the prevalence of eating disorders, they potentially become less aberrant from prevailing norms and more akin to a public health problem (3) rather than a strictly individualized pathology. Recent trends in the epidemiology of BED are noteworthy in this regard.

There is some concern that obesity prevention and treatment efforts may actually lead to the prototypical eating disorders of anorexia and nervosa; however, this concern is unfounded. The risk factors for eating disorders are well-documented and the adoption of health-promoting behaviors is not among them. Moreover, severe obesity shares many of the same risk factors with eating disorders (4). For example, food addiction may underlie of both subtypes of obesity and binge eating and other forms of overeating (5). So rather than one disorder causing the other, it seems more likely that obesity and eating disorders are two sides of the same coin.

Occasional or mildly disordered eating, related to cravings, aversions, and dissatisfaction with body image, is very prevalent, if not universal.

Bona fide eating disorders are considered principally psychopathologies, and management relies heavily on psychotherapy. Nonetheless, the disorders are expressed in interactions with food, requiring that dietary management be addressed as well.

OVERVIEW

The prevalence and public health importance of eating disorders has risen steeply since the 1970s, concurrent with a rapid rise in the prevalence of obesity. At the same time, societal concepts of beauty have increasingly prioritized thinness. Thus, although previously considered a consequence of family dysfunction and psychopathology, the link between eating disorders and prevailing imbalance between dietary goals and dietary practices seems self-evident. The biopsychosocial model is germane; social factors interact with biological (possibly genetic) and psychological vulnerability to culminate in the disordered pattern of eating behavior (6–8).

Dieting during adolescence appears to increase susceptibility to disordered eating (9,10). A population-based survey in Spain suggests that eating disorders occur against a backdrop of highly prevalent, less extreme, unhealthy eating practices (11), and a recent 10-year longitudinal follow-up found that adolescents who engaged in dieting and disordered eating behaviors were more likely to still engage in such behaviors 10 years later (12).

Exposure to Western culture and ideals of beauty is considered a risk factor for eating disorders (13). However, continued research has shown that eating disorders are not restricted to particular cultures or ethnicities (14–17). Eating disorders are perceived as conditions that overwhelmingly affect young women; however, there is increasing evidence that the disorders occur in men as well (6,18–26).

The risk factors for eating disorders are many and include psychological, biological, and cultural factors. Eating disorders of all types are associated with psychiatric comorbidities (27–30) and in particular eating disorders share features with depression and obsessive-compulsive disorder (31). Eating disorders are distinguished from these psychiatric comorbidities by the preoccupation with body weight. A personal history of obesity or perceived obesity is commonly reported as well, particularly in bulimia. Individuals encouraged to be preoccupied with weight control, such as models, actresses, dancers (32), and athletes (33,34), and type 1 diabetics (35–37) appear to be at increased risk. There is also evidence of increased risk for binge eating and unhealthful weight-control behaviors among teen vegetarians (38). Familial clustering and twin studies in particular suggest that genetic susceptibility is contributory (39,40). Additionally, candidate gene studies have identified genetic risk variants involved in the hypothalamic control of appetite and energy homeostasis that increase one's risk for anorexia (41,42). Diagnostic criteria for eating disorders have been codified in the *Diagnostic and Statistical Manual of Mental Disorders (DSM)* and the *International Classification of Diseases (ICD)*. The *DSM-V* was released in May 2013 and defines the most up-to-date diagnostic criteria for eating disorders.

Anorexia Nervosa

Fundamentally, AN is a morbid fear of becoming fat, an inability to gauge correctly the degree of thinness, and consequent self-starvation (43,44). According to the recently released *DSM-V* the criteria for AN include restriction of food intake leading to a "significantly low body weight," intense fear of weight gain, and distorted perception of body image. Notably, the criteria of amenorrhea and weight less than 85% of ideal body weight were eliminated in the new *DSM*. Diet is usually strictly controlled in anorexia, and the patient is apt to deny and genuinely not recognize that a problem exists. AN is further divided into two subtypes: in the restricting type, the individuals do not binge or purge as compared to the binge-eating/purging type in which the individuals engage in recurrent binging and purging (DSM-V). In the binge-eating/purging type, the distinction from bulimia rests on the degree of underweight (45).

AN most commonly occurs between the ages of 15 and 19; however, though rare, cases do develop in preteen children and in middle-aged adults (46).

Medical complications of anorexia are those of starvation. Basal metabolism is slowed, with potential hypotension and bradycardia. Amenorrhea due to reduced production of follicle-stimulating hormone and luteinizing hormone and reduced estrogen levels is common and may be one of the earliest indicators. Skin discoloration due to hypercarotenemia may occur, related to either dietary habits or metabolic dysfunction. Osteopenia is a frequent complication and results in an increased long-term risk of fractures. Adolescents with AN are at risk for impaired linear growth that may result in permanent short stature (47). Characteristic features of hypothyroidism often develop. Potentially irreversible bone loss may occur at a rate of up to 15% per year during periods of cachexia and amenorrhea. With protracted and severe starvation, visceral protein loss has the potential to become life threatening. Myocardial protein loss renders the anorexic susceptible to sudden cardiac death. The mortality rate in anorexia is approximately 5%, with one in five deaths attributed to suicide (48). The condition is often self-limited, however; the mean duration is generally thought to be between roughly 2 and 5 years (21,49).

Bulimia Nervosa

Bulimia is more common and more difficult to "cure" than anorexia. Data from the 2001–2003 National Comorbidity Survey Replication (NCS-R), which contains information about the mental health status of 9,282 people from across the United States, indicate that 0.9% of women and 0.3% of men had AN, while 1.5% of women and 0.5% of men had bulimia (21).

In bulimia, as in anorexia, there is preoccupation with body weight and fear of weight gain. *DSM-V* criteria include recurrent binges characterized by excessive calorie consumption and loss of control; recurrent inappropriate compensatory behavior to prevent weight gain; and undue preoccupation with body habitus. In order to meet the definition of BN, the binge eating and compensatory behaviors must occur at least once a week for 3 months and the episodes do not occur exclusively during times of AN. The distinguishing features of BN tend to be the degree of dietary control, which is strict in anorexia but poor in bulimia, and the related degree of thinness (43). Limited data suggest that impaired metabolism of cholecystokinin may contribute to lack of normal satiety signals (50,51). Between 30% and 50% of those with BN also abuse or are dependent on alcohol or drugs, and there is evidence that bulimia itself may represent an addictive disorder (52). Bulimics tend to binge eat and then "purge" by self-induced vomiting, use of laxatives, use of diuretics, calorie restriction, bouts of exercise, or some combination of these actions. Unlike anorexics, who appear unwell to any objective observer but tend to be unaware of a problem, bulimics generally appear well (unless the condition is advanced or decompensated) but tend to know their dietary behavior is pathological.

Most bulimics have had the condition for up to 5 years before seeking treatment, and they often get help only because of some acute disruption. The mean duration of bulimia is estimated at just over 8 years, comparable to that of BED. Survey data indicate that less than half of bulimics seek treatment specifically for their bulimia but rather are more likely to seek treatment for psychiatric comorbidities (21).

Bulimia generally manifests between the ages of 18 and 22 (21). Medical complications result from trauma to the gastrointestinal tract and electrolyte imbalance (53).

Since bulimics often appear well and tend to delay seeking treatment, diagnosis can be challenging. However, there are several warning signs and early medical complications that can guide the clinician in identifying this disorder. Russell sign, bruised knuckles as a result of self-inflicted vomiting, may be an early clue to the diagnosis. Repeated bouts of emesis erode dental enamel and can lead to tooth loss and dental caries. Loss of gastric acid can lead to hypochloremic alkalosis and hypokalemia, potentially inducing shock. These electrolyte disturbances in an otherwise healthy patient should prompt suspicion of bulimia. Other medical complications of bulimia include pancreatitis, which may occur following a binge. Enlargement of the parotid glands may be induced by a binge. Binging can lead to gastric rupture. Purging can result in esophagitis and esophageal tear or rupture. Ipecac taken in high doses is cardiotoxic, potentially leading to myocarditis and dysrhythmia. Laxatives can lead to renal tubular damage and can chronically impair gastrointestinal motility.

Binge-Eating Disorder

BED, formerly considered a sub-type of Eating Disorder Not Otherwise Specified, has now received its own category as an eating disorder in the new *DSM-V*. It is similar to bulimia in the commonly reported loss of impulse control that leads to a binging that occur at least once per week for 3 months. The distinction is that in BED, as opposed to BN, inappropriate compensatory behaviors, such as self-induced vomiting, do not occur. People with BED also tend to be middle aged, and as many as 25% are male (54). Binges tend to take place in private, with normal or even subnormal food intake in public. Recurrent binges contribute to the development of obesity over time. In obese patients with BED, it is recommended that the binge eating be treated before the patient attempts weight loss (55).

Recent survey data indicate that the prevalence of BED in the United States exceeds that of anorexia and bulimia combined (30). Some tendency to binge eat is common in most people, and indeed, in many species (see Chapter 44). The case has been made that BED may be more closely related to normal eating behaviors than the other disorders and the rising prevalence may be attributable to environmental and societal influences (56). If so, this may be analogous to the recent epidemiology of attention-deficit/hyperactivity disorder in children.

Other Specified Feeding or Eating Disorder

Other Specified Feeding or Eating Disorder is a new category in the *DSM-V*, replacing the former category of Eating Disorder Not Otherwise Specified. This category includes disorders that "cause clinically significant distress or impairment in social, occupational, or other important areas of functioning predominate but do not meet the full criteria for any of the disorders in the feeding and eating disorders diagnostic." Included in this category are atypical anorexia nervosa in which a patient meets all of the criteria for AN but is of a normal weight; BN and BED of low frequency or limited duration; purging disorder (a disorder of purging with no associated binging); and night eating syndrome (NES). NES is characterized by evening hyperphagia with nocturnal snacking, which causes significant impairment and distress (DSM-V). Unlike the 2,000 to 3,000 kcal binges typical of BED, nocturnal snacking in NES tends to be limited to roughly 400 kcal per episode, with multiple episodes throughout the night (57). It is estimated that up to 1.5% of the general population has the condition. Several studies of NES in obese individuals suggest extremely high rates in this population, ranging from about 10% to 15% of obesity clinic patients to 8% to 55% of patients seeking bariatric surgery (58–60).

Atypical Eating Disorders

States of aberrant eating behavior that do not meet criteria for anorexia, bulimia, or binge eating exist but receive limited attention in the medical literature. Such conditions include pica, and the newly defined avoidant/restrictive food intake disorder (ARFID) (DSM-V). Recognition of such disorders may be particularly important in sensitizing the primary care community to the prevalence and clinical impact of disordered eating.

Management: General Principles

The management of eating disorders is multidisciplinary and relies heavily on expert psychiatric or psychological care. Evidence is growing that selective serotonin reuptake inhibitors (SSRIs) may be useful in the treatment of patients with BN and BED (61–63). There is some evidence that SSRIs may help prevent relapse in patients with anorexia who achieve a normal weight The evidence on the use of the antipsychotic olanzapine in patients with anorexia is mixed (64–67), though the American Psychiatric Association suggest they may be useful in patients with "severe, unremitting resistance to gaining weight; severe obsessional thinking; and denial that assumes delusional proportions" (68). In addition to the primary care provider, the management team should generally involve a mental health specialist, dietitian, and social worker.

Cognitive-behavioral therapy is considered the treatment of choice for bulimia and BED (54,69,70). Individual psychotherapy may be helpful (71), and involving the family in the treatment of adolescents with anorexia may improve outcomes and prevent relapse (72,73). In adults

with anorexia, cognitive-behavioral therapy may prevent relapse in those who have achieved a normal weight (73).

The primary care provider has an important contribution to make in both preventing and managing eating disorders. A high index of suspicion is warranted to facilitate early detection. One screening tool that can be used by the primary care physician is the SCOFF questionnaire, a five question instrument that assesses the core psychopathology of anorexia and bulimia (74) (see Table 25-1). If a patient answers affirmatively for two or more of the questions, further investigation is warranted (75).

Recognition of psychopathology that contributes to disordered eating may allow for preemptive treatment. Efforts to contain societal influences that may propagate distorted body image among young people and to establish educational programs that encourage healthful eating and realistic perspectives on weight should derive support, if not leadership, from the primary care community (76–83).

Excellent and extensive literature is available on the various theories and approaches to the counseling of eating-disordered patients (see "Suggested Readings"). Dietary management per se is an important but limited aspect of the care plan.

Management: Diet

Severe anorexia may require hospitalization and enteral nutrition support, with meticulous management of electrolytes. A body mass index

---

TABLE 25.1

SCOFF Questionnaire

1. Do you make yourself sick because you feel uncomfortably full?
2. Do you worry you have lost control over how much you eat?
3. Do you believe yourself to be fat when others say you are too thin?
4. Have you recently lost more than fourteen pounds in a 3-month period?
5. Would you say that food dominates your life?

Note: If a patient answers affirmatively to two or more questions, further investigation is warranted.

Source: Reproduced from Morgan JF, Reid F, Lacey JH. The SCOFF questionnaire: assessment of a new screening tool for eating disorders. *BMJ.* 1999;319(7223):1467–1468. With permission from BMJ Publishing Group Ltd.

below 13, severe electrolyte imbalance, suicidality, and lack of improvement while in outpatient treatment are all indications for hospitalization. Refeeding should be gradual to avoid the refeeding syndrome, characterized by congestive heart failure, hypophosphatemia, and/or prolonged QT interval. Inpatient care should be supervised by a dietitian or another nutrition consultant.

Ambulatory care calls for close follow-up especially since drop-out from treatment is common (84). The principles of dietary counseling discussed in Chapter 47 are applicable. Nutritional management should begin with a dietary history (85). The history should include not only a description of current and past dietary behaviors but also the beliefs and motivations underlying them.

Weekly visits are appropriate until a consistent therapeutic response has been achieved. Weight monitoring should be routine. The patient should maintain a food diary, which should be reviewed at office visits. Because preoccupation with weight is predominant, patient education regarding healthy weight and dietary practices conducive to weight maintenance is essential.

Because the pathology is related to a very restrictive diet in anorexia, emphasis should be placed on a prudent but balanced and unrestricted diet. There is no single recommended nutritional regimen, as adequate caloric consumption is paramount (86). A similar goal is pertinent in the management of bulimia, with a need to emphasize that the disordered eating typically is a result of overly restrictive attitudes about food rather than overeating (85,87). Establishment of a consistent, moderate dietary pattern is helpful in resolving the tendencies to binge and purge.

If weight gain is indicated in anorexia, it should be gradual. The addition of approximately 500 kcal per day beyond what is required for maintenance will result in a weight gain of 1 lb per week. Involvement of a dietitian in the development of meal plans to facilitate weight gain or maintenance is indicated. In anorexia, the suppression of basal metabolism is such that seemingly modest intake of food energy may be sufficient to support weight maintenance or gradual weight gain. Rapid weight gain should be avoided, as much for its adverse psychological effects as for its physiologic effects.

A dietitian should determine the basal metabolic rate as a means of estimating caloric needs.

The diet should be advanced gradually to allay the patient's anxieties about excessive weight gain. In bulimia, stabilization of the dietary pattern and weight should be addressed initially. An effort should be made to identify foods associated with binges so that they can be avoided or their intake can be strictly controlled. There is also recent evidence that limiting food variety results in sensory-specific satiety and thus a more limited diet may help curb binge eating (88). If indicated, a diet for measured weight loss may be developed once the eating pattern has reliably stabilized. Dietary counseling (see Chapter 47) should be coupled to cognitive-behavioral therapy to ameliorate perceptions of body image and establish a sustainable dietary pattern that supports weight-control efforts.

An additional challenge to the physician is the concurrence of an eating disorder and a metabolic disease, such as diabetes mellitus. Girls with type 1 diabetes appear to be at least twice as likely to develop bulimia and BED as nondiabetic peers (89). Disordered eating in diabetics has been associated with greater frequency of medical complications including more frequent episode of ketoacidosis and acceleration of the development of retinopathy (37,90) in young women with insulin-dependent diabetes mellitus accelerates the development of retinopathy. Given the prevalence of both diabetes and eating disorders, the authors encourage consideration of concurrence whenever diabetes proves difficult to manage, especially in a young woman.

CLINICAL HIGHLIGHTS

A pervasive struggle with weight control, epidemic obesity, and fascination with thinness characterize modern society. A rising prevalence of eating disorders may be attributable to both individual susceptibility and environmental conditions. Increased awareness among clinicians with enhanced detection may also be contributory. The environmental contribution is such that every patient may reasonably be considered at some degree of risk for some degree of disordered eating. The incorporation of nutrition education and limited dietary counseling into primary care practice may support efforts at primary prevention of eating disorders, particularly by revealing the dietary habits imparted by parents to their children.

Eating disorders generally require a care team that includes a mental health specialist and dietitian. A therapeutic alliance between the patient and a primary care provider with a good working knowledge of nutrition is conducive to early detection and optimal management. Patients need education regarding healthy weight and dietary practices, as well as the adverse effects of disordered eating. A balanced but not overly restricted diet is conducive to overcoming eating disorders and to preventing excessive weight gain, which may precipitate recurrences of disordered eating. Contrary to an often-voiced concern, counseling to forestall obesity need not in any way contribute to eating disorders if delivered appropriately, with a focus on long-term health rather than short-term weight loss or thinness, per se.

A dietary pattern consistent with principles of health promotion and weight control (see Chapters 5 and 45) should be encouraged. Frequent follow-up, with monitoring of weight and dietary pattern, is essential until a therapeutic response is achieved and sustained.

REFERENCES

1. Sturm R. Increases in morbid obesity in the USA: 2000-2005. *Public Health* 2007;121(7):492–496.
2. Flegal KM, Carroll MD, Kit BK, et al. Prevalence of obesity and trends in the distribution of body mass index among US adults, 1999–2010. *JAMA* 2012;307(5):491–497.
3. Austin SB. A public health approach to eating disorders prevention: It's time for public health professionals to take a seat at the table. *BMC Public Health* 2012;12(1):854.
4. Haines J, Neumark-Sztainer D. Prevention of obesity and eating disorders: a consideration of shared risk factors. *Health Educ Res* 2006;21:770–782.
5. Corsica JA, Pelchat ML. Food Addiction: true or false? *Curr Opin Gastroenterol* 2010;26:165–169.
6. Ricciardelli LA, McCabe MP. A biopsychosocial model of disordered eating and the pursuit of muscularity in adolescent boys. *Psychol Bull* 2004;130:179–205.
7. Kirkley BG. Bulimia: clinical characteristics, development, and etiology. *J Am Diet Assoc* 1986;86:468–472,475.
8. Striegel-Moore RH, Bulik CM. Risk factors for eating disorders. *Am Psychol* 2007;62(3):181–198.
9. Howard CE, Porzelius LK. The role of dieting in binge eating disorder: etiology and treatment implications. *Clin Psychol Rev* 1999;19:25–44.
10. Spear BA. Does dieting increase the risk for obesity and eating disorders? *J Am Diet Assoc* 2006;106:523–525.
11. Martin AR, Nieto JM, Jimenez MA, et al. Unhealthy eating behaviour in adolescents. *Eur J Epidemiol* 1999;15:643–648.
12. Neumark-Sztainer D, Wall M, Larson NI, et al. Dieting and disordered eating behaviors from adolescence to young adulthood: findings from a 10-year longitudinal study. *J Am Diet Assoc* 2011;111(7):1004–1011.
13. Eddy KT, Hennessey M, Thompson-Brenner H. Eating pathology in East African women—the role of media exposure and globalization. *J Nerv Ment Dis* 2007;195(3):196–202.
14. Podar I, Allik J. A cross-cultural comparison of the eating disorder inventory. *Int J Eat Disord* 2009;42(4):346–355.
15. Soh NL, Touyz SW, Surgenor LJ. Eating and body image disturbances across cultures: a review. *Eur Eat Disord Rev* 2006;14:54–65.
16. Keel PK, Klump KL. Are eating disorders culture-bound syndromes? Implications for conceptualizing their etiology. *Psychol Bull* 2003;129:747–76.
17. Cummins LH, Simmons AM, Zane NWS. Eating disorders in Asian populations: a critique of current approaches to the study of culture, ethnicity, and eating disorders. *Am J Ortho psychiatry* 2005;75:553–574.
18. Cafri G, van den Berg P, Thompson JK. Pursuit of muscularity in adolescent boys: relations among biopsychosocial variables and clinical outcomes. *J Clin Child Adolesc Psychol* 2006;35:283–291.
19. Elgin J, Pritchard M. Gender differences in disordered eating and its correlates. *Eat Weight Disord* 2006;11:e96–e101.
20. Muris P, Meesters C, van de Blom W, et al. Biological, psychological, and sociocultural correlates of body change strategies and eating problems in adolescent boys and girls. *Eat Behav* 2005;6:11–22.
21. Hudson JI, Hiripi E, et al. The prevalence and correlates of eating disorders in the National Comorbidity Survey Replication. *Biol Psychiatry* 2007;61:348–358.
22. Dominé F, Berchtold A, Akré C, et al. Disordered eating behaviors: what about boys? *J Adolesc Health* 2009;44(2):111–117.
23. Striegel-Moore RH, Rosselli F, Perrin N, et al. Gender difference in the prevalence of eating disorder symptoms. *Int J Eat Disord* 2009;42(5):471–474.
24. Button E, Aldridge S, Palmer R. Males assessed by a specialized adult eating disorders service: patterns over time and comparisons with females. *Int J Eat Disord* 2008;41(8):758–761.
25. Raevuori A, Hoek HW, Susser E, et al. Epidemiology of anorexia nervosa in men: a Nationwide Study of Finnish Twins. *PLoS ONE* 2009;4(2):e4402.
26. Ousley L, Cordero ED, White S. Eating disorders and body image of undergraduate men. *J Am Coll Health* 2008;56(6):617–622.
27. Grilo CM, White MA, Masheb RM. DSM-IV psychiatric disorder comorbidity and its correlates in binge eating disorder. *Int J Eat Disord* 2009;42(3):228–234.
28. Spindler A, Milos G. Links between eating disorder symptom severity and psychiatric comorbidity. *Eat Behav* 2007;8(3):364–373.
29. O'Brien KM, Vincent NK. Psychiatric comorbidity in anorexia and bulimia nervosa: nature, prevalence, and causal relationships. *Clin Psychol Rev* 2003;23(1):57–74.
30. Swanson SA, Crow SJ, Le Grange D, et al. Prevalence and correlates of eating disorders in adolescents. Results from the national comorbidity survey replication adolescent supplement. *Arch Gen Psychiatry* 2011;68(7):714–723.
31. Stunkard AJ, Allison KC. Binge eating disorder: disorder or marker? *Int J Eat Disord* 2003;34:s107–s116.

32. Nascimento AL, Luna JV, Fontenelle LF. Body dysmorphic disorder and eating disorders in elite professional female ballet dancers. *Ann Clin Psychiatry* 2012;24(3):191–194.

33. Sundgot-Borgen J, Torstveit MK. Prevalence of eating disorders in elite athletes is higher than in the general population. *Clin J Sport Med* 2004;14(1):25–32.

34. Van Durme K, Goossens L, Braet C. Adolescent aesthetic athletes: a group at risk for eating pathology? *Eat Behav* 2012;13(2):119–122.

35. Mannucci E, Rotella F, Ricca V, et al. Eating disorders in patients with type 1 diabetes: a meta-analysis. *J Endocrinol Invest* 2005;28(5):417–419.

36. Goebel-Fabbri AE. Disturbed eating behaviors and eating disorders in type 1 diabetes: clinical significance and treatment recommendations. *Curr Diab Rep* 2009; 9(2): 133–139.

37. Larrañaga A, Docet MF, García-Mayor RV. Disordered eating behaviors in type 1 diabetic patients. *World J Diabetes* 2011;2(11):189–195.

38. Robinson-O'Brien R, Perry CL, Wall MM, et al. Adolescent and young adult vegetarianism: better dietary intake and weight outcomes but increased risk of disordered eating behaviors. *J Am Diet Assoc* 2009;109(4):648–655.

39. Strober M, Freeman R, Lampert C, et al. Controlled family study of anorexia nervosa and bulimia nervosa: evidence of shared liability and transmission of partial syndromes. *Am J Psychiatry* 2000;157:393–401.

40. Scherag S, Hebebrand J, Hinney A. Eating disorders: the current status of molecular genetic research. *Eur Child Adolesc Psychiatry* 2010;19(3):211–226.

41. Clarke TK, Weiss ARD, Berrettini WH. The genetics of anorexia nervosa. *Clin Pharmacol Ther* 2012;91(2): 181–188.

42. Hinney A, Scherag S, Hebebrand J. Genetic findings in anorexia and bulimia nervosa. *Prog Mol Biol Transl Sci* 2010;94:241–270.

43. Garfinkel PE. Classification and diagnosis of eating disorders. In: Brownell DK, Fairburn CG, eds. *Eating disorders and obesity. A comprehensive handbook*. New York, NY: Guilford Press, 1995.

44. Fairburn CG, Brownell, KD. *Eating disorders and obesity: a comprehensive handbook*, 2nd ed. New York, NY: Guilford Press, 2002.

45. American Psychiatric Association. *Diagnostic and statistical manual for mental disorders*, 4th ed. Washington, DC: American Psychiatric Association, 1994:61–76.

46. Smink FRE, van Hoeken D, Hoek HW. Epidemiology of eating disorders: incidence, prevalence and mortality rates. *Curr Psychiatry Rep* 2012;14(4):406–414.

47. Katzman DK. Medical complications in adolescents with anorexia nervosa: a review of the literature. *Int J Eat Disord* 2005;37(S1):s52–s59.

48. Arcelus J, Mitchell AJ, Wales J, et al. Mortality rates in patients with anorexia nervosa and other eating disorders. A meta-analysis of 36 studies. *Arch Gen Psychiatry* 2011;68(7):724–731.

49. Pope HG Jr, Lalonde JK, Pindyck LJ, et al. Binge eating disorder: a stable syndrome. *Am J Psychiatry* 2006; 163:2181–2183.

50. Tong J, D'Alessio D. Eating disorders and gastrointestinal peptides. *Curr Opin Endocrinol Diabetes Obes* 2011; 18(1):42–49.

51. Hannon-Engel S. Regulating satiety in bulimia nervosa: the role of cholecystokinin. *Perspect Psychiatr Care* 2012;48(1):34–40.

52. Umberg EN, Shader RI, Hsu LKG, et al. From disordered eating to addiction: the "food drug" in bulimia nervosa. *J Clin Psychopharmacol* 2012;32(3):376–389.

53. Mehler PS. Medical complications of bulimia nervosa and their treatments. *Int J Eat Disord* 2011;44(2):95–104.

54. Fairburn CG, Harrison PJ. Eating disorders. *Lancet* 2003;361:407–416.

55. Dingemans AE, Bruna MJ, van Furth EF. Bing eating disorder: a review. *Int J Obes* (London). 2002;26:299–307.

56. Katz DL. *Binge eating: back from the brink*. February 4, 2004. Available at http://www.davidkatzmd.com/admin/archives/brink%20of%20bingeing.Times.2-4-07.doc; accessed 2/4/07.

57. Stein K. It's 2:00 am, do you know where the snackers are? *J Am Diet Assoc* 2007;107:20–23.

58. Marshall HM, Allison KC, O'Reardon JP, et al. Night eating syndrome among nonobese persons. *Int J Eat Disord* 2004;35:217–222.

59. Allison KC, Wadden TA, Sarwer DB, et al. Night eating syndrome and binge eating disorder among persons seeking bariatric surgery: prevalence and related features. *Obesity* 2006;14:77s–82s.

60. Latner JD, Wetzler S, Goodman ER, et al. Gastric bypass in a low-income, inner-city population: eating disturbances and weight loss. *Obes Res* 2004;12:956–61.

61. Zhu AJ, Walsh BT. Pharmacologic treatment of eating disorders. *Can J Psychiatry* 2002;47:227–234.

62. American Dietetic Association. Position of the American Dietetic Association: nutrition intervention in the treatment of anorexia nervosa, bulimia nervosa, and other eating disorders. *J Am Diet Assoc* 2006;106:2073–2082.

63. McElroy SL, Guerdjikova AI, Mori N, et al. Current pharmacotherapy options for bulimia nervosa and binge eating disorder. *Expert Opin Pharmacother* 2012;13(14): 2015–2026.

64. Flament MF, Bissada H, Spettigue W. Evidence-based pharmacotherapy of eating disorders. *Int J Neuropsychopharmacol* 2012;15(02):189–207.

65. Powers PS, Santana CA, Bannon YS. Olanzapine in the treatment of anorexia nervosa: an open label trial. *Int J Eat Disord* 2002;32:146–154.

66. Malina A, Gaskill J, McConaha C, et al. Olanzapine treatment of anorexia nervosa: a retrospective study. *Int J Eat Disord* 2003;33:234–237.

67. Kishi T, Kafantaris V, Sunday S, et al. Are antipsychotics effective for the treatment of anorexia nervosa? Results from a systematic review and meta-analysis. *J Clin Psychiatry* 2012;73(6):e757–766.

68. American Psychiatric Association. Practice guideline for the treatment of patients with eating disorders (American Psychiatric Association). *Am J Psychiatry* 2006;157: 1–39.

69. Agras WS, Walsh BT, Fairburn CG, et al. A multicenter comparison of cognitive-behavioral therapy and interpersonal psychotherapy for bulimia nervosa. *Arch Gen Psychiatry* 2000;57:459–466.

70. Rosen DS. Identification and management of eating disorders in children and adolescents. *Pediatrics* 2010;126(6):1240–1253.

71. Hay P, Bacaltchuk J, Claudino A, et al. Individual psychotherapy in the outpatient treatment of adults with anorexia nervosa. *Cochrane Database Syst Rev* 2003; 4:CD003909–CD003909.

72. Fisher CA, Hetrick SE, Rushford N. Family therapy for anorexia nervosa. *Cochrane Database Syst Rev Online* 2010;(4):CD004780.

73. Bulik CM, Berkman ND, Brownley KA, et al. Anorexia nervosa treatment: a systematic review of randomized controlled trials. *Int J Eat Disord* 2007;40(4):310–320.

74. Morgan JF, Reid F, Lacey JH. The SCOFF questionnaire: assessment of a new screening tool for eating disorders. *BMJ* 1999;319(7223):1467–1468.

75. Luck AJ, Morgan JF, Reid F, et al. The SCOFF questionnaire and clinical interview for eating disorders in general practice: comparative study. *BMJ* 2002;325(7367):755–756.

76. Mijan de la Torre A, Perez-Garcia A, Martin de la Torre E, et al. Is an integral nutritional approach to eating disorders feasible in primary care? *Br J Nutr* 2006;96:s82–s85.

77. Mehler PS. Diagnosis and care of patients with anorexia nervosa in primary care settings. *Ann Intern Med* 2001;134:1048–1059.

78. Sayag S, Latzer Y. The role of the family physician in eating disorders. *Int J Adolesc Med Health* 2002;14:261–267.

79. Powers PS, Santana CA. Eating disorders: a guide for the primary care physician. *Prim Care* 2002;29:81–98.

80. Ebeling H, Tapanainen P, Joutsenoja A, et al. A practice guideline for treatment of eating disorders in children and adolescents. *Ann Med* 2003;35:488–501.

81. American Academy of Pediatrics, Committee on Adolescence. Identifying and treating eating disorders. *Pediatrics* 2003;111:204–211.

82. Sim LA, McAlpine DE, Grothe KB, et al. Identification and treatment of eating disorders in the primary care setting. *Mayo Clin Proc* 2010;85(8):746–751.

83. Williams PM, Goodie J, Motsinger CD. Treating eating disorders in primary care. *Am Fam Physician* 2008;77(2):187.

84. Dejong H, Broadbent H, Schmidt U. A systematic review of dropout from treatment in outpatients with anorexia nervosa. *Int J Eat Disord* 2012;45(5):635–647.

85. Beumont PJV, Touyz SW. The nutritional management of anorexia and bulimia nervosa. In: Brownell DK, Fairburn CG, eds. *Eating disorders and obesity. A comprehensive handbook.* New York, NY: Guilford Press, 1995.

86. Yager J, Anderson AE. Anorexia nervosa. *N Engl J Med* 2005;353:1481–1488.

87. Steiger H, Lehoux PM, Gauvin L. Impulsivity, dietary control and the urge to binge in bulimic syndromes. *Int J Eat Disord* 1999;26:261.

88. Raynor HA, Niemeier HM, Wing RR. Effect of limiting snack food variety on long-term sensory-specific satiety and monotony during obesity treatment. *Eat Behav* 2006;7(1):1–14.

89. Rodin G, Olmsted MP, Rydall AC, et al. Eating disorders in young women with type 1 diabetes mellitus. *J Psychosom Res* 2002;53:943–949.

90. Rydall AC, Rodin GM, Olmsted P, et al. Disordered eating behavior and microvascular complications in young women with insulin-dependent diabetes mellitus. *N Engl J Med* 1997;336:1849.

SUGGESTED READINGS

American Psychiatric Association. *Diagnostic and statistical manual of mental disorders*, 4th ed. Washington, DC: American Psychiatric Association, 1994.

Becker AE, Grinspoon SK, Klibanski A, et al. Eating disorders. *N Engl J Med* 1999;340:1092–1098.

Brownell DK, Fairburn CG, eds. *Eating disorders and obesity. A comprehensive handbook.* New York, NY: Guilford Press, 1995; the following chapters in particular: Andersen AE. Eating disorders in males; Beumont PJV. The clinical presentation of anorexia and bulimia nervosa; Cooper Z. The development and maintenance of eating disorders; Fairburn CG. The prevention of eating disorders; Halmi KA. Hunger and satiety in clinical eating disorders; Hsu LKG. Outcome of bulimia nervosa; Steinhausaen H-C. The course and outcome of anorexia nervosa.

Fairburn CG, Brownell KD, eds. *Eating disorders and obesity: a comprehensive handbook*, 2nd ed. New York, NY: Guilford Press, 2002.

Kaye WH, Gendall K, Kye C. The role of the central nervous system in the psychoneuroendocrine disturbances of anorexia and bulimia nervosa. *Psychiatr Clin North Am* 1998;21:381–396.

Mizes JS. Neglected topics in eating disorders: guidelines for clinicians and researchers. *Clin Psychol Rev* 1998;18:387–390.

Schebendach J, Nussbaum MP. Nutrition management in adolescents with eating disorders. *Adolesc Med* 1992;3:541.

Stunkard A. Eating disorders: the last 25 years. *Appetite* 1997;29:181.

Walsh BT, Devlin MJ. Eating disorders: progress and problems. *Science* 1998;29:1387.

World Health Organization. *International classification of diseases (ICD) 10. Classification of mental and behavioral disorders.* Geneva, Switzerland: World Health Organization, 1992.

CHAPTER 26

Malnutrition and Cachexia

Impaired functional status and anorexia (loss of appetite) of various etiologies may result in nutrient and energy intake inadequate for metabolic demand. Similarly, physiologic stresses including acute illness or injury may raise metabolic demand to a level not easily accommodated by a conventional diet. Often, impaired nutrient intake and increased metabolic demand are concurrent, as is the case in cancer, acquired immunodeficiency syndrome (AIDS), burns, or other acute and chronic disease states. Although there is little evidence to suggest that nutrient deficiency under such conditions strongly influences the course of illness or recovery over the first several days, nutritional status is fundamental to convalescence and health maintenance over time. Nutritional status influences immune function (see Chapter 11) and wound healing (see Chapter 23), both vital to recovery from acute and chronic illness or injury.

To achieve adequate nurture in the context of disease or disability, nutritional support may be indicated. Whenever possible, that support should be enteral, either by mouth or feeding tube. Parenteral nutrition can meet all metabolic need but at the cost of gastrointestinal (GI) atrophy and a risk of line sepsis. Adjuvant therapies, such as megestrol acetate or growth hormone, have been used with variable success to enhance appetite and promote preferential restitution of lean body mass. Increasingly, nutritional formulas tailored to a patient's particular condition and nutrient needs are available. There is a growing body of research to support the use of specific nutrient combinations to preserve and promote lean body mass. The selection and modification of nutrition support formulas generally should be overseen by a dietitian or other nutritionist; such consultation is typically readily available in the inpatient setting.

OVERVIEW

Decisions about nutritional support are based on the nutritional status of the patient as well as the clinical context. No single method or tool has proven sufficient to assess nutritional status with high sensitivity and specificity; instead, a combination of measurements is often used to develop the most accurate picture of a patient's nutritional risk (1). According to the European Society for Parenteral and Enteral Nutrition, the goal of nutritional assessment tools are to predict the probability of a positive or negative outcome due to nutrition and whether nutritional treatment would influence this outcome (2). The Subjective Global Assessment (SGA) is one of several clinical scoring tools that have been deemed useful for nutritional assessment in hospitalized patients (3). SGA incorporates medical history, functional assessment, and physical examination to identify patients with malnutrition who might benefit from nutritional support (1,4). In addition to SGA, another tool is The Malnutrition Universal Screening Tool (MUST; see Figure 26.1) which uses body mass index (BMI), unintentional weight loss, and effects of acute disease in order to determine adults who are either at risk of or are currently malnourished (5). It has been validated for primary care (predicting rate of hospital admissions and primary care physician visits) and inpatient care settings (predicting length of stay, mortality, and disposition after discharge) (2). Other clinical screening tools that have been validated include the Nutrition Risk Index, the Mini Nutritional Assessment, and the Nutrition Risk Score; these have all been reviewed by Delegge and Drake (1).

Nutritional status is evaluated using body weight, particularly in comparison with baseline weight, as well as dietary and medical history. The measure "percent usual body weight," actual body weight divided by usual body weight multiplied by 100, is often used in anthropometric assessment. Height can be measured along with weight to obtain BMI in adults (weight in kilograms divided by height in meters squared). Length and head circumference are useful in young children.

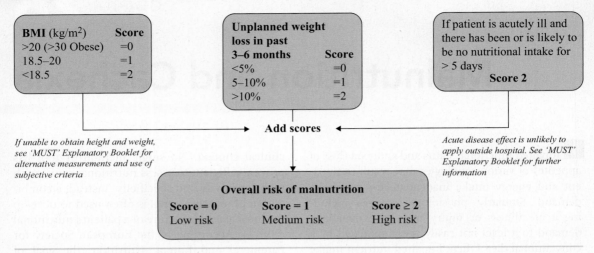

FIGURE 26.1 The 'MUST' Flowchart.

Source: The "Malnutrition Universal Screening Tool" is reproduced here with the kind permission of BAPEN (British Association for Parenteral and Enteral Nutrition). For further information on 'MUST' and management guidelines, see www.bapen.org.uk.

Calipers (typically Lange skin-fold calipers) can be used to measure skin-fold thickness and provide a measure of subcutaneous fat as compared with a reference standard; triceps skin-fold is used most often because the site is easy to reach and there is usually no edema. In men, a triceps skin-fold thickness less than 12.5 mm indicates malnutrition, whereas a thickness above 20 mm indicates over nutrition. The comparable values in women are 16.5 and 25 mm, respectively. Measurement of the mid-arm muscle circumference with a tape measure is also recognized as a proxy for body protein stores, with values under the 15th percentile indicative of under nutrition (6). Measures of body composition, including bioelectrical impedance and trans axial computed tomography, are useful in research settings but rarely applied clinically.

Biochemical indices of nutritional status include both somatic and visceral proteins

(see Table 26.1). The visceral proteins include albumin, transferrin, prealbumin, and retinol-binding protein. Albumin is used most commonly; its level varies consistently with the adequacy of protein stores. Albumin has a half-life of approximately 20 days and, therefore, cannot be used to measure acute states of malnutrition. Conversely, albumin levels tend to drop precipitously in septic states independent of nutritional status. An albumin level from 3.5 to 5.5 g per dL is considered normal, 2.8 to 3.5 g per dL is considered mild depletion, 2.1 to 2.7 g per dL is moderate depletion, and levels below 2.1 g per dL indicate severe depletion of visceral protein.

Transferrin, with a half-life of 8 to 10 days, can be used instead of albumin when acute nutritional perturbations are under evaluation. The half-life of prealbumin is approximately 2 days; like the level of albumin, the prealbumin

TABLE 26.1

Cutoff Values for Visceral and Somatic Protein Assays in Clinical Use

Level	Moderate Depletion Albumin (g/dL)	Transferrin (mg/dL)	Prealbumin (mg/dL)	Retinol-Binding Protein (mg/dL)	Urinary Creatinine (% of Reference Value)
Normal	3.5–5.5	250–300	15.7–29.6	2.6–7.6	>90
Mild Depletion	2.8–3.5	150–250	10–15	N/A	80–90
Moderate Depletion	2.1–2.7	100–150	5–10	N/A	60–80
Severe Depletion	<2.1	<100	<5	N/A	<60

level is acutely depressed by severe physiologic stress. The half-life of retinol-binding protein is approximately 10 hours, but its sensitivity to even minor stress limits the clinical utility of its measurement.

Somatic proteins are those that indicate the state of skeletal muscle mass. The most commonly used index is 24-hour urinary creatinine excretion. The index is expressed as milligrams of urinary creatinine in 24 hours for the patient per milligram of urinary creatinine in 24 hours by a normal subject of the same height and sex, multiplied by 100.

Functional testing—of muscle strength, for example—has advantages over biochemical and anthropometric assessments but is not used consistently. Other indicators of malnutrition include leukopenia and lymphopenia and skin-test anergy. Patients receiving home parenteral nutrition or those with fat malabsorption are at risk of essential fatty acid deficiency (EFAD) (7,8). This condition is diagnosed using the Holman Index, described as the plasma triene to tetraene ratio; a Holman Index of 0.2 is currently considered the upper limit of normal (9). Current preparations of parenteral nutrition used in the United States contain soybean and/or safflower oils. Concern that these formulations may contribute to liver disease in patients has spawned questions of whether fish oil preparations may be a better alternative. One study evaluated neonates who received fish oil based emulsion, showing that at proper dosages, fish oil emulsions contained adequate amounts of essential fatty acids to prevent EFAD (10).

Malnutrition results from deficient nutrient intake, impaired metabolism, excessive losses, or some combination of these factors. Clinical evaluation for malnutrition should include not only examination for signs of wasting (e.g., at the temples or in the hands) but also examination of hair for thinning or poor attachment, the skin for xerosis, and the mouth for inflammation, all indicative of macronutrient or micronutrient deficiencies (see Table 26.2).

Hospitalized patients are subject to marasmus (a term derived from a Greek word meaning "to waste"), a state of both protein and total energy malnutrition. Marasmus is distinguished from kwashiorkor, a Bantu word meaning "displaced child," which describes the state of protein deficiency despite adequate energy intake.

TABLE 26.2

Physical Findings Associated with Common Nutrient Deficiencies

Physical Finding	Responsible Nutrient Deficiency
Muscle wasting (temples, hands)	Protein; energy
Skin: xerosis scaling, bruising	Protein; energy; vitamins A, C, K
Hair: thinning, poor attachment, pigment changes	Protein; energy; vitamins A, E, B

Kwashiorkor occurs in babies weaned from the breast in many developing countries with subsistence diets. Kwashiorkor can be associated with a serum albumin as low as 1 g per dL as compared with the four-fold higher normal value, resulting in very low oncotic pressure and characteristic edema.

Approximately 25% of the body's protein reserves can be consumed to generate energy during starvation, sparing vital functions for a period as long as 50 days. In a well-nourished adult, nearly 3 kg of protein can be turned over to generate 12,000 kcal of energy.

Energy requirements in hospitalized patients can be estimated through application of the Harris-Benedict equation (see Section VIIA) or, when available, by use of indirect calorimetry. Limited evidence suggests the superiority of measurement versus estimation of energy requirements in the critically ill (11). One observational study evaluated various equations in calculating energy requirements for obese hospitalized patients. It found that the Harris-Benedict equation most accurately measured resting energy expenditure in this population within 10% in 50% of the patients. Yet authors concluded that indirect calorimetry is preferred for estimation of energy requirements (12). Protein requirements rise with metabolic stress. Baseline protein needs of approximately 0.8 g/kg/day nearly triple after a significant burn and rise to lesser degrees with all disease states. Hyperglycemia is a hazard associated with nutritional support; a recent Clinical Practice Guideline in review of pertinent literature concluded that tight glycemic control <180 in critically ill patients provided a mortality benefit (13).

NUTRITION SUPPORT

Dietary Supplements

Anorexia, or simply reduced appetite, may occur in patients with current nutritional deficiencies or patients at risk of developing them. Simple strategies to combat a persistently deficient appetite include frequent spacing of small meals and the prioritization of energy-dense (usually high-fat) foods. When energy-dense foods are proffered, there should still be attention to nutritional quality. Examples of foods rich in both nutrients and calories include nuts, seeds, nut butters, and avocado. Food supplements such as whey protein powder may also prove useful for concocting nutrient- and energy-dense dishes.

When efforts to modify the diet fail to provide adequate nutrition, powdered (for reconstitution) or liquid supplements may be indicated. A wide variety of commercial products are available; selection is often best based on the recommendations of an experienced dietitian and patient preference. Some of the available supplements (e.g., Ensure, Boost) are nutritionally complete and can be used, if needed, as the sole source of nutrients and energy.

Enteral Nutrition Support

Enteral nutrition support involves the administration of nutrient formulas into the GI tract through a tube. The weight of evidence clearly favors enteral over parenteral nutrition support whenever either is an option, leading to the axiom that the gut should be used whenever it works (14). When nutrients are not administered via the GI tract, mucosal atrophy occurs, as does dysfunction of the pancreatic/biliary system. Parenteral nutrition also appears to pose increased risk of infection compared to enteral feeding (15). Options in enteral nutrition have been enhanced over recent years with the development of low-risk procedures for tube insertion and the development of a variety of commercial preparations tailored to different clinical situations. For the most part, enteral feeding formulas are classified according to energy density, protein content, intended administration route, and molecular complexity.

Feeding Tubes

There are two types of feeding tubes: those that enter the GI tract through the nose or mouth and those that enter through the abdominal wall. Nasogastric tubes are used for short-duration feeding and when the risk of aspiration is low. Nasoduodenal and nasojejunal tubes are preferable for longer-term feeding and when the risk of aspiration is higher. The prevailing view is that the risk of aspiration falls the more distally the tube is placed. Several recent studies, however, seem to contradict this convention, finding no significant benefit of nasojejunal tubes over gastric feeding devices (16,17).

Tubes placed through the abdominal wall are more appropriate in general for long-term supplementation. Such tubes are less likely to kink or occlude, and they reduce the risk of aspiration (18). Gastrostomy and jejunostomy tubes can be inserted endoscopically, radiologically, or surgically (19). The percutaneous endoscopic gastrostomy (PEG) tube is generally most popular. Insertion requires an endoscopy laboratory and local anesthesia with sedation, and it is routinely done on an outpatient basis. Jejunostomy tubes, placed endoscopically or surgically, may be indicated when the risk of aspiration is considered particularly high. The technical difficulty is greater for jejunostomy tubes, and the complication rate is also higher (20). Advances in technique permit endoscopic tube placement in most circumstances, except when anatomy is distorted by surgery or pathology (21). A button gastrostomy is an option in particularly active patients for whom a tube gastrostomy is inconvenient or embarrassing (22).

Enteral Formulas

Conventional enteric formulas are polymeric, containing oligosaccharides, intact protein, and triglycerides. Commercial preparations are lactose free and can provide approximately 2,000 kcal per day. The energy density varies from 1 to 2 kcal per mL, with high-energy-density preparations indicated when fluid restriction is required. Formula proteins are derived from egg albumin, milk protein, or both. The fat is of vegetable origin. Such formulas can be delivered directly into the stomach, duodenum, or jejunum. Adding fiber, often in the form of soy polysaccharide or partially hydrolyzed guar gum, has become common practice; benefits include prevention of osmotic diarrhea and evening out of serum glucose responses (23). Monomeric formulas contain partially hydrolyzed protein and monosaccharides and disaccharides. Fat in the form of medium-chain triglycerides (MCTs) and long-chain triglycerides (LCTs) provides 5% or less of the total calories, compared to 30% to 40% in polymeric formulas. Monomeric formulas are available at higher cost and in general are not known to offer appreciable advantages over polymeric preparations. Theoretically, such solutions should be advantageous in states of impaired absorption, such as pancreatic insufficiency. Essential vitamins, minerals, and trace elements are routinely added to both polymeric and monomeric formulas in order to meet all nutrient requirements.

Targeted formulas are intended for use in particular disease states. Formulas specifically tailored for inborn errors of metabolism are of clear value in defined circumstances. Current recommendations for enteral feedings in patients with cystic fibrosis suggest using an elemental formula without enzyme replacement, administered in a slow continuous feeding; alternatively, polymeric formulas with enzyme supplementation may be given in one single-meal dose (24,25).

Tailored formulations for many conditions lack evidence of benefit compared with conventional preparations. Use of formulas tailored for hepatic dysfunction, containing a high ratio of branched-chain to aromatic amino acids, is supported by available evidence (26). Solutions based on essential amino acids have been developed for renal failure (27). In addition, children hospitalized in the pediatric intensive care unit may be more likely to develop acute kidney injury if underfed, thus stressing the importance of enteral feeding in the acute setting (28). Formulas tailored for pulmonary disease exploit the lower respiratory quotient (RQ) of fat and protein relative to carbohydrate. The RQ refers specifically to the molar ratio of carbon dioxide produced per oxygen consumed. The RQ is 1 for carbohydrate, 0.7 for fat, and approximately 0.8 for protein. Thus, fat and protein can be used to generate energy with less CO_2 production, which is of particular value in states of CO_2 retention (see Chapter 15).

There is some evidence that solutions using keto acids rather than amino acids can slow progression of chronic renal failure (27,29). Glycemic control can be improved with formulas tailored for diabetes (30,31). Supplementation of enteral nutrition with n-3 fatty acids (32) and other nutrients designed to enhance immune function have been shown to reduce infection rates, time spent on mechanical ventilation, and ICU lengths of stay (33). A recent randomized controlled trial evaluated antioxidant-enriched versus immune enhancing enteral nutrition in patients who had undergone esophagectomy for cancer. The results showed that there was no significant difference in nutritional markers after patients were given either formulation (34). There is increasing interest in the addition of glutamine to enteral solutions, as it is the preferred energy substrate of the GI tract (35). Preliminary studies of its use in enteral formulas are encouraging; there is also evidence to suggest increased benefit from high-dose parenteral glutamine (36). In mice with induced colitis, enteral formula enriched with glutamine, oligosaccharide, and fiber was found to decrease the level of inflammation in the intestine (37). This is a possible avenue for further research regarding enteral nutrition formulations and patients with ulcerative colitis.

Modular solutions are available to supplement commercial preparations so that nutrient composition can be tailored to the individual patient's need. There are more than 100 commercially available enteral feeding solutions. Selection is best based, other than for the nutrition specialist, on the advice of a consulting dietitian; inpatient use is constrained by the hospital formulary.

Enteral solutions can be delivered as bolus feeds or continuous infusions; bolus feeding is feasible only when the tube is in the stomach. Bolus feeds are more convenient, with infusions typically requiring a pump. Infusions into the small bowel generally can be tolerated at a rate up to 150 mL per hour.

Aspiration is the principal risk of enteral feeding. Risk is reduced by feeding with the torso at a 30- to 45-degree angle of inclination rather than supine (38). When the gag reflex is absent or impaired or gastric emptying is delayed, feeding into the jejunum is preferred. Diarrhea occurs not uncommonly, especially in patients taking antibiotics concomitantly. The risk generally is reduced by the use of iso-osmolar solutions.

Parenteral Nutrition Support

The delivery of nutrition directly into the bloodstream poses risks that enteral feeding does not, and it should be avoided when possible. Indications for parenteral feeding include states of severe malabsorption; such states occur in extensive bowel resection, radiation enteritis, and severe inflammatory bowel disease; disordered intestinal motility, obstruction, or persistent vomiting; premature birth; and states of extreme catabolism, such as extensive burns, for which enteral feeding may not be adequate.

Whereas enteral solutions are approved as foods, parenteral solutions must be approved by the Food and Drug Administration as drugs. Intravenous nutrient infusions are intended to meet energy and nutrient requirements completely (total parenteral nutrition; TPN) or incompletely (peripheral parenteral nutrition; PPN). PPN solutions can generally be delivered through a peripheral or central vein, but TPN requires central venous access. Near-complete nutrition support via peripheral access may be achievable in patients who can tolerate a high volume of isotonic solution. To meet energy needs while limiting the proportion of calories from fat, hypertonic carbohydrate solutions must be used, thus requiring TPN and central access.

Access for TPN is generally via the subclavian or jugular veins. Peripheral placement of long catheters threaded into the superior vena cava and creation of an arteriovenous fistula as in dialysis are alternatives. Surgical insertions are used to tunnel the catheter under the skin to reduce the risk of infection. Other vascular approaches are used less frequently. The risk of line sepsis is reduced by strict adherence to aseptic technique and infection control guidelines. Dedicated TPN lines can be maintained for months, if not years. Indwelling central venous catheters pose a risk not only of sepsis but also of thrombosis; antibiotic- and heparin-bonded catheters may help.

Various plastics are used for TPN delivery. There is some absorption of insulin by commonly used plastics, so the glucose levels of patients with diabetes should be monitored carefully, with adjustments in infused insulin made accordingly.

Parenteral nutrition is generally indicated only when intestinal absorption is impaired. Benefit is convincingly established only in the short bowel syndrome (39). Meta-analysis indicates that there is no net mortality benefit associated with use of TPN in surgical or critical care patients (40,41). A multicenter randomized controlled trial evaluated early versus late initiation (48 hours vs. greater than 8 days) of TPN in critically ill adults. The study found that late initiation was associated with less complications

and quicker recovery time (42). Lipid emulsions are generally provided as adjuvants to TPN formula. Micronutrient doses in TPN formulas are standardized, but they may need to be tailored in certain conditions. Evidence to date supports the use of glutamine-supplemented formulas in the critically ill (36,43,44). Glutamine is the preferred fuel of enterocytes.

There are clear disadvantages to over nutrition beyond those related to weight gain (45,46). In normal states, adults can oxidize glucose at a rate of up to approximately 14 mg/kg/min. This rate is reduced to as low as 5 mg/kg/min in burn patients. Glucose infused beyond this capacity is converted to fat, with elevation of the RQ to above 1 and loss of available energy due to metabolic demand and waste. Fatty liver may result over time from excessive hepatic synthesis of triglycerides.

Lipid emulsions administered with TPN become coated with apolipoproteins in circulation, much the same way as do endogenously produced lipoprotein particles. Because infused lipid particles differ from chylomicrons, they are metabolized differently, eliciting the formation of a novel lipoprotein (lipoprotein X). Emulsified lipid droplets are acted on by endothelial lipoprotein lipase and undergo metabolism much the way ingested fat does (see Chapter 2).

Because lipid solutions are highly susceptible to microbial growth, infusion times of less than 12 hours are recommended. Lipid mixed with the other components of TPN, known as total nutrient admixture, can allow lipid infusions over 24-hour periods but have disadvantages as well, among them catheter occlusions. Total nutrient admixture may be particularly useful in premature neonates, who may not tolerate standard lipid infusions.

Lipid infusions increase the risk of bacteremia and rarely can result in fat overload syndrome, which is characterized by fever, hepatosplenomegaly, and coagulopathy due to fat sludging. Impaired pulmonary function and interference with immune function by occupation of the reticuloendothelial system also occur. Structured lipid emulsions containing balanced mixtures of MCTs and LCTs apparently mitigate most of these complications (47,48).

The use of TPN in children is associated with metabolic bone disease. The etiology of the condition is likely multifactorial, with calcium and phosphate deficiencies playing an important but only partial role (49,50). Strategies to prevent onset of metabolic bone disease include supplementation with additional calcium and phosphorus, which helps avoid the development of chronic metabolic acidosis and subsequent hypercalciuria, and vitamin D supplementation (50).

Use of TPN is associated with gallstone formation due to stasis in the gallbladder (51,52). Protracted use of TPN warrants periodic evaluation of the gallbladder by ultrasound, with consideration of elective cholecystectomy if stones develop. Use of ursodeoxycholic acid and S-adenosyl-L-methionine (SAMe) have shown promise in preventing TPN-induced cholelithiasis (53,54). Both cholelithiasis (53,55) and immune dysfunction (56,57) associated with TPN may be reduced through "gut stimulation" with limited enteral feeds.

As is the case for enteral solutions, a variety of commercial parenteral formulas are available. The selection and constitution of parenteral solutions should be overseen by a dietitian or nutrition consult service.

Pancreatitis

Acute pancreatitis is an illness with high metabolic demand and an increased catabolic state. Patients can experience rapid nutritional deterioration especially in severe acute pancreatitis. As a result of these dramatic changes in body metabolic processes, much debate over method, formulation, and timing for feeding in acute pancreatitis has developed. Early refeeding via NG tube in severe acute pancreatitis has not been shown to increase mortality, hospital stay, or infection rate as compared with traditional methods of treatment for this condition (58). A recent meta-analysis showed that total enteral nutrition was superior to TPN in that it decreased mortality, infection, organ failure, and surgical intervention for patients with severe acute pancreatitis (59). In addition, a Cochrane systematic review also showed that patients receiving enteral nutrition over TPN with acute pancreatitis had decreased hospital length of stay (60).

Special Considerations

The progestational agent megestrol acetate (Megace) has been shown to improve appetite and weight gain in cancer-related cachexia (61–63). Results are also promising for megestrol as an appetite stimulant in AIDS patients (64–66). Megestrol

has also been evaluated for use in dialysis patients with malnutrition (as measured by low albumin levels). In dialysis patients, it improved appetite, but did not improve quality of life due to side effects of the medication (67). Although effective in stimulating appetite and supporting an increase in body mass, megestrol is associated with an increased risk of deep venous thrombosis.

Growth hormone has been shown to increase lean body mass in human immunodeficiency virus (HIV) wasting syndrome but at the cost of hypertriglyceridemia and hyperglycemia. A systematic review of HIV patients with HIV associated lipodystrophy treated with growth hormone axis medications showed an increase in lean body mass and decrease in visceral adipose tissue (68).

MCTs in either enteral or parenteral preparations may be useful in states of malabsorption. MCTs are more readily oxidized, whereas LCTs are needed to provide the essential fatty acid linoleic acid. Balanced mixtures of MCT and LCT may be particularly advantageous.

Use of both enteral and parenteral feeding may fail to suppress appetite completely because of the dependence of satiety in part on the sensations elicited during ingestion (69,70). A recent study found that supplementation of enteral feeds with pea-fiber and fructo-oligosaccharide led to higher reported fullness among subjects compared to those consuming enteral formulas with otherwise identical macronutrient composition (71).

Preoperative enteral nutrition support has proven benefit in patients with even moderate nutritional impairment (72,73), whereas parenteral nutrition preoperatively has no proven benefit and should be reserved for severely impaired patients in whom enteral nutrition is precluded (41). Postoperative TPN should be considered only if the period of needed support is likely to exceed one week (74,75). Although parenteral nutrition has been the convention in pediatric patients requiring extracorporeal membrane oxygenation, recent evidence suggests that enteral nutrition is both feasible and effective (76,77).

Nutritional intervention is indicated in patients with HIV who have lost more than 5% body weight in 3 months; oral nutritional supplements or enteral nutrition is preferable to parenteral delivery, if it is possible (78,79).

Cachexia is a specific form of malnutrition characterized by muscle wasting and loss of lean body mass. Commonly seen in cancer and AIDS patients, cachexia is associated with anorexia, but mere increase of nutrition intake is insufficient to reverse the changes associated with this condition (80). Increased protein breakdown is thought to be responsible for the muscle wasting of cachexia; recently, the leucine metabolite β-hydroxy-β-methylbutyrate (HMB) has emerged as a potential antagonist of this process. HMB is known to play an important role in protein synthesis (81) and has been used by athletes to help build muscle (see Chapter 32). In *previous* animal and human trials, HMB appeared to help prevent muscle wasting by preserving muscle mass and strength (82). Ross-Abbott Pharmaceuticals now produces an enteral supplement called Juven that combines HMB with arginine and glutamine, both of which appear to enhance protein synthesis (83). Preliminary evidence suggests benefit in reversing age-related muscle losses (84) and in accelerating wound repair (85). A recent randomized, double-blind, placebo-controlled trial was completed evaluating whether Juven improved cancer cachexia. The study experienced a large drop-out rate due to patient preference, but ultimately showed, after 8 weeks of treatment with Juven, no change in lean body mass (86).

Malnutrition is a consideration after bariatric surgery. Roux-en-Y gastric bypass surgery comprises 70% to 75% of bariatric surgery performed throughout the world today. This method of bariatric surgery intentionally causes decreased absorption by bypassing the distal stomach, duodenum, and proximal jejunum. Most commonly, patients may become deficient in iron, folic acid, calcium, and vitamins B_1, B_{12}, and D. Patients may be at increased long-term risk (12 months after surgery) of β-carotene and vitamins C and A deficiencies after Roux-en-Y gastric bypass surgery even after vitamin and mineral supplementation (87).

Nutrigenomic Considerations

Cachexia in cancer patients poses challenges for patients' quality of life and ability to recover from treatments. Certain cancers are more prone to causing cachexia, yet within the same subset of cancer types there remains a variation in the development of chronic wasting between patients. As a result of this paradox, researchers have questioned whether there are genetic variations (in the form of single nucleotide polymorphisms—SNPs)

present that result in higher risk for cachexia. At the present time, research shows that multiple polymorphisms may influence the development of wasting, but more investigation is required to elucidate the role of genetics in cancer cachexia (88).

Aging and Nutrition

Sarcopenia is defined as a decrease in appendicular muscle mass that falls below 2 standard deviations from the mean as compared to young, healthy adults of the same sex and ethnicity. Sarcopenia is an age-related process that increases as a patient grows older. It has been postulated that sarcopenia and dietary factors like consumption of antioxidant rich foods may be related. One study found that levels of vitamin A, C, E or selenium intake did not significantly affect the muscle mass of older men and women (89). The pathophysiology of aging and muscle mass is detailed further in Chapter 31.

The obesity epidemic has become a hot topic in recent years. The focus on normal BMI is based on studies showing that overweight and obese BMI increases morbidity and mortality for patients. Recent studies have called into question this association for the elderly population. As a person ages, it may be more "healthy" to have a BMI in the overweight category. One study highlights this by showing that elderly patients with overweight BMI resulted in lower mortality risk, whereas changes in BMI for an elderly patient whether increase or decrease increased mortality (90). Higher BMI may be indicative of a greater ability to utilize nutrients consumed or a decreased toll on the body from chronic medical illnesses.

■ CLINICAL HIGHLIGHTS

Clinical assessment for malnutrition can and should be routinely incorporated into the history and physical examination of both inpatients and outpatients. For chronically malnourished patients able to eat, dietary adjustments or supplements may permit restoration of nutritional adequacy. When eating is precluded by illness, enteral nutrition support is preferred to parenteral nutrition whenever the GI tract is functioning. Enteral formulas increasingly can be tailored to the condition and metabolic state of individual patients; dietary consultation is indicated to facilitate optimal choices. Feeding in acute pancreatitis has been debated; however, studies now show the superiority of enteral nutrition to parenteral nutrition in terms of mortality and hospital stay.

Parenteral nutrition support is riskier and costlier than enteral support but is indicated when the GI tract is nonfunctioning. Improvements in the composition of formulas and the techniques for vascular access offer the promise of TPN with lower rates of complication. Nutrition service consultation is always indicated when TPN is to be used.

Evidence is accruing that specific nutrients can be used to promote and protect lean body mass during times of acute stress, with potential enhancement of wound healing and overall recovery time. Proprietary preparations designed specifically for this application are available. There may be times when a higher BMI may actually be beneficial. In the elderly population, overweight BMI may be protective rather than harmful in terms of mortality (see Chapter 5).

REFERENCES

1. Delegge MH, Drake LM. Nutritional assessment. *Gastroenterol Clin North Am* 2007;36:1–22.
2. Anthony P. Nutrition screening tools for hospitalized patients. *Nutr Clin Pract* 2008;23:373.
3. Sungurtekin H, Sungurtekin U, Hanci V, et al. Comparison of two nutrition assessment techniques in hospitalized patients. *Nutrition* 2004;20:428–432.
4. Detsky AS, McLaughlin JR, Baker JP, et al. What is subjective global assessment of nutritional status? *JPEN* 1987;11:8.
5. Kvamme JM, Grønli O, Florholmen J, et al. Risk of malnutrition is associated with mental health symptoms in community living elderly men and women: the Tromsø Study. *BMC Psychiatry* 2011;11:112.
6. Frisancho AR. New norms of upper limb fat and muscle areas for assessment of nutritional status. *Am J Clin Nutr* 1981;34:2540–2545.
7. Ling P, Ollero M, Khaodhiar L, et al. Disturbances in essential fatty acid metabolism in patients receiving long-term home parenteral nutrition. *Dig Dis Sci* 2002;47:1679–1685.
8. Jeppesen PB, Hoy C-E, Mortensen PB. Essential fatty acid deficiency in patients receiving home parenteral nutrition. *Am J Clin Nutr* 1998;68:126–133.
9. Hamilton C, Austin T, Seidner DL. Essential fatty acid deficiency in human adults during parenteral nutrition. *Nutr Clin Pract* 2006;21:387–394.
10. De Meijer VE, Le HD, Meisel JA, et al. Parenteral fish oil as monotherapy prevents essential fatty acid deficiency in parenteral nutrition dependent patients. *J Pediatr Gastroenterol Nutr* 2010;50(2):212–218.
11. Reid CL. Poor agreement between continuous measurements of energy expenditure and routinely used prediction equations in intensive care unit patients. *Clin Nutr* 2007;26:649–657.
12. Anderegg BA, Worrall C, Barbour E, et al. Comparison of resting energy expenditure prediction methods with measured resting energy expenditure in obese, hospitalized adults. *JPEN* 2009;33(2):168–175.
13. Jacobi J, Bircher N, Krinsley J, et al. Guidelines for the use of an insulin infusion for the management of hyperglycemia in critically ill patients. *Crit Care Med* 2012;40(12):3251–3276.
14. Simpson F, Doig GS. Parenteral vs. enteral nutrition in the critically ill patient: a meta-analysis of trials using the intention to treat principle. *Intensive Care Med* 2005;31:12–23.
15. Braunschweig CL, Levy P, Sheean PM, et al. Enteral compared with parenteral nutrition: a meta-analysis. *Am J Clin Nutr* 2001;74:534–542.
16. Montejo JC, Grau T, Acosta J, et al. Multicenter, prospective, randomized, single-blind study comparing the efficacy and gastrointestinal complications of early jejunal feeding with early gastric feeding in critically ill patients. *Crit Care Med* 2002;30:796–800.
17. McClave SA, Lukan JK, Stefater JA, et al. Poor validity of residual volumes as a marker for risk of aspiration in critically ill patients. *Crit Care Med* 2005;33:324–330.
18. Vanek VW. Ins and outs of enteral access: part 2—long term access—esophagostomy and gastrostomy. *Nutr Clin Pract* 2003;18:50–74.
19. Ho SG, Marchinkow LO, Legiehn GM, et al. Radiological percutaneous gastrostomy. *Clin Radiol* 2001;56:902–910.
20. McClave SA, Chang W. Complications of enteral access. *Gastrointest Endosc* 2003;58:739–751.
21. Campos AC, Marchesini JB. Recent advances in the placement of tubes for enteral nutrition. *Curr Opin Clin Nutr Metab Care* 1999;2:265–269.
22. Schroder O, Hoepffner N, Stein J. Enteral nutrition by endoscopic means; I. techniques, indications, types of enteral feed. *Z Gastroenterol* 2004;42:1385–1392.
23. Slavin JL, Greenberg NA. Partially hydrolyzed guar gum: clinical nutrition uses. *Nutrition* 2003;19:549–552.
24. Erskine JM, Lingard CD, Sontag MK, et al. Enteral nutrition for patients with cystic fibrosis: comparison of a semi-elemental and nonelemental formula. *J Pediatr* 1998;132:265–269.
25. Erskine JM, Lingard C, Sontag M. Update on enteral nutrition support for cystic fibrosis. *Nutr Clin Pract* 2007;22:223–232.
26. Charlton M. Branched-chain amino acid enriched supplements as therapy for liver disease. *J Nutr* 2006;136:295s–298s.
27. Cano NJ, Fouque D, Leverve XM. Application of branched-chain amino acids in human pathological states: renal failure. *J Nutr* 2006;136:299s–307s.
28. Kyle UG, Akcan-Arikan A, Orellana RA, et al. Nutrition support among critically ill children with AKI. *Clin J Am Soc Nephrol* 2013;8(4):568–574.
29. Koretz RL. Does nutritional intervention in protein-energy malnutrition improve morbidity or mortality? *J Ren Nutr* 1999;9:119–121.
30. Coulston AM. Clinical experience with modified enteral formulas for patients with diabetes. *Clin Nutr* 1998;17:46–56.

31. Elia M, Ceriello A, Laube H, et al. Enteral nutritional support and use of diabetes-specific formulas for patients with diabetes: a meta-analysis. *Diabetes Care* 2005;28:2267–2279.

32. Singer P, Theilla M, Fisher H, et al. Benefit of an enteral diet enriched with eicosapentaenoic acid and gamma-linolenic acid in ventilated patients with acute lung injury. *Crit Care Med* 2006;34:1033–1038.

33. Montejo JC, Zarazaga A, Lopez-Martinez J, et al. Immunonutrition in the intensive care unit. A systematic review and consensus statement. *Clin Nutr* 2003;22:221–233.

34. Nagano T, Fujita H, Tanaka T, et al. A randomized controlled trial comparing antioxidant-enriched enteral nutrition with immune-enhancing enteral nutrition after esophagectomy for cancer: a pilot study. *Surg Today* 2013;43(11):1240–1249.

35. Griffiths RD. The evidence for glutamine use in the critically-ill. *Proc Nutr Soc* 2001;60:1–8.

36. Novak F, Heyland DK, Avenell A, et al. Glutamine supplementation in serious illness: a systematic review of the evidence. *Crit Care Med* 2002;30:2022–2029.

37. Joo E, Yamane S, Hamasaki A, et al. Enteral supplement enriched with glutamine, fiber, and oligosaccharide attenuates experimental colitis in mice. *Nutrition* 2013;29(3): 549–555.

38. Metheny NA. Preventing respiratory complications of tube feedings: evidence-based practice. *Am J Crit Care* 2006;15:360–369.

39. Koretz RL, Lipman TO, Klein S. AGA technical review on parenteral nutrition. *Gastroenterology* 2001;121: 970–1001.

40. Heyland DK, MacDonald S, Keefe L, et al. Total parenteral nutrition in the critically ill patient: a meta-analysis. *JAMA* 1998;280:2013–2019.

41. Koretz RL. Do data support nutrition support? Part I: intravenous nutrition. *J Am Diet Assoc* 2007;107:988–996.

42. Casaer MP, Mesotten D, Hermans G, et al. Early versus late parenteral nutrition in critically ill adults. *N Engl J Med* 2011;365(6):506–517.

43. Sacks GS. Glutamine supplementation in catabolic patients. *Ann Pharmacother* 1999;33:348–354.

44. Griffiths RD, Allen KD, Andrews FJ, et al. Infection, multiple organ failure, and survival in the intensive care unit: influence of glutamine-supplemented parenteral nutrition on acquired infection. *Nutrition* 2002;18:546–552.

45. Klein CJ, Stanek GS, Wiles CE 3rd. Overfeeding macronutrients to critically ill adults: metabolic complications. *J Am Diet Assoc* 1998;98:795–806.

46. Btaiche IF, Khalidi N. Metabolic complications of parenteral nutrition in adults, part 1. *Am J Health Syst Pharm* 2004;61:1938–1949.

47. Adolph M. Lipid emulsions in parenteral nutrition. *Ann Nutr Metab* 1999;43:1–13.

48. Chambrier C, Lauverjat M, Bouletreau P. Structured triglyceride emulsions in parenteral nutrition. *Nutr Clin Pract* 2006;21:342–350.

49. Klein GL. Metabolic bone disease of total parenteral nutrition. *Nutrition* 1998;14:149–152.

50. Ferrone M, Geraci M. A review of the relationship between parenteral nutrition and metabolic bone disease. *Nutr Clin Pract* 2007;22:329–339.

51. Moss RL, Amii LA. New approaches to understanding the etiology and treatment of total parenteral nutrition-associated cholestasis. *Semin Pediatr Surg* 1999;8:140–147.

52. Venneman NG, van Erpecum KJ. Gallstone disease: primary and secondary prevention. *Best Pract Res Clin Gastroenterol* 2006;20:1063–1073.

53. Amii LA, Moss RL. Nutritional support of the pediatric surgical patient. *Curr Opin Pediatr* 1999;11:237–240.

54. Lazaridis KN, Gores GJ, Lindor KD. Urodeoxycholic acid "mechanisms of action and clinical use in hepatobiliary disorders." *J Hepatol* 2001;35:134–146.

55. Guglielmi FW, Boggio-Bertinet D, Federico A, et al. Total parenteral nutrition-related gastroenterological complications. *Dig Liver Dis* 2006;38:623–642.

56. DeWitt RC, Kudsk KA. The gut's role in metabolism, mucosal barrier function, and gut immunology. *Infect Dis Clin North Am* 1999;13:465–481.

57. Schmidt H, Martindale R. The gastrointestinal tract in critical illness. *Curr Opin Clin Nutr Metab Care* 2001; 4:547–551.

58. Jiang K, Chen XZ, Xia Q, et al. Early nasogastric enteral nutrition for severe acute pancreatitis: a systematic review. *World J Gastroenterol* 2007;13(39):5253–5260.

59. Yi F, Ge L, Zhao J, et al. Meta-analysis: total parenteral nutrition versus total enteral nutrition in predicted severe acute pancreatitis. *Intern Med* 2012;51(6):523–530.

60. Al-Omran M, Albalawi ZH, Tashkandi MF, et al. Enteral versus parenteral nutrition for acute pancreatitis. *Cochrane Database Syst Rev* 2010;1:CD002837.

61. Loprinzi CL, Kugler JW, Sloan JA, et al. Randomized comparison of megestrol acetate versus dexamethasone versus fluoxymesterone for the treatment of cancer anorexia/cachexia. *J Clin Oncol* 1999;17:3299–3306.

62. De Conno F, Martini C, Zecca E, et al. Megestrol acetate for anorexia in patients with far-advanced cancer: a double-blind controlled clinical trial. *Eur J Cancer* 1998;34: 1705–1709.

63. Berenstein EG, Ortiz Z. Megestrol acetate for the treatment of anorexia-cachexia syndrome. *Cochrane Database Syst Rev* 2005;2:CD004310.

64. Tchekmedyian NS, Hickman M, Heber D. Treatment of anorexia and weight loss with megestrol acetate in patients with cancer or acquired immunodeficiency syndrome. *Semin Oncol* 1991;18:35–42.

65. Corcoran C, Grinspoon S. Treatments for wasting in patients with the acquired immunodeficiency syndrome. *N Engl J Med* 1999;340:1740–1750.

66. Nemechek PM, Polsky B, Gottlieb MS. Treatment guidelines for HIV-associated wasting. *Mayo Clin Proc* 2000; 75:386–394.

67. Gołębiewska JE, Lichodziejewska-Niemierko M, Aleksandrowicz-Wrona E, et al. Influence of megestrol acetate on nutrition, inflammation and quality of life in dialysis patients. *Int Urol Nephrol* 2012;44(4):1211–1222.

68. Sivakumar T, Mechanic O, Fehmie DA, et al. Growth hormone axis treatments for HIV-associated lipodystrophy: a systematic review of placebo-controlled trials. *HIV Med* 2011;12(8):453–462.

69. Stratton RJ, Elia M. The effects of enteral tube feeding and parenteral nutrition on appetite sensations and food intake in health and disease. *Clin Nutr* 1999;18:63–70.

70. Stratton RJ. The impact of nutritional support on appetite and food intake. *Clin Nutr* 2001;20:147–152.

71. Whelan K, Efthymiou L, Judd PA, et al. Appetite during consumption of enteral formula as a sole source

of nutrition: the effect of supplementing pea-fibre and fructo-oligosaccharides. *Br J Nutr* 2006;96:350–356.

72. McClave SA, Snider HL, Spain DA. Preoperative issues in clinical nutrition. *Chest* 1999;115:64s–70s.

73. Ochoa JB, Caba D. Advances in surgical nutrition. *Surg Clin North Am* 2006;86:1483–1493.

74. Waitzberg DL, Plopper C, Terra RM. Postoperative total parenteral nutrition. *World J Surg* 1999;23:560–564.

75. Salvino RM, Dechicco RS, Seidner DL. Perioperative nutrition support: who and how. *Cleve Clin J Med* 2004;71:345–351.

76. Pettignano R, Heard M, Davis R, et al. Total enteral nutrition versus total parenteral nutrition during pediatric extracorporeal membrane oxygenation. *Crit Care Med* 1998;26:358–363.

77. Hanekamp MN, Spoel M, Sharman-Koendjbiharie I, et al. Routine enteral nutrition in neonates on extracorporeal membrane oxygenation. *Pediatr Crit Care Med* 2005;6:275–279.

78. Kotler DP, Fogleman L, Tierney AR. Comparison of total parenteral nutrition and an oral, semielemental diet on body composition, physical function, and nutrition-related costs in patients with malabsorption due to acquired immunodeficiency syndrome. *JPEN* 1998;22:120–126.

79. Ockenga J, Grimble R, Jonkers-Schultema C, et al. ESPEN guidelines on enteral nutrition: wasting in HIV and other chronic infectious diseases. *Clin Nutr* 2006;25:319–329.

80. Argiles JM. Cancer-associated malnutrition. *Eur J Oncol Nurs* 2005;9:s39–s50.

81. Smith HJ, Greenburg NA, Tisdale MJ. Effect of eicosapentaenoic acid, protein and amino acids on protein synthesis and degradation in skeletal muscle of cachectic mice. *Br J Cancer* 1994;91:408–412.

82. Smith HJ, Mukerji PR, Tisdale M. Attenuation of proteasome-induced proteolysis in skeletal muscle by β-hydroxy-β-methylbutyrate in cancer-induced muscle loss. *Cancer Res* 2005;65:277–283.

83. Siddiqui R, Pandya D, Harvey K, et al. Nutrition modulation of cachexia/proteolysis. *Nutr Clin Pract* 2006;21:155–167.

84. Flakoll P, Sharp R, Baier S, et al. Effect of beta-hydroxy-beta-methylbutyrate, arginine, and lysine supplementation on strength, functionality, body composition, and protein metabolism in elderly women. *Nutrition* 2004;20:445–451.

85. Williams JZ, Abumrad N, Barbul A. Effect of a specialized amino acid mixture on human collagen deposition. *Ann Surg* 2002;236:369–375.

86. Berk L, James J, Schwartz A, et al. A randomized, double-blind, placebo-controlled trial of a beta-hydroxyl beta-methyl butyrate, glutamine, and arginine mixture for the treatment of cancer cachexia (RTOG 0122). *Support Care Cancer* 2008;16(10):1179–1188.

87. Donadelli SP, Junqueira-Franco MV, de Mattos Donadelli CA, et al. Daily vitamin supplementation and hypovitaminosis after obesity surgery. *Nutrition* 2012;28(4):391–396.

88. Tan BH, Ross JA, Kaasa S, et al., European Palliative Care Research Collaborative. Identification of possible genetic polymorphisms involved in cancer cachexia: a systematic review. *J Genet* 2011;90(1):165–177.

89. Chaput JP, Lord C, Cloutier M, et al. Relationship between antioxidant intakes and class I sarcopenia in elderly men and women. *J Nutr Health Aging* 2007;11(4):363–369.

90. Dahl AK, Fauth EB, Ernsth-Bravell M, et al. Body mass index, change in body mass index, and survival in old and very old persons. *J Am Geriatr Soc* 2013;61(4):512–518. doi: 10.1111/jgs.12158.

SUGGESTED READINGS

Bozzetti F, Gavazzi C, Mariani L, et al. Artificial nutrition in cancer patients: which route, what composition? *World J Surg* 1999;23:577–583.

Braga M, Gianotti L, Radaelli G, et al. Perioperative immunonutrition in patients undergoing cancer surgery: results of a randomized double-blind phase 3 trial. *Arch Surg* 1999;134:428–433.

Chan S, McCowen KC, Blackburn GL. Nutrition management in the ICU. *Chest* 1999;115:145s–148s.

Jolliet P, Pichard C, Biolo G, et al. Enteral nutrition in intensive care patients: a practical approach. *Clin Nutr* 1999;18:47–56.

Varella LD, Young RJ. New options for pumps and tubes: progress in enteral feeding techniques and devices. *Curr Opin Clin Nutr Metab Care* 1999;2:271–275.

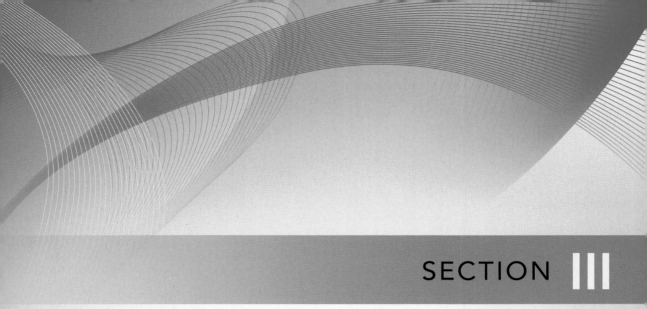

Special Topics in Clinical Nutrition

CHAPTER 27

Diet, Pregnancy, and Lactation

Optimal maternal nutrition during pregnancy and lactation is vitally important to the health of mother and infant. Nutritional needs rise during pregnancy (see Table 27.1) in response to the metabolic demand of the developing embryo as well as to changes in maternal physiology.

There is definitive evidence that periconceptional folate supplementation decreases the incidence of neural tube defects (NTD). The maternal diet is often deficient in calcium, iron, and other micronutrients, and supplementation with a prenatal vitamin throughout pregnancy is indicated. Vitamin A at doses of about 10,000 IU per day is potentially teratogenic and should be avoided during pregnancy. Carotenoids with vitamin A activity are safe. There is evidence supporting ω-3 fatty acid supplementation, generally in the form of fish oil, during both pregnancy and lactation (1). Caloric needs rise in pregnancy, and thus energy intake should be increased, but excessive weight gain is potentially disadvantageous to mother and fetus.

Under most circumstances, breast-feeding is the preferred nutritional source for neonates. The composition of human milk changes in response to maternal diet. A generous intake of dietary calcium and continued use of prenatal vitamins are indicated throughout the period of lactation. The pattern of macronutrient intake indicated for general health promotion is appropriate during pregnancy and lactation as well. Biologic maturity occurs on average 5 years after menarche. Before this time, a woman may still be growing herself, creating metabolic demands in conflict with the needs of pregnancy.

OVERVIEW

Diet

Maternal weight should be nearly ideal at the start of pregnancy to prevent complications that may arise from either maternal obesity or underweight. Underweight in the mother is associated with low birth weight, whereas maternal overweight is associated with many pregnancy increased risks of gestational hypertension, diabetes, and preeclampsia (2).

Babies of mothers with prepregnancy obesity appear to have an increased risk of spina bifida and other congenital anomalies, as well as increased incidence of macrosomia, low Apgar scores, shoulder dystocia, and childhood obesity (3,4). Maternal obesity is a major risk factor for childhood obesity, which persists into adulthood independent of other factors (5–8).

Physiologic changes during pregnancy alter nutritional requirements. Plasma volume expands nearly 50% during pregnancy. Total mass of red blood cells increases about 33% over prepregnancy levels. Basal metabolic rate is increased by 15% to 20% toward the end of gestation. These changes require increased intake of energy, nutrients, and fluid. The greater increase in plasma volume than in red cell mass will cause the hematocrit to fall during pregnancy; however, the mean corpuscular hemoglobin concentration (MCHC) should remain fairly constant, barring a concurrent anemia. Maternal hemoglobin during pregnancy should consistently be higher than 11 g per dL to ensure adequate oxygen delivery to the fetus. Nutritional causes of anemia should be considered if the hemoglobin level falls below this value and another explanation is not evident. A microcytic anemia suggests iron deficiency, whereas a macrocytic anemia suggests folate or vitamin B_{12} deficiency; the former is the more common.

Requirements for folate, calcium, iron, and zinc rise disproportionately during pregnancy. In general, intestinal nutrient absorption is enhanced during pregnancy as an adaptation to increased metabolic demands. Serum lipids tend to rise during pregnancy, due largely to the effects of progesterone.

Whereas electrolytes, fatty acids, and fat-soluble vitamins cross the placenta by simple

TABLE 27.1

Recommended Nutrient Intake Changes Associated with Pregnancy and Lactation[a]

Nutrient	Recommended Intake by Subject Category				Average US Dietary Intake in Adult Women	Content of Representative Prenatal Vitamin[b]
	Female (19–30 yr)	Female (31–50 yr)	Pregnancy	Lactation (Initial 6 mo)		
Calcium (mg)	1,000	1,000	1,000[c]	1,000[c]	530	250
Folate (μg)	400[b]	400	600[c]	500[c]	280–300	1,000
Iodine (μg)	150	150	220	290[d]	170	150
Iron (mg)	18	18	27[c]	9	10.7	60
Magnesium (mg)	310	320	350[c]	310[d]	207	25
n-3 fatty acids (g)	1.1	1.1	1.4	1.3		
Niacin (mg NE)	14	14	18	17[d]	16	20
Phosphorus (mg)	700	700	700[c]	700[c]	1,000	—
Protein (g)	46	50	60[d]	65[c]	70	—
Riboflavin (mg)	1.1	1.1	1.4[d]	1.6[d]	1.34	3.4
Selenium (μg)	55	55	60[d]	70[d]	108	—
Thiamin (mg)	1.1	1.1	1.4[d]	1.4[d]	1.05	3
Vitamin A (μg RE)	700	700	770	1,300[d]	1,170	1,500
Vitamin B$_{12}$ (μg)	2.4	2.4	2.6	2.8[d]	4.85	12
Vitamin B$_6$ (mg)	1.3	1.3	1.9[d]	2.0[d]	1.16	10
Vitamin C (mg)	75	75	85	120	77	100
Vitamin D (μg)	5	5	10[c]	10[c]	1.5	10
Vitamin E (mg TE)	15	15	15[d]	19[c]	7.1	22.2
Vitamin K (μg)	90	90	90	90	300–500	—
Zinc (mg)	8	8	11[d]	12[c]	10–15	25

[a]NE, niacin equivalent, which equals 1 mg of dietary niacin or 60 mg of dietary tryptophan; RE, retinol equivalent; TE, a-tocopherol equivalent.

[b]Intake of folate 400 μg per day is now recommended for all women of child-bearing age to ensure adequate stores at the time of conception.

[c]Maternal prenatal vitamins, Lederle Laboratories, 1997.

[d]Nutrient intake levels represent a 50% or more increase over recommendations for nonpregnant adult women.

Source: Adapted from the Dietary Reference Intakes and Food and Nutrition Board, Institute of Medicine. National Academy of Sciences DRI reports. Available at www.nap.edu; accessed 2/07.

diffusion, amino acids, water-soluble vitamins, sodium, calcium, and iron are actively transported across the placenta to the fetal circulation.

On average, pregnancy requires a calorie increase over baseline of approximately 300 kcal per day, and lactation requires 500 kcal per day. Nutrients for which the recommended dietary allowance is specifically raised in pregnancy include total protein, total energy, magnesium, iodine, zinc, selenium, vitamins E and C, thiamine, niacin, iron, calcium, and folate. Lactation requires additional increases in protein, zinc, vitamins A, E, C, and niacin; requirements for iron and folate decline (see Table 27.1).

Inadequate weight gain during pregnancy is associated with low birth weight and maternal

delivery complications (9), whereas excessive weight gain is associated with macrosomia, fetopelvic disproportion, and attendant complications of labor and delivery (10).

A study of more than 170,000 women demonstrated that weight gain during pregnancy in ranges recommended by the Institute of Medicine (IOM) decreased the incidence of low-birth-weight babies for lean white and Hispanic women. The data were less consistent with regard to black women. Low birth weight was uncommon among obese or high–body mass index (BMI) white and Hispanic women, and the benefit of recommended weight gain in these groups was unclear (11). Nutritional support of malnourished women during pregnancy is beyond the scope of this discussion, but in general is approached as is malnutrition under other circumstances (see Chapter 26). The topic has been reviewed elsewhere (12). The Women, Infants, and Children (WIC) program is designed to meet the nutritional needs of women and infants. The program assists nearly 1 million women annually in meeting nutritional needs during pregnancy. Because WIC supplements tend to be shared with family members, the nutrient intake of pregnant women in this population is often suboptimal and requires close scrutiny to ensure optimal pregnancy outcomes.

Maternal weight gain during pregnancy should occur predominantly during the second and third trimesters; total energy expenditure changes little in the first trimester but increases thereafter. Recent evidence suggests that in normal-BMI women, no increase in energy intake is required during the first trimester, while approximately 350 kcal per day should be added to the diet in the second trimester and 500 kcal per day in the third trimester (13). Pregnancy is thought to require an increase in energy consumption of 45,000 to 110,000 kcal over the level required for weight maintenance in the nonpregnant state; an 80,000 kcal increase is the standard estimate.

Gestational weight gain recommendations aim to optimize outcomes for the woman and the child. In 2009, the IOM published revised gestational weight gain guidelines that are based on prepregnancy BMI ranges for underweight, normal weight, overweight, and obese women recommended by the World Health Organization and are independent of age, parity, smoking history, race, and ethnic background weight gain recommendations for pregnancy vary with prepregnant weight. For women with a baseline BMI below 20, weight gain of 0.5 kg per week during the second and third trimesters is indicated. For overweight women (BMI of 25 to 29.9), weight gain of 0.3 kg per week during the same period is recommended. The IOM recommendations define obesity as a BMI of 30 or greater and do not differentiate between Class I obesity (BMI of 30 to 34.9), Class II obesity (BMI of 35 to 39.9), and Class III obesity (BMI of 40 or greater) (4). Given the limited data by class, the IOM recommendation for weight gain is 5 to 9.1 kg (0.2 to 0.3 kg per week) for all obese women (14). Weight gain of more than 1 kg per week at any time is generally excessive. Weight loss is always concerning

and weight gain of less than 1 kg per month, except for possibly during the first trimester, generally indicates inadequate nutrition. Obligatory added weight during pregnancy, attributable to fetal growth, placental growth, amniotic fluid production, uterine and breast enlargement, and expansion of the blood volume, accounts for approximately 7.5 kg on average. Weight gain in excess of this amount represents added maternal body weight, mostly in counterbalancing hip and gluteal fat, that the woman will need to lose following pregnancy to return to prepregnant weight and shape. Available evidence suggests that biologically immature women—i.e., those less than 5 years after beginning menarche—require on average an additional 150 kcal per day and an additional 3 kg weight gain to avoid having low-birth-weight babies.

Physical activity during pregnancy offers benefits to the mother at no cost to the fetus, provided that maternal tolerance is not taxed. Extreme exertion will result in elevated fetal temperature. Maintenance of moderate exercise during pregnancy is appropriate unless precluded by complications. Vigorous exercise before pregnancy and at least light-to-moderate activity during pregnancy may reduce risk for abnormal glucose tolerance and gestational diabetes mellitus (GDM) (15). Regular moderate-intensity exercise performed over the second-third trimesters of pregnancy can be used to attenuate important GDM-related adverse outcomes (16). Exercise with potential high impact (due to risk of blunt trauma) or at altitude (due to oxygenation) is to be avoided during pregnancy. Postpartum exercise facilitates desired weight loss.

A total of approximately 925 g of protein is incorporated into the developing fetus and other products of conception. Peak requirements during pregnancy add a need for 8.5 g of protein to basal requirements. Protein intake by women in the United States is typically about 70 g per day, a figure well in excess of minimal requirements for all stages of pregnancy. Therefore, no particular effort to raise protein intake during pregnancy is indicated unless the diet is atypical (e.g., strict veganism without adequate attention to protein adequacy and completeness). A recent study has been shown the association between dietary protein intake and GDM. Higher intake of animal protein, in particular red meat, was significantly associated with a greater risk of GDM. By contrast, higher intake of vegetable protein, specifically nuts, was associated with a significantly lower risk. Substitution of vegetable protein for animal protein, as well as substitution of some other animal protein sources for red meat, was associated with a lower risk of GDM (17).

The fetus gains approximately 30 g per day during the third trimester. Interventions to ensure term delivery are essential in maintaining this rate of development. Intensive care of premature infants can rarely sustain more than 20 g of growth per day.

The developing fetus uses glucose as its major energy source, and glucose is especially crucial for use by the fetal brain in the third trimester. Carbohydrate requirements therefore may increase to approximately 175 g per day in pregnancy.

Overall, the increased micronutrient requirements of pregnancy exceed the increased energy requirements. Therefore, vitamin supplementation during pregnancy is universally indicated, and the nutrient density of foods assumes increased importance.

The teratogenicity of vitamin A in high doses was revealed through the use of the vitamin A analogue isotretinoin for acne. Ingestion of 20,000 IU or more of vitamin A per day is thought to be potentially teratogenic. Carotenoid precursors of vitamin A provide adequate retinol while avoiding any known toxicity. Therefore, prenatal vitamin supplements typically provide vitamin A at well below the toxic threshold and generally in the form of the precursor β-carotene. On the other hand, in normal-weight mothers, dietary vitamin A intake during pregnancy below the recommended daily intake is significantly associated with an increased risk of a child with Congenital Diaphragmatic Hernia (18).

Immediately following birth for a period of approximately 3 to 5 days, the mother's mammary glands produce colostrum, a fluid rich in sodium, chloride, and immunoglobulins that confer passive immunity to the newborn. Colostrum is replaced by milk, which is rich in lactose and protein and comparatively low in sodium and chloride. Milk volume consumed by the neonate is 50 mL per day at birth, 500 mL by day 5, and 750 mL at 3 months.

Milk production is maintained by infant suckling, which suppresses hypothalamic dopamine production, thereby disinhibiting prolactin release. The first 4 months of lactation require, and convey to the infant, an amount of energy comparable to that of the entire gestational period. Human milk is both appropriate and optimal as the sole source of infant nutrition for the first 6 months of life, barring contraindication (e.g., active tuberculosis, Human immunodeficiency virus [HIV] infection). There is uncertainty whether milk meets all the infant's nutritional needs beyond this point (see Chapter 29). Multiple national and international medical and health organizations recommend exclusive breast-feeding as the preferred method of infant feeding for the first 4 to 6 months, with continued breast-feeding with complementary foods for at least 12 months (19–21). Increasing the proportion of infants who are breast-fed and of infants breast-feds until 6 months are the objectives of Healthy People 2010 (22).

The fatty acid composition of human milk varies with maternal dietary intake. With the exception of iodine and selenium, there is little evidence that the levels of minerals and trace elements in milk vary with maternal diet. In contrast, vitamin levels in milk are responsive to dietary intake, with the strength of the relationship varying by nutrient. The levels of both fat- and water-soluble vitamins in milk vary in proportion to maternal intake. Calcium and folate, and possibly other nutrients, are preserved in milk at the expense of maternal stores when maternal intake is less than daily requirements.

Recent work has shown that human colostrum and milk, which traditionally have been thought to be sterile, provides a continuous supply of commensal probiotic bacteria to the infant gut such as bifidobacteria and specific *Bifidobacterium* species (23). Milk also provides more than 100 different oligosaccharides, which serve not as food for this infant (still lacking the intestinal enzymes to digest them), but food for the newly introduced probiotics. There is current interest in the influence these probiotics and carbohydrates have on intestinal flora of the infant and their capacity to play a role in the prevention of infection, atopy, and various other diseases (24–26). Specific probiotic and prebiotic combinations during pregnancy and early feeding, via the mother or incorporated in early formula-feeding, may help shape the intestinal microbiota composition in infants and may be important determinants of later health (27,28).

As noted previously, maternal diet strongly influences the fatty acid and vitamin composition of breast milk, but it generally exerts a modest influence on minerals (29,30). Iodine and selenium are exceptions, varying substantially in response to maternal intake (31). Vitamins D and K are generally present at low levels in breast milk, and supplementation is recommended (32,33); however, there is some evidence that low vitamin D intake in breast-fed neonates may not adversely affect bone metabolism (34).

Breast-feeding is accompanied by a decline in maternal bone density, regardless of maternal calcium intake (35); however, studies show that bone mineral density is recovered fully after weaning (36). A study of 52 lactating women in the United States suggested that intake of calcium, zinc, folate, vitamins E and D, and pyridoxine may tend to be deficient in this group (37). Another study demonstrated that the transfer of fatty acids to breast milk occurs within several hours of ingestion, with the maximum effect varying with the particular fat source (38).

Breast milk and infant formulas differ substantially in a variety of nutrients (39). The significance of all of the differences has yet to be established. Although earlier studies suggested an association between breast-feeding and greater intelligence, a recent large prospective study by Der et al. (40) found no significant correlation when additional meta-analyses were conducted (see Chapter 29). In another recent cohort study, that evaluated the association between infant feeding and the development of overweight and obesity throughout life course, the use of infants formula was not associated with women's likelihood of becoming overweight or obese throughout life course. Although breast-feeding promotes the health of mother and child, it is unlikely to play an important role in controlling the obesity epidemic (41).

Energy requirements to sustain lactation are based on the caloric density of human milk (approximately 70 kcal per 100 mL), the metabolic cost of milk production, and total milk volume. The consensus view that lactation requires 500 kcal per day above the energy required to maintain maternal weight assumes that approximately 200 kcal per day of milk production energy will derive from pregnancy-related fat stores. Loss of 0.5 to 1 kg per month is common during lactation, whereas loss in excess of 2 kg per month implies inadequate nutrition. Weight

maintenance and weight gain during lactation are not uncommon. Weight loss of up to 2 kg per month appears to be safe during lactation, with preservation of energy transfer to breast milk. Prolactin levels tend to rise in response to maternal energy restriction during lactation, perhaps serving to preserve energy delivery to the neonate (42). Evidence suggests that energy restriction beginning 1 month postpartum can facilitate maternal weight loss without adverse effects on milk production or infant growth (43), but dietary restriction may lead to inadequate vitamin D and calcium intake (44). Judicious management of diet and weight throughout the gestational and postpartum periods, rather than a focus on energy restriction during lactation, is therefore clearly advisable (45).

Exercise during lactation, independent of energy restriction, is not known to pose any threat to mother or infant, and it offers a range of benefits. Lactation does not specifically aid in weight loss, despite the suggestion in folklore that it does. Women do tend to lose weight while breast-feeding (46), as is to be expected in the postpartum period. Generally, however, nonlactating women lose weight at least as readily as do their breast-feeding counterparts. Culturally defined mother-care practices probably play a role in weight change patterns among lactating women. This hypothesis should stimulate investigation into gestational weight gain and postpartum losses in different ethnocultural contexts (47).

There is interest in the role breast-feeding may play in preventing the development of atopy in the child, but the data are preliminary (48–50) (see Chapter 24). Evidence is convincing that breast-feeding confers protection against infections, although the mechanisms by which breast milk influences infant immunity remain under study (51–53).

Exclusive breast-feeding promotes an anti-inflammatory cytokine milieu, which is maintained throughout infancy. Such an immunological environment limits hyperresponsiveness and promotes tolerization, possibly prohibiting the onset of allergic disease (54). Erythropoietin in breast milk is apparently resistant to degradation in the infant gastrointestinal tract and may stimulate the newborn's marrow (55,56).

The amino acid pattern of breast milk is species specific, suggesting another way in which human milk might make unique contributions to early development (57). Maternal diet influences the flavor of breast milk and thereby serves as a means of introducing the neonate to a variety of taste experiences (58–60).

Strong flavors, and the familiarity or novelty of such flavors, may influence the feeding behaviors of infants. Ingestion of garlic by the mother has been shown to lengthen feeding at first but to shorten feeding when exposure is recurrent. The duration of breast-feeding may have an influence on sensory preference at the beginning of complementary feeding (61,62). Alcohol ingested by a breast-feeding woman is conveyed to breast milk and generally results in reduced feeding by the infant immediately after exposure to the alcohol, with compensatory increased feeding when alcohol is no longer present in the milk (63). Research by Mennella (64) and Mennella and Beauchamp (65) suggests that this effect is not due to the taste of alcohol per se but to some other effect of alcohol on the feeding experience. Contrary to folklore, maternal alcohol ingestion appears to decrease the sleep of a breast-feeding infant rather than increase it (66,67).

NUTRIENTS, NUTRICEUTICALS, AND FUNCTIONAL FOODS

Alcohol

Heavy alcohol ingestion during pregnancy is associated with the fetal alcohol syndrome, a condition of fetal developmental delay and cognitive deficits. The incidence of fetal alcohol syndrome in the United States among offspring of women consuming 1.5 to 8 drinks per week is approximately 10%. A "drink" contains on average 17 g of ethanol. An occasional alcoholic drink during pregnancy is not known to be harmful, but recommendations in the United States favor abstinence.

Caffeine/Coffee

Even though the World Health Organization recommendation and other major guidelines indicate that caffeine intake of up to 300 mg per day, the equivalent of up to five or six cups of coffee, is not harmful to mother or fetus. However, recent studies have suggested that coffee, but not caffeine intake, has been associated with decreased birth weight and increased odds of small for gestational age (68,69).

Calcium

The need for calcium supplementation was discussed earlier. There is some evidence that calcium supplementation may reduce the risk of pregnancy-induced hypertension and preterm delivery due to preeclampsia (70,71).

n-3 Fatty Acids

Available data suggest that high consumption of marine oils is associated with longer gestation (72) and that dietary supplementation with docosahexaenoic acid (DHA) via n-3 polyunsaturated oils may increase the proportion of term births in diverse populations (70,73). Maternal plasma DHA levels decrease significantly after delivery (74). A recent analysis found lower breast milk DHA content and lower seafood consumption to be associated with higher rates of postpartum depression in mothers across several countries (75). Preliminary evidence from several small open-label trials suggests beneficial effects of n-3 supplementation on symptoms of depression during pregnancy and the postpartum period (76,77).

There is evidence that n-3 fatty acids are important in the normal development of eye and brain function (78,79). A randomized trial found that the children born to mothers who had taken cod liver oil (rich in n-3 fatty acids) during pregnancy and lactation scored higher on a battery of intelligence tests at 4 years of age than children whose mothers had taken a non-n-3 oil supplement (80). A recent trial showed an association between fish and seafood intake during pregnancy and enhanced neurodevelopmental milestones and IQ in the offspring (81). Benefits were seen with up to 340 g (12 oz) of seafood intake per week as compared to none; higher intake levels showed neither decisive benefits nor harms compared to more moderate intake. Considerable evidence indicates that prenatal and neonatal long-chain polyunsaturated fatty acids (LCPUFA) status is associated with neurodevelopmental outcome, though the need for long-term longitudinal studies is still needed to prove this association (82). Though a recent systematic review on the effect of maternal ω-3 (n-3) LCPUFA supplementation during pregnancy on early childhood, cognitive and visual development does not conclusively support or refute that ω-3 LCPUFA supplementation in pregnancy improves cognitive or visual development (1).

The n-3 content of breast milk is mediated by maternal intake. Maternal supplementation with n-3 fatty acids instead of n-6 fatty acids during pregnancy and lactation has been shown to provide more DHA to the infant and decrease maternal plasma lipid levels (83). Increased consumption of n-3 fatty acids may therefore confer health benefits to both mother and baby. Relative to the prehistoric dietary pattern, the modern diet is deficient in n-3 fatty acids (84,85), lending the support of an evolutionary context to the hypothesis that increased intake may be beneficial.

Of note, while marine foods may provide n-3 fatty acids, several varieties are commonly contaminated with mercury, a potential neurotoxin. As a result, the U.S. Food and Drug Administration (FDA) advises pregnant women to avoid swordfish, tilefish, king mackerel, and shark. These species are all large predators, and they concentrate in their bodies the mercury accumulated by the smaller fish on which they feed. The FDA also cautions against albacore tuna, another large predatory fish; canned light tuna, made from smaller fish, contains much less mercury. The FDA recommends a total fish intake during pregnancy of up to 12 oz, or two to three meals, per week (86). Fish oil supplements can provide n-3 fatty acids while avoiding the risk of heavy metal contaminants (87).

Folate

The link between adequate folic acid intake and reduced risk of NTD is so definitive (88) that mandatory folic acid supplementation of refined grain products was instituted in the United States in 1998; studies show that the incidence of NTD declined by 20% to 30% following this public health measure (89). There is some controversy about whether fortification levels should be further increased to reduce NTD risk (90). Several recent studies have pointed to improved neurodevelopmental outcomes in children of mothers having higher folate concentrations or receiving folic acid supplements (91).

Surén et al. (92) evaluated 85,176 children from MoBa, including 114 who had autistic disorder. The authors reported an incidence of autistic disorder of 0.10% in offspring of mothers who took periconceptional folic acid supplements versus 0.21% in offspring of those who did not, for an adjusted odds ratio of 0.61 (95% CI, 0.41 to 0.90).

The findings suggest that periconceptional folic acid supplementation is associated with a reduced risk of autistic disorder in offspring, although certainly do not prove causality. Current recommendations suggest that all women capable of becoming pregnant supplement with approximately 400 μg of folic acid per day in addition to consuming a folate-rich diet. Pregnant women should increase supplementation to 600 μg per day. Ingestion of more than 1 mg per day of folate is generally not recommended. However, in women with prior pregnancies leading to NTD, the ingestion of up to 4 mg per day of folate may confer additional benefit.

Fluoride

Breast milk does not provide optimal fluoride levels to term infants, and supplementation is generally recommended (93).

Gingerroot

Ground gingerroot, at a dose of 250 mg four times daily, has been shown effective in the treatment of hyperemesis gravidarum (94,95). The combination of ginger and vitamin B_6 may be more effective than either used alone (96).

Iron

Anemia is the most common nutrient-related abnormality of pregnancy and is attributable to iron deficiency nearly 90% of the time, with the remainder due primarily to folate deficiency. Because of the cessation of menses, iron requirements drop during the first trimester. Demands increase over baseline in the second trimester and peak in the third trimester, at 4 mg per day.

Pregnancy consumes approximately 1,040 mg of iron in total, of which 200 mg is recaptured after pregnancy from the expanded red cell mass and 840 mg is permanently lost. The iron is lost to the fetus (300 mg), the placenta (50 to 75 mg), expanded red cell mass (450 mg), and blood loss at parturition (200 mg). Only about 10% of ingested iron is absorbed in the nonpregnant state, but pregnancy may enhance absorption by as much as 30%. Therefore, an intake between 13 and 40 mg per day is required during the third trimester. Multivitamin/multimineral supplements generally contain 30 mg of iron, and the diet provides an additional 15 mg, easily meeting the needs of most women without anemia.

Iron supplementation before conception will facilitate meeting the iron needs of pregnancy and lactation, which together result in a net loss between 420 and 1,030 mg of elemental iron. It is possible that iron supplementation in women with already adequate iron stores may increase risk of gestational diabetes and other maternal complications (97,98). Women with iron-deficiency anemia during pregnancy require increased intake to replenish bone marrow stores and still provide for the metabolic needs of the fetus. In this situation, daily iron intake between 120 and 150 mg is typically required. Iron supplementation should continue postpartum, both to provide iron for breast milk and to replenish losses due to bleeding at delivery. Routine iron supplementation for full-term, healthy breast-fed infants does not appear to be necessary (99).

Magnesium

The evidence that magnesium supplementation may prevent preeclampsia is mixed. Alternative medicine sources recommend supplements of about 500 mg per day, which appears to be safe. Conventional prenatal vitamins provide only 25 mg per day; as a result, intake is often below recommended levels. Magnesium supplementation may be a treatment option for women suffering from pregnancy-induced leg cramps.

Selenium

Based on the reported association between selenium deficiency and sudden infant death syndrome, as well as low birth weight, selenium supplementation of 200 μg per day is advocated in the complementary and alternative medicine literature (96). The benefits of selenium may be limited to individuals from areas with selenium-deficient soil. Selenium deficiency in the United States, where soil levels are high, is not generally considered a problem. Selenium in breast milk is very responsive to maternal intake, which distinguishes it from most other minerals (100).

Vitamin B$_6$

Other than its role in metabolism, supplemental B$_6$ is recommended for treatment of pregnancy-induced nausea based on the results of small randomized, double-blind trials (96,101). A dose range from 50 to 100 mg per day is advised, and this level exceeds the content of diet and prenatal vitamins combined.

Vitamin C

The naturopathic literature suggests that vitamin C supplementation of about 500 mg per day may play a role in the prevention of preeclampsia and premature rupture of membranes. However, a recent randomized placebo-controlled trial found no evidence of vitamins C and E prophylaxis for preeclampsia (102,103). This 500 mg per day dose is apparently safe. Third trimester maternal intake of ascorbic acid has been shown to influence the level of ascorbate in breast milk (104).

Vitamin D

Adequate vitamin D intake is important to ensure a healthy maternal response to neonatal calcium handling (105). Vitamin D supplementation in pregnancy and lactation has come under scrutiny in the past few years as a result of increased prevalence of vitamin D deficiency in Americans with more darkly pigmented skin. A recent review of the literature concluded that appropriate doses of vitamin D during pregnancy and lactation are not known but are likely higher than the current recommended intakes, especially in pregnant women and breast-feeding infants with darkly pigmented skin and those who do not live in sun-rich environments (106).

Zinc

Studies of zinc nutriture in relation to pregnancy outcome have shown mixed results. There is some evidence that zinc supplementation may extend pregnancy to term among women with low levels of serum zinc. Zinc supplementation may directly contribute to normal birth weight through its effects on protein metabolism, or the influence may be indirect as a result of extended gestation (70). Zinc levels in breast milk are not thought to vary readily with dietary intake. However, a cohort study in Spain suggests that low dietary zinc intake during the third trimester predicts relatively low levels in breast milk (104). Relative zinc deficiency among US adults has been reported.

SPECIAL CONSIDERATIONS

Diabetes/Gestational Diabetes

Diabetes during pregnancy should be controlled so that blood sugar is consistently in the normal range to prevent macrosomia and sacral agenesis (107). Pregnancy itself induces a state of mild insulin resistance and hyperinsulinemia, which predisposes some women to develop gestational diabetes. The dietary control of diabetes is discussed in Chapter 6.

Phenylketonuria

A history of phenylketonuria in the mother requires a return to a tyrosine-restricted diet during pregnancy to prevent related complication in the fetus (108).

Human Immunodeficiency Virus

HIV and other viruses are transmissible in breast milk. Breast-feeding is contraindicated in HIV-positive women (109).

CLINICAL HIGHLIGHTS

Dietary recommendations for pregnancy and lactation vary to some extent with the prepregnant weight, age, and nutritional status of individual women. Assuming near-optimal prepregnancy weight and nutritional status and biologic maturity at conception, most women following a prudent diet during pregnancy would be able to meet their macronutrient recommendations. In such a diet, 25% to 30% of calories come from fat, 45% to 60% from carbohydrate, and 15% to 25% from protein. Energy consumption should be increased approximately 300 kcal per day during pregnancy and 500 kcal per day during lactation.

The use of multivitamin/multimineral supplements beginning several months before conception and throughout pregnancy and lactation is indicated. An ω-3 fatty acid supplement, generally in the form of fish oil at 1 to 2 g per day, may be appropriate. Dairy products should be eaten regularly as a source of calcium (110), and lean red meat, shellfish, sardines, and other food with a high iron content should be eaten as a source of iron, provided that fat and protein intake is in compliance with guidelines. Vegetarian women may require iron supplementation in addition to a prenatal vitamin; such supplementation is generally not required in omnivorous women. Vegans may require calcium supplementation, as is true of other women without regular intake of dairy products (see Chapter 43).

Vitamin B_6 and gingerroot have been used with success in the management of pregnancy-related nausea and appear to be safe. A graded program of exercise and caloric restriction postpartum may be required to restore prepregnancy weight. Most women in the United States retain approximately 2.5 kg after each pregnancy, a factor contributing to the prevalence of obesity among women. Management of diet and the degree of weight gain during pregnancy are thought to be preferable to an exclusive focus on postpartum weight loss; obese women should try to lose weight before pregnancy to minimize adverse outcomes, but dieting to lose weight is not advised during pregnancy (111). When maternal weight gain is insufficient during pregnancy, the risk of low birth weight is increased; therefore, diet should be managed to ensure that energy intake is neither excessive nor deficient.

REFERENCES

1. Gould JF, Smithers LG, Makrides M. The effect of maternal omega-3 (n-3) LCPUFA supplementation during pregnancy on early childhood cognitive and visual development: a systematic review and meta-analysis of randomized controlled trials. *Am J Clin Nutr* 2013;97(3):531–544.
2. Athukorala C, Rumbold AR, Willson KJ, et al. The risk of adverse pregnancy outcomes in women who are overweight or obese. *BMC Pregnancy Childbirth* 2010;10:56. doi: 10.1186/1471-2393-10-56.
3. Catalano PM. Management of obesity in pregnancy. *Obstet Gynecol* 2007;109:419–433.
4. Watkins ML, Rasmussen SA, Honeru MA, et al. Maternal obesity and risk for birth defects. *Pediatrics* 2003;111:1152–1158.
5. Thangaratinam S, Rogozinska E, Jolly K, et al. Effects of interventions in pregnancy on maternal weight and obstetric outcomes: meta-analysis of randomised evidence. *BMJ* 2012;344:e2088. doi: 10.1136/bmj.e2088.
6. Hanley B, Dijane J, Fewtrell M, et al. Metabolic imprinting, programming and epigenetics—a review of present priorities and future opportunities. *Br J Nutr* 2010;104(suppl 1): S1–S25.
7. Waterland RA, Garza C. Potential mechanisms of metabolic imprinting that lead to chronic disease. *Am J Clin Nutr* 1999;69(2):179–197.
8. Heijmans BT, Tobi EW, Stein AD, et al. Persistent epigenetic differences associated with prenatal exposure to famine in humans. *Proc Natl Acad Sci USA* 2008;105(44): 17046–17049. doi: 10.1073/pnas.0806560105.

9. Ehrenberg HM, Dierker L, Milluzzi C, et al. Low maternal weight, failure to thrive in pregnancy, and adverse pregnancy outcomes. *Am J Obstet Gynecol* 2003;189:1726–1730.

10. Scotland NE, Cheng YW, Hopkins LM, et al. Gestational weight gain and adverse neonatal outcome among term infants. *Obstet Gynecol* 2006;108:635–643.

11. Schieve L, Cogswell M, Scanlon K. An empiric evaluation of the Institute of Medicine's pregnancy weight gain guidelines by race. *Obstet Gynecol* 1998;91:878–884.

12. Hamaoui E, Hamaoui M. Nutritional assessment and support during pregnancy. *Gastroenterol Clin North Am* 1998;27:89–121.

13. Butte NF, Wong WW, Treuth MS, et al. Energy requirements during pregnancy based on total energy expenditure and energy deposition. *Am J Clin Nutr* 2004;79:933–934.

14. ACOG. *Weight gain during Pregnancy.* Available at http://www.acog.org/Resources_And_Publications/Committee_Opinions/Committee_on_Obstetric_Practice/Weight_Gain_During_Pregnancy

15. Oken E, Ning Y, Rifas-Shiman SL, et al. Associations of physical activity and inactivity before and during pregnancy with glucose tolerance. *Obstet Gynecol* 2006;108:1200–1207.

16. Barakat R, Pelaez M, Lopez C, et al. Exercise during pregnancy and gestational diabetes-related adverse effects: a randomised controlled trial. *Br J Sports Med* 2013;47(10):630–636.

17. Bao W, Bowers K, Tobias DK, et al. Prepregnancy dietary protein intake, major dietary protein sources, and the risk of gestational diabetes mellitus: a prospective cohort study. *Diabetes Care* 2013;36(7):2001–2008.

18. Beurskens LW, Schrijver LH, Tibboel D, et al. Dietary vitamin A intake below the recommended daily intake during pregnancy and the risk of congenital diaphragmatic hernia in the offspring. *Birth Defects Res A Clin Mol Teratol* 2013;97(1):60–66.

19. American Academy of Pediatrics. Breastfeeding and the use of human milk. *Pediatrics* 2005;115:496–506.

20. US Department of Health and Human Services. *HHS blueprint for action on breastfeeding.* Washington, DC: US Department of Health and Human Services, Office on Women's Health, 2000.

21. World Health Organization. *Global strategy for infant and young child feeding.* Geneva, Switzerland: World Health Organization, 2003.

22. Websource Healthy People 2012 Objecives http://www.usbreastfeeding.org/LegislationPolicy/FederalPolicies Initiatives/HealthyPeople2020BreastfeedingObjectives/tabid/120/Default.aspx.

23. Fernández L, Langa S, Martin V, et al. The microbiota of human milk in healthy women. *Cell Mol Biol* (Noisy-le-grand). 2013;59(1):31–42.

24. McVeagh P, Miller J. Human milk oligosaccharides: only the breast. *J Paediatr Child Health* 1997;33:281–286.

25. Morrow AL, Ruiz-Palacios GM, Altaye M, et al. Human milk oligosaccharides are associated with protection against diarrhea in breast-fed infants. *J Pediatr* 2004;145:297–303.

26. Sjögren YM, Jenmalm MC, Böttcher MF, et al. Altered early infant gut microbiota in children developing allergy up to 5 years of age. *Clin Exp Allergy* 2009;39(4):518–526.

27. Grześkowiak Ł, Grönlund MM, Beckmann C, et al. The impact of perinatal probiotic intervention on gut microbiota: double-blind placebo-controlled trials in Finland and Germany. *Anaerobe* 2012;18(1):7–13.

28. Salminen S, Isolauri E. Opportunities for improving the health and nutrition of the human infant by probiotics. *Nestle Nutr Workshop Ser Pediatr Program* 2008;62:223–233; discussion 233–237. doi: 10.1159/000146350.

29. Emmett P, Rogers I. Properties of human milk and their relationship with maternal nutrition. *Early Hum Dev* 1997;49:s7–s28.

30. Bates C, Prentice A. Breast milk as a source of vitamins, essential minerals and trace elements. *Pharmacol Ther* 1994;62:193–220.

31. Picciano M. Human milk: nutritional aspects of a dynamic food. *Biol Neonate* 1998;74:84–93.

32. Jensen R, Ferris A, Lammi-Keefe C. Lipids in human milk and infant formulas. *Annu Rev Nutr* 1992;12:417–441.

33. Gartner LM, Greer FR. Section on breastfeeding and committee on nutrition. *Pediatrics* 2003;111:908–910.

34. Park M, Namgung R, Kim D, et al. Bone mineral content is not reduced despite low vitamin D status in breast milk-fed infants versus cow's milk based formula-fed infants. *J Pediatr* 1998;132:641–645.

35. Laskey M, Prentice A, Hanratty L, et al. Bone changes after 3 months of lactation: influence of calcium intake, breast-milk output, and vitamin D-receptor genotype. *Am J Clin Nutr* 1998;67:685–692.

36. Prentice A. Maternal calcium metabolism and bone mineral status. *Am J Clin Nutr* 2000;71:1312s–1316s.

37. Mackey A, Picciano M, Mitchell D, et al. Self-selected diets of lactating women often fail to meet dietary recommendations. *J Am Diet Assoc* 1998;98:297–302.

38. Francois C, Connor S, Wander R, et al. Acute effects of dietary fatty acids on the fatty acids of human milk. *Am J Clin Nutr* 1998;67:301–308.

39. Huisman M, Beusekom CV, Lanting C, et al. Triglycerides, fatty acids, sterols, mono- and disaccharides and sugar alcohols in human milk and current types of infant formula milk. *Eur J Clin Nutr* 1996;50:255–226.

40. Der G, Batty GD, Deary IJ. Effect of breast feeding on intelligence in children: prospective study, sibling pairs analysis, and meta-analysis. *BMJ* 2006;333:935.

41. Michels KB, Willett WC, Graubard BI, et al. A longitudinal study of infant feeding and obesity throughout life course. *Int J Obes* (Lond) 2007;31(7):1078–1085.

42. Dewey K. Effects of maternal caloric restriction and exercise during lactation. *J Nutr* 1998;128:386s–389s.

43. Lovelady C, Garner K, Moreno K, et al. The effect of weight loss in overweight, lactating women on the growth of their infants. *N Engl J Med* 2000;342:449–453.

44. Lovelady CA, Stephenson KG, Kuppler KM, et al. The effects of dieting on food and nutrient intake of lactating women. *J Am Diet Assoc* 2006;106:908–912.

45. Butte N. Dieting and exercise in overweight, lactating women. *N Engl J Med* 2000;342:502–503.

46. Winkvist A, Rasmussen K. Impact of lactation on maternal body weight and body composition. *J Mammary Gland Biol Neoplasia* 1999;4:309–318.

47. Onyango AW, Nommsen-Rivers L, Siyam A, et al., WHO Multicentre Growth Reference Study Group. Post-partum weight change patterns in the WHO Multicentre Growth Reference Study. *Matern Child Nutr* 2011;7(3):228–240. doi: 10.1111/j.1740-8709.2010.00295.x. Epub 2011 Feb 22.

48. Vandenplas Y. Myths and facts about breastfeeding: does it prevent later atopic disease? *Acta Paediatr* 1997;86: 1283–1287.

49. Kelly D, Coutts AG. Early nutrition and the development of immune function in the neonate. *Proc Nutr Soc* 2000;59:177–185.

50. Friedman NJ, Zeiger RS. The role of breast-feeding in the development of allergies and asthma. *J Allergy Clin Immunol* 2005;115:1238–1248.

51. Garofalo R, Goldman A. Cytokines, chemokines, and colony-stimulating factors in human milk: the 1997 update. *Biol Neonate* 1998;74:134–142.

52. Hamosh M. Protective function of proteins and lipids in human milk. *Biol Neonate* 1998;74:163–176.

53. Nauta AJ, Ben Amor K, Knol J, et al. Relevance of pre- and postnatal nutrition to development and interplay between the microbiota and metabolic and immune systems. *Am J Clin Nutr* 2013;98(2):586S–593S.

54. Kainonen E, Rautava S, Isolauri E. Immunological programming by breast milk creates an anti-inflammatory cytokine milieu in breast-fed infants compared to formula-fed infants. *Br J Nutr* 2013;109(11):1962–1970.

55. Kling P, Sullivan T, Roberts R, et al. Human milk as a potential enteral source of erythropoietin. *Pediatr Res* 1998;43:216–221.

56. Semba RD, Juul SE. Erythropoietin in human milk: physiology and role in infant health. *J Hum Lact* 2002; 18:252–261.

57. Sarwar G, Botting H, Davis T, et al. Free amino acids in milks of human subjects, other primates and non-primates. *Br J Nutr* 1998;79:129–131.

58. Mennella J. Mother's milk: a medium for early flavor experiences. *J Hum Lact* 1995;11:39–45.

59. Mennella J, Beauchamp G. Early flavor experiences: research update. *Nutr Rev* 1998;56:205–211.

60. Mennella JA, Jagnow CP, Beauchamp GK. Prenatal and postnatal flavor learning by human infants. *Pediatrics* 2001;107:E88.

61. Mennella J, Beauchamp G. The effects of repeated exposure to garlic-flavored milk on the nursling's behavior. *Pediatr Res* 1993;34:805–808.

62. Schwartz C, Chabanet C, Laval C, et al. Breast-feeding duration: influence on taste acceptance over the first year of life. *Br J Nutr* 2012;109(6):1154–1161.

63. Mennella JA. Regulation of milk intake after exposure to alcohol in mothers' milk. *Alcohol Clin Exp Res* 2001;25:590–593.

64. Mennella J. Infants' suckling responses to the flavor of alcohol in mothers' milk. *Alcohol Clin Exp Res* 1997; 21:581–585.

65. Mennella J, Beauchamp G. The transfer of alcohol to human milk. Effects on flavor and the infant's behavior. *N Engl J Med* 1991;325:981–985.

66. Mennella J, Gerrish C. Effects of exposure to alcohol in mother's milk on infant sleep. *Pediatrics* 1998;101:E2.

67. Mennella JA, Garcia-Gomez PL. Sleep disturbances after acute exposure to alcohol in mothers' milk. *Alcohol* 2001; 25:153–158.

68. Sengpiel V, Elind E, Bacelis J, et al. Maternal caffeine intake during pregnancy is associated with birth weight but not with gestational length: results from a large prospective observational cohort study. *BMC Med* 2013;11:42.

69. Bakker R, Steegers EA, Obradov A, et al. Maternal caffeine intake from coffee and tea, fetal growth, and the risks of adverse birth outcomes: the Generation R Study. 2010; 91(6):1691–1698.

70. Scholl T, Hediger M. Maternal nutrition and preterm delivery. In: Bendich A, Deckelbaum RJ, eds. *Preventive nutrition: the comprehensive guide for health professionals.* Totowa, NJ: Humana Press, 1997:387–404.

71. Hofmeyr GJ, Roodt A, Atallah AN, et al. Calcium supplementation to prevent pre-eclampsia—a systematic review. *S Afr Med J* 2003;93:224–228.

72. Olsen SF, Secher NJ. Low consumption of seafood in early pregnancy as a risk factor for preterm delivery: prospective cohort study. *BMJ* 2002;324:447.

73. Jensen CL. Effects of n-3 fatty acids during pregnancy and lactation. *Am J Clin Nutr* 2006;83:1452s–1457s.

74. Makrides M, Gibson RA. Long-chain polyunsaturated fatty acid requirements during pregnancy and lactation. *Am J Clin Nutr* 2000;71:307s–311s.

75. Hibbeln JR. Seafood consumption, the DHA content of mothers' milk and prevalence rates of postpartum depression: a cross-national, ecological analysis. *J Affect Disord* 2002;69:15–29.

76. Freeman MP, Hibbeln JR, Wisner KL, et al. An open trial of omega-3 fatty acids for depression in pregnancy. *Acta Neuropsychiatrica* 2006;18:21–24.

77. Freeman MP, Hibbeln JR, Wisner KL, et al. Randomized dose-ranging pilot trial of omega-3 fatty acids for postpartum depression. *Acta Psychiatr Scand* 2006;113:31–35.

78. Uauy R, Andraca ID. Human milk and breast feeding for optimal mental development. *J Nutr* 1995;125:2278s–2280s.

79. Lauritzen L, Jorgensen MH, Mikkelsen TB, et al. Maternal fish oil supplementation in lactation: effect on visual acuity and n-3 fatty acids content of infant erythrocytes. *Lipids* 2004;39:195–206.

80. Helland IB, Smith L, Saarem K, et al. Maternal supplementation with very-long-chain n-3 fatty acids during pregnancy and lactation augments children's IQ at 4 years of age. *Pediatrics* 2003;111:e39–e44.

81. Hibbeln JR, Davis JM, Steer C, et al. Maternal seafood consumption in pregnancy and neurodevelopmental outcomes in childhood (ALSPAC study): and observational cohort study. *Lancet* 2007;569:578–585.

82. Hadders-Algra M. Prenatal and early postnatal supplementation with long-chain polyunsaturated fatty acids: neurodevelopmental considerations. *Am J Clin Nutr* 2011; 94(6 suppl):1874S–1879S.

83. Helland IB, Saugstad OD, Saarem D, et al. Supplementation of n-3 fatty acids during pregnancy and lactation reduces maternal plasma lipid levels and provides DHA to the infants. *J Matern Fetal Neonatal Med* 2006;19:397–406.

84. Eaton S, Konner M. Paleolithic nutrition revisited: a twelve-year retrospective on its nature and implications. *Eur J Clin Nutr* 1997;51:207–216.

85. Denomme J, Stark KD, Holub BJ. Directly quantitated dietary (n-3) fatty acid intakes of pregnant Canadian women are lower than current dietary recommendations. *J Nutr* 2005;135:206–211.

86. US Food and Drug Administration. *While you're pregnant. Methylmercury: frequently asked questions.* Available at http://www.cfsan.fda.gov/~pregnant/whilmeth.html; accessed 2/18/07.

87. ConsumerLab.com. *Good news! These supplements have omega-3's without contaminants found in fish! but some are better than others. Find out now!* Available at http://www.consumerlab.com/results/omega3.asp; accessed 2/18/07.

88. MRC Vitamin Study Research Group. Prevention of neural tube defects (NTD): results of the Medical Research Council Vitamin Study. *Lancet* 1991;338:131–137.

89. Mills JL, Signore C. Neural tube defect rates before and after food fortification with folic acid. *Birth Defects Res A Clin Mol Teratol* 2004;70:844–845.

90. Wald NJ. Folic acid and the prevention of neural tube defects. *N Engl J Med* 2004;350:101–103.

91. Berry RJ, Crider KS, Yeargin-Allsopp M. Periconceptional folic acid and risk of autism spectrum disorders. *JAMA* 2013;309(6):611–613.

92. Surén P, Roth C, Bresnahan M, et al. Association between maternal use of folic acid supplements and risk of autism spectrum disorders in children. *JAMA* 2013;309(6):570–577.

93. Flynn A. Minerals and trace elements in milk. *Adv Food Nutr Res* 1992;36:209–252.

94. Fischer-Rasmussen W, Kjaer S, Dahl C, et al. Ginger treatment of hyperemesis gravidarum. *Eur J Obstet Gynecol Reprod Biol* 1990;38:19.

95. Borrelli F, Capasso R, Aviello G, et al. Effectiveness and safety of ginger in the treatment of pregnancy-induced nausea and vomiting. *Obstet Gynecol* 2005;105:849–856.

96. Murray M. *Encyclopedia of nutritional supplements.* Rocklin, CA: Prima, 1996.

97. Scholl TO. Iron status during pregnancy: setting the stage for mother and infant. *Am J Clin Nutr* 2005;81:1218s–1222s.

98. Helin A, Kinnunen TI, Raitanen J, et al. Iron intake, haemoglobin and risk of gestational diabetes: a prospective cohort study. *BMJ Open.* 2012; Sep 25;2(5):e001730.

99. Eglash A, Kendall SK, Fashner J. Clinical inquiries. What vitamins and minerals should be given to breastfed and bottle-fed infants? *J Fam Pract* 2005;54:1089–1091.

100. Alaejos MS, Romero CD. Selenium in human lactation. *Nutr Rev* 1995;53:159–166.

101. Jewell D, Young G. Interventions for nausea and vomiting in early pregnancy. *Cochrane Database Syst Rev* 2003;4:CD000145.

102. Poston L, Briley AL, Seed PT, et al. Vitamin C and vitamin E in pregnant women at risk for pre-eclampsia: randomized placebo-controlled trial. *Lancet* 2006;367:1145–1154.

103. Briley AL, Poston L, Shennan AH. Vitamins C and E and the prevention of preeclampsia. *N Engl J Med* 2006;355:1065–1066.

104. Ortega R, Andres P, Martinez R, et al. Zinc levels in maternal milk: the influences of nutritional status with respect to zinc during the third trimester of pregnancy. *Eur J Clin Nutr* 1997;51:253–258.

105. Specker B. Vitamin D requirements during pregnancy. *Am J Clin Nutr* 2004;80:1740s–1747s.

106. Hollis BW, Wagner CL. Assessment of dietary vitamin D requirements during pregnancy and lactation. *Am J Clin Nutr* 2004;79:717–726.

107. Jovanovic L, Pettitt DJ. Gestational diabetes mellitus. *JAMA* 2001;286:2516–2518.

108. American College of Obstetricians and Gynecologists Committee on Genetics. ACOG Committee Opinion No. 449: Maternal phenylketonuria. *Obstet Gynecol* 2009; 114(6):1432–1433.

109. Shapiro RL, Lockman S, Kim S, et al. Infant morbidity, mortality, and breast milk immunologic profiles among breast-feeding HIV-infected and HIV-uninfected women in Botswana. *J Infect Dis* 2007;196:562–569.

110. Chan GM, McElligott K, McNaught T, et al. Effects of dietary calcium intervention on adolescent mothers and newborns: a randomized controlled trial. *Obstet Gynecol* 2006;108:565–571.

111. Yu CK, Teoh TG, Robinson S. Obesity in pregnancy. *BJOG* 2006;113:1117–1125.

SUGGESTED READINGS

Czeizel A. Folic acid-containing multivitamins and primary prevention of birth defects. In: Bendich A, Deckelbaum RJ, eds. *Preventive nutrition: the comprehensive guide for health professionals.* Totowa, NJ: Humana Press, 1997; 351–372.

Dietz WH, Stern L, eds. *American Academy of Pediatrics guide to your child's nutrition.* New York, NY: Villard Books, 1999.

Duffy VB, Bartoshuk LM, Striegel-Moore R, et al. Taste changes across pregnancy. *Ann N Y Acad Sci* 1998;855:805–809.

Institute of Medicine. *Nutrition during lactation.* Washington, DC: National Academy Press, 1991.

Institute of Medicine. *Nutrition during pregnancy.* Washington, DC: National Academy Press, 1990.

Kleinman RE, ed. *Committee on Nutrition, American Academy of Pediatrics. Pediatric nutrition handbook,* 4th ed. Elk Grove Village, IL: American Academy of Pediatrics, 1998.

Koletzko B, Aggett PJ, Bindels JG, et al. Growth, development and differentiation: a functional food science approach. *Br J Nutr* 1998;80:s5–s45.

Locksmith G, Duff P. Preventing neural tube defects: the importance of periconceptual folic acid supplements. *Obstet Gynecol* 1998;91:1027–1034.

Picciano MF, McDonald SS. Lactation. In: Shils ME, Shike M, Ross AC, et al., eds. *Modern nutrition in health and disease,* 10th ed. Philadelphia, PA: Lippincott Williams & Wilkins, 2006:784–796.

Tamborlane WV, ed. *The Yale guide to children's nutrition.* New Haven, CT: Yale University Press, 1997.

CHAPTER 28

Diet and the Menstrual Cycle

Variations in food intake and preference occur during the normal menstrual cycle. Hormonal variation during the menstrual cycle induces changes in taste perception, nutrient metabolism, and the thermic effect of food. Such variations are characteristic of normal physiology but may manifest to a greater extreme as symptoms of the premenstrual syndrome (PMS) and premenstrual dysphoric disorder (PMDD). Dietary management and certain nutritional supplementation may alleviate symptoms of PMS/PMDD.

OVERVIEW

The normal menstrual cycle is approximately 28 days in length and consists of three phases: menstruation, the follicular phase, and the luteal phase. During menstruation, levels of the pituitary gonadotropins luteinizing hormone (LH) and follicle-stimulating hormone (FSH) as well as the ovarian hormones estradiol and progesterone are at baseline levels. When the endometrium has sloughed completely, the follicular phase begins and estradiol levels begin to rise. Estradiol levels peak just before the midpoint of the cycle (day 14), inducing a surge in levels of the gonadotropins. This surge, in turn, induces a transient fall in estradiol levels. Progesterone levels rise slowly throughout the follicular phase. Ovulation, induced by the mid-cycle surge in gonadotropins, occurs on or about day 14 and represents the division between the follicular and luteal phases. In the luteal phase, gonadotropin levels return quickly to baseline, as estradiol levels begin to rise again while progesterone levels continue to rise, now at a somewhat accelerated rate. Estradiol peaks for a second time, and progesterone for the first time, at or near the midpoint of the luteal phase. If implantation occurs, progesterone levels are maintained and continue to rise. In the absence of implantation, levels of both estradiol and progesterone fall toward baseline, inducing menstruation approximately 14 days after ovulation. The phases of the menstrual cycle are summarized in Table 28.1.

Diet

The recurrent hormonal fluctuations associated with the menstrual cycle interact with diet in important ways: Variation in eating pattern and appetite is a well-recognized occurrence even in normal menstrual cycles. Basal metabolic rate varies throughout the cycle, increasing by up to 15% during the luteal (premenstrual) phase (1).

Appetite, hunger, satiety, cravings, and aversions also vary with the cycle. There is evidence that with variation in steroid hormone levels, there is corresponding, albeit modest, variation in taste thresholds (2,3). For example, one study examining the influence of the menstrual cycle on salt preference found that women preferred unsalted popcorn in the menstrual phase but expressed greater preference for highly salted popcorn in the luteal phase (4). The extent to which seemingly subtle alterations in taste perception govern the variations in food preference and intake throughout the menstrual cycle is currently uncertain. Also uncertain at present is whether gustatory thresholds change more profoundly in women with PMS.

Nutrient analysis of dietary intake of women experiencing PMS compared to that of women not meeting PMS criteria has shown that women with PMS significantly increase total energy intake premenstrually, with significant increases in intake of fat and total carbohydrate, and particularly simple sugars. This phenomenon could potentially be a contributing factor for some women experiencing difficulties adhering to suggested dietary modification and should be considered when counseling premenopausal women (5).

Leptin levels have been shown to vary throughout the menstrual cycle, suggesting a role in the

TABLE 28.1

Phases of the Prototypical Menstrual Cycle[a]

Phase	Approximate Timing	Gonadotrophins (LH and FSH)	Estradiol	Progesterone
Menstruation	Days 1–3	Baseline level	Baseline level	Baseline level
Follicular phase	Days 3–14	Baseline level	Gradual rise/peak	Gradual rise
Ovulation	Day 14	Surge	Abrupt fall	Gradual rise
Luteal phase	Days 14–28	Baseline level	Gradual rise/second peak followed by a decline to baseline	Faster rise/peak followed by a decline to baseline

[a]FSH, follicle-stimulating hormone; LH, luteinizing hormone.

changes in appetite and occurrence of cravings. In an observational study, however, Paolisso et al. (6) found that although both leptin and food intake varied throughout the menstrual cycle in 16 healthy women, no significant correlations between food intake values and fasting plasma leptin concentration at all menstrual phases were found. A recent analysis of eating patterns and hormonal fluctuations in women with diagnosed bulimia nervosa found increases in binge eating to be significantly correlated with the luteal phase of the menstrual cycle, a finding consistent with animal studies that have suggested links between decreases in estradiol/increases in progesterone and binge eating (7).

Isoflavones in soy and other foods are known to exert selective estrogenic effects, generating clinical and popular interest in such foods as a natural means to replace ovarian hormones or modify disease risk. In a randomized crossover study of 14 premenopausal women, Duncan et al. (8) found that even high-level isoflavone supplementation induced no significant changes in menstrual cycle length, endometrial histology, or plasma estrogen levels. Using similar methods in 12 healthy premenopausal women, Xu et al. (9) found that soy protein supplementation decreased urinary excretion of endogenous estrogens while increasing excretion of soy phytoestrogens. A significant increase in the ratio of 2-hydroxyestrone to 16α-hydroxyestrone was observed, suggesting a mechanism by which phytoestrogens might reduce cancer risk (9); this remains a controversial area (see Chapters 12 and 33). A double-blind, placebo-controlled, crossover intervention study in women with confirmed PMS found soy protein containing soy isoflavones to significantly

reduce specific premenstrual symptoms from baseline compared to placebo (10).

SPECIAL CONSIDERATIONS

PMS and PMDD

PMS is a constellation of monthly physical and psychological symptoms occurring during the luteal phase of the cycle when fluctuations occur in levels of estrogen, progesterone, aldosterone, and prolactin. It has been estimated that up to 80% of women of reproductive age experience some degree of physical or emotional changes premenstrually; approximately half of those with symptoms have them to a degree that would fit criteria for PMS (11,12). Approximately 3% to 5% of all women in this age group experience more severe psychological symptoms recently characterized as a diagnostic variant of PMS called PMDD. Survey data suggest that the majority of these women are receiving suboptimal care from primary care physicians (13).

Although some women with PMS may experience a variety of emotional and physical symptoms, one potentially valuable approach to management, described in the early 1980s by Abraham (14), involves understanding which of several subtypes—which may correlate with differing physiological imbalances—a woman is experiencing. Most commonly, anxiety and irritability are predominant; this symptom cluster has been associated with elevated serum estrogen and low serum progesterone, and it may respond well to pyridoxine (vitamin B$_6$) supplementation. Hyperhydration, a second subtype associated with elevated aldosterone levels, can induce fluid retention and the commonly experienced premenstrual symptoms of abdominal bloating, breast tenderness, and weight gain; avoidance of caffeine and nicotine, restriction of sodium, and supplementation with pyridoxine and vitamin E have been advocated. Increased appetite and cravings for sugar and other refined carbohydrates during the luteal phase have been shown to respond to magnesium supplementation. Finally, a fourth subtype of PMS involves more severe symptoms of depression, and women in this category may meet diagnostic criteria for PMDD. Physical activity has consistently been reported to confer modest benefit for all subtypes.

Treatment strategies for PMS remain controversial, as most available evidence is inconclusive. For example, in a study of the hyperhydration variant of PMS, Olson et al. (15) found the syndrome to be associated with urinary sodium loss rather than retention; sodium restriction was not found to be beneficial. A trial of progesterone supplementation failed to show any benefit with regard to cyclical craving of chocolate and/or sweets (16). Nonetheless, timing of therapy may be critical. Perchere et al. (17) showed that the renal response to salt differs markedly in women investigated in luteal versus follicular phases. In the follicular phase, the renal response to a sustained increase in sodium intake is characterized by no change in renal hemodynamics and decreases in both proximal and distal sodium reabsorption. In contrast, during the luteal phase, increasing sodium intake leads to a renal vasodilation, a marked sodium escape from the distal nephron, and no change in proximal sodium reabsorption. Therefore a reduction in salt consumption during the luteal phase may be beneficial to prevent some of the premenstrual symptoms.

Understanding of the pathophysiology of the several subtypes of PMS is still quite limited. The possibility that the variants are mechanistically distinct suggests that intervention trials that failed to target a particular PMS variant were treating a heterogeneous group and, therefore, subject to type II error. Studies of PMS are increasingly focusing on subject groups homogeneous with regard to symptom complex.

Dietary manipulation may be helpful in alleviating symptoms; high-fat, low-fiber diets—which may contribute to the higher estrogen levels thought to be a factor in premenstrual symptoms—are discouraged in favor of dietary intake that is lower in fat and high in fiber (18,19).

Serotonin levels are thought to be related to symptoms of PMS (see Chapter 34), a hypothesis that would account for the carbohydrate craving experienced by some women. The rate of brain serotonin synthesis normally depends on its concentration of tryptophan, serotonin's essential amino acid precursor. Brain tryptophan concentrations and the flux of tryptophan from blood to brain depend, in turn, partly on plasma tryptophan and partly on plasma concentrations of other large neutral amino acids (LNAAs), namely, tyrosine, phenylalanine, leucine, isoleucine, valine, and methionine, which compete with tryptophan for blood–brain barrier transport.

Carbohydrate stimulates insulin secretion; this diminishes plasma levels of other LNAAs, thus increasing tryptophan's flux across the blood–brain barrier and its brain levels increasing the synthesis of serotonin. Consistent with this theory is evidence that selective serotonin reuptake inhibitors (SSRIs) relieve symptoms in many women and apparently more effectively than other commonly used classes of medications or nutriceuticals (20). The benefit of SSRIs apparently is greatest when dysphoric or depressive symptoms are predominant (21); SSRIs are considered a safe and effective therapy for PMDD when administered continuously or intermittently (22,23,24). Based on this theory, L-tryptophan, a precursor of 5-hydroxytryptophan may be used for the prevention of PMS symptoms (25). Further studies are needed to prove the effectiveness of L-tryptophan supplementation.

Although oral contraceptive pills have not previously been reported to be effective for treatment of PMDD, an oral contraceptive formulation containing drospirenone and ethinyl estradiol in a 24/4 cycle (rather than the usual 21/7 regimen) may help improve symptoms associated with PMDD (26).

The evidence supporting a therapeutic role for vitamin B$_6$ (pyridoxine) has been criticized for its methodologic limitations. Nonetheless, one double-blinded randomized controlled trial found pyridoxine to reduce both overall PMS symptoms and specific psychiatric symptoms compared to baseline and placebo (27). In a systematic review, Wyatt et al. (28) found evidence supporting use of up to 100 mg per day of vitamin B$_6$ in the treatment of PMS, particularly with depressive symptoms. In the Nurses' Health Study II Cohort, Chocano Bodoya et al. (29) showed a lower risk of PMS in women with higher intakes of other B vitamins (thiamine and riboflavin), but from food sources only. Further research is needed to evaluate the effects of B vitamins in the development of PMS.

Evidence appears to be strongest for the role of calcium in PMS. Ovarian hormones, including estrogen, are known to influence calcium, magnesium, and vitamin D metabolism, processes that vary across the menstrual cycle. In 1995, Thys-Jacobs and Alvir (30) demonstrated that although total and ionized calcium levels varied predictably throughout the menstrual cycle in subjects with PMS and in matched controls, only the subjects with PMS experienced a mid-cycle surge in levels of intact parathyroid hormone. The authors interpreted these data to indicate that a transient, secondary hyperparathyroid state was implicated in the pathogenesis of PMS. Interestingly, symptoms of PMS are remarkably similar to those of hypocalcemia (31). Following up on this finding, Thys-Jacobs et al. (32) conducted a randomized trial of calcium supplementation involving more than 450 women. Compared with placebo, supplementation with 1,200 mg per day of elemental calcium resulted in a significant reduction in all symptoms of PMS. A recent study also found that women reporting the highest intake of vitamin D and calcium from food sources were significantly less likely to develop PMS over 10 years of follow-up compared to women with the lowest intake of these nutrients (33).

Related evidence suggests that impaired calcium homeostasis may be an important element in the pathophysiology of polycystic ovarian syndrome (34). While foods rich in calcium appear to decrease risk for symptomatic kidney stones, supplemental calcium may increase it (35). Similarly, there is evidence that calcium supplementation, but not dietary intake, particularly in excess of 500 mg daily, may increase the risk of cardiovascular events such as myocardial infarction, coronary revascularization, death from coronary heart disease, and stroke (36,37).

Although in the aggregate less compelling than the evidence for calcium, there is evidence of a therapeutic effect of magnesium as well (38). Facchinetti et al. (39) studied a high-magnesium yeast product (Sillix Donna) in a double-blind, placebo-controlled, randomized trial and found a statistically and clinically significant reduction in PMS symptoms over the 6-month study

period. Walker et al. (40) found that a daily dose of 200 mg of magnesium oxide reduced symptoms of hyperhydration by the second month of administration in a randomized, double-blind, crossover trial of 38 women; no significant effect was seen on other symptom categories. Cocoa, and therefore chocolate, is a relatively rich source of magnesium, suggesting one possible reason why chocolate craving is apparently common both in PMS and the normal menstrual cycle. There is suggestive evidence of a role for manganese supplementation as well (41).

There has been interest in the use of essential fatty acids in the treatment of PMS, and evening primrose oil, which is rich in γ-linolenic acid, has been advocated. However, clinical trials have not shown clear significant benefit over placebo (42).

Studies on fatty acids are still controversial. In a randomized crossover trial, Collins et al. (43) found no benefit of essential fatty acid supplementation in 27 women with PMS. Nevertheless more recent studies have shown that ω-3 fatty acids may improve PMS symptomatology. Rocha Filho et al. (44) showed that the administration of 1 or 2 g of fatty acids (γ-linolenic acid, oleic acid, and linoleic acid) results in a significant reduction of PMS symptoms. Also Krill oil, rich in n-3 (ω-3) polyunsaturated fatty acids (PUFAs) incorporated in phosphatidylcholine, has been reported to reduce the PMS symptomatic and dysmenorrhoe (45).

Menstrual Cycle Irregularities

Competitive athletics in adolescent girls is associated with amenorrhea due to the energy demands of training and, in some, associated eating disorders thought to be induced by the pressure to remain thin; the concurrence of disordered eating, amenorrhea, and resultant osteoporosis is known as the "female athlete triad" (46). Of note, the occurrence of menstrual irregularities in female athletes without disordered eating is also well established; the term "exercise-related menstrual irregularities" has been applied (47). Although it was previously thought that the amenorrhea was primarily due to reduction of body fat from intense training that disrupted the menstrual cycle via effects on estrogen metabolism (48), negative energy balance is thought to lead to low levels of circulating leptin, a metabolic signal that provides negative feedback in the regulation of body weight homeostasis; suppression of leptin may in turn act as a link between adipose tissue, energy availability, and the reproductive axis, inducing hypothalamic changes that lead to amenorrhea when insufficient energy is available to compensate for exercise-related energy costs (49). The nutritional requirements associated with competitive athletics are discussed in Chapter 32; the prevention of osteoporosis is discussed in Chapter 14. Amenorrhea in adolescent girls is a clear indication of a risk for potentially irreversible osteopenia. Although management should focus on the restoration of adequate nutrition and energy balance, oral contraceptives are indicated when the patient is resistant to such interventions or when primary or secondary amenorrhea persists despite these actions.

Vegetarianism has been reported to be associated with an increased propensity for amenorrhea, oligomenorrhea, and anovulation. However, studies to date have been limited by sampling bias (50,51), and it may be that some women with disordered eating adopt vegetarian diets as a way to incur significant weight loss. Weight loss can cause menstrual disturbances in omnivores as well. Indeed, no menstrual cycle disturbances have been associated with weight-stable vegetarians with a normal BMI (52). (see Chapter 43 for more on vegetarianism.)

Dysmenorrhea is a common problem in adolescent girls and women of reproductive age. To date, there is no clear association between dietary pattern and the risk of dysmenorrhea (53). However, there is some evidence of symptomatic benefit with the use of thiamine, vitamin E, and fish oil supplements (54). A small study testing the effects of a low-fat vegetarian diet found associations of the diet with increased serum sex-hormone binding globulin concentration, reductions in body weight, and reductions in dysmenorrheal duration and intensity; the authors concluded that their results may have stemmed from dietary influence on estrogen activity (55).

CLINICAL HIGHLIGHTS

The normal menstrual cycle produces changes in metabolism and taste that result in variations in food intake pattern. This tendency becomes extreme in the craving variant of PMS. Such cravings may respond to supplemental magnesium in particular, although data are preliminary. All

variants of PMS may respond to calcium supplementation, which should be attempted in most patients, given its safety and other potential benefits. Supplementation with calcium and magnesium, and a multivitamin with minerals, appears appropriate given available evidence. Available evidence suggests that a daily dose of calcium in the range of 1,000 to 1,500 mg along with 200 to 400 mg of magnesium are appropriate for a therapeutic trial.

If this strategy is ineffective, a trial of pyridoxine of approximately 100 mg per day appears to be justified; whether such intervention should be combined or applied separately has not yet been fully resolved and must rely on clinical judgment. Combination therapy is not precluded by any potential toxicity. A diet rich in complex carbohydrates may be beneficial in ameliorating depressive symptoms of PMS through a serotonergic mechanism. When depressive symptoms are pronounced or refractory to dietary interventions, SSRIs should be used as indicated. Physical activity, a diet rich in fruit and vegetables, avoidance of nicotine, and restricted intake of saturated fat, salt, and caffeine may offer benefit in PMS and are indicated on other grounds. By judiciously selecting and combining available therapies, clinicians may hope to alleviate symptoms in the great majority of patients with PMS.

REFERENCES

1. McNeil J, Doucet É. Possible factors for altered energy balance across the menstrual cycle: a closer look at the severity of PMS, reward driven behaviors and leptin variations. *Eur J Obstet Gynecol Reprod Biol* 2012;163:5–10.
2. Kuga M, Ikeda M, Suzuki K. Gustatory changes associated with the menstrual cycle. *Physiol Behav* 1999;66: 317–322.
3. Alberti-Fidanza A, Fruttini D, Servili M. Gustatory and food habit changes during the menstrual cycle. *Int J Vitam Nutr Res* 1998;68:149–153.
4. Verma P, Mahajan KK, Mittal S, et al. Salt preference across different phases of menstrual cycle. *Indian J Physiol Pharmacol* 2005;49:99–102.
5. Cross GB, Marley J, Miles H, et al. Changes in nutrient intake during the menstrual cycle of overweight women with premenstrual syndrome. *Br J Nutr* 2001;85:475–482.
6. Paolisso G, Rizzo MR, Mazziotti G, et al. Lack of association between changes in plasma leptin concentration and in food intake during the menstrual cycle. *Eur J Clin Invest* 1999;29:490–495.
7. Edler C, Lipson SF, Keel PK. Ovarian hormones and binge eating in bulimia nervosa. *Psychol Med* 2007;37:131–141.
8. Duncan AM, Merz BE, Xu X, et al. Soy isoflavones exert modest hormonal effects in premenopausal women. *J Clin Endocrinol Metab* 1999;84:192.

9. Xu X, Duncan AM, Merz BE, et al. Effects of soy isoflavones on estrogen and phytoestrogen metabolism in premenopausal women. *Cancer Epidemiol Biomarkers Prev* 1998;7:1101.

10. Bryant M, Cassidy A, Hill C, et al. Effect of consumption of soy isoflavones on behavioural, somatic and affective symptoms in women with premenstrual syndrome. *Br J Nutr* 2005;93:731–739.

11. Ugarriza DN, Klingner S, O'Brien S. Premenstrual syndrome: diagnosis and intervention. *Nurse Pract* 1998;23: 40, 45, 49–52.

12. Singh BB, Berman BM, Simpson RL, et al. Incidence of premenstrual syndrome and remedy usage: a national probability sample study. *Altern Ther Health Med* 1998;4:75–79.

13. Kraemer GR, Kraemer RR. Premenstrual syndrome: diagnosis and treatment experiences. *J Womens Health* (Larchmt). 1998;7:893.

14. Abraham GE. Nutritional factors in the etiology of the premenstrual tension syndromes. *J Reprod Med* 1983;28:446–464.

15. Olson BR, Forman MR, Lanza E, et al. Relation between sodium balance and menstrual cycle symptoms in normal women. *Ann Intern Med* 1996;125:564–567.

16. Michener W, Rozin P, Freeman E, et al. The role of low progesterone and tension as triggers of perimenstrual chocolate and sweets craving: some negative experimental evidence. *Physiol Behav* 1999;67:417–420.

17. Pechère-Bertschi A, Maillard M, Stalder H, et al. Renal segmental tubular response to salt during the normal menstrual cycle. *Kidney Int* 2002;61:425–431.

18. Nagata C, Hirokawa K, Shimizu N, et al. Soy, fat and other dietary factors in relation to premenstrual symptoms in Japanese women. *Br J Obstet Gynecol* 2004;111:594–599.

19. Low Dog T. Integrative treatments for premenstrual syndrome. *Altern Ther Health Med* 2001;7:32–39.

20. Diegoli MS, da Fonseca AM, Diegoli CA, et al. A double-blind trial of four medications to treat severe premenstrual syndrome. *Int J Gynaecol Obstet* 1998;62:63–67.

21. Yonkers KA, Halbreich U, Freeman E, et al. Symptomatic improvement of premenstrual dysphoric disorder with sertraline treatment. A randomized controlled trial. Sertraline premenstrual dysphoric collaborative study group. *JAMA* 1997;278:983–988.

22. Dimmock PW, Wyatt KM, Jones PW, et al. Efficacy of selective serotonin-reuptake inhibitors in premenstrual syndrome. *Lancet* 2000;356:1131–1136.

23. Brown J, O'Brien PM, Marjoribanks J, et al. Selective serotonin reuptake inhibitors for premenstrual syndrome. *Cochrane Database Syst Rev* 2009;2:CD001396.

24. Marjoribanks J, Brown J, O'Brien PM, et al. Selective serotonin reuptake inhibitors for premenstrual syndrome. *Cochrane Database Syst Rev* 2013;6:CD001396.

25. Steinberg S, Annable L, Young SN, et al. A placebo-controlled clinical trial of L-tryptophan in premenstrual dysphoria. *Biol Psychiatry* 1999;45:313–320.

26. Pearlstein TB, Bachmann GA, Zacur HA, et al. Treatment of premenstrual dysphoric disorder with a new drospirenon-containing oral contraceptive formulation. *Contraception* 2005;72:414–421.

27. Kashanian M, Mazinani R, Jalalmanesh S. Pyridoxine (vitamin B$_6$) therapy for premenstrual syndrome. *Int J Gynaecol Obstet* 2007;96:43–44.

28. Wyatt KM, Dimmock PW, Jones PW, et al. Efficacy of vitamin B$_6$ in the treatment of premenstrual syndrome: a systematic review. *BMJ* 1999;318:1375–1381.

29. Chocano-Bedoya PO, Manson JE, Hankinson SE, et al. Dietary B vitamin intake and incident premenstrual syndrome. *Am J Clin Nutr* 2011;93:1080–1086.

30. Thys-Jacobs S, Alvir MJ. Calcium-regulating hormones across the menstrual cycle: evidence of a secondary hyperparathyroidism in women with PMS. *J Clin Endocrinol Metab* 1995;80:2227–2232.

31. Thys-Jacobs S. Micronutrients and the premenstrual syndrome: the case of calcium. *J Am Coll Nutr* 2000;19: 220–227.

32. Thys-Jacobs S, Starkey P, Bernstein D, et al. Calcium carbonate and the premenstrual syndrome: effects on premenstrual and menstrual symptoms. Premenstrual Syndrome Study Group. *Am J Obstet Gynecol* 1998;179:444–452.

33. Bertone-Johnson ER, Hankinson SE, Bendich A, et al. Calcium and vitamin D intake and risk of incident premenstrual syndrome. *Arch Intern Med* 2005;165:1246–1252.

34. Thys-Jacobs S, Donovan D, Papadopoulos A, et al. Vitamin D and calcium dysregulation in the polycystic ovarian syndrome. *Steroids* 1999;64:430–435.

35. Curhan GC, Willett WC, Speizer FE, et al. Comparison of dietary calcium with supplemental calcium and other nutrients as factors affecting the risk for kidney stones in women. *Ann Intern Med* 1997;126:497–504.

36. Bolland MJ, Avenell A, Baron JA et al. Effect of calcium supplements on risk of myocardial infarction and cardiovascular events: meta-analysis. *BMJ* 2010;341:c3691.

37. Bolland MJ, Grey A, Avenell A, et al. Calcium supplements with or without vitamin D and risk of cardiovascular events: reanalysis of the Women's Health Initiative limited access dataset and meta-analysis. *BMJ* 2011;342:d2040.

38. Facchinetti F, Borella P, Sances G, et al. Oral magnesium successfully relieves premenstrual mood changes. *Obstet Gynecol* 1991;78:177–181.

39. Facchinetti F, Nappi RE, Sances MG, et al. Effects of a yeast-based dietary supplementation on premenstrual syndrome. A double-blind placebo-controlled study. *Gynecol Obstet Invest* 1997;43:120–124.

40. Walker AF, De Souza MC, Vickers MF, et al. Magnesium supplementation alleviates premenstrual symptoms of fluid retention. *J Womens Health* (Larchmt). 1998;7:1157–1165.

41. Penland JG, Johnson PE. Dietary calcium and manganese effects on menstrual cycle symptoms. *Am J Obstet Gynecol* 1993;168:1417–1423.

42. Dante G, Facchinetti F. Herbal treatments for alleviating premenstrual symptoms: a systematic review. *J Psychosom Obstet Gynaecol* 2011;32:42–51.

43. Collins A, Cerin A, Coleman G, et al. Essential fatty acids in the treatment of premenstrual syndrome. *Obstet Gynecol* 1993;81:93–98.

44. Rocha Filho EA, Lima JC, Pinho Neto JS, et al. Essential fatty acids for premenstrual syndrome and their effect on prolactin and total cholesterol levels: a randomized, double blind, placebo-controlled study. *Reprod Health* 2011;8:2. doi: 10.1186/1742-4755-8-2.

45. Sampalis F, Bunea R, Pelland MF, et al. Evaluation of the effects of Neptune Krill Oil on the management of premenstrual syndrome and dysmenorrhea. *Altern Med Rev* 2003;8:171–179.

46. Gabel KA. Special nutritional concerns for the female athlete. *Curr Sports Med Rep* 2006;5:187–191.

47. De Cree C. Sex steroid metabolism and menstrual irregularities in the exercising female. A review. *Sports Med* 1998;25:369–406.

48. Warren MP, Stiehl AL. Exercise and female adolescents: effects on the reproductive and skeletal systems. *J Am Med Womens Assoc* 1999;54:115–130.

49. Thong FSL, McLean C, Graham TE. Plasma leptin in female athletes: relationship with body fat, reproductive, nutritional, and endocrine factors. *J Appl Physiol* 2000; 88:2037–2044.

50. Barr SI. Vegetarianism and menstrual cycle disturbances: is there an association? *Am J Clin Nutr* 1999;70:549s–554s.

51. Griffith J, Omar H. Association between vegetarian diet and menstrual problems in young women: a case presentation and brief review. *J Pediatr Adolesc Gynecol* 2003;16:319–323.

52. Rajaram S, Dyett PA, Sabaté J. Nutrition and vegetarianism. In: Klimis-Zacas D, Wolinsky I, eds. *Nutritional concerns of women.* Boca Raton, FL: CRC Press, 2004:419–456.

53. Di Cintio E, Parazzini F, Tozzi L, et al. Dietary habits, reproductive and menstrual factors and risk of dysmenorrhoea. *Eur J Epidemiol* 1997;13:925–930.

54. French L. Dysmenorrhea. *Am Fam Physician* 2005;71: 285–291.

55. Barnard ND, Scialli AR, Hurlock D, et al. Diet and sex-hormone binding globulin, dysmenorrheal, and premenstrual symptoms. *Obstet Gynecol* 2000;95:245–250.

SUGGESTED READINGS

Barnhart KT, Freeman EW, Soundheimer SJ. A clinician's guide to the premenstrual syndrome. *Med Clin North Am* 1995;79:1457–1472.

Bhatia SC, Bhatia SK. Diagnosis and treatment of premenstrual dysphoric disorder. *Am Fam Physician* 2002;66: 1239–1248, 1253–1254.

Dye L, Blundell JE. Menstrual cycle and appetite control: implications for weight regulation. *Hum Reprod* 1997;12:1142–1151.

Freeman EW, Halbreich U. Premenstrual syndromes. *Psychopharmacol Bull* 1998;34:291.

Girman A, Lee R, Kligler B. An integrative medicine approach to premenstrual syndrome. *Am J Obstet Gynecol* 2003;188:s56–s65.

CHAPTER 29

Diet and Early Development: Pediatric Nutrition

hysical and cognitive development are rapid during infancy and early childhood, which imposes extreme metabolic demands. The provision of adequate nutrition from birth is fundamental to the maintenance of normal growth and development. Infants are subject to certain specific micronutrient deficiencies, and they have requirements different from those of adults for macronutrients, particularly protein.

The health benefits of breast-feeding (see Chapter 27) during the first 6 months of life are increasingly clear. Although the principal goal of nutrition management in early childhood is the preservation of optimal growth and development, children in the United States and other developed countries are increasingly susceptible to the adverse effects of dietary excess, particularly obesity (see Chapter 5). As a result, there is intense interest regarding the age at which dietary restrictions might first be safely imposed.

In general, restriction of macronutrients (saturated fat being of particular concern) is discouraged before age 2, with increasing evidence that restrictions comparable to those recommended for adults may be safe and appropriate after age 2. The establishment of health-promoting diet and activity patterns in childhood may be of particular importance, as preferences established early in life tend to persist (see Chapters 38 and 44).

OVERVIEW

Diet Nutrient Recommendations

The importance of adequate nutrition to normal growth and development during the neonatal period and early childhood is well established and largely self-evident. Basal metabolic rate is higher in infants and children than in adults; the nutritional needs to support growth are superimposed on the higher basal metabolism, resulting in considerably higher energy and nutrient requirements per unit body weight.

The average-term infant triples in weight and doubles in length during the first year of life. Consequently, energy requirements in early childhood are very high. Newborns require three to four times more energy per unit body weight than do adults: 100 to 110 kcal/kg/day (1) compared to 25 to 30 kcal/kg/day for adults (2). Inefficiency of intestinal absorption contributes to this difference.

As a result of a child's rapid growth, protein requirements are higher in infancy than in adulthood. Total protein requirement is greater than the additive needs for essential amino acids by a factor of two to three. Protein intake of 1.5g/kg/day is recommended for infants and 1.1g/kg/day for children 1 to 3 years of age, compared with 0.8 to 1.0 g/kg/day for adults who engage in moderate levels of physical activity (3).

Infants require protein of high biologic value to ensure adequate consumption of essential amino acids (leucine, isoleucine, valine, threonine, methionine, phenylalanine, tryptophan, lysine, and histidine). Cysteine and tyrosine also are recognized as essential dietary proteins in infancy, although not beyond the first 6 months of life. The reason is unclear in the case of tyrosine, whereas for cysteine, there is a well-characterized delay in the maturity of the enzymatic pathway that converts methionine to cysteine. The minimal intake necessary to provide the indicated amounts of all essential amino acids would provide half or less of total protein requirements, indicating the importance of both quantity and quality of dietary protein.

The protein composition of human milk is ideal for infants. Breast milk provides on average 1 g of protein per 100 mL. Therefore, to achieve the recommended intake of 1.5g/kg/day, infants need to consume approximately 150 mL of breast milk per kg per day. This level may exceed the intake of many infants, yet protein deficiency generally does not occur in breast-fed infants. Apparently, any limitations in the quantity of breast milk protein consumed are compensated by the digestibility and quality of protein in breast milk (see Chapter 27). Currently available infant formulas contain all amino acids essential for infants and, therefore, provide protein of comparable quality to that of breast milk.

Need for carbohydrate and fat in infancy is restricted to those levels necessary to prevent ketosis and fatty acid deficiency, respectively. Total intake of carbohydrate and fat generally are adequate whenever total energy intake is appropriate.

Recommended dietary allowances (RDAs) have been established for essential nutrients for both the first and second 6-month intervals of life (see Table 29.1). Iron deficiency is the most common nutrient deficiency in early childhood,

TABLE 29.1

Recommended Dietary Allowances (or Adequate Intakes) in Infancy/Childhood[a]

Nutrient	Age			
	0–6 Mo	7–12 Mo	1–3 Yr	4–8 Yr
Protein (g)	9.1	11	13	19
Vitamin A (μg RE)	400	500	300	400
Vitamin D (μg)	10	10	15	15
Vitamin E (mg TE)	4	5	6	7
Vitamin K (μg)	2	2.5	30	55
Vitamin C (mg)	40	50	15	25
Thiamine (mg)	0.2	0.3	0.5	0.6
Riboflavin (mg)	0.3	0.4	0.5	0.6
Niacin (mg NE)	2	4	6	8
Vitamin B_6 (mg)	0.1	0.3	0.5	0.6
Folate (μg)	65	80	150	200
Vitamin B_{12} (μg)	0.4	0.5	0.9	1.2
Calcium (mg)	200	260	700	1,000
Phosphorus (mg)	100	275	460	500
Magnesium (mg)	30	75	80	130
Iron (mg)	0.27	11	7	10
Zinc (mg)	2	3	3	5
Iodine (μg)	110	130	90	90
Selenium (μg)	15	20	20	30
Biotin (μg)	5	6	8	12
Pantothenic acid (mg)	1.7	1.8	2	3
Copper (μg)	200	220	340	440
Manganese (mg)	0.003	0.6	1.2	1.5
Fluoride (mg)	0.01	0.5	0.7	1.0
Chromium (μg)	0.2	5.5	11	15
Molybdenum (μg)	2	3	17	22

[a]NE, niacin equivalent, which equals 1 mg of dietary niacin or 60 mg of dietary tryptophan; RE, retinol equivalent; TE, α-tocopherol equivalent.

Source: Dietary Reference Intakes (DRIs): Recommended Dietary Allowances and Adequate Intakes, Vitamins. Food and Nutrition Board, Institute of Medicine, National Academies. Available at: http://iom.edu/Activities/Nutrition/SummaryDRIs/~/media/Files/Activity%20Files/Nutrition/DRIs/RDA%20and%20AIs_Vitamin%20and%20Elements.pdf. Accessed on 6/11/2013.

with a prevalence of 4% deficiency at 6 months and 12% at 1 year of age (4). The adequate intake of iron is 0.27 mg per day from birth to 6 months of age and then increases to 11 mg per day from 7 to 12 months of age. Infants born at full-term usually have iron stores until approximately 4 to 6 months. For this reason, preterm infants that are breast-fed should be supplemented with 2 mg/kg/day of elemental iron starting at 1 month and continuing through 12 months to prevent deficiency. Iron supplementation of 1 mg/kg/day for exclusively breast-fed infants is recommended beginning at 4 months until complementary foods fortified with iron are introduced (4). Micronutrient fortified milk and cereal products have been found to reduce iron-deficiency anemia in children up to 3 years of age. (5). Increased use of iron-fortified infant formula among babies who were not breast-fed has substantially reduced the incidence of iron deficiency in this age group. Vitamin deficiencies are rare in adequately nourished infants. Vitamin K is provided by injection at or near the time of birth to prevent neonatal hemorrhage; subsequently, deficiency is uncommon.

An intake of 75 to 100 mL fluid per kg per day is considered adequate for the first years of life, but 150 mL is preferred as a defense against dehydration. A well-nourished infant generally easily meets the recommended intake with either breast milk or formula.

The nutrient recommendations for infants 6 to 12 months of age are based largely on extrapolation from the first 6-month period; less is known about the nutrient needs of infants 6 to 12 months old. There is currently debate regarding the optimal level of energy intake, with some recommending a reduction to 80 to 85 kcal/kg/day (1). Adequate growth apparently is maintained at the lower energy-intake level.

By 6 months of age, gastrointestinal physiology is substantially mature, and infants metabolize most nutrients comparably to adults. Nutrient needs can be met with breast milk or formula, but most authorities advocate the gradual introduction of solid foods beginning at or around 6 months. As infant foods begin to replace breast milk or formula, the nutrient density of the diet is apt to decline, and the introduction of a multivitamin supplement may be indicated. Of note, a recent study found an inverse association between early multivitamin supplementation, before the age of 4, and sensitization to food allergens and allergic rhinitis. No association was found in children that were supplemented with multivitamins after the age of 5 (6). Completion of weaning to solid food by 1 year of age is common practice and is appropriate.

Breast-Feeding

Breast milk is widely considered the optimal means of nourishing newborns, barring contraindications such as communicable disease in the mother. The properties of breast milk are discussed in greater detail in Chapter 27. Breast milk has lower calcium and phosphorus than does bovine milk. Compared to formula-fed infants, breast-fed infants have a less mineralized skeleton at several months of age, but there is no evidence that this is harmful. Bone density during the first several months of life is lower in breast-fed than in formula-fed infants because of the lower calcium and phosphorus of breast milk. Differences in bone density do not persist beyond infancy. Breast-feeding is also associated with transient hyperbilirubinemia during the first few days of life; if extreme, phototherapy is indicated to prevent kernicterus.

The protein content of breast milk seems lower than ideal, yet, as noted, breast-fed infants rarely display evidence of protein deficiency. The particular advantages of breast-feeding relate to the development of immune function and resistance to infection, development of the intestinal tract, and psychological bonding between mother and infant (see Chapter 27). There is increasing evidence that breast-feeding reduces the risk of infant and childhood infections (7,8). A recent study found that full breast-feeding for 6 months of life was associated with reduced risk of hospital admission for infections in the first year of life (9). Breast-feeding also likely protects against food allergy and intolerance as well, as discussed in Chapter 24.

An increasing body of evidence points to prolonged breast-feeding as protective against later obesity (10,11). The meta-analysis of several observational studies determined the risk of obesity for school-aged children was reduced by 15% to 25% in children who were breast-fed compared to children that were formula fed (12). Other studies have had similar results (13,14). One hypothesized mechanism for this is that mothers who breast-feed develop less restrictive feeding behavior and are more responsive to infant cues of hunger and satiety (15). A relationship has also been found between children who were breast-fed with improved appetite regulation during early childhood (16). The duration of breast-feeding has also been associated with a reduced risk of overweight dose-dependently. It was found that 1 month of breast-feeding was associated with a 4% decrease in overweight risk (OR, 0.96 per month of breast-feeding; 95% CI: 0.94, 0.98) (17).

The principal hazard of breast-feeding is the issue of supply; infants must be followed closely during the first few days to weeks of life to ensure normal growth. The adequacy of breast-feeding can be assessed by preprandial and postprandial weighings; every milliliter of milk consumed should add 1 g of weight.

Inclusion of cow's milk in the diets of infants 6 to 12 months old appears to be fairly common practice in the United States. There are concerns about converting from breast milk to bovine milk, rather than formula, as the principal source of nutrition after 6 months as this can result in protein and sodium intake well above recommendations. The substitution of bovine milk for formula also tends to reduce the iron level in the diet, and skim milk will reduce the intake of linoleic acid below recommended levels. Deficiency of essential fatty acids is the most significant concern regarding the use of bovine milk (whole or reduced fat) as the staple after 6 months. The substitution of skim or reduced-fat milk for whole milk in this age group does not confer any known benefit, nor does it appear to reduce total energy intake as a result of compensation for the missing calories (18,19).

Formulas are generally based on either unmodified or modified bovine milk protein. Bovine milk can be modified so that the whey-to-casein ratio approximates that of human milk. There is no clear evidence that either is superior. For infants intolerant of bovine milk protein, the protein can be hydrolyzed, or soy protein can be substituted. Soy-based formulas are appropriate for infants with lactose intolerance (see Chapter 18).

Formulas based on bovine milk protein typically provide 1.5 g of protein per 100 mL, or 50% more protein than breast milk. The nutrient composition of commercial formulas is otherwise very comparable to that of breast milk (see Table 29.2). Provided that a sanitary water supply is available, the safety of formula generally is not of concern. Properly nourished, a healthy infant should double in weight by 4 to 5 months of age and triple in weight by 12 months. Demand feeding is the preferred method of ensuring adequate energy intake.

Parental Feeding Practices

Children over the age of 1 year tend to eat an appropriate variety of foods/nutrients when provided access to them. Balance may not be achieved on any given day; however, provided that the child continues to be provided reasonable food choices, balance will be achieved over several days' time. Parents should be reassured that a balanced diet need not be measured on a per-meal or even per-day basis. A reasonable approach is to avoid any major distinction between snacks and meals so that healthy food can be eaten when the child is hungry, and meal size can be adjusted to account for snacking (20).

The food environment parents provide during childhood may have an effect on eating behaviors and weight later in the child's life. The foods provided during mealtime as well as parents eating style can both have an influence on the child's intake. Restriction and pressure can eventually lead to overeating, food dislikes, or disordered eating (21). One study analyzed four different parenting styles (authoritative, authoritarian, permissive, and neglectful), with the risk of having an overweight child. The authoritarian (strict disciplinarian) parenting style was determined to have the highest prevalence of overweight children (17.1%). Neglectful (emotionally uninvolved) and permissive (indulgent, without discipline) parenting had a 9.8% to 9.9% rate of overweight children. The authoritative parents (respectful of child's opinion, but maintain clear boundaries) were found to have the lowest prevalence of overweight children (3.9%) (22). This study as well as several others demonstrate the relationship between feeding styles and children's weight (23,24). A recent issue of the journal *Childhood Obesity* is devoted to this topic (see http://online.liebertpub.com/toc/chi/9/s1).

Childhood Overweight and Obesity

The prevalence of childhood and adolescent obesity in the United States from 2009 to 2010 was 16.9% (25). Although the incidence of obesity

TABLE 29.2

Composition of Commonly Available Commercial Formulas Compared to that of Breast Milk

Nutrient (Quantity Per Liter)	Nestle Good Start DHA & ARA	Human Milk	Similac with Iron (Abbott)	Enfamil Lipil (Mead Johnson)	Enfamil Prosobee Lipil[a] (Mead Johnson)	Similac Isomil[a] (Abbott)
Energy (kcal)	670	680	676	680	680	676
Protein (g)	15	10.5	14	14.2	16.9	16.55
Fat (g)	34	39	36.5	36	36	36.9
Percent polyunsaturated	22	14.2	26	20	20	27
Percent monounsaturated	33	41.6	40	37	37	40
Percent saturated	45	44.2	34	43	43	33
Carbohydrate (g)	75	72	73	74	72	69.6
Calcium (mg)	449	280	528	530	710	710
Phosphorus (mg)	255	140	284	290	470	507
Magnesium (mg)	47	35	41	54	74	50.7
Iron (mg)	10	0.3	12.2	12.2	12.2	12.2
Zinc (mg)	5	1.2	5.1	6.8	8.1	5.07
Manganese (μg)	101	6	34	101	169	169
Copper (μg)	536	252	609	510	510	507
Iodine (μg)	80	110	41	68	101	101
Sodium (mEq)	8	179.4	7.1	8	10.4	12.9
Chloride, (mEq)	12		12.4	12.1	15.2	11.8
Potassium (mEq)	19	526.5	18.2	18.7	21	18.7
Vitamin A (IU)	2,010	675	2,029	2,000	2,000	2,029
Vitamin D (IU)	402	0.5	406	410	410	406
Vitamin E (IU)	13	4	10.1	13.5	13.5	10.1
Vitamin K (μg)	54	2.1	54	54	54	74
Thiamine (μg)	670	210	676	540	540	406
Riboflavin (μg)	938	350	1,014	950	610	609
Pyridoxine (μg)	503	205	406	410	410	406
Vitamin B$_{12}$ (μg)	2	0.5	1.7	2.0	2.0	3.04
Niacin (mg)	7	1.5	7.1	6.8	6.8	9.13
Folic Acid (μg)	101	50	101	108	108	101
Pantothenic acid (mg)	3	1.8	3.04	3.4	3.4	5.1
Vitamin C (mg)	60	40	61	81.2	81	61
Biotin (μg)	29	4	29.8	20	20	30.4
Choline, mg	161		108	162	162	81
Inositol, mg	40		31.8	41	41	33.8

[a]Soy-based formulas.

Source: Values are derived from the 6th Edition of the Pediatric Handbook from the American Academy of Pediatrics, 2009.

has begun to level off over the past decade in the United States, childhood obesity still continues to be a worldwide epidemic requiring the focus of health professionals (26). Childhood obesity is associated with serious health problems including hypertension, dyslipidemia, type 2 diabetes, as well as quality of life issues (27). Many factors may lead to overweight or obese children including newborn feeding practices and parenting styles mentioned above, as well as the timing of the introduction of solid foods, increased portion sizes, increased intake of calories from sugar-sweetened beverages and high energy-dense foods, and lack of physical activity (28–32) (see Chapter 5).

The Institute of Medicine's (IOM) Committee on Obesity Prevention for Young Children recommends following the Dietary Guidelines for Americans for children 2 years of age and older and the American Academy of Pediatrics for children younger than 2. The IOM also suggests using "responsive feeding" practices in which parents provide healthy foods and children control the amount they eat using hunger and fullness cues. To further prevent obesity, the IOM also recommends limiting screen time to less than 2 hours per day for children ages 2 to 5, advises appropriate sleep duration for age, and promotes increasing physical activity (33). In 2011, the USDA replaced MyPyramid with MyPlate to better illustrate portion sizes for each food group with suggestions about how to prepare a healthy plate (34). The Dietary Guidelines for Americans and MyPlate recommend a healthy diet focusing on fruits, vegetables, whole grains, fat-free or low-fat milk and milk products, lean meats, and low in saturated fat, trans fat, cholesterol, salt, and added sugars (35).

Cardiovascular Disease

Studies show that children today are consuming a significantly greater volume of food and beverages than children did decades ago (29,36), as well as large amounts of soft drinks and fast foods not compensated for by physical activity (30,37). Most children still consume saturated and trans fat in excess of recommendations and fail to consume the recommended quantities of fruits and vegetables. National surveys have revealed excessive intake of both total and saturated fat in children over the age of 1 year (38,39). Dietary fat intake was excessive in children as young as 6 months in the Bogalusa Heart Study, which also demonstrated important racial differences in dietary patterns in young children, with African American children consuming more total energy and fat than their white counterparts (40,41). The increased prevalence of overweight and hypertension has also been observed to be disproportionately great among ethnic minority children (42).

A pathology study of adolescents and young adults who died of trauma demonstrated that elevated serum lipids, as well as smoking, influence the development of early signs of atherosclerosis in adolescents; the Bogalusa Heart Study found that childhood measures of low-density lipoprotein (LDL) cholesterol and body mass index (BMI) were predictive of carotid intima-media thickness, an important predictive measure of future atherosclerotic events (43). Elevated serum lipids probably contribute to early lesions of atherosclerosis in children 10 to 14 years old and may begin to do so in children between the ages of 3 and 9 years (44). Dietary intervention has been shown to lower the high cholesterol levels common among children in Finland, with levels rising again on resumption of the habitual diet (45). A follow-up study, The Special Turku Coronary Risk Factor Intervention Project (STRIP), was used to determine the possibility of reducing the effects of coronary risk factors using dietary counseling from 7 months to 19 years of age. Families met with a nutritionist who recommended an intake of fat between 30% and 35% with a ratio of 1:2 of saturated to monounsaturated/polyunsaturated fat and cholesterol intake less than 200 mg per day. Individualized counseling was also provided based on the children's food records, and recommendations were made for improved consumption. Study findings showed that low-fat dietary counseling started during infancy was found to have a positive effect on serum LDL-cholesterol levels and various lipoprotein measures, especially among boys, without negatively effecting children's growth (46,47). Therefore, from a population perspective, there appears to be little potential harm and considerable potential gain in promoting the dietary pattern recommended for adults to school-aged children as well (48).

The prudence of advocating the same diet for adults and children has been challenged. There is still only limited evidence that dietary restrictions in childhood prevent chronic disease in adults (49). Obtaining such evidence, however, is a daunting challenge. Indirect, epidemiological, and inferential evidence may be the best guidance available (50). Over the past decade, there has been controversy over the safety and efficacy of fat restriction after age 2 (51); proponents of the restriction of dietary fat beginning at age 2 cite evidence that atherosclerosis begins in childhood and that a diet with not more than 30% of calories from fat beginning at age 2 is compatible with optimal growth (52); others argue for a gradual transition to lower fat intake and attention to the type and distribution of dietary fat, as has been recommended in Canada (53).

Further support for advocating dietary fat restriction in particular for young children comes from epidemiological data in Italy. A recent rise in the consumption of saturated fat has been noted in a population with a traditionally health-promoting "Mediterranean" diet (54). A study of 100 Finnish school-aged children demonstrated that the intake of several important nutrients tended to be lower among the children with the highest fat intake (55). Further, this study suggested that the diets of young children are quite diverse, so that offering dietary recommendations was unlikely to "disrupt" a traditional dietary pattern chosen by families for their young children.

Efforts to resolve the debate regarding the safety of fat restriction in early childhood have resulted in controlled intervention studies (56–58). One earlier intervention trial (the Child and Adolescent Trial for Cardiovascular Health [CATCH]) examined the effects of a multidisciplinary program emphasizing change in school nutrition on cardiac risk factors in children beginning in third grade (59). The study lowered fat intake significantly and lowered serum cholesterol minimally. Growth and development were unaffected. Another study using the CATCH program also showed a significant effect in slowing the increased risk of overweight/obesity in low-income elementary schools serving primarily Hispanic students (60).

The Dietary Intervention Study in Children (DISC) randomly assigned 8- to 10-year-old children with LDL cholesterol above the 80th percentile to either usual care or a dietary intervention with 28% of energy from total fat, less than 8% from saturated fat, up to 9% from polyunsaturated fat, and less than 75 mg per 1,000 kcal cholesterol per day. After approximately 7 years of follow-up, children in the intervention group were found to have greater reductions in LDL-cholesterol levels compared to the usual care group, and they had no adverse effects on growth and development (61). Results of a long-term follow-up study, 9 years after the end of the original DISC study, showed that the consumption of a low-fat diet in childhood may contribute to significant blood pressure and glycemic control in adulthood (62).

In addition to the Dietary Guidelines for Americans and MyPlate recommendations mentioned above, the American Heart Association (AHA) guidelines for promoting cardiovascular health includes eating a variety of fruits and vegetables while limiting juice intake, choosing whole grain/high-fiber bread and cereals, and keeping fat intake between 30% to 35% of calories for children 2 to 3 years of age and between 25% to 35% above 3 years of age. Dairy products should include fat-free and low-fat; children ages 1 to 8 need 2 cups of milk or its equivalent per day and 3 cups per day for children from 9 to 18 years of age (63). It is hoped that these dietary modifications will not only constitute primary prevention, limiting the development of cardiovascular disease, but also act as primordial prevention, a term now used to describe the prevention of the development of cardiovascular risk factors (64). Furthermore, data from studies encourage a common eating pattern for families, with the implication that the fat content in the diets of children might decline, and all sources encourage the promotion of regular physical activity and fruit and vegetable consumption during childhood (65).

There is increasing evidence that efforts to modify the diets of children to reduce long-term cardiovascular risk are likely to be safe. Whether such diets reduce long-term risk is less clear. Obviously, evidence of long-term outcome effects is difficult to obtain. To be considered in the debate is the importance of providing a single, consistent dietary pattern for a family, as well as the issue of dietary patterns tracking over time. Data from the Bogalusa Heart Study and the Muscatine Study demonstrate that there is tracking through early childhood and adolescence of dietary pattern, physical fitness, and cardiovascular risk factors (66,67).

In light of these considerations, it appears that the recommendation in the United States to advocate a similar diet for everyone over the age of 2 years is reasonable and safe, and it may offer long-term benefits (68). Although there is some evidence that a comparable diet may be safe even before age 2 (69), consensus opinion in the United States and prudence argue against the imposition of macronutrient restrictions in this age group. Conclusive evidence of benefit from early dietary modification efforts will accrue very slowly.

Type 2 Diabetes

The prevalence of type 2 diabetes, formerly considered to be an adult-onset disease, among children and adolescents has been rising (see Chapter 6).

The cause of this disease in children is similar to adults as it includes factors such as obesity, metabolic syndrome, physical inactivity, and inflammation (70). Children at greatest risk for type 2 diabetes include children with BMI > 85th percentile, family history of DM, signs of insulin resistance such as dyslipidemia, hypertension, acanthosis nigricans, and polycystic ovary syndrome (71). Nutritional management is an important aspect of treatment in children with type 2 diabetes. The International Society for Pediatric and Adolescent Diabetes recommendations include eliminating sugar-sweetened beverages, reducing total and saturated fat intake, increasing fiber intake, portion control, and increased physical activity (71).

NUTRIENTS, NUTRICEUTICALS, AND FUNCTIONAL FOODS

n-3 Fatty Acids

Long-chain polyunsaturated fatty acids are particularly concentrated in the brain and retina. Eicosapentaenoic acid and docosahexaenoic acid (DHA) are relatively abundant in human breast milk and prominently incorporated into the developing brain (72,73). DHA in particular is considered essential to healthy brain development (74). Impaired cognitive development in premature infants may be related in part to insufficient availability of DHA during a critical period of brain development (75,76).

Breast-feeding has been associated with enhancement of IQ and visual acuity in infants (77,78), though recent evidence suggests that the evidence for an effect on intelligence may have been confounded by maternal IQ (79). The apparent health benefits of breast-feeding relative to formula feeding may be related in part to the DHA content of breast milk. Increasingly, long-chain polyunsaturated fatty acids, including DHA, are being added to commercial formulas (80). One recent double-blind, randomized trial compared DHA and arachidonic acid supplementation of infant formula to breast milk; at 4 years of age, children who had been fed either the DHA- and AHA-supplemented formula had visual acuity and verbal IQ scores similar to those who were breast-fed, while the control group had poorer visual acuity and poorer verbal IQ scores (81). Although the essential fatty acid *α*-linolenic acid is a precursor to DHA as well

as to eicosapentaenoic acid, conversion to DHA in particular appears to be limited and variable. The putative benefits of DHA apparently require that it be administered directly in the diet (82). Although health benefits of DHA supplementation are likely on the basis of confluent lines of evidence, the benefits are not yet conclusive (83).

Relevant Nutrigenomic Considerations

An association between children's environment and its effect on overweight and obesity has been found, but there may also be a genetic connection. A variant in the FTO (fat mass and obesity-associated) gene has been linked to obesity and BMI in several studies (84–86). Research has revealed that the FTO gene may play a role in the regulation of feeding and energy homeostasis (87). A study also determined that children with the A allele had a significantly higher weight, greater BMI, and consumed more energy-dense food at meals when compared to the noncarriers (88). As this nutrient–gene interaction research advances, future studies will be able to shed more light in its influence on health promotion and disease prevention.

SPECIAL CONSIDERATIONS

Hygiene Hypothesis

Over the past several decades, there has been a rise of several chronic inflammatory disorders, specifically allergies (asthma), autoimmune diseases (type 1 diabetes and multiple sclerosis), and inflammatory bowel disease (IBD), along with improvements in hygiene in developed and developing countries (89). The hygiene hypothesis, first formulated by Strachan in 1989, claims a patient's exposure to viral and bacterial infections as well as to microbials in the environment may decrease their risk of developing allergies and have an effect on their innate and adaptive immune response. The timing of exposure and genetics may also have an influence on immunity (90). Studies have found that children living on a farm who are exposed to a large amount of microbials have significantly lower rates of asthma and hay fever (91). A link between damaged regulatory T cells (Treg) and autoimmune disease has also been found (92). An association between *Helicobacter pylori*, helminthes, breast-feeding, and family size with the development of IBD was also indicated (93).

Low-Birth-Weight Infants

Approximately 7% of all infants born in the United States weigh less than 2,500 g at birth. The energy reserves of a term infant of normal size are enough to withstand nearly 1 month of starvation, whereas those of a 1,000 g infant would last only 4 to 5 days. Adequate nutrition is likely to be critical to normal cognitive development in premature and low-birth-weight (LBW) infants in particular. The caloric and protein density of formula generally allows for more rapid catch-up growth, but evidence to date suggests that breast milk may reduce the risk of infections and confer a range of other benefits as well, including superior visual acuity and cognition. In order to maximize the benefits of both, human milk is now often supplemented with protein for use in premature and LBW infants (94).

Energy needs of LBW infants are estimated to be 120 kcal/kg/day. Protein intake and weight gain are directly related in LBW infants; a protein intake of about 3 g/kg/day is recommended. For a variety of reasons, insensible water loss of LBW infants tends to be approximately twice that of term infants; fluid intake of approximately 140 mL/kg/day is recommended. Higher fluid intake can increase the risk of patent ductus arteriosus. A team of specialists is invariably involved in the nutritional management of LBW infants, and the details of such management are beyond the scope of this text.

CLINICAL HIGHLIGHTS

The provision of optimal nutrition during infancy and early childhood is of vital importance to growth and development and is likely related to a wide array of health outcomes later in life. The establishment of good nutriture for an infant begins while in utero, during which time maternal dietary practices may influence fetal metabolism (see Chapter 27).

The most reliable way to ensure optimal nutrition for a newborn is breast-feeding. Therefore, clinicians should routinely encourage breast-feeding for a period of 6 months unless the practice is contraindicated by communicable disease. This advice is based on the confluence of multiple lines of evidence.

The maintenance of salutary maternal nutrition during lactation is of importance to the health of both mother and baby (see Chapter 27). As evidence of the importance of DHA and other essential fatty acids continues to accrue, the composition of most commercial formulas has been revised to mimic levels found in breast milk.

Weaning to solid food generally should begin at approximately 6 months (see Chapter 24). Weaning from breast milk or formula is generally complete by around 12 months, although such practices are culturally determined; medically, weaning at 12 months is appropriate.

Children generally will self-select foods that meet micronutrient requirements when provided with an array of healthy food choices; this practice is to be encouraged. Children also reliably meet their energy needs, although energy intake may vary considerably by meal and even day. Parents should be reassured in this regard and discouraged from placing too great an emphasis on "plate cleaning;" whether or not such a practice contributes to later obesity is unknown, but an association is plausible. In addition, parental feeding practices have been associated with a child's eating behavior and weight status. Parents who use authoritative approach (respectful of child's opinion, but maintain clear boundaries) were found to have the lowest prevalence of overweight children.

Controversy persists regarding the optimal timing for approximating adult dietary guidelines in children. There is evidence that adult dietary recommendations are safe for children as young as 7 months of age, although few in the United States would endorse such a practice. Evidence is more definitive that the imposition of such guidelines beginning at age 2 is safe and reasonable. Taking this approach provides the added benefit of unifying family dietary practices earlier. There is evidence that dietary preferences established in childhood tend to persist (see Chapter 38), highlighting the importance of establishing a prudent dietary pattern early. Therefore, the diet that should be advocated to adults and older children to promote health (see Chapter 45) may be provided promptly, or approximated gradually, in children beginning at age 2. Micronutrient supplementation with a multivitamin/multimineral tailored for children is a reasonable practice. Regular consumption of fish should be encouraged. The consistent intake of DHA may offer considerable health benefits, which is supported by preliminary, but accumulating, evidence.

REFERENCES

1. FAO. Food and Nutrition Technical Report Series, Human Energy Requirements. *Energy requirements of infants from birth to 12 months.* Available at: http://www.fao.org/docrep/007/y5686e/y5686e05.htm; accessed 5/28/13.

2. Beach PS, Revai K , Niebuhr V. *Nutrition in infancy, childhood and youth: foundations for life.* Available at: http://www.utmb.edu/pedi_ed/CORE/Nutrition/page_08.htm; accessed 5/28/13.

3. Food and Nutrition Board of the Institute of Medicine. Dietary reference intakes for energy, carbohydrate. fiber, fat, fatty acids, cholesterol, protein, and amino acids (2002/2005). Available at: http://www.iom.edu/Global/News%20Announcements/~/media/C5CD2DD7840544979A549EC47E56A02B.ashx; accessed 5/28/13.

4. Baker R, Greer F. Diagnosis and prevention of iron deficiency and iron-deficiency anemia in infants and young children (0–3 years of age). *Pediatrics* 2010;126(5):1040–1050.

5. Eichler K, Wieser S, Ruthemann I, et al. Effects of micronutrient fortified milk and cereal food for infants and children: a systematic review. *BMC Public Health* 2012;12:506.

6. Marmsjö K, Rosenlund H, Bergström A, et al. Use of multivitamin supplements in relation to allergic disease in 8-y-old children. *Am J Clin Nutr* 2009;90(6):1693–1698.

7. Oddy WH, Sly PD, de Klerk NH, et al. Breast feeding and respiratory morbidity in infancy: a birth cohort study. *Arch Dis Child* 2003;88:224–228.

8. Duijts L, Jaddoe V, Hofman A, et al. Prolonged and exclusive breastfeeding reduces the risk of infectious diseases in infancy. *Pediatrics* 2010;126(1):e18–e25.

9. Ladomenou F, Moschandreas J, Kafatos A, et al. Protective effect of exclusive breastfeeding against infections during infancy: a prospective study. *Arch Dis Child* 2010;95(12):1004–1008.

10. Metzger MW, McDade TW. Breastfeeding as obesity prevention in the United States: a sibling difference model. *Am J Hum Biol* 2010;22(3):291–296.

11. Burke V, Beilin LJ, Simmer K, et al. Breastfeeding and overweight: longitudinal analysis in an Australian birth cohort. *J Pediatr* 2005;147:56–61.

12. Koletzko B, von Kries R, Grote V, et al. Can infant feeding choices modulate later obesity risk? *Am J Clin Nutr* 2009;89(5):1502S–1508S.

13. Toschke AM, Vignerova J, Lhotska L, et al. Overweight and obesity in 6- to 14-year-old Czech children in 1991: protective effect of breast-feeding. *J Pediatr* 2002;141:764–769.

14. Armstrong J, Reilly JJ. Breastfeeding and lowering the risk of childhood obesity. *Lancet* 2002;359:2003–2004.

15. Taveras EM, Scanlon KS, Birch L, et al. Association of breastfeeding with maternal control of infant feeding at age 1 year. *Pediatrics* 2004;114:e577–e583.

16. Disantis K, Collins B, Fisher J, et al. Do infants fed directly from the breast have improved appetite regulation and slower growth during early childhood compared with infants fed from a bottle? *Int J Behav Nutr Phys Act* 2011;8:89.

17. Harder T, Bergmann R, Kallischnigg G, et al. Duration of breastfeeding and risk of overweight: a meta-analysis. *Am J Epidemiol* 2005;162(5):397–403.

18. Wosje KS, Specker BL, Giddens J. No differences in growth or body composition from age 12 to 24 months between toddlers consuming 2% milk and toddlers consuming whole milk. *J Am Diet Assoc* 2001;101:53–56.

19. Huh S, Rifas-Shiman S, Rich-Edwards J, et al. Prospective association between milk intake and adiposity in preschool-aged children. *J Am Diet Assoc* 2010;110(4):563–570.

20. Allen RE, Myers AL. Nutrition in toddlers. *Am Fam Physician* 2006;74:1527–2532.

21. Scaglioni S, Salvioni M, Galimberti C. Influence of parental attitudes in the development of children eating behaviour. *Br J Nutr* 2008;99(suppl 1):S22–S25.

22. Rhee K, Lumeng J, Appugliese D, et al. Parenting styles and overweight status in first grade. *Pediatrics* 2006;117(6):2047–2054.

23. Hurley K, Cross M, Hughes S. A systematic review of responsive feeding and child obesity in high-income countries. *J Nutr* 2011;141(3):495–501.

24. Stang J, Loth KA. Parenting style and child feeding practices: potential mitigating factors in the etiology of childhood obesity. *J Am Diet Assoc* 2011;111:1301–1305.

25. Ogden C, Carroll M, Kit B, et al. Prevalence of obesity and trends in body mass index among US children and adolescents, 1999–2010. *JAMA* 2012;307(5):483–490.

26. de Onis M, Blössner M, Borghi E. Global prevalence and trends of overweight and obesity among preschool children. *Am J Clin Nutr* 2010;92(5):1257–1264.

27. Reedy J, Krebs-Smith S. Dietary sources of energy, solid fats, and added sugars among children and adolescents in the United States. *J Am Diet Assoc* 2010;110(10):1477–1484.

28. Huh S, Rifas-Shiman S, Taveras E, et al. Timing of solid food introduction and risk of obesity in preschool-aged children. *Pediatrics* 2011;127(3):e544–e551.

29. Piernas C, Popkin B. Increased portion sizes from energy-dense foods affect total energy intake at eating occasions in US children and adolescents: patterns and trends by age group and sociodemographic characteristics, 1977–2006. *Am J Clin Nutr* 2011;94(5):1324–1332.

30. Wang Y, Bleich S, Gortmaker S. Increasing caloric contribution from sugar-sweetened beverages and 100% fruit juices among US children and adolescents, 1988–2004. *Pediatrics* 2008;121(6):e1604–e1614.

31. Vernarelli J, Mitchell D, Hartman T, et al. Dietary energy density is associated with body weight status and vegetable intake in U.S. children. *J Nutr* 2011;141(12):2204–2210.

32. Metallinos-Katsaras E, Freedson P, Fulton J, et al. The association between an objective measure of physical activity and weight status in preschoolers. *Obesity* (Silver Spring, Md.). 2007;15(3):686–694.

33. Insitute of Medicine. *Early childhood obesity prevention policies.* Available at http://www.iom.edu/Reports/2011/Early-Childhood-Obesity-Prevention-Policies.aspx; accessed 5/4/13.

34. USDA. Choose a Food Group. Available at: http://www.choosemyplate.gov/foodgroups/. Accessed on May 4, 2013.

35. USDA. Dietary Guidelines. Available at: http://www.choosemyplate.gov/dietary-guidelines.html. Accessed on May 4, 2013.

36. Nicklas TA, Demory-Luce D, Yang S, et al. Are children consuming more food today than yesterday? *FASEB J* 2002;16:494–516.

37. St-Onge M-P, Keller KL, Heymsfield SB. Changes in childhood food consumption patterns: a cause for concern in light of increasing body weights. *Am J Clin Nutr* 2003;78:1068–1073.

38. Kimm S, Gergen P, Malloy M, et al. Dietary patterns of US children: implications for disease prevention. *Prev Med* 1990;19:432.

39. Nicklas TA, Elkasabany A, Srinivasan SR, et al. Trends in nutrient intake of 10-year-old children over two decades (1973–1994). *Am J Epidemiol* 2001;153:969–977.

40. Nicklas T, Farris R, Major C, et al. Dietary intakes. *Pediatrics* 1987;80:797.

41. Nicklas T, Morales M, Linares A, et al. Children's meal patterns have changed over a 21-year period: the Bogalusa Heart Study. *J Am Diet Assoc* 2004;104:753–761.

42. Sorof JM, Lai D, Turner J, et al. Overweight, ethnicity, and the prevalence of hypertension in school-aged children. *Pediatrics* 2004;113:475–482.

43. Shengxu L, Chen W, Srinivasan S, et al. Childhood cardiovascular risk factors and carotid vascular changes in adulthood. *JAMA* 2003;290:2271–2276.

44. Magnussen C, Niinikoski H, Raitakari O, et al. When and how to start prevention of atherosclerosis? Lessons from the Cardiovascular Risk in the Young Finns Study and the Special Turku Coronary Risk Factor Intervention Project. *Pediatr Nephrol* 2012;27(9):1441–1452.

45. Vartiainen E, Puska P, Pietinen P, et al. Effects of dietary fat modifications on serum lipids and blood pressure in children. *Acta Paediatr Scand* 1986;75:396.

46. Simell O, Niinikoski H, Viikari J, et al. Cohort Profile: the STRIP Study (Special Turku Coronary Risk Factor Intervention Project), an Infancy-onset Dietary and Life-style Intervention Trial. *Int J Epidemiol* 2009;38(3):650–655.

47. Niinikoski H, Pahkala K, Raitakari O, et al. Effect of repeated dietary counseling on serum lipoproteins from infancy to adulthood. *Pediatrics* 2012;129(3):e704–e713.

48. Kennedy E, Powell R. Changing eating patterns of American children: a view from 1996. *J Am Coll Nutr* 1997;16:524.

49. Lifshitz F. Children on adult diets: is it harmful? Is it healthful? *J Am Coll Nutr* 1992;11:84s.

50. Celermajer DS, Ayer JGJ. Childhood risk factors for adult cardiovascular disease and primary prevention in childhood. *Heart* 2006;92:1701–1706.

51. Taras HL, Nader P, Sallis JF, et al. Early childhood diet: recommendations of pediatric health care. *J Am Diet Assoc* 1988;88:1417.

52. Kleinman R, Finberg L, Klish W, et al. Dietary guidelines for children: US recommendations. *J Nutr* 1996;126:1028s.

53. Lifshitz F, Tarim O. Considerations about dietary fat restrictions for children. *J Nutr* 1996;126:1031s.

54. Greco L, Musmarra R, Franzese C, et al. Early childhood feeding practices in southern Italy: is the Mediterranean diet becoming obsolete? Study of 450 children aged 6–32 months in Campania, Italy. *Acta Paediatr* 1998;87:250.

55. Rasanen L, Ylonen K. Food consumption and nutrient intake of one- to two-year-old Finnish children. *Acta Paediatr* 1992;81:7.

56. Niinikoski H, Viikari J, Ronnemaa T, et al. Prospective randomized trial of low-saturated-fat, low-cholesterol diet during the first 3 years of life. The STRIP Baby Project. *Circulation* 1996;94:1386.

57. Niinikoski H, Lapinleimu H, Viikari J, et al. Growth until 3 years of age in a prospective, randomized trial with reduced saturated fat and cholesterol. *Pediatrics* 1997;99:687.

58. Kaitosaari T, Ronnemaa T, Raitakari O, et al. Effect of a 7-year infancy-onset dietary intervention on serum lipoproteins and lipoprotein subclasses in healthy children in the prospective, randomized Special Turku Coronary Risk Factor Intervention Project for Children (STRIP) Study. *Circulation* 2003;108:672.

59. Luepker R, Perry C, McKinlay S, et al. Outcomes of a field trial to improve children's dietary patterns and physical activity. The Child and Adolescent Trial for Cardiovascular Health (CATCH). *JAMA* 1996;275:768.

60. Coleman K, Tiller C, Dzewaltowski D, et al. Prevention of the epidemic increase in child risk of overweight in low-income schools: the El Paso coordinated approach to child health. *Arch Pediatr Adolesc Med* 2005;159(3):217–224.

61. Obarzanek E, Kimm SYS, Barton BA, et al. Long-term safety and efficacy of a cholesterol-lowering diet in children with elevated low-density lipoprotein cholesterol: seven-year results of the Dietary Intervention Study in Children (DISC). *Pediatrics* 2001;107:256–264.

62. Dorgan JF, Liu L, Barton BA, et al. Adolescent diet and metabolic syndrome in young women: results of the dietary intervention study in children (DISC) follow-up study. *J Clin Endocrinol Metab* 2011;96(12):E1999–E2008.

63. American Heart Association. Dietary Recommendations for Healthy Children. Available at:http://www.heart.org/HEARTORG/GettingHealthy/Dietary-Recommendations-for-Healthy-Children_UCM_303886_Article.jsp; accessed 5/4/13.

64. Weintraub WS, Daniels SR, Burke LE, et al. Value of primordial and primary prevention for cardiovascular disease: a policy statement from the American Heart Association. *Circulation* 2011;124:967–990.

65. Zlotkin S. A review of the Canadian "Nutrition Recommendations Update: Dietary Fat and Children." *J Nutr* 1996;126:1022s.

66. Srinivasan S, Myers L, Berenson G. Changes in metabolic syndrome variables since childhood in prehypertensive and hypertensive subjects: the Bogalusa Heart Study. *Hypertension* 2006;48(1):33–39.

67. Burns T, Letuchy E, Paulos R, et al. Childhood predictors of the metabolic syndrome in middle-aged adults: the Muscatine study. *J Pediatr* 2009;155(3):S5.e17–e26.

68. American Heart Association. Dietary recommendations for children and adolescents: consensus statement from the American Heart Association. *Circulation* 2005;112:2061–2075.

69. Talvia S, Lagstrom H, Rasanen M, et al. A randomized intervention since infancy to reduce intake of saturated fat: calorie (energy) and nutrient intakes up to the age of 10 years in the Special Turku Coronary Risk Factor Intervention Project. *Arch Pediatr Adolesc Med* 2004;158:41–47.

70. Kempf K, Rathmann W, Herder C. Impaired glucose regulation and type 2 diabetes in children and adolescents. *Diabetes Metab Res Rev* 2008;24(6):427–437.

71. Rosenbloom A, Silverstein J, Amemiya S, et al. Type 2 diabetes in children and adolescents. *Pediatr Diabetes* 2009;10 (suppl 12):17–32.

72. Wainwright PE. Dietary essential fatty acids and brain function: a developmental perspective on mechanisms. *Proc Nutr Soc* 2002;61:61–70.

73. Auestad N, Scott D, Janowsky J, et al. Visual, cognitive, and language assessments at 39 months: a follow-up study of children fed formulas containing long-chain polyunsaturated fatty acids to 1 year of age. *Pediatr* 2003;112:e177–e183.

74. Innis S. Dietary (n-3) fatty acids and brain development. *J Nutr* [serial online]. 2007;137(4):855–859.

75. Georgieff M, Innis S. Controversial nutrients that potentially affect preterm neurodevelopment: essential fatty acids and iron. *Pediatr Res* 2005;57(5 pt 2):99R–103R.

76. Crawford MA, Golfetto I, Ghebremeskel K, et al. The potential role for arachidonic and docosahexaenoic acids in protection against some central nervous system injuries in preterm infants. *Lipids* 2003;38:303–315.

77. Caspi A, Williams B, Moffitt T, et al. Moderation of breastfeeding effects on the IQ by genetic variation in fatty acid metabolism. *Proc Natl Acad Sci USA* 2007; 104(47):18860–18865.

78. Kramer M, Aboud F, Shapiro S, et al. Breastfeeding and child cognitive development: new evidence from a large randomized trial. *Arch Gen Psychiatry* 2008;65(5):578–584.

79. Der G, Batty GD, Deary IJ. Effect of breast feeding on intelligence in children: prospective study, sibling pairs analysis, and meta-analysis. *BMJ* 2006;333:945.

80. Qawasmi A, Landeros-Weisenberger A, Leckman J, et al. Meta-analysis of long-chain polyunsaturated fatty acid supplementation of formula and infant cognition. *Pediatrics* 2012;129(6):1141–1149.

81. Birch EE, Garfield S, Castaneda Y, et al. Visual acuity and cognitive outcomes at 4 years of age in a double-blind, randomized trial of long-chain polyunsaturated fatty acid-supplemented infant formula. *Early Hum Dev* 2007;83: 279–284.

82. Gerster H. Can adults adequately convert alpha-linolenic acid (18:3n-3) to eicosapentaenoic acid (20:5n-3) and docosahexaenoic acid (22:6n-3)? *Int J Vitam Nutr Res* 1998;68:159.

83. Morley R. Nutrition and cognitive development. *Nutrition* 1998;14:752–754.

84. Frayling T, Timpson N, McCarthy M, et al. A common variant in the FTO gene is associated with body mass index and predisposes to childhood and adult obesity. *Science (New York, NY)*. 2007;316(5826):889–894.

85. Dina C, Meyre D, Gallina S, et al. Variation in FTO contributes to childhood obesity and severe adult obesity. *Nat Genet* 2007;39:724–726.

86. Scuteri A, Sanna S, Chen WM, et al. Genome-wide association scan shows genetic variants in the FTO gene are associated with obesity-related traits. *PLoS Genet* 2007;3:e115.

87. Fredriksson R, Hagglund M, Olszewski PK, et al. The obesity gene, FTO, is of ancient origin, upregulated during food deprivation and expressed in neurons of feeding-related nuclei of the brain. *Endocrinology* 2008;149:2062–2071.

88. Cecil J, Tavendale R, Watt P, et al. An obesity-associated FTO gene variant and increased energy intake in children. *N Engl J Med* 2008;359(24):2558–2566.

89. Okada H, Kuhn C, Feillet H, et al. The 'hygiene hypothesis' for autoimmune and allergic diseases: an update. *Clin Exp Immunol* 2010;160(1):1–9.

90. von Mutius E. Allergies, infections and the hygiene hypothesis—the epidemiological evidence. *Immunobiology* 2007;212(6):433–439.

91. Riedler J, Braun-Fahrländer C, Eder W, et al. Exposure to farming in early life and development of asthma and allergy: a cross-sectional survey. *Lancet* 2001;358:1129–1133.

92. Guarner F, Bourdet-Sicard R, Rook G, et al. Mechanisms of disease: the hygiene hypothesis revisited. *Nat Clin Pract Gastroenterol Hepatol* 2006;3(5):275–284.

93. Koloski N, Bret L, Radford-Smith G. Hygiene hypothesis in inflammatory bowel disease: a critical review of the literature. *World J Gastroenterol* 2008;14(2):165–173.

94. Kuschel CA, Harding JE. Protein supplementation of human milk for promoting growth in preterm infants. *Cochrane Database Syst Rev* 2000;2:CD000433.

SUGGESTED READINGS

American Academy of Pediatrics. *Pediatric nutrition handbook*, 6th ed. Elk Grove Village, IL: American Academy of Pediatrics, 2009.

Dietz WH, Stern L, eds. *Guide to your child's nutrition. American Academy of Pediatrics.* New York, NY: Random House, 1999.

Dobrin-Seckler B, Deckelbaum R. Safety of the American Heart Association step 1 diet in childhood. *Ann N Y Acad Sci* 1991;623:263.

Koletzko B, Aggett PJ, Bindels JG, et al. Growth, development and differentiation: a functional food science approach. *Br J Nutr* 1998;80:s5–s45.

Lanting CI, Boersma ER. Lipids in infant nutrition and their impact on later development. *Curr Opin Lipidol* 1996;7:43.

Otten JJ, Hellwig JP, Meyers LD, eds. *Dietary reference intakes. The essential guide to nutrient requirements.* Washington, DC: National Academies Press, 2006.

Tamborlane WV, ed. *The Yale guide to children's nutrition.* New Haven, CT: Yale University Press, 1997.

Writing Group for the DISC collaborative research group. Efficacy and safety of lowering dietary intake of fat and cholesterol in children with elevated low-density lipoprotein cholesterol. The Dietary Intervention Study in Children (DISC). *JAMA* 1995;273:1429.

CHAPTER 30

Diet and Adolescence

T he nutritional requirements of adolescence differ from those of childhood by virtue of the adolescent's larger body size and the advent of sexual maturation. They differ as well from those of adulthood because of the metabolic demands of rapid growth. As a result, the recommended dietary allowances (RDAs), and now dietary reference intakes (DRIs), for adolescence differ from those of other periods of the life cycle (see Table 30.1). Nutrients of particular importance to all adolescents appear to be magnesium, zinc, and calcium. With the advent of menses, adolescent girls become particularly subject to iron deficiency.

Specific aspects of diet, health, and adolescence relate to physical activity patterns and issues of body image. Relatively sedentary adolescents are at risk of obesity because nutrient energy intake exceeds need. Adolescent obesity anticipates adult obesity. Similarly, the combination of inactivity and a diet excessive in processed and fast food high in saturated fat, sugar, salt, and calories predisposes to elevations of cholesterol, insulin, and possibly blood pressure.

Many adolescents participate in competitive sports and, therefore, are at potential risk of inadequate nutrient intake. Inadequate nutrients and energy are particularly problematic in those participating in sports requiring low body weight, such as wrestling, crew, gymnastics, and ballet.

In addition to the pressure to excel on the sports stage, with the increasing competitive nature in academics and college admissions, adolescents often feel the need to excel in the classroom. Teens continue to stay up late, consuming poor diets and unregulated supplements such as energy drinks with the goal of better concentration, performance, and stamina.

Body image is of particular importance to adolescents and may result in extreme efforts to control or modify diet. The adoption of vegetarianism by an adolescent may mask a weight-loss effort and, if so, may result in a nutritionally unbalanced diet. Eating disorders, considered psychiatric rather than truly nutritional disorders, are typically manifest in adolescence.

OVERVIEW

Factors influencing changes in dietary pattern in adolescence are both physiologic and social. Physiologically, energy and nutrient requirements are driven up by increasing body size and the advent of sexual maturation, including menarche in girls. Socially, adolescence affords opportunity for food selection independent of parental guidance, often for the first time. Such choices are often made on the basis of prevailing patterns in peer groups. Adolescents are particularly resistant to health promotion messages, likely a consequence of the need to exercise autonomy. Typical dietary patterns in adolescents are influenced by targeted advertising and industry promotions and, therefore, emphasize commercial products, such as sodas and fast foods, rather than unprocessed foods.

These poor eating patterns and newfound autonomy are manifest in the adolescent skipping meals. Adolescents may often skip any meal of the day; however, the most common meal skipped is breakfast. They describe sleeping late and therefore not having time to eat breakfast, poor appetite, and even trying to avoid weight gain by avoiding "excess calories" as common reasons for skipping. The process of skipping breakfast is thought to contribute to a reflex overcompensation of calories at later meals, but also limits important nutrients into the adolescent diet that are often associated with the first meal of the day such as vitamins A, B_6, B_{12}, iron, and calcium (1). Recent data have challenged many of these theories surrounding breakfast skipping. One recent study at Cornell University had students either

TABLE 30.1

Dietary Reference Intakes: Recommended Dietary Allowances/Adequate Intake for Adolescents[a]

Nutrient Energy[b]	Ages 9–13 Yr		Ages 14–18 Yr		Ages 19–30 Yr	
	Female	Male	Female	Male	Female	Male
Kcal (Sedentary lifestyle)	1,400–1,600	1,600–2,000	1,800	2,000–2,400	1,800–2,000	2,400–2,600
Kcal (Moderately Active)	1,600–2,000	1,800–2,200	2,000	2,400–2,800	2,000–2,200	2,600–2,800
Protein (g)	34	34	46	52	46	56
Sodium[c,h] (mg) (AI)	<1,500	<1,500	<1,500	<1,500	<1,500	<1,500
Vitamin A[d] (μg RAE)	600	600	700	900	700	900
Vitamin D (IU)	600	600	600	600	600	600
Vitamin E (mg TE)	11	11	15	15	15	15
Vitamin K (μg)(AI)	60	60	75	75	90	120
Vitamin C[d,e] (mg)	45	45	65	75	75	90
Thiamine (mg)	0.9	0.9	1.0	1.2	1.1	1.2
Riboflavin (mg)	0.9	0.9	1.0	1.3	1.1	1.3
Niacin (mg NE)	12	12	14	16	14	16
Vitamin B$_6$ (mg)	1.0	1.0	1.2	1.3	1.3	1.3
Folate[f] (μg)	300	300	400	400	400	400
Vitamin B$_{12}$ (μg)	1.8	1.8	2.4	2.4	2.4	2.4
Calcium[d,g] (mg)	1,300	1,300	1,300	1,300	1,000	1,000
Phosphorus (mg)	1,250	1,250	1,250	1,250	700	700
Magnesium (mg)	240	240	360	410	310	400
Iron[d,h] (mg)	8	8	15	11	18	8
Zinc[d] (mg)	8	8	9	11	8	11
Iodine (μg)	120	120	150	150	150	150
Selenium (μg)	40	40	55	55	55	55
Copper (μg)	700	700	890	890	900	900

[a]NE, niacin equivalent, which equals 1 mg of dietary niacin or 60 mg of dietary tryptophan; RAE, retinol activity equivalent; TE, α-tocopherol equivalent.

[b]Energy intake is expressed based on activity levels and requirement needed to maintain calorie balance, using average height and weight.

[c]These values represent AI (Adequate Intake) for sodium. The upper limit is 2200–2300. But recent guidelines have recommended further reducing intake of all African-Americans, those with hypertension, diabetes, or chronic kidney disease to <1500 mg. AIs are believed to cover the needs of healthy individuals, but lack data to define the percentage of individuals covered by this intake.

[d]Nutrients for which adolescent intake is most likely to fall short of recommendations.

[e]The recommended intake of vitamin C has been increased for adults from 60 to 200 mg per day.

[f]Daily intake of about 400 μg is recommended before conception to prevent neural tube defects. This intake is advisable in adolescent girls planning on becoming or at risk of becoming pregnant.

[g]Calcium supplementation may be particularly important in adolescent girls unless the diet is very calcium dense. An intake of 1,500 mg per day may be better than the RDA of 1,200 mg. During pregnancy and lactation, the calcium requirements of adolescent girls are even higher.

[h]Iron supplementation in adolescent girls may be indicated. Monitoring of the complete blood count after menarche is indicated but has low sensitivity for early iron deficiency. If an individual adolescent is believed to be at risk of deficiency, serum ferritin should be assayed.

Source: Adapted from Institute of Medicine. Dietary reference intakes: Recommended intakes for individuals. National Academy of Sciences, recently updated 2010. Available at http://www.iom.edu/Activities/Nutrition/SummaryDRIs/~/media/Files/Activity%20Files/Nutrition/DRIs/5_Summary%20Table%20Tables%201-4.pdf; accessed 4/10/13; U.S. Department of Agriculture and US. Department of Health and Human Services. Dietary guidelines for Americans, 7th ed. Washington, DC: U.S. Government Printing Office, 2010.

eat or skip breakfast and found the daily total caloric intake was 408 calories less in the breakfast skipping group indicating no overall daily reflex overcompensation (2). Overall, breakfast is associated with healthier body weights; the literature on cognitive effects in adolescents is limited, but benefits are clearly seen with individuals who are undernourished (3).

Although adolescents often voluntarily choose to skip sources of good nutrition, the problem of food insecurity cannot be overlooked. The WHO defines food security to be "when all people at all times have access to sufficient, safe, nutritious food to maintain a healthy and active life." The number of children and adolescents experiencing food insecurity in 2008 was about 11% of households (4). Children and adolescents spend a large majority of their time in the school setting, so with the passing of the Healthy Hunger-Free Kids Act of 2010, school districts that receive federal funding for specific meal programs are increasing the standards for nutrient-rich school foods and allowing students to access these foods in the comfort of their school (5).

As a consequence, dietary patterns established in adolescence may initiate susceptibility to obesity, hyperlipidemia, hypertension, and other chronic disease. The common preoccupation with body image during adolescence (particularly among girls), along with the psychosocial pressures of this period, is related to the development of eating disorders. Both anorexia and bulimia nervosa are typically first revealed in adolescence; these, along with binge eating disorder, are discussed further in Chapter 25.

Topics of importance in the dietary management of health during adolescence include obesity, hypertension, metabolic syndrome, attention deficit hyperactivity disorder (ADHD), diabetes, osteoporosis, vegetarian diets, athletic activity, school performance, and eating disorders (see Chapters 5, 6, 8, 14, 25, 32, and 43), as well as the nutritional demands of rapid growth. Although adolescents' energy requirements are high because of their rapid growth, the recommended dietary pattern is the same as that for adults. Recommendations call for calories predominantly from complex carbohydrates, but adolescents in developed countries tend to have diets particularly high in fat and sugar, a phenomenon that has led to markedly increased prevalence of

overweight and obesity in recent years (6) (see Chapter 5). The short-term risks of such a dietary pattern are modest, but the persistence of this pattern beyond adolescence is common and clearly is associated with the prevailing chronic diseases of adulthood.

In the United States, there continues to be a downward trend in pubertal age for children and adolescents. A variety of factors are linked to early puberty including higher meat consumption, increased dairy intake, and less vegetable consumption (7–9). One study evaluated female food consumption using food frequency questionnaires at 3, 7, and 10 years of age. Increased total and animal protein consumption weekly was associated with 49% of girls starting earlier puberty compared to 35% of girls with lower meat consumptions (7). The maximal rate of growth in height for girls occurs between the ages of 10 and 13, whereas for boys it is between the ages of 12 and 15 (10). In girls, peak height velocity usually occurs 0.5 years prior to menarche, with African American and Hispanic girls more commonly reaching these milestones earlier than Caucasian girls (11,12). The adolescent growth spurt contributes approximately 15% to 20% to adult height and 45% to 50% to adult weight. The growth during adolescence reduces the proportion of total body mass contributed by adipose tissue in boys but increases it in girls. Body fat in girls rises during adolescence from 10% to between 20% and 24%. A divergence in adiposity at adolescence contributes to the diverging nutritional requirements of males and females at this stage of life. By the end of adolescence, lean body mass in males on average is double that of females.

In girls, peak calorie intake typically occurs in the year of menarche. In boys, calorie intake continues to rise throughout the growth spurt, generally peaking near 3,400 kcal at about age 16. The divergence in lean body mass results in a marked divergence in macronutrient needs. The average daily caloric requirement per unit height rises during adolescence for boys, and it actually falls for girls because of the increasing proportion and lower metabolic demand of body fat.

The adequacy of energy intake in adolescents can be assessed through determination of body mass index and comparison to age-appropriate reference ranges (13). Inadequate energy intake in adolescents, if mild, tends to delay the growth spurt rather than prevent attainment of normal height. While RDAs were developed and DRIs are being developed on the basis of chronologic age, the developmental stage is a more reliable index of actual needs. The Tanner scale of sexual maturity is widely used and can guide nutritional recommendations to adolescents.

Protein intake in adolescents in the United States is more likely to exceed than to fall short of recommendations. However, if protein deficiency is suspected because of dietary restrictions, prealbumin and retinol-binding proteins are useful laboratory assays that provide high sensitivity for subclinical protein malnutrition.

National data suggest that in the United States, the average adolescent consumes a diet deficient in several key vitamins and minerals, most prominently calcium, iron, folate, vitamins A and E, zinc, and magnesium (14). Inadequate calcium intake is both common and of great concern in adolescents, as it contributes to the risk of osteoporosis and fractures in later life (see Chapter 14). Rapid growth and expansion of both blood volume and muscle mass lead to increased iron requirements in adolescence; with the onset of menarche, girls become further susceptible to iron deficiency. Serum ferritin is the most reliable measure of iron stores. Iron deficiency commonly leads to anemia, defined in adolescents as a hemoglobin level below 11.8 g per dL at ages 12 to 14.9 years and below 12.0 g per dL at 15 years and older. Adolescents have increased requirements for folate; supplementation may therefore be warranted. This is especially true for sexually active young women, given the demonstrated benefits of folate supplementation in reducing risk of neural tube defects if taken early in pregnancy (15) (see Chapter 27). Nominal zinc and magnesium deficiency are common in US adolescents, and inclusion in the diet of foods rich in these minerals (see Section VIIE) or supplementation (in a multivitamin/multimineral) is appropriate.

Micronutrient deficiencies have weakly associated with ADHD, specifically iron and zinc deficiency. Behavioral treatment and medications are still considered first line for treatment of adolescents with ADHD, but multiple dietary recommendations have been suggested. Recommendations include elimination diets (oligoantigenic diet and removal of additives/preservatives), supplementation of needed micronutrients, restricted refined sugars, and fatty acid supplementation. The elimination diets are considered burdensome on families, but these other more practical recommendations may show some future promise as the literature continues to become more robust (16,17).

In general, the dietary fiber intake of the US population is well below recommendations. Although there has been concern that high fiber intake could interfere with micronutrient absorption and adequate caloric intake among growing children and adolescents, the current recommendation of "age+5"—that is, fiber intake equal to age plus 5 to 10 g per day—is both safe and sufficient for disease prevention (18,19).

Excess energy and fat intake is common in children and adolescents in the United States, contributing to obesity, type 2 diabetes, and adult risk of cardiac events (20–22). Consumption of sugar-sweetened drinks such as soda (23) and increased sedentary activities—particularly television/video and computer use—have also been found to be associated with increased risk of obesity (24). As severity of obesity increases, the requirement for alternative strategies for control must be entertained. One strategy consists of adolescent bariatric surgery, still very rare, which account for 0.7% of national procedures. The most common procedure is the Roux-en Y gastric bypass accounting for 90% of the documented cases (25). Although it is still considered throughout the world as a morally challenging decision, lacking high-quality evidence, and typically a last resort, due to the severe health consequences of morbid obesity, it is important to evaluate this strategy as an option when alternative strategies continue to fail (26). The past two decades have witnessed a dramatic increase in the incidence of type 2 diabetes among obese children and adolescents (27). One syndrome correlated with obesity in adults is the metabolic syndrome, also known as syndrome X, or the insulin-resistance syndrome. This syndrome is often linked with hyperinsulinemia and is the term given to a constellation of symptoms including abnormalities in waist circumference, body weight, Triglycerides, high-density lipoprotein, blood pressure, and glucose levels. In adults, these risk factors have been inextricably tied with obesity and with worsening cardiac disease, hypertension, and most certainly type 2 diabetes (28,29). However, in adolescents the correlations are less apparent for a variety of reasons, including the numerous changes that occur during the development of adolescents through puberty, and changes in insulin resistance with hormonal variation (30). There continues to be no general consensus definition for metabolic syndrome in adolescents, but many national organizations have attempted to define criteria most notably in 2007, the International Diabetes Foundation for children between ages 10 and 16 years (>16 years old may use adult criteria). These criteria require central obesity and two additional risk factors (31). Although the long-term outcomes are less firmly established when associated with the cluster of risk factors, it is clear that the prevalence of metabolic syndrome is higher amongst obese adolescents, which in itself has clear associations with cardiovascular disease, diabetes, and insulin resistance (32,33).

The past three decades have witnessed a dramatic increase in the incidence of type 2 diabetes among obese children and adolescents. Now, approximately 1 in 3 new cases of diabetes mellitus in children <18 years old is type 2 DM, and as a result, primary care clinicians are being forced to provide care for many adult complications at an earlier age (34). Although medicines such as metformin are being attempted earlier to quell some of these complications of hyperinsulinemia and impaired glucose tolerance, most of these medications have not been tested for safety and efficacy in adolescents <18 years old (35). Cardiac risk factors established in adolescence or earlier are known to track into adulthood. Diabetes screenings as well as assessment of tobacco use and serum lipids, body mass index, blood pressure, physical activity level, and habitual diet are indicated in adolescence to reverse or prevent developing risk for cardiovascular disease in adulthood (36). Hypertension in adolescents poses increased long-term health risks; prompt identification and management are therefore warranted (37). A 2006 meta-analysis of controlled trials assessing effects of salt restriction on blood pressure in children found that modest reductions in dietary salt intake resulted in significant reduction in systolic blood pressure (38) (see Chapter 8).

On average, adolescents typically sleep about 7 hours nightly, while recommendations range from 8.5 to 9.5 hours (39). The decreased sleep duration has been attributed to many factors including social and school obligations and early school time. With adolescents staying up later at night, they are increasingly exposed to the toxic obesegenic environment and increased snacking (40). In addition, the hormone dysregulation associated with short sleep duration includes decreased leptin and increased ghrelin levels leading to increased hunger and overconsumption of calories throughout the day. Overall, short sleep duration in adolescents is strongly correlated with etiology and maintenance of obesity (41). Another method adolescents use to alter sleep is consumption of energy drinks. As mentioned earlier, energy drinks are becoming a popular supplement for teens for a variety of reasons. Introduced in Austria in 1987 (i.e., Red Bull) and brought to the United States in 1997, children, adolescents and young adults make up half of the energy drink consumption market (42). These drinks are marketed heavily toward youth for improving energy, athletic performance and concentration using catchy slogans, and compelling adolescent risk taking behavior (43). Self-surveys report 30% to 50% of adolescents and young adults consume energy drinks, primarily to compensate for insufficient sleep, to increase energy, and to "have more fun" (44,45). Energy drinks contain a variety of "secret" ingredients that tend to include caffeine and sugar most importantly, but also contains some combination of taurine, B vitamins, sugars, guarana, ginseng, ginkgo biloba, L-carnitine (46). Because energy drinks are considered a "natural dietary supplement" and not a "food," the regulations placed by the Food and Drug Administration are quite limited and safety determinations are put in the hands of the manufacturers (42). The most potent ingredient in these drinks is caffeine, and the lack of regulation poses a poignant danger. Small amounts of caffeine can have some clear benefits such as improving physical performance, reaction time, slowing fatigue, and increasing auditory vigilance; however, these effects are dose dependent, variable, and usually generated by adult studies. A recent pediatric policy recommended that adolescents and children should not exceed 100 mg per day of caffeine or 2.5 mg/kg/day (47). Another pediatric policy affirmed that stimulant-containing energy drinks have no place in the diets of children and adolescents (48). Translating recommendations into practice may be particularly difficult with adolescent patients (see Chapter 47). Dietary counseling in adolescence is most likely to be influential if it emphasizes current health, current activities, and/or appearance rather than long-term health effects to which adolescents generally feel relatively invulnerable. Dietary health promotion in the school setting may be particularly important (49,50), and there is some evidence that school-based interventions can help modify activity and nutrition behaviors (51–53). Home environment may also play a role: An association has been shown between adolescents who eat dinner with their families and more healthful dietary intake patterns, illustrating the importance of parental involvement as well (54,55).

In general, physical activity is beneficial to health and complementary to the health-promoting effects of prudent diet. Competitive athletics in adolescent girls, however, can lead to a syndrome known as the female athlete triad, which consists of osteoporosis, disordered eating, and menstrual disorders (56). Though initially thought to stem from low adiposity, menstrual disturbances in female adolescents are now believed to result principally from inadequate energy availability, which causes hypothalamic-pituitary hormone dysfunction (57,58) (see Chapters 29 and 34). Amenorrhea in particular is associated with reduced peak bone mass, stress fractures, and increased risk of osteoporosis in later years. In the treatment of adolescent amenorrhea, reductions in training or increases in energy intake or both and use of oral contraceptives may be indicated to restore menses and maintain normal bone mineralization (57,59).

Another potential risk related to athletics in adolescents is overconsumption of sports drinks, which can worsen overweight/obesity and dental erosion. In general, water is the most effective choice for hydration during sports unless there is a need for more rapid replenishment for prolonged periods (>1hr) of vigorous physical activity at which time sports drinks are perfectly appropriate (48).

Although the subject is of considerable interest to adolescents and their parents, there is no convincing evidence of a direct link between diet and acne. However, there may be an association between obesity and insulin resistance—conditions potentially modifiable through diet—with hyperandrogenism and risk of acne (59).

CLINICAL HIGHLIGHTS

In the United States, the average adolescent is at greater risk of nutritional excess and obesity than of macronutrient deficiencies. But even in the context of overnutrition, deficiencies of select micronutrients appear to be quite common. Deficiencies of iron, calcium, zinc, and vitamins A and C are particularly common, although other nutrients probably are not consumed at truly optimal levels. ω-3 Fatty acids tend to be deficient in the diets of children and adults alike. Although a balanced diet provides needed micronutrients, social pressures at adolescence tend to favor a particular pattern of dietary imbalance, with excessive intake of processed and fast foods and, consequently, sugar, salt, and fat. A multivitamin/multimineral supplement is an appropriate recommendation, although clearly not compensatory for an imprudent dietary pattern.

Energy requirements of athletes may not be met. This is particularly problematic for girls, who as a result may develop endocrinological disturbances and even amenorrhea. The resultant disruption of bone mineralization may be irreversible. Calcium supplementation, control of energy expenditure, and supplemental energy intake are all indicated to maintain menses and protect the bones of female athletes. In extreme cases, oral contraceptives should be used as well. Screening for iron-deficiency anemia is also recommended for menstruating girls.

Eating disorders often emerge at adolescence, and a high level of suspicion facilitates early detection. Management is specialized, relying in particular on expert and often multidisciplinary psychiatric care.

Risk factors for cardiovascular disease often develop during adolescence and, when they do, track into adulthood. Therefore, efforts to identify and modify risk factors for cardiovascular and other chronic disease in adolescents are clearly indicated, as are screening for hypertension, lipid disorders, and diabetes.

Modification of adolescent dietary patterns to promote health will be most effective if environmental as well as behavioral factors are addressed. Clinicians should educate their patients on proper

LIVERPOOL JOHN MOORES UNIVERSITY
LEARNING SERVICES

dietary habits and good sleep hygiene to decrease their dependence on "stimulant-seeking behaviors." Clinicians should be aware of the potential dangers of energy drink consumption. They should also include screening for episodic/chronic energy drink consumption. Children with cardiac conditions should be especially counseled on the risk of consuming caffeine-containing beverages including arrhythmias, syncope, and sudden death. The same overall dietary pattern recommended for health promotion in adults (see Chapter 45) is appropriate for adolescents, but translating such recommendations into practice represents a particular challenge with this age group.

REFERENCES

1. Deshmukh-Taskar PR, Nicklas TA, O'Neil CE, et al. The relationship of breakfast skipping and type of breakfast consumption with nutrient intake and weight status in children and adolescents: the National Health and Nutrition Examination Survey 1999–2006. *J Am Diet Assoc* 2010;110: 869–878.
2. Levitsky DA, Pacanowski CR. Effect of skipping breakfast on subsequent energy intake. *Physiol Behav* 2013;119:9–16.
3. Hoyland A, Dye L, Lawton CL. A systematic review of the effect of breakfast on the cognitive performance of children and adolescents. *Nutr Res Rev* 2009;22:220–243.
4. Nord M. *Food insecurity in households with children: prevalence, severity, and household characteristics.* Economic Information Bulletin 56. Economic Research Service: U.S. Department of Agriculture. 2009.
5. Food and Nutrition Service, USDA. National School Lunch Program and School Breakfast Program: nutrition standards for all foods sold in school as required by the Healthy, Hunger-Free Kids Act of 2010. Interim final rule. *Fed Regist* 2013;78:39067–39120.
6. Ogden CL, Carroll MD, Curtin LR, et al. Prevalence of overweight and obesity in the United States, 1999–2004. *JAMA* 2006;295:1549–1555.
7. Rogers IS, Northstone K, Dunger DB, et al. Diet throughout childhood and age at menarche in a contemporary cohort of British girls. *Public Health Nutr* 2010;13:2052–2063.
8. Gunther AL, Karaolis-Danckert N, Kroke A, et al. Dietary protein intake throughout childhood is associated with the timing of puberty. *J Nutr* 2010;140:565–571.
9. Wiley AS. Milk intake and total dairy consumption: associations with early menarche in NHANES 1999–2004. *Public Libr Sci One* 2011;6:e14685.
10. Tanner JM, Davies PS. Clinical longitudinal standards for height and height velocity for North American children. *J Pediatr.* 1985;107:317–329.
11. Biro FM, Huang B, Crawford PB, et al. Pubertal correlates in black and white girls. *J Pediatr* 2006;148:234–240.
12. Biro FM, Galvez MP, Greenspan LC, et al. Pubertal assessment method and baseline characteristics in a mixed longitudinal study of girls. *Pediatrics* 2010;126:e583–e590.
13. American Academy of Pediatrics. *Pediatric nutrition handbook*, 4th ed. Elk Grove Village, IL: American Academy of Pediatrics, 1998.
14. Gleason P, Suitor C. *Children's diets in the mid-1990s: dietary intake and its relationship with school meal participation, DCN-01-CD1.* Alexandra, VA: US Department of Agriculture, Food and Nutrition Service, 2001.
15. Institute of Medicine. *Nutrition during pregnancy: part I, weight gain: part II, nutrient supplements.* Washington, DC: National Academy Press, 1990.
16. Millichap JG, Yee MM. The diet factor in attention-deficit/ hyperactivity disorder. *Pediatrics* 2012;129:330–337.
17. Subcommittee on Attention-Deficit/Hyperactivity Disorder, Steering Committee on QualityImprovement and Management. ADHD: clinical practice guideline for the diagnosis, evaluation, and treatment of attention-deficit/ hyperactivity disorder in children and adolescents. *Pediatrics* 2011;128:1007–1022.
18. Williams CL, Bollella M, Wynder EL. A new recommendation for dietary fiber in childhood. *Pediatrics* 1995;96:985–988.
19. Williams CL. Dietary fiber in childhood. *J Pediatr* 2006;149: s121–s130.
20. Berenson GS, Srinivasan SR, Nicklas TA. Atherosclerosis: a nutritional disease of childhood. *Am J Cardiol* 1998; 82:22t–29t.
21. Bronner YL. Nutritional status outcomes for children: ethnic, cultural, and environmental contexts. *J Am Diet Assoc* 1996;96:891–903.
22. Groner JA, Joshi M, Bauer JA. Pediatric precursors of adult cardiovascular disease: noninvasive assessment of early vascular changes in children and adolescents. *Pediatrics* 2006;118:1683–1691.
23. Ludwig DS, Peterson KE, Gortmaker SL. Relation between consumption of sugar-sweetened drinks and childhood obesity: a prospective, observational analysis. *Lancet* 2001;357:505–508.
24. Utter J, Neumark-Sztainer D, Jeffery R, et al. Couch potatoes or French fries: are sedentary behaviors associated with body mass index, physical activity, and dietary behaviors among adolescents? *J Am Diet Assoc* 2003;103:1298–1305.
25. Tsai WS, Inge TH, Burd RS. Bariatric surgery in adolescents: recent national trends in use and in-hospital outcome. *Arch Pediatr Adolesc Med* 2007;161:217–221.
26. Hofmann B. Bariatric surgery for obese children and adolescents: a review of the moral challenges. *BMC Medical Ethics* 2013;14:18.
27. Hannon TS, Rao G, Arslanian SA. Childhood obesity and type 2 diabetes mellitus. *Pediatrics* 2005;116:473–480.
28. Eckel RH, Grundy SM, Zimmet PZ. The metabolic syndrome. *Lancet* 2005;365:1415–1428.
29. Ferrannini E. Metabolic syndrome: a solution in search of a problem. *J Clin Endocrinol Metab* 2007;92:396–398.
30. Moran A, Jacobs Jr DR, Steinberger J, et al. Changes in insulin resistance and cardiovascular risk during adolescence: establishment of differential risk in males and females. *Circulation* 2008;117:2361–2368.
31. Zimmet P, Alberti KG, Kaufman F, et al; IDF Consensus Group. The metabolic syndrome in children and adolescents – an IDF consensus report. *Pediatr Diabetes* 2007;8:299–306.

LIVERPOOL JOHN MOORES UNIVERSITY
LEARNING SERVICES

32. Weiss R, Dziura J, Burgert TS, et al. Obesity and the metabolic syndrome in children and adolescents. *N Engl J Med* 2004;350:2362–2374.

33. Cook S, Auinger P, Li C, et al. Metabolic syndrome rates in United States adolescents, from the national health and nutrition examination survey, 1999–2002. *J Pediatr* 2008;152:165–170.

34. Springer SC, Silverstein J, Copeland K, et al. Management of type 2 diabetes mellitus in children and adolescents. *Pediatrics* 2013;131:e648–e664.

35. Kane MP, Abu-Baker A, Busch RS. The utility of oral diabetes medications in type 2 diabetes of the young. *Curr Diabetes Rev* 2005;1:83–92.

36. Gidding SS. Preventive pediatric cardiology. Tobacco, cholesterol, obesity, and physical activity. *Pediatr Clin North Am* 1999;46:253–262.

37. Luma GB, Spiotta RT. Hypertension in children and adolescents. *Am Fam Physician* 2006;73:1558–1568.

38. He FJ, MacGregor GA. Importance of salt in determining blood pressure in children: meta-analysis of controlled trials. *Hypertension* 2006;48:861–869.

39. Eaton DK, McKnight-Eily LR, Lowry R, et al. Prevalence of insufficient, borderline, and optimal hours of sleep among high school students – United States, 2007. *J Adolesc Health* 2010;4:399–401.

40. Klingenberg L, Chaput JP, Holmbäck U, et al. Sleep restriction is not associated with a positive energy balance in adolescent boys. *Am J Clin Nutr* 2012;96:240–248.

41. Hart CN, Cairns A, Jelalian E. Sleep and obesity in children and adolescents. *Pediatr Clin North Am* 2011;58:715–733.

42. Reissig CJ, Strain EC, Griffiths RR. Caffeinated energy drinks – a growing problem. *Drug Alcohol Depend* 2009;99;1–10.

43. Miller, KE. Wired: energy drinks, jock identity, masculine norms, and risk taking. *J Am Coll Health* 2008;56:481–489.

44. O'dea JA. Consumption of nutritional supplements among adolescents: usage and perceived benefits. *Health Educ Res* 2003;18:98–107.

45. Malinauskas BM, Aeby VG, Overton RF, et al. A survey of energy drink consumption patterns among college students. *Nutr J* 2007;6:35.

46. Higgins JP, Tuttle TD, Higgins CL. Energy beverages: content and safety. *Mayo Clin Proc* 2010;85:1033–1041.

47. Seifert SM, Schaechter JL, Hershorin ER, et al. Health effects of energy drinks on children, adolescents, and young adults. *Pediatrics* 2011;127:511–528.

48. Committee on nutrition and the council on sports medicine and fitness. Sports drinks and energy drinks for children and adolescents: are they appropriate? *Pediatrics* 2011;127:1182–1189.

49. Lytle LA. Lessons from the Child and Adolescent Trial for Cardiovascular Health (CATCH): interventions with children. *Curr Opin Lipidol* 1998;9:29–33.

50. Centers for Disease Control and Prevention. Guidelines for school health programs to promote lifelong healthy eating. *MMWR* 1996;45:1–41.

51. Kong AS, Sussman AL, Yahne C, et al. School-based health center intervention improves body mass index in overweight and obese adolescents. *J Obes* 2013;2013:575016.

52. Sharma M. School-based interventions for childhood and adolescent obesity. *Obes Rev* 2006;7:261–269.

53. Summerbell CD, Waters E, Edmunds LD, et al. Interventions for preventing obesity in children. *Cochrane Database Syst Rev* 2005;3: CD001871.

54. Hammons AJ, Fiese BH. Is frequency of shared family meals related to the nutritional health of children and adolescents? *Pediatrics* 2011;127:e1565–e1574.

55. Gillman MW, Rifas-Shiman SL, Frazier AL, et al. Family dinner and diet quality among older children and adolescents. *Arch Fam Med* 2000;9:235.

56. Birch K. Female athlete triad. *BMJ* 2005;330:244–246.

57. Warren MP, Stiehl AL. Exercise and female adolescents: effects on the reproductive and skeletal systems. *J Am Womens Assoc* 1999;54:115.

58. Loucks A, Vurdun M, Heath E. Low energy availability, not stress of exercise, alters LH pulsatility in exercising women. *J Appl Physiol* 1998;84:37–46.

59. American Academy of Pediatrics Committee on Sports Medicine and Fitness. Medical concerns in the female athlete. *Pediatrics* 2000;106:610–613.

■ SUGGESTED READINGS

Dietz WH, Stern L, eds. *American Academy of Pediatrics guide to your child's nutrition.* New York, NY: Villard Books, 1999.

Jacobson MS, Rees JM, Golden NH, et al., eds. Adolescent nutritional disorders. Prevention and treatment. In: *Annals of the New York Academy of Sciences*, Volume 817. New York, NY: The New York Academy of Sciences, 1997.

Neinstein Ls, Gordon C, Katzman D, et al., eds. *Adolescent health care: a practical guide*, 5th ed. Philadelphia, PA: Lippincott Williams & Wilkins, 2007.

Neumark-Sztainer D, Story M, Perry C, et al. Factors influencing food choices of adolescents: findings from focus-group discussion with adolescents. *J Am Diet Assoc* 1999;99: 929–937.

Riley M, Bluhm B. High blood pressure in children and adolescents. *Am Fam Physician* 2012;85:693–700.

Stang J, Story M, eds. Nutrition needs of adolescents. In: *Guidelines for adolescent nutrition services.* Minneapolis, MN: University of Minnesota, 2005:21–34.

Story M, Neumark-Sztainer D. Promoting healthy eating and physical activity in adolescents. *Adoles Med* 1999;10:109.

Marie-Pierre S, Keler K. Nutrition in adolescence. In: Ross CA, Benjamin C, Cousins RJ, et al., eds. *Modern nutrition in health and disease*, 11th ed. Philadelphia, PA: Lippincott Williams & Wilkins, 2012:734–744.

McNaughton SA. Understanding the eating behaviors of adolescents: application of dietary patterns methodology to behavioral nutrition research. *J AM Diet Assoc* 2011;111:226–229.

Tamborlane WV, ed. *The Yale guide to children's nutrition.* New Haven, CT: Yale University Press, 1997.

CHAPTER 31

Diet and Senescence

Nutritional factors play important roles in the process of aging. Requirements for energy and specific nutrients change as a result of altered metabolism, diminished energy expenditure, and changes in behavioral patterns. The optimal adjustments in micronutrient intake for individuals older than 65 or the "older old," greater than age 80, are uncertain, but progress is being made in this area of study, and new recommendations are being generated.

Even more fundamental than the modified energy needs of older age is the role nutrition appears to play in the physiology of aging. Oxidation is emerging as an important aspect of cellular aging; therefore, dietary pro-oxidants and antioxidants may influence the nature and pace of the aging process itself. Research into the metabolic pathways that regulate longevity is well underway, and the SIRT1 complex, AMPK, and mTOR are emerging as key players that are modulated by caloric restriction. Animal studies demonstrate convincing extension of the lifespan with reduced energy intake, provided that micronutrient adequacy is maintained; the implications of this for humans are at present as speculative as tantalizing, but our understanding of the physiology is advancing.

Nutritional recommendations may be made with some confidence both to older patients trying to maintain health and to younger patients seeking ways to forestall the effects of aging. The importance of optimal nutrition for the elderly population continues to increase with the size of this population and the prolongation of life expectancy.

OVERVIEW

Diet

Life expectancy is steadily increasing and may soon reach 85 to 90 years (1). Current projections suggest that by the year 2030, as much as 20% of the US population will be 65 or older (2).

Assigning particular physiologic characteristics to the process of aging is a complex and controversial process. Cellular degradation, the accumulation of oxidative stress, and a putative limit to the replicative capacity of DNA appear to be key components. Recent study into the antiaging effects of resveratrol, a compound concentrated in the skin of grapes, has suggested the governance of aging processes by a discrete cluster of genes and their products, including SIRT1, SIRT3, SIRT4, PBEF, and FoxOs (3–5). Whatever the natural pace of aging might be, it is clearly influenced, in humans and other species, by environmental stressors. Among such stressors are not only infectious disease and trauma but also nutrient excess and deficiency, psychological stress, sleep quality and quantity, environmental toxins, and an array of other factors (6,7).

Daily energy consumption is driven largely by resting metabolic rate (RMR), which accounts for 60% to 75% of the total (8). An additional 10% is accounted for by postprandial thermogenesis, the thermic effect of food. The energy consumed as fuel for physical activity can vary by nearly 30-fold, from a low of approximately 100 kcal per day (8).

Aging is associated with reductions in RMR, postprandial thermogenesis, and physical activity, with declines in activity disproportionately responsible for reduced energy expenditure (8,9). People older than 65 initially are subject to weight gain and obesity because they tend to maintain the energy intake of their younger years and reduce their expenditure. On the other hand, the older old greater than 80 are increasingly subject to weight loss and the sequelae of malnutrition as a result of reduced intake. The decline in RMR associated with aging is the result of reduced fat-free body mass, as well as the effects of reduced physical activity (10). Studies suggest that the association between age and declining RMR begins at around age 40 in men (8).

Use of the doubly labeled water method suggests that energy requirements of the elderly may, in general, have been underestimated (11,12). Such methods also suggest that an age-related increase in body fat may be largely attributable to reduced physical activity (11,13). The potential hazards of both undernutrition and overnutrition in the elderly have been noted (14). Energy requirements generally decline with age, predominantly because of a loss of lean body mass and associated change in metabolic rate, as well as reductions in energy expenditure in physical activity (15,16). There is evidence that basal metabolic rate declines with age to some degree; some reduction in RMR not attributable to declines in physical activity or fat-free mass is apparent (17).

A regimen of regular physical activity can, to varying degrees, preserve lean body mass in the elderly and will naturally result in higher energy requirements, while conferring a host of health benefits as is true in younger age groups. A study of 11 healthy women with a mean age of 73 revealed that, with maintenance of physical activity, energy expenditure was not reduced as a product of age (18). Evidence suggests that the effects of aging on energy requirements and body composition are quite variable and modified substantially by general health and physical activity (18,19). A longitudinal evaluation of elderly subjects found that higher levels of physical activity were associated with higher muscle mass (20).

Although in general energy requirements decline with age, in part or whole because of diminished physical activity and consequent loss of lean body mass, there is evidence that energy intake goes down disproportionately. Consequently, many elderly, particularly those living alone and homebound, are undernourished (21,22). One multinational study estimated that over a fifth of all elderly are malnourished, with higher prevalence of undernutrition in the rehabilitation and hospital settings (23). Factors influencing reduced energy intake in elderly individuals include changes in olfaction or taste, poor dentition, dysphagia, constipation, anorexia, as well as several comorbid conditions such as cancer, infection, or delirium (see Chapter 38) (24). Of note, inadequate nutrition was found to predict future health care costs and risk of future hospitalizations (25).

Aging is associated with a substantial increase in proportional body fat, along with a loss of lean body mass up to age 65 or so, after which body fat content declines as well. As overall life expectancy increases, sarcopenia, the age-related degenerative loss of muscle size and strength, is emerging as a major health concern (26). Similar to osteoporosis, sarcopenia is exacerbated by inactivity and counteracted by exercise. Diet and protein consumption may also play a role. As people age, negative energy balance and particularly negative nitrogen balance becomes more significant. As energy intake falls, protein requirements to avoid negative nitrogen balance rise (27). Protein requirements tend to rise in the elderly, especially those with limited mobility. Both inactivity and reduced muscle mass tend to result in negative nitrogen balance, requiring increased protein consumption to compensate (28). A recent randomized crossover trial found that amino acid supplementation in elderly sarcopenic patients showed improved nutritional status as well as increased muscle strength (29). Likewise, a recent review of 17 studies concluded that nutritional supplementation was an effective treatment for age-related sarcopenia, particularly when combined with exercise (30). One formulation of β-hydroxy-β-methylbutyrate, glutamine, and arginine was found to decrease the rate of muscle breakdown in patients with cachexia-inducing conditions (31,32).

Protein requirements remain relatively stable in elderly people whose functional status and activity are preserved. Whereas protein deficiency appears not to be a problem in most elderly people who live independently, protein malnutrition is common among those living in institutions (33). Increased protein is needed particularly when demands rise in the context of injury or illness, both of which are common in the elderly. There is no evidence that protein intake above 0.8 g per kg accelerates a decline in renal function in elderly people who show no evidence of renal insufficiency (15). For elderly people in whom renal insufficiency is established, protein restriction may be indicated (see Chapter 16).

Because many protein-rich foods have a high nutrient content in general, their consumption by elderly should be encouraged (15). Protein intake in the elderly in the United States is generally near the recommended 0.8 to 1 g/kg/day. The maintenance of nitrogen balance is strongly influenced by total energy intake. When energy intake is inadequate, negative nitrogen balance occurs even with putatively adequate protein intake. Inadequate protein intake can lead to suppressed immune function, poorer healing, and increased recovery time from illness (28).

Even when a person's weight stays consistent, energy requirements decline with advancing age, whereas protein requirements remain fairly constant or increase (33). Therefore, the maintenance of adequate protein nutriture requires the percentage of calories from protein to rise over time. For example, 56 g per day of protein would be required to provide 0.8 g/kg/day to a 70 kg individual. At an energy intake of 2,500 kcal, protein would constitute 9% of calories. At a reduced energy intake of 1,800 kcal, protein would constitute over 12% of calories (33). Carbohydrate and fat intake guidelines for the elderly do not differ from those for younger adults.

Whereas the maintenance of adequate nutritional intake in the elderly is a priority, calorie restriction over time is associated with longevity in most species studied (34). In virtually all species studied to date, caloric restriction appears to lower body temperature, reduce basal metabolic rate, and reduce signs of oxidative injury to cells, organelles, and DNA (35). Although several mechanisms have been proposed, one leading hypothesis is that the reduction in mitochondrial free radical generation underlies the markedly reduced oxidative damage (a major factor in the pathological aging process) seen in caloric restriction (36).

The effects of restricted energy intake result not only in optimizing survival (i.e., raising mean survival to nearer the predicted maximum) but in extending the natural lifespan as well. Preliminary studies of caloric restriction in primates suggest that the same effects seen in rodents and other species also occur in primates (37). Caloric restriction appears to affect longevity via multiple signaling pathways involving modulation of inflammation, cellular survival, stress defense, autophagy, and protein synthesis (38). Emerging research involves the AMPK/mTOR pathway that is modulated by both metformin and rapamycin. The pathways involving SIRT1 are also a topic of special interest as SIRT1 is activated by resveratrol, a compound found in the skin of grapes and in red wine. Studies examining the effects of resveratrol on protein expression and enzymatic activity are yielding insights into the potential mechanisms by which calorie restriction promotes longevity (39,40).

Sparking significant debate, recent evidence supporting the "obesity paradox" suggests that being overweight (BMI of 25 to 29.9) or being classified as having stage 1 obesity (BMI of 30 to 34.9) was associated with a decrease in all-cause mortality (41). This paper built upon prior work showing that obesity poses less risk of premature mortality to older subjects than to younger (42). However, only those individuals who have already avoided early mortality live to experience obesity late in life, and obesity at earlier ages, including middle age, is clearly associated with increased risk of premature mortality (43) (see Chapter 5). Obesity has been shown time and time again to cause serious medical complications and exacerbate age-related functional declines in older adults (44). Weight loss in older, obese adults associated with diet and exercise has been shown to improve physical function (45). The study by Flegal et al. (41) also cautions that obesity in general is related to a significant increase in mortality (see Chapter 5).

There is, to date, no confirmatory evidence in humans that energy restriction directly extends survival, although it does appear to improve biomarkers of longevity (46). A recent randomized trial found that after 6 months on a very-low-calorie diet, overweight adult male subjects had significantly decreased levels of fasting insulin and body temperature (47). Nonetheless, there is no evidence that caloric restriction initiated in old age is beneficial (48). If calorie restriction is beneficial in humans, energy restriction must be accompanied by nutrient supplementation to prevent deficiencies. Other hurdles to caloric restriction involve quality of life issues like decreased bone density, decreased muscle mass, hunger, lethargy, and feelings of cold (49).

Arguments for modifying the contributions of various fats to the diet are made throughout this text (see Chapters 5, 7, and 45). As the maintenance of adequate energy and micronutrient intake in the elderly is often of paramount importance, efforts to restrict fat intake in elderly patients whose fat intake was not previously restricted are likely to be justified only when in response to some specific health risk or need. In elderly subjects already adhering to a fat-restricted diet, there is likely to be little reason to increase fat intake, provided that weight maintenance is satisfactory (15). In either case, supplementation of fat-soluble vitamins is likely to be prudent.

The reduction in physical activity associated with age and resultant decline in energy consumption leads to reduced intake of micronutrients unless the nutrient density of the diet is intentionally altered. The decline in micronutrient intake places the elderly at risk of subtle deficiencies, with potentially important implications for health (33). In the population over 65 years old, 80% have one or more chronic medical conditions requiring use of prescription drugs. Both the disease state and the pharmacotherapy may influence metabolism (33), and polypharmacy is associated with increased risk of malnutrition (50). The wide variation in the state of health and the rate of aging, producing extreme heterogeneity among the elderly with regard to energy and nutrient requirements, limits the utility of broad, age-specific recommendations (33).

Skeletal muscle is approximately 40% less at age 70 than during early adulthood (33), resulting in declines in RMR of 1% to 2% per decade beginning at age 25. Between ages 25 and 75, a person would have to reduce energy consumption by 25% to maintain energy balance and avoid excessive body fat. But the maintenance of a comparably nutrient-dense diet over time would then result in a corresponding 25% reduction in the intake of micronutrients.

For some nutrients, intake is generally sufficiently abundant so that such a reduction would preserve adequacy. For others, such a reduction might lower intake below the desired threshold. Intake levels of copper, zinc, chromium, calcium, and vitamin D during adulthood typically do not allow for a 25% reduction, thus placing the elderly at risk of deficiency (see Nutrients, Nutriceuticals, and Functional Foods).

Between 1997 and 2002, the Food and Nutrition Board of the Institute of Medicine released a set of nutrition recommendations for all age groups. Unlike previous guidelines that focused on avoiding dietary deficiencies, the new recommendations reflect an emphasis on health promotion and disease prevention. In addition, there are now age-specific recommendations for adults age 51 to 70 and adults over 70 years of age, based on the growing recent literature examining nutritional issues in the elderly (51). The recommended dietary allowances (RDAs) for these two age groups are shown in Table 31.1, and are accessible online (52).

There is evidence that deficiencies of vitamins C, B_6, and B_{12} are fairly prevalent among the elderly in the United States. On this basis, supplementation, at least with the doses provided by a multivitamin, seems prudent (15).

TABLE 31.1

Recommended Dietary Allowance (in Bold) or Adequate Intake (in Regular Font) for Certain Vitamins and Minerals for Males and Females Aged 51 to 70 and Over Age 70[a]

Nutrient	Females			Males		
	Age 31–50	Age 51–70	Age >70	Age 31–50	Age 51–70	Age >70
Vitamin A (μg/d)	**700**	**700**	**700**	**900**	**900**	**900**
Vitamin C (mg/d)	**75**	**75**	**75**	**90**	**90**	**90**
Vitamin D (μg/d[b])	15	15	20	15	15	20
Vitamin E (mg/d)	**15**	**15**	**15**	**15**	**15**	**15**
Vitamin B_6 (mg/d)	**1.3**	**1.5**	**1.5**	**1.3**	**1.7**	**1.7**
Vitamin B_{12} (μg/d)	**2.4**	**2.4**	**2.4**	**2.4**	**2.4**	**2.4**
Folate (μg/d)	**400**	**400**	**400**	**400**	**400**	**400**
Calcium (mg/d)	1,000	1,200	1,200	1,000	1,000	1,200
Chromium (μg/d)	25	20	20	35	30	30
Selenium (μg/d)	**55**	**55**	**55**	**55**	**55**	**55**
Zinc (mg/d)	**8**	**8**	**8**	**11**	**11**	**11**

[a]The RDA for younger adults is shown for comparison.

[b]Each μg of cholecalciferol = 40 IU of vitamin D.

Source: Data derived from Otten JJ, Hellwig JP, Meyers LD, eds. *Dietary reference intakes. The essential guide to nutrient requirements.* Washington, DC: National Academies Press, 2006; Institute of Medicine. *Dietary Reference Intakes for Calcium and Vitamin D.* Washington, DC: National Academy Press, 2011.

In general, deficiency of fat-soluble vitamins is infrequent because of large tissue stores. One exception in the elderly appears to be vitamin D, the levels of which decline with age because of decreased consumption, decreased sun exposure, and decreased efficiency of the body's ability to convert provitamin D to the active form (15). Recent evidence suggests that higher doses of vitamin D than previously advised may confer a range of health benefits (see Chapter 12). The Institute of Medicine recommends supplementation of 600 IU of vitamin D in the elderly through age 70 and increased supplementation to 800 IU beyond 70 (53).

Although most mineral requirements do not appear to change with aging per se, metabolic disturbances associated with disease or treatment (e.g., diuretic use) may alter certain nutrient needs. Iron requirements tend to decline somewhat with age, especially in postmenopausal women; elderly women in particular may benefit from increased calcium intake (54). The RDA for vitamin A may be too high for the elderly, as absorption appears to increase with age (33).

In a 1997 review of the nutritional needs of the elderly, Blumberg (55) recommended eggs as a dietary source of the macronutrients and micronutrients often deficient in older adults. Recent studies suggesting that egg consumption is unlikely to adversely affect cardiovascular risk lend support (see Chapter 7). Nutrient density is of particular importance in the diets of the elderly, given reduced energy intake and largely preserved or increased micronutrient and protein requirements (55,56).

In 1998, Saltzman and Russell (57) reviewed age-dependent changes in gastrointestinal (GI) physiology. The principal changes cited include achlorhydria secondary to *Helicobacter pylori*-induced atrophic gastritis and lactose intolerance. The former can impair absorption of iron, folate, calcium, and vitamins K and B_{12}, whereas the latter may contribute to poor calcium nutriture. With these exceptions, GI function is well preserved with aging and generally is not the limiting factor in the maintenance of optimal nutritional status (51).

Serum glucose levels tend to rise with age, and suggestions have been made for age-specific thresholds for defining fasting hyperglycemia (15). Age-related glucose intolerance may be compensated by relative restriction of simple sugar intake. Hyperglycemia even in the absence of diabetes may be associated with increased mortality. One cohort study found that HbA(1c) was associated with increased mortality in nondiabetic kidney disease (58). Nonenzymatic glycosylation (NEG) of in vivo proteins is believed to play an important role in the process of senescence (59).

Complex carbohydrates should be prioritized as a source of fiber, both soluble and insoluble, and of micronutrients. Dietary fiber intake in the United States is approximately 12 g per day among adults, whereas the recommended amount is 25 to 30 g per day. Reductions of energy consumption by elderly patients are likely to result in low fiber intake as well. The elderly are particularly susceptible to constipation and are apt to benefit from increased consumption of dietary fiber.

The more rapid intestinal transit time that comes with increased fiber consumption, however, may reduce mineral absorption, increasing the risk of deficiencies in the elderly. Therefore, increased nutrient density or supplementation is indicated when fiber intake is augmented (33). Fruits, vegetables, and cereal grains may offer protection against constipation, diverticulosis, and nutrient deficiencies. Dentition should be assessed in making such recommendations; ability to eat fruit and vegetables may be impaired in elderly patients with poor dentition (15,60).

Aging is associated with a decline in immune function, as well as greater susceptibility to an array of micronutrient deficiencies. In a study of institutionalized elderly individuals with evidence of micronutrient deficiencies, multivitamin supplementation (B complex, vitamins C and E, and β-carotene) for a period of 10 weeks significantly enhanced immune function, as gauged by cutaneous hypersensitivity reactions to injected antigens (61). While multivitamins have not been shown to decrease rates of infection (62), they have been shown to decrease the length of infections (63).

The effects of aging on cell-mediated immunity are accentuated in individuals with nutritional deficiencies (64). Mazari and Lesourd (65) studied the effects of age and nutritional status on cell-mediated immunity. Although T-cell function was reduced in elderly people compared with young adults, the differences were much greater among the elderly with one or more indications of nutritional impairment. The authors conclude that some of what has traditionally been considered an age-dependent decline in immune function is, in fact, nutrition dependent.

Elderly patients are particularly subject to dehydration and its sequelae because of reduced body water, diminished renal concentrating ability, diminished thirst, insensitivity to antidiuretic hormone, and susceptibility to orthostatic hypotension due to reduced autonomic tone. Thirst is not a very reliable index of hydration status among the elderly.

Recommendations to maintain optimal fluid status are for fluid intake of 30 mL per kg of actual weight, 1 mL per kcal consumed, or 1,500 mL per day, whichever is highest; this is generally appropriate under conditions of typical daily activity (15,33). A study examining the prevalence of dehydration in community-dwelling older adults reported virtually no evidence of dehydration in those subjects ingesting six or more glasses of fluid per day (66).

Kerstetter et al. (33) offer a practical approach that does not require patients to measure their fluid intake so precisely. Maximal concentration of urine at age 90 is estimated at 800 mosmol per L, down from 1,200 mosmol per L at younger age. Therefore, in the elderly, fluid intake should be maintained at a level that allows for the excretion of approximately 1,200 mosmol of solute waste per day. This amount would require at least 1.5 L of urine produced per day for the very elderly. At this concentration, the urine appears light yellow. Therefore, a level of fluid intake that results in urine that is consistently light yellow implies adequate hydration status.

In an article on the potential benefits of complementary medicine to an aging population, Bland (67) characterizes the functional declines of aging in discrete categories, such as impaired mitochondrial function related to oxidative stresses, glycation of functional proteins, chronic inflammation, and impaired methylation. Many of the physiologic changes of aging are nutrient responsive. Mitochondrial function may be influenced by a range of nutrients, including ubiquinone, n-acetylcysteine, lipoic acid, creatine, vitamin E, and n-acetylcarnitine (67,68).

Glycation may be reduced by improved glucose tolerance, potentially influenced by intake of chromium, magnesium, and other nutrients (67) (see Chapter 6). Inflammation may be reduced by augmenting intake of n-3 fatty acids and by other interventions. Methylation is supported by adequate intake of B vitamins and can be tracked by the level of plasma homocysteine (67). Although the evidence for various nutritional interventions in efforts to curtail adverse effects of aging varies, many "complementary" or "alternative" practices are consistent with the weight of available evidence in the scientific literature.

Elderly patients are more likely to be taking medications and are typically more susceptible to adverse effects related to food–drug interactions. Coumarin-based anticoagulants are commonly taken to prevent life-threatening clot formation. It is important to note that foods rich in vitamin K such as spinach, kale, or other greens can render such anticoagulants inactive (69). Likewise tetracycline antibiotics should not be taken with dairy products or foods rich in divalent cations calcium, magnesium, iron, or zinc, as they can decrease bioavailability through physicochemical binding (70). Certain food–drug interactions can also make medications too effective. For example, monoamine oxidase inhibitors (MAO-I), medications used to treat depression and Parkinson's symptoms, may be associated with increased adverse effects when taken with tyramine containing foods like cheese or aged wines.

Food intake, especially foods high in fat content, can slow the rate of gastric emptying. Medication bioavailability can often vary in response to whether the stomach is empty or full. Taking some medications like nonsteroidal anti-inflammatory drugs with food may decrease GI upset or irritation. Such variation highlights the importance of carefully reading and following medication labels.

NUTRIENTS, NUTRICEUTICALS, AND FUNCTIONAL FOODS

Vitamin D

Actual or suspected lactose intolerance, as well as prevailing social patterns, tends to limit milk consumption by the elderly. Fortified dairy products and fatty fish—intake of which tends to be low among the elderly—are the principal dietary sources of vitamin D. The skin's ability to manufacture vitamin D with exposure to sunlight becomes less efficient with age, and the elderly tend to reduce their amount of sun exposure. Therefore, vitamin D deficiency appears to be fairly widespread among the older population, and a recent study of more than 1,200 independent, community-dwelling older persons found that nearly 50% were vitamin D deficient or insufficient at the onset of the trial. Moreover, those with baseline vitamin D deficiency were at significantly greater risk of future nursing home admission than were equivalent individuals with high vitamin D levels (71). Low levels of vitamin D may also be associated with increased diabetes, hypertension, hyperlipidemia, and peripheral vascular disease (72). Deficiency of vitamin D leads to impaired calcium absorption, compounding the generally inadequate calcium intake in this age group. Current recommendations suggest supplementation with 600 IU of vitamin D alone or as part of a multivitamin as a prudent precaution against deficiency and accelerated osteopenia. Even higher doses, of 800 IU, are recommended for adults over the age of 71 and those at high risk of deficiency (53). High-dose supplementation in this range appears to reduce the risk of both falls (73) and fractures (74). A growing body of research is also supporting an inverse and dose-dependent relationship with colorectal cancer. A meta-analysis of 18 prospective studies found that each 10 ng/ml increment in vitamin D levels was associated with a RR of 0.74 for colorectal cancer (75) (see Chapter 12).

Vitamin C

The RDA for vitamin C is currently 75 to 90 mg per day (76). There is no specific evidence that deficiency occurs more commonly among the elderly than among younger people, but specific populations, such as those who have dementia or reside in nursing homes, appear to have reduced intakes of vitamin C, and smokers of any age have increased requirements to compensate for the oxidative damage of smoking. High-dose supplementation is not known to be particularly beneficial, but there is some evidence that maintaining adequate stores of vitamin C (whether through diet or supplementation) may be a valuable preventive health measure (77). For the same reasons that intake up to 500 mg per day (see Chapter 45 and Section VIIE) may be beneficial to other age groups, intake in this range may offer benefits to the elderly as well.

Vitamin B$_6$

The current RDA for vitamin B$_6$ is 1.5 mg in females and 1.7 mg in males over the age of 51. Recent evidence suggests that even this revised level

is too low. Intake of vitamin B$_6$ among the elderly often fails to meet the RDA. Low intake of vitamin B$_6$ may contribute to elevations of serum homocysteine and accelerated atherosclerosis. A vitamin B$_6$ supplement of 2 mg per day is indicated for the elderly; most multivitamins provide this dose.

Vitamin B$_{12}$

Atrophic gastritis is more prevalent in the elderly than in others and, therefore, so is vitamin B$_{12}$ deficiency. In individuals with atrophic gastritis, vitamin B$_{12}$ must be supplemented parenterally because intrinsic factor is lacking. Less severe vitamin B$_{12}$ deficiency due to poor diet may also occur and may contribute to cognitive impairment, anemia, or elevated homocysteine levels in older people. Vitamin B$_{12}$ supplementation in a multivitamin is reasonable and appropriate for elderly individuals.

Folate

Folate deficiency does not appear to be a particular problem associated with aging. However, low folate intake will occur when the diet is poor and may contribute to elevations in homocysteine. Folate supplementation in the form of a multivitamin is appropriate. Note that symptoms of vitamin B$_{12}$ deficiency, a much more common problem in this population, may be masked by high folate consumption; folate supplements should therefore also include vitamin B$_{12}$, and the index of suspicion for vitamin B$_{12}$ deficiency should be high so that it is detected early if it occurs.

Calcium

Calcium intake throughout life tends to be lower than recommended, especially for women (see Chapter 14). In the elderly, the discrepancy between recommended and actual intake is more pronounced with calcium than perhaps any other micronutrient. Calcium absorption declines with age, particularly after age 60 or so (33,78). This decline in function is compounded by vitamin D deficiency. Marginal intake of both vitamin D and calcium contributes to age-related bone loss and the risk of fracture (79). The elderly are particularly susceptible to osteoporosis and related fracture. Adequate calcium intake may forestall osteoporotic fracture (80), but it cannot restore bone density already lost. Calcium intake is also associated with reduced risk of colon cancer (see Chapter 12) and reduction in blood pressure (see Chapter 8). Reduced-fat dairy products are preferable as dietary sources of calcium, but supplementation with up to 1,000 to 1,200 mg per day may offer benefits.

One recent study suggests a modest association between calcium supplementation and risk of cardiovascular disease (81). This study, a subgroup analysis from the Women's Health Initiative, did not control for known risk factors for cardiovascular events (82). At this time, current research supports continued supplementation with calcium (83).

Copper

The current RDA for copper is 0.9 mg per day for both younger and older adults. Copper intake is often inadequate in the elderly due to decreased total caloric intake. Copper is needed for hematopoiesis, and deficiency can result in both anemia and neutropenia, particularly in tube-fed institutionalized elderly patients. Idiopathic myopathy in adults may also be a result of unrecognized copper deficiency (84).

Chromium

The typical American diet provides approximately 15 μg per 1,000 kcal of chromium. At the prevailing level of chromium density, at least 2,000 kcal per day would be required to meet recommended intake, placing the elderly at particular risk for deficiency. Deficiency of chromium impairs glucose and insulin metabolism, produces elevations of serum triglycerides, and is associated with peripheral neuropathy (33). Older adults with, or at risk for, type 2 diabetes may particularly benefit from chromium supplementation (85,86).

Zinc

Zinc intake is below the recommended level for adults in the United States, and the gap is greater for the elderly. Zinc appears to affect immunity. As immune dysfunction is characteristic of aging and may result in life-threatening infections, efforts to maintain optimal immune function are important.

Consumption of less than 10 mg per day by elderly individuals may impair immunity, wound healing, and the acuity of taste and smell (33). The average diet provides approximately 5 mg of zinc per 1,000 kcal; therefore, 3,000 kcal would be required to provide the recommended 12 to 15 mg per day.

Zinc is abundant in poultry, fish, and meat, and diets rich in these sources may provide a greater density of zinc. However, increased meat consumption generally is precluded by efforts to limit fat intake and promote fruit and vegetable consumption. Zinc supplementation of 15 mg per day is a reasonable precaution; this level is provided by most multivitamin/multimineral supplements. A randomized controlled trial found that daily supplementation of 45 mg of zinc in elderly subjects reduced incidence of infections and levels of oxidative stress markers compared to placebo (87).

Iron

Iron requirements decline with age for women because of the cessation of monthly blood loss following menopause (54). Even though iron absorption declines with age, iron stores tend to increase (33).

Magnesium

Magnesium intake in developed countries is often marginal in all age groups. Whereas intake in the range of 4 mg/kg/day is common, 6 mg/kg/day is considered more appropriate (88). Deficiency is particularly likely among the elderly, due to reduced intake, depletion associated with chronic disease states such as type 2 diabetes mellitus, and impaired GI absorption (89). Clinical consequences may include sleep disturbance, cognitive impairment, and myalgias (88). Although the results of trials demonstrating sustained benefit of magnesium supplementation are lacking to date, the use of diet or supplements to achieve an intake level greater than 5 mg/kg/day appears justified (88). Of note, use of magnesium-containing laxatives among the elderly may lead to hypermagnesemia.

Resveratrol

Resveratrol is an antioxidant concentrated in the skin of grapes, and thus in red wine. Animal research suggests potent effects on enzyme systems of vital importance to diverse processes of aging, in particular cellular oxygen consumption (40,90). High-dose administration in rodent models appears to forestall aging (39). Encouraging studies in humans show that resveratrol supplementation may improve inflammatory biomarkers and decrease expression of proatherosclerotic factors (91,92). Supplementation, however, is not currently advised, but the topic is of clear interest and warrants close attention.

Coenzyme Q_{10}

Coenzyme Q_{10} or CoQ_{10} is an antioxidant found in mitochondria that inhibits the oxidation of both lipids and proteins. Oral supplementation with CoQ_{10} appears to be safe and well tolerated at doses as high as 3,600 mg daily, although the observed safety level is 1,200 mg per day. One study published in 2004 showed that supplementation with CoQ_{10} reduced oxidation of and breaks in DNA (93). It also showed a modest increase in lifespan in rats with controlled diet and CoQ_{10} supplementation. Follow-up studies, however, have not found effective lengthening of lifespan or slowing of aging in mice with supplementation (94–96). CoQ_{10} supplementation may have a role in specific diseases like CHF or migraine, but does not appear to have any clear effect on longevity.

CLINICAL HIGHLIGHTS

Aging is associated with a loss of lean body mass and an increase in body fat up until the sixth decade. Thereafter, both lean mass and fat mass diminish. Energy requirements tend to decline with age, in part because of reduced physical activity and in part because of the loss of metabolically active tissue. Nutrient and energy intake, however, tend to decline disproportionately to energy needs, so that many elderly are undernourished.

Energy deficiency in the elderly results in negative nitrogen balance with accelerated muscle loss. Deficiencies of micronutrients, particularly of B vitamins, vitamin D, and certain minerals, such as zinc, are very common. Use of prescription medications may compound age-related changes in olfaction, taste, and GI motility, contributing to poor dietary intake.

Emphasis in primary care should be on the maintenance of weight and especially preservation of lean body mass, whether through nutrient-dense diet, nutritional supplementation, or by exercise.

The decrease in all-cause mortality evidenced by the obesity paradox likely supports the avoidance of malnourishment and the maintenance of lean body mass more than the promotion of obesity per se. Elderly people should be encouraged to become or remain physically active as their functional status permits. Periodic assessment of dietary intake, informally or via referral to a dietitian, may be helpful in ensuring maintenance of adequate nurture. A multivitamin/multimineral supplement is a low-cost and safe means of protecting elderly patients against several common micronutrient deficiencies, although specific evidence of benefit from such a practice is lacking.

An effort to increase the nutrient density of the diet is a valid, although more difficult, alternative, and the two practices are complementary rather than mutually exclusive. Common sequelae of aging, such as cognitive and immunologic deficits, may be due in part to nutrient deficiencies and, therefore, are potentially preventable or reversible. There is convincing evidence to support supplementing the diets of elderly patients with zinc, chromium, magnesium, calcium, and possibly copper, along with vitamins. There is some suggestive evidence that nutrients not traditionally included on the RDA lists, such as ubiquinone (coenzyme Q_{10}) and lipoic acid, may offer benefits for elderly patients.

As patients age, the short-term functional benefits of adequate nurture may need to be compared with any long-term consequences of specific dietary practices. For example, whereas the cholesterol content of eggs may be a relevant consideration in younger adults at long-term risk for coronary disease, the nutrient density of eggs may provide benefits in excess of any risks for elderly patients. A diet rich in a variety of fruits and vegetables offers the same array of benefits to the elderly as to younger age groups.

Specific nutriceutical practices to confer longevity are of tantalizing interest, and our understanding of the basic science behind how such supplements could work continues to develop. Evidence guiding clinical practice, however, is still in progress.

REFERENCES

1. Olshansky SJ, Carnes BA, Cassel CK. In search of Methuselah: estimating the upper limits to human longevity. *Science* 1990;250:634.
2. Roush W. Live long and prosper? *Science* 1996;273:42.

3. Baur JA, Pearson KJ, Price NL, et al. Resveratrol improves health and survival of mice on a high-calorie diet. *Nature* 2006;444:337–342.

4. Nemoto S, Fergusson MM, Finkel T. SIRT1 functionally interacts with the metabolic regulator and transcriptional coactivator PGC-1(alpha). *J Biol Chem* 2005;280:16456–16460.

5. Mukherjee S, Lekli I, Gurusamy N, et al. Expression of the longevity proteins by both red and white wines and their chemoprotective components, resveratrol, tyrosol, and hydroxytyrosol. *Free Radic Biol Med* 2009;46(5):573–578.

6. Sehl ME, Yates FE. Kinetics of human aging: I. Rates of senescence between ages 30 and 70 years in healthy people. *J Gerontol A Biol Sci Med Sci* 2001;56:B198–B208.

7. Bortz WM. Biological basis of determinants of health. *Am J Public Health* 2005;95:389–392.

8. Poehlman ET. Energy expenditure and requirements in aging humans. *J Nutr* 1992;122:2057.

9. Elia M, Ritz P, Stubbs RJ. Total energy expenditure in the elderly. *Eur J Clin Nutr* 2000;54:s92–s103.

10. Ritz P. Factors affecting energy and macronutrient requirements in elderly people. *Public Health Nutr* 2001;4:561–568.

11. Roberts SB, Dallal GE. Effects of age on energy balance. *Am J Clin Nutr* 1998;68:975s.

12. Seale JL, Klein G, Friedmann J, et al. Energy expenditure measured by doubly labeled water, activity recall, and diet records in the elderly. *Nutrition* 2002;18:568–573.

13. Roberts SB, Young VR, Fuss P, et al. What are the energy needs of elderly adults? *Int J Obes* (Lond) 1992;16:969.

14. Hosoya N. Nutrient requirements of the elderly: an overview. *Nutr Rev* 1992;50:447.

15. Chernoff R. Effects of age on nutrient requirements. *Clin Geriatr Med* 1995;11:641.

16. Roberts SB, Dallal GE. Energy requirements and aging. *Public Health Nutr* 2005;8:1028–1036.

17. Pannemans DLE, Westerterp KR. Energy expenditure, physical activity and basal metabolic rate of elderly subjects. *Br J Nutr* 1995;73:571.

18. Reilly JJ, Lord A, Bunker VW, et al. Energy balance in healthy elderly women. *Br J Nutr* 1993;69:21.

19. Mitchell D, Haan MN, Steinberg FM, et al. Body composition in the elderly: the influence of nutritional factors and physical activity. *J Nutr Health Aging* 2003;7:130–139.

20. Raguso CA, Kyle U, Kossovsky MP, et al. A 3-year longitudinal study on body composition changes in the elderly: role of physical exercise. *Clin Nutr* 2006;25:573–580.

21. Ausman LM, Russell RM. Nutrition in the elderly. In: Shils ME, Olson JA, Shike M, eds. *Modern nutrition in health and disease*, 8th ed. Philadelphia, PA: Lea & Febiger, 1994:770–780.

22. Wakimoto P, Block G. Dietary intake, dietary patterns, and changes with age: an epidemiological perspective. *J Gerontol A Biol Sci Med Sci* 2001;56:65–68.

23. Kaiser MJ, Bauer JM, Rämsch C, et al. Frequency of malnutrition in older adults: a multinational perspective using the mini nutritional assessment. *J Am Geriatr Soc* 2010;58:1734.

24. Mudge AM, Ross LJ, Young AM, et al. Helping understand nutritional gaps in the elderly (HUNGER): a prospective study of patient factors associated with inadequate nutritional intake in older medical inpatients. *Clin Nutr* 2011;30:320.

25. Baumeister SE, Fischer B, Döring A, et al. The Geriatric Nutritional Risk Index predicts increased healthcare costs and hospitalization in a cohort of community-dwelling older adults: results from the MONICA/KORA Augsburg cohort study, 1994–2005. *Nutrition* 2011;27:534.

26. Muscaritoli M, Anker S, Argilés J, et al. Consensus definition of sarcopenia, cachexia and pre-cachexia: Joint document elaborated by Special Interest Groups (SIG) cachexia-anorexia in chronic wasting diseases and nutrition in geriatrics. *Clin Nutr* 2010;29:154–159.

27. Roberts SB. Effects of aging on energy requirements and the control of food intake in men. *Gerontol* 1995; 50A:101.

28. Chernoff R. Protein and older adults. *J Am Coll Nutr* 2004;23:627s–630s.

29. Rondanelli M, Opizzi A, Antoniello N, et al. Effect of essential amino acid supplementation on quality of life, amino acid profile and strength in institutionalized elderly patients. *Clin Nutr* 2011;30:571.

30. Malafarina V, Uriz-Otano F, Iniesta R, et al. Effectiveness of nutritional supplementation on muscle mass in treatment of sarcopenia in old age: a systematic review. *J Am Med Dir Assoc* 2013;14(1):10–17.

31. May PE, Barber A, D'Olimpio JT, et al. Reversal of cancer-related wasting using oral supplementation with a combination of beta-hydroxy-beta-methylbutyrate, arginine, and glutamine. *Am J Surg* 2002;183(4):471–479.

32. Marcora S, Lemmey A, Maddison P. Dietary treatment of rheumatoid cachexia with beta-hydroxy-beta-methylbutyrate, glutamine and arginine: a randomized controlled trial. *Clin Nutr* 2005;24(3):442–454.

33. Kerstetter JE, Holthausen BA, Fitz PA. Nutrition and nutritional requirements for the older adult. *Dysphagia* 1993;8:51.

34. Masoro EJ. Caloric restriction. *Aging Clin Exp Res* 1998;10:173.

35. Weindruch R, Sohal RS. Caloric intake and aging. *N Engl J Med* 1997;337:986.

36. Gredilla R, Gustavo B. Minireview: the role of oxidative stress in relation to caloric restriction and longevity. *Endocrinology* 2005;146:3713–3717.

37. Ingram DK, Young J, Mattison JA. Calorie restriction in nonhuman primates: assessing effects on brain and behavioral aging. *Neuroscience* 2007;145;1359–1364.

38. Barzilai N, Huffman DM, Muzumdar RH, et al. The critical role of metabolic pathways in aging. *Diabetes* 2012; 1315–1322.

39. Baur JA, Sinclair DA. Therapeutic potential of resveratrol: the in vivo evidence. *Nat Rev Drug Discov* 2006;5:493–506.

40. Ingram DK, Zhu M, Mamcarz J, et al. Calorie restriction mimetics: an emerging research field. *Aging Cell* 2006; 5:97–108.

41. Flegal KM, Kit BK, Orpana H, et al. Association of all-cause mortality with overweight and obesity using standard body mass index categories: a systematic review and meta-analysis. *JAMA* 2013;309(1):71–82.

42. Bender R, Jockel KH, Trautner C, et al. Effect of age on excess mortality in obesity. *JAMA* 1999;281:1498–1504.

43. Adams KF, Schatzkin A, Harris TB, et al. Overweight, obesity, and mortality in a large prospective cohort of persons 50 to 71 years old. *N Engl J Med* 2006;355:763–778.

44. Villareal DT, Apovian CM, Kushner RF, et al. Obesity in older adults: technical review and position statement of the American Society for Nutrition and NAASO, the Obesity Society. *Am J Clin Nutr* 2005;82:923–934.

45. Villareal DT, Chode S, Parimi N, et al. Weight loss, exercise, or both and physical function in obese older adults. *N Engl J Med* 2011;364:1218.

46. Walford RL, Mock D, Verdery R, et al. Calorie restriction in Biosphere 2: alterations in physiologic, hematologic, hormonal, and biochemical parameters in humans restricted for a 2-year period. *J Gerontol A Biol Sci Med Sci* 2002;57:b211–b224.

47. Heilbronn LK, de Jonge L, Frisard MI, et al. Effect of 6-month calorie restriction on biomarkers of longevity, metabolic adaptation, and oxidative stress in overweight individuals. *JAMA* 2006;295:1539–1548.

48. Forster MJ, Morris P, Sohal RS. Genotype and age influence the effect of caloric intake on mortality in mice. *FASEB J* 2003;17:690–692.

49. Speakman JR, Hambly C. Starving for life: what animal studies can and cannot tell us about the use of caloric restriction to prolong human lifespan. *J Nutr* 2007;137:1078–1086.

50. Frazier SC. Health outcomes and polypharmacy in elderly individuals: an integrated literature review. *J Gerontol Nurs* 2005;31:4–11.

51. Russell RM. The aging process as a modifier of metabolism. *Am J Clin Nutr* 2000;72:529s–532s.

52. Institute of Medicine. *Dietary reference intakes*. Available at http://www.iom.edu/Activities/Nutrition/SummaryDRIs/DRI-Tables.aspx; accessed 12/1/13.

53. Institute of Medicine. Report at a Glance, Report Brief: Dietary reference intakes for calcium and vitamin D, released 11/30/2010. http://www.iom.edu/Reports/2010/Dietary-Reference-Intakes-for-Calcium-and-Vitamin-D/Report-Brief.aspx; accessed 12/20/12.

54. Chernoff R. Micronutrient requirements in older women. *Am J Clin Nutr* 2005;81:1240s–1245s.

55. Blumberg J. Nutritional needs of seniors. *J Am Coll Nutr* 1997;16:517.

56. Rigler S. A clinical approach to proper nutrition in the elderly. *Kans Med* 1998;98:20.

57. Saltzman JR, Russell RM. The aging gut. Nutritional issues. *Gastroenterol Clin North Am* 1998;27:309.

58. Menon V, Greene T, Pereira AA, et al. Glycosylated hemoglobin and mortality in patients with nondiabetic chronic kidney disease. *J Am Soc Nephrol* 2005;16:3411–3417.

59. Sullivan R. Contributions to senescence: non-enzymatic glycosylation of proteins. *Arch Physiol Biochem* 1996;104:797–806.

60. Hung HC, Willett W, Ascherio A, et al. Tooth loss and dietary intake. *J Am Dent Assoc* 2003;134:1185–1192.

61. Buzina-Suboticanec K, Buzina R, Stavljenic A, et al. Aging, nutritional status and immune response. *Int J Vitam Nutr Res* 1998;68:133.

62. Liu BA, McGeer A, McArthur MA, et al. Effect of multivitamin and mineral supplementation on episodes of infection in nursing home residents: a randomized, placebo-controlled study. *J Am Geriatr Soc* 2007;55:35.

63. El-Kadiki A, Sutton AJ. Role of multivitamins and mineral supplements in preventing infections in elderly people: systematic review and meta-analysis of randomised controlled trials. *BMJ* 2005;330:871.

64. Lesourd B. Nutrition: a major factor influencing immunity in the elderly. *J Nutr Health Aging* 2004;8:28–37.

65. Mazari L, Lesourd BM. Nutritional influences on immune response in healthy aged persons. *Mech Ageing Dev* 1998;104:25.

66. Lindeman RD, Romero LJ, Liang HC, et al. Do elderly persons need to be encouraged to drink more fluids? *J Gerontol A Biol Sci Med Sci* 2000;55:M361–M365.

67. Bland JS. The use of complementary medicine for healthy aging. *Altern Ther Health Med* 1998;4:42–48.

68. Sethumadhavan S, Chinnakannu P. L-carnitine and alpha-lipoic acid improve age-associated decline in mitochondrial respiratory activity of rat heart muscle. *J Gerontol A Biol Sci Med Sci* 2006;61:650–659.

69. Ansell J, Hirsh J, Hylek E, et al. Pharmacology and management of the vitamin K antagonists: American College of Chest Physicians evidence-based clinical practice guidelines (8th Edition). *Chest* 2008;133(6 suppl):160S–198S.

70. Schmidt LE and Dalhoff K. Food-drug interactions. *Drugs* 2002;62(10):1481–502.

71. Visser M, Deeg DJ, Puts MT, et al. Low serum concentrations of 25-hydroxyvitamin D in older persons and the risk of nursing home admission. *Am J Clin Nutr* 2006;84:616–622.

72. Anderson JL, May HT, Horne BD, et al. Relation of vitamin D deficiency to cardiovascular risk factors, disease status, and incident events in a general healthcare population. *Am J Cardiol* 2010;106:963.

73. Bischoff-Ferrari HA, Dawson-Hughes B, Willett WC, et al. Effect of vitamin D on falls: a meta-analysis. *JAMA* 2004;291:1999–2006.

74. Bischoff-Ferrari HA, Willett WC, Wong JB, et al. Fracture prevention with vitamin D supplementation: a meta-analysis of randomized controlled trials. *JAMA* 2005;293:2257–2264.

75. Ma Y, Zhang P, Wang F, et al. Association between vitamin D and risk of colorectal cancer: a systematic review of prospective studies. *Am Soc Clin Oncol* 2011;3775–3782.

76. Institute of Medicine. *Dietary reference intakes for vitamin C, vitamin E, selenium and carotenoids*. Washington DC: National Academy Press, 2000.

77. Fletcher AE, Breeze E, Shetty PS. Antioxidant vitamins and mortality in older persons: findings from the nutrition add-on study to the Medical Research Council Trial of Assessment and Management of Older People in the Community. *Am J Clin Nutr* 2003;78:999–1010.

78. Nordin BE, Need AG, Morris HA, et al. Effect of age on calcium absorption in postmenopausal women. *Am J Clin Nutr* 2004;80:998–1002.

79. Nieves JW. Osteoporosis: the role of micronutrients. *Am J Clin Nutr* 2005;81:1232s–1239s.

80. Gass M, Dawson-Hughes B. Preventing osteoporosis-related fractures: an overview. *Am J Med* 2006;119:s3–s11.

81. Bolland MJ, Grey A, Avenell A, et al. Calcium supplements with or without vitamin D and risk of cardiovascular events: reanalysis of the Women's Health Initiative limited access dataset and meta-analysis. *BMJ* 2011;342:d2040.

82. Heaney RP, Kopecky S, Maki KC, et al. A review of calcium supplements and cardiovascular disease risk. *Adv Nutr* 2012;3(6):763–771.

83. Downing L and Islam MA. Influence of calcium supplements on the occurrence of cardiovascular events. *Am J Health Syst Pharm* 2013;70(13):1132–1139.

84. Kumar N, Gross JB Jr, Ahlskog JE. Copper deficiency myelopathy produces a clinical picture like subacute combined degeneration. *Neurology* 2004;63:33–39.

85. Anderson RA, Cheng N, Bryden NA, et al. Elevated intakes of supplemental chromium improve glucose and insulin variables in individuals with type 2 diabetes. *Diabetes* 1997;46:1786–1791.

86. Cefalu WT, Hu FB. Role of chromium in human health and in diabetes. *Diabetes Care* 2004;27:2741–2751.

87. Prasad AS, Beck FW, Bao B, et al. Zinc supplementation decreases incidence of infections in the elderly: effect of zinc on generation of cytokines and oxidative stress. *Am J Clin Nutr* 2007;85:837–844.

88. Durlach J, Bac P, Durlach V, et al. Magnesium status and ageing: an update. *Magnes Res* 1998;11:25–42.

89. Vaquero MP. Magnesium and trace elements in the elderly: intake, status and recommendations. *J Nutr Health Aging* 2002;6:147–153.

90. Koo SH, Montminy M. In vino veritas: a tale of two sirt1s? *Cell* 2006;127:1091–1093.

91. Agarwal B, Campen MJ, Channell MM, et al. Resveratrol for primary prevention of atherosclerosis: clinical trial evidence for improved gene expression in vascular endothelium. *Int J Cardiol* 2013;166:246–248.

92. Tomé-Carneiro J, Gonzálvez M, Larrosa M, et al. One-year consumption of a grape nutraceutical containing resveratrol improves the inflammatory and fibrinolytic status of patients in primary prevention of cardiovascular disease. *Am J Cardiol* 2012;110(3):356–363.

93. Hathcock JN, Shao A. Risk assessment for coenzyme Q_{10} (Ubiquinone). *Regul Toxicol Pharmacol* 2006;45(3):282–288.

94. Quiles J, Ochoa JJ, Huertas JR, et al. Coenzyme Q supplementation protects from age-related DNA double-strand breaks and increases lifespan in rats fed on a PUFA-rich diet. *Exp Gerontol* 2004;39(2):189–94.

95. Lee C, Pugh TD, Klopp RG, et al. The impact of α-lipoic acid, coenzyme Q_{10} and caloric restriction on life span and gene expression patterns in mice. *Free Radic Biol Med* 2004;36(8):1043–57.

96. Rajindar SS, Sergey K, Nathalie S, et al. Effect of coenzyme Q_{10} intake on endogenous coenzyme Q content, mitochondrial electron transport chain, antioxidative defenses, and life span of mice. *Free Radic Biol Med* 2006;40(3):480–487.

SUGGESTED READINGS

Hetherington MM. Taste and appetite regulation in the elderly. *Proc Nutr Soc* 1998;57:625.

Morley JE, Glick Z, Rubenstein LZ, eds. *Geriatric nutrition. A comprehensive review*, 2nd ed. New York, NY: Raven Press, 1995.

Rolls BJ. Do chemosensory changes influence food intake in the elderly? *Physiol Behav* 1999;66:193.

Yeh SS, Schuster MW. Geriatric cachexia: the role of cytokines. *Am J Clin Nutr* 1999;70:18.

CHAPTER 32

Ergogenic Effects of Foods and Nutrients: Diet and Athletic Performance & Sports Nutrition

The role of diet in optimizing athletic performance has long been a topic of considerable interest, a natural extrapolation of efforts to optimize dietary health. Diet provides the fuel that is burned to sustain physical activity, and it seems reasonable that alterations in the fuel will influence the efficiency of that combustion. Optimal nutrition plays a direct role in optimizing physical activity, athletic performance, and recovery from exercise. Macronutrient composition of meals, selection of foods and fluids, timing of intake, and use of ergogenic substances and micronutrient supplements are all variables, albeit with varying degrees of scientific support, relevant to achieving peak physical performance.

Ideally, the well-established link between diet and physical prowess in athletes would foster a general appreciation for the importance of diet to vitality. Indeed, the optimal diet of an "athlete" is quite similar to the well-balanced diet of any physically active person. Instead, all too often, this link is misused to develop marketing schemes, misleading messages, and misguided practices, such as the consumption of sports drinks and energy bars by masses of consumers far more subject to obesity and nutritional excesses than to dehydration and depletion. The clinician has a role to play both in guiding the athlete toward optimal nutrition and guiding the more typical and sedentary patient away from eating like an athlete without acting like one.

OVERVIEW

Diet

In general, the US population engages in too little physical activity and consumes too many calories. Therefore, although sufficient calorie intake is a fundamental requirement to maintain physical activity, it is not a concern for the majority of patients. It is helpful for both patients and providers to understand the activity level of the patient in order to gauge caloric needs. The resting metabolic rate (RMR) is an estimate of the caloric expenditure with no physical activity, meaning the energy required by an animal to stay alive with no activity. Key determinants of RMR include age, sex, weight, height, and fat-free body mass. Calculating RMR is the first step in calculating real metabolic rate. RMR can then be combined with the caloric expenditure through physical activity to provide a working estimate of total daily energy expenditure.

Your Metabolic Rate = Your RMR + Estimated Energy Consumed by Your Daily Activities

Numerous tools exist online to assist in performing this calculation and determining a working estimate of metabolic rate. Table 32.1 provides a list of common physical activities and corresponding caloric expenditures that may be useful for estimating activity-related energy consumption. For comparison, the average number

TABLE 32.1

Energy Expenditure of Some Representative Physical Activities[a] and Representative Food Equivalents[b]

Activity	Mets (Multiples of RMR)[c]	KCAL (Calories) Burned Per Minute	Maximum KCAL (Calories) Burned Per Hour (Approximate)	Common Fast Food Equivalent in Number of Calories (Approximate)
Resting (sitting or lying down)	1.0	1.2–1.7	100	Wendy's 4 piece spicy chicken nuggets
Sweeping	1.5	1.8–2.6	150	Jack in the box egg roll—1 piece
Driving a car	2.0	2.4–3.4	200	32 oz bottle of Gatorade
Walking slowly (2 mph)	2.0–3.5	2.8–4.0	240	Coke 20 fl oz bottle
Cycling slowly (6 mph)	2.0–3.5	2.8–4.0	240	McDonald's hamburger
Horseback riding (at a walk)	2.5	3.0–4.2	250	16 oz Starbucks vanilla latte
Volleyball	3.0	3.5	210	1/3 order of Arby's curly fries
Mopping	3.5	4.2–6.0	360	2 krispy kreme original glazed donuts
Golf	4.0–5.0	4.2–5.8	350	Dunkin donuts medium strawberry fruit Coolatta
Swimming slowly	4.0–5.0	4.2–5.8	350	IHOP pork sausage links (4 pieces)
Walking moderately fast (3 mph)	4.0–5.0	4.2–5.8	350	Dairy Queen chili cheese dog
Baseball	4.5	5.4–7.6	450	Panera chicken Caesar salad
Cycling moderately fast (12 mph)	4.5–9.0	6.0–8.3	500	Au Bon Pain blueberry muffin
Dancing	4.5–9.0	6.0–8.3	500	1/2 Order of TGI Fridays sesame Jack chicken strips
Skiing	4.5–9.0	6.0–8.3	500	Coldstone "Love it" chocolate dipped strawberry ice cream
Skating	4.5–9.0	6.0–8.3	500	Panda Express Chow Mein
Walking fast (4.5 mph)	4.5–9.0	6.0–8.3	500	1/2 Cinnabon caramel pecanbon
Swimming moderately fast	4.5–9.0	6.0–8.3	500	Chick Fil A waffle fries (large)
Tennis (singles)	6.0	7.7	500	1/2 of a chipotle burrito with chicken, white rice, black beans, salsa, sour cream, and cheese
Chopping wood	6.5	7.8–11.0	660	Sonic peanut butter shake
Shoveling	7.0	8.4–12.0	720	Pizza Hut 6" personal pepperoni lover's pizza
Digging	7.5	9.0–12.8	770	Taco Bell volcano burrito
Cross-country skiing	7.5–12.0	8.5–12.5	750	3 Popeye's biscuits
Jogging	7.5–12.0	8.5–12.5	750	Subway footlong steak and cheese sub
Football	9.0	9.1	550	Burger King rib sandwich

(continued)

TABLE 32.1

Energy Expenditure of Some Representative Physical Activities[a] and Representative Food Equivalents[b] (continued)

Activity	Mets (Multiples of RMR)[c]	KCAL (Calories) Burned Per Minute	Maximum KCAL (Calories) Burned Per Hour (Approximate)	Common Fast Food Equivalent in Number of Calories (Approximate)
Basketball	9.0	9.8	590	1/2 of a Domino's small cheese pizza
Running	15.0	12.7–16.7	1000	2 McDonald's big macs
Running at 4-min. mile pace	30.0	36.0–51.0	3060	2 chili's club sandwiches w/fries
Swimming (crawl) fast	30.0	36.0–51.0	3060	2 orders of BAJA FRESH steak quesadillas

[a]All values are estimates and based on a prototypical 70 kg male. Energy expenditure generally is lower in women and higher in larger individuals. MET and kilocalorie values derived from different sources may not correspond exactly.

[b]Calorie values for the recommended serving size of common food items were ascertained from the company's website and this value was then used to calculate the amount of food equal to the maximum number of calories burned per hour doing the corresponding physical activity

[c]A MET is the rate of energy expenditure at rest, attributable to the resting (or basal) metabolic rate (RMR). Whereas resting energy expenditure varies with body size and habitus, a MET generally is accepted to equal approximately 3.5 mL/kg/min of oxygen consumption. The energy expenditure at 1 MET generally varies over the range of 1.2 to 1.7 kcal/min. The intensity of exercise can be measured relative to the RMR in METs.

Source: Derived from Ensminger AH, Ensminger M, Konlande J, et al. *The concise encyclopedia of foods and nutrition.* Boca Raton, FL: CRC Press, 1995; Wilmore JH, Costill DL. *Physiology of sport and exercise. Human kinetics.* Champaign, IL: 1994; American College of Sports Medicine. *Resource manual for guidelines for exercise testing and prescription,* 2nd ed. Philadelphia, PA: Williams & Wilkins, 1993; Burke L, Deakin V, eds. *Clinical sports nutrition.* Sydney, AU: McGraw-Hill Book Company, 1994; and McArdle WD, Katch FI, Katch VL. *Sports exercise nutrition.* Baltimore, MD: Lippincott Williams & Wilkins, 1999.

of calories burned per hour is compared to the equivalent number of calories in a popular fast food choice for means of a common reference for all to appreciate. The health care provider can use this as a benchmark and a resource to educate patients about caloric intake versus caloric expenditure.

For the most part, little evidence exists that the dietary pattern for physically active individuals should be altered from that generally recommended for health promotion (see Chapter 45). However, there is evidence that certain deviations from and additions to current dietary recommendations may be beneficial in cases of intense physical activity and caloric expenditure. Individuals engaging in extremely intense physical activity for extended periods, particularly competitive endurance athletes, may actually need to make an effort to meet energy requirements. There is also the potential for dangerous and even life-threatening dehydration and nutrient depletion when protracted and arduous exertion is combined with stressful environmental conditions. Under such conditions, specialized dehydration formulas (e.g., Gatorade), sports drinks, and energy bars offer potentially important advantages (1). However, undue reliance on such products by patients at modest levels of exertion is apt to contribute to a disadvantageous excess of calories and sugar.

Macronutrient composition of meals may need to be adjusted to meet caloric needs and to accelerate recovery. The role of increasing dietary protein in augmenting muscle mass and supporting recovery remains controversial. The current recommended dietary allowance remains at 0.8 g per kg of protein of body weight due to a lack of evidence that additional protein is beneficial for strength and endurance athletes (2). For years, however, sports enthusiasts and competitive athletes have perceived a need for increased protein intake. Recent studies have demonstrated benefit with protein intake three or more times this recommended dietary allowance. Consensus is emerging that a moderate increase in protein intake may be indicated for some athletes (3). Intake in the range 1.2 to 1.4 g/kg/day is recommended for endurance athletes, 1.7 to 1.8 g/kg/day for athletes engaged in strength training, and 1.3 to 1.8 g/kg/day for vegetarian athletes (4). The US and Canadian Dietetic Association now recommends 1.2 to 1.7 g/kg/day of protein intake for endurance and strength trained athletes (5). This position is based on research showing that increased protein intake is necessary to maintain nitrogen balance in endurance training and to sustain muscle growth in strength training.

These levels of intake may be optimal in terms of the athletic effort, but the long-term effects of such a diet on specific health outcomes and chronic disease risk have not been adequately studied. Therefore, an athlete should prepare to modify dietary intake to meet prevailing recommendations whenever he or she tapers the level of physical activity. The use of amino acid beverages and supplementation with specific classes of amino acids are popular practices, but the evidence of beneficial effects is equivocal (6–9).

The acceptable macronutrient distribution range for fat is 20% to 35% of energy intake (2). In general, those who engage in strenuous physical activity should follow these general recommendations even if total caloric intake must increase to meet energy demand. Fat is the most calorically dense macronutrient, and fat restriction may be untenable in athletes with high energy expenditure. The average calorie requirements of a sedentary, 70 kg male adult are estimated at approximately 2,400 kcal. Studies in elite human athletes have demonstrated 24-hour expenditures of more than 10,000 calories, and a maximal sustainable expenditure of up to 12,000 kcal is estimated on the basis of animal research (10). High fat intake is the most efficient means for meeting very high energy requirements associated with extreme exertion, such as endurance training or mountain-climbing expeditions. The health hazards to the general public of excessive dietary fat intake should be borne in mind, and recommendations for individual athletes to increase dietary fat intake should be made judiciously, with a clear emphasis on the distinctions among fatty acid classes.

Evidence in other areas suggests the virtue of prioritizing intake of monounsaturated fatty acids and a mixture of n-3 and n-6 polyunsaturates in a ratio of 1:1 to 1:4. Saturated and trans-fatty acid intake should be kept proportionally low (see Chapters 2, 7, and 45). Studies characterizing the ideal profile of fatty acids in a high-fat diet and the proper timing of fat intake for optimal athletic performance are lacking to date; the evidence for a role of high-fat diets in influencing athletic performance other than by meeting high energy requirements is equivocal (11,12). When energy requirements are high and increased fat intake is desirable, nuts, seeds, nut butters, avocado, fatty fish such as salmon, and olives all represent salutary means to the desired ends.

In addition to the ideal composition of diet for physical performance, the issue of timing—when to eat certain macronutrients in relation to exercise or competition—deserves mention. An explicit prescription of what and when to eat prior to exercise is lacking, presumably due to individual variation regarding type of exercise, hunger level, metabolic function, and digestive sensitivity. The majority of research on nutrient timing looks at the ingestion of carbohydrates after exercise to best facilitate recovery. Exercise induces a greater sensitivity and responsiveness to the biochemical events controlled by insulin (13). In vitro and in vivo studies have shown increased insulin-mediated glucose uptake in response to muscle contraction (14,15). Exercise lowers basal and postprandial insulin concentrations, improves insulin sensitivity, and reduces glycosylated hemoglobin levels (16). Rigorous physical training catabolizes glycogen and diverts amino acids away from protein synthesis. Hence, proper nutrient timing for recovery involves utilizing the insulin response from exercise to optimize postexercise glycogen repletion and muscle repair. Immediate carbohydrate consumption, particularly those that are easily digestible and provide a high glycemic response, accelerates glycogen repletion as compared to carbohydrate consumption 2+ hours postexercise (17). Combining a rapidly digesting protein source with the carbohydrate immediately after exercise enhances accretion of whole body protein and promotes muscle repair via the exercise-induced insulin response (18–20). In addition to nutrient timing for post-exercise recovery, more recent studies suggest that ingestion of free amino acids plus carbohydrates before exercise results in a superior anabolic response to exercise than if ingested after exercise alone (21). With particular consideration of resistance training, most have shown that supplementation with protein, particularly a fast digesting whey protein, and carbohydrates immediately after and possibly before and during resistance exercise can enhance the muscle hypertrophy response to resistance training in healthy adults (22–24). More research is necessary to delineate the optimal dose-response combination of nutrients and timing for various types of desired training adaptations.

Competing Dietary Claims Pertaining to Athletic Performance

Carbohydrate is generally the predominant energy source in the human diet and is readily oxidized to support physical activity. Studies generally suggest that monosaccharides and polysaccharides are comparable energy sources, although glucose is metabolized somewhat more efficiently than are other sugars. Preliminary studies suggest that carbohydrate sources with a low glycemic index/load, such as lentils, may support endurance better than foods with a high glycemic index, such as potatoes, when consumed prior to exercise (see Chapter 6). The low-glycemic-index foods are absorbed more slowly into the bloodstream, thereby providing a steady and gradual energy supply to support prolonged exercise. In contrast, a source of high-glycemic-index carbohydrate immediately after exercise appears to promote glycogen storage, greater glucose and insulin responses, and enhanced recovery (25).

Carbohydrate loading apparently is of no benefit for exercise of short or moderate duration. When high-intensity exercise lasts for more than 90 minutes, muscle glycogen depletion tends to occur. A modest benefit of carbohydrate loading under such circumstances is probable (26,27), although it may be due to neuroprotective effects on perception of fatigue rather than changes in glycogen or protein metabolism (28,29). Sustained elevations in muscle glycogen following several days of carbohydrate loading have been reported (30,31). There is some evidence that the effects of carbohydrate loading differ by gender, with less evidence of benefit in women, but these limited findings may be explained in part by lower carbohydrate intakes by women or menstrual cycle fluctuations in glycogen storage (32–34). Overall, the preponderance of evidence generally supports the prevailing practice of carbohydrate loading for extreme endurance sports such as marathon running.

Controversy persists regarding optimal alterations of diet for the enhancement of sustained, high-intensity exercise and fast recovery. Over recent years, different diet theories, supplementation regimens, and fueling strategies have arisen, purporting to optimize athletic performance. These trends range from excess consumption of certain macronutrients while completely avoiding others to only consuming foods that are cultivated in certain ways. Patients, whether competitive athletes or not, will undoubtedly hear about these trends and will seek expert advice regarding dietary experimentation strategies. We address some of the most common trends here in an effort to better equip health care professionals with evidence to better guide their patients toward optimal health and performance.

Dietary protein is of particular interest to bodybuilders and other athletes involved in strength training and is the most commonly used ergogenic aid (6). A high-protein diet is often recommended by bodybuilders and nutritionists to repair muscle damage after anaerobic training and to aid in muscle growth and fat loss. An intake of 3 g of protein for every 4 g of carbohydrate is touted to promote health and enhance athletic performance in the book *Enter the Zone* by Sears and Lawren (35). Despite its popularity, the Zone diet is not supported by evidence accessible in the peer-reviewed literature. An evaluation by Cheuvront (36) suggested that the Zone diet is more likely to compromise than enhance athletic performance. Some studies show that the body is more primed to absorb and utilize amino acids for muscle growth immediately after anaerobic exercise, presumably due to catabolism during training (37). There is also evidence that high protein intake may better support muscle growth when compared to moderate protein intake; on the contrary, there are studies which fail to show a translation between higher protein intake and muscle gain (38). It is clear, however, that consistent underconsumption of protein causes a decline in lean muscle mass even with adequate caloric intake (39). Therefore, it seems reasonable to prescribe current dietary guidelines of protein intake (0.8 g per kg of protein of body weight per day) for sedentary individuals with the recommendation of boosting protein intake to 1.2 to 1.7 g/kg/day for those who are physically active, particularly those engaging in strength training.

A high-protein diet is not synonymous with low-carbohydrate diets such as the original Atkin's diet, which did not control for calories, and instead, substituted large amounts of fat for carbohydrates. Those engaging in exercise while on the low-carbohydrate diets experienced more fatigue, more negative affect, and less positive affect in response to exercise than those who were not restricting carbohydrates (40). With respect to athletic performance, there have been reports and observations that consuming a carbohydrate-restricted diet may improve performance. There is some suggestion that a short period of high fat intake may enhance fat oxidation, spare carbohydrate, and delay fatigue (41,42). Original theories explaining the purported benefits centered on the fact that fat oxidation increases, thereby sparing muscle glycogen. While endurance training enhances fatty acid utilization in muscle (10), there is little evidence that high fat intake actually enhances performance (43). While low-carbohydrate, high-fat diets may elicit changes in body composition, this diet compromises the ability to maintain high-intensity training when compared with consumption of more carbohydrates (44). Concern has been raised about fat loading, both on the basis of limited and contrary evidence and because the practice is potentially at odds with dietary practices for health promotion, although that depends in part on the variety of fat ingested (34,45).

The Paleolithic diet that gained widespread following in recent years and has been popularized as a viable strategy for athletes and those engaging in intense physical training. The nutrition plan is based on the presumed ancient diet of wild plants, animals, and fruits that hominid species consumed during the Paleolithic era, before the development of agriculture and grain-based diets. In the book The Paleo Diet for Athletes: A Nutritional Formula for Peak Athletic Performance, Loren Cordain and Joe Friel study the diets of our ancestors and today's top athletes to provide meticulous evidence that this nutrition plan can improve and sustain optimal performance (46). While the diet has been shown to improve metabolic biomarkers in preliminary investigations (47,48), there are no controlled studies to date showing a demonstrable improvement in athletic performance.

Also of interest is the rise in vegan diets among athletes and its compatibility with optimal training and performance. Scientific data in the literature investigating vegetarian diets for athletes are sparse. Emerging evidence from those working with elite vegan athletes provides evidence that the vegan athlete can compete effectively at a high level by focusing the diet on micronutrient-rich whole plant foods and avoiding potential deficiencies. It is possible to maintain a strict vegan high-protein diet. However, vegans must increase food intake to absorb and assimilate protein due to the lower nutrient density of plant-based foods as compared to animal products. This requires careful construction of the diet, paying attention to the higher-protein plant foods. Additionally, supplemental B_{12}, riboflavin, vitamin D, iron, zinc, docosahexaenoic acid (DHA), and possibly taurine are likely beneficial (5,49).

Hydration

One realm in which a general consensus exists is that hydration is essential. Replenishment of water and electrolytes before and during exercise is vital for maintaining homeostasis and health (50). Dehydration can degrade aerobic performance, increase risk of heat exhaustion, and may also lead to cognitive impairment. Exact sweat losses vary by individual, type of activity, and other environmental variables, ranging from 0.5 to 2.0 L per hour of activity (51). Drinking only water or other hypotonic solutions during prolonged or strenuous exercise may lead to hyponatremia, especially among women (52); consumption of isotonic fluids containing electrolytes, as well as avoiding overhydration at a rate exceeding sweat losses, can help prevent symptomatic hyponatremia (53). It has been recommended that fluid replacement beverages contain approximately 20 to 30 mEq per L sodium chloride to replace electrolyte losses, stimulate thirst, and promote fluid retention; 2 to 5 mEq per L potassium to replace electrolyte losses; and 5% to 10% carbohydrate for energy (54). Consumption of beverages containing electrolytes and carbohydrates can help sustain fluid and electrolyte balance and endurance exercise performance. High intensity and long duration of exercise, particularly in hot and humid conditions, should guide the need for replacement fluids and electrolytes (5,51).

The "sports drink" market has used this formula to grow into a multibillion-dollar industry, with numerous products available that claim to optimize athletic performance and improve health. Most sports drinks contain a combination of simple carbohydrates, including glucose, sucrose, fructose, and maltodextrins; there is little evidence to suggest the superiority of any one sports drink over another (55). Companies like Gatorade are now promoting a series of drinks designed to optimize preworkout priming, midworkout performance and endurance, and post-workout recovery. This is based on recommendations from sports nutritionists that team-sport athletes participating in intermittent high-intensity exercise for ≥1 hour consume 1 to 4 g carbohydrate per kg 1 to 4 hours before, 30 to 60 g carbohydrate per hour during, and 1 to 1.2 g carbohydrate/kg/hour and 20 to 25 g protein as soon as possible after exercise (56). To date, there have been no studies demonstrating clear performance advantages with this recipe, and more importantly, this prescription applies to elite athletes exercising in oppressive conditions for over an hour per day. Although these drinks may be helpful in replenishing nutrient and water loss and preventing excess muscle breakdown during strenuous training, they are nonetheless high-calorie sugared drinks; as such, they become virtually indistinguishable from other obesigenic sugared beverages such as soda when consumed in quantity by nonexercising individuals. The aggressive marketing of sports drinks to the population at large, particularly children, is a dubious practice at best, that may contribute to the negative health consequences of overweight and obesity if consumed in excess of energy expenditure (57).

Recently, coconut water has enjoyed increasing popularity under the premise that it is low in calories, fat and cholesterol free, high in potassium, and effective as a super rehydrating fluid. The industry claims that the electrolytes and vitamins found in coconut water improve circulation, slow the aging process, fight viruses, boost immunity, and reduce the risk of stroke, heart disease, and cancer. A Merill Lynch analysis in 2009 showed that with aggressive branding and marketing, investment by large beverage companies, and celebrity endorsements, coconut water sales went from virtually zero sales in 2005 to $30 to $35 million annually in 5 years. Health claims aside, the hard evidence shows that coconut water contains easily digestible carbohydrate in the form of sugar and electrolytes. It has fewer calories, less sodium, and more potassium than a sports drink. Ounce per ounce, most unflavored coconut water contains approximately 6 calories, 0.8 g sugar, 76 mg of potassium, and 32 mg of sodium compared to Gatorade, which has 8 calories, 1.6 g of sugar, 5 mg of potassium, and 12mg of sodium. (Source: USDA National Nutrient Database for Standard Reference, Release 26) Anecdotally, the ample potassium in coconut water may help prevent cramping during prolonged, rigorous exercise in excessive heat. However, one gaping hole in the coconut water nutrition profile is the absence of protein, which is essential for optimal performance and recovery. It also may be devoid of adequate sodium for optimal electrolyte replenishment, particularly for those who perspire heavily and exercise rigorously for an extended time period. Sweating makes people lose more sodium than potassium, and coconut water alone cannot replace this lost sodium. Summing up the evidence to date, it appears that coconut water may be a valid and natural way to hydrate, reduce sodium, and add potassium to the diet. Beyond this, however, there is a paucity of supportive evidence in the scientific literature to substantiate claims about coconut water's ability to prevent and cure diseases, to counteract aging with antioxidant effects, and to improve hydration status beyond that of plain water and sports drinks (58,59). The same holds true for the multitude of new drinks that contain vitamins and other health-promoting supplements, many of which are loaded with excess sugar.

The reality is that for the average exerciser, exercising in a temperate environment for an hour or less, water is an appropriate source of rehydration (51). It is important that qualified health care professionals educate consumers about the composition and appropriate use of sports drinks, gels, and bars, empowering the consumer to make appropriate health choices.

NUTRIENTS, NUTRICEUTICALS, AND FUNCTIONAL FOODS

That the overall quality of diet can influence physical performance in an athlete, as well as in general, is beyond dispute. Yet, since ancient times, a proclivity to seek performance enhancement through dietary supplementation has existed. In antiquity, such practices were rooted in what is easily seen today as superstition, such as the belief that eating the heart of an enemy would impart courage (6). Whereas modern practices are more likely to derive from science than superstition, interest in performance-enhancing dietary regimens consistently runs ahead of available evidence. A variety of micronutrients that play defined roles in energy metabolism have received attention as potential enhancers of athletic performance, among them carnitine, creatine, boron, coenzyme Q_{10}, and other nutriceutical agents, such as dehydroepiandrosterone (DHEA). Although evidence of enhanced athletic performance with supplementation is accumulating for some of these substances, the research is generally of marginal quality and the findings are inconsistent to date. These so-called ergogenic aids are often promoted on the basis of animal or in vitro data, before human interventions can be conducted (60). The financial imperative and loose regulation driving the promotion of such products warrant cautious skepticism (61,62).

Creatine

Creatine phosphate serves as an immediate energy reserve in muscle by donating phosphate to adenosine diphosphate to reconstitute adenosine triphosphate. The intent of creatine supplementation is to increase energy storage in muscle as a means to enhance performance. There is some evidence of benefit in high-intensity, short-term exercise, but currently there is little evidence of benefit in endurance activities (60,63). A double-blind, randomized trial in college football players demonstrated significant benefits of creatine supplementation in muscle mass and sprint performance. Adverse effects with common doses appear to be minimal, limited largely to gastrointestinal cramping and weight gain (64). Several studies of weight lifters have demonstrated significant increases in repetitions following short-term creatine supplementation (65,66). The preponderance of evidence suggests some benefit in high-intensity, repetitive activities and in muscle building (67–69). Creatine appears to be safe in doses commonly used (69) (see Section VIIE).

Carnitine

Carnitine participates in the transport of long-chain fatty acids into mitochondria and is thought to spare muscle glycogen by facilitating fat oxidation (60). Carnitine supplementation may also increase levels of coenzyme A, enhancing the efficiency of the Krebs cycle (70). Preliminary studies suggest that carnitine may suppress accumulation of lactic acid during high-intensity exercise, enhance performance and quicker recovery (71), and even upregulate androgen receptors (72).

However, despite many trials documenting benefits, the overall evidence to date suggesting that carnitine may enhance athletic performance is inconsistent (60,73) (see Section VIIE).

Bicarbonate

Sodium bicarbonate loading is used as an ergogenic aid in the belief that it will buffer lactic acid accumulated in muscle and prevent or delay muscle fatigue and dysfunction. The evidence suggests that bicarbonate does enhance performance, provided that the activity is brief (i.e., several minutes) and intense, but not too brief (e.g., 30 seconds), and that the dose of bicarbonate is adequate (300 mg per kg sodium bicarbonate) (60,74–76). In particular, bicarbonate loading may enhance recovery time between repeated bouts of short, high-intensity activity, such as sprinting, by neutralizing muscle lactate (60,77). Sodium citrate may have similar effects, though the evidence is preliminary. A double-blind crossover trial on well-trained college runners found that the ingestion of 0.5 g per kg body mass of sodium citrate significantly improved 5k run times and reduced post-run lactate concentration compared with placebo (78). There is some suggestion that the benefit attributed to bicarbonate may instead be due to the effects of a sodium load on intravascular volume (60).

β-Hydroxy-β-Methylbutyrate

β-hydroxy-β-methylbutyrate (HMB), a metabolite of the amino acid leucine, is a relatively new ergogenic aid. One placebo-controlled study found short-term HMB use to be associated with significant increases in strength during resistance training (79). Early trials have shown potential benefit for resistance and endurance training, but the evidence is insufficient to establish safety and efficacy at this time.

Dehydroepiandrosterone

DHEA is a steroid hormone with potential for both estrogenic and androgenic effects (80). There is interest in the role of DHEA in enhancing athletic performance, but to date no reliable data on which to base a conclusion are available (81). There is a general consensus that data from human intervention trials with DHEA are inadequate to support its use as a supplement for an ergogenic effect (82,83). Levels of DHEA decline significantly over the course of adulthood, suggesting theoretical benefit for supplementation in the elderly. One randomized controlled trial found beneficial effect of DHEA replacement in increasing muscle mass and strength during weight training by elderly individuals (84). However, it remains uncertain whether or not DHEA or low-dose testosterone replacement in elderly people has a physiologically appreciable impact on body composition, physical performance, insulin sensitivity, or quality of life (85).

Caffeine

Caffeine, taken alone, is considered a drug rather than a nutrient and is banned by the International Olympic Committee. Caffeine functions as a stimulant via adenosine receptor blockade and possibly by increasing adrenergic tone (86). It may enhance fat oxidation and sparing of muscle glycogen. Alternatively, caffeine may lower the threshold for exercise-induced β-endorphin and cortisol release, hormones that produce the so-called "runner's high" (87). Evidence suggesting that endurance is increased by short-term caffeine supplementation is convincing (60,88); however, long-term caffeine supplementation may have little to no ergogenic effect (89,90). Overall, data show that consumption of caffeine prior to exercise improves endurance during physical exercise.

Caffeine is the main component of virtually all energy drinks, performance enhancers, and weight-loss supplements. These products are targeted at individuals interested in athletics and an active lifestyle and represent one of the fastest growing sectors in the fitness industry. Most of these supplements feature caffeine and a combination of other components, including taurine, sucrose, guarana, ginseng, niacin, and cyanocobalamin. Ergogenic benefits are likely due to caffeine and glucose content. As with any pharmacoactive substance, however, these products are associated with adverse effects, most notably insomnia, nervousness, headache, tachycardia, and increased blood pressure. Additionally, these products often contain excess sugars, consumption of which is associated with development of obesity and insulin resistance (91). There are increasing reports of caffeine abuse, intoxication, and dependence, all of which pose serious threat to physical and mental health (92,93). Practitioners should beware of the adverse effects of these loosely regulated products and help to educate and monitor those most likely to consume them.

Chromium Picolinate

Chromium functions as a cofactor in the metabolism of glucose and protein, principally by enhancing insulin action. Picolinic acid is a natural derivative of tryptophan and is thought to enhance the uptake and bioavailability of chromium. Chromium picolinate is reputed to enhance energy metabolism in muscle and thereby improves strength and stamina while promoting weight loss. No convincing evidence exists to date, however, of enhanced athletic performance, muscle growth, or fat loss attributable to chromium supplementation (94). There is evidence from randomized and crossover trials of the failure of chromium supplementation to enhance the effects of resistance training on muscle size and strength (95–98). Claims that chromium picolinate supplementation aids in reducing *insulin resistance*, particularly in *diabetics*, are equivocal with a recent reviews and *meta-analysis* showing no association between chromium and glucose or insulin concentrations for nondiabetics, and inconclusive results for diabetics (99,100). Thus, the popular notion that chromium picolinate is an ergogenic aid must be considered unsubstantiated (101). Other more likely benefits are discussed in Chapter 7.

Coenzyme Q$_{10}$

Coenzyme Q$_{10}$ functions in mitochondrial electron transfer and therefore is fundamental to energy metabolism in all cells. There is interest in the potential role of coenzyme Q$_{10}$ supplementation in the enhancement of athletic performance. Although the evidence is relatively strong for a therapeutic role of coenzyme Q$_{10}$ in certain pathologic states (see Chapter 7 and Section VIIE), evidence of ergogenic effect remains equivocal (102).

Fish Oil

Fish oil contains the ω-3 fatty acids and eicosapentaenoic acid (EPA) and DHA, precursors of certain eicosanoids that are known to reduce inflammation throughout the body and confer multiple health benefits. Studies on fish oil supplements and athletic performance are scarce. Those that do exist indicate that fish oil may help reduce the stress caused by exercise by facilitating the immune system and combating inflammation (103). Additionally, those who suffer from exercise-induced bronchoconstriction may also benefit from the protective effect of fish oil supplementation (104).

Antioxidants

Intense exercise can increase production of reactive oxygen species, which damage cells (105,106). Supplementation with Vitamins C and E and other antioxidants may reduce symptoms and biomarkers of exercise-induced oxidative stress. Trained athletes who receive antioxidant supplementation show evidence of reduced oxidative stress (107). Whether or not the body's inherent antioxidant products are sufficient to combat this level of oxidative stress or if antioxidant supplementation is truly protective has yet to be determined. Likely, a diet rich in antioxidants is adequate to confer this same level of protection.

Amino Acids Supplements

Individual amino acids, most notably branched-chain amino acids, glutamine, and arginine are marketed as supplements for muscle growth in weightlifting, bodybuilding, endurance, and other sports. In theory, branched-chain amino acids provide and alternative energy source once glycogen stores have been depleted. Glutamine, an important fuel for some cells of the immune system, such as lymphocytes and macrophages, may be immunoprotective after prolonged exercise and in instances of overtraining. Arginine supplementation is theorized to be ergogenic because it is a substrate for the synthesis of nitric oxide, a potent endogenous vasodilator that increases blood flow and endurance capacity. Overall, the studies of amino acid supplementation on athletic performance are equivocal as shown in recent review articles (108,109).

CLINICAL HIGHLIGHTS

Interest in the potential for dietary manipulations to enhance athletic performance is widespread and long-standing. On the whole, the evidence of such effects is relatively sparse. Small deviations from a health-promoting diet, however, may be conducive to enhancements in strength or endurance. Although the recommended protein intake for healthy adults is approximately 0.8 g/kg/day, a level twice that much may support muscle development with resistance training and clearly is safe over the short term. A protein intake up to 2 g/kg/day may support strength as opposed to endurance training, and there is limited evidence that an intake as high as 2.5 g/kg/day may facilitate bodybuilding. The long-term health effects of protein intake at this level are uncertain; a return to more moderate intake once the period of intense training is over is indicated. Although the protein consumed should be of high biologic value (see Chapter 3), there is no evidence to support the use of protein formulas or modified commercial protein products over whole foods other than for matters of convenience and portability.

Studies of putatively ergogenic nutrients have largely been negative, although there is some evidence of improved endurance with creatine supplementation. The evidence that bicarbonate loading enhances tolerance of short bouts of high-intensity exercise is fairly convincing. Caffeine enhances endurance; of note, the International Olympic Committee considers it a drug rather than a nutrient. High carbohydrate ingestion for several days before an endurance event seems likely to delay fatigue by sustaining muscle glycogen stores, with the evidence of benefit more convincing in men than in women. Fluid replenishment with isotonic fluids is recommended, particularly during high-intensity endurance exercise. Patients engaged in only modest physical activity (i.e., an hour or less per day) should generally be dissuaded from use of sports drinks and energy bars, which can readily contribute more calories to the diet than are being utilized in such exertions; the scientific support for such products pertains to the serious athlete involved in intense competition with multiple training sessions per day.

Ultimately, a dietary pattern associated with health promotion (see Chapter 45) is, for the most part, associated with optimal functional status as well. There should not be many extreme deviation between the optimal diet of a serious athlete and the optimal diet of any other healthy, active human being. In order to better optimize the health and performance of their patients, physicians must be knowledgeable about dietary trends, marketing gimmicks, leading research in order to sift the kernels of truth amidst the mountains of myth.

REFERENCES

1. Vandenbogaerde TJ, Hopkins WG. Effects of acute carbohydrate supplementation on endurance performance: a meta-analysis. *Sports Med* 2011;41:773–792.

2. Institute of Medicine, Food and Nutrition Board. *Dietary reference intakes for energy, carbohydrate, fiber, fat, fatty acids, cholesterol, protein, and amino acids.* Washington, DC: National Academies Press, 2005.

3. Tipton KD, Witard OC. Protein requirements and recommendations for athletes: relevance of ivory tower arguments for practical recommendations. *Clin Sports Med* 2007;26:17–36.

4. Lemon W. Is increased dietary protein necessary or beneficial for individuals with a physically active lifestyle? *Nutr Rev* 1996;54:s169–s175.

5. American Dietetic Association; Dietitians of Canada; American College of Sports Medicine, Rodriguez NR, Di Marco NM, Langley S. American College of Sports Medicine position stand. Nutrition and athletic performance. *Med Sci Sports Exerc* 2009;41:709–731.

6. Applegate E, Grivetti L. Search for the competitive edge: a history of dietary fads and supplements. *J Nutr* 1997;127:869s–873s.

7. Paddon-Jones D, Borsheim E, Wolfe RR. Potential ergogenic effects of arginine and creatine supplementation. *J Nutr* 2004;2888s–2894s.

8. Nosaka K, Sacco P, Mawatari K. Effects of amino acid supplementation on muscle soreness and damage. *Int J Sport Nutr Exerc Metab* 2006;16:620–635.

9. Coyle EF. Fluid and fuel intake during exercise. *J Sports Sci* 2004;22:39.

10. Buskirk E. Exercise. In: Ziegler E, Filer FJ, eds. *Present knowledge in nutrition*, 7th ed. Washington, DC: ILSI Press, 1996.

11. Burke LM, Kiens B. Fat adaptation for athletic performance: the nail in the coffin? *J Appl Physiol* 2006;100:7–8.

12. Stephens BR, Braun B. Impact of nutrient intake timing on the metabolic response to exercise. *Nutr Rev* 2008;66:473–476.

13. Wasserman DH, Geer RJ, Rice DE, et al. Interaction of exercise and insulin action in humans. *Am J Physiol Endocrinol Metab* 1991;260:E37–E45.

14. Richter EA, Garetto LP, Goodman MN, et al. Enhanced muscle glucose metabolism after exercise: modulation by local factors. *Am J Physiol Endocrinol Metab* 1984;246:E476–E482.

15. Mikines KJ, Sonne B, Farrell PA, et al. Effect of physical exercise on sensitivity and responsiveness to insulin in humans. *Am J Physiol Endocrinol Metab* 1988;254:E248–E259.

16. Devlin J, Horton E. Effect of prior high-intensity exercise on glucose metabolism in normal and insulin-resistant man. *Diabetes* 1985;34:973–979.

17. Ivy JL, Katz AL, Cutler CL, et al. Muscle glycogen synthesis after exercise: effect of time of carbohydrate ingestion. *J Appl Physiol* 1988;64:1480–1485.

18. Levenhagen DK, Carr C, Carlson MG, et al. Postexercise protein intake enhances whole-body and leg protein accretion in humans. *Med Sci Sports Exerc* 2002;34:828–837.

19. Beelen M, Koopman R, Gijsen AP, et al. Protein co-ingestion stimulates muscle protein synthesis during resistance-type exercise. *Am J Physiol Endocrinol Metab* 2008;295:E70–E77.

20. Beelen M, Burke LM, Gibala MJ, et al. Nutritional strategies to promote postexercise recovery. *Int J Sport Nutr Exerc Metab* 2010;20:515–532.

21. Tipton KD. Role of protein and hydrolysates before exercise. *Int J Sport Nutr Exerc Metab* 2007;17(suppl):S77–S86.

22. Hulmi JJ, Kovanen V, Selänne H, et al. Acute and long-term effects of resistance exercise with or without protein ingestion on muscle hypertrophy and gene expression. *Amino Acids* 2009;37:297–308.

23. Tipton KD, Elliott TA, Cree MG, et al. Stimulation of net muscle protein synthesis by whey protein ingestion before and after exercise. *Am J Physiol Endocrinol Metab* 2007;292:E71–E76.

24. Hulmi JJ, Lockwood CM, Stout JR. Effect of protein/essential amino acids and resistance training on skeletal muscle hypertrophy: a case for whey protein. *Nutr Metab (Lond)* 2010;7:51.

25. Siu PM, Wong SH. Use of the glycemic index: effects on feeding patterns and exercise performance. *J Physiol Anthropol Appl Human Sci* 2004;23:1–6.

26. Hawley J, Schabort E, Noakes T, et al. Carbohydrate-loading and exercise performance. An update. *Sports Med* 1997;24:73–81.

27. Bussau VA, Fairchild TJ, Rao A, et al. Carbohydrate loading in human muscle: an improved 1 day protocol. *Eur J Appl Physiol* 2002;87:290–295.

28. van Zant RV, Lemon P. Preexercise sugar feeding does not alter prolonged exercise muscle glycogen or protein catabolism. *Can J Appl Physiol* 1997;22:268–279.

29. Lambert EV, Goedecke JH. The role of dietary macronutrients in optimizing endurance performance. *Curr Sports Med Rep* 2003;2:194–201.

30. Goforth HJ, Arnall D, Bennett B, et al. Persistence of supercompensated muscle glycogen in trained subjects after carbohydrate loading. *J Appl Physiol* 1997;82:342–347.

31. Arnal DA, Nelson AG, Quigley J, et al. Supercompensated glycogen loads persist 5 days in resting trained cyclists. *Eur J Appl Physiol* 2007;99:251–256.

32. Tarnopolsky M, Atkinson S, Phillips S, et al. Carbohydrate loading and metabolism during exercise in men and women. *J Appl Physiol* 1995;78:1360–1368.

33. Tarnopolsky MA, Zawada C, Richmond LB, et al. Gender differences in carbohydrate loading are related to energy intake. *J Appl Physiol* 2001;91:225–230.

34. Burke L. Nutrition strategies for the marathon: fuel for training and racing. *Sports Med* 2007;37:344–347.

35. Sears B, Lawren B. Enter the zone. New York, NY: Regan Books, 1995.

36. Cheuvront S. The zone diet and athletic performance. *Sports Med* 1999;27:213–228.

37. Rasmussen BB, Tipton KD, Miller SL, et al. An oral essential amino acid-carbohydrate supplement enhances muscle protein anabolism after resistance exercise. *J Appl Physiol* 2000;88:386–392.

38. Tipton KD, Wolfe RR. Protein and amino acids for athletes. *J Sports Sci* 2004;22:65–79.

39. Bray GA, Smith SR, de Jonge L, et al. Effect of dietary protein content on weight gain, energy expenditure, and body composition during overeating: a randomized controlled trial. *JAMA* 2012;307:47–55.

40. Butki BD, Baumstark J, Driver S. Effects of a carbohydrate-restricted diet on affective responses to acute exercise

among physically active participants. *Percept Mot Skills* 2003;96:607–615.

41. Lambert E, Hawley J, Goedecke J, et al. Nutritional strategies for promoting fat utilization and delaying the onset of fatigue during prolonged exercise. *J Sports Sci* 1997;15: 315–324.

42. Burke LM, Hawley JA, Angus DJ, et al. Adaptations to short-term high-fat diet persist during exercise despite high carbohydrate availability. *Med Sci Sports Exerc* 2002; 34:83–91.

43. Havemann L, West SJ, Goedecke JH, et al. Fat adaptation followed by carbohydrate loading compromises high-intensity sprint performance. *J Appl Physiol* 2006;100:194–202.

44. Cook CM, Haub MD. Low-carbohydrate diets and performance. *Curr Sports Med Rep* 2007;6:225–229.

45. Sherman W, Leenders N. Fat loading: the next magic bullet? *Int J Sport Nutr* 1995;5:s1–s12.

46. Cordain L, Friel J, eds *The paleo diet for athletes: a nutritional formula for peak athletic performance*, 2005 Rodale Books, New York, NY.

47. Frassetto LA, Schloetter M, Mietus-Synder M, et al. Metabolic and physiologic improvements from consuming a paleolithic, hunter-gatherer type diet. *Eur J Clin Nutr* 2009;63:947–955.

48. Jönsson T, Granfeldt Y, Ahrén B, et al. Beneficial effects of a Paleolithic diet on cardiovascular risk factors in type 2 diabetes: a randomized cross-over pilot study. *Cardiovasc Diabetol* 2009;8:35.

49. Fuhrman J, Ferreri DM. Fueling the vegetarian (vegan) athlete. *Curr Sports Med Rep* 2010;9:233–241.

50. Aoi W, Naito Y, Yoshikawa T. Exercise and functional foods. *Nutr J* 2006;5:15.

51. American College of Sports Medicine, Sawka MN, Burke LM, et al. American College of Sports Medicine position stand. Exercise and fluid replacement. *Med Sci Sports Exerc* 2007;39:377–390.

52. Almond CS, Shin AY, Fortescue EB, et al. Hyponatremia among runners in the Boston Marathon. *N Engl J Med* 2005;352:1550–1556.

53. Montain SJ, Cheuvront SN, Sawka MN. Exercise-associated hyponatremia: quantitative analysis for understand the aetiology. *Br J Sports Med* 2006;40:98–106.

54. Institute of Medicine. *Fluid replacement and heat stress.* Washington, DC: National Academies Press, 1994.

55. Coombes JS, Hamilton KL. The effectiveness of commercially available sports drinks. *Sports Med* 2000;29:181–209.

56. Baker LB, Heaton LE, Nuccio RP, et al. Dietitian-observed macronutrient intakes of young skill and team-sport athletes: adequacy of pre, during, and post-exercise nutrition. *Int J Sport Nutr Exerc Metab* 2013; Oct 2 [Epub ahead of print].

57. Harris JL, Schwartz M, Brownell K, et al. *Sugary drink facts: evaluating sugary drink nutrition and marketing to youth.* 2011. Available at http:// www.sugarydrinkfacts.org/ resources/SugarydrinkFACTS_Report.pdf

58. Saat M, Singh R, Sirisinghe RG, et al. Rehydration after exercise with fresh young coconut water, carbohydrate-electrolyte beverage and plain water. *J Physiol Anthropol Appl Human Sci* 2002;21:93–104.

59. Ismail I, Singh R, Sirisinghe RG. Rehydration with sodium-enriched coconut water after exercise-induced dehydration. *Southeast Asian J Trop Med Public Health* 2007;38:769–85.

60. Clarkson P. Nutrition for improved sports performance. Current issues on ergogenic aids. *Sports Med* 1996;21: 393–401.

61. Beltz S, Doering P. Efficacy of nutritional supplements used by athletes. *Clin Pharm* 1993;12:900–908.

62. Bernstein A, Safirstein J, Rosen JE. Athletic ergogenic aids. *Bull Hosp Jt Dis* 2003;61:164–171.

63. Jones AM, Carter H, Pringle JSM, et al. Effect of creatine supplementation on oxygen uptake kinetics during submaximal cycle exercise. *J Appl Physiol* 2002;92: 2571–2577.

64. Greenwood M, Farris J, Kreider R, et al. Creatine supplementation patterns and perceived effects in select division I collegiate athletes. *Clin J Sport Med* 2000;10:191–194.

65. Tokish JM, Kocher MS, Hawkins RJ. Ergogenic aids: a review of basic science, performance, side effects, and status in sports. *Am J Sports Med* 2004;32:1543–1553.

66. Antonio J, Ciccone V. The effects of pre versus post workout supplementation of creatine monohydrate on body composition and strength. *J Int Soc Sports Nutr* 2013;10:36.

67. Volek J, Kraemer W. Creatine supplementation: its effect on human muscular performance and body composition. *J Strength Cond Res* 1996;10:200–210.

68. Bemben MG, Lamont HS. Creatine supplementation and exercise performance. *Sports Med* 2005;35:107–125.

69. Williams MH, Branch JD. Creatine supplementation and exercise performance: an update. *J Am Coll Nutr* 1998;17: 216–234.

70. Karlic H, Lohninger A. Supplementation of L-carnitine in athletes: does it make sense? *Nutrition* 2004;20:709–715.

71. Volek JS, Kraemer WJ, Rubin MR, et al. L-carnitine L-tartrate supplementation favorably affects markers of recovery from exercise stress. *Am J Physiol Endocrinol Metab* 2002;282:E474.

72. Kraemer WJ, Spiering BA, Volek JS, et al. Androgenic responses to resistance exercise: effects of feeding and L-carnitine. *Med Sci Sports Exerc* 2006;38:1288–1296.

73. McNaughton L, Backx K, Palmer G, et al. Effects of chronic bicarbonate ingestion on the performance of high-intensity work. *Eur J Appl Physiol* 1999;80:333–336.

74. McNaughton L, Dalton B, Palmer G. Sodium bicarbonate can be used as an ergogenic aid in high-intensity, competitive cycle ergometry of 1 h duration. *Eur J Appl Physiol* 1999;80:64–69.

75. Bishop D, Edge J, Davis C, et al. Induced metabolic alkalosis affects muscle metabolism and repeated-sprint ability. *Med Sci Sports Exerc* 2004;36:807–813.

76. Van Montfoort MC, Van Dieren L, Hopkins WG, et al. Effects of ingestion of bicarbonate, citrate, lactate, and chloride on sprint running. *Med Sci Sports Exerc* 2004;36: 1239–1243.

77. Requena B, Zabala M, Padial P, et al. Sodium bicarbonate and sodium citrate: ergogenic aids? *J Strength Cond Res* 2005;19:213–224.

78. Oopik V, Saaremets I, Medijainen L, et al. Effects of sodium citrate ingestion before exercise on endurance performance in well trained college runners. *Br J Sports Med* 2003;37:485–489.

79. Jowko E, Ostaszewski P, Jank M, et al. Creatine and beta-hydroxy-beta-methylbutyrate (HMB) additively increase lean body mass and muscle strength during a weight-training program. *Nutrition* 2001;17:558–566.

80. Ebeling P, Koivisto V. Physiological importance of dehydroepiandrosterone. *Lancet* 1994;343:1479–1481.

81. Bernstein A, Safirstein J, Rosen JE. Athletic ergogenic aids. *Bull Hosp Jt Dis* 2003;61:164–171.

82. Katz S, Morales A. Dehydroepiandrosterone (DHEA) and DHEA-sulfate (DS) as therapeutic options in menopause. *Semin Reprod Endocrinol* 1998;16:161–170.

83. Khorram O. DHEA: a hormone with multiple effects. *Curr Opin Obstet Gynecol* 1996;8:351–354.

84. Villareal DT, Holloszy JO. DHEA enhances effects of weight training on muscle mass and strength in elderly women and men. *Am J Phsyiol Endocrinol Metab* 2006;291: e1003–e1008.

85. Nair KS, Rizza RA, O'Brien P, et al. DHEA in elderly women and DHEA or testosterone in elderly men. *N Engl J Med* 2006;355:1647–1659.

86. Magkos F, Kavouras SA. Caffeine use in sports, pharmacokinetics in man, and cellular mechanisms of action. *Crit Rev Food Sci Nutr* 2005;45:535–562.

87. Laurent D, Schneider KE, Prusaczyk WK, et al. Effects of caffeine on muscle glycogen utilization and the neuroendocrine axis during exercise. *J Clin Endocrinol Metab* 2000;85(6):2170–2175.

88. Keisler BD, Armsey TD 2nd. Caffeine as an ergogenic aid. *Curr Sports Med Rep* 2006;5:215–219.

89. Crowe MJ, Leicht AS, Spinks WL. Physiological and cognitive responses to caffeine during repeated, high-intensity exercise. *Int J Sport Nutr Exerc Metab* 2006;16: 528–544.

90. Malek MH, Housh TJ, Coburn JW, et al. Effects of eight weeks of caffeine supplementation and endurance training on aerobic fitness and body composition. *J Strength Cond Res* 2006;20:751–755.

91. Graham, TE. Caffeine and exercise: metabolism, endurance and performance. *Sports Med* 2001;31:785–807.

92. Higgins JP, Tuttle TD, Higgins CL. Energy beverages: content and safety. *Mayo Clin Proc* 2010;85:1033–1041.

93. Reissig CJ, Strain EC, Griffiths RR. Caffeinated energy drinks—a growing problem. *Drug Alcohol Depend* 2009;99: 1–10.

94. Vincent JB. The potential value and toxicity of chromium picolinate as a nutritional supplement, weight loss agent and muscle development agent. *Sports Med* 2003;33:213–230.

95. Campbell W, Joseph L, Davey S, et al. Effects of resistance training and chromium picolinate on body composition and skeletal muscle in older men. *J Appl Physiol* 1999;86:29–39.

96. Hallmark M, Reynolds T, DeSouza C, et al. Effects of chromium and resistive training on muscle strength and body composition. *Med Sci Sports Exerc* 1996;28:139–144.

97. Walker L, Bemben M, Bemben D, et al. Chromium picolinate effects on body composition and muscular performance in wrestlers. *Med Sci Sports Exerc* 1998; 30:1730–1737.

98. Davis JM, Welsh RS, Alerson NA. Effects of carbohydrate and chromium ingestion during intermittent high-intensity exercise to fatigue. *Int J Sport Nutr Exerc Metab* 2000;10:476–485.

99. Althuis MD, Jordan NE, Ludington EA, et al. Glucose and insulin responses to dietary chromium supplements: a meta-analysis. *Am J Clin Nutr* 2002;76:148–155.

100. Balk EM, Tatsioni A, Lichtenstein AH, et al. Effect of chromium supplementation on glucose metabolism and lipids: a systematic review of randomized controlled trials. *Diabetes Care* 2007;30:2154–2163.

101. Federal Trade Commission. *Companies advertising popular dietary supplement chromium picolinate can't substantiate weight loss and health claims, says FTC.* FTC web page (http://www.ftc.gov) news release on commission actions. November 7, 1996.

102. Rosenfeldt F, Hilton D, Pepe S, et al. Systematic review of effect of coenzyme Q10 in physical exercise, hypertension and heart failure. *Biofactors* 2003;18:91–100.

103. Venkatraman JT, Pendergast DR. Effect of dietary intake on immune function in athletes. *Sports Med* 2002;32(5): 323–337.

104. Mickleborough TD, Rundell KW. Dietary polyunsaturated fatty acids in asthma- and exercise-induced bronchoconstriction. *Eur J Clin Nutr* 2005;59: 1335–1346.

105. Ji LL. Oxidative stress during exercise: implication of antioxidant nutrients. *Free Radic Biol Med* 1995;18: 1079–86.

106. Clarkson PM. Antioxidants and physical performance. *Clin Rev Food Sci Nutr* 1995;35:131–41.

107. Clarkson PM, Thompson HS. Antioxidants: what role do they play in physical activity and health? *Am J Clin Nutr* 2000;72:637S–46S.

108. Williams M. Dietary supplements and sports performance: amino acids. *J Int Soc Sports Nutr* 2005;2:63–67.

109. Wagenmakers AJ. Amino acid supplements to improve athletic performance. *Curr Opin Clin Nutr Metab Care* 1999;2(6):539–544.

SUGGESTED READINGS

Burke L, Deakin V, eds. *Clinical sports nutrition.* Sydney, AU: McGraw-Hill, 1994.

Kreider R, Ferreira M, Wilson M, et al. Effects of creatine supplementation on body composition, strength, and sprint performance. *Med Sci Sports Exerc* 1998;30:73–82.

McArdle WD, Katch FI, Katch VL. *Sports exercise nutrition.* Baltimore, MD: Lippincott Williams & Wilkins, 1999.

Svensson M, Malm C, Tonkonogi M, et al. Effect of Q_{10} supplementation on tissue Q_{10} levels and adenine nucleotide catabolism during high-intensity exercise. *Int J Sport Nutr* 1999;9:166–180.

CHAPTER 33

Endocrine Effects of Diet: Phytoestrogens

Natural constituents of foods with hormonal effects are widespread. Phytoestrogens are a diverse group of naturally occurring plant-derived chemicals with varying degrees of estrogen agonism and antagonism. There is particular interest in use of phytoestrogens, in food or as concentrated supplements, to modify both the symptoms and sequelae associated with menopause. Isoflavones in soy have been studied most extensively to date.

OVERVIEW

The principal classes of phytoestrogens include isoflavones, lignans, and coumestans. Both soybeans and flaxseeds are particularly rich sources of phytoestrogens. Phytoestrogens are widespread in plants; their distribution has been reviewed elsewhere (1,2). The presence of phytoestrogens in whole-grain products may be responsible for some of the health benefits associated with their regular consumption (3–5).

The various effects of phytoestrogens, a mix of estrogen agonism and antagonism, mimic those of synthetic selective estrogen receptor modulators (SERMs), raising the possibility that natural products could be used as substitutes for synthetic SERMs (6–8). Isoflavones in soy and other foods are known to exert selective estrogen effects, generating both clinical and popular interest in such foods as a natural means to replace ovarian hormones, alleviate symptoms of menopause, or modify disease risk (9). Use of hormone replacement therapy (HRT) has declined since the release of the Women's Health Initiative results, leading to a concomitant increase in the interest and use of nonhormonal therapies by peri- and postmenopausal women (10). Trials of phytoestrogens for the amelioration of menopausal symptoms have yielded mixed results to date (11,12), warranting further studies with rigorous design (13,14).

A review by Kronenberg and Fugh-Berman (15) suggests that isoflavone preparations, the form used in the majority of trials, may be less effective than soy foods; greater benefit may also be achieved by dividing soy or supplements into several doses, taken throughout the day (16). A recent study has shown that preparations containing isoflavones should be standardized for the isoflavone aglycone content, to facilitate the prediction of theoretical hormonal activity, facilitate the intake of a controlled amount of isoflavones, and ensure greater product reliability (17).

A randomized controlled trial of two isoflavone-containing red clover extracts on recently postmenopausal women found that the higher-dose supplement Promensil (82 mg total isoflavones per day) reduced hot flashes more rapidly than either the lower-dose Rimostil (57 mg total isoflavones per day) or placebo (18). Many herbs are used to treat aspects of women's health related to hormonal function; the mechanism by which such herbs exert their effects is often through agonism or antagonism of estrogen receptors (19,20). Chinese herbal preparations traditionally used for management of menopause-related symptoms have been found to contain phytoestrogens. In some instances, the potency is commensurate with that of conventional HRT (21,22). The evidence available suggests that up to two-thirds of women experience some relief from hot flashes by using phytoestrogenic supplements, although relatively few can be expected to gain relief from vaginal dryness (23,24). Consumption of soy products in the premenopausal state may have a protective effect against vasomotor symptoms of menopause (25). Jacobs A. et al. (26) in a recent review have suggested a positive trend, but no conclusive evidence of the benefit of soy isoflavones on hot flash frequency or severity.

The mixed agonist/antagonist properties of many estrogenic herbs have led to much investigation into their potential influence on the risk of breast cancer. In vitro studies using breast cancer cell lines have shown that high doses of isoflavones and lignans can inhibit cell growth (27,28), tumor progression, and angiogenesis (29), via both estrogen-dependent and estrogen-independent mechanisms (30–33).

There are an increasing number of in vitro and animal studies that are showing how isoflavones interact with epigenetic modifications, such as hypermethylation of tumor suppressor genes (34–36). These studies are providing new evidence on potential epigenetic mechanisms by which the isoflavones genistein, daidzein, and their derivatives might contribute to the prevention of breast cancer. These effects may also be one means by which fruits and vegetables in the diet mitigate cancer risk (37) (see Chapter 12).

A recent systematic review of both observational studies and randomized control trial that aimed to assess the impact of soy, red clover, or isoflavones from these plants on the risk of primary breast cancer or the risk of recurrence suggests that soy consumption may protect against the development of breast cancer and less so breast cancer recurrence and mortality (38). Also flaxseed intake has been associated with a reduction in breast cancer risk. In the Ontario Women's Diet and Health Study, an observational study, consumption of flaxseed was associated with a significant reduction in breast cancer risk (odds ratio [OR], 0.82; 95% confidence interval [CI], 0.69 to 0.97), as was consumption of flax bread (OR, 0.77; 95% CI, 0.67 to 0.89) (39).

Despite the wealth of epidemiological observations that populations in countries with high dietary intake of soy and other phytoestrogen-rich foods have significantly lower levels of breast and prostate cancer than others (40), evidence from clinical trials has been conflicting (41–43). Recent literature has attempted to address this issue, and several possible explanations have begun to emerge.

The timing, duration, and amount of soy intake may each be relevant to breast cancer prevention. Wu AH. et al. (44) have shown in a population-based, case-control trial investigating the association between dietary soy intake and breast cancer risk that Asian- American subjects who were the highest soy consumers during adolescence and adult life showed much lower risk (OR, 0.53; 95% CI, 0.36 to 0.78) compared to subjects who were low soy consumers during those periods. These results have been corroborated by a more recent population-based cohort study, the Shangai Women's Health Study, in which a cohort of 73,223 Chinese women has been followed over a mean of 7.4 year. The women who consumed a high amount of soy foods consistently during adolescence and adulthood had a substantially reduced risk of breast cancer (RR, 0.57; 95% CI: 0.34, 0.97) (45). These data support a growing speculation that early and substantial exposure to isoflavones in childhood and adolescence, regardless of adult intake, may be what provides the majority of the protective effects against breast cancer (46,47).

Genistein, a phytoestrogen derived from soy, appears to have a biphasic effect in vitro, inhibiting breast cancer cell growth when applied in high doses (48) but stimulating cancer growth at low doses; this has generated concern for the safety of soy food consumption by women with breast cancer. Thus far, animal and human studies have been reassuring, with no evidence that increased dietary soy or isoflavone supplements adversely affect breast tissue density in pre- or postmenopausal women; although further studies are clearly necessary, it may be that the effects of soy in vivo differ from those in vitro (49,50). Still, other hormones commonly have different and even opposite effects in vivo at different concentrations; some degree of non–dose-dependence in the endocrine system may be the rule. Soy and phytoestrogen intake may also have biologic activity leading to decreased risk of prostate cancer (51,52) and even lung cancer (53), though there are limited data to support these hypotheses to date. Animal studies have shown promising evidence that dietary genistein may have a dose-dependent effect on reducing the incidence of prostate cancer (54), but human trials are lacking.

More research is needed to elucidate the effects of soy and isoflavones on both breast cancer risk and survival of breast cancer patients (41). To date results are still controversial (55,56). For now, soy supplementation cannot be recommended for cancer prevention, but the inclusion of soy in the diet is of likely benefit. Given soy's wide use as a meat substitute, it may be that its protective effects stem not only exclusively from what it provides to the diet but also from what it removes from the diet; a high-soy-food diet is more likely to contain less meat and subsequently less associated with cancer risk. Larger, long-term trials are needed to better define these effects. In particular, research is needed to more clearly identify possible subgroups of women that may differentially benefit from soy or not, based on receptor status and/or use of antiestrogen therapy.

There is preliminary evidence of cardiovascular benefits of soy phytoestrogens, apparently with comparable effects in men and women (57). In 1999, the FDA approved a health claim stating that including 25 g of soy protein in a low-fat, low-cholesterol diet may reduce the risk of heart disease (58). Specific mechanisms include lowering of low-density lipoprotein, raising of high-density lipoprotein and apoprotein A-1, inhibition of low-density lipoprotein oxidation, and salutary effects on vascular reactivity (57,59,60). In a randomized crossover trial of 60 healthy postmenopausal, Welty et al. (61) demonstrated reductions in blood pressure and low-density lipoprotein cholesterol levels in women who substituted soy nuts for non-soy dietary protein, with greater effects observed in hypertensive subjects compared to normotensive subjects. In another study, adding soy nuts to the diet for 8 weeks significantly improved glycemic control and lipid profiles in postmenopausal women with the metabolic syndrome (62). A randomized crossover trial testing soy isoflavone protein, soy lecithin, and the combination of the two found significant improvements in subjects' lipid profiles after 4 weeks of treatment. Effects on cardiovascular risk indices suggest a probable reduction of cardiac risk, but this hypothesis is as yet unproved. The ability of raloxifene (a SERM) to enhance endothelial-mediated dilation (63) constitutes a possible mechanism for its cardioprotective effects, and recent studies suggest similar action with soy supplementation (60).

Isoflavones appear to be specifically involved in the lipid-lowering effects of soy; trials comparing soy formulations with varying amounts of isoflavone content only found efficacy with those containing isoflavones (64). Trials using semi-purified isoflavone supplements found no lipid-lowering effect (65) suggesting that intact, minimally processed soy protein may be required for cardiovascular benefit (66). The effects of isoflavones on serum lipid are still controversial. A recent randomized control trial has shown that soy protein and isoflavone (either alone or together) did not impact serum lipids or inflammatory markers. In this randomized control trial, 131 healthy women older than 60 years were randomized into 1 of 4 intervention groups: soy protein (18 g per day) and isoflavone tablets (105 mg per day isoflavone aglycone equivalents), soy protein and placebo tablets, control protein and isoflavone tablets, or control protein and placebo tablets. Tests were used to assess differences between equol and nonequol producers. The study has shown that after 1 year, in the entire population, there were either no or little effects on serum lipids and inflammatory markers, regardless of treatment group. Equol producers, when analyzed separately, had significant improvements in total cholesterol/high-density lipoprotein and low-density lipoprotein/high-density lipoprotein ratios (-5.9%, $P = 0.02$; -7.2%, $P = 0.04$, respectively) (67,68).

Phytoestrogens have been identified in hops (69), and consequently beer (70), and grapes, and consequently wine (71,72). Some of the putative health benefits of moderate alcohol consumption may be attributable to phytoestrogen effects (73) (see Chapter 40).

Increasingly, studies have shown that isoflavones, via diet or supplementation, may have a protective effect on postmenopausal bone loss (74,75). In one double-blind, randomized controlled trial, women aged 49 to 65 receiving a red clover-derived isoflavone supplement for 1 year demonstrated significantly reduced loss of bone mineral content and density compared to women receiving a placebo (76). Similar results were achieved with increased dietary soy products (77,78) and the natural phytoestrogen genistein (79). Recent studies of young premenopausal (80) and older postmenopausal (81) women have not found significant effects of soy supplementation on bone mineral density. There are conflicting data about the potential benefits of the synthetic isoflavone analogue ipriflavone (82,83), and at this point, the relationship between isoflavones and bone health is still far from fully understood (84,85) (see Chapter 14). To date, although there is considerable variability in study design and duration, study population, type of soy isoflavone employed in the intervention, and study outcomes, the evidence points to a lack of a protective role of soy isoflavones in the prevention of postmenopausal bone loss (86).

Phytoestrogens have been shown to influence sexual differentiation and fertility in animal models (13). Even though some soy-based infant formulas are very rich in phytoestrogens, no adverse effects in humans have been reported (13,87). Human breast milk contains negligible concentrations of isoflavones (88); however, there is evidence that maternal soy consumption significantly increases urinary isoflavone levels in breast-feeding infants (89). There is speculation that early exposure to soy phytoestrogens may reduce the risk of certain chronic diseases later in life (88,90).

A recent cross-sectional study of postmenopausal women found significant associations between phytoestrogen exposure and circulating sex hormone levels in a large group of postmenopausal women. The same investigators also found evidence of phytoestrogen–gene interactions among subjects, lending support to the hypothesis that certain people may gain more or less benefit from phytoestrogens (91). In vitro studies of cultured adrenal cortical cells suggest that phytoestrogen consumption reduces cortisol production (92), an effect seen with a lactovegetarian diet (93). A recent study of 35 healthy young men found that soy protein consumption decreased dihydrotestosterone (DHT) and testosterone levels (94).

One of the limiting factors in efforts to gauge the potential benefits of phytoestrogens has been their exclusion from standard measures of diet composition (95,96). Using the recently released U.S. Department of Agriculture Isoflavone Database (97), Chun et al. (96) have estimated a total daily isoflavone intake of approximately 1.1 to 1.3 mg among US adults; lignans appear to be the most abundant source of phytoestrogens in the American diet (98).

It is unknown whether these levels are sufficient to produce any of the health effects associated with phytoestrogens (99). The highest intake of phytoestrogens has been reported in Japanese and Chinese populations, with estimations of intakes up to 50 times those of most Americans (100); Wu et al. (101) estimated that isoflavone intakes in Asian Americans falls between levels consumed by typical American and Asian populations.

The discovery of equol has provided a new understanding of the variance in reported evidence of the health benefits of soy. Equol is a nonsteroidal estrogen of the isoflavone class, produced exclusively by intestinal bacterial metabolism of dietary isoflavones. Among humans, 30% to 55% have the bacteria capable of producing equol. Factors that influence the capacity to produce equol are not clearly established; however, gut physiology, host genetics, and diet appear to contribute to interindividual differences in conversion of daidzein to equol. Equol appears to be the most potent of the isoflavones, and evidence of equol production can be measured in urinary excretion; it is estimated that up to 50% of the adult population does not excrete equol after soy consumption (102). Preliminary evidence from clinical studies suggests that compared to these "nonequol producers," "equol producers" may be a subpopulation that can maximally benefit from soy isoflavones (103,104).

Many clinical studies have been carried out to determine the health benefits of soy protein and the isoflavones contained in soy. In those intervention studies in which plasma S-equol levels were determined, a concentration of >5 to 10 ng per mL has been associated with a positive outcome for vasomotor symptoms, osteoporosis (as measured by an increase in bone mineral density), prostate cancer, and the cardiovascular risk (105). Several studies of soy supplementation and bone density suggest that soy products may be more effective in maintaining bone density in equol-producing individuals (106). As mentioned previously, equol producers, compared with nonequol producers, have a significant improvements in total cholesterol/high-density lipoprotein and low-density lipoprotein/high-density lipoprotein ratios (67). In a recent randomized controlled trial to assess the effect of isoflavones on endothelial function in postmenopausal women with type 2 diabetes mellitus (T2DM), Curtis et al. (107) have shown that equol producers had larger reductions in diastolic BP, mean arterial pressure, and pulse wave velocity (-2.24 ± 1.31 mm Hg, -1.24 ± 1.30 mm Hg, and -0.68 ± 0.40 m/s, respectively; $p < 0.01$) compared with nonequol producers (n = 30). The association between equol production and cancer risk in humans has not been extensively characterized (108). In European populations, two large studies conducted in the European Prospective Investigation into Cancer and Nutrition (EPIC) cohorts reported no association between equol measures and overall breast cancer risk (42); however, among estrogen receptor-positive cases in the Norfolk cohort, urinary equol was associated with a slightly higher risk (OR [95% CI] = 1.07 [1.01–1.112]; $P = 0.013$) in the 95 cases compared with the 329 controls (109). The results of in vitro and animal studies are still controversial. Equol such as other phytoestrogens may have an impact on the expression of oncosuppresor genes. In a recent study, Bosviel et al. (36) have shown that equol increases the level of expressed oncosuppressors BRCA1 and BRCA2 genes in breast cancer cell lines. Niculescu et al. showed a stronger effect of isoflavone supplementation (900 mg day for 84 days) on estrogen-responsive genes in peripheral lymphocytes among postmenopausal women who were equol producers (110). Understanding the pathways through which the equol-producer phenotype modifies response to isoflavones may clarify the role of equol itself. More studies are needed that are designed to address a priori the effect of the equol-producer phenotype on disease risk (111).

CLINICAL HIGHLIGHTS

Phytoestrogens act as selective estrogen receptor agonists and antagonists, in much the same way as SERMs. The possibility that foods containing phytoestrogens, or concentrated supplements, could be used to ameliorate symptoms and sequelae of menopause is supported by available evidence, much of which is preliminary. A diet rich in a variety of plant foods, particularly soybeans, flaxseeds, and whole grains, is advisable on other grounds and will provide a rich supply of the best-studied phytoestrogens. Such a diet, via the effects of both phytoestrogens and other beneficial constituents, appears likely to reduce the risk of breast cancer, prostate cancer, cardiovascular disease, and possibly other cancers and osteoporosis, but effects with regard to phytoestrogens specifically may depend to a large extent on an individual's distribution of gut bacteria and the ability to generate equol. Phytoestrogens may be an alternative for the management of menopausal symptoms, though evidence is still preliminary. For patients interested in the use of phytoestrogens as an alternative to HRT, dosing is a matter of conjecture. Clinical benefits have been seen with daily doses of soy protein of 60 g and with 30 to 40 mg of soy isoflavones. While there may be some cause for concerns about the risk/benefit trade-off of supplementation with soy or other phytoestrogen source, the benefits of making whole-soy foods a part of the diet, particularly when used as an alternative to meat, are generally both persuasive and reassuring.

REFERENCES

1. Mazur W. Phytoestrogen content in foods. *Baillieres Clin Endocrinol Metab* 1998;12:729–742.
2. Fletcher RJ. Food sources of phyto-oestrogens and their precursors in Europe. *Br J Nutr* 2003;89:s39–s43.
3. Slavin J, Martini M, Jacobs DJ, et al. Plausible mechanisms for the protectiveness of whole grains. *Am J Clin Nutr* 1999;70:459s–463s.
4. Slavin JL. Mechanisms for the impact of whole grain foods on cancer risk. *J Am Coll Nutr* 2000;19:300s–307s.
5. Truswell AS. Cereal grains and coronary heart disease. *Eur J Clin Nutr* 2002;56:1–14.
6. Brzezinski A, Debi A. Phytoestrogens: the "natural" selective estrogen receptor modulators? *Eur J Obstet Gynecol Reprod Biol* 1999;85:47–51.
7. Fitzpatrick L. Selective estrogen receptor modulators and phytoestrogens: new therapies for the postmenopausal women. *Mayo Clin Proc* 1999;74:601–607.
8. Basly JP, Lavier MC. Dietary phytoestrogens: potential selective estrogen enzyme modulators? *Planta Med* 2005;71:287–294.
9. Newton KM, Buist DS, Keenan NL, et al. Use of alternative therapies for menopause symptoms: results of a population-based survey. *Obstet Gynecol* 2002;100:18–25.
10. Brett K, Keenan NL. Complementary and alternative medicine use among midlife women for reasons including menopause in the United States: 2002. *Menopause* 2006;14:300–307.
11. Krebs EE, Ensrud KE, MacDonald R, et al. Phytoestrogens for treatment of menopausal symptoms: a systematic review. *Obstet Gynecol* 2004;104:824–836.
12. Nelson HD, Vesco KK, Haney E, et al. Nonhormonal therapies for menopausal hot flashes: systematic review and meta-analysis. *JAMA* 2006;295:2057–2071.
13. Whitten P, Naftolin F. Reproductive actions of phytoestrogens. *Baillieres Clin Endocrinol Metab* 1998;12:667–690.
14. Nedrow A, Miller J, Walker M, et al. Complementary and alternative therapies for the management of menopause-related symptoms: a systematic evidence review. *Arch Intern Med* 2006;166:1453–1565.
15. Kronenberg F, Fugh-Berman A. Complementary and alternative medicine for menopausal symptoms: a review of randomized, controlled trials. *Ann Intern Med* 2002;137: 805–813.
16. Kurzer MS. Phytoestrogen supplement use by women. *J Nutr* 2003;133:1983s–1986s.
17. Reiter E, Beck V, Medjakovic S, et al. Comparison of hormonal activity of isoflavone-containing supplements used to treat menopausal complaints. *Menopause* 2009;16(5):1049–1060.
18. Tice JA, Ettinger B, Ensrud K, et al. Phytoestrogen supplement for the treatment of hot flashes: the Isoflavone Clover Extract (ICE) Study: a randomized controlled trial. *JAMA* 2003;290:207–214.

19. Wade C, Kronenberg F, Kelly A, et al. Hormone-modulating herbs: implications for women's health. *J Am Med Womens Assoc* 1999;54:181–183.

20. Usui T. Pharmaceutical prospects of phytoestrogens. *Endocr J* 2006;53:7–20.

21. Shiizaki K, Goto K, Ishige A, et al. Bioassay of phytoestrogen in herbal medicine used for postmenopausal disorder using transformed MCF-7 cells. *Phytother Res* 1999;13:498–503.

22. Wang X, Wu J, Chiba H, et al. Puerariae radix prevents bone loss in ovariectomized mice. *J Bone Miner Metab* 2003;21:268–275.

23. Eden J. Phytoestrogens and the menopause. *Baillieres Clin Endocrinol Metab* 1998;12:581–587.

24. North American Menopause Society. Treatment of menopause-associated vasomotor symptoms: position statement of the North American Menopause Society. *Menopause* 2004;11:11–33.

25. Nagata C, Takatsuka N, Kawakami N. Soy product intake and hot flashes in Japanese women: results from a community-based prospective study. *Am J Epidemiol* 2001;153:790–793.

26. Jacobs A, Wegewitz U, Sommerfeld C, et al. Efficacy of isoflavones in relieving vasomotor menopausal symptoms – a systematic review. *Mol Nutr Food Res* 2009;53(9):1084–1097.

27. Dixon-Shanies D, Shaikh N. Growth inhibition of human breast cancer cells by herbs and phytoestrogens. *Oncol Rep* 1999;6:1383–1387.

28. Le Bail J, Champavier Y, Chulia A, et al. Effects of phytoestrogens on aromatase 3b and 17b-hydroxysteroid dehydrogenase activities and human breast cancer cells. *Life Sci* 2000;66:1281–1291.

29. Dabrosin C, Chen J, Wang L, et al. Flaxseed inhibits metastasis and decreases extracellular vascular endothelial growth factor in human breast cancer xenografts. *Cancer Lett* 2002;185:31–37.

30. Magee PJ, Rowland IR. Phyto-oestrogens, their mechanism of action: current evidence for a role in breast cancer. *Br J Nutr* 2004;91:513–531.

31. Krazeisen A, Breitling R, Möller G, et al. Phytoestrogens inhibit human 17 beta-hydroxysteroid dehydrogenase type 5. *Mol Cell Endocrinol* 2001;171(1–2):151–162.

32. Saarinen NM, Power K, Chen J, et al. Flaxseed attenuates the tumor growth stimulating effect of soy protein in ovariectomized athymic mice with MCF-7 human breast cancer xenografts. *Int J Cancer* 2006;119(4):925–931.

33. Levis S, Strickman-Stein N, Ganjei-Azar P, et al. Soy isoflavones in the prevention of menopausal bone loss and menopausal symptoms: a randomized, double-blind trial. *Arch Intern Med* 2011;171(15):1363–1369.

34. Dagdemir A, Durif J, Ngollo M, et al. Histone lysine trimethylation or acetylation can be modulated by phytoestrogen, estrogen or anti-HDAC in breast cancer cell lines. *Epigenomics* 2013;5(1):51–63. doi: 10.2217/epi.12.74.

35. Bosviel R, Dumollard E, Déchelotte P, et al. Can soy phytoestrogens decrease DNA methylation in BRCA1 and BRCA2 oncosuppressor genes in breast cancer? *OMICS* 2012;16(5):235–244. doi: 10.1089/omi.2011.0105.

36. Bosviel R, Durif J, Déchelotte P, et al. Epigenetic modulation of BRCA1 and BRCA2 gene expression by equol in breast cancer cell lines. *Br J Nutr* 2012;108(7):1187–1193.

37. Fotsis T, Pepper M, Montesano R, et al. Phytoestrogens and inhibition of angiogenesis. *Baillieres Clin Endocrinol Metab* 1998;12:649–666.

38. Fritz H, Seely D, Flower G, et al. Soy, red clover, and isoflavones and breast cancer: a systematic review. *PLoS One*. 2013;8(11):e81968.

39. Lowcock EC, Cotterchio M, Boucher BA. Consumption of flaxseed, a rich source of lignans, is associated with reduced breast cancer risk. *Cancer Causes Control* 2013;24(4):813–816. doi: 10.1007/s10552-013-0155-7.

40. Pisani P, Bray F, Parkin DM. Estimates of the world-wide prevalence of cancer for 25 sites in the adult population. *Int J Cancer* 2002;97:72–81.

41. Messina M, McCaskill-Stevens W, Lampe JW. Addressing the soy and breast cancer relationship: review, commentary, and workshop proceedings. *J Natl Cancer Inst* 2006;98:1275–1284.

42. Verheus M, van Gils CH, Keinan-Boker L, et al. Plasma phytoestrogens and subsequent breast cancer. *J Clin Oncol* 2007;25:648–655.

43. Keinan-Boker L, van Der Schouw YT, Grobbee DE, et al. Dietary phytoestrogens and breast cancer risk. *Am J Clin Nutr* 2004;79:282–288.

44. Wu AH, Wan P, Hankin J, et al. Adolescent and adult soy intake and risk of breast cancer in Asian-Americans. *Carcinogenesis* 2002;23:1491–1496.

45. Lee SA, Shu XO, Li H, et al. Adolescent and adult soy food intake and breast cancer risk: results from the Shanghai Women's Health Study. *Am J Clin Nutr* 2009;89(6):1920–1926. doi: 10.3945/ajcn.2008.27361.

46. Shu XO, Jin F, Dai Q, et al. Soyfood intake during adolescence and subsequent risk of breast cancer among Chinese women. *Cancer Epidemiol Biomarkers Prev* 2001;10:483–488.

47. Lamartiniere CA. Timing of exposure and mammary cancer risk. *J Mammary Gland Biol Neoplasia* 2002;7:67–76.

48. Tanos V, Brzezinski A, Drize O, et al. Synergistic inhibitory effects of genistein and tamoxifen on human dysplastic and malignant epithelial breast cells in vitro. *Eur J Obstet Gynecol Reprod Biol* 2002;102:188–194.

49. Messina MJ, Loprinzi CL. Soy for breast cancer survivors: a critical review of the literature. *J Nutr* 2001;131:3095s–3108s.

50. Maskarinec G, Meng L. An investigation of soy intake and mammographic characteristics in Hawaii. *Breast Cancer Res* 2001;3:134–141.

51. Messina MJ. Merging evidence on the role of soy in reducing prostate cancer risk. *Nutr Rev* 2003;61:117–131.

52. Magee PJ, Rowland IR. Phyto-oestrogens, their mechanism of action: current evidence for a role in breast and prostate cancer. *Br J Nutr* 2004;91:513–531.

53. Schabath MB, Hernandez LM, Wu X, et al. Dietary phytoestrogens and lung cancer risk. *JAMA* 2005;294:1493–1504.

54. Mentor-Marcel R, Lamartiniere C, Eltoum I-E, et al. Genistein in the diet reduces the incidence of poorly differentiated prostatic adenocarcinoma in transgenic mice (TRAMP). *Cancer Res* 2001;61:6777–6782.

55. Shu XO, Zheng Y, Cai H, et al. Soy food intake and breast cancer survival. *JAMA* 2009;302(22):2437–2443.

56. Chi F, Wu R, Zeng YC, et al. Post-diagnosis soy food intake and breast cancer survival: a meta-analysis of cohort studies. *Asian Pac J Cancer Prev* 2013;14(4):2407–2412.

57. Clarkson T, Anthony M. Phytoestrogens and coronary heart disease. *Baillieres Clin Endocrinol Metab* 1998;12:589–604.

58. Food and Drug Administration. Food labeling: health claims; soy protein and coronary heart disease. *Fed Regist* 1999;64:57700–57733.

59. Cassidy A, Griffin B. Phyto-oestrogens: a potential role in the prevention of CHD? *Proc Nutr Soc* 1999;58:193–199.

60. Evans M, Njike VY, Hoxley M, et al. Effect of soy isoflavone protein and soy lecithin on endothelial function in healthy postmenopausal women. *Menopause* 2007;14:141–149.

61. Welty FK, Lee KS, Lew NS, et al. Effect of soy nuts on blood pressure and lipid levels in hypertensive, prehypertensive, and normotensive postmenopausal women. *Arch Intern Med* 2007;167:1060–1067.

62. Azadbakht L, Kimiagar M, Mehrabi Y, et al. Soy inclusion in the diet improves features of the metabolic syndrome: a randomized crossover study in postmenopausal women. *Am J Clin Nutr* 2007;85:735–741.

63. Sarrel PM, Nawaz H, Chan W, et al. Raloxifene and endothelial function in healthy postmenopausal women. *Am J Obstet Gynecol* 2003;188:304–309.

64. Gardner CD, Newell KA, Cherin R, et al. The effect of soy protein with or without isoflavones relative to milk protein on plasma lipids in hypercholesterolemic postmenopausal women. *Am J Clin Nutr* 2001;73:728–735.

65. Dewell A, Hollenbeck CB, Bruce B. The effects of soy-derived phytoestrogens on serum lipids and lipoproteins in moderately hypercholesterolemic postmenopausal women. *J Clin Endocrinol Metab* 2002;87:118–121.

66. Kurzer MS. Phytoestrogen supplement use by women. *J Nutr* 2003;133:1983s–1986s.

67. Mangano KM, Hutchins-Wiese HL, Kenny AM, et al. Soy proteins and isoflavones reduce interleukin-6 but not serum lipids in older women: a randomized controlled trial. *Nutr Res* 2013;33(12):1026–1033.

68. van der Schouw YT, Kreijkamp-Kaspers S, Peeters PH, et al. Prospective study on usual dietary phytoestrogen intake and cardiovascular disease risk in Western women. *Circulation* 2005;111:465–471.

69. Milligan S, Kalita J, Pocock V, et al. Oestrogenic activity of the hop phyto-oestrogen, 8-prenylnaringenin. *Reproduction* 2002;123:235–242.

70. Milligan S, Kalita J, Heyerick A, et al. Identification of a potent phytoestrogen in hops (*Humulus lupulus L.*) and beer. *J Clin Endocrinol Metab* 1999;84:2249–2252.

71. Calabrese G. Nonalcoholic compounds of wine: the phytoestrogen resveratrol and moderate red wine consumption during menopause. *Drugs Exp Clin Res* 1999;25:111–114.

72. Li X, Phillips FM, An HS, et al. The action of resveratrol, a phytoestrogen found in grapes, on the intervertebral disc. *Spine* (Phila Pa 1976) 2008;33(24):2586–2595.

73. Stevens JF, Page JE. Xanthohumol and related prenylflavonoids from hops and beer: to your good health! *Phytochemistry* 2004;65:1317–1330.

74. Ming LG, Lv X, Ma XN, et al. The prenyl group contributes to activities of phytoestrogen 8-prenylnaringenin in enhancing bone formation and inhibiting bone resorption in vitro. *Endocrinology* 2013;154(3):1202–1214.

75. Ming LG, Chen KM, Xian CJ. Functions and action mechanisms of flavonoids genistein and icariin in regulating bone remodeling. *J Cell Physiol* 2013;228(3):513–521.

76. Atkinson C, Compston JE, Day NE, et al. The effects of phytoestrogen isoflavones on bone density in women: a double-blind, randomized, placebo-controlled trial. *Am J Clin Nutr* 2004;79:326–333.

77. Alekel DL, Germain AS, Peterson CT, et al. Isoflavone-rich soy protein isolate attenuates bone loss in the lumbar spine of perimenopausal women. *Am J Clin Nutr* 2000;72:844–885.

78. Lydeking-Olsen E, Beck-Jensen JE, Setchell KD, et al. Soymilk or progesterone for prevention of bone loss—a 2 year randomized, placebo-controlled trial. *Eur J Nutr* 2004;43:246–257.

79. Morabito N, Crisafulli A, Vergara C, et al. Effects of genistein and hormone-replacement therapy on bone loss in early postmenopausal women: a randomized double-blind placebo-controlled study. *J Bone Miner Res* 2002;17:1904–1912.

80. Anderson JJB, Chen X, Boass A, et al. Soy isoflavones: no effects on bone mineral content and bone mineral density in healthy, menstruating young adult women after one year. *J Am Coll Nutr* 2002;21:388–393.

81. Kreijkamp-Kaspers S, Kok L, Grobbee DE, et al. Effect of soy protein containing isoflavones on cognitive function, bone mineral density, and plasma lipids in postmenopausal women. *JAMA* 2004;292:65–74.

82. Scheiber M, Rebar R. Isoflavones and postmenopausal bone health: a viable alternative to estrogen therapy? *Menopause* 1999;6:233–241.

83. Alexandersen P, Toussaint A, Christiansen C, et al. Ipriflavone in the treatment of postmentopausal osteoporosis. *JAMA* 2001;285:1482–1488.

84. Weaver CM, Cheong MK. Soy isoflavones and bone health: the relationship is still unclear. *J Nutr* 2005;135:1243–1247.

85. Cheong JMK, Martin BR, Jackson GS, et al. Soy isoflavones do not affect bone resorption in postmenopausal women: a dose-response study using a novel approach with ^{41}Ca. *J Clin Endocrinol Metab* 2007;92:577–582.

86. Lagari VS, Levis S. Phytoestrogens for menopausal bone loss and climacteric symptoms. *J Steroid Biochem Mol Biol* 2014;139:294–301.

87. Mitchell J, Cawood E, Kinniburgh D, et al. Effect of a phytoestrogen food supplement on reproductive health in normal males. *Clin Sci* (Lond) 2001;100:613–618.

88. Setchell K, Zimmer-Nechemias L, Cai J, et al. Isoflavone content of infant formulas and the metabolic fate of these phytoestrogens in early life. *Am J Clin Nutr* 1998;68:1453s–1461s.

89. Franke AA, Halm BM, Custer LJ, et al. Isoflavones in breastfed infants after mothers consume soy. *Am J Clin Nutr* 2006;84:406–413.

90. Bonacasa B, Siow RC, Mann GE. Impact of dietary soy isoflavones in pregnancy on fetal programming of endothelial function in offspring. *Microcirculation* 2011;18(4):270–285.

91. Low Y-L, Dunning AM, Dowsett M, et al. Phytoestrogen exposure is associated with circulating sex hormone levels in postmenopausal women and interact with ESR1 and NR1I2 gene variants. *Cancer Epidemiol Biomarkers Prev* 2007;16:1009–1016.

92. Mesiano S, Katz S, Lee J, et al. Phytoestrogens alter adrenocortical function: genistein and diadzein suppress glucocorticoid and stimulate androgen production by cultured adrenal cortical cells. *J Clin Endocrinol Metab* 1999;84:2443–2448.

93. Remer T, Pietrzik K, Manz F. Short-term impact of a lactovegetarian diet on adrenocortical activity and adrenal androgens. *J Clin Endocrinol Metab* 1998;83: 2132–2137.

94. Dillingham BL, McVeigh BL, Lampe JW, et al. Soy protein isolates of varying isoflavone content exert minor effects on serum reproductive hormones in healthy young men. *J Nutr* 2005;135:584–591.

95. Pillow P, Duphorne C, Chang S, et al. Development of a database for assessing dietary phytoestrogen intake. *Nutr Cancer* 1999;33:3–19.

96. Chun OK, Chung SJ, Song WO. Estimated dietary flavonoid intake and major food sources of US adults. *J Nutr* 2007;137:1244–1252.

97. Agricultural Research Service. *USDA–Iowa State University database on the isoflavone content of foods, Release 1.3.* Washington, DC: US Department of Agriculture, 2002.

98. de Kleijn MJ, van der Schouw YT, Wilson PW, et al. Intake of dietary phytoestrogens is low in postmenopausal women in the United States: the Framingham study. *J Nutr* 2001;131:1826–1832.

99. Messina M. Western soy intake is too low to produce health effects. *Am J Clin Nutr* 2004;80:528–529.

100. Beecher GR. Overview of dietary flavonoids: nomenclature, occurrence and intake. *J Nutr* 2003;133: 3248s–3254s.

101. Wu AH, Wan P, Hankin J, et al. Adolescent and adult soy intake and risk of breast cancer in Asian-Americans. *Carcinogenesis* 2002;23:1491–1496.

102. Setchell KD, Brown NM, Lydeking-Olsen E. The clinical importance of the metabolite equol—a clue to the effectiveness of soy and its isoflavones. *J Nutr* 2002;132: 3577–3584.

103. Lydeking-Olsen E, Jensen J-BE, Damhus M, et al. Isoflavone-rich soymilk prevents bone-loss in the lumbar spine of postmenopausal women. A 2 year study. *J Nutr* 2002;132:581s.

104. Adlercreutz H. Phyto-oestrogens and cancer. *Lancet* 2002;3:364–373.

105. Jackson RL, Greiwe JS, Schwen RJ. Emerging evidence of the health benefits of S-equol, an estrogen receptor β agonist. *Nutr Rev* 2011;69(8):432–448.

106. Frankenfeld CL, McTiernan A, Thomas WK, et al. Postmenopausal bone mineral density in relation to soy isoflavone-metabolizing phenotypes. *Maturitas* 2006; 53(3):315–324.

107. Curtis PJ, Potter J, Kroon PA, et al. Vascular function and atherosclerosis progression after 1 y of flavonoid intake in statin-treated postmenopausal women with type 2 diabetes: a double-blind randomized controlled trial. *Am J Clin Nutr* 2013;97(5):936–942.

108. Lampe JW. Emerging research on equol and cancer. *J Nutr* 2010;140(7):1369S–1372S. doi: 10.3945/jn.109.118323.

109. Ward H, Chapelais G, Kuhnle GG, et al. European Prospective into Cancer-Norfolk cohort. Breast cancer risk in relation to urinary and serum biomarkers of phytoestrogen exposure in the European Prospective into Cancer-Norfolk cohort study. *Breast Cancer Res* 2008;10:R32.

110. Niculescu MD, Pop EA, Fischer LM, et al. Dietary isoflavones differentially induce gene expression changes in lymphocytes from postmenopausal women who form equol as compared with those who do not. *J Nutr Biochem* 2007;18:380–390.

111. Lampe JW. Is equol the key to the efficacy of soy foods? *Am J Clin Nutr* 2009;89(5):1664S–1667S. doi: 10.3945/ ajcn.2009.26736T.

SUGGESTED READINGS

Albertazzi P, Pansini F, Bottazzi M, et al. Dietary soy supplementation and phytoestrogen levels. *Obstet Gynecol* 1999; 94:229–231.

Anderson J, Garner S. Phytoestrogens and bone. *Baillieres Clin Endocrinol Metab* 1998;12:543–557.

Davis SR, Dalais FS, Simpson ER, et al. Phytoestrogens in health and disease. *Recent Prog Horm Res* 1999;54:185.

Duncan A, Merz B, Xu X, et al. Soy isoflavones exert modest hormonal effects in premenopausal women. *J Clin Endocrinol Metab* 1999;84:192–197.

Garner D, Olmstead M, Bohr Y, et al. The eating attitudes test: psychometric features and clinical correlates. *Psychol Med* 1982;12:871–878.

Griffiths K, Denis L, Turkes A, et al. Phytoestrogens and diseases of the prostate gland. *Baillieres Clin Endocrinol Metab* 1998;12:625–647.

Humfrey CD. Phytoestrogens and human health effects: weighting up the current evidence. *Nat Toxins* 1998;6:51.

Keller C, Fullerton J, Mobley C. Supplemental and complementary alternatives to hormone replacement therapy. *J Am Acad Nurse Pract* 1999;11:187.

Moyad M. Soy, disease prevention, and prostate cancer. *Semin Urol Oncol* 1999;17:97–102.

Setchell KD. Phytoestrogens: the biochemistry, physiology, and implications for human health of soy isoflavones. *Am J Clin Nutr* 1998;68:1333s.

Setchell KD, Cassidy A. Dietary isoflavones: biological effects and relevance to human health. *J Nutr* 1999;129:758s.

Stephens F. The rising incidence of breast cancer in women and prostate cancer in men. Dietary influences: a possible preventive role for nature's sex hormone modifiers—the phytoestrogens. *Oncol Rep* 1999;6:865–870.

Washburn S, Burke G, Morgan T, et al. Effect of soy protein supplementation on serum lipoproteins, blood pressure, and menopausal symptoms in perimenopausal women. *Menopause* 1999;6:7–13.

CHAPTER 34

Diet, Sleep–Wake Cycles, and Mood

A potential role for both macronutrients and micronutrients in the regulation of the sleep–wake cycle and mood is of clinical and popular interest. The interaction between diet and mood has the potential to ameliorate or compound affective disorders, eating disorders, and weight gain/obesity. Dietary patterns may influence the quality of nighttime sleep, the propensity for daytime somnolence, vigilance, and concentration.

The role of dietary protein and carbohydrate in the metabolism of serotonin is of particular importance. Pharmacologic manipulation of brain serotonin levels using selective serotonin reuptake inhibitors (SSRIs) has the potential to influence food cravings and dietary patterns as well as affect. Although the literature on nutrition, sleep, and mood is extensive, most studies involve small numbers of subjects. The importance of diet to sleep and mood is increasingly clear, whereas evidence to support specific therapeutic interventions remains largely preliminary to date. There is now persuasive evidence that sleep deprivation may often be an important contributing factor to weight gain/obesity by several means, including neuroendocrine effects (see Chapter 5).

OVERVIEW

In a variety of ways, dietary pattern and nutrients can influence somnolence, alertness, and the adequacy of sleep. The specific neural mechanisms controlling patterns of sleep and wakefulness are under active investigation (1–5). Alterations in levels of neurotransmitters, particularly serotonin (6), as well as dopamine, acetylcholine, and glutamate, are clearly involved and influenced by diet.

Diet and Neurotransmitters

Tryptophan and Serotonin

The amino acid tryptophan is converted into serotonin, which plays an important role in regulating sleep and mood, with implications for obesity as discussed later in the chapter. Tryptophan is relatively abundant in meat and fish, and it is thought to be the soporific substance in the time-honored glass of warm milk. α-lactalbumin, a milk whey protein, contains a higher content of tryptophan than does any other protein food source (7). Tryptophan supplements were available and then banned by the Food and Drug Administration (FDA) following an outbreak of the eosinophilia-myalgia syndrome induced by contaminated batches of L-tryptophan from Japan. However, restrictions on sales were lifted after 2002 as the FDA stated that it could not necessarily conclude that the occurrences of EMS occurred from the content of L-tryptophan; thus, some high-quality supplements are now available (8). Experimentally induced tryptophan depletion has been shown to disrupt the pattern of the sleep electroencephalogram (9,10) and lead to irritability (11). There is also evidence that tryptophan loading is effective in improving mood and sleep in some adults with mood and sleep disturbances, though the effects of tryptophan loading in healthy subjects is less clear (12).

The ingestion of carbohydrate triggers an insulin release that facilitates the deposition of circulating amino acids into skeletal muscle. However, the effect is selective, causing the levels of branched-chain amino acids in circulation to fall by as much as 40%, while negligibly affecting levels of tryptophan (see Chapter 3). The level of tryptophan in the brain is determined in part by its competition with other amino acids; the lower the level of other neutral amino acids presented to the blood–brain barrier, the greater the brain uptake of tryptophan. Since tryptophan hydroxylase, the rate-limiting enzyme of serotonin synthesis, is not saturated at physiological brain tryptophan concentrations, the greater the uptake of tryptophan, the more serotonin is produced (13). Elevations in serotonin enhance mood and promote sleepiness. High-carbohydrate, low-protein meals appear to elevate tryptophan levels (14), with an even greater serotonergic response with high-glycemic-index carbohydrates (15). Afaghi et al. (16) have shown that consumption of a high-carbohydrate, high-glycemic-index evening meal significantly shortens sleep onset latency. The combination of such foods with a concentrated source of tryptophan may be particularly soporific. A tryptophan-rich diet may also alleviate depression (17).

Dopamine

Dopamine, an important transmitter involved in reward and pleasure, is also influenced by diet (18). Studies have shown that dietary fat and sugar reduce dopamine receptor signaling (19), a high-fat diet alters dopamine-related gene expression (20), and the long-term consumption of a low-protein, high-carbohydrate diet decreases dopamine receptor density (21). Striatal dopamine levels were increased in rats supplemented with strawberry, spinach, or vitamin E (22).

The synthesis of catecholamines, including dopamine and norepinephrine, also varies with the availability of the precursor amino acid L-tyrosine. However, the rate of catecholamine synthesis appears to be less influenced by precursor levels than serotonin formation is affected by levels of tryptophan (23).

Acetylcholine

Choline is the precursor to the neurotransmitter acetylcholine, which plays a role in attention and arousal. Choline has been considered a required dietary nutrient since 1998, and experimental data suggest an appropriate intake in adults would be 1 to 2 g of choline chloride daily. However, given that it is ubiquitous in the diet (with a greater presence in organ meats), this is of more relevance for patients who would benefit from the inclusion of choline in parenteral nutrition (24).

Acetylcholine is of particular clinical relevance for Alzheimer's disease and Myasthenia Gravis, though there are no studies looking at the potential role of choline in sleep or mood in these disorders.

Glutamate

The excitatory neurotransmitter glutamate is implicated in the energy balance regulation by the mediobasal hypothalamus. In a study looking at rat models, feeding is associated with rapid release of glutamate, with a greater release of glutamate by foods that stimulate obesity (25).

Diet and Sleep

There are several micronutrients and macronutrients that contribute to sleep. L-theanine, a non-protein amino acid (γ-glutamylethylamide) that occurs naturally in green tea leaves (*Camellia sinensis*), may play a role in sleep quality. In a randomized trial of objectively measured sleep quality in a population of 98 boys diagnosed with attention deficit hyperactivity disorder (ADHD), 400 mg of L-theanine daily was found to be safe and effective in improving the percentage of time in restful sleep, with fewer bouts of nocturnal activity (26). Vitamins also have a role in sleep. Vitamin B_{12} has also been shown to contribute to the secretion of melatonin, a hormone that regulates sleep and wake cycles (27). The last step of the conversion of tryptophan to serotonin is dependent on vitamin B_6, and vitamin B_6 also has some influence on sleep as it was found to increase cortical arousal during rapid eye movement (REM) sleep and to increase the vividness of the dreams (28). Vitamin B_3 (niacin) suppresses the activity of tryptophan 2,3-dioxygenase, a key enzyme in the conversion of tryptophan to niacin. Therefore B_3 supplementation can reduce the "loss" of tryptophan to niacin versus to serotonin and melatonin (27).

The effects of macronutrient distribution on somnolence remain under investigation. The recent discovery of orexin (hypocretin), a hypothalamic peptide involved in both sleep/wakefulness and energy expenditure, has further elucidated the interconnectedness of sleep and satiety (29). In a study of intragastric infusions in nine healthy adult subjects, Wells et al. (30) demonstrated the induction of sleepiness by infusion of lipid as compared with either sucrose or saline. In a crossover trial of 16 adults, somnolence was induced by both a high-fat and a high-carbohydrate test meal (31). In a study of 10 adults, Orr et al. (32) found that sleep latency was reduced by a solid meal, regardless of composition, compared with an isocaloric liquid meal or water. However, some evidence suggests that high-fat meals induce more somnolence, possibly related to the release of cholecystokinin (33). There is also evidence that a low-carbohydrate, high-fat diet decreases the amount of REM sleep, also possibly related to the release of cholecystokinin (34).

There may be considerable interindividual variability in susceptibility to postprandial somnolence (35). When a midday meal was compared to a fast in 21 healthy men, time to onset of sleep was comparable, but sleep duration was longer in the fed state (36). There is suggestive evidence that high-fat meals may induce a particular decline in postprandial alertness and concentration (37) as compared with isocaloric meals higher in carbohydrate. A high-carbohydrate meal has been shown to counter the stimulatory effects of a bout of exercise (38). Although obstructive sleep apnea occurs in normal-weight individuals, it is more common in the obese. While the sleep fragmentation and other sequelae of the syndrome may be ascribed in large measure to excess energy intake (39), new evidence suggests that sleep deprivation may itself lead to neuroendocrine dysregulation, resulting in increased hunger and weight gain, and it may represent a risk factor for type 2 diabetes (40–42).

Alcohol and caffeine ingestion can interfere with sleep, particularly in the elderly (43,44). Low alcohol consumption may enhance sleep induction and deepen sleep initially, but this effect may reverse over the course of the night (45); higher alcohol intake and withdrawal from regular consumption are known to disrupt sleep patterns. Alcohol in breast milk alters the sleep–wake pattern and generally reduces the total duration of sleep in infants (46,47). See Chapter 41 for more about the potential health effects of caffeine.

In addition to diet's influence on sleep, disordered sleep can lead to changes in diet. The night-eating syndrome consists of insomnia, hyperphagia at night, and anorexia in the morning. The condition has been shown to be associated with a blunted nocturnal rise in melatonin and leptin levels and elevated levels of plasma cortisol (48). Features of somnambulism and disordered eating may be concurrent (49), and treatment for both may be indicated. A serotonergic mechanism may also be involved; a recent trial found significant symptomatic improvement and weight loss with SSRI treatment (50).

A study examining the relationship between sleep patterns and adiposity in young adult women showed that inconsistent sleep patterns and poor sleep efficiency are related to adiposity, leading the authors to conclude that consistent sleep patterns including sufficient sleep may be important in modifying risk of excess body fat in young adult women (51). There is also increasing evidence linking sleep deprivation to childhood obesity, with a meta-analysis demonstrating a stronger association between short sleep duration and obesity risk in children than in adults (52). Studies also show a stronger and more consistent findings regarding sleep and weight status in younger children (53,54), with some evidence that boys with short sleep duration were at greater risk of being overweight than girls with short sleep duration (55,56).

Night-shift workers have been found to have increased cardiovascular risk factors compared to day workers (57); circadian rhythms in glucose tolerance and energy metabolism, leading to peaks in glucose and triacylglycerol at night, may be involved (58). There is also some evidence suggesting that the morning chronotype (individual circadian rhythm) is associated with a greater intake of calcium and vitamin B_6 versus the evening chronotype, which is associated with a greater energy intake from alcohol, fat, confections, and meat (59). In a study of night-shift workers, Paz and Berry (60) found only modest differences in mood and performance when meal composition was varied. Mood and performance were optimized by meals containing a macronutrient distribution (55% carbohydrate, 18% protein, and 27% fat) closely matching prevailing nutritional guidelines, as compared with meals higher in either protein or carbohydrate (60).

Diet and Mood

There is evidence linking a healthy diet to a lower incidence of mental health. In a cross-sectional population-based study from Australia (61), a healthy diet was associated with a lower likelihood of depressive and anxiety disorders, while an unhealthy diet was associated with a higher likelihood of psychological symptoms and disorders, independent of confounding variables including age, socioeconomic status, and lifestyle factors. In Spain, a prospective study following a cohort of initially healthy university graduates has found a potential protective role of a Mediterranean dietary pattern in regard to the prevention of depressive disorders (62).

There is a tendency of patients to use carbohydrate and fat to influence serotonin production and thus mood. In a comparison of 24 stress-prone to 24 control subjects, Markus et al. (63) demonstrated that a high-carbohydrate meal, leading to increased brain serotonin levels, mitigated the effects of induced stress in the predisposed subjects. In a randomized crossover trial comparing carbohydrate-craving obese subjects to matched controls, however, Toornvliet et al. (64) found no evidence of mood enhancement with high-carbohydrate meals.

Another example is seen with seasonal affective disorder (SAD), which tends to result in a craving for carbohydrate. The condition is associated with elevated levels of tyrosine and impaired serotonin metabolism. Melatonin was initially implicated, but more recent data refute that concept (65,66). Sunlight exposure and concentrated light therapy constitute the most effective known treatments (67). St. John's wort or intake of complex carbohydrates to elevate levels of serotonin may also be helpful. Evidence for benefit of vitamin D supplementation in SAD is inconsistent (68,69), but it may be helpful in individuals at high risk for deficiency.

The intake of carbohydrates and fats to influence serotonin production is associated with weight gain and obesity (70). In a study of nine women with a history of food cravings, Gendall et al. (71) found that subjects who ate high-protein meals experienced a greater tendency to binge on carbohydrate than after consuming a high-carbohydrate or mixed meal. The authors suggest that sensory-specific satiety or a serotonergic mechanism might be involved. The use of SSRIs may be helpful in the management of obesity in select patients, particularly those with symptoms of depression and carbohydrate craving (70,72). The FDA approved the use of lorcaserin, a selective serotonin receptor agonist that acts as an appetite suppressant, for weight loss for adults with a body mass index of 27 or greater who have at least one weight-related health condition (73–75).

Chocolate is associated with a stronger pleasure response than most other foods (see Chapter 39). Chocolate craving in some women, particularly associated with menstrual cycle variations (see Chapter 28), is strong enough to have been labeled "addiction." Although chocolate ingestion in self-labeled "chocolate addicts" is pleasurable, the guilt associated with ingestion obviates any genuine mood enhancement (76,77). While both serotonergic and dopaminergic systems have been implicated in the mechanism of chocolate craving, recent evidence suggests that this phenomenon is more often a result of emotional eating patterns than a substance-specific "addiction" (78). Similarly, there is ongoing discussion as to what extent sugar more generally is an addiction (79,79a). There is some evidence that it may be addictive for some individuals when consumed in a "binge-like" manner as it has neurochemical effects similar to those of drug intake, albeit in smaller magnitude for sugar (80).

Popular diet books emphasize the restriction of dietary carbohydrate, and especially sugar, in efforts to improve weight control and overall health. However, Surwit et al. (81) demonstrated that with comparable caloric restriction, high- and low-sucrose diets for 6 weeks resulted in comparable degrees of weight loss in obese women, with no discernible differences in emotional affect between groups. Depression, hunger, and negative mood decreased in both groups, and vigilance and positive mood increased, suggesting that these benefits may result from weight loss per se. Restriction of all carbohydrates, as has been advocated by fad high-protein diet regimens, has been shown to increase fatigue and negatively impact mood in physically active individuals (82).

Several studies suggest a potential role for dietary fat and serum lipids in mood regulation; in particular, associations have been demonstrated between low consumption or serum levels of long-chain polyunsaturated fatty acids and depression (83), bipolar disorder (84), and risk of suicide (85). Wells et al. (86) found that converting subjects from a 41% fat-energy to a 25% fat-energy diet for a period of 1 month was associated with adverse changes in mood, including more anger/hostility. These effects were independent of any change in plasma cholesterol. Such effects are likely referable to indiscriminate reductions of fat intake that do not facilitate a balanced intake of fatty acid classes (see Chapters 2 and 45).

Pain perception has been shown to be attenuated in the fed as compared with the fasting state, with dietary fat apparently particularly effective at mitigating pain (87,88). The fasted, or energy-restricted state, however, has not produced consistently deleterious effects. A study in soldiers has shown that 30 days of relative calorie deficiency had no adverse effects on mood or performance as compared with a control condition (89). Similarly, in a study of healthy female volunteers, Green et al. (90) showed that a fast for up to 24 hours has minimal effects on concentration and cognitive function.

Deficiencies of B-complex vitamins are associated with neuropsychiatric disturbances, including delirium and psychosis. Nominal deficiencies may be involved in mood disturbance; low levels of folate and vitamin B_{12} have been observed in studies of depressed patients (91). Evidence of B vitamin deficiencies in the US population has been increasing; nutrient-poor diets high in refined carbohydrate and processed sugar are particularly likely to induce such B vitamin deficiency states. The avoidance of such patterns, and compensation with a daily multivitamin, may confer benefit to mood in susceptible individuals (92).

Dietary Supplements for Sleep and Mood

Melatonin, a hormone produced by the pineal gland, is available exogenously as a dietary supplement with reported benefits for people with sleep disturbances. A recent meta-analysis found significant shortening of sleep latency along with increases in sleep efficiency and duration with administration of melatonin (93); however, the available evidence does not support its efficacy in treating secondary sleep disorders such as shift work disorder (94). Melatonin appears to be both safe and modestly effective in alleviating jet lag when crossing multiple time zones (95). Ramelteon, a melatonin-receptor agonist, has been approved for use in insomnia (96). However, long-term safety studies may still be lacking (97).

Valerian is an herb traditionally used to make tea for treating insomnia. Apparently effective as a mild tranquilizer (98), the sleep-inducing chemical in valerian is as yet unidentified (99). The tea has a bitter and rather unpleasant taste. Valerian root extract is available; 150 to 300 mg approximately 30 minutes before bedtime is recommended. However, adverse reactions in the liver have been suggested between valerian and the antipsychotic haloperidol (100).

Magnesium, a γ-aminobutyric acid (GABA) agonist, may help with age-related sleep difficulty (101); some alternative medicine sources recommend 500 mg of magnesium taken 30 minutes before bedtime, or 250 mg of magnesium in conjunction with melatonin and zinc (102). Some traditional somnolents may exert only a placebo effect. In a double-blind, placebo-controlled study of lemongrass, a common ingredient in sleep-promoting herbal tea, no sedative-hypnotic effects were demonstrated (103).

The herb St. John's wort, or hypericum, has been advocated for use in depression. St. John's wort has been shown in multiple randomized controlled trials to have efficacy equivalent to conventional antidepressants in the treatment of mild to moderate depression (104–107); studies of patients with severe depression have generated conflicting results. The active ingredient, hypericum, appears to inhibit the reuptake of serotonin, dopamine, and norepinephrine (106). The suggested daily intake is approximately 900 mg, divided into either two or three doses (107). The clinical trial evidence remains inconclusive (108–111). St. John's wort is also a potent inducer of enzymes that metabolize other medications, and comedication can result in decreased plasma concentrations of drugs including amitriptyline, cyclosporine, digoxin, indinavir, irinotecan, warfarin, phenprocoumon, alprazolam, dextromethorphan, simvastatin, and oral contraceptives. This effect correlates strongly with the amount of hyperforin found in the product (112). However, a Cochrane review suggests that the hypericum extracts tested in the included trials are superior to placebo in patients with major depression, are similarly effective as standard antidepressants, and have fewer side effects than standard antidepressants (113). A beneficial role of ω-3 fatty acids in affective disorders is suggested but not yet confirmed by the some evidence (114–116); however, a recent meta-analysis did show strong evidence that bipolar depressive symptoms may be improved by adjunctive use of ω-3, though the evidence does not support its adjunctive use in attenuating mania (117). The probability of beneficial effects, the general low risk, and the likely benefits to general health (see Chapter 45) make supplementation as a matter of routine reasonable, if not advisable.

Antidepressant effects have also been attributed to vitamin B_6. A review of the pertinent literature suggests possible effects when depression occurs in premenopausal women, with little evidence of effect in other populations (118).

Nutrigenomics

Folate metabolism genetic polymorphisms have been studied in regard to age of onset, occurrence, and response to treatment for depression. One study looking at late life depression found that there were no significant genetic differences that predicted age of onset of depression or occurrence of depression, but there is a genotype (the MTRR A66G) that does predict response to SSRI antidepressants (119). Given mixed results on whether folic acid and B_{12} supplementation potentiates antidepressant medication (120), further studies on the nutrigenomics in regard to folate metabolism and depression will be helpful to determine whether the effects are in fact limited to certain clinical populations.

■ CLINICAL HIGHLIGHTS

Diet and nutrients influence mood, somnolence, and wakefulness in a variety of ways, many of which are poorly understood at present. The role of food intake on levels of serotonin in the brain has emerged as a mechanism of particular importance. What is known of this pathway suggests that a diet rich in complex carbohydrates, consistent with prevailing recommendations, is appropriate to maintain appropriate serotonin levels. Perturbations in serotonin metabolism may account for both affective and eating disorders, and in such situations, pharmacotherapy with SSRIs may be indicated.

Contrary to the view advanced by many popular diet books, high levels of dietary protein have not been shown to enhance energy levels or sense of well-being. Meals high in fat are associated with particularly pronounced postprandial somnolence. Animal research suggests that extreme dietary fat restriction, however, resulting in reduced plasma lipoprotein levels, may favor aggressiveness. Such findings would support the macronutrient distribution advocated throughout the text, with approximately 55% to 60% of calories from predominantly complex carbohydrate, 20% to 25% from fat, and 15% to 20% from protein (see Chapter 45).

Sleep adequate in quantity and quality is supported by the avoidance of excess caffeine or alcohol in the diet. Sleep apnea is often consequent to obesity; therefore, avoidance of excess energy consumption and overweight is important in efforts to ensure normal sleep patterns. A large midday meal induces postprandial somnolence independent of meal composition, whereas smaller snacks throughout the day actually tend to promote alertness. Thus, the food intake pattern conducive to daytime alertness is that supported by other lines of evidence (see Chapters 5, 6, and 38, indicating the value of distributing calories in small meals). At the same time, some conflicting evidence does show that lower tendency for eating during conventional eating hours and greater snack dominance over meals are related to higher intakes of fat and sweets for energy and lower intakes of fruits and vegetables; thus, there are clearly multiple factors at play (121).

Finally, mood may be influenced by intense cravings for food, sharing characteristics of addiction; chocolate appears to be the most important example. Chocolate craving varies with the phase of the menstrual cycle, as discussed in Chapters 28 and 39. In general, control of such cravings is facilitated by consistent, moderate consumption of the craved food in a fed rather than fasted state.

Various micronutrients may influence affect, but overall, the literature is limited. There is strongest support for ω-3 fatty acids, specifically eicosapentaenoic acid and docosahexaenoic acid (122), also (see Chapter 2) at a dose of 1 to 2 g daily as fish oil. However, there is also new support linking vegetarian diets, with reduced intake of arachidonic acid, as well as eicosapentaenoic acid and docosahexaenoic acid, with improved mood (123). Nonetheless, because supplementation is generally advisable on general principles, this recommendation may be made routinely, barring contraindications.

■ REFERENCES

1. Kayama Y, Koyama Y. Brainstem neural mechanisms of sleep and wakefulness. *Eur Urol* 1998;33:12–15.
2. Xi M, Morales F, Chase M. Evidence that wakefulness and REM sleep are controlled by a GABAergic pontine mechanism. *J Neurophysiol* 1999;82:2015–2019.
3. Gottesmann C. The neurophysiology of sleep and waking: intracerebral connections, functioning and ascending influences of the medulla oblongata. *Prog Neurobiol* 1999;59:1–54.

4. Harris CD. Neurophysiology of sleep and wakefulness. *Respir Care Clin N Am* 2005;11:567–586.

5. Markov D, Goldman M. Normal sleep and circadian rhythms: neurobiologic mechanisms underlying sleep and wakefulness. *Psychiatr Clin North Am* 2006;841–853.

6. Ursin R. Serotonin and sleep. *Sleep Med Rev* 2002;6:55–69.

7. Markus CR, Jonkman LM, Lammers J, et al. Evening intake of alpha-lactalbumin increases plasma tryptophan availability and improves morning alertness and brain measures of attention. *Am J Clin Nutr* 2005;81:1026–1033.

8. Center for Food Safety and Applied Nutrition, Office of Nutritional Products, Labeling, and Dietary Supplements (2001-02-01). FDA/CFSAN – Information Paper on L-tryptophan and 5-hydroxy-L-tryptophan. U.S. Food and Drug Administration.

9. Voderholzer U, Hornyak M, Thiel B, et al. Impact of experimentally induced serotonin deficiency by tryptophan depletion on sleep EEG in healthy subjects. *Neuropsychopharmacology* 1998;18:112–124.

10. Bell CJ, Hood SD, Nutt DJ. Acute tryptophan depletion. Part II: clinical effects and implications. *Aust N Z J Psychiatry* 2005;39:565–574.

11. Young SN, Leyton M. The role of serotonin in human mood and social interaction. Insight from altered tryptophan levels. *Pharmacol Biochem Behav* 2002;71:857–865.

12. Silber BY, Schmitt JAJ. Effects of tryptophan loading on human cognition, mood and sleep. *Neuro Bio Rev* 2010;34:387–407.

13. Le Floc'h N. Tryptophan metabolism, from nutrition to potential therapeutic applications. *Amino Acids* 2011;41:1195–1205.

14. Wurtman RJ, Wurtman JJ, Regan MM, et al. Effect of normal meals rich in carbohydrates or proteins on plasma tryptophan and tyrosine rations. *Am J Clin Nutr* 2003;77:128–132.

15. Lyons PM, Truswell AS. Serotonin precursor influenced by type of carbohydrate meal in healthy adults. *Am J Clin Nutr* 1988;47:433–439.

16. Afaghi A, O'Connor H, Chow CM. High-glycemic-index carbohydrate meals shorten sleep onset. *Am J Clin Nutr* 2007;85:426–430.

17. Shabbir F, Patel A, Mattison C et al. Effect of diet on serotonergic neurotransmission in depression. *Neurochem Int* 2013;62:324–329.

18. Lopresti AL, Hood SD, Drummond PD. A review of lifestyle factors that contribute to important pathways associated with major depression: Diet, sleep and exercise. *J Affect Disord* 2013;148:12–27.

19. Pritchett CE, Hajnal A. Obesogenic diets may differentially alter dopamine control of sucrose and fructose intake in rats. *Physiol Behav* 2011;104:111–116.

20. Vucetic Z, Carlin JL, Totoki K, et al. Epigenetic dysregulation of the dopamine system in diet-induced obesity. *J Neurochem* 2012;120:891–898.

21. Hamdi A, Onavivi ES, Prasad C. A low protein-high carbohydrate diet decreases D2 dopamine receptor density in rat brain. *Life Sci* 1992;50:1529–1534.

22. Martin A, Prior R, Shukitt-Hale B, et al. Effect of fruits, vegetables, or vitamin E-rich diet on vitamins E and C distribution in peripheral and brain tissues: implications for brain function. *J Gerontol Ser A Biol Sci Med Sci* 2000;55:B144–B151.

23. Fernstrom JD. Effects on the diet on brain neurotransmitters. *Metabolism* 1977;26:207–223.

24. Buchman A. The addition of choline to parenteral nutrition. *Gastroenterology* 2009;137:S119–S128.

25. Guyenet SJ, Matsen ME, Morton GJ, et al. Rapid glutamate release in the mediobasal hypothalamus accompanies feeding and is exaggerated by an obesogenic food. *Mol Metab* 2013;2(2):116–122.

26. Lyon MR, Kapoor MP, Juneja LR. The effects of L-theanine (Suntheanine®) on objective sleep quality in boys with attention deficit hyperactivity disorder (ADHD): a randomized, double-blind, placebo-controlled clinical trial. *Altern Med Rev* 2011;16:348–354.

27. Peuhkuri K, Sihvola N, Korpela R. Diet promotes sleep duration and quality. *Nutr Res* 2012;32:309–319.

28. Ebben M, Lequerica A, Spielman A. Effects of pyridoxine on dreaming: a preliminary study. *Percept Mot Skills* 2002;94:135–140.

29. Sakurai T. Roles of orexin/hypocretin in regulation of sleep/wakefulness and energy homeostasis. *Sleep Med Rev* 2005;9:231–241.

30. Wells A, Read N, Macdonald I. Effects of carbohydrate and lipid on resting energy expenditure, heart rate, sleepiness, and mood. *Physiol Behav* 1998;63:621–628.

31. Wells A, Read N, Idzikowski C, et al. Effects of meals on objective and subjective measures of daytime sleepiness. *J Appl Physiol* 1998;84:507–515.

32. Orr W, Shadid G, Harnish M, et al. Meal composition and its effect on postprandial sleepiness. *Physiol Behav* 1997;62:709–712.

33. Wells A, Read N, Uvnas-Moberg K, et al. Influences of fat and carbohydrate on postprandial sleepiness, mood, and hormones. *Physiol Behav* 1997;61:679–686.

34. Afaghi A, O'Connor H, Chow CM. Acute effects of the very low carbohydrate diet on sleep indices. *Nutr Neurosci* 2008;11:146–54.

35. Monk T, Buysse D, Reynolds CR, et al. Circadian determinants of the postlunch dip in performance. *Chronobiol Int* 1996;14:123–133.

36. Zammit G, Kolevzon A, Fauci M, et al. Postprandial sleep in healthy men. *Sleep* 1995;18:229–231.

37. Wells A, Read N, Craig A. Influences of dietary and intraduodenal lipid on alertness, mood, and sustained concentration. *Br J Nutr* 1995;74:115–123.

38. Verger P, Lagarde D, Betejat D, et al. Influence of the composition of a meal taken after physical exercise on mood, vigilance, performance. *Physiol Behav* 1998;64:317–322.

39. Day R, Gerhardstein R, Lumley A, et al. The behavioral morbidity of obstructive sleep apnea. *Prog Cardiovasc Dis* 1999;41:341–354.

40. Spiegel K, Knutson K, Leproult R, et al. Sleep loss: a novel risk factor for insulin resistance and type 2 diabetes. *J Appl Physiol* 2005;99:2008–2019.

41. Leproult R, Van Cauter E. Role of sleep and sleep loss in hormonal release and metabolism. *Endocr Dev* 2010;17:11–21.

42. St-Onge MP, Roberts AL, Chen J et al. Short sleep duration increases energy intake but does not change energy expenditure in normal-weight individuals. *Am J Clin Nutr* 2011;94:410–416.

43. Neubauer D. Sleep problems in the elderly. *Am Fam Physician* 1999;59:2551–2558, 2559–2560.

44. Wolkove N, Elkholy O, Baltzan M, et al. Sleep and aging: 1. Sleep disorders commonly found in older people. *CMAJ* 2007;176:1299–1304.

45. Feige B, Gann H, Brueck R, et al. Effects of alcohol on polysomnographically recorded sleep in healthy subjects. *Alcohol Clin Exp Res* 2006;30:1527–1537.

46. Mennella J, Gerrish C. Effects of exposure to alcohol in mother's milk on infant sleep. *Pediatrics* 1998;101:E2.

47. Mennella J. Alcohol's effect on lactation. *Alcohol Res Health* 2001;25:230–234.

48. Birketvedt G, Florholmen J, Sundsfjord J, et al. Behavioral and neuroendocrine characteristics of the night-eating syndrome. *JAMA* 1999;282:657–663.

49. Winkelman J. Clinical and polysomnographic features of sleep-related eating disorder. *J Clin Psychiatry* 1998;59:14–19.

50. O'Reardon JP, Allison KC, Martino NS, et al. A randomized, placebo-controlled trial of sertraline in the treatment of night eating syndrome. *Am J Psychiatry* 2006;163:893–898.

51. Bailey BW, Allen MD, Lecheminant JD, et al. Objectively measured sleep patterns in young adult women and the relationship to adiposity. *Am J Health Promot* 2013;(epub ahead of print.)

52. Hart CN, Lawton J, Fava JL, et al. Changes in children's eating behaviors following increases and decreases in their sleep duration. *Ann Behav Med* 2012;43:s77.

53. Chen X, Beydoun MA, Wang Y. Is sleep duration associated with childhood obesity? A systematic review and meta-analysis. *Obesity* (Silver Spring) 2008;16:265–274.

54. Bell JF, Zimmerman FJ. Shortened nighttime sleep duration in early life and subsequent childhood obesity. *Arch Pediatr Adolesc Med* 2010;164:840–845.

55. Cappuccio FP, Taggart FM, Kandala NB, et al. Meta-analysis of short sleep duration and obesity in children and adults. *Sleep* 2008;31:619–626.

56. Shi Z, Taylor AW, Gill TK, et al. Short sleep duration and obesity among Australian children. *BMC Public Health* 2010;10:609.

57. Di Lorenzo L, De Pergola G, Zocchetti C, et al. Effect of shift work on body mass index: results of a study performed in 319 glucose-tolerant men working in a southern Italian industry. *Int J Obes Relat Metab Disord* 2003;27:1353–1358.

58. Holmback U, Forslund A, Forslund J, et al. Metabolic responses to nocturnal eating in med are affected by sources of dietary energy. *J Nutr* 2002;132:1892–1899.

59. Sato-Mito N, Sasaki S, Murakami K, et al. Freshmen in Dietetic Courses Study II group. The midpoint of sleep is associated with dietary intake and dietary behavior among young Japanese women. *Sleep Med* 2011;12:289–94.

60. Paz A, Berry E. Effect of meal composition on alertness and performance of hospital night-shift workers. Do mood and performance have different determinants? *Ann Nutr Metab* 1997;41:291–298.

61. Jacka FN, Pasco JA, Mykletun A, et al. Association of Western and traditional diets with depression and anxiety in women. *Am J Psychiatry* 2010;167(3):305–311.

62. Sanchez-Villegas A, Delgado-Rodriguez M, Alonso A, et al. Association of the Mediterranean dietary pattern with the incidence of depression: the Seguimiento Universidad de Navarra/University of Navarra follow-up (SUN) cohort. *Arch Gen Psychiatry* 2009;66(10):1090–1098.

63. Markus CR, Panhuysen G, Tuiten A, et al. Does carbohydrate-rich, protein-poor food prevent a deterioration of mood and cognitive performance of stress-prone subjects when subjected to a stressful task? *Appetite* 1998;31:49.

64. Toornvliet A, Pijl H, Tuinenberg J, et al. Psychological and metabolic responses of carbohydrate craving obese patients to carbohydrate, fat, and protein-rich meals. *Int J Obes Relat Metab Disord* 1997;21:860–864.

65. Partonen T, Lonnqvist J. Seasonal affective disorder. *Lancet* 1998;352:1369–1374.

66. Partonen T, Vakkuri O, Lonnqvist J. Suppression of melatonin secretion by bright light in seasonal affective disorder. *Biol Psychiatry* 1997;42:509–513.

67. Miller AL. Epidemiology, etiology, and natural treatment of seasonal affective disorder. *Altern Med Rev* 2005;10:5–13.

68. Lansdowne A, Provost S. Vitamin D_3 enhances mood in healthy subjects during winter. *Psychopharmacology* (Berl) 1998;135:319–323.

69. Dumville JC, Miles JN, Porthouse J, et al. Can vitamin D supplementation prevent winter-time blues? A randomized trial among older women. *J Nutr Health Aging* 2006;10:151–153.

70. Wurtman R, Wurtman J. Brain serotonin, carbohydrate-craving, obesity and depression. *Obes Res* 1995;3:477s–480s.

71. Gendall K, Joyce P, Abbott R. The effects of meal composition on subsequent cravings and binge eating. *Addict Behav* 1999;24:305–315.

72. Halford JC, Harrold JA, Lawton CL, et al. Serotonin (5-HT) drugs: effects on appetite expression and use for the treatment of obesity. *Curr Drug Targets* 2005;6:201–213.

73. Smith SR, Weissman NJ, Anderson CM, et al. Multicenter, placebo-controlled trial of lorcaserin for weight management. *NEJM* 2010;363:245–256.

74. Fidler MC, Sanchez M, Raether B, et al. A one-year randomized trial of lorcaserin for weight loss in obese and overweight adults: the BLOSSOM trial. *J Clin Endocrinol Metab* 2011;96:3067–3077.

75. O'Neil PM. Randomized placebo-controlled clinical trial of lorcaserin for weight loss in type 2 diabetes mellitus: the BLOOM-DM study. *Obesity* 2012;20:1426–1436.

76. Macdiarmid J, Hetherington M. Mood modulation by food: an exploration of affect and cravings in "chocolate addicts." *Br J Clin Psychol* 1995;34:129–138.

77. Rogers PJ, Smit HJ. Food craving and food "addiction": a critical review of the evidence from a biopsychosocial perspective. *Pharmacol Biochem Behav* 2000;66:3–14.

78. Parker G, Parker I, Brotchie H. Mood state effects of chocolate. *J Affect Disord* 2006;92:149–159.

79. Ziauddeen H, Fletcher PC. Is food addiction a valid and useful concept? *Obesity Rev* 2013;14:19–28.

79a. DiLeone RJ, Taylor JR, Picciotto MR. The drive to eat: comparisons and distinctions between mechanisms of food reward and drug addiction. *Nat Neurosci*. 2012;15:1330–5.

80. Avena NM, Rada P, Hoebel BG. Evidence for sugar addiction: behavioral and neurochemical effects of intermittent, excessive sugar intake. *Neurosci Biobehav Rev* 2008;32:20–39.

81. Surwit R, Feinglos M, McCaskill C, et al. Metabolic and behavioral effects of a high-sucrose diet during weight loss. *Am J Clin Nutr* 1997;65:908–915.

82. Butki BD, Baumstark J, Driver S. Effects of a carbohydrate-restricted diet on affective responses to acute exercise among physically active participants. *Percept Mot Skills* 2003;96:607–615.

83. Tanskanen A, Hibbeln JR, Tuomilehto J, et al. Fish consumption and depressive symptoms in the general population in Finland. *Psychiatr Serv* 2001;52:529–531.

84. Noaghiul S, Hibbeln JR. Cross-national comparisons of seafood consumption and rates of bipolar disorders. *Am J Psychiatry* 2003;160:2222–2227.

85. Sublette ME, Hibbeln JR, Galfalvy H, et al. Omega-3 polyunsaturated essential fatty acid status as a predictor of future suicide risk. *Am J Psychiatry* 2006;163:1100–1102.

86. Wells A, Read N, Laugharne J, et al. Alterations in mood after changing to a low-fat diet. *Br J Nutr* 1998;79:23–30.

87. Zmarzty S, Wells A, Read N. The influence of food on pain perception in healthy human volunteers. *Physiol Behav* 1997;62:185–191.

88. Beauchamp GK, Keast RS, Morel D, et al. Ibuprofen-like activity in extra-virgin olive oil. *Nature* 2005;437;45–46.

89. Shukitt-Hale B, Askew E, Lieberman H. Effects of 30 days of undernutrition on reaction time, moods, and symptoms. *Physiol Behav* 1997;62:783–789.

90. Green M, Elliman N, Rogers P. Lack of effect of short-term fasting on cognitive function. *J Psychiatr Res* 1995;29:245–253.

91. Coppen A, Bolander-Gouaille C. Treatment of depression: time to consider folic acid and vitamin B_{12}. *J Psychopharmacol* 2005;19:59–65.

92. Taylor MJ, Carney S, Geddes J, et al. Folate for depressive disorders. *Cochrane Database Syst Rev* 2003;2:CD 003390.

93. Brzezinski A, Vangel MG, Wurtman RJ, et al. Effects of exogenous melatonin on sleep: a meta-analysis. *Sleep Med Rev* 2005;9:41–50.

94. Buscemi N, Vandermeer B, Hooton N, et al. Efficacy and safety of exogenous melatonin for secondary sleep disorders and sleep disorders accompanying sleep restriction: meta-analysis. *BMJ* 2006;332:385–393.

95. Herxheimer A, Petrie KJ. Melatonin for the prevention and treatment of jet lag. *Cochrane Database Syst Rev* 2002;2:CD001520.

96. Kato K, Hirai K, Nishiyama K, et al. Neurochemical properties of ramelteon (TAK-375), a selective MT_3/MT_2 receptor agonist. *Neuropharmacology* 2005;48:301–310.

97. Cardinali DP, Srinivasan V, Brzezinski A, et al. Melatonin and its analogs in insomnia and depression. *J Pineal Res* 2012;52:365–375.

98. Hadley S, Petry JJ. Valerian. *Am Fam Physician* 2003;67:1755–1758.

99. Houghton PJ. The scientific basis for the reputed activity of Valerian. *J Pharm Pharmacol* 1999;51:505–512.

100. Dalla Corte CL, Fachinetto R, Colle D, et al. Potentially adverse interactions between haloperidol and valerian. *Food Chem Toxicol* 2008;46:2369–2375.

101. Held K, Antonijevic IA, Kunzel H, et al. Oral Mg(2+) supplementation reverses age-related neuroendocrine and sleep EEG changes in humans. *Pharmacopsychiatry* 2002;35:135–143.

102. Rondanelli M, Opizzi A, Monteferrario F, et al. The effect of melatonin, magnesium, and zinc on primary insomnia in long-term care facility residents in Italy: a double-blind, placebo-controlled clinical trial. *J Am Geriatr Soc.* 2011;59:82–90.

103. Leite J, Seabra Mde L, Maluf E, et al. Pharmacology of lemongrass (*Cymbopogon citratus Stapf*). III. Assessment of eventual toxic, hypnotic and anciolytic effects on humans. *J Ethnopharmacol* 1986;17:75–83.

104. Schrader E. Equivalence of St John's wort extract (Ze 117) and fluoxetine: a randomized, controlled study in mild-moderate depression. *Int Clin Psychopharmacol* 2000;15:61–68.

105. Brenner R, Azbel V, Madhusoodanan S, et al. Comparison of an extract of hypericum (LI 160) and sertraline in the treatment of depression: a double-blind, randomized pilot study. *Clin Ther* 2000;22:411–419.

106. Muller WE. Current St John's wort research from mode of action to clinical efficacy. *Pharmacol Res* 2003;47:101–109.

107. Lawvere S, Mahoney MC. St. John's wort. *Am Fam Physician* 2005;72:2249–2254.

108. Thachil AF, Mohan R, Bhugra D. The evidence base of complementary and alternative therapies in depression. *J Affect Disord* 2007;97:23–35.

109. Clement K, Covertson CR, Johnson MJ, et al. St. John's wort and the treatment of mild to moderate depression: a systematic review. *Holist Nurs Pract* 2006;20:197–203.

110. Fava M, Alpert J, Nierenberg AA, et al. A double-blind, randomized trial of St John's wort, fluoxetine, and placebo in major depressive disorder. *J Clin Psychopharmacol* 2005;25:441–447.

111. Linde K, Mulrow CD, Berner M, et al. St John's wort for depression. *Cochrane Database Syst Rev* 2005;2:CD 000448.

112. Madabushi R, Frank B, Drewelow B et al. Hyperforin in St. John's wort drug interactions. *Eur J Clin Pharmacol* 2006;62:225–233.

113. Linde K, Berner MM, Kriston L. St. John's wort for major depression. *Cochrane Database Syst Rev* 2008;8:CD 000448.

114. Do omega-3 fatty acids help in depression? *Drug Ther Bull* 2007;45:9–12.

115. Parker G, Gibson NA, Brotchie H, et al. Omega-3 fatty acids and mood disorders. *Am J Psychiatry* 2006;163:969–978.

116. Williams AL, Katz D, Ali A, et al. Do essential fatty acids have a role in the treatment of depression? *J Affect Disord* 2006;93:117–123.

117. Sarris J, Mischoulon D, Schweitzer I. Omega-3 for bipolar disorder: meta-analyses of use in mania and bipolar depression. *J Clin Psychiatry* 2012;73:81–86.

118. Williams AL, Cotter A, Sabina A, et al. The role for vitamin B-6 as treatment for depression: a systematic review. *Fam Pract* 2005;22:532–537.

119. Jamerson BD, Payne ME, Garrett ME, et al. Folate metabolism genes, dietary folate and response to antidepressant medications in late-life depression. *Int J Geriatr Psychiatry* 2013;28(9):925–932.

120. Christensen H, Aiken A, Batterham PJ, et al. No clear potentiation of antidepressant medication effects by folic acid + vitamin B12 in a large community sample. *J Affect Disord* 2011;130:37–45.

121. Kim S, DeRoo LA, Sandler DP, et al. Eating patterns and nutritional characteristics associated with sleep duration. *Public Health Nutr* 2010;14:889–895.

122. Sinn N, Milte CM, Street SJ, et al. Effects of n-3 fatty acids, EPA v. DHA, on depressive symptoms, quality of life, memory and executive function in older adults with mild cognitive impairement: a 6 month randomized controlled trial. *Br J Nutr* 2012;107:1682–1693.

123. Beezhold BL, Johnston CS. Restriction of meat, fish and poultry in omnivores improves mood: a pilot randomized controlled trial. *Nutr J* 2012;11:9.

SUGGESTED READINGS

Avery D, Lenz M, Landis C. Guidelines for prescribing melatonin. *Ann Med* 1998;30:122–130.

Bellisle F, Blundell JE, Dye L, et al. Functional food science and behavior and psychological functions. *Br J Nutr* 1998;80:s173–s193.

Breakey J. The role of diet and behavior in childhood. *J Paediatr Child Health* 1997;33:190–194.

Christensen L. The effect of carbohydrates on affect. *Nutrition* 1997;13:503–514.

Deltito J, Beyer D. The scientific, quasi-scientific and popular literature on the use of St. John's wort in the treatment of depression. *J Affect Disord* 1998;51:345–351.

Garcia-Garcia F, Drucker-Colin R. Endogenous and exogenous factors on sleep–wake cycle regulation. *Prog Neurobiol* 1999;58:297–314.

Kanarek R. Psychological effects of snacks and altered meal frequency. *Br J Nutr* 1997;77:s105–s120.

Kaplan J, Muldoon M, Manuck S, et al. Assessing the observed relationship between low cholesterol and violence-related mortality. Implications for suicide risk. *Ann N Y Acad Sci* 1997;836:57–80.

Keenan SA. Normal human sleep. *Respir Care Clin N Am* 1999;5:319–331.

Kirkwood CK. Management of insomnia. *J Am Pharm Assoc (Wash DC)* 1999;39:688–696.

Kurzer MS. Women, food, and mood. *Nutr Rev* 1997;55:268–276.

Spitzer R, Terman M, Williams J, et al. Jet lag: clinical features, validation of a new syndrome-specific scale, and lack of response to melatonin in a randomized, double-blind trial. *Am J Psychiatr* 1999;156:1392–1396.

Toornvliet AC, Pijl H, Tuinenburg JC, et al. Psychological and metabolic responses of carbohydrate craving obese patients to carbohydrate, fat and protein-rich meals. *Int J Obes Metab Disord* 1997;21:860–864.

Tuomisto T, Heterington M, Morris M, et al. Psychological and physiological characteristics of sweet food "addiction." *Int J Eat Disord* 1999;25:169–175.

Diet and Cognitive Function

The importance of nutritional status in the development of the brain and normal cognitive function is indisputable. Although there is considerable interest in the role of diet in the age-related decline in mental capacity, the evidence linking specific dietary patterns and practices to the prevention or promotion of such decline is at best suggestive. More definitive evidence of such associations is likely to accrue quite slowly.

The study of diet and cognition is hampered by difficulty in the establishment of temporal relationships (i.e., change in mental status may influence diet rather than the other way around) and the difficulty in obtaining accurate dietary intake data from individuals with cognitive deficits. Despite these limitations, available data support general recommendations for maintenance of lean body mass (i.e., the prevention of ongoing weight loss), intake of adequate but not excessive calories, and abundant intake of antioxidant vitamins, B vitamins, and minerals.

There is evidence supporting increased consumption of fruits and vegetables, as well as n-3 fatty acids from fish. Intake of total fat, saturated fat, and cholesterol should be moderate. Although the strength of these associations in the literature on cognitive function is modest, such recommendations may be made on the basis of evidence in other areas of health promotion and maintenance.

OVERVIEW

Diet

Antiaging properties of antioxidant nutrients have stimulated interest in the role these nutrients might play in the enhancement and preservation of cognitive ability. Further, oxidative injury is recognized in neurodegenerative conditions (1). Animal studies suggest that dietary supplementation with fruit or vegetable extracts rich in antioxidants, or with isolated vitamin E, may retard age-related declines in cognitive function and basic neurophysiology (2,3). Despite promising epidemiological evidence, experimental evidence of benefit of dietary antioxidants in preservation of neurocognitive function in humans is still inconsistent and limited to date (4,5).

Suggestion of benefit from mouse models and observational studies has emerged for vitamins E and C (6,7). One prospective study found that the combined daily use of 400 IU vitamin E with 500 mg vitamin C was associated with the reduction of both prevalence and incidence of Alzheimer's disease (AD) (8). Another population-based prospective cohort study also found a modest decrease in risk of dementia with vitamin E supplementation (9). A 15-year cohort study also found that vitamin E supplementation in patients with AD extended survival (10). However, subsequent randomized clinical trials have not found convincing evidence of benefit for vitamin E in improving cognitive outcomes in older adults (11–14). Given concern over potential risks of high-dose vitamin E supplementation in patients with preexisting vascular disease or diabetes mellitus, vitamin E supplements are not currently recommended for primary or secondary prevention of AD (15), although diets rich in foods containing antioxidants can still be recommended with enthusiasm on general principles. A study found that elderly adults who drank fruit or vegetable juices at least three times per week were significantly less likely to develop AD compared to those who drank juices less than once per week (hazard ratio [HR], 0.24; 95% CI, 0.09 to 0.61), even after adjusting for possible confounders. Of note, this study found a greater reduction in risk among the subjects with the apolipoprotein E4 allele, and it did not find any association with vitamins E and C, β-carotene, or tea consumption (16).

Difficulties in assessing the relationship between antioxidants and cognitive impairment include the possibility that cognitive impairment alters dietary intake (17), as well as the inherent difficulty in obtaining accurate dietary intake data from cognitively impaired individuals. In addition, many of the cross-sectional studies demonstrating positive associations between nutrient intake and cognitive function use food-frequency questionnaires, which only measure intake of whole foods, to estimate intake of specific micronutrients.

Some evidence suggests that AD may have more in common with vascular dementia than has previously been thought (18). It now appears that AD may also stem from vascular insufficiency, and known preventive measures for vascular dementia may therefore also reduce the risk of developing AD (19). Hypercholesterolemia and hypertension have been shown to increase the risk for AD (20), and there is some evidence that a diet high in saturated or trans fats may be associated with cognitive decline in the elderly (21). In one study of long-term antihypertensive therapy in patients with preexisting systolic hypertension and no dementia at baseline, therapy was found to reduce the risk of dementia by 55% when compared with the non-treatment controls (22).

Studies have also found a strong association between AD and diabetes (see Chapter 6), where risk of AD is approximately doubled in people with diabetes (23,24). This relationship is even stronger in people with APOE epsilon 4 gene (25). It is thought that insulin signaling plays a key role in the health of neurons, including the development of neurotransmitters, memory formation, and importantly, regulation of the phosphorylation of tau proteins (26,27). Disruption of insulin signaling in the brain seen in patients with AD mimics peripheral disruption of insulin signaling found in diabetes (26), and some have proposed referring to AD as "Type 3 Diabetes" (28). If AD represent a form of diabetes selective to the brain, it may be possible to alter or even prevent incidence of AD by modifying diabetes risk factors. Perlmutter has published a recent mainstream book entitled *Grain Brain*, arguing that strict glycemic control may be the key to preventing cognitive decline and AD (29). He cites research demonstrating that diets high in carbohydrates appeared to promote the development of AD, whereas diets rich in healthy fats appeared to decrease incidence (30).

Another recent study based on theoretical predictions estimated that by reducing vascular disease risk factors like hypertension, diabetes, and inactivity by 10% to 25%, up to one half of all Alzheimer Disease cases could be prevented (31). While prudent to treat patients with hypertension with antihypertensive medications and patients with diabetes with anti-diabetes medications, administration of these medications for primary dementia prevention is not currently recommended (32).

The evidence linking cigarette smoking to cognitive decline in either men or women is mixed (33,34). A potential beneficial effect of moderate alcohol intake, especially wine, on cognitive function and progression to dementia has been reported (35). One study that followed 121 patients with mild cognitive impairment for 3.5 years found that those with moderate daily wine intake (approximately 15 g of alcohol) had a significantly lower rate of progression to dementia than those who did not drink alcohol (HR, 0.15; 95% CI, 0.03 to 0.77) (36,37), with no additional protection apparent with more than one drink per day. Another study followed women over 34 years, tracking alcohol intake and dementia incidence, and found that wine was associated with a decreased risk of dementia, whereas other alcoholic beverages were associated with unchanged or even increased risk (38). The mechanism for such effects is conjectured to be inhibition or promotion of atherosclerosis in the cerebrovasculature (see Chapter 10).

The association between overall dietary pattern and cognitive function has been assessed in several population studies, using the healthy diet index (HDI) established by the World Health Organization as a summary of dietary pattern. Evidence to date suggests that overall "healthier" diets are associated with better cognitive performance in the elderly (39,40). Several studies have now explored the cognitive effects of the Mediterranean diet, a diet rich in fruits, vegetables, nuts, and olive oil. Known to dramatically lower risk for cardiovascular disease and overall mortality, the Mediterranean diet has also been found to decrease cognitive decline and risk of dementia (41–44). High intake of vegetables, especially green leafy vegetables, has been associated with slower cognitive decline in several populations of aging adults (45).

It seems that some of the items popularly touted as "brain foods" may indeed support cognitive function as part of a healthy diet. For example, preliminary evidence from in vitro and animal studies suggests that foods rich in polyphenols, such as green tea (46) and blueberries (47,48), may have neuroprotective effects (49).

There is evidence that high intake of linoleic acid (polyunsaturated, n-6) may accelerate cognitive decline, whereas fish consumption and consequent n-3 polyunsaturated fat intake may be protective (50–52). One randomized controlled trial (RCT), which randomized patients with AD to daily intake of 1.7 g docosahexaenoic acid (DHA) and 0.6 g eicosapentaenoic acid (EPA) or placebo for 6 months, found a significant reduction in cognitive decline rate among a subgroup of patients with milder dementia (Mini-Mental State Exam >27 out of 30 possible points) but no significant benefit in patients with more advanced dementia (53). A prospective study of elderly participants in the Chicago Health and Aging Project found that individuals who consumed fish weekly had a 10% to 13% slower rate of cognitive decline over 6 years of follow-up compared to those who consumed fish less than weekly; of note, this observed effect became less significant when adjusting for intake of other types of fat, indicating a possibility that it was not the fish itself but rather the reduced saturated-fat diet of regular fish eaters that made the difference (54). However, follow-up analysis on 899 men and women in the Framingham Heart Study did find a significant inverse relationship between plasma DHA levels and development of dementia, with a relative risk of 0.53 of developing all-cause dementia among subjects in the highest quartile of baseline plasma DHA levels (95% CI, 0.29 to 0.97) (55); the authors suggest that DHA, found in concentrated amounts in brain tissue, may play a specific role in cognitive function and the development of dementia (56).

More recent studies, however, have not found any significant benefit in ω-3 supplementation on the cognitive function in healthy, elderly adults (57). The authors comment that supplementation of ω-3 fatty acids is generally well-tolerated and perhaps longer trials are needed to discern benefit. An 18-month trial of DHA supplementation in 295 patients with mild-moderate AD found no benefit when compared to placebo (58).

Associations have been reported between caloric restriction in the context of intentional weight loss and deficits in cognitive function. Several studies have found that individuals on a severely calorie-restricted weight loss plan demonstrate deficits in memory, attention, processing speed, and concentration (59,60). However, the data of recent RCTs found no clear evidence of this (61,62), and there is increasing speculation that deficits in recall and task planning among dieters may be associated with preoccupation with dieting and body habitus rather than calorie restriction (60,63).

Conversely, several cohort studies have revealed a significant positive association between total calorie intake and cognitive decline (64,65). Caloric restriction has been shown in animal models to increase life span and decrease inflammatory processes. Current research is well on its way to elucidating the mechanism for these effects (see Chapter 31). This phenomenon is thought to occur in part via decreased oxidative damage, one of the putative mechanisms involved in the pathogenesis of dementia. Investigation has therefore ensued to examine whether total caloric intake might be involved in the development of dementia, in particular AD. One cohort study that followed 980 elderly, nondemented individuals found that those falling into the highest quartile of total caloric intake had an increased risk of developing AD over the 4 years of follow-up compared to individuals in the lowest quartile (HR, 1.5; 95% CI, 1.0 to 2.2); moreover, this association was significantly more pronounced among the subgroup of individuals with the apolipoprotein E4 allele (HR, 2.3; 95% CI, 1.1 to 4.7), a known predictor for AD (66). It has recently been determined that SIRT1, a key regulatory protein in producing the effects observed in caloric restriction, may have direct actions on β-amyloid accumulation (67).

Despite the enticing potential of caloric restriction, the reality is that many older adults develop unintentionally calorie-restricted diets that are not nutritionally balanced, and malnutrition can ensue. There is fairly consistent evidence that iron-deficiency anemia, the most common anemia in the United States, is associated with cognitive impairment (see Chapter 13). In a study of 14 obese women, Kretsch et al. (68) demonstrated that severe caloric restriction for 15 weeks resulted in signs of iron deficiency despite supplementation. A placebo-controlled study on reproductive-age women found both that subjects with adequate iron levels at baseline performed better and faster on cognitive tasks than those with baseline iron deficiency and that treatment of iron-deficient subjects restored cognitive performance significantly. Furthermore, the investigators found that increased serum ferritin saturation was related to a five- to sevenfold improvement in cognitive performance, and increased hemoglobin was related to enhanced speed of task completion (69).

Elevated levels of homocysteine, considered a marker for folate and vitamin B_{12} deficiency, is a well-established risk factor for vascular disease (see Chapter 7); evidence from prospective trials points to hyperhomocysteinemia as a strong, independent risk factor for the development of dementia and AD as well (70,71). Furthermore, elevated plasma homocysteine levels have been correlated with cerebral white matter changes in patients with AD, leading to speculation of a direct pathogenic mechanism of homocysteine (72). Nevertheless, data from recent RCTs examining the potential cognitive benefits of folic acid or vitamin B_{12} supplementation, have not shown a benefit in improving cognitive function or slowing decline in patients with AD or in patients with normal cognition (73–76).

Epidemiological studies have suggested a link between hormone changes at menopause and the development of dementia (77), indicating potential benefit of hormone replacement therapy (78); however, data from the Women's Health Initiative Memory Study refuted this hypothesis (79), and estrogen replacement is not currently recommended for prevention of dementia in postmenopausal women (80,81). A recent review concluded that different hormone replacement therapies overall had no major impact on cognition outcomes (82).

The effects of dietary carbohydrate on tryptophan levels have been linked to both stress tolerance and short-term cognition (83), and early evidence suggests that cognitive performance can be enhanced with dietary carbohydrate ingestion (84,85). Responding to stress is associated with activity in the serotonergic systems in the brain. Low levels of serotonin are implicated in disorders of mood (see Chapter 34) and are associated with certain aspects of cognition as

well. Dietary tryptophan serves as a precursor to serotonin; thus, serum tryptophan can influence the quantity of serotonin in the brain. Insulin facilitates the entry of large neutral amino acids, with the exception of tryptophan, into skeletal muscle. In response to carbohydrate ingestion and an insulin spike, the ratio of tryptophan to other large amino acids rises, theoretically raising the relative availability of tryptophan for use by the brain; ingestion of protein will tend to have the opposite effect (86). The Cochrane review on the subject concludes that without trial data, further studies are required for definitive recommendations (85).

Diet and childhood development is discussed in Chapter 29. There appear to be implications for adult cognition and cognitive deficits of childhood nutriture. Advantages of breast-feeding in the cognitive development of both preterm and term infants have been reported (87) but are uncertain (88). The developmental effects of breast milk seem to pertain in particular to its composition of essential fatty acids, both n-3 and n-6 (86,88). Breast milk is discussed in greater detail in Chapter 27.

NUTRIENTS, NUTRICEUTICALS, AND FUNCTIONAL FOODS

Dehydroepiandrosterone

Dehydroepiandrosterone (DHEA) and its sulphate, DHEAS, have become extremely popular supplements among patients based on theoretical possibility of their neuroprotective effects. However, although there is no evidence of adverse effects, there is also no convincing evidence to date that supplementation with DHEA or DHEAS can significantly attenuate cognitive decline in the elderly (89). Further long-term, high-quality trials are warranted before reliable clinical recommendations can be made.

Ginkgo Biloba

Ginkgo biloba is extracted from the leaves of the ginkgo tree, which can live as long as 4,000 years (90). Leaf extract, which has been used as a tonic in China for more than 1,000 years, contains antioxidant flavonoids and terpenoids. One of the constituents of standard preparations, ginkgolide B, exerts an inhibitory effect on platelets (91) by antagonizing platelet-activating factor. This moiety is responsible for the principal toxicity of the extract, an increased bleeding propensity, particularly in patients taking aspirin (91). Nevertheless, available evidence suggests that coadministration of ginkgo and aspirin does not constitute a safety risk (92).

Standardized ginkgo biloba leaf extract has been shown to inhibit β-amyloid oligomers, a main compound implicated in the pathogenicity of AD, in both in vitro (93) and in vivo (94) studies. The benefits of ginkgo biloba in dementia have been demonstrated with varying consistency in RCTs (95-97). Effects on brain function are supported by evidence from electroencephalography of a stimulatory effect of the extract (95).

Several recent trials have found no difference between ginkgo treatment and placebo, and although these results are not evident of null effect for all populations, the most recent Cochrane review concluded that ginkgo biloba has uncertain effect on cognition and inconsistent effects on dementia (98). A large, multi-center RCT placebo-controlled study of ginkgo biloba in adults over 75 years found no significant effect in reducing incidence of dementia or cognitive decline in individuals with normal or impaired cognition (99,100).

Ginseng

Ginseng is an adaptogenic herb that comes from the roots of plants in the Panax genus. Traditionally, it has been used as a stimulant, an aphrodisiac, or a "cure all" supplement. In review of five RCTs, ginseng was found to have mild improvement in cognitive function and quality of life with no serious adverse effects (101). Most common side effects of ginseng include insomnia, headaches, nausea, diarrhea, and nose bleeds (102). The authors conclude that there is little convincing evidence of cognitive enhancement in either healthy patients or patients with dementia, and that more clinical trials are needed.

Choline

Choline is an essential nutrient found in foods like meats, eggs, and cruciferous vegetables (103). Choline serves as a precursor for acetylcholine, an important neurotransmitter which facilitates muscle control and memory. Choline is also found

in the phospholipid phosphatidylcholine (PC), a molecule found in cell membranes. The Institute of Medicine recommends intake of 550 mg of choline for males and 425 mg of choline for females per day (104). Recommendations for pregnant and lactating females are increased to 450 mg and 550 mg, respectively. One egg contains 113 mg of choline, a pound of broccoli contains 182 mg, and a quart of 1% milk has 173 mg (105). One study from the National Health and Nutrition Examination Survey found that amongst postmenopausal women, a mere 2% consumed the recommended amount of choline (106).

Choline supplementation comes in the form of lecithin, a soy or egg derivative, as well as in phospholipid form, PC. A commonly endorsed supplement, PC is thought to promote synthesis and transmission of neurotransmitters (107). A review of PC found that 600 to 1,000 mg daily supplementation in patients with cognitive impairment or dementia was associated with a positive effect on memory in the short and medium term (108). There is yet no conclusive evidence of effect in adults without dementia.

■ CLINICAL HIGHLIGHTS

Overall evidence linking dietary practices to cognitive function or decline is limited in quality and quantity, and the progression from positive observational studies to randomized trials has been convoluted with null and negative results. Regardless, common-sense practices and well-studied recommendations for deficiency avoidance can guide patient education. Patients should be encouraged to establish stable dietary patterns that facilitate maintenance of near-ideal body weight; both obesity and persistent efforts at weight loss appear to be disadvantageous. The health benefits of weight loss in overweight patients, however, more than justify any modest impairment of cognitive function such efforts may impose (see Chapter 5).

Generous intake of vegetables and fruits appears to be beneficial, perhaps because of multiple effects. Supplements of vitamin E or C (or both) at moderate doses, if indicated for other purposes, may contribute to preservation of cognitive function. Smoking should be avoided, but moderate alcohol consumption may confer modest benefit. Systematic modification of risk factors for cardiovascular disease (see Chapter 7) and cerebrovascular disease (see Chapter 10) appears to be important in the maintenance of cognitive ability. Specific foods, such as blueberries, green tea, and fish, may confer cognitive benefits, largely by contributing to overall health and vascular health in particular. "Brain food" and healthful food are much the same.

Beneficial effects of ginkgo biloba, ginseng, and choline may exist but, if so, are likely modest. Gingko extract should be used cautiously in patients taking aspirin or anticoagulants, to avoid increased risk of bleeding.

REFERENCES

1. Christen Y. Oxidative stress and Alzheimer disease. *Am J Clin Nutr* 2000;71:621s–629s.

2. Joseph J, Shukitt-Hale B, Denisova N, et al. Long-term dietary strawberry, spinach, or vitamin E supplementation retards the onset of age-related neuronal signal-transduction and cognitive behavioral deficits. *J Neurosci* 1998;18:8047–8055.

3. Kolosova NG, Shcheglova TV, Sergeeva SV, et al. Long-term antioxidant supplementation attenuates oxidative stress markers and cognitive deficits in senescent-accelerated OXYS rats. *Neurobiol Aging* 2006;27:1289–1297.

4. Daviglus ML, Bell CC, Berrettini W, et al. National Institutes of Health State-of-the-Science Conference statement: preventing Alzheimer disease and cognitive decline. *Ann Intern Med* 2010;153:176.

5. Del Parigi A, Panza F, Capurso C, et al. Nutritional factors, cognitive decline, and dementia. *Brain Res Bull* 2006;69:1–19.

6. Engelhart MJ, Geerlings MI, Ruitenberg A, et al. Dietary intake of antioxidants and risk of Alzheimer disease. *JAMA* 2002;287:3223–3229.

7. Morris MC, Evans DA, Bienias JL, et al. Dietary intake of antioxidant nutrients and the risk of incident Alzheimer disease in a biracial community. *JAMA* 2002;287:3230–3237.

8. Zandi PP, Anthony JC, Khachaturian AS, et al. Reduced risk of Alzheimer disease in users of antioxidant vitamin supplements. *Arch Neurol* 2004;61:82–88.

9. Devore EE, Grodstein F, van Rooij FJ, et al. Dietary antioxidants and long-term risk of dementia. *Arch Neurol* 2010;67:819.

10. Pavlik VN, Doody RS, Rountree SD, et al. Vitamin E use is associated with improved survival in an Alzheimer's disease cohort. *Demen Geriatr Cogn Disord* 2009;28(6):536–540.

11. Kang JH, Cook N, Manson J, et al. A randomized trial of vitamin E supplementation and cognitive function in women. *Arch Intern Med* 2006;166:2462–2468.

12. Luchsinger JA, Tang MX, Shea S, et al. Antioxidant vitamin intake and risk of Alzheimer disease. *Arch Neurol* 2003;60:203–208.

13. Peterson RC, Thomas RG, Grundman M, et al. Vitamin E and donepezil for the treatment of mild cognitive impairment. *N Engl J Med* 2005;352:2379–2388.

14. Dunn JE, Weintraub S, Stoddard AM, et al. Serum alpha-tocopherol, concurrent and past vitamin E intake, and mild cognitive impairment. *Neurology* 2007;68:670.

15. Boothby LA, Doering PL. Vitamin C and vitamin E for Alzheimer's disease. *Ann Pharmacother* 2005;39: 2073–2079.

16. Dai Q, Borenstein AR, Wu Y, et al. Fruit and vegetable juices and Alzheimer's disease: the Kame Project. *Am J Med* 2006;119:751–759.

17. Hays NP, Roberts SB. The anorexia of aging in humans. *Physiol Behav* 2006;88:257–266.

18. de la Torre JC. Vascular basis of Alzheimer's pathogenesis. *Ann N Y Acad Sci* 2002;977:196–215.

19. Kilander L, Nyman H, Boberg M, et al. Cognitive function, vascular risk factors and education. A cross-sectional study based on a cohort of 70-year-old men. *J Intern Med* 1997;242:313–321.

20. Crisby M, Carlson LA, Winblad B. Statins in the prevention and treatment of Alzheimer disease. *Alzheimer Dis Assoc Disord* 2002;16:131–136.

21. Morris MC, Evans DA, Bienias JL, et al. Dietary fat intake and 6-year cognitive change in an older biracial community population. *Neurology* 2004;62:1573–1579.

22. Forette F, Seux ML, Staessen JA, et al. The prevention of dementia with antihypertensive treatment: new evidence from the Systolic Hypertension in Europe (Syst-Eur) Study. *Arch Intern Med* 2002;162:2046–2052.

23. Ohara T, Doi Y, Ninomiya T et al. Glucose tolerance status and risk of dementia in the community. *Neurology* 2011;77:1126–1134.

24. Xu WL, von Strauss E, Qiu CX, et al. Uncontrolled diabetes increase the risk of Alzheimer's disease: a population-based cohort study. *Diabetologia* 2009;52:1031–1039.

25. Irie F, Fitzpatrick AL, Lopez OL, et al. Enhanced risk for Alzheimer disease in persons with type 2 diabetes and APOE epsilon4: the Cardiovascular Health Study Cognition Study. *Arch Neurol* 2008;65(1):89–93.

26. Liu Y, Liu F, Grundke-Iqbal I, et al. Deficient brain insulin signalling pathway in Alzheimer's disease and diabetes. *J Pathol* 2011;225:54–62.

27. Mosconi L, Pupi A, De Leo MJ. Brain glucose hypometabolism and oxidative stress in preclinical Alzheimer's disease. *Ann N Y Acad Sci* 2008;1147:180–95.

28. Steen E, Terry BM, Rivera EJ, et al. Impaired insulin and insulinlike growth factor expression and signaling mechanisms in Alzheimer's disease—is this type 3 diabetes? *J Alzheimers Dis* 2005;7:63–80.

29. Perlmutter D. *Grain brain: the surprising truth about wheat, carbs, and sugary—your brain's silent killers.* Boston, MA: Little, Brown and Company, 2013.

30. Roberts RO, Roberts LA, Geda YE, et al. Relative intake of macronutrients impacts risk of cognitive impairment or dementia. *J Alzheimers Dis* 2012;32:329–339.

31. Barnes DE, Yaffe K. The projected effect of risk factor reduction on Alzheimer's disease prevalence. *Lancet Neurol* 2011;10:819.

32. McGuinness B, Todd S, Passmore P, et al. The effects of blood pressure lowering on development of cognitive impairment and dementia in patients without apparent prior cerebrovascular disease. *Cochrane Database Syst Rev* 2006;(2):CD004034.

33. Edelstein S, Kritz-Silverstein D, Barrett-Connor E. Prospective association of smoking and alcohol use with cognitive function in an elderly cohort. *J Womens Health* (Larchmt) 1998;7:1271–1281.

34. Lindsay J, Laurin D, Verreault R, et al. Risk factors for Alzheimer's disease: a prospective analysis from the Canadian Study of Health and Aging. *Am J Epidemiol* 2002;156:445–453.

35. Espeland MA, Gu L, Masaki KH, et al. Association between reported alcohol intake and cognition: results from the Women's Health Initiative Memory Study. *Am J Epidemiol* 2005;161:228–238.

36. Launer L, Feskens E, Kalmijn S, et al. Smoking, drinking, and thinking. The Zutphen Elderly Study. *Am J Epidemiol* 1996;143:219–227.

37. Solfrizzi V, D'Introno A, Colacicco AM, et al. Alcohol consumption, mild cognitive impairment, and progression to dementia. *Neurology* 2007;68:1790–1799.

38. Mehlig K, Skoog I, Guo X, et al. Alcoholic beverages and incidence of dementia: 34-year follow-up of the prospective population study of women in Goteborg. *Am J Epidemiol* 2008;167:684.

39. Huijbregts P, Feskens E, Rasanen L, et al. Dietary patterns and cognitive function in elderly men in Finland, Italy and The Netherlands. *Eur J Clin Nutr* 1998;52:826–831.

40. Correa Leite ML, Nicolosi A, Cristina S, et al. Nutrition and cognitive deficit in the elderly: a population study. *Eur J Clin Nutr* 2001;55:1053–1058.

41. Scarmeas N, Stern Y, Tang MX, et al. Mediterranean diet and risk for Alzheimer's disease. *Ann Neurol* 2006;59:912–921.

42. Féart C, Samieri C, Rondeau V, et al. Adherence to a Mediterranean diet, cognitive decline, and risk of dementia. *JAMA* 2009;302:638.

43. Scarmeas N, Stern Y, Mayeux R, et al. Mediterranean diet and mild cognitive impairment. *Arch Neurol* 2009;66:216.

44. Gu Y, Nieves JW, Stern Y, et al. Food combination and Alzheimer disease risk: a protective diet. *Arch Neurol* 2010;67:699.

45. Kang JH, Ascherio A, Grodstein F. Fruit and vegetable consumption and cognitive decline in aging women. *Ann Neurol* 2005;57:713–720.

46. Bastianetto S, Yao ZX, Papadopoulos V, et al. Neuroprotective effects of green and black teas and their catechin gallate esters against beta-amyloid-induced toxicity. *Eur J Neurosci* 2006;23:55–64.

47. Gemma C, Mesches MH, Sepesi B, et al. Diets enriched in foods with high antioxidant activity reverse age-induced decreases in cerebellar beta-adrenergic function and increases in proinflammatory cytokines. *J Neurosci* 2002;22:6114–6120.

48. Wang Y, Chang CF, Chou J, et al. Dietary supplementation with blueberries, spinach, or spirulina reduces ischemic brain damage. *Exp Neurol* 2005;193:75–84.

49. Ramassamy C. Emerging role of polyphenolic compounds in the treatment of neurodegenerative diseases: a review of their intracellular targets. *Eur J Pharmacol* 2006;545:51–64.

50. Kalmijn S, Feskens E, Launer L, et al. Polyunsaturated fatty acids, antioxidants, and cognitive function in very old men. *Am J Epidemiol* 1997;145:33–41.

51. Barberger-Gateau P, Letenneur L, Deschamps V, et al. Fish, meat, and risk of dementia: cohort study. *BMJ* 2002;325:932–933.

52. Morris MC, Evans DA, Bienias JL, et al. Consumption of fish and n-3 fatty acids and risk of incident Alzheimer disease. *Arch Neurol* 2003;60:940–946.

53. Freund-Levi Y, Eriksdotter-Jonhagen M, Cederholm T, et al. N-3 fatty acid treatment in 174 patients with mild to moderate Alzheimer disease: OmegAD study. *Arch Neurol* 2006;63:1402–1408.

54. Morris MC, Evans DA, Tangney CC, et al. Fish consumption and cognitive decline with age in a large community study. *Arch Neurol* 2005;62:1849–1853.

55. Schaefer EJ, Bongard V, Beiser AS, et al. Plasma phosphatidylcholine docosahexaenoic acid content, and risk of dementia and Alzheimer's disease: the Framingham Study. *Arch Neurol* 2006;63:1527–1528.

56. Johnson EJ, Schaefer EJ. Potential role of dietary n-3 fatty acids in the prevention of dementia and macular degeneration. *Am J Clin Nutr* 2006;83:1494s–1498s.

57. Sydenham E, Dangour AD, Lim WS. Omega 3 fatty acid for the prevention of cognitive decline and dementia. *Cochrane Database Syst Rev* 2012;(6):CD005379.

58. Quinn JF, Raman R, Thomas RG, et al. Docosahexaenoic acid supplementation and cognitive decline in Alzheimer disease: a randomized trial. *JAMA* 2010;304:1903.

59. Kretsch M, Green M, Fong A, et al. Cognitive effects of a long-term weight reducing diet. *Int J Obes* (Lond) 1997;21:14–21.

60. Green M, Rogers P. Impairments in working memory associated with spontaneous dieting behaviour. *Psychol Med* 1998;28:1063–1070.

61. Martin CK, Anton SD, Han H, et al. Examination of cognitive function during six months of calorie restriction: results of a randomized controlled trial. *Rejuvenation Res* 2007;10:179–189.

62. Halyburton AK, Brinkworth GD, Wilson CJ, et al. Low- and high-carbohydrate weight-loss diets have similar effects on mood but not cognitive performance. *Am J Clin Nutr* 2007;86:580–587.

63. Kemps E, Tiggemann M. Working memory performance and preoccupying thoughts in female dieters: evidence for a selective central executive impairment. *Br J Clin Psychol* 2005;44:357–366.

64. Fraser G, Singh P, Bennett H. Variables associated with cognitive function in elderly California Seventh-day Adventists. *Am J Epidemiol* 1996;143:1181–1190.

65. Luchsinger JA, Tang MX, Mayeux R. Glycemic load and risk of Alzheimer's disease. *J Nutr Health Aging* 2007;11:238–241.

66. Luchsinger JA, Tang M-X, Shea S, et al. Caloric intake and the risk of Alzheimer disease. *Arch Neurol* 2002;59:1258–1263.

67. Qin W, Yang T, Ho L, et al. Neuronal SIRT1 activation as a novel mechanism underlying the prevention of Alzheimer disease amyloid neuropathology by calorie restriction. *J Biol Chem* 2006;281:21745–21754.

68. Kretsch M, Fong A, Green M, et al. Cognitive function, iron status, and hemoglobin concentration in obese dieting women. *Eur J Clin Nutr* 1998;52:512–518.

69. Murray-Kolb LE, Beard JL. Iron treatment normalizes cognitive functioning in young women. *Am J Clin Nutr* 2007;85:778–787.

70. Seshadri S, Beiser A, Selhub J, et al. Plasma homocysteine as a risk factor for dementia and Alzheimer's disease. *N Engl J Med* 2002;346:476–483.

71. Duthie SJ, Whalley LF, Collins AR, et al. Homocysteine, B vitamin status, and cognitive function in the elderly. *Am J Clin Nutr* 2002;75:908–913.

72. Hogervorst E, Ribeiro HM, Molyneux A, et al. Plasma homocysteine levels, cerebrovascular risk factors, and cerebral white matter changes (leukoaraiosis) in patients with Alzheimer disease. *Arch Neurol* 2002;59:787–793.

73. Malouf M, Grimley EJ, Areosa SA. Folic acid with or without vitamin B12 for cognition and dementia. *Cochrane Database Syst Rev* 2003;4:CD004514.

74. Aisen PS, Schneider LS, Sano M, et al. High-dose B vitamin supplementation and cognitive decline in Alzheimer disease: a randomized controlled trial. *JAMA* 2008;300:1774.

75. Ford AH, Flicker L, Alfonso H, et al. Vitamins B(12), B(6), and folic acid for cognition in older men. *Neurology* 2010;75:1540.

76. Balk EM, Raman G, Tatsioni A, et al. Vitamin B6, B12, and folic acid supplementation and cognitive function: a systematic review of randomized trials. *Arch Intern Med* 2007;167(1):21–30.

77. Fillit HM. The role of hormone replacement therapy in the prevention of Alzheimer disease. *Arch Intern Med* 2002;162:1934–1942.

78. LeBlanc ES, Janowsky J, Chan BK, et al. Hormone replacement therapy and cognition: systematic review and meta-analysis. *JAMA* 2001;285:1489–1499.

79. Espeland MA, Rapp SR, Shumaker SA, et al. Conjugated equine estrogens and global cognitive function in postmenopausal women: Women's Health Initiative Memory Study. *JAMA* 2004;291:2959–2968.

80. Schneider LA. Estrogen and dementia: insights from the Women's Health Initiative Memory Study. *JAMA* 2004;291:3005.

81. Shah S, Bell RJ, Davis SR. Homocysteine, estrogen and cognitive decline. *Climacteric* 2006;9:77–87.

82. Maki PM. Minireview: effects of different HT formulations on cognition. *Endocrinology* 2012;153(8):3564–3570.

83. Markus C, Panhuysen G, Tuiten A, et al. Does carbohydrate-rich, protein-poor food prevent a deterioration of mood and cognitive performance of stress-prone subjects when subjected to a stressful task? *Appetite* 1998;31:49–65.

84. Kaplan RJ, Greenwood CE, Winocur G, et al. Cognitive performance is associated with glucose regulation in healthy elderly persons and can be enhanced with glucose and dietary carbohydrates. *Am J Clin Nutr* 2000;72:825–836.

85. Ooi CP, Loke SC, Yassin Z, at al. Carbohydrates for improving the cognitive performance of independent-living older adults with normal cognition or mild cognitive impairment. *Cochrane Database Syst Rev* 2011;(4):CD007220. doi: 10.1002/14651858.CD007220.pub2.

86. Gordon N. Nutrition and cognitive function. *Brain Dev* 1997;19:165–170.

87. Der G, Batty GD, Deary IJ. Effect of breast feeding on intelligence in children: prospective study, sibling pairs analysis, and meta-analysis. *BMJ* 2006;333:935.

88. Helland IB, Smith L, Saarem K, et al. Maternal supplementation with very-long-chain n-3 fatty acids during pregnancy and lactation augments children's IQ at 4 years of age. *Pediatrics* 2003;111:e39–e44.

89. Grimley EJ, Malouf R, Huppert F, et al. Dehydroepiandrosterone (DHEA) supplementation for cognitive function in healthy elderly people. *Cochrane Database Syst Rev* 2006;4:CD006221.

90. Pang Z, Pan F, He S. Ginkgo biloba L.: history, current status, and future prospects. *J Altern Complement Med* 1996;2:359–363.

91. Sierpina VS, Wollschlaeger B, Blumenthal M. Ginkgo Biloba. *Am Fam Physician.* 2003;68(5):923–926.

92. Wolf HR. Does *Ginkgo biloba* special extract EGb761 provide additional effects on coagulation and bleeding when added to acetylsalyclic acid 500 mg daily? *Drugs R D* 2006;7:163–172.

93. Luo Y, Smith JV, Paramasivam V, et al. Inhibition of amyloid-beta aggregation and caspase-3 activation by the *Ginkgo biloba* extract EGb761. *Proc Natl Acad Sci USA* 2002;99:12197–12202.

94. Wu Y, Wu Z, Butko P, et al. Amyloid-beta-induced pathological behaviors are suppressed by *Ginkgo biloba* extract EGb761 and ginkgolides in transgenic *Caenorhabditis elegans*. *J Neurosci* 2006;26:13102–13113.

95. Maurer K, Ihl R, Dierks T, et al. Clinical efficacy of *Ginkgo biloba* special extract Egb 761 in dementia of the Alzheimer type. *J Psychiatr Res* 1997;31:645–655.

96. Napryeyenko O, Borzenko I. *Ginkgo biloba* special extract in dementia with neuropsychiatric features. A randomized, placebo-controlled trial. *Arzneimittelforschung* 2007;57:4–11.

97. Carlson JJ, Farquhar JW, DiNucci E, et al. Safety and efficacy of a ginkgo biloba-containing dietary supplement on cognitive function, quality of life, and healthy, cognitively intact older adults. *J Am Diet Assoc* 2007;107: 422–432.

98. Birks J, Grimley EV, Evans J. *Ginkgo biloba* for cognitive impairment and dementia. *Cochrane Database Syst Rev* 2007;2:CD003120.

99. DeKosky ST, Williamson JD, Fitzpatrick AL, et al. *Ginkgo biloba* for prevention of dementia: a randomized controlled trial. *JAMA* 2008;300:2253.

100. Snitz BE, O'Meara ES, Carlson MC, et al. *Ginkgo biloba* for preventing cognitive decline in older adults: a randomized trial. *JAMA* 2009;302:2663.

101. Geng J, Dong J, Ni H, et al. Ginseng for cognition. *Cochrane Database Syst Rev* 2010;(12):CD007769. doi: 10.1002/14651858.CD007769.pub2.

102. Kiefer D, Pantuso T. Panax ginseng. *Am Fam Physician* 2003;68(8):1539–1542.

103. Zeisel SH, DaCosta KA. Choline: an essential nutrient for public health. *Nutrition Reviews* 2009;67(11): 615–623.

104. Institute of Medicine. *Dietary reference intakes.* Available at http://www.iom.edu/Activities/Nutrition/Summary-DRIs/DRI-Tables.aspx; accessed 12/1/13.

105. United States Department of Agriculture. Database for the choline content of common foods, release 2. http://www.ars.usda.gov/services/docs.htm?docid=6232, accessed 12/31/13.

106. Fischer LM, Da Costa KA, Kwock L, et al. Dietary choline requirements of women: effects of estrogen and genetic variation. *Am J Clin Nutr* 2010;92(5): 1113–1119.

107. Serby MJ, Yhap C, Landron EY. A study of herbal remedies for memory complaints. *J Neuropsychiatry Clin Neurosci* 2010;22(3):345–347.

108. Fioravanti M, Yanagi M. Cytidinediphosphocholine (CDP-choline) for cognitive and behavioural disturbances associated with chronic cerebral disorders in the elderly. *Cochrane Database Syst Rev* 2005;2:CD000269.

SUGGESTED READINGS

Capurso A, Solfrizzi V, Panza F, et al. Dietary patterns and cognitive functions in elderly subjects. *Aging Clin Exp Res* 1997;9:45–47.

Jama J, Launer L, Witteman J, et al. Dietary antioxidants and cognitive function in a population-based sample of older persons. The Rotterdam Study. *Am J Epidemiol* 1996;144: 275–280.

LeBars P, Katz M, Berman N, et al. A placebo-controlled, double-blind, randomized trial of an extract of *Ginkgo biloba* for dementia. *JAMA* 1997;278:1327–1332.

McCaddon A, Davies G, Hudson P, et al. Total serum homocysteine in senile dementia of Alzheimer type. *Int J Geriatr Psychiatry* 1998;13:235–239.

Ortega R, Requejo A, Andres P, et al. Dietary intake and cognitive function in a group of elderly people. *Am J Clin Nutr* 1997;66:803–809.

Paleologos M, Cumming R, Lazarus R. Cohort study of vitamin C intake and cognitive impairment. *Am J Epidemiol* 1998;148:45–50.

Sano M, Ernesto C, Thomas R, et al. A controlled trial of selegiline, alpha-tocopherol, or both as treatment for Alzheimer's disease. *N Engl J Med* 1997;336:1216–1222.

Spindler A, Renvall M, Nichols J, et al. Nutritional status of patients with Alzheimer's disease: a 1-year study. *J Am Diet Assoc* 1996;96:1013–1018.

CHAPTER 36

Diet and Vision

The two leading causes of visual impairment in older adults are age-related macular degeneration (AMD) and cataracts. More than 10% of individuals over age 80 have impaired vision due to AMD, and about 50% in this age group have cataracts that impair vision (1–4). Younger populations do fare better than the elderly. According to NHANES data analysis from the years 2005–2008 by Chou et al. (5), the prevalence of visual impairment not due to refractive errors in US adults over the age of 40 is 2.0% and is significantly increased among those with AMD. As the population ages, the public health impact of these conditions is rising.

Photocoagulation is effective for treatment of advanced macular degeneration in only a minority of patients. Because it is safe and generally effective, cataract extraction has become the most common surgery performed in people over age 60 in the United States and thus represents an enormous public health burden. Cataract is both more prevalent and more disabling in developing than in developed countries; worldwide, cataract accounts for 50% of all blindness (6). There is, therefore, well-founded interest in preventive strategies for both diseases.

Both conditions have been linked to cumulative oxidative injury. In the lens, reactive oxygen species damage crystallin proteins. In the macula, peroxidation of polyunsaturated fatty acids in photoreceptor cells may lead to degeneration. Dietary factors have the potential to accelerate or retard the development of impaired visual acuity and blindness with aging. Studies of antioxidants in diet and supplement form suggest a possible benefit.

Ocular complications of diabetes mellitus resulting in impaired vision may be forestalled by dietary practices that improve glycemic control. This topic is addressed in Chapter 6.

OVERVIEW

The lens is composed of proteins that are retained throughout life, migrating toward the lens center or nucleus. Damage to the proteins from exposure to light and oxygen accumulates over time. Vitamin C is concentrated in the lens (2), and levels in the lens and eye compartments are apparently responsive to dietary intake (1). Levels generally decline with aging, and low levels have been associated with cataract formation (2).

Overall, the evidence linking specific nutrients to cataract prevention is preliminary. The evidence is suggestive for vitamins C and E, as well as the carotenoids (7). However, randomized trials of individual vitamin C and/or E supplements have thus far been inconclusive. Yoshida et al. (8) found a significant difference between onset of cataracts in association with varying levels of dietary vitamin C, while Zheng et al. (9) found a statistically significant increase in the risk of developing cataracts among older men (older than age 65) who took high-dose vitamin C supplements. These same authors found an increased hazard ratio of older men taking high-dose vitamin E supplements. These same risks were not seen with multivitamins and/or multiple single vitamin supplements. Further muddying the waters, McNeil et al. (10) found no protective effect of daily vitamin E on cataract formation after 4 years of supplementation, while the Roche European American Cataract Trial demonstrated a significant reduction in cataract formation among subjects taking a combination of β-carotene and vitamins C and E for 3 years (11). The evidence of a protective effect is more convincing for a diet rich in fruits and vegetables than for specific nutrients (2). Smoking and folate deficiency have both been implicated in cataract formation (12). Dietary and lifestyle recommendations that may be made with confidence for other reasons, such as smoking cessation and increased fruit and vegetable consumption, offer the promise of reduced cataract risk as well (2,13).

Although not definitive, the evidence suggests that vitamin C supplementation in the range of 500 mg per day may offer benefit. The results of ongoing and future intervention trials will be required before more definitive recommendations can be made with security.

The retina, in general, and the macula, in particular, may be susceptible to oxidative injury because of their concentration of unsaturated fatty acids, high use of oxygen, and frequent exposure to intense light (14). The antioxidant effects of vitamins C and E, the carotenoids, and zinc, copper, and selenium may play a role in protecting the macula from injury caused by singlet oxygen, which is generated by light absorption (1). According to Zeng et al. (15), they may also affect angiogenesis and endothelial–macrophage interactions. Zinc and copper are cofactors to superoxide dismutase; selenium is needed for the action of glutathione peroxidase.

Evidence derived from animal models, case-control, observational-cohort, and occasional randomized trials clearly supports a role for nutritional factors in the course of macular degeneration. The Age-Related Eye Disease Study (AREDS) of patients with existing macular degeneration found that subjects randomized to receive supplementation with zinc plus an antioxidant combination had a 25% reduced risk of disease progression compared with placebo (16). The evidence is most convincing that, among the antioxidants, lutein and zeaxanthin are protective (1,17,18). Lutein and zeaxanthin are carotenoids found abundantly in dark green vegetables; they have no provitamin A activity, but they have been associated with protection against macular degeneration; they are preferentially taken up by the macula and are key components of macular pigment (1,14). As such, they are thought to play a role in the prevention of progression of the disease (19,20).

Carotenoids are a diverse family of pigments, some with and some without provitamin A activity (see Section VIIE). Both β-carotene and α-carotene are moderate antioxidants with provitamin A activity. Although essential for eye function as a component of rhodopsin, which is the visual pigment of rod cells in the retina, vitamin A does not appear to play a role in the development or prevention of macular degeneration.

Preliminary evidence supports a protective role of zinc supplementation (with cupric oxide) in combination with other antioxidants or in people at high risk of zinc deficiency (21). Deficiencies in habitual intake of several nutrients were reported in an evaluation of a representative population of elderly subjects (ages 65 to 85) in Maryland; zinc deficiency was particularly common (22). Risk factors, dietary and other, for coronary artery disease are correlated with the risk of macular degeneration as well (23). Furthermore, the AREDS showed that the intermediate form of nonneovascular AMD in one or both eyes or with advanced AMD or vision loss due to AMD in one eye improved with supplementation of high-dose antioxidants (vitamins C and E and β-carotene) and zinc (24).

Postmenopausal estrogen replacement appears to be protective, as does intake of n-3 fatty acid (1,25,26). There is interest in the possible role of dietary supplementation with long-chain polyunsaturated fatty acids, especially of the n-3 class, in the development and protection of the macula (27–31). A large prospective cohort study by Cho et al. (32) found that frequent consumption of fish containing n-3 fatty acids was associated with reduced risk of developing macular degeneration and high plasma total ω-3 fatty acid levels were also associated with a reduced risk for developing late AMD in the Alienor study in Bordeaux, France (33,34). As such, the evidence in support of dietary n-3 fatty acids is growing but is still inconclusive (28,35,36). Surprisingly, despite the epidemic lack of ω-3 fatty acids in the American diet, the prevalence of AMD amongst people aged 40 and older decreased by approximately 3% between the 1994–1998 and the 2005–2008 NHANES studies (4).

Although the nutrient-specific data to date are preliminary, general dietary recommendations for the prevention of macular degeneration may be made with some confidence. A diet rich in green leafy vegetables provides abundant lutein and zeaxanthin and should be encouraged. Other fruits and vegetables may provide additional benefits and should be consumed to promote health in any event. A large, population-based study of visually impaired subjects in Finland revealed a convincing association between eye disease, particularly macular degeneration, and cancer (37). The authors concluded that age-related eye disease and various cancers share risk factors, particularly smoking and diet. Another large population-based study in Korea found associations between AMD and low serum high-density lipoprotein (HDL) level, HBsAg serum positivity, history of ever smoking, and elevated systolic blood pressure (23), and a cross-sectional study of more than 3,500 patients in an Indian hospital found a significant risk reduction of AMD amongst those patients with high intakes of dietary lutein, zeaxanthin, and β-carotene (38). Similar associations between high intake of lutein and zeaxanthin and prevention of AMD or decreased progression of AMD have been found by other authors (39–41).

The benefit of vitamin E or C and of several minerals remains uncertain, but multivitamin/multimineral supplementation, advocated on other grounds, may confer protection against macular degeneration. Cardiovascular disease risk factor modification, including smoking cessation and postmenopausal hormone replacement therapy, may be protective of the macula as well. Studies suggest that intake of high-glycemic-index (GI) carbohydrates can increase the risk of AMD and cataract development (42–47), whereas intake of cereal fibers, breads, and grains decreased risk of developing soft drusen (48). One study of over 2,300 12-year-old students in Sydney, Australia, showed a significant decrease in the retinal vessel width amongst kids who drank one or more sodas (a very high-GI drink) a day in comparison to those who did not drink soda (49), indicating direct damage to retinal blood vessels from beverages of high GI. In their prospective study, Chiu et al. estimated that 7.8% of new advanced AMD cases would be prevented in 5 years if people consumed a low-GI diet (45,50). Current research does not delineate whether or not sugar or starch alone versus total carbohydrate load contribute to the development of AMD or cataracts.

Chiu and Taylor (3) reviewed the literature on prevention of macular degeneration and cataract. Cross-sectional, case-control, prospective observational studies produced variable results but were generally compatible with a modest benefit of high antioxidant intake in the form of supplements or food on age-related eye disease. A Cochrane review of clinical trials involving vitamin supplementation for the prevention and/or delay of progression of AMD by Evans and Lawrenson concluded a moderate beneficial effect (51). Conversely, a systematic review

of studies pertaining to lifestyle modification, nutrition, supplements, and eye health by Sin, Liu, and Lam failed to find any further clinical trials beyond the AREDS study showing a risk reduction of progression to advanced AMD with vitamins A, C, and E and zinc with copper supplements (13). Another systematic review of 10 studies on zinc supplementation for prevention and treatment of AMD was inconclusive (52).

On the topic of cataract formation, The Australian Blue Mountain Study found multivitamin and vitamin A use protected against cataract formation in their cohort while vitamins E and C did not impact cataract formation (53). Multivitamin use was also noted to decrease the risk of cataract (defined by self-report and/or cataract surgery) by 27% in the Physician's Health Study (54). More conclusive evidence, and specification of nutrient and dose, awaits clarification from further randomized trials (55). Brown et al. (56) reviewed the same literature and offered specific "reasonable" doses for daily supplementation that may offer benefit to eye health with little risk of toxicity. Suggested supplements include 1 mg of vitamin A, 500 to 1,000 mg of vitamin C, up to 300 mg of vitamin E, and 20 mg of zinc; other recommendations mirror the recommended dietary allowances. The Nurses' Health Study and Health Professionals Follow-up Study reported no strong association between the risk of primary open-angle glaucoma and antioxidant use (57).

Nutrigenomics and Eye Health

Two genes (LIPC and LPL) that metabolize HDL molecules have been associated with AMD due to the HDL molecules' transport mechanism for the carotenoids lutein and zeaxanthin. Merle et al. (58) made this association in their population-based prospective study of 963 elderly people in Bordeaux, France. In their study, the TT genotype of the LIPC rs493258 variant was found to be associated with a decreased risk for developing AMD. The LPL genotype variant was associated with early AMD. A study by Seddon et al. (59) at Tufts Medical Center conferred an association of the TT genotype of the LIPC variant with a decreased risk of AMD, regardless of environmental and demographic factors.

Other possible contributing polymorphisms for AMD include the rs754203 C allele in the CYP46A1 gene, which has been associated with a higher risk for developing exudative AMD according to research done by Fourgeux et al. (60), and the SNP rs2872060 in the IGF1 receptor gene. This SNP was found to be associated with the development of advanced AMD (61).

Nutriceuticals/Functional Foods for Eye Health

Lutein

As discussed above, lutein appears to play an important role in decreasing the risk of AMD. It is postulated that lutein neutralizes free radicals that can damage the eye thus preventing photooxidation. Thus, individuals with diets high in lutein may be less likely to develop AMD or cataracts, the two most common causes of vision loss in adults. Supplements containing lutein and other carotenoids are now being heavily marketed in health food stores; however, there is some concern that lutein in supplement form may not provide the same benefit as that found naturally in foods such as leafy green vegetables (7.4 mg per 100 g) and cooked cabbage (14.4 mg per 100 g). Other sources of lutein are parsley, egg yolks, salmon, spinach, and kale (62).

The National Eye Institute of the NIH released a statement on lutein and its role in eye disease in the year 2000 stating, "Claims made about an association between lutein and eye health should be approached with caution. The possible benefits of lutein on the eye remain uncertain." In addition, the AREDS study found no significant effect of the risk of cataract development or progression with the ingestion of high doses of vitamins C and E and β-carotene versus placebo over 6.3 years (63). On the other hand, high dietary intake of lutein and zeaxanthin had a 22% risk reduction for cataract surgery in The Nurse's Health Study (64,65), and amongst a Finnish cohort of elderly men and women, high plasma lutein and zeaxanthin levels were associated with a decreased risk of developing nuclear cataracts (66). Another cross-sectional cohort study assessing antioxidant intake from vegetables in Congolese subjects with type 2 diabetes found a significant decrease in the rate of cataract development in those subjects stating they had high daily intakes of red beans and vegetables (three or more) per day (67).

Further research on the possible beneficial effects of lutein on preventing eye disease is still warranted (51,65,68–71).

Ginkgo biloba

Another popular nutriceutical/supplement that shows promise for eye health is the herb *Ginkgo biloba*. It is thought to be a potent antioxidant and blood thinner (by means of decreasing blood viscosity and increasing erythrocyte deformation) (57). One small, nongeneralizable study (N = 20) found a statistically significant improvement in visual acuity after 6 months of randomized treatment compared with placebo versus 80 mg twice daily *Ginkgo biloba* supplementation (72). The herb has also been reported to increase ophthalmic artery blood flow, thus decreasing, at least in theory, intraocular pressure in patients with glaucoma (73). More research is needed to elucidate *Gingko*'s potential benefit on eye health.

Bilberry fruit is also considered helpful for night vision and general eye health; however, there are no clinical studies that support this claim (57).

CLINICAL HIGHLIGHTS

Definitive evidence of nutrient-specific protection of the lens or macula is as yet unavailable, although evidence from various sources strongly suggests that generous antioxidant intake from diet is protective. A diet rich in green leafy vegetables should be recommended as primary prevention of age-related eye disease. Smoking cessation is clearly indicated for this and other clinical goals. Multivitamin/multimineral supplementation may be beneficial, especially in those over age 50 or with less-than-judicious diets.

As discussed elsewhere (see Chapter 11 and Section VIIE), zinc deficiency may be widespread in the United States; use of a daily mineral supplement is supported by the potential role of zinc in protection of both the macula and the lens. Patients with a particular interest in prevention of eye disease should consider supplementation with vitamin C at 500 mg, vitamin E at 200 IU, and lutein at 3 mg, although evidence of benefit is at best suggestive.

Inclusion in the diet of n-3 fatty acids from fish or plant sources is advisable on general principles and may prove to be of benefit to vision (see Chapter 45). Intake of this class of fat may be particularly important to the eyes, as it appears to be for cognitive development, during infancy (see Chapters 27 and 29). The dietary pattern tentatively associated with protection of vision, rich in fruits and vegetables, is advisable on general principles and may be recommended with conviction.

REFERENCES

1. Hung S, Seddon J. The relationship between nutritional factors and age-related macular degeneration. In: Bendich A, Deckelbaum R, eds. *Preventive nutrition.* Totowa, NJ: Humana Press, 1997:245–266.
2. Taylor A, Jacques P. Antioxidant status and risk for cataract. In: Bendich A, Deckelbaum R, eds. *Preventive nutrition.* Totowa, NJ: Humana Press, 1997:267–284.
3. Chiu CJ, Taylor A. Nutritional antioxidants and age-related cataract and maculopathy. *Exp Eye Res* 2007;84:229–245.
4. Klein R, Chou CF, Klein BE, et al. Prevalence of age-related macular degeneration in the US population. *Arch Ophthalmol* 2011;129(1):75–80.
5. Chou CF, Cotch MF, Vitale S, et al. Age-related eye diseases and visual impairment among U.S. adults. *Am J Prev Med* 2013;45(1):29–35. doi: 10.1016/j.amepre.2013.02.018.
6. Javitt J, Wang F, West S. Blindness due to cataract: epidemiology and prevention. *Annu Rev Public Health* 1996;17:159–177.
7. Christen WG, Liu S, Glynn RJ, et al. Dietary carotenoids, vitamins C and E, and risk of cataract in women: a prospective study. *Arch Ophthalmol* 2008;126(1):102–109.
8. Yoshida M, Takashima Y, Inoue M, et al. Prospective study showing that dietary vitamin C reduced the risk of age-related cataracts in a middle-aged Japanese population. *Eur J Nutr* 2007;46(2):118–124.
9. Zheng Selin J, Rautiainen S, Lindblad BE, et al. High-dose supplements of vitamins C and E, low-dose multivitamins, and the risk of age-related cataract: a population-based prospective cohort study of men. *Am J Epidemiol* 2013;177(6):548–555. doi: 10.1093/aje/kws279.
10. McNeil JJ, Robman L, Tikellis G, et al. Vitamin E supplementation and cataract randomized controlled trial. *Ophthalmology* 2004;111:75–84.
11. Chylack LT Jr, Brown NP, Bron A, et al. The Roche European American Cataract Trial (REACT) a randomized clinical trial to investigate the efficacy of an oral antioxidant micronutrient mixture to slow progression of age-related cataract. *Ophthalmic Epidemiol* 2002;9:49–80.
12. Chen KJ. Association between folate status, diabetes, antihypertensive medication and age-related cataracts in elderly Taiwanese. *J Nutr Health Aging* 2011;15(4):304–310.
13. Sin HP, Liu DT, Lam DS. Lifestyle modification, nutritional and vitamins supplements for age-related macular degeneration. *Acta Ophthalmol* 2013;91(1):6–11. doi: 10.1111/j.1755-3768.2011.02357.x.
14. Hogg R, Chakravarthy U. Mini-Review. *Curr Eye Res* 2004; 29:387–401.
15. Zeng S, Hernández J, Mullins RF. Effects of antioxidant components of AREDS vitamins and zinc ions on endothelial cell activation: implications for macular degeneration. *Invest Ophthalmol Vis Sci* 2012;53(2):1041–1047. doi: 10.1167/iovs.11-8531.
16. Age-Related Eye Disease Study Research Group. A randomized, placebo-controlled, clinical trial of high-dose supplementation with vitamins C and E, beta carotene, and zinc for age-related macular degeneration and vision loss AREDS report no. 8. *Arch Ophthalmol* 2001;119:1417–1436.
17. Krinsky NI, Landrum JT, Bone RA. Biologic mechanisms of the protective role of lutein and zeaxanthin in the eye. *Annu Rev Nutr* 2003;23:171–201.
18. Koh HH, Murray IJ, Nolan D, et al. Plasma and macular responses to lutein supplement in subjects with and without age-related maculopathy: a pilot study. *Exp Eye Res* 2004;79:21–27.
19. Ma L, Yan SF, Huang YM, et al. Effect of lutein and zeaxanthin on macular pigment and visual function in patients with early age-related macular degeneration. *Ophthalmology* 2012;119(11):2290–2297. doi: 10.1016/j.ophtha.2012.06.014.
20. Weigert G, Kaya S, Pemp B, et al. Effects of lutein supplementation on macular pigment optical density and visual acuity in patients with age-related macular degeneration. *Invest Ophthalmol Vis Sci* 2011;52(11):8174–8178. doi: 10.1167/iovs.11-7522.
21. Seddon J. Multivitamin-multimineral supplements and eye disease: age-related macular degeneration and cataract. *Am J Clin Nutr* 2007;85:304s–307s.
22. Cid-Ruzafa J, Calulfield L, Barron Y, et al. Nutrient intakes and adequacy among an older population on the eastern shore of Maryland: the Salisbury Eye Evaluation. *J Am Diet Assoc* 1999;99:564–571.
23. Cho BJ, Heo JW, Kim TW, et al. Prevalence and risk factors of age-related macular degeneration in Korea: the Korean National Health and Nutrition Examination Survey. *Invest Ophthalmol Vis Sci* 2014;55(2):1101–1108. doi: 10.1167/iovs.13-13096.
24. Cheung LK, Eaton A. Age-related macular degeneration. *Pharmacotherapy* 2013;33(8):838–855. doi: 10.1002/phar.1264.
25. Seddon J, George S, Rosner B. Cigarette smoking, fish consumption, omega-3 fatty acid intake, and associations with age-related macular degeneration. The US twin study of age-related macular degeneration. *Arch Ophthalmol* 2006;124:995–1001.
26. Christen WG, Schaumberg DA, Buring JE, et al. Dietary ω-3 fatty acid and fish intake and incident age-related macular degeneration in women. *Arch Ophthalmol* 2011;129(7):921–929. doi:10.1001/archophthalmol.2011.34.
27. Birch E, Hoffman D, Uauy R, et al. Visual acuity and the essentiality of docosahexaenoic acid and arachidonic acid in the diet of term infants. *Pediatr Res* 1998;44:201–209.
28. Gibson R, Makrides M. Polyunsaturated fatty acids and infant visual development: a critical appraisal of randomized clinical trials. *Lipids* 1999;34:179.
29. SanGiovanni JP, Chew EY; the Age Related Eye Disease Study Research Group. The relationship of dietary ω-3 long-chain polyunsaturated fatty acid intake with incident age-related macular degeneration AREDS Report No. 23. *Arch Ophthalmol* 2008;126(9):1274–1279.
30. Augood C, Chakravarthy U, Young I, et al. Oily fish consumption, dietary docosahexaenoic acid and eicosapentaenoic acid intakes, and associations with neovascular age-related macular degeneration. *Am J Clin Nutr* 2008;88(2):398–406.
31. Mance TC, Kovacević D, Alpeza-Dunato Z, et al. The role of omega6 to omega3 ratio in development and progression of age-related macular degeneration. *Coll Antropol* 2011;35(suppl 2):307–310.

32. Cho E, Hung S, Willett WC, et al. Prospective study of dietary fat and the risk of age-related macular degeneration. *Am J Clin Nutr* 2001;73:209–218.

33. Merle B, Delyfer MN, Korobelnik JF, et al. Dietary omega-3 fatty acids and the risk for age-related maculopathy: the Alienor Study. *Invest Ophthalmol Vis Sci* 2011;52(8):6004–6011. doi: 10.1167/iovs.11-7254.

34. Merle BM, Delyfer MN, Korobelnik JF, et al. High concentrations of plasma n3 fatty acids are associated with decreased risk for late age-related macular degeneration. *J Nutr* 2013;143(4):505–511. doi: 10.3945/jn.112.171033.

35. Hodge WG, Schachter HM, Barnes D, et al. Efficacy of n-3 fatty acids in preventing age-related macular degeneration: a systematic review. *Ophthalmology* 2006;113:1165–1173.

36. Lawrenson JG, Evans JR. Omega 3 fatty acids for preventing or slowing the progression of age-related macular degeneration. *Cochrane Database Syst Rev* 2012;11:CD010015. doi: 10.1002/14651858.CD010015.pub2.

37. Pukkala E, Verkasalo P, Ojamo M, et al. Visual impairment and cancer: a population-based cohort study in Finland. *Cancer Causes Control* 1999;10:13–20.

38. Nidhi B, Mamatha BS, Padmaprabhu CA, et al. Dietary and lifestyle risk factors associated with age-related macular degeneration: a hospital based study. *Indian J Ophthalmol* 2013;61(12):722–727.

39. Ma L, Dou HL, Huang YM, et al. Improvement of retinal function in early age-related macular degeneration after lutein and zeaxanthin supplementation: a randomized, double-masked, placebo-controlled trial. *Am J Ophthalmol* 2012;154(4):625–634.e1. doi: 10.1016/j.ajo.2012.04.014.

40. Ma L, Dou HL, Wu YQ, et al. Lutein and zeaxanthin intake and the risk of age-related macular degeneration: a systematic review and meta-analysis. *Br J Nutr* 2012;107(3):350–359. doi: 10.1017/S0007114511004260.

41. Johnson EJ. Age-related macular degeneration and antioxidant vitamins: recent findings. *Curr Opin Clin Nutr Metab Care* 2010;13(1):28–33. doi: 10.1097/MCO.0b013e32833308ff.

42. Weikel KA, Garber C, Baburins A, et al. Nutritional modulation of cataract. *Nutr Rev* 2014;72(1):30–47.

43. Chiu CJ, Taylor A. Dietary hyperglycemia, glycemic index and metabolic retinal diseases. *Prog Retin Eye Res* 2011;30(1):18–53. doi: 10.1016/j.preteyeres.2010.09.001.

44. Chiu C-J, Liu S, Willett WC, et al. Informing food choices and health outcomes by use of the dietary glycemic index. *Nutr Rev* 2011;69:231–242. doi: 10.1111/j.1753-4887.2011.00382.x.

45. Chiu CJ, Milton RC, Klein R, et al. Dietary carbohydrate and the progression of age-related macular degeneration: a prospective study from the Age-Related Eye Disease Study. *Am J Clin Nutr* 2007;86(4):1210–1218.

46. Chiu CJ, Klein R, Milton RC, et al. Does eating particular diets alter the risk of age-related macular degeneration in users of the Age-Related Eye Disease Study supplements? *Br J Ophthalmol* 2009;93(9):1241–1246. doi: 10.1136/bjo.2008.143412.

47. Tan J, Wang JJ, Flood V, et al. Carbohydrate nutrition, glycemic index, and the 10-y incidence of cataract. *Am J Clin Nutr* 2007;86(5):1502–1508.

48. Kaushik S, Wang JJ, Flood V, et al. Dietary glycemic index and the risk of age-related macular degeneration. *Am J Clin Nutr* 2008;88:1104–1110.

49. Gopinath B, Flood VM, Wang JJ, et al. Carbohydrate nutrition is associated with changes in the retinal vascular structure and branching pattern in children. *Am J Clin Nutr* 2012;95(5):1215–1222. doi: 10.3945/ajcn.111.031641.

50. Chiu CJ, Robman L, McCarty CA, et al. Dietary carbohydrate in relation to cortical and nuclear lens opacities in the Melbourne visual impairment project. *Invest Ophthalmol Vis Sci* 2011;52(6):3593.

51. Evans JR, Lawrenson JG. Antioxidant vitamin and mineral supplements for slowing the progression of age-related macular degeneration. *Cochrane Database Syst Rev* 2012;11:CD000254. doi: 10.1002/14651858.CD000254.pub3.

52. Vishwanathan R, Chung M, Johnson EJ. A systematic review on zinc for the prevention and treatment of age-related macular degeneration. *Invest Ophthalmol Vis Sci* 2013;54(6):3985–3998. doi: 10.1167/iovs.12-11552.

53. Kuzniarz M, Mitchell P, Cumming RG, et al. Use of vitamin supplements and cataract: the Blue Mountains Eye Study. *Am J Ophthalmol* 2001;132:19–26.

54. Seddon JM, Christen WG, Manson JE, et al. The use of vitamin supplements and the risk of cataract among US male physicians. *Am J Public Health* 1994;84:788–792.

55. Christen W. Antioxidant vitamins and age-related eye disease. *Proc Assoc Am Physicians* 1999;111:16–21.

56. Brown N, Bron A, Harding J, et al. Nutrition supplements and the eye. *Eye* 1998;12:127–133.

57. West AL, Oren GA, Moroi SE. Evidence for the use of nutritional supplements and herbal medicines in common eye diseases. *Am J Ophthalmol* 2006;141(1):157–166.

58. Merle BM, Maubaret C, Korobelnik JF, et al. Association of HDL-related loci with age-related macular degeneration and plasma lutein and zeaxanthin: the Alienor Study. *PLoS One* 2013;8(11):e79848. doi: 10.1371/journal.pone.0079848.

59. Seddon JM, Reynolds R, Rosner B. Associations of smoking, body mass index, dietary lutein, and the LIPC gene variant rs10468017 with advanced age-related macular degeneration. *Mol Vis* 2010;16:2412–2424.

60. Fourgeux C, Dugas B, Richard F, et al. Single nucleotide polymorphism in the cholesterol-24S-hydroxylase (CYP46A1) gene and its association with CFH and LOC387715 gene polymorphisms in age-related macular degeneration. *Invest Ophthalmol Vis Sci* 2012;53(11):7026–7033. doi: 10.1167/iovs.12-9652.

61. Chiu CJ, Conley YP, Gorin MB, et al. Associations between genetic polymorphisms of insulin-like growth factor axis genes and risk for age-related macular degeneration. *Invest Ophthalmol Vis Sci* 2011; 52(12):9099–9107. doi: 10.1167/iovs.11-7782.

62. El-Sayed M, Abdel-Aal, Humayoun Akhtar, et al. Dietary sources of lutein and zeaxanthin carotenoids and their role in eye health. *Nutrients* 2013;5(4):1169–1185. doi: 10.3390/nu5041169.

63. Age-related Eye Disease Study Group. A randomized, placebo- controlled, clinical trial of high-dose supplementation with vitamins C and E and beta carotene for age-related cataract and vision loss: AREDS report no. 9. *Arch Ophthalmol* 2001;119:1439–1452.

64. Chasan-Taber L, Willett WC, Seddon JM, et al. A prospective study of vitamin supplement intake and cataract extraction among US women. *Epidemiology* 1999; 10:679–684.

65. Chasan-Taber L, Willett WC, Seddon JM, et al. A prospective study of carotenoid and vitamin A intakes and risk of cataract extraction in US women. *Am J Clin Nutr* 1999;70:509–516.

66. Karppi J, Laukkanen JA, Kurl S. Plasma lutein and zeaxanthin and the risk of age-related nuclear cataract among the elderly Finnish population. *Br J Nutr* 2012;108(1): 148–154. doi: 10.1017/S0007114511005332.

67. Mvitu M, Longo-Mbenza B, Tulomba D, et al. Regular, high, and moderate intake of vegetables rich in antioxidants may reduce cataract risk in Central African type 2 diabetics. *Int J Gen Med* 2012;5:489–493. doi: 10.2147/ IJGM.S28588.

68. Mares-Perlman JA, Millen AE, Ficek TL, et al. The body of evidence to support a protective role for lutein and zeaxanthin in delaying chronic disease. Overview. *J Nutr* 2002;132:518s–524s.

69. Seddon JM, Ajani UA, Sperduto RD, et al. Dietary carotenoids, vitamins A, C, and E and advanced age-related macular degeneration. Eye disease case-control study group. *J Am Med Assoc* 1994;272:1413–1420.

70. Brown L, Rimm EB, Seddon JM, et al. A prospective study of carotenoid intake and risk of cataract extraction in US men. *Am J Clin Nutr* 1999;70:517–524.

71. Mares-Perlman JA. Too soon for lutein supplements. *Am J Clin Nutr* 1999;70:431–432.

72. Lebuisson DA, Leroy L, Rigal G. Treatment of senile macular degeneration with *Ginkgo biloba* extract: a preliminary double-blind drug vs. placebo study [in French]. *Presse Med* 1986;15:1556–1558.

73. Quaranta L, Bettelli S, Uva MG, et al. Effect of *Ginkgo biloba* extract on preexisting visual field damage in normal tension glaucoma. *Ophthalmology* 2003;110: 359–364.

CHAPTER 37

Diet and Dentition

The associations among diet, the oral cavity, and health are diverse and bidirectional. A variety of nutrient deficiencies are reflected in the oral cavity, with inflammation of the buccal and glossal mucous membranes. Nutrition influences immunocompetence (see Chapter 11), which in turn influences the degree to which bacteria in the oral cavity contribute to tooth decay and caries. Poor dentition, particularly in the elderly, may play a role in malnutrition, with restriction in the variety and quantity of food attributable to mechanical limitations. Nutrition, through site-specific and systemic effects, plays a role in the development and maintenance of dental health.

OVERVIEW

Diet

Teeth are composed of an outer layer of enamel and an inner layer of dentin surrounding the pulp. Erosion of the outer mineralized layers leads to the formation of cavities, or caries. Dental caries, an infectious disease of the oral cavity and teeth, remains a considerable public health problem, despite declines over recent decades attributable primarily to fluoridation of the water supply and of dentifrices; it is the most common, chronic infectious disease of humans. At least 50% of children still develop dental caries, and the prevalence of the disease rises with age, so that very few adults are caries free.

The pathogenesis of dental caries involves demineralization of the tooth surface, a period of equilibration, and remineralization. The process appears to span nearly 18 months; therefore, the opportunity exists to arrest and reverse caries before a clinically overt cavity is formed. However, too much fluoride during this time period can lead to fluorosis of the teeth (a condition during which teeth become mottled and discolored permanently) or bone, during which bones and joints are damaged and become painful (1,2).

More about fluoridation of water is discussed below in the Nutriceuticals section.

The four factors influencing the development of caries, other than genetically induced susceptibility, are mouth bacteria, fermentable dietary carbohydrate, deficient exposure to fluoride and other dietary minerals, and the volume and composition of saliva. Plaque is composed of oral bacterial flora, polysaccharides, and salivary proteins. The predominant bacterial species is *Streptococcus mutans*, although current research shows that salivary levels of bifidobacteria directly correlate with formation of caries in children (3). Plaque bathes and—without consistent oral hygienic practice—adheres to teeth.

Ingested carbohydrate is metabolized (fermented) to organic acids, including lactic, butyric, acetic, formic, and propionic. A decline in plaque pH ensues, with dissolution of tooth surface enamel at a pH between 5.3 and 5.7. Any acid can lead to tooth demineralization and the formation of caries. Eating disorders that include purging (self-induced vomiting) have serious consequences for dental health because of the frequent exposure of teeth to gastric acid (4). This issue is addressed in Chapter 25.

A variety of epidemiological studies, including the natural experiments imposed by periods of shortage (e.g., World War II), reveal that dietary sugars are implicated in the etiology of dental caries. Plaque formation is accelerated when sucrose is present. *S. mutans* elaborates polysaccharides in the presence of sucrose that facilitate adhesion of bacteria to dental surfaces. Other commonly ingested sugars behave like sucrose and precipitate a comparable fall in the pH of plaque.

According to dental surveys of Kalahari Bushmen (5) and other hunter-gatherer populations (6), these groups display a remarkable absence of caries. The absence is explained by the repetitive annual abstinence of fermentable sugars in their diet, with a consequent inability to build a cariogenic oral load.

Because of several properties, dried fruits, cereals, cookies, crackers, chips, and breads all contribute to the formation of caries. Although they contain concentrated sugars, fresh fruits tend to be of low cariogenic potential because of their high water content and the presence of citric acid, which is a sialagogue. Foods containing citrate stimulate saliva production and may be beneficial if only moderate citrate is ingested.

Saliva plays an important role in the prevention of caries; xerostomic patients develop caries at particularly high rates. Saliva mobilizes food particles, directly buffers acid in plaque, depresses bacterial counts, and promotes remineralization by transporting calcium, phosphorus, and fluoride. The acid content of fruit may inhibit bacterial fermentation, but when high, as in lemons and oranges, it may directly erode enamel.

Meats, hard cheeses, nuts, and most vegetables appear to be uninvolved in the formation of caries. Cheese has been shown to enhance remineralization of enamel, and certain hard cheeses prevent dietary sugar from lowering plaque pH; these effects may be due to activation of protective saliva and release of calcium and phosphorus from cheese during mastication (7). The implication is that certain foods may specifically protect tooth enamel from the effects of sugars in other foods.

The adherence of starchy foods to the teeth contributes to cariogenesis; processed foods high in starch tend to adhere to teeth for protracted periods and thus may contribute disproportionately to cavity formation (8). Refined and processed grains contain modified starch susceptible to the action of salivary amylase. The release of maltose results, and its fermentation lowers plaque pH and contributes to demineralization. Of note, dietary starch present in vegetables is noncariogenic. It appears that complex starches eaten in the context of a low-sugar diet have low cariogenicity, while the processed starches typically found in modern diets, combined with high sugar consumption, are particularly inductive of caries (6,9).

The frequency of meals or snacks containing starch or sugar correlates directly with the formation of caries. Foods that adhere to teeth and which are eaten between meals increase the risk in particular. Food sequence is influential as well. When sugar-containing foods are consumed at the end of a meal or snack, they produce the most

protracted fall in plaque pH; other foods eaten after sources of starch or sugar can immediately attenuate their effects.

Although sugar in solution adheres less to teeth surfaces than does sugar from solids, sweetened drinks are associated with increased risk of caries (10,11). The risk appears to be most significant with sodas and sugar-based powdered beverages; 100% fruit juices may be slightly less cariogenic (11,12). Soda consumption may compromise dental health independently of the cariogenic effects of sugar; phosphoric acid may exert an erosive influence on enamel (10,13). In a small cross-sectional study by Ismail et al., a correlation between soda consumption and the development of severe early childhood caries (ECC) was found. Dental caries were also found to be more prevalent in low-income African American children. More research by this author showed a positive correlation between the prevalence of caries in caregivers and the prevalence of caries in their children (14,15). This research has been replicated (16–18) and has influenced the development of cavity screening guidelines for health care practitioners and dentists (19).

There is some evidence to show that development of childhood caries in kids younger than 5 years of age is significantly impacted by their mothers' gestational intake of fats and sugars (20), as well as by maternal oral health and oral flora during pregnancy (21,22). One study of 315 Japanese mother-child pairs found a significantly decreased risk of childhood dental caries among mothers who consumed more cheese but not milk or other dairy products during pregnancy (23). Small studies have found that poor maternal periodontal health can also significantly increase the risk of delivering a low-birth-weight infant or going in to preterm labor, although the evidence is not clear insofar (24,25). Thus, various factors beyond genetic predisposition and behavioral factors greatly influence dental health (20,26).

The potential benefits of artificial sweeteners are under investigation (see Chapter 42). Although less cariogenic because of their lack of sugar (27), sugar substitutes, such as xylitol used in chewing gums and aspartame used in diet sodas, may generate false security because people may automatically believe that sugar-free products are safe on teeth (28).

Diet sodas that are acidic, and generally contain aspartame, may be as damaging to teeth as nondiet varieties; the acid content contributes directly to demineralization (28,29). A similar process appears to occur with energy drinks and to a much lesser degree with sports drinks. One study, in which teeth were submerged in a variety of popular sports and energy drinks, showed a disproportionate degree of enamel dissolution. Energy drinks had significantly higher titratable acidity levels (lower pHs) and significantly increased resultant enamel dissolution (two times higher) than did sports drinks. High titratable acidity in drinks serve as a significant predictor of enamel dissolution. Thus, enamel weight loss varies inversely with the pH of the drink. Given the high usage rates of these types of drinks (it is currently estimated that up to 30% to 50% of American teens use energy drinks and up to 62% drink sports drinks at least once a day), this may be one area of intervention for public health organizations (30,30a).

Sugar alcohols, such as mannitol and sorbitol, are fermented more slowly than monosaccharides and disaccharides, and they are less cariogenic, although bacterial acclimation appears to occur if habitual intake is high. Lactose does not appear to be cariogenic, and milk consumption is associated with a slightly reduced risk of caries (31).

Xylitol is not cariogenic, and saccharin has been found to inhibit tooth decay in animal studies. Animal studies of aspartame indicate that it plays no role in the development of caries. Chewing gum sweetened with noncariogenic substances such as xylitol has a protective effect by stimulating the production and flow of saliva that neutralizes bacterial acids, dislodging trapped food particles, and reducing plaque. Xylitol-sweetened gum has been shown in studies to inhibit growth of *S. mutans* in both children (32) and adults (33). However, the Xylitol for Adult Caries Trial (X-ACT), a 33-month double-blinded, placebo controlled interventional trial that tested the effectiveness of daily xylitol lozenge use (up to 5 g per day) versus placebo lozenge use to prevent caries in adults at elevated risk of experiencing caries, showed no significant differences between the prevalence of caries in the intervention and placebo groups (34). Thus, xylitol is not currently recommended for use in the prevention of caries. A more promising sugar substitute investigated for preventing dental caries is erythritol. In a 3-year long intervention trial assessing dental plaques in 7- and 8-year-old children chewing candies containing erythritol versus xylitol or sorbitol-containing candies, the intervention group was noted to have reduced plaque growth, lowered levels of plaque acetic acid and propionic acid, and reduced oral counts of mutans (35).

Although moderation of dietary sugar intake may be beneficial to dental health and is advisable on other grounds, greater benefit to dentition may be achieved by consistently brushing with a fluoride toothpaste at least twice per day (19,36). One Cochrane review involving 79 trials on 73,000 children concluded that toothpastes containing at least 1,000 parts per million (ppm) fluoride are effective at preventing tooth decay in children (37). This dose supports the current international standard level recommended. The authors note that none of the trials in the review assessed for fluorosis or teeth mottling, which are both important risk factors when supplementing with fluoride. Naturally, these practices need not be mutually exclusive, and their benefits are likely to be additive.

During tooth development, protein/calorie malnutrition can retard tooth eruption and reduce tooth size. Vitamin A deficiency during development results in malformed teeth. Deficiencies of vitamin D, calcium, or phosphorus impair tooth mineralization. The availability of fluoride in sufficient but not excessive quantity strengthens tooth enamel; excess mottles the teeth. However, for some children (those considered to be at high risk of tooth decay by their dentist), the benefits to health of preventing tooth decay outweighs the risk of fluorosis (38). Iodine deficiency delays tooth eruption and alters growth patterns. Protein/calorie malnutrition and vitamins A and D, calcium, fluoride, and iodine deficiencies are all implicated in the development of caries. Vitamin C deficiency has been implicated in impaired tooth development and possibly in the development of caries.

Childhood and adolescent obesity is another possible contributor to the formation of dental caries, as it has been associated with earlier eruption of teeth in children and increased gingival inflammation, respectively (39). Earlier rupture of teeth may put children at higher risk of caries due to the extended length of time exposed in the oral cavity (40). Indications of increased gingival inflammation in obese adolescents included lower salivary secretion rate and higher sIgA levels. This is an important public health concern as rates of obesity among children, adolescents, and adults have reached epidemic levels (see chapter 5).

Infants and toddlers between the ages of 1 and 2 are at risk of baby-bottle tooth decay (41), which results when they are allowed to fall asleep drinking milk or formula from a bottle. The pooling of sugar-containing fluid around the teeth produces a characteristic, and sometimes severe, pattern of tooth decay. The condition is avoided by limiting nighttime and naptime fluid intake to water after the teeth have erupted. Human breast milk is apparently not cariogenic (42,43), whereas bovine milk and infant formulas (both milk and soy-based) have been shown to induce enamel erosion and higher levels of lactobacilli in study participants, and are thus not considered noncariogenic (44,45). A recent cross-sectional study of over 1,500 Scottish children found that a higher intake of non-milk extrinsic sugars (NMES), but not total sugar, increased the risk of having had treatment for decay, even after controlling for brushing their teeth twice a day (16). The diet to which infants are weaned is considered to influence dentition over both the short term and long term. An emphasis in the literature has been placed on the avoidance of sugar-containing beverages between meals and at bedtime (46,47).

There is some evidence in the literature demonstrating that dietary interventions in dental offices can improve dental health behaviors (48). Based on NHANES data, Nunn et al. found that children with healthier eating habits as measured by the Health Eating Index (HEI) developed fewer severe childhood caries than those in the lower tertiles of the HEI, suggesting that healthier eating habits can prevent such dental developments (49). This information may help guide clinicians and researchers in the development of interventions for preventing ECC. More research in this area is needed to elucidate more specifically which types of interventions are most effective.

Older adults with receding gingiva are at risk for caries over exposed surfaces of tooth roots. These surfaces lack enamel and are susceptible to caries at an accelerated rate. Implicated foods include sweetened beverages and starches. Care of the gingiva is fundamental to the prevention of this condition.

Gingivitis, inflammation of the gums, and periodontitis, a more serious infectious process involving the attachment apparatus of the tooth, are thought to be influenced by nutritional status, but evidence for specific associations is still limited (50). Because both processes are infectious and inflammatory, nutritional adequacy with regard to immune function (see Chapter 11) likely plays a role in the health of the gingiva and periodontal tissues, indirectly if not directly. The evidence that periodontal disease correlates with systemic inflammation and contributes to conditions such as coronary atherosclerosis, metabolic syndrome, and hypertension is now persuasive (51–53). Additionally, diabetes mellitus, a widespread phenomenon mostly of industrialized nations, is associated with progression of periodontal disease including a greater number of exposed root surfaces at risk for root caries, putting diabetics at even greater risk of systemic infection, and microvascular complications (54–56). Proper oral hygiene in this unique population is likely beneficial as some researchers are finding a correlation between the number of caries identified and hyperglycemia in study populations (57).

Tooth decay and loss affects nutritional status (58–60). Approximately 40% of adults over the age of 65 in the United States are edentulous. Many medications reduce saliva production, and for this reason, as many as 50% of the elderly have iatrogenically induced reductions in saliva production. Reduction of saliva can accelerate tooth decay and interfere with the functioning of dentures if already placed. The stimulation of saliva through the use of chewing gums containing xylitol may be compensatory (61).

Maintenance of oral health is essential to maintaining good nutritional patterns and thereby reducing risk for a variety of chronic diseases in elderly adults (62,63). Masticatory ability in individuals with partial or complete dentures generally is reduced to approximately 20% of normal; this may cause individuals to modify their diets to exclude potentially nutritious foods with challenging consistencies (64). Specifically, orofacial pain and sore gums, symptoms often experienced in this general population, have been associated with poorer general health (65). Data from an observational study of more than 1,200 male veterans indicate that poor dentition is associated with reduced intake of many vitamins, minerals, protein, and fiber. The diets of those with compromised and intact dentition differed both qualitatively and quantitatively. The study revealed that subjects with compromised dentition avoid eating nutrient-dense foods considered difficult to chew, including fruits, vegetables, nuts, and meats.

A recent epidemiological assessment of NHANES data examined nutritional status in elderly people with full and partial dentition. It, too, showed decreases in specific vitamin and nutrient intakes among the elderly in direct correlation with the number of natural teeth in place. Elderly women with partial or incomplete dentition were found to have lower β-carotene intake than their control counterparts having complete natural dentition, and elderly men with partial or incomplete dentition were found to have decreased vitamin C and overall caloric intake when compared to the control group (66). A second study showed a direct correlation between severe tooth loss in an elderly population and an inability to meet standard dietary recommendations (67). More serious concerns were raised by a population-based assessment of 1,803 participants living in Germany. Subjects who had nine or more unreplaced teeth were found to have a significant increase in all-cause mortality and cardiovascular mortality, even after adjusting for smoking, alcohol consumption, physical activity, obesity, hypertension, diabetes, and dyslipidemia in all subjects (68).

Fortunately, for a variety of reasons, the prevalence of tooth loss in the elderly is decreasing over time. Dental health correlates to some extent with education level and the consistency of dental care (20). Krall et al. (69) suggest that some variation in diet previously attributed to education level may be confounded by dentition status.

POLYMORPHISMS RELEVANT TO DENTITION

Common polymorphisms in the sweet taste receptor (TAS1R2) and glucose transporter (GLUT2) genes are associated with dental caries according to an 80-subject cohort study of healthy Caucasian individuals aged 21 to 32 years. Subjects were genotyped for the above polymorphisms, stratified accordingly into four groups, and then assessed for dental caries. Carriers of the Ile allele for GLUT2 showed increased amounts of decayed, missing, and filled teeth, while those with the Val allele for TAS1R2 demonstrated lower caries scores. This research indicates that there are important genetic factors that need to be

taken into account when assessing and caring for patients with dental caries (70). Clearly, further research is needed in this area.

NUTRIENTS, NUTRICEUTICALS, AND FUNCTIONAL FOODS

Calcium and Vitamin D

Adequate intake of calcium and vitamin D may be necessary for the maintenance of healthy gingiva (71–75). Vitamin D and calcium supplementation is associated with a decreased risk of periodontal disease in patients undergoing periodontal maintenance therapy (76).

Fluoride

A reduction in the rate of dental caries attributable to water and dentifrice fluoridation is irrefutable (77). Fluoride is incorporated into the hydroxyapatite of teeth, rendering tooth mineral less susceptible to demineralization. Fluoride also inhibits the replication and enzymes of S. mutans. A substantial decrease in the risk of caries for both children and adults is associated with fluoride at a dose of 1 part per million in the drinking water. This dose, studied extensively, is not associated with any known adverse health effects, although critics of systemic fluoridation claim it is the cause of increased rates of osteosarcoma, osteopenia, and other disorders of bone metabolism. These claims are not supported by current epidemiologic evidence (78,79). One epidemiologic review in Iran, however, did find a significantly positive correlation between high ground water levels of fluoride and hypertension (80); thus, more research is needed. A careful balance between prophylaxis of caries with fluoride and fluorosis must be attained to maximize benefit of this compound. Fluoride treatments of public water sources, table salt, fluoridated toothpaste, sealants, and even milk are recommended for both children and adults as they have been found to be safe and effective means of decreasing risk of dental caries (81–86). The incorporation of fluoride into skeletal bone may also confer benefit (see Chapter 14).

Bottled water, used increasingly in this country, may or may not have adequate fluoride concentration (87). When water is not fluoridated, fluoride supplementation for children (either in tablet, drop or lozenge form) is indicated; the dose recommended is 0.05 mg/kg/day (77). Fluoride supplementation is recommended for infants breast-fed beyond 6 months, beginning at that age, as the fluoride content of breast milk is low. Prenatal supplementation is of uncertain benefit (88). Because young children will swallow a portion of toothpaste used, small amounts should be dispensed to prevent excess fluoride ingestion. A systematic review by Santos, Oliviera, and Nadanovsky showed that low-fluoride toothpastes significantly increased the risk of dental caries in preschoolers but did not decrease the risk of developing sequelae of fluorosis in upper anterior permanent teeth. The authors do not recommend the use of low-fluoride toothpastes for these reasons (89).

Cranberry

Cranberry (*Vaccinium macrocarpon*), a fruit long touted as a treatment for urinary tract infections, is currently being investigated for its potential preventive characteristics in regards to dental caries. In studies, the polyphenols of these small fruits, including proanthocyanidins and anthocyandins, demonstrate inhibition of *Streptococcus* bacterial adhesion to hydroxyapatite pellets pretreated with saliva (90). Other studies also suggest that cranberry extracts prevent the formation of biofilms by cariogenic streptococci, implying that cranberry extracts slow the development of dental plaque (91,92). Among other effects, cranberry extract is also thought to inhibit acid production by cariogenic bacteria as well as their proteolytic activities, thus leading to less potential for the development of caries and periodontal disease (93).

Coenzyme Q$_{10}$

There has long been interest in a potential role for coenzyme Q$_{10}$ (ubiquinol) in the prevention and treatment of periodontal disease (94). And interest has grown further over recent years. Yoneda et al. found a significant decrease in osteoclast activity and age-related inflammatory reactions in periodontal tissue of rats treated with topical reduced coenzyme Q$_{10}$ (95). Solitary application of coQ$_{10}$ to the gingiva of 30 subjects with plaque-induced gingivitis showed marked reductions in their gingival, bleeding, and plaque scores according to a RCT by Chatterjee et al. (96). These findings have been replicated both in vivo and in vitro (97–100). Overall, evidence on the usefulness of

CoQ$_{10}$ for prevention and treatment of periodontal disease is promising.

Probiotics

A relatively new field (bacteriotherapy with probiotics) is showing promise of being beneficial for oral health. Probiotics (or microorganisms with beneficial health benefits) have been shown to decrease the pH of the oral cavity so that plaque bacteria (generally thought to be *mutans streptococci* species) cannot form the dental plaque that causes periodontal disease (101). In their review of meta-analyses on effects of probiotics on teeth in children, Twetman & Stecksén-Blicks found six studies showing a hampering effect on mutans streptococci and/or yeast in the mouth with ingestion of lactobacilli- or bifidobacteria-derived probiotics (102). Different strains, however, may have differing cariogenic potential as outlined by a study comparing the effects of two differing *Lactobacillus reuteri* strains on the biofilm (103). Despite these different effects, probiotics produce antioxidants which prevent plaque formation by neutralizing free electrons needed for mineral formation (104). Probiotics have also been found to break down foul odors in the mouth by converting volatile gases to those needed for metabolism, thus improving halitosis (105,106). Few randomized controlled trials have been completed in this area of study and are needed to elucidate the potential benefit of probiotics for oral health (107).

Iron

Multiple studies have found a significant association between low serum iron levels and ECC among children (108,109). Children with more ECCs were also found to have low serum ferritin levels in one case-controlled study and in a separate population study. These children were subsequently at greater risk of being anemic (110,111), which has advanced public health implications, including permanent effects on growth and development. Further research should be done to evaluate the clinical relevance of low serum iron levels in the development of ECC.

Xylitol

As previously mentioned, xylitol has been evaluated for the treatment of dental caries. The X-ACT, a 33-month double-blinded, placebo controlled interventional trial that tested the effectiveness of daily xylitol lozenge use (up to 5 g per day) versus placebo lozenge use to prevent caries in adults at elevated risk of experiencing caries, showed no significant differences between the prevalence of caries in the intervention and placebo groups (34). Thus, xylitol is not currently recommended for use in the prevention of caries.

CLINICAL HIGHLIGHTS

Diet influences dentition, and dentition and the health of the oral cavity influence diet, as well as the overall state of health. The dietary factors most important in the pathogenesis of dental caries are the sugar and starch content of the diet, the conclusion of meals and snacks with foods high in processed starch or sugar, and the frequency of snacks containing such foods.

The incidence of dental caries can be reduced by limiting sugar intake, avoiding sugary or starchy snacks, using chewing gum sweetened with xylitol or other nonfermentable sweeteners, and frequent brushing to remove trapped food particles. Dietary adequacy in general is important to optimize immune function and the health of the buccal and lingual mucosae. A multivitamin supplement may be of benefit, particularly in individuals past the age of 50.

Fluoride intake over years greatly influences susceptibility to caries. The fluoride content of patients' drinking water should be addressed in primary care; physicians should advise supplementation when the water fluoride is low. Virtually all municipal or public water supplies are fluoridated; private wells generally, of course, are not. Children should be weaned to diets that are moderate in sugar content and, in particular, should not be allowed to take a sweetened beverage to bed. Careful attention to the dentition of aging adults is essential to the preservation of native teeth, which in turn influences the adequacy, in terms of quality and quantity, of the overall diet.

REFERENCES

1. Buzalaf MA, Levy SM. Fluoride intake of children: considerations for dental caries and dental fluorosis. *Monogr Oral Sci* 2011;22:1–19. doi:10.1159/000325101.
2. Namkaew M, Wiwatanadate P. Association of fluoride in water for consumption and chronic pain of body parts in residents of San Kamphaeng district, Chiang Mai, Thailand. *Trop Med Int Health* 2012;17(9):1171–1176. doi:10.1111/j.1365-3156.2012.03061.x.
3. Kaur R, Gilbert SC, Sheehy EC, et al. Salivary levels of Bifidobacteria in caries-free and caries-active children. *Int J Paediatr Dent* 2013;23(1)32–38.
4. Milosevic A, Brodie D, Slade P. Dental erosion, oral hygiene, and nutrition in eating disorders. *Int J Eat Disord* 1997;21:195–199.
5. Clement AJ, Fosdick LL, Plotkin R. The formation of lactic acid in dental plaques. II. Oral conditions of primitive Bushmen of the Western Kalahari Desert. *J Dent Res* 1956;35,786–791.
6. Larsen CS. Biological changes in human populations with agriculture. *Annu Rev Anthropol* 1995;24,185–213.
7. Ahola AJ, Yli-Knuuttila H, Suomalainen T, et al. Short-term consumption of probiotic-containing cheese and its effect on dental caries risk factors. *Arch Oral Biol* 2002;47:799–804.
8. Kashket S, Zhang J, Houte JV. Accumulation of fermentable sugars and metabolic acids in food particles that become entrapped on the dentition. *J Dent Res* 1996;75: 1885–1891.
9. Lingstrom P, van Houte J, Kashket S. Food starches and dental caries. *Crit Rev Oral Biol Med* 2000;11:366–380.
10. Levine RS, Nugent ZJ, Rudolf MC, et al. Dietary patterns, toothbrushing habits and caries experience of schoolchildren in West Yorkshire, England. *Community Dent Health* 2007;24(2):82–87.
11. Dugmore CR, Rock WP. A multifactorial analysis of factors associated with dental erosion. *Br Dent J* 2004;196; 283–286.
12. Marshall TA, Levy SM, Broffitt B, et al. Dental caries and beverage consumption in young children. *Pediatrics* 2003;112:e184–e191.
13. Van Eygen I, Vannet BV, Wehrbein H. Influence of a soft drink with low pH on enamel surfaces: an in vitro study. *Am J Orthod Dentofacial Orthop* 2005;128:372–377.
14. Ismail AI, Lim S, Sohn W, et al. Determinants of early childhood caries in low-income African American young children. *Pediatr Dent* 2008;30(4):289–296.
15. Reisine S, Tellez M, Willem J, et al. Relationship between caregiver's and child's caries prevalence among disadvantaged African Americans. *Community Dent Oral Epidemiol* 2008;36(3):191–200. doi:10.1111/j.1600-0528. 2007.00392.x.
16. Masson LF, Blackburn A, Sheehy C, et al. Sugar intake and dental decay: results from a national survey of children in Scotland. *Br J Nutr* 2010;104(10):1555–1564.
17. Wigen TI, Espelid I, Skaare AB, et al. Family characteristics and caries experience in preschool children. A longitudinal study from pregnancy to 5 years of age. *Community Dent Oral Epidemiol* 2011;39(4):311–317.
18. Huew R, Waterhouse PJ, Moynihan PJ, et al. Dental erosion and its association with diet in Libyan schoolchildren. *Eur Arch Paediatr Dent* 2011;12(5):234–240.
19. American Academy of Pediatric Dentistry Council on Clinical Affairs. *Guideline on caries-risk assessment and management for infants, children, and adolescents. Council on clinical affairs.* Revised 2011. Available at http://www.aapd.org/media/Policies_Guidelines/G_CariesRisk Assessment.pdf; accessed 1/14/13.
20. Wigen TI, Wang NJ. Maternal health and lifestyle, and caries experience in preschool children. A

longitudinal study from pregnancy to age 5 yr. *Eur J Oral Sci* 2011;119(6):463–468.

21. Boggess KA, Edelstein BL. Oral health in women during preconception and pregnancy: implications for birth outcomes and infant oral health. *Matern Child Health J* 2006;10(suppl 1):169–174.

22. Boggess KA. Maternal oral health in pregnancy. *Obstet Gynecol* 2008;111(4):976–986.

23. Tanaka K, Miyake Y, Sasaki S, et al. Dairy products and calcium intake during pregnancy and dental caries in children. *Nutr J* 2012;11:33.

24. Dasanayake AP. Poor periodontal health of the pregnant woman as a risk factor for low birth weight. *Ann Periodontol* 1998;3(1):206–212.

25. Offenbacher S, Jared HL, O'Reilly PG, et al. Potential pathogenic mechanisms of periodontitis associated pregnancy complications. *Ann Periodontol* 1998;3(1):233–250.

26. Edelstein BL, Chinn CH. Update on disparities in oral health and access to dental care for America's children. *Acad Pediatr* 2009;9(6):415–419. doi:10.1016/j.acap.2009.09.010.

27. Forshee RA, Storey ML. Evaluation of the association of demographics and beverage consumption with dental caries. *Food Chem Toxicol* 2004;42:1805–1816.

28. Nadimi H, Wesamaa H, Janket SJ, et al. Are sugar-free confections really beneficial for dental health? *Br Dent J* 2011;211(7):E15. doi:10.1038/sj.bdj.2011.823.

29. Thomas B. *Nutrition in primary care. A handbook for health professionals*. Oxford, UK: Blackwell Science, 1996.

30. Jain P, Hall-May E, Golabek K, et al. A comparison of sports and energy drinks—Physiochemical properties and enamel dissolution. *Gen Dent* 2012;60(3):190–197.

30a. Conley, M. Energy, Sports Drinks Destroys Teeth, Study Says. http://abcnews.go.com/blogs/health/2012/05/03/energy-sports-drinks-destroy-teeth-says-study/; accessed on 1/13/13.

31. Moynihan PJ. The role of diet and nutrition in the etiology and prevention of oral diseases. *Bull World Health Organ* 2005;83:694–699.

32. Makinen K, Bennett C, Hujoel P, et al. Xylitol chewing gums and caries rates: a 40-month cohort study. *J Dent Res* 1995;74:1904–1913.

33. Haresaku S, Hanioka T, Tsutsui A, et al. Long-term effect of xylitol gum use on mutans streptococci in adults. *Caries Res* 2007;41:198–203.

34. Bader JD, Vollmer WM, Shugars DA, et al. Results from the Xylitol for Adult Caries Trial (X-ACT). *J Am Dent Assoc* 2013;144(1):21–30.

35. Runnel R, Mäkinen KK, Honkala S, et al. Effect of three-year consumption of erythritol, xylitol and sorbitol candies on various plaque and salivary caries-related variables. *J Dent* 2013;41(12):1236–1244. doi:10.1016/j.jdent.2013.09.007.

36. Gibson S, Williams S. Dental caries in pre-school children: association with social class, toothbrushing habit and consumption of sugars and sugar-containing foods. Further analysis of data from the National Diet and Nutrition Survey of children aged 1.5–4.5 years. *Caries Res* 1999;33:101–113.

37. Walsh T, Worthington HV, Glenny A-M, et al. Fluoride toothpastes of different concentrations for preventing dental caries in children and adolescents. *Cochrane Database Syst Rev* 2010;1:CD007868. doi:10.1002/14651858.CD007868.pub2.

38. Wong MCM, Glenny A-M, Tsang BWK, et al. Topical fluoride as a cause of dental fluorosis in children. *Cochrane Database Syst Rev* 2010;(1):CD007693. doi:10.1002/14651858.CD007693.pub2.

39. Fadel HT, Pliaki A, Gronowitz E, et al. Clinical and biological indicators of dental caries and periodontal disease in adolescents with or without obesity. *Clin Oral Investig* 2014;18(2):359–368.

40. Must A, Phillips SM, Tybor DJ, et al. The association between childhood obesity and tooth eruption. *Obesity* (Silver Spring) 2012; 20(10):2070–2074. doi:10.1038/oby.2012.23.

41. Sonis A, Castle J, Duggan C. Infant nutrition: implications for somatic growth, adult onset disease, and oral health. *Curr Opin Pediatr* 1997;9:289–297.

42. Erickson P, Mazhari E. Investigation of the role of human breast milk in caries development. *Pediatr Dent* 1999;21:86–90.

43. World Health Organization. *Diet, nutrition and the prevention of chronic diseases*. WHO Technical Report Series, No. 916. Geneva, Switzerland: World Health Organization, 2003.

44. de Mazer Papa AM, Tabchoury CP, Del Bel Cury AA, et al. Effect of milk and soy-based infant formulas on in situ demineralization of human primary enamel. *Pediatr Dent* 2010;32(1):35–40.

45. Muñoz-Sandoval C, Muñoz-Cifuentes MJ, Giacaman RA, et al. Effect of bovine milk on *Streptococcus mutans* biofilm cariogenic properties and enamel and dentin demineralization. *Pediatr Dent* 2012;34(7):197–201.

46. Holt R, Moynihan P. The weaning diet and dental health. *Br Dent J* 1996;181:254–259.

47. Nainar SM, Mohummed S. Diet counseling during the infant oral health visit. *Pediatr Dent* 2004;26:459–462.

48. Harris R, Gamboa A, Dailey Y, et al. One-to-one dietary interventions undertaken in a dental setting to change dietary behaviour. *Cochrane Database Syst Rev* 2012; (3):CD006540.

49. Nunn ME, Braunstein NS, Krall Kaye EA, et al. Healthy eating index is a predictor of early childhood caries. *J Dent Res* 2009;88(4):361–366.

50. Enwonwu CO, Phillips RS, Falkler WA Jr. Nutrition and oral infectious diseases: state of the science. *Compend Contin Educ Dent* 2002;23:431–434.

51. Bensley L, VanEenwyk J, Ossiander EM. Associations of self-reported periodontal disease with metabolic syndrome and number of self-reported chronic conditions. *Prev Chronic Dis* 2011;8(3):A50.

52. Humphrey LL, Fu R, Buckley DI, et al. Periodontal disease and coronary heart disease incidence: a systematic review and meta-analysis. *J Gen Intern Med* 2008; 23(12):2079–2086.

53. Tonetti MS. Periodontitis and risk for atherosclerosis: an update on intervention trials. *J Clin Periodontol* 2009; 36(suppl 10):15–19.

54. Bajaj S, Prasad S, Gupta A, et al. Oral manifestations in type-2 diabetes and related complications. *Indian J Endocrinol Metab* 2012;16(5):777–779. doi:10.4103/2230-8210.100673.

55. Garton BJ, Ford PJ. Root caries and diabetes: risk assessing to improve oral and systemic health outcomes. *Aust Dent J* 2012;57(2):114–122. doi:10.1111/j.1834-7819.2012.01690.x.

56. Tu YK, D'Aiuto F, Lin HJ, et al. Relationship between metabolic syndrome and diagnoses of periodontal diseases among participants in a large Taiwanese cohort. *J Clin Periodontol* 2013;40(11):994–1000. doi:10.1111/jcpe.12157.

57. Lalla E, Cheng B, Kunzel C, et al. Dental findings and identification of undiagnosed hyperglycemia. *J Dent Res* 2013;92(10):888–892. doi:10.1177/0022034513502791.

58. Ettinger R. Changing dietary patterns with changing dentition: how do people cope? *Spec Care Dent* 1998;18:33–39.

59. Papas A, Palmer C, Rounds M, et al. The effects of denture status on nutrition. *Spec Care Dent* 1998;18:17–25.

60. Walls AW, Steele JG, Sheiham A, et al. Oral health and nutrition in older people. *J Public Health Dent* 2000;60:304–307.

61. Makinen KK, Isotupa KP, Kivilompolo T, et al. The effect of polyol-combinant saliva stimulants on *S. mutans* levels in plaque and saliva of patients with mental retardation. *Spec Care Dentist* 2002;22:187–193.

62. Saunders M. Nutrition and oral health in the elderly. *Dent Clin North Am* 1997;41:681–698.

63. Ritchie CS, Joshipura K, Hung HC, et al. Nutrition as a mediator in the relation between oral and systemic disease: associations between specific measures of adult oral health and nutrition outcomes. *Crit Rev Oral Biol Med* 2002;13:291–300.

64. N'gom PI, Woda A. Influence of impaired mastication on nutrition. *J Prosthet Dent* 2002;87:667–673.

65. Brennan DS, Singh KA. Dietary, self-reported oral health and socio-demographic predictors of general health status among older adults. *J Nutr Health Aging* 2012;16(5):437–441.

66. Ervin RB, Dye BA. Number of natural and prosthetic teeth impact nutrient intakes of older adults in the United States. *Gerodontology* 2012;29(2):e693–e702.

67. Savoca MR, Arcury TA, Leng X, et al. Severe tooth loss in older adults as a key indicator of compromised dietary quality. *Public Health Nutr* 2010;13(4):466–474.

68. Schwahn C, Polzer I, Haring R, et al. Missing, unreplaced teeth and risk of all-cause and cardiovascular mortality. *Int J Cardiol* 167(4):1430–1437.

69. Krall E, Hayes C, Garcia R. How dentition status and masticatory function affect nutrient intake. *J Am Dent Assoc* 1998;129:1261–1269.

70. Kulkarni GV, Chng T, Eny KM, et al. Association of GLUT2 and TAS1R2 genotypes with risk for dental caries. *Caries Res* 2013;47(3):219–225. doi:10.1159/000345652.

71. Millen AE, Hovey KM, Lamonte MJ, et al. Plasma 25-hydroxyvitamin D concentrations and periodontal disease in postmenopausal women. *J Periodontol* 2013;84(9):1243–1256.

72. Yao SG, Fine JB. A review of vitamin D as it relates to periodontal disease. *Compend Contin Educ Dent* 2012;33(3):166–171; quiz 172, 182.

73. Zhou X, Han J, Song Y, et al. Serum levels of 25-hydroxyvitamin D, oral health and chronic obstructive pulmonary disease. *J Clin Periodontol* 2012;39(4):350–356.

74. Stein SH, Tipton DA. Vitamin D and its impact on oral health—an update. *J Tenn Dent Assoc* 2011;91(2):30–33; quiz 34–35.

75. Dietrich T, Joshipura KJ, Dawson-Hughes B, et al. Association between serum concentrations of 25-hydroxyvitamin D_3 and periodontal disease in the US population. *Am J Clin Nutr* 2004;80(1):108–113.

76. Miley DD, Garcia MN, Hildebolt CF, et al. Cross-sectional study of vitamin d and calcium supplementation effects on chronic periodontitis. *J Periodontology* 2009;80(9):1433–1439.

77. Tubert-Jeannin S, Auclair C, Amsallem E, et al. Fluoride supplements (tablets, drops, lozenges or chewing gums) for preventing dental caries in children. *Cochrane Database Syst Rev* 2011;(12):CD007592.

78. Levy M, Leclerc BS. Fluoride in drinking water and osteosarcoma incidence rates in the continental United States among children and adolescents. *Cancer Epidemiol* 2012;36(2):e83–e88. doi:10.1016/j.canep.2011.11.008.

79. Comber H, Deady S, Montgomery E, et al. Drinking water fluoridation and osteosarcoma incidence on the island of Ireland. *Cancer Causes Control* 2011;22(6):919–924. doi:10.1007/s10552-011-9765-0.

80. Amini H, Taghavi Shahri SM, Amini M, et al. Drinking water fluoride and blood pressure? An environmental study. *Biol Trace Elem Res* 2011;144(1–3):157–163. doi:10.1007/s12011-011-9054-5.

81. Palmer CA, Gilbert JA; Academy of Nutrition and Dietetics. Position of the Academy of Nutrition and Dietetics: the impact of fluoride on health. *J Acad Nutr Diet* 2012;112(9):1443–1453. doi:10.1016/j.jand.2012.07.012.

82. Harding MA, O'Mullane DM. Water fluoridation and oral health. *Acta Med Acad* 2013;42(2):131–139. doi:10.5644/ama2006-124.81.

83. Parnell C, Whelton H, O'Mullane D. Water fluoridation. *Eur Arch Paediatr Dent* 2009;10(3):141–148.

84. Yengopal V, Chikte UM, Mickenautsch S, et al. Salt fluoridation: a meta-analysis of its efficacy for caries prevention. *SADJ* 2010;65(2):60–64, 66–67.

85. Mariño R, Fajardo J, Morgan M. Cost-effectiveness models for dental caries prevention programmes among Chilean schoolchildren. *Community Dent Health* 2012;29(4):302–308.

86. Marinho VC. Cochrane reviews of randomized trials of fluoride therapies for preventing dental caries. *Eur Arch Paediatr Dent* 2009;10(3):183–191.

87. Warren JJ, Levy SM. Current and future role of fluoride in nutrition. *Dent Clin North Am* 2003;47:225–243.

88. Leverett DH, Adair SM, Vaughan BW, et al. Randomized clinical trial of the effect of prenatal fluoride supplements in preventing dental caries. *Caries Res* 1997;31:174–179.

89. Santos AP, Oliveira BH, Nadanovsky P. Effects of low and standard fluoride toothpastes on caries and fluorosis: systematic review and meta-analysis. *Caries Res* 2013;47(5):382–390. doi:10.1159/000348492.

90. Yamanaka A, Kimizuka R, Kato T, et al. Inhibitory effects of cranberry juice on attachment of oral streptococci and biofilm formation. *Oral Microbiol Immunol* 2004;19(3):150–154.

91. Duarte S, Gregoire S, Singh AP, et al. Inhibitory effects of cranberry polyphenols on formation and acidogenicity of *Streptococcus mutans* biofilms. *FEMS Microbiol Lett* 2006;257(1):50–56.

92. Yamanaka-Okada A, Sato E, Kouchi T, et al. Inhibitory effect of cranberry polyphenol on cariogenic bacteria. *Bull Tokyo Dent Coll* 2008;49(3):107–112.

93. Bonifait L, Grenier D. Cranberry polyphenols: potential benefits for dental caries and periodontal disease. *J Can Dent Assoc* 2010;76:a130.

94. Watts TL. Coenzyme Q_{10} and periodontal treatment: is there any beneficial effect? *Br Dent J* 1995;178:209–213.

95. Yoneda T, Tomofuji T, Ekuni D, et al. Anti-aging effects of co-enzyme Q10 on periodontal tissues. *J Dent Res* 2013;92(8):735–739. doi:10.1177/0022034513490959. Epub 2013 May 21.

96. Chatterjee A, Kandwal A, Singh N, et al. Evaluation of Co-Q10 anti-gingivitis effect on plaque induced gingivitis: a randomized controlled clinical trial. *J Indian Soc Periodontol* 2012;16(4):539–542. doi:10.4103/0972-124X.106902.

97. Hans M, Prakash S, Gupta S. Clinical evaluation of topical application of perio-Q gel (Coenzyme Q(10)) in chronic periodontitis patients. *J Indian Soc Periodontol* 2012;16(2):193–199. doi:10.4103/0972-124X.99261.

98. Brzozowska TM, Flisykowska AK, OEwitkowska MW, et al. Healing of periodontal tissue assisted by Coenzyme Q10 with Vitamin E: clinical and laboratory evaluation. *Pharmacol Rep* 2007;59:257–60.

99. Shizukuishi S, Hanioka T, Tsunemitsu A, et al. Clinical effect of Coenzyme 10 on periodontal disease; evaluation of oxygen utilisation in gingiva by tissue reflectance spectrophotometry. In: Shizukuishi S, Hanioka T, Tsunemitsu A, eds. *Biomedical and clinical aspects of Coenzyme Q*, Vol. 5. Amsterdam: Elsevier, 1986;359–368.

100. McRee JT, Hanioka T, Shizukuishi S, et al. Therapy with Coenzyme Q10 for patients with periodontal disease. 1. Effect of Coenzyme Q10 on subgingival microorganisms. *J Dent Health* 1993;43:659–666.

101. Shivamanjunath RG. Benefits of live microorganisms (probiotics) in periodontal health. *Int J Contemp Dent* 2011;2:97–100.

102. Twetman S, Stecksén-Blicks C. Probiotics and oral health effects in children. *Int J Paediatr Dent* 2008;18(1):3–10.

103. Jalasvuori H, Haukioja A, Tenovuo J. Probiotic *Lactobacillus reuteri* strains ATCC PTA 5289 and ATCC 55730 differ in their cariogenic properties in vitro.

Arch Oral Biol 2012;57(12):1633–1638. doi:10.1016/j.archoralbio.2012.07.014.

104. Chopra R, Mathur S. Probiotics in dentistry: a boon or sham. *Dent Res J* (Isfahan) 2013;10(3): 302–306.

105. Kang MS, Kim BG, Chung J, et al. Inhibitory effect of *Weissella cibaria* isolates on the production of volatile sulphur compounds. *J Clin Periodontol* 2006;33:226–232.

106. Burton JP, Chilcott CN, Moore CJ, et al. A preliminary study of the effect of probiotic *Streptococcus salivarius* K12 on oral malodour parameters. *J Appl Microbiol* 2006; 100:754–764.

107. Anilkumar K, Monisha AL. Role of friendly bacteria in oral health–a short review. *Oral Health Prev Dent* 2012; 10(1):3–8.

108. Tang RS, Huang MC, Huang ST. Relationship between dental caries status and anemia in children with severe early childhood caries. *Kaohsiung J Med Sci* 2013; 29(6):330–336. doi:10.1016/j.kjms.2012.10.003.

109. Sadeghi M, Darakhshan R, Bagherian A. Is there an association between early childhood caries and serum iron and serum ferritin levels? *Dent Res J* (Isfahan) 2012;9(3):294–298.

110. Schroth RJ, Levi J, Kliewer E, et al. Association between iron status, iron deficiency anaemia, and severe early childhood caries: a case-control study. *BMC Pediatr* 2013;13:22. doi:10.1186/1471-2431-13-22.

111. Clarke M, Locker D, Berall G, et al. Malnourishment in a population of young children with severe early childhood caries. *Pediatr Dent* 2006;28(3):254–259.

SUGGESTED READINGS

DePaola DP, Touger-Decker R, Rigassio-Radler D, et al. Nutrition and dental medicine. In: Shils ME, Shike M, Ross AC, et al., eds. *Modern nutrition in health and disease*, 10th ed. Philadelphia, PA: Lippincott Williams & Wilkins, 2006:1152–1178.

Rugg-Dunn AJ, Nunn JH. *Nutrition, diet, and oral health*. Oxford, UK: Oxford University Press, 1999.

CHAPTER 38

Hunger, Appetite, Taste, and Satiety

ontrol over the process of energy and nutrient intake is vital to the survival of an individual and a species. Minimally, food intake is influenced by *hunger*, the sensations induced by a deficit in readily metabolizable energy sources. But it is also influenced by *appetite*, a desire for food influenced by cravings for specific tastes and/or nutrients, and the palatability, familiarity, and availability of specific foods. Also important is *satiety*, the sensation that the impulses that have led to food consumption have been satisfied (see Table 38.1).

In humans, food intake is the product of physiologic, psychological, and sociologic factors that defy simple classification. The conditions of endemic and epidemic obesity that are increasingly common in industrialized countries, while ascribable to an imbalance in the regulation of energy intake, are less readily ascribed to a particular component of the complex governing systems. There is evidence that redundant processes in humans govern energy intake, a state that may have conferred survival benefit throughout human prehistory, when the adequacy of dietary energy was often in question.

TABLE 38.1

Fundamental Factors Governing Energy Intake and Balance

Factor	Definition/Influence
Hunger	The various sensations associated with a deficit in the body's supply of "fuel"; a physical compulsion to eat
Appetite	A desire for a particular food or craving for a particular taste; may not involve hunger at all
Satiety	The effect that eating now has on eating later; how long the state of feeling full and satisfied lasts

The properties of specific foods and the physiologic responses evoked by their consumption appear to have implications for the regulation of energy intake, although simple explanations are elusive and perhaps ill advised. Sufficient insights and evidence have accumulated to permit clinical recommendations that may be expected to contribute to salutary energy balance. While the primary care clinician need not be truly expert in the pathways regulating appetite and energy balance, a familiarity with these pathways should foster more insightful and compassionate counseling. Several discrete and fairly simple dietary adjustments may be espoused that offer the promise of facilitating fullness and satisfaction on fewer calories, an important potential contributor to sustainable weight control.

OVERVIEW

Physiologic defenses against undernutrition are far more robust than those against overnutrition (1). The case may even be made that *Homo sapiens* has no native defense against caloric excess, never having needed one throughout most of our history. Even so, were physiology alone responsible for nutrient energy consumption, food intake would begin with hunger and end with satiety. The characteristic physical sensations of hunger and fullness, however, are one part of a complex interplay of physiologic and nonphysiologic factors governing the quantity, frequency, and variety of food intake (2–4).

Social, environmental, psychological, economic, and biological factors all influence our intake of food (5–8). Most creatures have a fairly simple and straightforward relationship with food: Eat to live. Whether or not humans live to eat is debatable, but our relationship with food is certainly a lot more complicated than eat to live (9). Humans eat for almost every reason imaginable: to reward ourselves, punish ourselves, console ourselves (10); celebrate and commemorate; sustain and satisfy ourselves; and often, perhaps, just because we can.

Dietary choices are very much influenced by cultural norms (11). Such norms are influenced by the familiarity of food, the accessibility of food, and the convenience, cost, and context of food. There is no real rhyme or reason to eating certain foods for breakfast and other foods for dinner, for example; it's all a matter of what a given culture considers normative.

How much people eat is influenced by the volume of food, the number of ingredients, the timing, the form (liquid vs. solid), and even the packaging (shape and size) and ambient lighting (12). Food intake can be influenced by something as trivial as how much food is set in front of a person at any given time (13–15). The evidence is strong that portion size influences food consumption (16,17). In our era of super-sized portions, this influence on our patients is pervasive and adverse. The concept of "mindless eating" refers to the empirical finding that, each day, people make twenty times more decisions about food than they are aware of, and thus, can be subconsciously influenced by numerous environmental cues—"family and friends, packages and plates, names and numbers, labels and lights, colors and candles, shapes and smells, distractions and distances, cupboards and containers." Seemingly inconsequential decisions about how we interact with, store, and serve food all influence how much and how often we eat (18).

People eat to address a wide array of emotional needs, some of them as profound as depression, some as superficial as wanting a brief feeling of comfort or reward (19). Social factors also strongly influence dietary patterns (20), as do environmental settings (21). Palatability—how tasty and pleasant food is—and social norms and expectations interact to influence the amount of food consumed at any given occasion (22).

Cost incentives around the world tend to drive people toward more energy-dense food (23,24). Highly processed foods tend to be low in volume but high in calories and therefore energy dense. Such foods are widely available, highly palatable, and generally inexpensive, and they therefore play a role in financial hardship, leading so often toward obesity.

The composition of foods can be manipulated considerably by manufacturers without consumers even being aware (25,26). This is done routinely in ways that may influence appetite and food consumption (27,28), such as the addition of salt to sweet foods or sugar to salty foods. Both the energy density of food and portion size influence the calories taken in at any given meal; modifications of either can help produce satiety with fewer calories or stimulate appetite and caloric intake (29). Taste also exerts a powerful influence on appetite (30–32), an influence independent of the need for any particular nutrient (33). The composition of snack foods in particular can and is being manipulated in various ways to increase how much we eat (34).

The Gut–Brain Axis in the Regulation of Food Intake

Complex signals influencing hunger, appetite, and satiety produced in brain interact with those signals produced in the gastrointestinal tract, all of which vary based on current energy status, external cues, genetic factors, and the specific composition of foods (35,36). A basic understanding of gut–brain axis biology provides a useful framework for understanding the interplay between hunger and satiety. Ultimately, food ingestion and fasting trigger a release of hormones produced by the gastrointestinal tract, adipose tissue, and the brain to promote energy balance (37).

The hypothalamus is the main regulatory center of human appetite. The ventromedial hypothalamus appears to be important in the generation of satiety, whereas hunger is in part regulated by the lateral hypothalamus. When the body is in need of fuel, the hypothalamus produces and releases neuropeptide Y, which in turn raises levels of insulin and glucocorticoids. Neuropeptide Y is coexpressed with agouti related protein, which works synergistically to increase appetite and decrease metabolism and energy expenditure. These master hormones work from the top down to stimulate hunger, the physical sensation of needing food for energy. Hunger then manifests as appetite, the motivation to eat food. In turn, the stomach, produces the hormone ghrelin, which interacts with neuropeptide Y secreting neurons in the brain to stimulate appetite. Other chemicals that stimulate appetite include galanin, melanin-concentrating hormone, and norepinephrine, glucocorticoids, and the orexins/hypocretins (I and II) (38). Additionally, hypothalamocortical and hypothalamolimbic projections contribute to the awareness of hunger, and somatic processes controlled by the hypothalamus—vagal tone, stimulation of the thyroid, and the hypothalamic–pituitary–adrenal axis—impact energy balance.

Following a meal, insulin release triggers a release of the hormone leptin from adipocytes, which contributes to satiety, and especially leptin, inhibit release of neuropeptide Y, enabling adipocytes to signal repletion to the brain. The communication between body fat, the gastrointestinal tract, and the brain plays a major role in appetite and weight regulation over time (39). Adipose tissue releases leptin, which triggers satiety, and adiponectin and resistin, which contribute to appetite. Fat is a very active hormone-producing organ, in constant communication with the hypothalamus, and potentially fighting hard to stay just where it is (40)—validating the well-known lament about the difficulties involved in permanently losing excess body fat.

Satiety is also immediately driven by signals from stretch receptors in the stomach and by the delivery of nutrient energy to the duodenum. The effects of ingestion on satiety are mediated by the vagus nerve and by gut hormones. A litany of gut hormones has been shown to influence satiety, including cholecystokinin, glucagon-like peptide-1, oxyntomodulin, pancreatic polypeptide,

somatostatin, calcitonin, gastrin-releasing peptide, obestatin, neuromedin C, and peptide YY3-36 (PYY) (41,42). The best studied satiety hormone to date is cholecystokinin, which shortens the duration of feeding. The entry of gastric chyme into the duodenum is a stimulus for the release of cholecystokinin. Cholecystokinin slows gastric emptying, increasing the signals to gastric stretch receptors and contributing to a sense of satiety. Cholecystokinin may also provide direct signaling of satiety to the brain. Macronutrient absorption in the small bowel stimulates the vagus nerve, which also signals satiety to the brain. The pace at which food is consumed, and whether the food is consumed in solid or liquid form also influences the rate of absorption, and hence, the effect on satiety (43,44).

The signals of satiety delivered before or during nutrient absorption are reinforced by postabsorptive signals. Nutrient entry into the portal vein results in signals of satiety from the liver to the brain via the vagus nerve. The mechanisms of signal exchange between the liver and central nervous system are not yet fully known. Circulating levels of glucose, insulin, and amino acids may all feed back to the brain to confer the sensation of satiety (see Figure 38.1).

In essence, the control of appetite and energy balance is tightly regulated by a complex neuronal

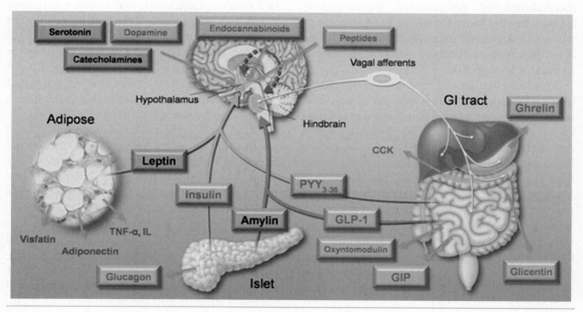

FIGURE 38.1 Peripheral and central signals: Regulation of food intake, body weight, and metabolism. (TNF-α = Tumor necrosis factor-alpha; IL= interleukin; PYY$_{3-36}$ = peptide YY$_{3-36}$; GIP = gastric inhibitory polypeptide; GLP-1 = glucagon-like peptide-1; CCK = cholecystokinin.) (Adapted from Badman MK, Flier JS. Science 2005;307(5717):1909–1914. With permission from AAAS.)

network in the brainstem and hypothalamus that receive inputs from the periphery via nutrients, hormones, and afferent nerve fibers (45). Hormones produced in the gut feed back to the hypothalamus to modify the hypothalamic response. Processes from other cerebral loci are involved as well. Information from the limbic system and the cerebral cortex is relayed directly to the hypothalamus to modify appetite. Appetite regulation is an immensely complex process involving the gastrointestinal tract, many hormones, and both the central and autonomic nervous systems. Redundancy in central regulation of energy intake may confer a survival advantage but obviously complicates efforts to isolate genetic or metabolic defects responsible for perturbations of energy balance, such as those leading to obesity or severe anorexia.

A variety of homeostatic, external sensory, hedonic, and genetic factors influence the gut–brain interactions to tip the scale back and forth between hunger and satiety. Body energy requirements are clearly one factor driving ghrelin release and subsequent hunger and appetite. The availability of nutrient energy is reflected in diet-induced thermogenesis, the generation of heat for a period of approximately 6 hours following ingestion due to the metabolic work of digestion and activation of the sympathetic nervous system. A rise in body temperature due to diet-induced, or postprandial, thermogenesis signals the adequacy of nutrient energy supplies, whereas a decline in temperature between meals is an indication of declining energy supplies and a stimulus for appetite.

An interaction among core body temperature, heat generation by brown adipose tissue, and serum glucose levels has been theorized to influence hunger and consequent energy intake. When core temperature falls, heat generation by brown fat increases, with resultant extraction of glucose from serum. Relative hypoglycemia is likely a stimulus for ingestion. With ingestion, core temperature rises, reducing the metabolic activity of brown fat, providing a stimulus for meal termination. Postprandial thermogenesis may influence the initiation and termination of meals, as well as their size and frequency. The evidence for the role of this mechanism in the control of food intake is preliminary.

Taste, texture, temperature, and visual cues all contribute to the effects that food has on appetite and satiety. Food enters the mouth, where at least three chemicals are involved in perception of taste and responses to it: substance P, cholecystokinin, and opioids (36). The flavor of foods is perceived as the combination of taste, smell, and chemical stimuli, each activating different systems. Taste is mediated by taste buds, clustered in fungiform papillae over the anterior tongue and foliate papillae on the posterior tongue. The gustatory system is innervated by branches of the seventh and tenth cranial nerves. While there are myriad flavors, there are seven widely accepted flavor categories: sweet, sour, salty, bitter, savory, astringent, and umami.

A large volume of research and anecdotal clinical evidence indicate that taste is a malleable sensation as taste buds respond and adapt to available foods. Taste perception is influenced by food intake. By choosing foods that are more nutritious and allowing time to acclimate to this new taste, we can actually come to prefer the healthier foods over those loaded with sugar, salt, and fat. Recent studies have shown that obese children and adolescents have less sensitive taste buds when compared to their leaner counterparts (46). Regardless of whether or not this is a cause or a consequence of the obesity epidemic, the opportunity exist to reverse engineer this taste insensitivity. This concept of "taste bud rehab" requires time and patience necessary to learn to prefer more nutritious foods through habituation, and then to rely on these foods to help facilitate satiety. Substituting options with less sugar, salt, and fat may be unappealing at first, but within a few weeks, this new taste and texture becomes the new normal and the health benefits follow suit.

Olfaction is mediated by neurons in the nasal cavities that are components of the first cranial nerve and lead directly to the olfactory bulb in the brain. The chemical properties and physiologic responses that permit the discernment of diverse smells remain speculative.

There is also a somatosensory component to taste, responsible for the perception of chemical irritants such as capsaicin. This system is subtended primarily by the trigeminal nerve. There may be some overlap between the perception of chemical irritants and the perception of temperature in the oral cavity (e.g., spicy is perceived as "hot," and menthol is perceived as "cold").

Whereas the function of the chemosensory tissues influences food intake, nutritional status also influences the activity of these tissues, which are metabolically active and have a high rate of cellular turnover.

The visual system is also intimately involved in recognizing and categorizing food cues in the environment in anticipation of consumption. Brain regions involved in object recognition, attention, reward processing, and executive decision-making respond differentially to visual cues of food compared with nonfood objects (47–49). Functional neuroimaging techniques reveal an attenuation of activity in the brain's reward area in response to visual food stimuli when humans are fed. This suggests that the physiological state of hunger influences the reward valuation of food (50). This same attenuation can be recreated in the fasted state by the administration of anorectic gut hormones. Furthermore, differences in the brain activity between obese and lean individuals are now providing additional insight into the complex etiology of overeating (51).

This discussion introduces the distinction between the metabolically regulated, more automatic appetite, controlled by homeostatic mechanisms, and the dimension of food intake that is cognitive-behavioral in nature. As discussed, the gut along with numerous peripheral signals influences feeding behavior by generating hunger and satiety signals that are conveyed to the brain. Characterization of the biochemical signals involved in hunger, meal initiation, and satiety has been the subject of extensive research for many years. More recent research reflects the notion that an increasing proportion of human food consumption is driven by pleasure—the hedonic side of food intake. Increased attention is being directed toward the influence of reward sensitivity, the brain's dopaminergic reward pathways, mechanisms of executive function and inhibitory control, and the neurobiology of liking and wanting. In an obesogenic environment, it is abundantly clear that the hedonic response to food stimuli can overwhelm the careful homeostatic balance of the gut–brain axis (52).

Food intake does not follow the neat energy balance paradigm described by the yin and yang of appetite and satiety. Consumption may be in excess of that required to meet energy needs when the food is particularly palatable or the social context is conducive to overindulgence. Food intake may fail to meet the demands of hunger, even when ingestible energy is abundantly available, if the food is unfamiliar or unpalatable. Cravings, for example, represent an extreme expression of appetite, not necessarily driven by physiologic hunger, but usually occurring in a particular social or physiologic context, such as during pregnancy, at a party, or at a particular stage of the menstrual cycle. The predominant example of food craving is for chocolate (see Chapter 39). Many theories have been advanced to account for various food cravings under various circumstances, but none is entirely conclusive. Cognitive processing of chemosensory properties of food interfacing with the brain's mesolimbic reward pathways determines the hedonic properties, or the capacity of food to induce pleasure. Neuroimaging data show that many of the most pleasurable foods activate the same dopaminergic neural circuits that underlie addictive behaviors (53). The cornerstone ingredients of our obesogenic environment—sugar, salt, and fat—may be undermining the prefrontal executive control that allows us to make rational, healthy choices (54).

The role of genetic factors in regulating energy balance, and consequently body weight, remains a subject of intense interest. The ob gene, originally identified in mice in 1994, has been cloned from humans. The gene encodes for leptin, a protein produced by adipocytes that acts as a satiety signal (55). Whereas obese mice homozygous for ob gene mutations are deficient in leptin (56), in obese humans, leptin levels correlate positively with percentage of body fat (57). Originally dubbed as "the obesity gene," the ob gene is now one of dozens of genes implicated in weight regulation in humans (see Chapter 5).

Neuropeptide Y stimulates appetite by elevating levels of insulin and glucocorticoids. In turn, insulin and cortisol stimulate release of leptin, completing an inhibitory feedback pathway between adipose tissue and the hypothalamus. Insensitivity to leptin appears to be the defect resulting from ob gene mutation in humans and is a potential contributor to disordered energy regulation and obesity (58) (see Chapter 5). While many of the factors influencing dietary intake patterns appear to be heritable (59), it is clear that the motivation toward energy intake is multifactorial.

Physical activity can induce an energy deficit comparable to fasting. However, the effects of physical activity on appetite appear to be distinct. Limited evidence suggests that fasting increases hunger, whereas exercise may not (60,61). In fact, evidence indicates that active people have sharper hunger-satiety mechanisms, and hence, improved control of appetite (62). Contrary to popular belief that physical activity increases appetite and caloric intake, men and women can tolerate exercise-induced energy deficits and without compensating by overeating (63). Conversely, it has been shown that reducing physical activity does not induce a compensatory decrease in energy increase, thereby promoting a positive energy balance (64). However, studies on the immediate metabolic impact of physical activity are limited by short duration and poor dietary assessments.

Aging is associated with apparently minor reductions in taste and smell sensitivity in healthy individuals, but memory deficits, comorbidity, and medication use are issues that compound dietary patterns in older people. The elderly may be subject to nutritional deficiencies due to declines in taste, olfaction, or the regulation of appetite, complicated by social factors that may limit dietary diversity (65).

Dietary preferences are also strongly influenced by cultural factors (66). The physiology of appetite regulation interacts with an array of social and behavioral influences on dietary selection in producing a particular dietary pattern (2). There is reason to believe that early food exposures may play an important role in establishing lifelong preferences, possibly during specific developmental periods (67), although much remains uncertain to date.

Despite this dynamic array of influences, the evidence for central control of appetite and food intake is clear and compelling (68). The complex array of neurochemical signals that influence appetite and satiety appear to converge at the hypothalamus (36,37,68–76). Considering how fundamental food choice is to survival, it is unsurprising that brain regions are demonstrably committed to this function. Even social and environmental factors that influence eating do so, ultimately, by affecting neurophysiology (77) (see Figure 38.2). However, it is now clear that in addition to the homeostatic mechanisms of energy balance, the hedonic influence of reward and pleasure are at play. These central mechanisms governing appetite evolved in a world of relative caloric scarcity, and their functioning is reflective of that (78). That physiology does not clearly facilitate portion control in the modern world should thus come as no surprise. We are genetically hard wired to seek, eat, and covet food as essential means of survival and reproduction. Indeed, food and sex subserve the intrinsic reward system of the brain and are the very reason that the phenomenon of addiction exists!

Ideally, many of the modern-world factors (79) that contribute to widespread overeating and weight gain could, and should, be managed by making significant changes in the modern environment so that eating well and being active become the path of least resistance (11,80–83). Until or unless such environmental changes accumulate, the patient is obligated to overcome the obesigenic challenges of the modern world or succumb to them. The clinician's understanding of the interaction between environmental and physiologic factors influencing appetite and food intake is the starting point for constructive exchanges and productive counseling (see Chapter 47). Current thinking is that to gain permanent mastery over appetite, our patients must manage their personal food environment in a way that fosters healthful choices but still allows for flexibility in food choices (12,84). The dietary intake of even children can be influenced just by changing what is conveniently available in the home (85). A book for lay readers offers comprehensive guidance in establishing a "safe" nutritional environment in the home responsive to these considerations (86).

Diet

Foods directly from nature—such as vegetables and fruits—tend to be relatively high in volume and low in calories. Processed foods, in contrast, cram an abundance of calories into minimal space. Numerous studies, predominantly by Dr. Barbara Rolls and her colleagues at Penn State, have demonstrated the importance of food volume to appetite and satiety (87,88). Decreasing food volume contributes to overeating. Simply increasing the volume of foods facilitates satiety when total calories are held constant (89,90).

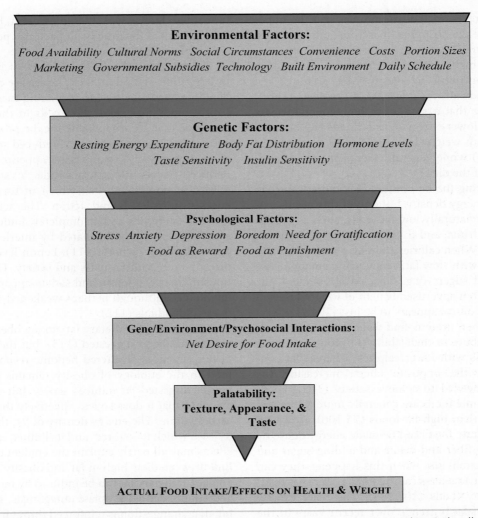

FIGURE 38.2 The confluence of factors influencing hunger, appetite, and satiety. Ultimately, all such influences must converge to exert an effect on the appetite center in the hypothalamus.

Source: Information derived from Hetherington MM. The physiological–psychological dichotomy in the study of food intake. *Proc Nutr Soc* 2002;61:497–507.

This important concept is the basis for Dr. Rolls's excellent book *The Volumetrics Weight-Control Plan: Feel Full on Fewer Calories* (91).

One way to increase food volume is to increase fluid content, by eating soups and stews. However, controversy persists regarding the effects of shifting calories from solids to liquids (92); in some situations, more liquid calories can actually increase total consumption. Others have not consistently been able to replicate Dr. Rolls's work (93).

Energy density is related to volume because it refers to the number of calories per given serving size. A food is energy dense if it packs a lot of calories into a relatively small serving. Highly energy-dense foods likely lead to increased over-consumption (94–97).

Foods high in fat content are the most energy dense, but processed foods with a high sugar content come in a close second. Many processed foods are dense in both fat and sugar and thus are a concentrated load of calories. Because fiber takes up space in food but provides no calories, it has been suggested that simply increasing fiber intake could help control appetite and weight (98). The highly processed food supply has just the opposite influence, stripping fiber from grain products, such as breads, cereals, crackers, and chips.

Diets high in energy-dense foods almost certainly contribute to obesity (99), although not every study affirms this (100,101). Most authorities agree that a shift from high-energy-density foods to lower-energy-density foods can be helpful to both weight loss and weight maintenance (102,103) while generally enhancing the healthfulness of the diet.

Reducing the fat content of the diet can help reduce energy density, but only if this means eating more naturally low-fat foods, such as vegetables and fruits, and if highly processed foods are avoided. When calories from fat are removed and replaced with "low fat," yet equally energy-dense processed sugars (e.g., SnackWell cookies), the all-too-often advertised benefit of weight loss and appetite control appears to be lost (104).

The fiber, protein, and water content of foods all contribute to their ability to produce a sense of fullness with fewer calories, whereas fat content has the opposite effect, increasing the calories needed to achieve satiety (105). High-carbohydrate foods are generally more filling and satiating than high-fat foods (75,106). However, carbohydrate foods can be made energy dense by removing fiber and water and adding sugar and refined starch, and when this happens, they can contribute to excess calorie intake almost as readily as fatty foods (107,108). These are exactly the food supply trends over recent years in the United States and ostensibly the reason carbohydrate is implicated in epidemic obesity (see Chapter 5). While sugar and fat substitutes can be used to take calories out of foods, it's not at all clear that they can be relied upon to help with weight control (see Chapter 42). The tendency to compensate for these "missing" calories by eating more at other times appears to prevail (109). First the trend was to cut out fat with "low-fat" diets that actually increased waistlines with processed carbohydrates. Now the trend is to restrict carbohydrates in order to lose weight. Ultimately, it appears that a middle ground with a balanced diet consisting of filling foods with high fiber, water, and protein content may be the winner—a trend toward the middle.

All calories are not created equally. Calories from different macronutrients, the properties of individual foods, and the interaction between food groups differentially impact the perceived senses of appetite and satiety.

The lipostatic theory links stores of body fat to regulation of food intake. The release of leptin by adipocytes may be the mediating messenger. Leptin binds to receptors on cells in the hypothalamus that are responsible for the production and release of neuropeptide Y; reduced secretion of neuropeptide Y suppresses appetite (110). Reduced levels of neuropeptide Y stimulate release of norepinephrine, which in turn influences insulin levels and action. The actions of leptin are complex and incompletely understood; some effects may be mediated by interleukin 1, prostaglandins, or both (111). Leptin levels vary directly both with fat mass and satiety. The relationship between leptin and satiety apparently is maintained, although perhaps weakened, even in obese individuals (112).

A preference for dietary fat among obese individuals has been suggested (113), but the role of taste differences or altered hedonic responses to food in the etiology of obesity remains controversial. Ingested fat induces satiety, but there is evidence that it does so less effectively than does carbohydrate. The energy density of fat, the facility with which it is stored, and its limited satiating effects may all partly explain the epidemiological link between diets high in fat and obesity. A preference for dietary fat can be induced by morphine and suppressed with opiate antagonists, indicating that fat ingestion is reinforced through endogenous opiate production (114).

Physiologic habituation to high fat intake, in the form of enhanced oxidation, has been demonstrated in animals, suggesting that dietary fat may be more rewarding when habitual intake is high (115). In addition to physiologic adaptation, the familiarity of a high-fat diet has been shown to produce preference (116). Postingestive effects of dietary fat have also been shown to influence preference (117). In humans, both sugar and dairy fat have been shown to induce dose-dependent pleasure ratings, with the fat not producing an upper threshold (118). The association of sugar and fat in the diet may contribute to excess energy intake, with sugar serving as a vehicle for the caloric density of fat (119).

Calorie-for-calorie, protein is the most satiating (filling) of the nutrient classes (120), followed by complex carbohydrate, then simple carbohydrate, and, finally, fat (106,121–124). Thus, it takes more calories from fat than from either carbohydrate or protein to feel comparably full. Because fat is the least "satiating" of the nutrient classes, high-fat foods can contribute to overconsumption of calories (125–133).

Given the potent satiety-inducing effect of protein, increasing protein intake—as is recommended in some popular diets—may be of use in weight control (134,135). The aminostatic theory posits that protein status dominates in control of appetite. There is interest in tryptophan as a precursor to serotonin synthesis and in tyrosine and histidine as precursors to catecholamines and histamine, respectively, as these compounds suppress appetite. To date, no direct evidence has been established of specific amino acid effects on satiety. When a diverse source of nutrients is available, protein intake generally constitutes approximately 15% of total calories, suggesting that a protein-specific appetite may be operative. The need for amino acid ingestion would be the putative teleologic basis for a protein appetite.

There is a clear difference between the satiating power of simple and complex carbohydrates (136), and there are very compelling reasons for this. For one thing, complex carbohydrate sources such as vegetables, fruits, and whole grains tend to be rich in fiber, water, or both and thus are high-volume foods. Fiber content may be particularly important because fiber increases food volume without the addition of calories and also can slow the absorption of nutrients into the bloodstream, thereby lowering blood glucose and stabilizing blood insulin levels (137). For lasting weight control, it makes far more sense to choose carbohydrate foods wisely than to abandon them altogether (138).

Some studies have shown that foods with a high glycemic index tend to be less filling than foods with a low glycemic index when calories are matched (139,140), although other studies have failed to confirm this (94,107). (For further discussion of the glycemic index and the glycemic load, see Chapters 5 and 6.)

Carbohydrate is less readily stored than fat, less calorically dense, and generally more satiating; nonetheless, ingestion of carbohydrate may contribute substantially to obesity. Sugar, in particular, may stimulate appetite and be subject to a higher satiety threshold than other nutrients (141). Individuals with depression, and particularly those with seasonal affective disorder, may develop carbohydrate craving. This tendency has been postulated to be a response to low levels of brain serotonin. Low serotonin may be causally related to both depression and excessive hunger (see Chapter 34). Carbohydrate ingestion increases brain uptake of tryptophan, a serotonin precursor.

It has also been suggested that different types of simple carbohydrates have a differential impact on satiety and hunger. In a recent study, glucose reduced cerebral blood flow to brain regions that regulate appetite and reward while fructose did not. Likewise, glucose increased the subjects' feelings of fullness and satiety while fructose did not (142). In any case, it is clear that simple sugars do not curb appetite and hence contribute to caloric surplus and obesity.

There are many reasons complex carbohydrates would have a favorable influence on appetite and weight control, and simple, highly processed carbohydrates would tend to have the opposite effects. In general, slowly absorbed carbohydrates that result in small, sustained elevations of glucose and insulin are more satiating than rapidly absorbed carbohydrates. This fact suggests that carbohydrate sources rich in fiber, and especially soluble fiber, are more satiating in general than low-fiber sources. Overall, the evidence that whole grains tend to result in a lasting feeling of fullness is quite convincing (143,144). There is evidence that lowering the glycemic load of the diet can help in achieving weight control without hunger (145). A diet with a low glycemic load is limited in highly processed foods and rich in vegetables, fruits, whole grains, and lean protein sources. Again, despite trends toward the extremes, the evidence indicates that a diet that is based on healthful, wholesome foods within each nutrient class facilitates both health and lasting weight control (146). Anecdotal evidence, both from widespread use of the Nuval scoring system and from work with individual patients indicates that the more nutritious the food, the higher the level of satiety. A higher satiety index is intrinsic to better nutrition. It is, therefore, possible to slim down without starving oneself by trading up for more nutritious food choices and leveraging satiety to fill up on fewer calories.

Simply adjusting the levels of various macronutrients in the diet is unlikely to exert a significant influence on total calories consumed over time (124,147–150). When foods are mixed together, as they always are in any reasonable diet, the satiating influence of each macronutrient class is mitigated by that of each of the other classes (151). There is evidence that the pattern, or distribution, of foods within meals and throughout the day can also influence satiety (152–156).

Overall, the literature on appetite indicates that restricting or emphasizing a single nutrient class is unlikely to have a major influence on appetite or weight, although modest benefits are plausible. Because a balance among the macronutrients—and, more importantly, foods—is required for optimal health, there are bounds imposed upon this strategy by other, overriding considerations (see Chapter 45).

Among the forces that influence appetite is *sensory-specific satiety*, the declining pleasure we experience when eating the same food or flavor over time. Our ancestors struggled to achieve the dietary diversity needed to meet nutrient requirements, as discussed in Chapter 44. Some nutritionally challenged populations still do (157). The result is that the human appetite center is specifically adapted to encourage a variety of foods. In nutritionally challenged populations, dietary diversity is desirable. Populations in industrialized countries, however, are victims of our successful efforts to make an abundant and diverse food supply continuously available.

The specific evidence for the influence of sensory-specific satiety on dietary intake is strong (158–161). There is scientific evidence that repeated exposure to the same, or even similar food, results in achieving satiety on fewer calories (153). Raynor et al. (162–165) have conducted several trials suggesting that voluntary limits on food variety are associated with weight control and that imposed restrictions on food variety may be a useful strategy for facilitating weight loss and maintenance. The group advises further study of this strategy. Another study involved a 12-week trial of a meal plan predicated on a purposeful distribution of flavors (i.e., designed to exploit sensory-specific satiety) and providing consistent, high standards of overall nutrition, in 20 overweight adults. The mean weight loss at 12 weeks was 16 lb, and improvements in blood pressure, lipids, serum glucose, and endothelial function were all significant (166).

Independent of other factors, variety in the diet can apparently contribute to excess intake and weight gain (167–171). Energy density and volume potentially alter the point at which sensory-specific satiety is reached (89), suggesting that appetite/satiety influences interact. Flavor may exert a particularly strong influence (172,173).

NUTRIENTS, NUTRICEUTICALS, AND FUNCTIONAL FOODS

Levels of vitamins and minerals derived from our natural diet can have a profound impact on effect on our sense of taste and perception of hunger and satiety.

Vitamin A

Vitamin A deficiency is associated with impairment of taste and smell that may lead to or exacerbate malnutrition. The condition is reversible with vitamin A supplementation (174).

B Vitamins

Atrophy of taste buds occurs with various B vitamin deficiencies, as does glossitis. The condition is quickly reversed with B vitamin supplementation.

Chromium

As addressed in Chapters 5 and 6, chromium supplementation may ameliorate insulin resistance. There is some evidence that chromium may suppress hunger in some patients (175). The author's anecdotal experience suggests a favorable influence of chromium supplementation on hunger and cravings in insulin-resistant patients.

Copper

Copper deficiency is associated with reduced sensitivity to the taste of salt and a relative salt craving. Copper repletion reverses the condition.

Zinc

Zinc deficiency may impair taste, but definitive evidence in humans is lacking.

Salt

Preferences for salt have been proved malleable in response to habitual exposure. Exposure to high- or low-salt diets over a period of 6 to 8 weeks has been shown to alter preferences.

Nutraceuticals

A nutraceutical is a product isolated or purified from foods that is generally sold in medicinal forms and not usually associated with foods. Many nutraceuticals have a demonstrated or claimed physiologic benefit to aid in appetite suppression and weight loss. Some of the most popular nutraceuticals are reviewed here.

Hoodia Gordonii

Extracts from the plant *Hoodia gordonii* have received considerable media attention as a potential weight loss aid. Chewed by indigenous people of the Kalahari Desert, the plant is purported to suppress appetite. Studies of the plant and its extracts are as yet insufficient to permit any evidence-based conclusion, however (176,177).

Caffeine

Caffeine may slightly boost weight loss or prevent weight gain, but there is no sound evidence indicating that this effect is generalizable or long term. One theory underlying the possible weight loss and caffeine connection is appetite suppression. Caffeine may temporarily blunt the desire to eat (178). Research also indicates that caffeine, capsaicin, and various teas have the potential to produce significant impact on metabolic targets such as satiety, thermogenesis, and fat oxidation (179).

Sugar Substitutes

Marketed for their ability to promote healthy weight maintenance and weight loss, accumulating evidence now suggests that these substances may not help, and may actually undermine weight loss goals (180,181). Research in animal models suggests that sugar substitutes actually increase appetite for sweet foods and promote overeating, perhaps by uncoupling sweetness and energy and blunting the body's ability to gauge caloric intake (182). The dissociation between sweet taste and caloric consequences diminishes the ability of sweet tastes to evoke physiologic responses that regulate energy balance. This model is complemented by a study showing that real sugar is more potent than low-calorie sweetener in stimulating brain areas related to satisfactions and satiety (183). The research is currently hindered by the lack of a physiologically relevant model to explain the biologic mechanism underlying these observations. To date, there is currently no official recommendation about using artificial sweeteners as a tool for weight control.

Mangosteen/Garcinia Mangostan

Mangosteen is a tropical evergreen tree that produces the mangosteen fruit—sweet and tangy, juicy, and somewhat fibrous with an inedible, deep reddish-purple colored rind. Mangosteen is touted for its antioxidants, especially xanthones, and it is promoted to support microbiological balance, help the immune system, improve joint flexibility, and provide mental support. Various parts of the plant have been used in traditional medicine for its anti-inflammatory properties in the treatment of skin infections, wounds, dysentery, and urinary tract infections. Products containing its fruits are now sold widely as "liquid botanical supplements," but evidence for the health benefits of these products is still lacking (184), although evidence from in vitro and animal studies demonstrates that xanthones inhibit proliferation of a wide range of human tumor cell types by modulating various targets and signaling transduction pathways (185). The American Cancer Society maintains that "there is no reliable evidence that mangosteen juice, puree, or bark is effective as a treatment for cancer in humans" (186). With regard to its ability to promote satiety, the high fiber content may indeed work to this effect, although this is based solely on anecdotal evidence and opinion at this time.

Green Coffee Bean Extract

Green coffee beans are coffee beans that have not yet been roasted and therefore have a higher level of chlorogenic acid—a polyphenol antioxidant—compared to regular, roasted coffee beans. Chlorogenic acid is thought to have health benefits for heart disease, diabetes, and weight loss by reducing the absorption of fat and glucose in the gut and lowering insulin levels to improve metabolic function. Although this product has received much attention in the popular media, few published studies have examined the extract's effects on weight loss and none over the long term. Results from a study funded by a company that manufactures green coffee bean extract found that subjects who took the extract lost about 18 lb on average (187). However, a 2011 review found that green coffee bean extract only lowers body weight by an average of 5.5 lb compared to placebo, and these studies may be compromised by poor quality and design. Moreover, the ingestion of too much chlorogenic acid may actually raise the risk of heart disease by elevating homocysteine levels (188). Given the relatively modest weight loss and lack of long-term data and side effect profile, the verdict is still out and consumers should approach with caution.

Functional Foods

Functional foods are those foods which are intended to be consumed as part of the normal diet and that contain biologically active components which offer the potential of enhanced health or reduced risk of disease (189). In other words, these foods contain specific minerals, vitamins, fatty acids, dietary fiber, and/or biologically active substances such as phytochemicals or other antioxidants and probiotics that have physiological benefits and/or reduce the risk of chronic disease beyond basic nutritional functions. In the supermarket, functional foods are ubiquitous, including calcium-fortified orange juice, bread fortified with iodine and folate, margarine that lowers cholesterol, and yogurt with probiotics.

Satiety is a weapon in the war on weight, and sales of satiety-promoting functional foods are skyrocketing. Euromonitor International health and wellness statistics showed that retail value sales of fortified/functional products amounted to almost $246 billion in 2012, accounting for one third of health and wellness-positioned packaged foods and beverages. As a category, fortified/functional products also demonstrated the most dynamism over the 2007–2012 review periods. Many of these products, such as yogurts and cereals, come with added protein and fiber blends. Flavored water drinks are now sold as replacements for sugared drinks/juices to those trying to lose weight. Calorie-burning drinks have become wildly popular as well.

In the pipeline, a new range of breakfast cereals with a low glycemic index and double the fiber content is coming to market and catering to the rapidly growing diabetic population worldwide. Studies suggesting a possible neuroprotective effect of DHA ω-3 fatty acids, caffeine, and vitamin D (190,191) have encouraged the development of nutritional products promoting brain health in the aging population. And then, of course, there is the research investigating the connection between the microbiome and chronic diseases (192), which has the potential to spawn numerous products, such as probiotics, designed to manipulate the bacteria that influence our physiologic processes and improve health status. Whether or not these products will have a measureable impact to reduce the chronic disease burden has yet to be determined, but the future is ripe for further research.

Other

The identification of hormones involved in the regulation of appetite, hunger, and satiety is fostering investigation into synthetic compounds that mimic or block these effects. Some examples are discussed in Chapter 5. Most recently, pramlintide, a synthetic analogue of the pancreatic hormone amylin, has been approved by the Food and Drug Administration for diabetes management. A 6-week clinical trial showed evidence of suppressed appetite and food intake and facilitated weight loss (193). This literature is evolving rapidly and requires continuous monitoring.

PATIENT RESOURCES OF PARTICULAR RELEVANCE

The following four books address specific strategies for appetite control while adhering to high standards of overall nutrition for health promotion:

- *The Way to Eat* (86): Provides an overview of strategies for appetite control.
- *The Flavor Point Diet* (166): Explains sensory-specific satiety and offers a 6-week, family-friendly meal plan.
- *The Volumetrics Weight-Control Plan* (91): Provides appetite control guidance and a meal plan based on food volume.
- *Mindless Eating: Why We Eat More Than We Think* (18): Provides insights about diverse influences on food intake.

CLINICAL HIGHLIGHTS

The capacity of clinicians to influence health outcomes in their patients by means of dietary manipulation is ultimately dependent on the patients' capacity to change dietary patterns. This capacity, in turn, is dependent on the factors that govern dietary patterns and dietary preferences in the first place. Appetite, hunger, and satiety are mediated by a complex array of biopsychosocial factors.

Although neither patient nor clinician is able to directly control much of the physiology of appetite, compensations may be built into dietary practices to defend against specific vulnerabilities. When the principal threat to health is excess dietary intake, diet may be manipulated to optimize its satiating properties and minimize the stimulation of appetite. Among the many pertinent strategies (see Chapters 5 and 47) are increasing intake of fiber and complex carbohydrate, avoiding excessive variety within a given day or meal, optimizing protein intake, and restricting dietary fat intake. The effects of volume on satiety support the common practice of drinking water before a meal to help curb appetite. Conversely, when appetite is poor and dietary intake is inadequate, restricting fiber, increasing variety, and increasing fat intake may provide some compensation (see Chapter 26).

Efforts should be made to encourage parents to establish judicious eating habits in their children early, as dietary habits may be increasingly resistant to change over time. Creativity in the use of ingredients can be used to reduce the fat, sugar, salt, and calorie content of foods while preserving familiar aspects of the diet important in the provision of pleasure (see Section VIIJ).

A short list of strategies that are supportive of appetite and weight control, and of overall nutritional health, may be confidently conveyed to patients. These include increasing mean food volume by eating naturally high-volume foods such as vegetables and fruits as well as soups and stews; consuming lean protein foods toward the high end of the recommended intake range; consuming an abundance of fiber in whole grains, beans, lentils, vegetables, and fruits; and avoiding an excessive variety of foods and flavors at any given meal or snack.

Patients who have been provided with information about the physiology of appetite may be able to make better use of nutrition labels to guard against manipulative food industry marketing schemes. A shared understanding between patient and clinician of the complex and largely involuntary nature of appetite and satiety is supportive of counseling that is practical, productive, and compassionate (see Chapter 47).

REFERENCES

1. Blundell J, King N. Overconsumption as a cause of weight gain: behavioural-physiological interactions in the control of food intake (appetite). *Ciba Found Symp* 1996;201:138–154.
2. Nestle M, Wing R, Birch L, et al. Behavioral and social influences on food choice. *Nutr Rev* 1998;56:s50–s74.
3. Glanz K, Basil M, Maibach E, et al. Why Americans eat what they do: taste, nutrition, cost, convenience, and weight control concerns as influences on food consumption. *J Am Diet Assoc* 1998;98:1118–1126.
4. Drewnowski A. Taste preferences and food intake. *Annu Rev Nutr* 1997;17:237–253.
5. Nestle M, Wing R, Birch L, et al. Behavioral and social influences on food choice. *Nutr Rev* 1998;56:s50–s64; discussion s64–s74.
6. Blass EM. Biological and environmental determinants of childhood obesity. *Nutr Clin Care* 2003;6:13–19.
7. Shepherd R. Social determinants of food choice. *Proc Nutr Soc* 1999;58:807–812.
8. French SA. Pricing effects on food choices. *J Nutr* 2003;133: 841s–843s.
9. Mela DJ. Food choice and intake: the human factor. *Proc Nutr Soc* 1999;58:513–521.
10. Macht M, Simons G. Emotions and eating in everyday life. *Appetite* 2000;35:65–71.
11. Nestle M, Jacobson MF. Halting the obesity epidemic: a public health policy approach. *Public Health Rep* 2000;115:12–24.
12. Wansink B. Environmental factors that increase the food intake and consumption volume of unknowing consumers. *Annu Rev Nutr* 2004;24:455–479.
13. Rozin P, Kabnick K, Pete E, et al. The ecology of eating: smaller portion sizes in France than in the United States help explain the French paradox. *Psychol Sci* 2003;14:450–454.
14. Levitsky DA, Youn T. The more food young adults are served, the more they overeat. *J Nutr* 2004;134:2546–2549.
15. Painter JE, Wansink B, Hieggelke JB. How visibility and convenience influence candy consumption. *Appetite* 2002; 38:237–238.
16. Rolls BJ, Roe LS, Kral TV, et al. Increasing the portion size of a packaged snack increases energy intake in men and women. *Appetite* 2004;42:63–69.
17. Rolls BJ, Morris EL, Roe LS. Portion size of food affects energy intake in normal-weight and overweight men and women. *Am J Clin Nutr* 2002;76:1207–1213.
18. Brian Wansink, ed. *Mindless eating: why we eat more than we think.* New York, NY: Bantam Books, 2006; 1.
19. Wansink B, Cheney MM, Chan N. Exploring comfort food preferences across age and gender. *Physiol Behav* 2003;79:739–747.
20. Herman CP, Roth DA, Polivy J. Effects of the presence of others on food intake: a normative interpretation. *Psychol Bull* 2003;129:873–886.

21. Weber AJ, King SC, Meiselman HL. Effects of social interaction, physical environment and food choice freedom on consumption in a meal-testing environment. *Appetite* 2004;42:115–118.

22. Pliner P, Mann N. Influence of social norms and palatability on amount consumed and food choice. *Appetite* 2004;42:227–237.

23. Darmon N, Ferguson E, Briend A. Do economic constraints encourage the selection of energy dense diets? *Appetite* 2003;41:315–322.

24. Drewnowski A, Specter SE. Poverty and obesity: the role of energy density and energy costs. *Am J Clin Nutr* 2004;79:6–16.

25. Stubbs RJ, Mullen S, Johnstone AM, et al. How covert are covertly manipulated diets? *Int J Obes Relat Metab Disord* 2001;25:567–573.

26. Zandstra EH, Stubenitsky K, De Graaf C, et al. Effects of learned flavour cues on short-term regulation of food intake in a realistic setting. *Physiol Behav* 2002;75:83–90.

27. Prescott J. Effects of added glutamate on liking for novel food flavors. *Appetite* 2004;42:143–150.

28. Davidson TL, Swithers SE. A Pavlovian approach to the problem of obesity. *Int J Obes Relat Metab Disord* 2004;28:933–935.

29. Kral TV, Rolls BJ. Energy density and portion size: their independent and combined effects on energy intake. *Physiol Behav* 2004;82:131–138.

30. French S, Robinson T. Fats and food intake. *Curr Opin Clin Nutr Metab Care* 2003;6:629–634.

31. Wansink B, Westgren R. Profiling taste-motivated segments. *Appetite* 2003;41:323–327.

32. Nasser J. Taste, food intake and obesity. *Obes Rev* 2001;2:213–218.

33. Yeomans MR, Blundell JE, Leshem M. Palatability: response to nutritional need or need-free stimulation of appetite? *Br J Nutr* 2004;92:s3–s14.

34. Green SM, Blundell JE. Subjective and objective indices of the satiating effect of foods. Can people predict how filling a food will be? *Eur J Clin Nutr* 1996;50:798–806.

35. French SJ. The effects of specific nutrients on the regulation of feeding behaviour in human subjects. *Proc Nutr Soc* 1999;58:533–539.

36. Kalra SP, Kalra PS. Overlapping and interactive pathways regulating appetite and craving. *J Addict Dis* 2004;23:5–21.

37. Hellstrom PM, Geliebter A, Naslund E, et al. Peripheral and central signals in the control of eating in normal, obese and binge-eating human subjects. *Br J Nutr* 2004;92:s47–s57.

38. Vila G, Grimm G, Resl M, et al. B-type natriuretic peptide modulates ghrelin, hunger, and satiety in healthy men. *Diabetes* 2012;61:2592–2596.

39. Konturek SJ, Konturek JW, Pawlik T, et al. Brain-gut axis and its role in the control of food intake. *J Physiol Pharmacol* 2004;55:137–154.

40. Meier U, Gressner AM. Endocrine regulation of energy metabolism: review of pathobiochemical and clinical chemical aspects of leptin, ghrelin, adiponectin, and resistin. *Clin Chem* 2004;50:1511–1525.

41. Small CJ, Bloom SR. Gut hormones and the control of appetite. *Trends Endocrinol Metab* 2004;15:259–263.

42. Wynne K, Stanley S, Bloom S. The gut and regulation of body weight. *J Clin Endocrinol Metab* 2004;89:2576–2582.

43. Andrade AM, Kresge DL, Teixeira PJ, et al. Does eating slowly influence appetite and energy intake when water intake is controlled? *Int J Behav Nutr Phys Act* 2012;9:13.

44. Houchins JA, Tan SY, Campbell WW, et al. Effects of fruit and vegetable, consumed in solid vs beverage forms, on acute and chronic appetitive responses in lean and obese adults. *Int J Obes* (Lond) 2013;37(8):1109–1115.

45. Murphy KG, Dhillo WS, Bloom SR. Gut peptides in the regulation of food intake and energy homeostasis. *Endocr Rev* 2006;27:719–727.

46. Overberg J, Hummel T, Krude H, et al. Differences in taste sensitivity between obese and non-obese children and adolescents. *Arch Dis Child* 2012;97:1048–1052.

47. Killgore WD, Young AD, Femia LA, et al. Cortical and limbic activation during viewing of high- versus low-calorie foods. *Neuroimage* 2003;19:1381–1394.

48. van der Laan LN, de Ridder DT, Viergever MA, et al. The first taste is always with the eyes: a meta-analysis on the neural correlates of processing visual food cues. *Neuroimage* 2011;55:296–303.

49. Schur EA, Kleinhans NM, Goldberg J, et al. Activation in brain energy regulation and reward centers by food cues varies with choice of visual stimulus. *Int J Obes* (Lond) 2009;33:653–661.

50. Mehta S, Melhorn SJ, Smeraglio A, et al. Regional brain response to visual food cues is a marker of satiety that predicts food choice. *Am J Clin Nutr* 2012;96(5):989–999.

51. De Silva A, Salem V, Matthews PM, et al. The use of functional MRI to study appetite control in the CNS. *Exp Diabetes Res* 2012;2012:764017.

52. Joseph RJ, Alonso-Alonso M, Bond DS, et al. The neurocognitive connection between physical activity and eating behaviour. *Obes Rev* 2011;12(10):800–812.

53. Volkow ND, Wang GJ, Tomasi D, et al. The Addictive dimensionality of obesity. *Biol Psychiatry* 2013;73(9):811–818.

54. Kessler D. *The end of overeating Rodale Inc,* 2009 New York, NY.

55. Coleman R, Herrmann T. Nutritional regulation of leptin in humans. *Diabetologia* 1999;42:639–646.

56. Rohner-Jeanrenaud F, Jeanrenaud B. Obesity, leptin, and the brain. *N Engl J Med* 1996;334:324–332.

57. Considine R, Sinha M, Heiman M, et al. Serum immunoreactive-leptin concentrations in normal-weight and obese humans. *N Engl J Med* 1996;334:292–295.

58. Castro JD. Behavioral genetics of food intake regulation in free-living humans. *Nutrition* 1999;15:550–554.

59. Hubert P, King N, Blundell J. Uncoupling the effects of energy expenditure and energy intake: appetite response to short-term energy deficit induced by meal omission and physical activity. *Appetite* 1998;31:9–19.

60. King N. What processes are involved in the appetite response to moderate increases in exercise-induced energy expenditure? *Proc Nutr Soc* 1999;58:107–113.

61. Martins C, Morgan L, Truby H. A review of the effects of exercise on appetite regulation: an obesity perspective. *Int J Obes* 2008;32:1337–1347.

62. Blundell JE, Stubbs RJ, Hughes DA, et al. Cross-talk between physical activity and appetite control: does PA stimulate appetite? *Proc Nutr Soc* 2003;62:651–661.

63. Stubbs RJ, Hughes DA, Johnstone AM, et al. A decrease in physical activity affects appetite, energy, and nutrient balance in lean men feeding ad libitum. *Am J Clin Nutr* 2004;79:62–69.

64. Rolls B. Do chemosensory changes influence food intake in the elderly? *Physiol Behav* 1999;66:193–197.

65. Axelson M. The impact of culture on food-related behavior. *Annu Rev Nutr* 1986;6:345–363.

66. Mennella J, Beauchamp G. Early flavor experiences: research update. *Nutr Rev* 1998;56:205–211.

67. Druce M, Bloom SR. Central regulators of food intake. *Curr Opin Clin Nutr Metab Care* 2003;6:361–367.

68. Neary NM, Goldstone AP, Bloom SR. Appetite regulation: from the gut to the hypothalamus. *Clin Endocrinol* (Oxf) 2004;60:153–160.

69. Bray GA. Afferent signals regulating food intake. *Proc Nutr Soc* 2000;59:373–384.

70. Leibowitz SF, Alexander JT. Hypothalamic serotonin in control of eating behavior, meal size, and body weight. *Biol Psychiatry* 1998;44:851–864.

71. de Graaf C, Blom WA, Smeets PA, et al. Biomarkers of satiation and satiety. *Am J Clin Nutr* 2004;79:946–961.

72. Romon M, Lebel P, Velly C, et al. Leptin response to carbohydrate or fat meal and association with subsequent satiety and energy intake. *Am J Physiol* 1999;277:e855–e861.

73. Dallman MF, la Fleur SE, Pecoraro NC, et al. Minireview: glucocorticoids—food intake, abdominal obesity, and wealthy nations in 2004. *Endocrinology* 2004;145:2633–2638.

74. Berthoud HR. Mind versus metabolism in the control of food intake and energy balance. *Physiol Behav* 2004; 81:781–793.

75. Holt S, Brand J, Soveny C, et al. Relationship of satiety to postprandial glycaemic, insulin and cholecystokinin responses. *Appetite* 1992;18:129–141.

76. Hetherington MM. The physiological–psychological dichotomy in the study of food intake. *Proc Nutr Soc* 2002;61:497–507.

77. Flatt JP. Macronutrient composition and food selection. *Obes Res* 2001;9:256s–262s.

78. Mela DJ. Determinants of food choice: relationships with obesity and weight control. *Obes Res* 2001;9:249s–255s.

79. Swinburn BA, Caterson I, Seidell JC, et al. Diet, nutrition and the prevention of excess weight gain and obesity. *Public Health Nutr* 2004;7:123–146.

80. Hill JO, Wyatt HR, Reed GW, et al. Obesity and the environment: where do we go from here? *Science* 2003;299:853–855.

81. French SA, Story M, Jeffery RW. Environmental influences on eating and physical activity. *Annu Rev Public Health* 2001;22:309–335.

82. de Castro JM. How can eating behavior be regulated in the complex environments of free-living humans? *Neurosci Biobehav Rev* 1996;20:119–131.

83. de Castro JM. Genes, the environment and the control of food intake. *Br J Nutr* 2004;92:s59–s62.

84. Lowe MR. Self-regulation of energy intake in the prevention and treatment of obesity: is it feasible? *Obes Res* 2003;11:44s–59s.

85. Cullen KW, Baranowski T, Owens E, et al. Availability, accessibility, and preferences for fruit, 100% fruit juice, and vegetables influence children's dietary behavior. *Health Educ Behav* 2003;30:615–626.

86. Katz DL, Gonzalez MH. The way to eat. Naperville, IL: Sourcebooks, Inc., 2002.

87. Rolls BJ, Castellanos VH, Halford JC, et al. Volume of food consumed affects satiety in men. *Am J Clin Nutr* 1998;67:1170–1177.

88. Rolls BJ, Bell EA, Waugh BA. Increasing the volume of a food by incorporating air affects satiety in men. *Am J Clin Nutr* 2000;72:361–368.

89. Bell EA, Roe LS, Rolls BJ. Sensory-specific satiety is affected more by volume than by energy content of a liquid food. *Physiol Behav* 2003;78:593–600.

90. Rolls BJ, Bell EA, Thorwart ML. Water incorporated into a food but not served with a food decreases energy intake in lean women. *Am J Clin Nutr* 1999;70:448–455.

91. Rolls BJ, Barnett RA. The volumetrics weight-control plan: feel full on fewer calories. New York, NY: Perennial Currents, 2000.

92. Almiron-Roig E, Chen Y, Drewnowski A. Liquid calories and the failure of satiety: how good is the evidence? *Obes Rev* 2003;4:201–212.

93. Gray RW, French SJ, Robinson TM, et al. Increasing preload volume with water reduces rated appetite but not food intake in healthy men even with minimum delay between preload and test meal. *Nutr Neurosci* 2003;6:29–37.

94. Holt SH, Brand-Miller JC, Stitt PA. The effects of equal-energy portions of different breads on blood glucose levels, feelings of fullness and subsequent food intake. *J Am Diet Assoc* 2001;101:767–773.

95. Rolls BJ. The role of energy density in the overconsumption of fat. *J Nutr* 2000;130:268s–271s.

96. Rolls BJ, Bell EA. Intake of fat and carbohydrate: role of energy density. *Eur J Clin Nutr* 1999;53:s166–s173.

97. Rolls BJ, Bell EA, Castellanos VH, et al. Energy density but not fat content of foods affected energy intake in lean and obese women. *Am J Clin Nutr* 1999;69:863–871.

98. Drewnowski A. Energy density, palatability, and satiety: implications for weight control. *Nutr Rev* 1998;56:347–353.

99. Howarth NC, Saltzman E, Roberts SB. Dietary fiber and weight regulation. *Nutr Rev* 2001;59:129–139.

100. Prentice AM, Jebb SA. Fast foods, energy density and obesity: a possible mechanistic link. *Obes Rev* 2003;4:187–194.

101. Phillips SM, Bandini LG, Naumova EN, et al. Energy-dense snack food intake in adolescence: longitudinal relationship to weight and fatness. *Obes Res* 2004;12:461–472.

102. Drewnowski A. Sensory control of energy density at different life stages. *Proc Nutr Soc* 2000;59:239–244.

103. Westerterp-Plantenga MS. Analysis of energy density of food in relation to energy intake regulation in human subjects. *Br J Nutr* 2001;85:351–361.

104. Drewnowski A. The role of energy density. *Lipids* 2003;38:109–115.

105. Poppitt SD, Prentice AM. Energy density and its role in the control of food intake: evidence from metabolic and community studies. *Appetite* 1996;26:153–174.

106. Holt SH, Miller JC, Petocz P, et al. A satiety index of common foods. *Eur J Clin Nutr* 1995;49:675–690.

107. Holt SH, Brand Miller JC, Petocz P. Interrelationships among postprandial satiety, glucose and insulin responses and changes in subsequent food intake. *Eur J Clin Nutr* 1996;50:788–797.

108. Blundell JE, Stubbs RJ. High and low carbohydrate and fat intakes: limits imposed by appetite and palatability and their implications for energy balance. *Eur J Clin Nutr* 1999;53:s148–s165.

109. Rolls BJ, Miller DL. Is the low-fat message giving people a license to eat more? *J Am Coll Nutr* 1997;16:535–543.

110. Stubbs RJ, Whybrow S. Energy density, diet composition and palatability: influences on overall food energy intake in humans. *Physiol Behav* 2004;81:755–764.

111. Lonnqvist F, Nordfors L, Schalling M. Leptin and its potential role in human obesity. *J Intern Med* 1999; 245:643–652.

112. Luheshi G, Gardner J, Rushforth D, et al. Leptin action on food intake and body temperature are mediated by IL-1. *Proc Natl Acad Sci USA* 1999;96:7047–7052.

113. Heini A, Lara-Castro C, Kirk K, et al. Association of leptin and hunger-satiety ratings in obese women. *Int J Obes Relat Metab Disord* 1998;22:1084–1087.

114. Drewnowski A. Why do we like fat? *J Am Diet Assoc* 1997;97:s58–s62.

115. Reed D, Tordoff M. Enhanced acceptance and metabolism of fats by rats fed a high-fat diet. *Am J Physiol* 1991;261: r1084–r1088.

116. Warwick Z, Schiffman S, Anderson J. Relationship of dietary fat content to food preferences in young rats. *Physiol Behav* 1990;48:581–586.

117. Lucas F, Sclafani A. Flavor preferences conditioned by intragastric fat infusions in rats. *Physiol Behav* 1989; 46:403–412.

118. Drewnowski A, Greenwood M. Cream and sugar: human preferences for high-fat foods. *Physiol Behav* 1983; 30:629–633.

119. Emmett P, Heaton K. Is extrinsic sugar a vehicle for dietary fat? *Lancet* 1995;345:1537–1540.

120. Anderson GH, Moore SE. Dietary proteins in the regulation of food intake and body weight in humans. *J Nutr* 2004;134:974s–979s.

121. Stubbs J, Ferres S, Horgan G. Energy density of foods: effects on energy intake. *Crit Rev Food Sci Nutr* 2000;40:481–515.

122. Crovetti R, Porrini M, Santangelo A, et al. The influence of thermic effect of food on satiety. *Eur J Clin Nutr* 1998;52:482–488.

123. Westerterp-Plantenga MS, Rolland V, Wilson SA, et al. Satiety related to 24 h diet-induced thermogenesis during high protein/carbohydrate vs high fat diets measured in a respiration chamber. *Eur J Clin Nutr* 1999;53:495–502.

124. Raben A, Agerholm-Larsen L, Flint A, et al. Meals with similar energy densities but rich in protein, fat, carbohydrate, or alcohol have different effects on energy expenditure and substrate metabolism but not on appetite and energy intake. *Am J Clin Nutr* 2003;77:91–100.

125. Green SM, Wales JK, Lawton CL, et al. Comparison of high-fat and high-carbohydrate foods in a meal or snack on short-term fat and energy intakes in obese women. *Br J Nutr* 2000;84:521–530.

126. Green SM, Burley VJ, Blundell JE. Effect of fat- and sucrose-containing foods on the size of eating episodes and energy intake in lean males: potential for causing overconsumption. *Eur J Clin Nutr* 1994;48:547–555.

127. Blundell JE, Burley VJ, Cotton JR, et al. Dietary fat and the control of energy intake: evaluating the effects of fat on meal size and postmeal satiety. *Am J Clin Nutr* 1993;57:772s–777s.

128. Green SM, Blundell JE. Effect of fat- and sucrose-containing foods on the size of eating episodes and energy intake in lean dietary restrained and unrestrained

females: potential for causing overconsumption. *Eur J Clin Nutr* 1996;50:625–635.

129. Blundell JE, MacDiarmid JI. Fat as a risk factor for overconsumption: satiation, satiety, and patterns of eating. *J Am Diet Assoc* 1997;97:s63–s69.

130. Golay A, Bobbioni E. The role of dietary fat in obesity. *Int J Obes Relat Metab Disord* 1997;21:s2–s11.

131. Rolls BJ. Carbohydrates, fats, and satiety. *Am J Clin Nutr* 1995;61:960s–967s.

132. Blundell JE, Lawton CL, Cotton JR, et al. Control of human appetite: implications for the intake of dietary fat. *Annu Rev Nutr* 1996;16:285–319.

133. Saris WH. Sugars, energy metabolism, and body weight control. *Am J Clin Nutr* 2003;78:850s–857s.

134. Westerterp-Plantenga MS, Lejeune MP, Nijs I, et al. High protein intake sustains weight maintenance after body weight loss in humans. *Int J Obes Relat Metab Disord* 2004;28:57–64.

135. Poppitt SD, McCormack D, Buffenstein R. Short-term effects of macronutrient preloads on appetite and energy intake in lean women. *Physiol Behav* 1998;64:279–285.

136. Liu S, Willett WC, Manson JE, et al. Relation between changes in intakes of dietary fiber and grain products and changes in weight and development of obesity among middle-aged women. *Am J Clin Nutr* 2003;78:920–927.

137. Bjorck I, Elmstahl HL. The glycaemic index: importance of dietary fibre and other food properties. *Proc Nutr Soc* 2003;62:201–206.

138. Wylie-Rosett J, Segal-Isaacson CJ, Segal-Isaacson A. Carbohydrates and increases in obesity: does the type of carbohydrate make a difference? *Obes Res* 2004;12: 124s–129s.

139. Ball SD, Keller KR, Moyer-Mileur LJ, et al. Prolongation of satiety after low versus moderately high glycemic index meals in obese adolescents. *Pediatrics* 2003;111:488–494.

140. Brand-Miller JC, Holt SH, Pawlak DB, et al. Glycemic index and obesity. *Am J Clin Nutr* 2002;76:281s–285s.

141. Drewnowski A. Energy intake and sensory properties of food. *Am J Clin Nutr* 1995;62:1081s–1085s.

142. Page KA, Chan O, Arora J, et al. Effects of fructose vs. glucose on regional cerebral blood flow in brain regions involved with appetite and reward pathways. *JAMA* 2013;309:63–70.

143. Pasman WJ, Blokdijk VM, Bertina FM, et al. Effect of two breakfasts, different in carbohydrate composition, on hunger and satiety and mood in healthy men. *Int J Obes Relat Metab Disord* 2003;27:663–668.

144. Holt SH, Delargy HJ, Lawton CL, et al. The effects of high-carbohydrate vs high-fat breakfasts on feelings of fullness and alertness, and subsequent food intake. *Int J Food Sci Nutr* 1999;50:13–28.

145. Ebbeling CB, Leidig MM, Sinclair KB, et al. A reduced-glycemic load diet in the treatment of adolescent obesity. *Arch Pediatr Adolesc Med* 2003;157:773–779.

146. Hung T, Sievenpiper JL, Marchie A, et al. Fat versus carbohydrate in insulin resistance, obesity, diabetes and cardiovascular disease. *Curr Opin Clin Nutr Metab Care* 2003;6:165–176.

147. Jequier E. Pathways to obesity. *Int J Obes Relat Metab Disord* 2002;26:s12–s17.

148. Gerstein DE, Woodward-Lopez G, Evans AE, et al. Clarifying concepts about macronutrients' effects on satiation and satiety. *J Am Diet Assoc* 2004;104:1151–1153.

149. Vozzo R, Wittert G, Cocchiaro C, et al. Similar effects of foods high in protein, carbohydrate and fat on subsequent spontaneous food intake in healthy individuals. *Appetite* 2003;40:101–107.

150. Marmonier C, Chapelot D, Louis-Sylvestre J. Effects of macronutrient content and energy density of snacks consumed in a satiety state on the onset of the next meal. *Appetite* 2000;34:161–168.

151. Lang V, Bellisle F, Oppert JM, et al. Satiating effect of proteins in healthy subjects: a comparison of egg albumin, casein, gelatin, soy protein, pea protein, and wheat gluten. *Am J Clin Nutr* 1998;67:1197–1204.

152. Speechly DP, Rogers GG, Buffenstein R. Acute appetite reduction associated with an increased frequency of eating in obese males. *Int J Obes Relat Metab Disord* 1999;23:1151–1159.

153. Plantenga MS, IJedema MJ, Wijckmans-Duijsens NE. The role of macronutrient selection in determining patterns of food intake in obese and non-obese women. *Eur J Clin Nutr* 1996;50:580–591.

154. Rolls BJ, Roe LS, Meengs JS. Salad and satiety: energy density and portion size of a first-course salad affect energy intake at lunch. *J Am Diet Assoc* 2004;104:1570–1576.

155. de Castro JM. The time of day of food intake influences overall intake in humans. *J Nutr* 2004;134:104–111.

156. De Graaf C, De Jong LS, Lambers AC. Palatability affects satiation but not satiety. *Physiol Behav* 1999;66:681–688.

157. Torheim LE, Ouattara F, Diarra MM, et al. Nutrient adequacy and dietary diversity in rural Mali: association and determinants. *Eur J Clin Nutr* 2004;58:594–604.

158. Johnson J, Vickers Z. Factors influencing sensory-specific satiety. *Appetite* 1992;19:15–31.

159. Guinard JX, Brun P. Sensory-specific satiety: comparison of taste and texture effects. *Appetite* 1998;31:141–157.

160. de Graaf C, Schreurs A, Blauw YH. Short-term effects of different amounts of sweet and nonsweet carbohydrates on satiety and energy intake. *Physiol Behav* 1993;54:833–843.

161. Vickers Z. Long-term acceptability of limited diets. *Life Support Biosph Sci* 1999;6:29–33.

162. Raynor HA, Niemeier HM, Wing RR. Effect of limiting snack food variety on long-term sensory-specific satiety and monotony during obesity treatment. *Eat Behav* 2006;7:1–14.

163. Raynor HA, Jeffery RW, Phelan S, et al. Amount of food group variety consumed in the diet and long-term weight loss maintenance. *Obes Res* 2005;13:883–890.

164. Raynor HA, Wing RR. Effect of limiting snack food variety across days on hedonics and consumption. *Appetite* 2006;46:168–176.

165. Raynor HA, Jeffery RW, Tate DF, et al. Relationship between changes in food group variety, dietary intake, and weight during obesity treatment. *Int J Obes Relat Metab Disord* 2004;28:813–820.

166. Katz DL, Katz CS. *The flavor point diet.* Emmaus, PA: Rodale, Inc., 2005.

167. Kennedy E. Dietary diversity, diet quality, and body weight regulation. *Nutr Rev* 2004;62:s78–s81.

168. Sorensen LB, Moller P, Flint A, et al. Effect of sensory perception of foods on appetite and food intake: a review of studies on humans. *Int J Obes Relat Metab Disord* 2003;27:1152–1166.

169. Raynor HA, Epstein LH. Dietary variety, energy regulation, and obesity. *Psychol Bull* 2001;127:325–341.

170. McCrory MA, Suen VM, Roberts SB. Biobehavioral influences on energy intake and adult weight gain. *J Nutr* 2002;132:3830s–3834s.

171. McCrory MA, Fuss PJ, McCallum JE, et al. Dietary variety within food groups: association with energy intake and body fatness in men and women. *Am J Clin Nutr* 1999;69:440–447.

172. Snoek HM, Huntjens L, Van Gemert LJ, et al. Sensory-specific satiety in obese and normal-weight women. *Am J Clin Nutr* 2004;80:823–831.

173. Poothullil JM. Regulation of nutrient intake in humans: a theory based on taste and smell. *Neurosci Biobehav Rev* 1995;19:407–412.

174. Mattes RD, Kare MR. Nutrition and the chemical senses. In: Shils ME, Olson JA, Shike M, eds. *Modern nutrition in health and disease,* 8th ed. Philadelphia, PA: Lea & Febiger, 1994.

175. Docherty JP, Sack DA, Roffman M, et al. A double-blind, placebo-controlled, exploratory trial of chromium picolinate in atypical depression: effect on carbohydrate craving. *J Psychiatr Pract* 2005;11:302–314.

176. Dall'acqua S, Innocenti G. Steroidal glycosides from *Hoodia gordonii.* Steroids 2007;72:559–568.

177. Rader JI, Delmonte P, Trucksess MW. Recent studies on selected botanical dietary supplement ingredients. *Anal Bioanal Chem* 2007;389:26–35.

178. Carter BE, Drewnoski A. Beverages containing soluble fiver, caffeine, and green tea catechins suppress hunger and lead to less energy consumption at the next meal. *Appetite* 2012;59:755–761.

179. Hursel R, Westerterp-Plantenga MS. Thermogenic ingredients and body weight regulation. *Int J Obes* (Lond) 2010;34:659–669.

180. Hampton T. Sugar substitutes linked to weight gain. *JAMA* 2008;299:2137–2138.

181. Bellisle F, Drewnowski A. Intense sweeteners, energy intake and the control of body weight. *Eur J Clin Nutr* 2007;61:691–700.

182. Swithers SE, Davidson TL. A role for sweet taste: calorie predictive relations in energy regulation by rats. *Behav Neurosci* 2008;122:161–173.

183. Frank GK, Oberndorfer TA, Simmons AN, et al. Sucrose activates human taste pathways differently from artificial sweetener. *Neuroimage* 2008;39:1559–1569.

184. Obolskiy D, Pischel I, Siriwatanametanon N, et al. *Garcinia mangostana* L.: a phytochemical and pharmacological review. *Phytother Res* 2009;23:1047–1065.

185. Shan T, Ma Q, Guo K, et al. Xanthones from mangosteen extracts as natural chemopreventive agents: potential anticancer drugs. *Curr Mol Med* 2011;11:666–677.

186. American Cancer Society. *Mangosteen Juice.* November 2008. Retrieved October 2013.

187. Vinson JA, Burnham BR, Nagendran MV. Randomized, double-blind, placebo-controlled, linear dose, crossover study to evaluate the efficacy and safety of a green coffee bean extract in overweight subjects. *Diabetes Metab Syndr Obes* 2012;5:21–27.

188. Onakpoya I, Terry R, Ernst E. The use of green coffee extract as a weight loss supplement: a systematic review and meta-analysis of randomised clinical trials. *Gastroenterol Res Pract* 2011;2011:382852.

189. Scientific concepts of functional foods in Europe. Consensus document. *Br J Nutr* 1999;81 (suppl 1):s1–s27.

190. Mizwicki MT, Liu G, Fiala M, et al. 1α,25-dihydroxy-vitamin D3 and resolvin D1 retune the balance between amyloid-β phagocytosis and inflammation in Alzheimer's disease patients. *J Alzheimers Dis* 2013;34:155–170.

191. Cao C, Loewenstein DA, Lin X, et al. High blood caffeine levels in MCI linked to lack of progression to dementia. *J Alzheimers Dis* 2012;30:559–572.

192. Le Chatelier E, Nielsen T, Qin J. Richness of human gut microbiome correlates with metabolic markers. *Nature* 2013;500:541–546.

193. Smith SR, Blundell J, Burns C, et al. Pramlintide treatment reduces 24-hour caloric intake and meal sizes, and improves control of eating in obese subjects: a 6-week translational research study. *Am J Physiol Endocrinol Metab* 2007;293:e620–e627.

SUGGESTED READINGS

Bellisle F. Why should we study human food intake behaviour? *Nutr Metab Cardiovasc Dis* 2003;13:189–193.

Bernstein DM, Laney C, Morris EK, et al. False beliefs about fattening foods can have healthy consequences. *Proc Natl Acad Sci USA* 2005;102:13724–13731.

Blundell JE, Stubbs RJ. High and low carbohydrate and fat intakes: limits imposed by appetite and palatability and their implications for energy balance. *Eur J Clin Nutr* 1999;53:s148–s165.

Coppola A, Liu ZW, Andrews ZB, et al. A central thermogenic-like mechanism in feeding regulation: an interplay between arcuate nucleus T3 and UCP2. *Cell Metab* 2007;5:21–33.

de Graaf C, Blom WA, Smeets PA, et al. Biomarkers of satiation and satiety. *Am J Clin Nutr* 2004;79:946–961.

de Graaf C, De Jong LS, Lambers AC. Palatability affects satiation but not satiety. *Physiol Behav* 1999;66:681–688.

Drewnowski A. Energy density, palatability, and satiety: implications for weight control. *Nutr Rev* 1998;56:347–353.

Drewnowski A. Intense sweeteners and energy density of foods: implications for weight control. *Eur J Clin Nutr* 1999;53:757–763.

Duffy VB, Bartoshuk LM, Striegel-Moore R, et al. Taste changes across pregnancy. *Ann N Y Acad Sci* 1998;855:805–809.

Eertmans A, Baeyens F, Van den Bergh O. Food likes and their relative importance in human eating behavior: review and preliminary suggestions for health promotion. *Health Educ Res* 2001;16:443–456.

Flatt JP. What do we most need to learn about food intake regulation? *Obes Res* 1998;6:307–310.

French SA. Pricing effects on food choices. *J Nutr* 2003;133:841s–843s.

French S, Robinson T. Fats and food intake. *Curr Opin Clin Nutr Metab Care* 2003;6:629–634.

Gendall K, Joyce P, Abbott R. The effects of meal composition on subsequent cravings and binge eating. *Addict Behav* 1999;24:305–315.

Gibson E, Desmond E. Chocolate craving and hunger state: implications for the acquisition and expression of appetite and food choice. *Appetite* 1999;32:219–240.

Hetherington MM. Taste and appetite regulation in the elderly. *Proc Nutr Soc* 1998;57:625–631.

Holt S, Miller J, Petocz P, et al. A satiety index of common foods. *Eur J Clin Nutr* 1995;49:675–690.

Holt S, Delargy H, Lawton C, et al. The effects of high-carbohydrate vs. high-fat breakfasts on feelings of fullness and alertness, and subsequent food intake. *Int J Food Sci Nutr* 1999;50:13–28.

Kostas G. Low-fat and delicious: can we break the taste barrier? *J Am Diet Assoc* 1997;97:s88–s92.

Lin SL, Wilber JF. Appetite regulation. In: DeGroot LJ, Jameson JL, eds. *Endocrinology*, 4th ed. Philadelphia: W.B. Saunders, 2001:600–604.

Louis-Sylvestre J, Tournier A, Verger P, et al. Learned caloric adjustment of human intake. *Appetite* 1989;1:95–103.

MacBeth H, ed. *Food preferences and taste*. Providence, RI: Berghahn Books, 1997.

Melanson K, Westerterp-Plantenga M, Saris W, et al. Blood glucose patterns and appetite in time-blinded humans: carbohydrate vs. fat. *Am J Physiol* 1999;277:r337–r345.

Nestle M, Wing R, Birch L, et al. Behavioral and social influences on food choice. *Nutr Rev* 1998;56:s50–s64.

Poppitt S, McCormack D, Buffenstein R. Short-term effects of macronutrient preloads on appetite and energy intake in lean women. *Physiol Behav* 1998;64:279–285.

Porrini M, Crovetti R, Riso P, et al. Effects of physical and chemical characteristics of food on specific and general satiety. *Physiol Behav* 1995;57:461–468.

Reed DR, Bachmanov AA, Beauchamp GK, et al. Heritable variation in food preferences and their contribution to obesity. *Behav Genet* 1997;27:373–387.

Rogers PJ. Eating habits and appetite control: a psychobiological perspective. *Proc Nutr Soc* 1999;58:59–67.

Rolls B. Experimental analyses of the effects in a meal on human feeding. *Am J Clin Nutr* 1985;42:932–939.

Rolls B. Sensory-specific satiety. *Nutr Rev* 1986;44:93–101.

Rolls BJ, Bell EA. Intake of fat and carbohydrate: role of energy density. *Eur J Clin Nutr* 1999;53:s166–s173.

Rolls B, Castellanos V, Halford J, et al. Volume of food consumed affects satiety in men. *Am J Clin Nutr* 1998;67:1170–1177.

Rolls ET. Taste and olfactory processing in the brain and its relation to the control of eating. *Crit Rev Neurobiol* 1997;11:263–287.

Sclafani A. Psychobiology of food preferences. *Int J Obes Relat Metab Disord* 2001;25:s13–s16.

Seeley RJ, Schwartz MW. Neuroendocrine regulation of food intake. *Acta Paediatr Suppl* 1999;88:58–61.

Stubbs R. Peripheral signals affecting food intake. *Nutrition* 1999;15:614–625.

Stubbs RJ, Johnstone AM, Mazlan N, et al. Effect of altering the variety of sensorially distinct foods, of the same macronutrient content, on food intake and body weight in men. *Eur J Clin Nutr* 2001;55:19–28.

Wardle J. Hunger and satiety: a multidimensional assessment of responses to caloric loads. *Physiol Behav* 1987;40:577–582.

Westerterp-Plantenga M, Rolland V, Wilson S, et al. Satiety related to 24 h diet-induced thermogenesis during high protein/carbohydrate vs. high fat diets measured in a respiration chamber. *Eur J Clin Nutr* 1999;53:495–502.

World Health Organization. *Obesity and overweight*. Available at http://www.whoint/dietphysicalactivity/publications/facts/obesity/en; accessed 11/7/07.

CHAPTER 39

Health Effects of Chocolate

T he epitome of nutritional indulgence (see Chapter 38), chocolate has over recent years attracted increasing attention because of its health effects. The predominant saturated fatty acid in cocoa butter, stearic acid (18:0), has been found to be nonatherogenic (1–3). Dark chocolate with cocoa content of approximately 60% or more is, in general, a highly concentrated—if not the most highly concentrated—source of bioflavonoid antioxidants as compared to other commonly available foods. Dark chocolate is a relatively concentrated source of fiber as well. Studies have demonstrated benefits of dark chocolate consumption on blood pressure, insulin sensitivity, lipids, and endothelial function; there is observational evidence of a beneficial effect on susceptibility to heart disease. While much about both the allure and the health effects of chocolate remain to be elucidated, the available evidence makes a fairly strong case for the inclusion of dark chocolate in a healthful diet and a decisive case for the substitution of dark chocolate for milk chocolate. Chocolate serves as a particularly good demonstration of the principle that eating well is best achieved by making well-informed choices within any given food category rather than abandoning categories of foods. That even an indulgence can be health promoting belies the oft-heard lament that "if it's good, it can't be good for you." Dark chocolate, by most accounts, is both.

OVERVIEW

While modern confections containing a great many ingredients are often referred to as "chocolates," chocolate, per se, is a product of the seeds of the cacao tree, indigenous to Central and South America. Initially used by mesoamerican peoples to brew a bitter drink, chocolate has been in the human diet for over 2,000 years. The origins of chocolate as a sweet delicacy can be traced to the sixteenth century and conquest of Central America and Mexico by the Spanish. Cacao was among the spoils of war and thus introduced to European epicures. The addition of sugar to cacao likely first occurred in Spain. Sweet preparations of chocolate were popular among Spanish aristocracy, who had privileged access until sometime after the turn of the seventeenth century. Chocolate then became a delicacy sought by all the royal courts of Europe; the rest, as the saying goes, is history.

The uniquely alluring, if not addictive, attributes of chocolate are well recognized but only partially understood. Chocolate has a nutritional composition that explains part of its appeal; it is a concentrated source of both fat and, in most commercial preparations, sugar, which are associated with hedonic responses. The texture of chocolate may enhance its appeal, with melting in the mouth serving to distribute and enhance flavor. Of particular interest is variation in chocolate craving associated with the menstrual cycle.

Chocolate craving could be partly explained by biologically active constituents of chocolate, including methylxanthines, biogenic amines, and cannabinoid-like fatty acids, along with a potential influence of chocolate consumption on levels of both serotonin and dopamine (4). Rozin et al. (5) found evidence of stronger chocolate craving in females than in males, with menstrual cycle variation. Some have hypothesized that chocolate craving associated with the menstrual cycle is a learned behavior that functions as a strategy for coping with perimenstrual symptoms (6). Hormes and Timko offer an alternative explanation (7). In their study, women reporting chocolate cravings related to the menstrual cycle exhibited different eating behaviors and attitudes compared with women reporting noncyclic chocolate cravings. Menstrual cravers had significantly higher body mass indices and reported greater feelings of guilt, greater levels of dietary restraint, and lower flexible control over intake compared with noncyclic cravers. The authors speculate that menstrual cravings for chocolate may be the result of dietary restriction in attempt to manage cyclic weight fluctuations. On the other hand, a study by Zellner et al. suggests that menstrual cravings may be largely mediated by culture (8). The work of Rozin et al. suggests that it is the sensory properties of chocolate, rather than neurochemical effects of its xanthine constituents, that account for the cravings it elicits. A 2006 review by Parker and colleagues also concluded that chocolate's sensory properties and palatability are the most likely explanation for its psychoactive properties (9). Because chocolate craving is apparently both potent and rather common, whatever the mechanism, the identification of healthful formulations of chocolate is of genuine clinical significance.

Composition of Chocolate

The nutritional properties of products called "chocolate" naturally vary with their composition. Cacao itself is a fairly concentrated source of caffeine and another related stimulant, theobromine. The attribution of energy-boosting properties to chocolate is likely justified, although it provides less of a jolt than the extract of the coffee bean. While the caffeine content of chocolate is considerably lower than that of coffee (see Section VIE), chocolate is still a relatively concentrated source of the compound. The level of caffeine intake

associated with chocolate in the diet is unlikely to pose a health threat to individuals with normal caffeine tolerance, including pregnant women. Highly sensitive individuals and those with cardiac rhythm abnormalities may be adversely affected by caffeine from chocolate (10).

The oil in cacao, referred to as cocoa butter (the name "cocoa" is apparently an early adulteration of "cacao"), is a mixture of predominantly monounsaturated and saturated fatty acids. In the monounsaturated fraction, oleic acid predominates, as it does in olive oil. Roughly 20% of the fat in dark chocolate is monounsaturated.

The saturated fat content in cocoa butter is the most noteworthy. In solid dark chocolate, nearly 80% of the fat is saturated. The predominant fatty acid in cocoa butter is stearic acid (see Chapter 2 and Tables 39.1 and 39.2), an 18-carbon molecule. Whereas shorter-chain saturated fatty acids such as myristic acid (14:0) and palmitic acid (16:0) are associated with increases in low-density lipoprotein (LDL) cholesterol and atherogenesis, stearic acid is not (1). Thus, the fat in dark chocolate is at worst neutral with regard to health effects, if it is not actually salubrious. The nonatherogenic nature of stearic acid was specifically acknowledged by the 2010 Dietary Guidelines Advisory Committee (11), though it was not mentioned in the *Dietary Guidelines for Americans, 2010.*

TABLE 39.1		
Salient Features of the Nutritional Composition of Common Formulations of Milk Chocolate and Dark Chocolate		
Nutrient	Milk Chocolate, 44 g (1.55 Oz) Bar	Dark Chocolate, 44 g (1.55 Oz) Bar, Special Dark
Energy	235.0 kcal	233.0 kcal
Fat	13.0 g	13.0 g
Saturated fat	6.3 g	10.8 g
Myristic acid (14:0)	0.3 g	—
Palmitic acid (16:0)	2.6 g	—
Stearic acid (18:0)	2.7 g	—
Monounsaturated fat	5.8 g	2.0 g
Polyunsaturated fat	0.4 g	0.2 g
Fiber	1.5 g	2.7 g
Calcium	83.0 mg	12.0 mg
Magnesium	28.0 mg	13.0 mg
Arginine	0.1 g	Not provided
Bioflavonoids	Not provided	Not provided

Source: Data from US Department of Agriculture Agricultural Research Service. *Nutrient data laboratory.* Available at http://www.nal.usda.gov/fnic/foodcomp/search; accessed 11/7/07.

TABLE 39.2

Fatty Acids in Cocoa Butter, Dark Chocolate, Milk Chocolate, and Milk Fat[a]

	Product			
	Cocoa Butter[b]	Dark Chocolate[b]	Milk Chocolate[c]	Milk Fat[b]
Saturated Fatty Acids				
4.0				3.5
6.0				2.1
8.0				1.2
10.0				2.8
12.0				3.1
C4.0–C12.0	0.0	0.0	1.3	12.7
14.0	0.1	0.1	1.6	11.0
15.0	0.0	0.0	0.0	0.0
16.0	26.9	25.7	25.4	28.9
17.0	0.0	0.2	0.0	0.0
18.0	35.2	34.9	32.3	13.4
20.0	0.0	0.9	1.0	0.0
22.0	0.0	0.1	0.0	0.0
24.0	0.0	0.0	0.0	0.0
Monounsaturated Fatty Acids				
14.1	0.0	0.0	0.0	0.0
16.1	0.2	0.2	0.4	2.4
18.1	34.5	34.6	31.6	27.6
20.1	0.0	0.0	0.0	0.0
Polyunsaturated Fatty Acids				
18.2	3.0	3.2	3.0	2.4
18.3	0.1	0.2	0.4	1.5
Other	0.0	0.0	3.2	0.0
Total	**100.0**	**100.0**	**100.0**	**100.0**

[a]Dark and milk chocolate samples represented are industry averages. Fatty acids are expressed as a percentage of total; all columns add up to 100%.

[b]Values derived from US Department of Agriculture, Agricultural Research Service. *Nutrient data laboratory.* Available at http://www.ars.usda.gov/ba/bhnrc/ndl.

[c]Values derived from Hurst WJ, Tarka SM, Dobson G, et al. Determination of conjugated linoleic acid (CLA) concentrations in milk chocolate. *J Agric Food Chem* 2001;49:1264–1265.

The reasons for this omission are not obvious, but because the development of the Dietary Guidelines is often influenced by politics and must take into account feasibility and utility of messages for the general population, the continued inclusion of stearic acid under the umbrella of harmful solid fats is likely not due to a lack of scientific evidence. Milk chocolate is slightly more concentrated in palmitic and myristic acid than dark chocolate by virtue of higher milk fat content (the addition of some milk fat to dark chocolate is permitted under the current standards of identity in order to soften the bite of the chocolate) (12), but these differences are modest. The marked divergence in health effects of milk and dark chocolate is most convincingly attributed to the difference in antioxidant content.

Whereas the fat content of dark chocolate is at worst neutral in its health effects, other constituents of cocoa render it decidedly favorable in its overall health impact. Salient among these are the bioflavonoid content and antioxidant capacity of dark chocolate. Based on the oxygen radical absorbance capacity (ORAC) as a measure of overall antioxidant potential, dark chocolate is a more concentrated source of antioxidants than most fruits, and it offers more than twice the antioxidant potency of milk chocolate (13).

Along with wine and tea, dark chocolate is a concentrated source of polyphenols that are widely distributed but generally less concentrated in fruits, vegetables, and cereal grains. Animal and cell culture studies suggest protective effects of polyphenolic antioxidants against cardiovascular diseases (CVD), cancers, neurodegenerative diseases, diabetes, and osteoporosis, although definitive human studies in vivo are as yet lacking for the most part (14).

Dark chocolate with 60% cocoa or higher is the most concentrated food source of antioxidants readily available, with a higher antioxidant capacity than green tea (15). The flavonoids in chocolate contribute to its bitterness (16). It is worth noting that cocoa powder that has been treated with alkali, or "Dutched," contains significantly reduced concentrations of flavanols (17–18). Miller and colleagues compared the flavanol content of commercially available natural (nonalkalized) and Dutched cocoa powders, and found that flavanol content was reduced by 60% to 78% depending on the level of alkalization (18). In addition to flavonoids, dark chocolate is a concentrated source of magnesium, fiber, and the amino acid arginine (see Table 39.1). As discussed elsewhere (see Chapter 7 and Section VIE), arginine may contribute directly to vasodilatory capacity and enhanced endothelial function.

While most research on the topic attributes health effects to the bioflavonoids in dark chocolate, the occasional study diverges from this consensus. Record et al. (19) found a comparable reduction in free radicals in fecal water following 4 weeks of ingestion of either high- or low-flavanol chocolate in 18 healthy adult volunteers. These authors postulate that something other than flavanols may account for the antioxidant activity of chocolate.

Cardiovascular Health and Glucose Metabolism

Epidemiologic Studies

Studies of dark chocolate have quite consistently suggested health benefits (20–22), attributed largely to the flavanol content (23). In their recent meta-analysis of 10 observational studies, Zhang et al. reported a 25% reduced risk of CVD outcomes associated with the highest versus lowest

level of chocolate intake (24). Epidemiologic studies have found inverse associations between more frequent chocolate or cocoa consumption and myocardial infarction (25), stroke (25,26), CHD (27), cardiac mortality (28–29), all-cause mortality (28), and diabetes (30). Although observational studies do not typically differentiate between types of chocolate (i.e., white, milk, or dark chocolate) when assessing chocolate consumption, it is likely that dark chocolate provides the most benefit because it is the most concentrated source of cocoa flavanols.

Experimental Trials

The effects of chocolate or cocoa consumption on blood pressure are perhaps the most well-documented. A 2012 Cochrane review of 20 short-term randomized controlled trials reported a small but significant reduction in blood pressure associated with consumption of flavanol-rich chocolate or cocoa compared with low-flavanol or flavanol-free control products (31). In the included studies, intervention groups received a mean of 545.5 mg of flavanols in cocoa products daily, with a wide range of 30 to 1,080 mg. Mean reductions in systolic and diastolic blood pressures were 2.77 mmHg and 2.20 mmHg, respectively.

Grassi et al. (32) showed both blood pressure reduction and enhanced insulin sensitivity following dark chocolate ingestion in a short-term crossover trial of 15 healthy adults. The test dose in this study was 100 g of dark chocolate, providing roughly 500 mg of polyphenols. These investigators also compared 100 g of dark chocolate providing 88 mg of flavanols to white chocolate for 7 days in a crossover trial of 20 adults with untreated essential hypertension (33). The study showed significant improvements in blood pressure, endothelial function, and measures of insulin sensitivity (e.g., HOMA-IR) following dark chocolate treatment.

Innes et al. (34) found that 100 g of dark chocolate, but not milk or white chocolate, acutely inhibited platelet aggregation in healthy adults. In a study of 32 healthy adults, daily ingestion of 234 mg of cocoa flavanols daily for 4 weeks significantly inhibited platelet aggregation (35).

Improvement in endothelial function has been seen in healthy adults (36–39,86), and in smokers (40), medicated diabetic patients (41), hypertensives (33), and adults with cardiac risk factors (42). The author's lab has demonstrated improved endothelial function with both daily and single-dose ingestion of flavonoid-rich liquid cocoa, as well as with acute ingestion of solid dark chocolate, by otherwise healthy, overweight adults (38,39). Among subjects with established CVD, study findings are mixed, but suggestive of beneficial effects of cocoa products. Farouque et al. (43) did not see beneficial effects on vascular function among subjects with established coronary artery disease (CAD) following 6 weeks of daily dark chocolate ingestion. However, Heiss et al. (44) observed improved endothelial function in CAD patients after 30 days of twice daily high-flavanol cocoa ingestion, compared with low-flavanol cocoa ingestion. In a randomized, controlled trial, Flammer and colleagues reported beneficial short-term effects (2 hours after ingestion) of flavanol-rich chocolate on both vascular function and platelet adhesion in patients with congestive heart failure and sustained effects (over a 4-week period) on vascular function (45).

Effects of cocoa products on the lipid panel and oxidative stress are also somewhat unclear. Engler et al. (46) demonstrated improvement in endothelial function following dark chocolate ingestion by healthy adults but did not observe between-group differences in measures of oxidative stress or the lipid profile. In contrast, Wan et al. (47) showed reduced LDL oxidation, increased high-density lipoprotein (HDL), and increased total antioxidant capacity in serum with a dark chocolate–supplemented diet in 23 healthy adults over a 2-week period. Fraga et al. (48) demonstrated reduction in both blood pressure and LDL cholesterol in young adult male athletes following consumption of flavanol-rich dark chocolate daily for 2 weeks, with no such changes observed when milk chocolate low in flavanols was consumed. A 2010 meta-analysis of eight trials summarized the short-term impact of cocoa consumption on blood lipids (49). The data from these trials indicate that cocoa may significantly reduce LDL cholesterol, and may also reduce total cholesterol in individuals with cardiovascular risk factors. This meta-analysis supports a lipid-lowering effect of cocoa, but it is limited by the small total sample (n = 215), the paucity of well-designed trials, and the heterogeneity of the studies included. Whether cocoa products substantially improve lipid levels in the blood remains unclear. There is, however, convincing evidence that consumption of chocolate in most forms has at worst a neutral effect on the lipid profile. This evidence should allay fears that the high saturated fat content of chocolate would negate the effects of its other health-promoting compounds.

Other Health Effects

While the effects of cocoa products on cardiometabolic health are well studied, additional health effects are being newly explored. Weisburger (50) has suggested a possible role for chocolate and cocoa in the prevention of cancer, while acknowledging the need for more research before this benefit can be asserted with confidence. The potential for cocoa flavanols to influence immune function, (51) inflammation, (52) antioxidant status, (53) and apoptosis (54) has been demonstrated and could at least theoretically influence cancer risk.

Desideri and colleagues have demonstrated improvement in cognitive function among elderly individuals with mild cognitive impairment after an 8-week high-flavanol cocoa drink intervention; an effect the authors speculate may be mediated in part by improvement in insulin sensitivity (55).

Jenkins et al. (56) have published data suggesting that chocolate-flavored cocoa bran has comparable effects on fecal bulk as wheat bran and improves lipid ratios. The authors propose that cocoa bran might be useful in efforts to increase fiber intake in general and to prevent or manage constipation and hyperlipidemia.

Several studies have suggested that cocoa flavanols may protect skin from damage from UV light (57–59). Twelve weeks of high-flavanol cocoa consumption decreased erythema induced by UV light by 25% in one study (58). In another, specially produced high-flavanol chocolate, but not commercially available chocolate, more than doubled the dose of UV light necessary to produce erythema (57).

Finally, there is an emerging body of research on the effects of cocoa products during pregnancy. Triche and colleagues assessed the association between consumption of cocoa or chocolate during pregnancy and subsequent risk of preeclampsia (60). Chocolate intake, measured by self-report and by cord theobromine levels, was inversely associated with preeclampsia risk. Klebanoff et al. conducted a similar study assessing maternal serum theobromine levels, but not diet, and did not confirm these findings (61). Saftlas et al.

found that chocolate intake in the first trimester was associated with reduced odds of both pre-eclampsia and gestational hypertension, whereas chocolate intake in the third trimester was associated with reduced odds of preeclampsia only (62). Two randomized, controlled trials have now been completed to evaluate the effects of regular chocolate consumption during pregnancy (63,64). Di Renzo and colleagues randomized 90 pregnant women at approximately 12 weeks gestation to receive either a 30 g portion of dark chocolate daily or no intervention for the duration of pregnancy (64). They found that the intervention group had significantly lower blood pressure and lower levels of liver enzymes at multiple time points throughout pregnancy, compared with the control group. Despite the additional 160 calories provided by the chocolate, there was no difference in weight gain between the groups. In contrast, Mogollon et al. did not find any effect of daily consumption of 20 g high-flavanol dark chocolate for 12 weeks on endothelial function or blood pressure in pregnant women, compared with low-flavanol chocolate (63). This study was shorter in duration and had a smaller sample size (N = 44) than the study by Di Rienzo et al. Additional trials will be necessary to determine whether regular consumption of cocoa or chocolate during pregnancy can reduce the risk of hypertension, preeclampsia, or other related pregnancy complications.

Mechanisms of Action

Kris-Etherton and Keen (65) reviewed the evidence for health benefits associated with antioxidant flavonoids in both tea and chocolate. The literature is suggestive of an array of potential benefits, including reduced inflammation, inhibition of atherogenesis, improved endothelial function, reduced thrombosis, and interference with cellular adhesion molecules. In general, such effects have been seen with between 150 and 500 mg of flavonoids. This translates into between 1 and 3.5 cups of tea and from 40 to 125 g of flavonoid-rich chocolate.

Consumption of chocolate has been shown to reduce oxidation products in human plasma (66). Potent anti-inflammatory effects of cocoa extracts have been demonstrated in vitro, with inhibition of interleukin-2 expression in particular (67).

Dark chocolate purportedly inhibits platelet aggregation by several mechanisms (68). Cocoa polyphenols may increase the concentration of HDL cholesterol as well as modify the fatty acid composition of LDL cholesterol and make it more resistant to oxidative damage (69,70). Theobromine may also play a role in increasing HDL concentrations (71).

Potential Risks

Data from the Zutphen Elderly Study (28) reveal an inverse association between cocoa intake, blood pressure, cardiovascular mortality, and all-cause mortality over 15 years. But the evidence base for long-term health effects, and optimal dosing, is quite limited, and thus more research will be required to define precisely the role for dark chocolate in a health-promoting diet (14).

Among the perennial concerns regarding chocolate ingestion, for adolescents at least, is a putative link to acne vulgaris. The scientific literature on the topic is considered indecisive, but overall, there is scant evidence that chocolate does in fact contribute to exacerbations of acne (72,73). Heartburn and migraines are sometimes believed to be adverse effects of chocolate consumption, but evidence for a causal relationship between chocolate consumption and these maladies is lacking (74–76).

Of course, the health benefits of chocolate may nevertheless come at a cost. Chocolate of any variety is a concentrated source of calories (see Table 39.1). Whereas dark chocolate may offer four times the flavonoid content of green tea, tea is generally a very low-calorie source of antioxidants (77). This trade-off between nutrient value and energy density should be considered when making room for chocolate in a healthful and reasonably apportioned diet. Despite the reasonable concern that the caloric density of chocolate could cause weight gain, there is some preliminary evidence suggesting that chocolate could actually have a beneficial effect on body weight by promoting satiety and suppressing appetite (78). In one study in rats, cocoa prevented weight gain associated with a high-fat diet and favorably influenced the expression of genes involved in lipid metabolism (79). Another study in mice found that cocoa supplementation reduced the rate of weight gain and reduced inflammation, insulin resistance, and the severity of fatty liver disease in mice fed a high-fat diet (80). However, cocoa does not have the high fat and calorie content of chocolate; it is plausible that these negative attributes of chocolate would neutralize or even outweigh the benefits of cocoa. In a small study in women, Massolt and colleagues found that smelling or eating dark chocolate decreased appetite acutely (81). Sørensen and Astrup compared the appetite suppressing effects of milk chocolate and dark chocolate in a crossover study in men (82). They found that 100 g of dark chocolate decreased appetite and energy intake at an ad libitum meal compared with an equal quantity of milk chocolate. After adjusting for a difference in energy content between the two types of chocolate, energy intake was 8% lower in the dark chocolate condition. The authors speculate that the more intense flavor of the dark chocolate may have contributed to greater feelings of satiety. This explanation is consistent with previous study findings indicating that a chocolate bar rated as intense in flavor produced more sensory-specific satiety than other less intense snack items (83).

Although there is currently little evidence of an antiobesity effect of chocolate, there is also no clear indication that moderate chocolate consumption leads to weight gain. One cross-sectional study found an inverse relationship between frequency of chocolate consumption and body mass index among healthy adults (84). In contrast, Greenberg and Buijsse observed a significant dose-response relationship between higher frequency of chocolate consumption and greater weight gain during a 6-year follow-up period in a large prospective cohort study (85). However, randomized trials have not typically found an increase in weight after sustained consumption of small amounts of cocoa (38,41–43) or dark chocolate (46). In one study, a daily dose of 25 g (125 kcal) of dark chocolate slightly increased body weight after 3 months, but a 6 g dose (30 kcal) was not associated with any weight change. Both doses were effective in reducing blood pressure (87). To minimize the potential for weight gain, identification of the smallest effective dose of chocolate for a particular condition and population group should be a goal of future research.

Environmental Concerns

The impact of cocoa farming practices on the environment and human rights has drawn some attention (88–90). Large forested areas are often cleared to plant cocoa trees that can grow in full sun, increasing short-term yields, but dramatically reducing biodiversity. Shaded growing systems retain some, but not all, of the biodiversity of an undisturbed forest. Full sun growing conditions also contribute to increased fertilizer and pesticide use and produce yields for a shorter period of time than shaded systems. Franzen and Mulder have provided a thorough review of pertinent issues in cocoa production (91). Also of concern is the use of child labor on cocoa farms in West Africa. Child labor and associated exposure to pesticides and other hazards of physical work have been relatively well-documented (92,93). Cases of slavery have also been reported (89).

Consumers who are aware of these issues may understandably have reservations about consuming chocolate for health benefits or may be confused about how to find chocolate that has been sourced in a way that is ethical and environmentally responsible. There is no simple solution to these concerns. Some brands of chocolate may carry labels like "Organic," "Fair Trade" (94), or "Rainforest Alliance Certified," (95) but no single certification guarantees that the chocolate's production did not involve any child labor, unfair pay to farmers, or harm to the environment. In response to the pitfalls of third-party certification, some companies are turning to direct trade with cocoa farmers, in what has been called a "bean-to-bar" movement (96). This approach allows chocolate manufacturers to ensure that farmers are paid well and are using sustainable farming methods and fair labor practices.

Nutrigenomic and Metabolomic Considerations

At present, there are no known studies of diet–genome interactions pertaining to cocoa and chocolate consumption. However, there is some evidence that individual characteristics may modulate the effects of chocolate. For example, Martin and colleagues observed different metabolic profiles and response to dark chocolate consumption in individuals who reported high levels of anxiety compared with those who reported low anxiety (97). The concentrations of several metabolites in urine were significantly different between the groups at baseline. After the dark chocolate intervention, these differences were reduced such that the metabolic profiles of high-anxiety participants more closely resembled those of low-anxiety participants. Specifically, urine concentrations of catecholamines, corticosterone, and cortisol all decreased during the intervention period in participants who reported high levels of anxiety. In a subsequent study, Martin et al. also identified specific metabolic profiles associated with habitual chocolate consumption, suggesting that long-term exposure to chocolate influences gut bacterial metabolism (98). After 1 week of twice-daily dark chocolate consumption, a significant increase in HDL was observed in both habitual chocolate consumers and nonconsumers. However, only the habitual chocolate consumers experienced reduced triglyceride concentrations. It is now becoming clear that the gut microbiome influences the metabolism of cocoa polyphenols (99). Interindividual differences in the production of metabolites by microbiota from the molecular components of cocoa are relevant because these metabolites may lead to observable health effects. However, the complex relationship between the many phenolic metabolites of cocoa and their physiological effects is not yet fully understood.

CLINICAL HIGHLIGHTS

It is virtually idiomatic for the public at large that foods that taste good are bad for health. Yet accruing evidence suggests that one of the most widely preferred of all foods—chocolate—belies this notion, provided that the chocolate is chosen wisely.

Accumulating evidence of the health benefits of dark chocolate is quite convincing. A dose of 1 to 2 ounces of dark chocolate (60% cocoa content or higher) several times per week appears to be sufficient to confer benefit. Current evidence strongly supports improvement in cardiovascular risk factors, and blood pressure in particular. Recent studies suggest that dark chocolate may reduce blood pressure during pregnancy, when the effects of hypertension are especially perilous. There is also preliminary evidence for a protective effect on cognitive function, metabolic health, immune function, and carcinogenesis. The most salient potential risk of chocolate consumption is weight gain, but such risk is largely theoretical. Additional studies are needed to establish benefits of cocoa and chocolate beyond cardiovascular protection, to confirm a null effect on body weight, and to determine whether the

physiological effects of cocoa vary by individual characteristics such as genotype.

REFERENCES

1. Sanders TA, Berry SE. Influence of stearic acid on postprandial lipemia and hemostatic function. *Lipids* 2005;40:1221–1227.
2. Hunter JE, Zhang J, Krist-Etherton PM. Cardiovascular disease risk of dietary stearic acid compared with trans, other saturated, and unsaturated fatty acids: a systematic review. *Am J Clin Nutr* 2010;91(1):46–63.
3. Denke MA. Dietary fats, fatty acids, and their effects on lipoproteins. *Curr Atheroscler Rep* 2006;8(6):466–471.
4. Bruinsma K, Taren DL. Chocolate: food or drug? *J Am Diet Assoc* 1999;99:1249–1256.
5. Rozin P, Levine E, Stoess C. Chocolate craving and liking. *Appetite* 1991;17:199–212.
6. Rogers PJ, Smit HJ. Food craving and food addiction: a critical review of the evidence from a biopsychosocial perspective. *Pharmacol Biochem Behav* 2000;66(1):3–14.
7. Hormes JM, Timko CA. All cravings are not created equal: correlates of menstrual versus non-cyclic chocolate craving. *Appetite* 2011;57(1):1–5.
8. Zellner DA, Garriga-Trillo A, Centeno S, et al. Chocolate craving and the menstrual cycle. *Appetite* 2004;42:119–121.
9. Parker G, Parker I, Brotchie H. Mood state effects of chocolate. *J Affect Disord* 2006;92:149–159.
10. Nawrot P, Jordan S, Eastwood J, et al. Effects of caffeine on human health. *Food Addit Contam* 2003;20:1–30.
11. United States Department of Agriculture. *Report of the Dietary Guidelines Advisory Committee on the Dietary Guidelines for Americans*, 2010.
12. Stuart DA, director, Nutrition & Natural Product Sciences, The Hershey Company (personal communication).
13. Miller KB, Hurst WJ, Flannigan N, et al. Survey of commercially available chocolate- and cocoa-containing products in the United States. 2. Comparison of flavan-2-ol content with nonfat cocoa solids, total polyphenols, and percent cacao. *J Agric Food Chem* 2009;57:9169–9180.
14. Scalbert A, Manach C, Morand C, et al. Dietary polyphenols and the prevention of diseases. *Crit Rev Food Sci Nutr* 2005;45:287–306.
15. Keen CL. Chocolate: food as medicine/medicine as food. *J Am Coll Nutr* 2001;20:436s–439s; discussion 440s–442s.
16. Lesschaeve I, Noble AC. Polyphenols: factors influencing their sensory properties and their effects on food and beverage preferences. *Am J Clin Nutr* 2005;81:330s–335s.
17. McShea A, Ramiro-Puig E, Munro SB, et al. Clinical benefit and preservation of flavanols in dark chocolate manufacturing. *Nutr Rev* 2008;66:630–641.
18. Miller KB, Hurst WJ, Payne MJ, et al. Impact of alkalization on the antioxidant and flavanol content of commercial cocoa powders. *J Agric Food Chem* 2008;56(18):8527–8533.
19. Record IR, McInerney JK, Noakes M, et al. Chocolate consumption, fecal water antioxidant activity, and hydroxyl radical production. *Nutr Cancer* 2003;47:131–135.
20. Steinberg FM, Bearden MM, Keen CL. Cocoa and chocolate flavonoids: implications for cardiovascular health. *J Am Diet Assoc* 2003;103:215–223.

21. Engler MB, Engler MM. The emerging role of flavonoid-rich cocoa and chocolate in cardiovascular health and disease. *Nutr Rev* 2006;64:109–118.

22. Katz DL, Doughty K, Ali A. Cocoa and chocolate in human health and disease. *Antioxid Redox Signal* 2011; 15(10):2779–2811.

23. Keen CL, Holt RR, Oteiza PI, et al. Cocoa antioxidants and cardiovascular health. *Am J Clin Nutr* 2005;81:298s–303s.

24. Zhang Z, Xu G, Liu X. Chocolate intake reduces risk of cardiovascular disease: evidence from 10 observational studies. *Int J Cardiol* 2013;168(6):5448–5450.

25. Buijsse B, Weikert C, Drogan D, et al. Chocolate consumption in relation to blood pressure and risk of cardiovascular disease in German adults. *Eur Heart J* 2010;31:1616–1623.

26. Larsson SC, Virtamo J, Wolk A. Chocolate consumption and risk of stroke: a prospective cohort of men and meta-analysis. *Neurology* 2012;79(12):1223–1229.

27. Djousse L, Hopkins PN, North KE, et al. Chocolate consumption is inversely associated with prevalent coronary heart disease: The National Heart, Lung, and Blood Institute Family Heart Study. *Clin Nutr* 2011;30(2):182–187.

28. Buijsse B, Feskens EJ, Kok FJ, et al. Cocoa intake, blood pressure, and cardiovascular mortality: the Zutphen elderly study. *Arch Intern Med* 2006;166:411–417.

29. Janszky I, Mukamal KJ, Ljung R, et al. Chocolate consumption and mortality following a first acute myocardial infarction: the Stockholm Heart Epidemiology Program. *J Intern Med* 2009;266:248–257.

30. Oba S, Nagata C, Nakamura K, et al. Consumption of coffee, green tea, oolong tea, black tea, chocolate snacks and the caffeine content in relation to risk of diabetes in Japanese men and women. *Br J Nutr* 2010;103:453–459.

31. Ried K, Sullivan TR, Fakler P, et al. Effect of cocoa on blood pressure. *Cochrane Database Syst Rev* 2012;8:CD008893.

32. Grassi D, Lippi C, Necozione S, et al. Short-term administration of dark chocolate is followed by a significant increase in insulin sensitivity and a decrease in blood pressure in healthy persons. *Am J Clin Nutr* 2005;81:611–614.

33. Grassi D, Necozione S, Lippi C, et al. Cocoa reduces blood pressure and insulin resistance and improves endothelium-dependent vasodilation in hypertensives. *Hypertension* 2005;46:398–405.

34. Innes AJ, Kennedy G, McLaren M, et al. Dark chocolate inhibits platelet aggregation in healthy volunteers. *Platelets* 2003;14:325–327.

35. Murphy KJ, Chronopoulos AK, Singh I, et al. Dietary flavonols and procyanidin oligomers from cocoa (*Theobroma cacao*) inhibit platelet function. *Am J Clin Nutr* 2003;77:1466–1473.

36. Vlachopoulos C, Aznaouridis K, Alexopoulos N, et al. Effect of dark chocolate on arterial function in healthy individuals. *Am J Hypertens* 2005;18:785–791.

37. Fisher ND, Hughes M, Gerhard-Herman M, et al. Flavanol-rich cocoa induces nitric-oxide-dependent vasodilation in healthy humans. *J Hypertens* 2003;21:2281–2286.

38. Njike VY, Faridi Z, Shuval K, et al. Effects of sugar-sweetened and sugar-free cocoa on endothelial function in overweight adults. *Int J Cardiol* 2011;149(1):83–88.

39. Faridi Z, Njike VY, Dutta S, et al. Acute dark chocolate and cocoa ingestion and endothelial function: a randomized controlled crossover trial. *Am J Clin Nutr* 2008; 88(1):58–63.

40. Heiss C, Finis D, Kleinbongard P, et al. Sustained increase in flow-mediated dilation after daily intake of high-flavanol cocoa drink over 1 week. *J Cardiovasc Pharmacol* 2007;49:74–80.

41. Balzer J, Rassaf T, Heiss C, et al. Sustained benefits in vascular function through flavanol-containing cocoa in medicated diabetic patients: a double-masked, randomized, controlled trial. *J Am Coll Cardiol* 2008;51(22):2141–2149.

42. Heiss C, Dejam A, Kleinbongard P, et al. Vascular effects of cocoa rich in flavan-3-ols. *JAMA* 2003;290(8):1030–1031.

43. Farouque HM, Leung M, Hope SA, et al. Acute and chronic effects of flavonol-rich cocoa on vascular function in subjects with coronary artery disease: a randomized, double-blind, placebo-controlled study. *Clin Sci (Lond)* 2006;111:71–80.

44. Heiss C, Jahn S, Taylor M, et al. Improvement of endothelial function with dietary flavanols is associated with mobilization of circulating angiogenic cells in patients with coronary artery disease. *J Am Coll Cardiol* 2010;56(3):218–224.

45. Flammer AJ, Sudano I, Wolfrum M, et al. Cardiovascular effects of flavanol-rich chocolate in patients with heart failure. *Eur Heart J* 2012;33(17):2172–2180.

46. Engler MB, Engler MM, Chen CY, et al. Flavonoid-rich dark chocolate improves endothelial function and increases plasma epicatechin concentrations in healthy adults. *J Am Coll Nutr* 2004;23:197–204.

47. Wan Y, Vinson JA, Etherton TD, et al. Effects of cocoa powder and dark chocolate on LDL oxidative susceptibility and prostaglandin concentrations in humans. *Am J Clin Nutr* 2001;74:596–602.

48. Fraga CG, Actis-Goretta L, Ottaviani JI, et al. Regular consumption of a flavanol-rich chocolate can improve oxidant stress in young soccer players. *Clin Dev Immunol* 2005;12:11–17.

49. Jia LLX, Bai YY, Li SH, et al. Short-term effect of cocoa product consumption on lipid profile: a meta-analysis of randomized controlled trials. *Am J Clin Nutr* 2010;92(1):218–225.

50. Weisburger JH. Chemopreventive effects of cocoa polyphenols on chronic diseases. *Exp Biol Med (Maywood)* 2001;226:891–897.

51. Mackenzie GG, Carrasquedo F, Delfino JM, et al. Epicatechin, catechin, and dimeric procyanidins inhibit PMA-induced NF-kappaB activation at multiple steps in Jurkat T cells. *FASEB J* 2004;18:167–169.

52. Monagas M, Khan N, Andres-Lacueva C, et al. Effect of cocoa powder on the modulation of inflammatory biomarkers in patients at high risk of cardiovascular disease. *Am J Clin Nutr* 2009;90:1144–1150.

53. Maskarinec G. Cancer protective properties of cocoa: a review of the epidemiologic evidence. *Nutr Cancer* 2009;61:573–579.

54. Arlorio M, Bottini C, Travaglia F, et al. Protective activity of *Theobroma cacao* L. phenolic extract on AML12 and MLP29 liver cells by preventing apoptosis and inducing autophagy. *J Agric Food Chem* 2009;57:10612–10618.

55. Desideri G, Kwik-Uribe C, Grassi D, et al. Benefits in cognitive function, blood pressure, and insulin resistance through cocoa flavanol consumption in elderly subjects with mild cognitive impairment: the Cocoa, Cognition, and Aging (CoCoA) study. *Hypertension* 2012;60(3): 794–801.

56. Jenkins DJ, Kendall CW, Vuksan V, et al. Effect of cocoa bran on low-density lipoprotein oxidation and fecal bulking. *Arch Intern Med* 2000;160:2374–2379.

57. Williams S, Tamburic S, Lally C. Eating chocolate can significantly protect the skin from UV light. *J Cosmet Dermatol* 2009;8:169–173.

58. Heinrich U, Neukam K, Tronnier H, et al. Long-term ingestion of high flavanol cocoa provides photoprotection against UV-induced erythema and improves skin condition in women. *J Nutr* 2006;136:1565–1569.

59. Neukam K, Stahl W, Tronnier H, et al. Consumption of flavanol-rich cocoa acutely increases microcirculation in human skin. *Eur J Nutr* 2007;46:53–56.

60. Triche EW, Grosso LM, Belanger K, et al. Chocolate consumption in pregnancy and reduced likelihood of preeclampsia. *Epidemiology* 2008;19(3):459–464.

61. Klebanoff MA, Zhang J, Zhang C, et al. Maternal serum theobromine and the development of preeclampsia. *Epidemiology* 2009;20(5):727–732.

62. Saftlas AF, Triche EW, Beydoun H, et al. Does chocolate intake during pregnancy reduce the risks of preeclampsia and gestational hypertension? *Ann Epidemiol* 2010;20(8):584–591.

63. Mongollon JA, Bujold E, Lemieux S, et al. Blood pressure and endothelial function in healthy, pregnant women after acute and daily consumption of flavanol-rich chocolate: a pilot, randomized controlled trial. *Nutr J* 2013;12(1):41.

64. Di Renzo GC, Brillo E, Romanelli M, et al. Potential effects of chocolate on human pregnancy: a randomized controlled trial. *J Matern Fetal Neonatal Med* 2012;25(10):1860–1867.

65. Kris-Etherton PM, Keen CL. Evidence that the antioxidant flavonoids in tea and cocoa are beneficial for cardiovascular health. *Curr Opin Lipidol* 2002;13:41–49.

66. Rein D, Lotito S, Holt RR, et al. Epicatechin in human plasma: *in vivo* determination and effect of chocolate consumption on plasma oxidation status. *J Nutr* 2000;130:2109s–2114s.

67. Mao TK, Powell J, Van de Water J, et al. The effect of cocoa procyanidins on the transcription and secretion of interleukin 1 beta in peripheral blood mononuclear cells. *Life Sci* 2000;66:1377–1386.

68. Pearson DA, Holt RR, Rein D, et al. Flavonols and platelet reactivity. *Clin Dev Immunol* 2005;12:1–9.

69. Mursu J, Voutilainen S, Nurmi T, et al. Dark chocolate consumption increases HDL cholesterol concentration and chocolate fatty acids may inhibit lipid peroxidation in healthy humans. *Free Radic Biol Med* 2004;37:1351–1359.

70. Osakabe N, Baba S, Yasuda A, et al. Daily cocoa intake reduces the susceptibility of low-density lipoprotein to oxidation as demonstrated in healthy human volunteers. *Free Radic Res* 2001;34:93–99.

71. Neufingerl N, Zebregs YE, Schuring EA, et al. Effect of cocoa and theobromine consumption on serum HDL-cholesterol concentrations: a randomized controlled trial. *Am J Clin Nutr* 2013;97(6):1201–1209.

72. Magin P, Pond D, Smith W, et al. A systematic review of the evidence for "myths and misconceptions" in acne management: diet, face-washing and sunlight. *Fam Pract* 2005;22:62–70.

73. Fries JH. Chocolate: a review of published reports of allergic and other deleterious effects, real or presumed. *Ann Allergy* 1978;41:195–207.

74. Kaltenbach T, Crockett S, Gerson LB. Are lifestyle measures effective in patients with gastroesophageal reflux disease? An evidence-based approach. *Arch Intern Med* 2006;166: 965–971.

75. Wober C, Holzhammer J, Zeitlhofer J, et al. Trigger factors of migraine and tension-type headache: experience and knowledge of the patients. *J Headache Pain* 2006;7:188–195.

76. Marcus DA, Scharff L, Turk D, et al. A double-blind provocative study of chocolate as a trigger of headache. *Cephalalgia* 1997;17:855–862; discussion 800.

77. Arts IC, Hollman PC, Kromhout D. Chocolate as a source of tea flavonoids. *Lancet* 1999;354:488.

78. Farhat G, Drummond S, Fyfe L, et al. Dark chocolate: an obesity paradox or a culprit for weight gain? *Phytother Res* 2013.

79. Matsui N, Ito R, Nishimura E, et al. Ingested cocoa can prevent high-fat diet-induced obesity by regulating the expression of genes for fatty acid metabolism. *Nutrition* 2005;21(5):594–601.

80. Gu Y, Yu S, Lambert JD. Dietary cocoa ameliorates obesity-related inflammation in high fat-fed mice. *Eur J Nutr* 2014 Feb;53(1):149–58.

81. Massolt ET, van Haard PM, Rehfeld JF, et al. Appetite suppression through smelling of dark chocolate correlates with changes in ghrelin in young women. *Regul Pept* 2010;161(1–3):81–86.

82. Sørensen LB, Astrup A. Eating dark and milk chocolate: a randomized crossover study of effects on appetite and energy intake. *Nutr Diabetes* 2011;1(12):e21.

83. Weijzen PLG, Zandstra EH, Alfieri C, et al. Effects of complexity and intensity on sensory specific satiety and food acceptance after repeated consumption. *Food Qual Pref* 2008;19:349–359.

84. Golomb BA, Koperski S, White HL. Association between more frequent chocolate consumption and lower body mass index. *Arch Intern Med* 2012;172(6):519–521.

85. Greenberg JA, Buijsse B. Habitual chocolate consumption may increase body weight in a dose-response manner. *PLoS One* 2013;8(8):370271.

86. Davison K, Coates AM, Buckley JD, et al. Effect of cocoa flavanols and exercise on cardiometabolic risk factors in overweight and obese subjects. *Int J Obes (Lond)* 2008;32:1289–1296.

87. Desch S, Kobler D, Schmidt J, et al. Low vs. higher-dose dark chocolate and blood pressure in cardiovascular high-risk patients. *Am J Hypertens* 2010;23(6):694–700.

88. http://green.blogs.nytimes.com/2012/12/11/reshaping-the-future-of-cocoa-in-africa/?_php=true&_type=blogs&_r=0. Last accessed 5/11/14.

89. http://www.foodispower.org/slavery-chocolate/. Last accessed 5/11/14.

90. http://grist.org/food/a-guide-to-ethical-chocolate/ Last accessed 5/11/14.

91. Franzen M, Mulder MB. Ecological, economic and social perspectives on cocoa production worldwide. *Biodivers Conserv* 2007;16:3835–3849.

92. International Cocoa Initiative. *Child labour in cocoa growing.* http://www.cocoainitiative.org/images/stories/pdf/ICI_Leaflets_presentations/ICI_Information_Kit_-_April_2012_-_Child_Labour_in_Cocoa_Growing.pdf; accessed 10/31/13.

93. Mull DL, Kirkhorn SR. Child labor in Ghana cocoa production: focus upon agricultural tasks, ergonomic

exposures, and associated injuries and illnesses. *Public Health Rep* 2005;120(6):649–656.

94. Fair Trade USA. http://www.fairtradeusa.org/; accessed 10/31/2003.

95. Rainforest Alliance. Certification, verification, and validation services. http://www.rainforest-alliance.org/certification-verification; accessed 10/31/13.

96. Shute N. *Bean-to-bar chocolate makers dare to bare how it's done.* http://www.npr.org/blogs/thesalt/2013/02/13/171891081/bean-to-bar-chocolate-makers-dare-to-bare-how-its-done; accessed 10/31/13.

97. Martin FP, Rezzi S, Peré-Trepat E, et al. Metabolic effects of dark chocolate consumption on energy, gut microbiota, and stress-related metabolism in free-living subjects. *J Proteome Res* 2009;8(12):5568–5579.

98. Martin FJ, Montoliu I, Nagy K, et al. Specific dietary preferences are linked to differing gut microbial metabolic activity in response to dark chocolate intake. *J Proteome Res* 2012;11(12):6252–6263.

99. Moco S, Martin FP, Rezzi S. Metabolomics view on gut microbiome modulation by polyphenol-rich foods. *J Proteome Res* 2012;11(10):4781–4790.

CHAPTER 40

Health Effects of Ethanol

E thanol ingestion epitomizes for clinical and public health nutrition the concept of the double-edged sword. The harms of excessive alcohol consumption contribute mightily to the toll of preventable self-inflicted pathology. In a review of the causes of premature death in the world in the year 2004 by the World Health Organization (WHO), alcohol ranked third (1,1a). But the cardiovascular benefits of alcohol ingestion are also well characterized. This dichotomy is further compounded by the relatively narrow therapeutic window for ethanol and the fact that its dose-dependent risk/benefit ratio varies with circumstance (e.g., driving). There are thus ramifications related to the health effects of alcohol ingestion that pertain to public policy, law, and risk communication. Much of this is beyond the scope and intent of the current chapter. The focus here is limited to the common health effects, salutary and adverse, of dietary alcohol at or near recommended intake levels.

OVERVIEW

Alcoholic beverages vary widely in total nutrient composition. The common ingredient of particular interest is ethanol. Ethanol, otherwise known as ethyl alcohol, is one of several varieties of alcohol, and it is the predominant one in beverages. Ethanol, represented by the molecular formula C_2H_6O, is a fermentation product of sugar acted upon by several varieties of yeast in the absence of oxygen. Brewing refers to the process of combining yeast with fruits or germinated grains to produce ethanol.

Brewing per se can produce an alcohol concentration of up to approximately 25% by volume; more concentrated alcohol is toxic to the yeast. Alcoholic beverages are thus divided generally into fermented beverages and distilled beverages ("hard" alcohol). The ethanol concentration of fermented beverages, including beer and wine, is limited by the tolerance of yeast. Distilled

beverages, such as whiskey, gin, rye, vodka, and diverse spirits, concentrate alcohol well beyond the tolerance of yeast. The common term still refers to a device for the distillation, and thus concentration, of alcohol (2).

The concentration of alcohol in beverages is often expressed in terms of "proof" units, a designation of interesting but not relevant historical origin (3). In the United Kingdom, proof of 70 corresponds to an ethanol concentration by volume of roughly 40%; thus, conversion from proof to percentage calls for multiplication by 7/4. In the United States, proof is twice the percentage of alcohol content. By law, alcoholic beverages in the United States must indicate the percentage of alcohol content on the container.

Epidemiological study suggests that there are net health benefits from modest alcohol ingestion as compared to no intake at all. It is from this comparison that guidance for an advisable intake level derives. The Dietary Guidelines for Americans (4) advise, for those who choose to drink alcohol, an average daily intake of up to one drink for women and up to two drinks for men. A drink is defined as 10 to 15 g of ethanol contained in 12 oz beer, 5 oz wine, 3 oz fortified (dessert) wine, or 1.5 oz distilled spirits.

Evidence for a cardiovascular benefit of alcohol has been available for decades (5) and is very strong in the aggregate, although it is perhaps not definitive for want of long-term randomized trial data (6); such trials are precluded for fairly obvious reasons. Human epidemiological data from such sources as the Health Professionals Follow-Up Study in the United States (7) and the WHO's MONICA (Monitoring Trends and Determinants in Cardiovascular Disease Project) trial in Europe (8) suggest a reduction in cardiovascular mortality and morbidity with moderate alcohol intake and a reduction in all-cause mortality more specifically associated with red wine intake. The INTER-HEART study, a case-control study following 27,000 patients from 52 countries, found an association between regular alcohol consumption and a reduced incidence of myocardial infarction in both genders and in all age groups (9).

Evidence from population studies suggests that moderate alcohol intake may also reduce the risk of type 2 diabetes by as much as 40%, independent of other influences, although excessive intake actually increases such risk (10,11). This dose-dependent risk increase demonstrates a J-shaped curve as heavy alcohol use has been associated with increased mortality, in part, secondary to decreasing cardiac ejection fraction and progressive left ventricular hypertrophy (12,12a). The decrease in mortality begins to appear at intakes of more than two drinks daily in women and more than three drinks daily in men (13). Effects on stroke risk are unresolved, with available evidence suggesting neutral effects at recommended intake levels and harm with higher doses (14–17). Mechanisms for the beneficial effects of ethanol have been elucidated in human, animal, and cell culture studies (18). These include enhanced insulin sensitivity, increases in high-density lipoprotein (HDL) cholesterol, decreases in fibrinogen, increases in plasminogen and endogenous TPA, reduced inflammation, reduced platelet aggregation, reduced Lp(a), and improved endothelial function (8,13,19–21). Ethanol, when consumed by diabetic patients in small to moderate quantities with or immediately before the evening meal, has been shown to substantially reduce the glucose release following the meal (22,23). This important biologic phenomenon may play an important role in the epidemic of diabetes and obesity our nation currently faces. The biologic mechanism whereby alcohol improves insulin sensitivity is thought to involve the suppression of fatty acid release from adipose tissue, which decreases substrate competition in the Krebs cycle of skeletal muscles and facilitates glucose metabolism (13,22). Some studies suggest that ethanol is the primary explanation for such effects (21,24,25), whereas others have highlighted the potential importance of nutrients other than ethanol (26–29).

Red wine is one such beverage thought to offer health benefits for reasons other than its ethanol content (30–33). Bioflavonoid antioxidants are concentrated in the skins of grapes and are thus present in red wine. Several such nutrients, including proanthocyanidins and the flavonoids resveratrol and quercetin, are thought to contribute to the health profile of red wine. One paper (34) suggests that when highly concentrated, resveratrol, a compound found in red wine, may influence several key enzymes, such as SERT1 and genes involved in senescence, and may forestall aging in mice in a manner similar to calorie restriction. One study on the effects of a resveratrol-containing extract found higher levels of adiponectin, an anti-inflammatory compound, and lower levels of thrombogenic plasminogen activator inhibitor type 1 (PAI-1), an inflammatory compound, in the intervention group (35).

Another recent study found that 1-year consumption of a resveratrol-rich grape supplement improved the inflammatory and fibrinolytic status in patients who were on statins for primary prevention of CVD and at high CVD risk (36). Another study randomized 67 men with a high cardiovascular risk and randomly assigned them to consume red wine, dealcoholized red wine, and gin for 4 weeks. Both forms of wine were associated with decreases in markers of insulin resistance between 22% and 30%, while HDL levels in the groups who consumed alcohol (either red wine or gin) were statistically higher than those from the dealcoholized wine (33). Yet another study by Agarwal et al. found significantly decreased expression of proinflammatory markers (endothelial cell ICAM, VCAM, and IL-8) in patients who took a resveratrol supplement in comparison to placebo (37). The results of these studies collectively indicate that there are independent benefits from both wine (alcoholic or not) and the alcohol consumed (33). Of note, higher HDL-cholesterol levels have been linked to a significantly reduced risk for cancer (38).

Overall, wine consumption at prudent levels has been suggested to lower all-cause mortality rates by as much as 30% (39,40). Some researchers suggest that beneficial changes to hematologic parameters, such as whole blood viscosity and red blood cell deformability, contribute to these effects (41,42).

The harms of excessive ethanol ingestion are well established and are addressed to a limited extent in Chapter 17. There is some potential for harm at the recommended intake level as well (43). Such harms include increased risk for liver disease; pancreatitis; metabolic syndrome; and oropharyngeal, esophageal, colorectal, prostate, colorectal, and breast cancers (44–48). Overall, it is estimated that up to 4% of all breast cancers diagnosed in developed countries may be attributable to alcohol ingestion (49). Several large epidemiological studies suggest that alcohol increases the risk of estrogen receptor-positive breast cancer in a dose-dependent manner, with a relative risk increase of roughly 30% ascribed to moderate intake (50–52). A prospective observational study of over 105,000 women enrolled in the Nurses' Health Study followed over the course of 28 years evaluated the relative risk of developing invasive breast cancer and found that binge drinking, but not frequency of drinking, was associated with increased breast cancer risk after controlling for total alcohol intake. The authors noted that alcohol intake both earlier and later in adult life was independently associated with risk (53). In another large prospective study of over 87,000 women, Li et al. found an association between alcohol intake and hormone receptor-positive breast cancer of lobular type but not ductal type, when compared to nondrinkers (54). Interestingly, two published reports assessing alcohol intake as a risk factor for breast cancer recurrence and mortality found no increased association between modest alcohol intake and increased breast cancer events or mortality (55,56).

In addition, it has been noted that alcohol consumption is associated with increased prostate cancer risk, and this association is stronger among men with low folate intake (46), whereas a protective effect with light to moderate alcohol intake has been noted in association with renal cell carcinoma (57) and endometrial cancer (58). The mitigation of cancer risk with high folate levels also occurs with breast cancer risk, with higher folate levels being associated with lower cancer risk (59–62). Therefore, promoting diets rich in folate may be an important strategy for cancer prevention in both men and women who drink alcohol.

Colorectal cancer appears to be influenced by alcohol intake as well, with two meta-analyses showing a 50% increased risk for colon cancer and a 63% increase in rectal cancer in one analysis (63) and a 63% increase in risk for adenomas among higher alcohol consumers in the EPIC cohort (64). On a more positive note, dietary folate intake (but not supplemental folate) was found to have a protective effect on colon and rectal cancer risk among over 56,332 Danish subjects of the Danish Cohort Study who consumed more than 10 g of alcohol per day (65). The dose

at which ethanol confers net harm rather than benefit is highly variable, due at least in part to variations in genes for key alcohol-metabolizing enzymes, including alcohol dehydrogenase (66). A 2013 study by Barrio-Lopez et al. found an increased risk of developing metabolic syndrome in subjects consuming seven or more alcoholic beverages per week. These subjects were found to have elevated risks of hypertriglyceridemia as well as impaired fasting glucose. Beer consumption was independently associated with a higher risk for metabolic syndrome and hypertriglyceridemia (48). There are also individuals for whom any ethanol intake at all is more likely to do harm than good; these, of course, include anyone with a family history, and presumably the associated genetic polymorphisms, that predispose to alcoholism. Genetic polymorphisms likely also influence the probability of health benefit from moderate alcohol consumption (67).

Both the quantity and distribution of ethanol intake have health implications. Intermittent binges, even when the average daily intake is at recommended levels, have potentially adverse effects (44). Among these, the holiday heart syndrome, the induction of potentially lethal cardiac rhythm abnormalities following an alcohol binge (68,69), is noteworthy.

Overall, then, alcohol very clearly is a proverbial doubled-edged sword with regard to health effects, with potential to do both good and harm (44,10,14,70,71). The cumulative evidence of its effects has led many authors to recommend it with some enthusiasm (72,73) and others to urge caution (19).

Nutriceuticals

Resveratrol

As discussed in detail above, resveratrol is a well-studied, polyphenolic compound found in the skin of grapes. Initially used to treat cancer, it was noted to have many effects on various cardiovascular, metabolic, and cerebral disorders (74). It is found in higher concentrations in red grapes and is easily isolated for inclusion in supplement form. However, it's bioavailability is low and is generally an unstable molecule, with a short half-life is low and a prodrug addition may be necessary to reach adequate bioavailability in the body (75–77). Resveratrol is considered an antioxidant whose benefits include decreasing inflammatory markers (37), including but not limited to endothelial cell ICAM, VCAM, and IL-8, increasing HDL levels, and working to decrease markers of insulin resistance. It is thought to downregulate proinflammatory genes per research by Tomé-Carneiro et al. (35,36). A dose-dependent response has been noted in studies of flow-mediated dilation of the brachial artery in vivo with sustained effect after regular consumption (78). Due to its potent antiproliferative activity on cancer cells, resveratrol is being investigated for cancer treatment (79–82).

CLINICAL HIGHLIGHTS

The 2010 Dietary Guidelines for Americans (83) do not specifically recommend the consumption of alcohol as part of a health-promoting diet but rather specify the intake level advisable for those adults who choose to drink. That level is up to one drink (roughly 10 to 15 g of ethanol) per day for women and up to two drinks per day for men. A drink is defined as 12 oz beer, 5 oz wine, 3 oz fortified (dessert) wine, or 1.5 oz distilled spirits. The calorie range for a drink is generally 90 to 150 kcal. The Institute of Medicine, in its Dietary Reference Intakes (84), addresses the effects of alcohol on requirements for various nutrients but does not offer a recommended intake level for alcohol per se.

The case against a clear recommendation for alcohol consumption is predicated on several salient considerations. First, alcohol intake is neither recommended nor in many cases even legal for children. Second, alcohol is not an essential component of diet, nor does it, in its various forms, provide nutrients known to be essential and unavailable from other sources (85). Third, the toxicity of alcohol at excessive intake levels is clearly established (see Chapter 17), the therapeutic window separating healthful and harmful doses is relatively narrow, and the toxic dose varies substantially with individual vulnerability, predicated in part on variability in the activity of alcohol dehydrogenase and related enzymes (86–88). Fourth, the potential toxicity of alcohol varies with circumstance, and thus even a healthful intake level might be acutely harmful if ill timed. In lieu of high obesity rates and an ever-increasing caseloads of patients with metabolic syndrome, the energy density of alcohol might contribute a fifth, albeit lesser, indictment (48,89).

Despite these issues, however, a case can be made—and indeed has been made—for the explicit inclusion of alcohol in a health-promoting diet. Alcohol is featured along with fish, dark chocolate, fruits, vegetables, garlic, and almonds in a "polymeal" with the purported potential to reduce heart disease risk by more than 75% (72,35,36). Alcohol is prominent in the healthful Mediterranean diet and often invoked as a full or partial explanation for the "French paradox (90)."

Given the diverse implications of alcohol consumption for health, individualized clinical guidance is clearly warranted. In specific cases, some self-evident (e.g., a history of alcoholism or liver disease) and some more approximately toss-ups (e.g., a family history of breast cancer in a female patient), arguments against alcohol consumption will carry the day. Some argue that the potential for harm exceeds any potential benefit for the population at large (91). This view notwithstanding, a default recommendation for moderate intake of alcohol, and preferentially red wine, is reasonably well justified for the average patient (73,92).

REFERENCES

1. World Health Organization. *Global health risks: mortality and burden of disease attributable to selected major risks.* Available at http://www.who.int/healthinfo/global_burden_disease/GlobalHealthRisks_report_full.pdf; accessed 12/28/12.
1a. Mokdad AH, Marks JS, Stroup DF, et al. Actual causes of death in the United States, 2000. *JAMA* 2004;291:1238–1245.
2. Wikipedia. *Distillation.* Available at http://en.wikipedia.org/wiki/Distillation; accessed 11/6/07.
3. Wikipedia. *Proof (alcohol).* Available at http://en.wikipedia.org/wiki/Alcoholic_proof; accessed 11/6/07.
4. US Department of Health & Human Services. *Dietary guidelines for Americans, 2010.* Available at http://health.gov/dietaryguidelines/dga2010/DietaryGuidelines2010.pdf; accessed 12/28/12.
5. Hennekens CH, Willett W, Rosner B, et al. Effects of beer, wine, and liquor in coronary deaths. *JAMA* 1979;242:1973–1974.
6. Ruidavets JB, Bataille V, Dallongeville J, et al. Alcohol intake and diet in France, the prominent role of lifestyle. *Eur Heart J* 2004;25:1153–1162.
7. Harvard School of Public Health. *The Health Professionals Follow-Up Study (HPFS).* Available at http://www.hsph.harvard.edu/hpfs/. Last accessed date 5/11/14.
8. Imhof A, Woodward M, Doering A, et al. Overall alcohol intake, beer, wine, and systemic markers of inflammation in Western Europe: results from three MONICA samples (Augsburg, Glasgow, Lille). *Eur Heart J* 2004;25:2092–2100.

9. Yusuf S, Hawken S, Ounpuu S. INTER-HEART Study investigators: effect of potentially modifiable risk factors associated with myocardial infarction in 52 countries (the INTER-HEART study): case-control study. *Lancet* 2004; 364:937–952.

10. Conigrave KM, Rimm EB. Alcohol for the prevention of type 2 diabetes mellitus? *Treat Endocrinol* 2003;2:145–152.

11. Nilssen O, Averina M, Brenn T, et al. Alcohol consumption and its relation to risk factors for CV disease in the north-west of Russia: the Arkhangelsk study. *Int J Epidemiol* 2005; 34:781–788.

12. de Leiris J, de Lorgeril M, Boucher F. Ethanol and cardiac function. *Am J Physiol Heart Circ Physiol* 2006;291: H1027–H1028.

12a. Lucas DL, Brown RA, Wassef M, et al. Alcohol and the cardiovascular system. *J Am Coll Cardiol* 2005;45:1916–1924.

13. O'Keefe JH, Bybee KA, Lavie, CJ. Alcohol and health: the J-shaped curve. *Am Coll Cardiol* 2007;50(11):1009–1014.

14. Mukamal KJ, Ascherio A, Mittleman MA, et al. Alcohol and risk for ischemic stroke in men: the role of drinking patterns and usual beverage. *Ann Intern Med* 2005;142:11–19.

15. Mukamal KJ, Chung H, Jenny NS. Alcohol use and risk of ischemic stroke among older adults: the CV Health Study. *Stroke* 2005;36:1830–1834.

16. Mukamal KJ, Kuller LH, Fitzpatrick AL, et al. Prospective study of alcohol consumption and risk of dementia in older adults. *JAMA* 2003;289:1405–1413.

17. Klatsky AL. Alcohol and stroke: an epidemiological labyrinth. *Stroke* 2005;36:1835–1836.

18. Agarwal DP. Cardioprotective effects of light-moderate consumption of alcohol: a review of putative mechanisms. *Alcohol Alcohol* 2002;37:409–415.

19. Vogel RA. Alcohol, heart disease, and mortality: a review. *Rev Cardiovasc Med* 2002;3:7–13.

20. Ruf JC. Alcohol, wine and platelet function. *Biol Res* 2004;37:209–215.

21. Hansen AS, Marckmann P, Dragsted LO, et al. Effect of red wine and red grape extract on blood lipids, haemostatic factors, and other risk factors for cardiovascular disease. *Eur J Clin Nutr* 2005;59:449–455.

22. Greenfield JR, Samaras K, Hayward CS, et al. Beneficial postprandial effect of a small amount of alcohol on diabetes and CV risk factors: modification by insulin resistance. *J Clin Endocrinol Metab* 2005;90:661–672.

23. Turner BC, Jenkins E, Kerr D, et al. The effect of evening alcohol consumption on next-morning glucose control in type 1 diabetes. *Diabetes Care* 2001;24:1888–1893.

24. Mukamal KJ, Conigrave KM, Mittleman MA, et al. Roles of drinking pattern and type of alcohol consumed in coronary heart disease in men. *N Engl J Med* 2003;348:109–118.

25. Schroder H, Ferrandez O, Jimenez Conde J, et al. Cardiovascular risk profile and type of alcohol beverage consumption: a population-based study. *Ann Nutr Metab* 2005;49:100–106.

26. de Lange DW, van de Wiel A. Drink to prevent: review on the cardioprotective mechanisms of alcohol and red wine polyphenols. *Semin Vasc Med* 2004;4:173–186.

27. Constant J. Alcohol, ischemic heart disease, and the French paradox. *Coron Artery Dis* 1997;8:645–649.

28. Gronbaek M. Alcohol, type of alcohol, and all-cause and coronary heart disease mortality. *Ann N Y Acad Sci* 2002;957:16–20.

29. Sato M, Maulik N, Das DK. Cardioprotection with alcohol: role of both alcohol and polyphenolic antioxidants. *Ann N Y Acad Sci* 2002;957:122–135.

30. Burns J, Crozier A, Lean ME. Alcohol consumption and mortality: is wine different from other alcoholic beverages? *Nutr Metab Cardiovasc Dis* 2001;11:249–258.

31. Wu JM, Wang ZR, Hsieh TC, et al. Mechanism of cardioprotection by resveratrol, a phenolic antioxidant present in red wine (Review). *Int J Mol Med* 2001;8:3–17.

32. Quintieri AM, Baldino N, Filice E, et al. Malvidin, a red wine polyphenol, modulates mammalian myocardial and coronary performance and protects the heart against ischemia/reperfusion injury. *J Nutr Biochem* 2013; 24(7):1221–1231.

33. Chiva-Blanch G, Urpi-Sarda M, Ros E, et al. Effects of red wine polyphenols and alcohol on glucose metabolism and the lipid profile: a randomized clinical trial. *Clin Nutr* 2013;32(2):200–206.

34. Baur JA, Pearson KJ, Price NL, et al. Resveratrol improves health and survival of mice on a high-calorie diet. *Nature* 2006;444:337–342.

35. Tomé-Carneiro J, Gonzálvez M, Larrosa M, et al. Grape resveratrol increases serum adiponectin and downregulates inflammatory genes in peripheral blood mononuclear cells: a triple-blind, placebo-controlled, one-year clinical trial in patients with stable coronary artery disease. *Cardiovasc Drugs Ther* 2013;27(1):37–48.

36. Tomé-Carneiro J, Gonzalvez M, Larrosa M, et al. One-year consumption of a grape nutraceutical containing resveratrol improves the inflammatory and fibrinolytic status of patients in primary prevention of cardiovascular disease. *Am J Cardiol* 2012;110:356–363.

37. Agarwal B, Campen MJ, Channell MM, et al. Resveratrol for primary prevention of atherosclerosis: clinical trial evidence for improved gene expression in vascular endothelium, *Int J Cardiol* 2013;166(1):246–248; Available at http://dx.doi.org/10.1016/j.ijcard.2012.09.027. Last accessed on 5/11/14.

38. Jafri H, Alsheikh-Ali AA, Karas RH. Baseline and on-treatment high-density lipoprotein cholesterol and the risk of cancer in randomized controlled trials of lipid-altering therapy. *J Am Coll Cardiol* 2010;55(25):2846–2854.

39. Ruf JC. Overview of epidemiological studies on wine, health and mortality. *Drugs Exp Clin Res* 2003;29:173–179.

40. Renaud S, Lanzmann-Petithory D, Gueguen R, et al. Alcohol and mortality from all causes. *Biol Res* 2004;37: 183–187.

41. Toth A, Sandor B, Papp J, et al. Moderate red wine consumption improves hemorheological parameters in healthy volunteers. *Clin Hemorheol Microcirc* 2014;56(1):13–23.

42. Rabai M, Detterich JA, Wenby RB, et al. Effects of ethanol on red blood cell rheological behavior. *Clin Hemorheol Microcirc* 2014;56(2):87–99.

43. Bloss G. Measuring the health consequences of alcohol consumption: current needs and methodological challenges. *Dig Dis* 2005;23:162–169.

44. Taylor B, Rehm J, Gmel G. Moderate alcohol consumption and the gastrointestinal tract. *Dig Dis* 2005;23:170–176.

45. Gonzalez CA. Nutrition and cancer: the current epidemiological evidence. *Br J Nutr* 2006;96:s42–s45.

46. Kobayashi LC, Limburg H, Miao Q, et al. Folate intake, alcohol consumption, and the methylenetetrahydrofolate reductase (MTHFR) C677T gene polymorphism:

influence on prostate cancer risk and interactions. *Front Oncol* 2012;2:100.

47. Bagnardi V, Rota M, Botteri E, et al. Light alcohol drinking and cancer: a meta-analysis. *Ann Oncol* 2013;24(2): 301–308.

48. Barrio-Lopez MT, Bes-Rastrollo M, Sayon-Orea C, et al. Different types of alcoholic beverages and incidence of metabolic syndrome and its components in a Mediterranean cohort. *Clin Nutr* 2013;32(5):797–804.

49. Hamajima N, Hirose K, Tajima K, et al. Alcohol, tobacco and breast cancer collaborative reanalysis of individual data from 53 epidemiological studies, including 58,515 women with breast cancer and 95,067 women without the disease. *Br J Cancer* 2002;87:1234–1245.

50. Suzuki R, Ye W, Rylander-Rudqvist T, et al. Alcohol and postmenopausal breast cancer risk defined by estrogen and progesterone receptor status: a prospective cohort study. *J Natl Cancer Inst* 2005;97:1601–1608.

51. Petri AL, Tjonneland A, Gamborg M, et al. Alcohol intake, type of beverage, and risk of breast cancer in pre- and postmenopausal women. *Alcohol Clin Exp Res* 2004; 28:1084–1090.

52. Terry MB, Zhang FF, Kabat G, et al. Lifetime alcohol intake and breast cancer risk. *Ann Epidemiol* 2006;16:230–240.

53. Chen WY, Rosner B, Hankinson SE, et al. Moderate alcohol consumption during adult life, drinking patterns, and breast cancer risk. *JAMA* 2011;306(17):1884–1890.

54. Li CI, Chlebowski RT, Freiberg M, et al. Alcohol consumption and risk of postmenopausal breast cancer by subtype: the women's health initiative observational study. *J Natl Cancer Inst* 2010;102(18):1422–1431.

55. Flatt SW, Thomson CA, Gold EB, et al. Low to moderate alcohol intake is not associated with increased mortality after breast cancer. *Cancer Epidemiol Biomarkers Prev: a publication of the American Association for Cancer Research, cosponsored by the American Society of Preventive Oncology* 2010;19(3):681–688.

56. Hellmann SS, Thygesen LC, Tolstrup JS, et al. Modifiable risk factors and survival in women diagnosed with primary breast cancer: results from a prospective cohort study. *Eur J Cancer Prev* 2010;19(5):366–373.

57. Bellocco R, Pasquali E, Rota M, et al. Alcohol drinking and risk of renal cell carcinoma: results of a meta-analysis. *Ann Oncol* 2012;23(9):2235–2244.

58. Friedenreich CM, Speidel TP, Neilson HK, et al. Case-control study of lifetime alcohol consumption and endometrial cancer risk. *Cancer Causes Control* 2013;24(11):1995–2003. doi: 10.1007/s10552-013-0275-0.

59. Baglietto L, English DR, Gertig DM, et al. Does dietary folate intake modify effect of alcohol consumption on breast cancer risk? Prospective cohort study. *BMJ* 2005; 331(7520):807.

60. Rohan TE, Jain MG, Howe GR, et al. Dietary folate consumption and breast cancer risk. *J Natl Cancer Inst* 2000; 92(3):266–269.

61. Sellers TA, Kushi LH, Cerhan JR, et al. Dietary folate intake, alcohol, and risk of breast cancer in a prospective study of postmenopausal women. *Epidemiology* (Cambridge, MA) 2001;12(4):420–428.

62. Zhang SM, Willett WC, Selhub J, et al. Plasma folate, vitamin B6, vitamin B12, homocysteine, and risk of breast cancer. *J Natl Cancer Inst* 2003;95(5):373–380.

63. Moskal A, Norat T, Ferrari P, et al. Alcohol intake and colorectal cancer risk: a dose-response meta-analysis of published cohort studies. *Int J Cancer* 2007;120(3): 664–671.

64. Hermann S, Rohrmann S, Linseisen J. Lifestyle factors, obesity and the risk of colorectal adenomas in EPIC-Heidelberg. *Cancer Causes Control* 2009;20(8):1397–408.

65. Roswall N, Olsen A, Christensen J, et al. Micronutrient intake and risk of colon and rectal cancer in a Danish cohort. *Cancer Epidemiol* 2010;34(1):40–46.

66. Chase V, Neild R, Sadler CW, et al. The medical complications of alcohol use: understanding mechanisms to improve management. *Drug Alcohol Rev* 2005;24:253–265.

67. Li JM, Mukamal KJ. An update on alcohol and atherosclerosis. *Curr Opin Lipidol* 2004;15:673–680.

68. Fuenmayor AJ, Fuenmayor AM. Cardiac arrest following holiday heart syndrome. *Int J Cardiol* 1997;59:101–103.

69. Menz V, Grimm W, Hoffmann J, et al. Alcohol and rhythm disturbance: the holiday heart syndrome. *Herz* 1996;21:227–231.

70. Papadakis JA, Ganotakis ES, Mikhailidis DP. Beneficial effect of moderate alcohol consumption on vascular disease: myth or reality? *J R Soc Health* 2000;120:11–15.

71. Rehm J, Gmel G, Sempos CT, et al. Alcohol-related morbidity and mortality. *Alcohol Res Health* 2003;27:39–51.

72. Franco OH, Bonneux L, de Laet C, et al. The Polymeal: a more natural, safer, and probably tastier (than the Polypill) strategy to reduce cardiovascular disease by more than 75%. *BMJ* 2004;329:1447–1450.

73. Ellison RC. Balancing the risks and benefits of moderate drinking. *Ann N Y Acad Sci* 2002;957:1–6.

74. Carrizzo A, Forte M, Damato A, et al. Antioxidant effects of resveratrol in cardiovascular, cerebral and metabolic diseases. *Food Chem Toxicol* 2013;61:215–226. doi: 10.1016/j.fct.2013.07.021.

75. Santos JA, de Carvaho GS, Oliveira V, et al. Resveratrol and analogues: a review of antioxidant activity and applications to human health. *Recent Pat Food Nutr Agric* 2013;5(2):144–153.

76. Francioso A, Mastromarino P, Masci A, et al. Chemistry, stability and bioavailability of resveratrol. *Med Chem* 2014;10(3):237–245.

77. Biasutto L, Zoratti M. Prodrugs of quercetin and resveratrol: a strategy under development. *Curr Drug Metab* 2014;15(1):77–95.

78. Wong RH, Coates AM, Buckley JD, et al. Evidence for circulatory benefits of resveratrol in humans. *Ann N Y Acad Sci* 2013;1290:52–58. doi: 10.1111/nyas.12155.

79. Sala M, Chimento A, Saturnino C, et al. Synthesis and cytotoxic activity evaluation of 2,3-thiazolidin-4-one derivatives on human breast cancer cell lines. *Bioorg Med Chem Lett* 2013;23(17):4990–4995. doi: 10.1016/j.bmcl.2013.06.051.

80. Chimento A, Sala M, Gomez-Monterrey IM, et al. Biological activity of 3-chloro-azetidin-2-one derivatives having interesting antiproliferative activity on human breast cancer cell lines. *Bioorg Med Chem Lett* 2013;23(23):6401–6405. doi: 10.1016/j.bmcl.2013.09.054.

81. Aires V, Limagne E, Cotte AK, et al. Resveratrol metabolites inhibit human metastatic colon cancer cells progression and synergize with chemotherapeutic drugs to induce cell death. *Mol Nutr Food Res* 2013;57(7):1170–1181. doi: 10.1002/mnfr.201200766.

82. Amiot MJ, Romier B, Dao TM, et al. Optimization of trans-resveratrol bioavailability for human therapy. *Biochimie* 2013;95(6):1233–1238. doi: 10.1016/j.biochi.2013.01.008.

83. US Department of Health & Human Services. (Chapter 9: dalcoholic beverages) *Dietary Guidelines for Americans.* Available at http://www.health.gov/dietaryguidelines/dga2005/document/html/chapter9.htm; accessed 11/6/07.

84. Otten JJ, Hellwig JP, Meyers LD, eds. *Dietary reference intakes: the essential guide to nutrient requirements.* Washington, DC: National Academies Press, 2006.

85. Suter PM. Alcohol and mortality: if you drink, do not forget fruits and vegetables. *Nutr Rev* 2001;59:293–297.

86. Thomasson HR, Crabb DW, Edenberg HJ, et al. Alcohol and aldehyde dehydrogenase polymorphisms and alcoholism. *Behav Genet* 1993;23:131–136.

87. Tanaka F, Shiratori Y, Yokosuka O, et al. Polymorphism of alcohol-metabolizing genes affects drinking behavior and alcoholic liver disease in Japanese men. *Alcohol Clin Exp Res* 1997;21:596–601.

88. Couzigou P, Coutelle C, Fleury B, et al. Alcohol and aldehyde dehydrogenase genotypes, alcoholism and alcohol related disease. *Alcohol Alcohol Suppl* 1994;2:21–27.

89. Saris WH, Tarnopolsky MA. Controlling food intake and energy balance: which macronutrient should we select? *Curr Opin Clin Nutr Metab Care* 2003;6(6):609–613.

90. de Lange DW. From red wine to polyphenols and back: a journey through the history of the French Paradox. *Thromb Res* 2007;119:403–406.

91. Lieber CS. Alcohol and health: a drink a day won't keep the doctor away. *Cleve Clin J Med* 2003;70:945–946,948,951–953.

92. Hendriks HF, van Tol A. Alcohol. *Handb Exp Pharmacol* 2005;170:339–361.

CHAPTER 41

Health Effects of Coffee

C offee is one of the most widely consumed beverages around the world, and caffeine from coffee, tea, and chocolate constitutes the world's most popular psychoactive substance. Although known mostly for its caffeinated properties, coffee contains multiple bioactive compounds with potential health effects. Recent evidence supports an inverse association between coffee consumption and total as well as cause-specific mortality, including deaths from heart disease, respiratory disease, stroke, injuries and accidents, diabetes, and infection. Coffee consumption also has an inverse association with risk of a wide variety of chronic diseases, including type 2 diabetes mellitus, Parkinson's disease, and alcohol-related liver disease. Moderate coffee consumption appears to be safe for most individuals, but caution is advised for pregnant women, the elderly, and those with cardiovascular disease. Further research is warranted to help elucidate the precise mechanisms and extent of the potential health benefits of coffee.

OVERVIEW

Coffee contains a number of components with potential impact on human health (1), including caffeine, antioxidants, magnesium, potassium, and niacin (2). The major active ingredient in regular coffee is caffeine, a xanthine alkaloid compound. The main dietary sources of caffeine include coffee, tea, soft drinks, chocolate, and increasingly a wide variety of energy drinks (see Table 41.1). Though known to be mildly addictive, caffeine is considered by the Food and Drug Administration as a multiple-purpose GRAS (generally regarded as safe) substance (3).

Caffeine acts as a stimulant to the central nervous system, primarily through antagonism of adenosine receptors (4), leading to increased activity of dopamine and the experiential effects of enhanced alertness and reduced physical fatigue. Caffeine is rapidly absorbed from

TABLE 41.1

Amounts of Caffeine in Common Sources of Dietary Caffeine

Product (Serving Size)	Caffeine Content per Serving (mg)
Brewed coffee (8 oz)	137
Espresso (2 oz)	100
Instant coffee (8 oz)	76
Hot black tea (8 oz)	48
Caffeinated soft drink (12 oz)	37
Dark chocolate (1 bar, 1.45 oz)	30
Milk chocolate (1.55 oz bar)	11
Hot cocoa (12 oz)	8–12
Energy Drinks (8–16 oz)	50–300

Source: Adapted from US Department of Agriculture, 2000. Data obtained from the USDA Nutrient Data Laboratory: http://www.nal.usda.gov/fnic/foodcomp/search/.

the gastrointestinal tract, and maximum serum caffeine concentrations peak within 90 minutes after ingestion. Caffeine metabolism is carried out by the liver's cytochrome P450 1A2 enzyme (CYP1A2). Variations in individual's response to caffeine may be explained by genetic polymorphisms in CYP1A2 gene. In particular, people with defects in CYP1A2 may have impaired metabolism and prolonged effects, both desired and undesired (5). It is estimated that mean dietary caffeine consumption among adults in the United States is approximately 106 to 170 mg per day (6), well within the daily limit of 400 to 450 mg proposed by members of the Canadian Bureau of Chemical Safety (7).

High-dose caffeine consumption and withdrawal from regular consumption can lead to adverse effects. Consumption of caffeine in excess of 250 mg at one time (approximately 2 to 3 cups of brewed coffee) may lead to a distressing set of symptoms that include palpitations, insomnia, anxiety, psychomotor agitation, and gastrointestinal distress. The Diagnostic and

Statistical Manual of Mental Disorders includes diagnostic criteria for four related psychiatric disturbances: caffeine intoxication, caffeine-induced sleep disorder, caffeine-induced anxiety disorder, and caffeine-related disorder not otherwise specified (NOS) (8). In contrast, caffeine withdrawal can induce headaches, drowsiness, depression, and irritability. Both caffeinated and decaffeinated coffee may cause or exacerbate symptoms of peptic ulcer disease, erosive esophagitis, and gastroesophageal reflux disease (see Chapter 19). Moderate to high amounts of caffeine intake in those with bladder symptoms may be associated with an increased risk of detrusor instability and urinary incontinence (9,10).

Caffeine appears to cause a slight negative shift in calcium balance (11). High caffeine intake in older adults with preexisting vitamin D or calcium deficiencies may increase the risk of hip fracture (12), although an overall effect of caffeine or coffee on bone mineral density or development of osteoporosis has not been clearly established (13,14) (see Chapter 14).

Coffee consumption was first associated with increased blood pressure in the 1930s (15). Both caffeinated and decaffeinated coffee have been shown to raise blood pressure acutely by as much as 10 mmHg in nonhabitual caffeine consumers (16), with greater effects seen in individuals with preexisting hypertension (17); however, these effects are all but eliminated with regular caffeine consumption (16).

Results from long-term studies are showing that chronic coffee intake may not increase the risk for hypertension over time, as was previously thought (18). A prospective cohort study of 155,594 US women found no linear association between caffeine or coffee intake and incident hypertension. Of note, in subgroup analysis of individual classes of caffeinated beverages, the investigators did find an increased risk of hypertension associated with consumption of sugared or diet cola beverages (19) (see Chapter 8).

Case reports have documented the development of clinically significant cardiac arrhythmias following the ingestion of extremely high doses of caffeine, especially in those with underlying cardiac disease (20). Reports of adverse events related to energy drinks and supplements continue to be collected by the Food and Drug Administration and include several deaths and hospitalizations. While energy drinks have yet to be studied

in depth (21), they should be consumed with caution, especially in children and young teenagers.

The evidence to date does not support an association between moderate doses of caffeine and increased risk of atrial (22) or ventricular (23) arrhythmias, even among patients with existing arrhythmias (24). One large meta-analysis including over 115,000 individuals found that low-dose caffeine may even have a protective effect (25).

Evidence to date does not support a clear association between coffee intake and increased risk of coronary heart disease (26,27). In fact, recent studies have found that when controlling for associated factors like increased smoking, coffee consumption may result in a modest decrease in cardiovascular mortality (28,29). However, coffee consumption may be associated with increased incidence of cardiovascular risk factors, which may indirectly affect cardiovascular health. For example, two substances in unfiltered coffee, kaweol and cafestol, have been shown to raise serum total cholesterol levels and low-density lipoprotein levels (30). The difference in preparation method has become more relevant as unfiltered coffee has increased in prevalence. More studies distinguishing preparation method, comparing boiling, filtering, french press, and brewed are warranted. The effects of cafestol and kahweol can generally be avoided by switching from unfiltered to paper-filtered coffee (31).

Caffeine crosses the placenta, and there is some evidence suggesting possible adverse effects on fetal growth and development (32). Evidence for an association between caffeine consumption and increased risk of spontaneous abortion is mixed (33–35); Signorello and McLaughlin (36) reviewed the evidence in 2004 and concluded that although many studies to date had found evidence of an association between caffeine intake and miscarriage, the methodological limitations and biases inherent in a majority of the studies precluded clear causal inferences. The 2013 Cochrane review also found insufficient evidence from randomized trials to either confirm or refute the potential for caffeine avoidance or consumption to affect pregnancy outcomes (37). The American College of Obstetricians and Gynecologists developed an updated consensus statement in 2013 that less than 200 mg of caffeine, classified as "moderate intake," was not associated with miscarriage or preterm birth. They concluded that data regarding more than moderate intake were inconclusive (38).

Similarly, there is some evidence that high caffeine intake during pregnancy may be associated with infants of low birth weight or small for gestational age (39,40), though other studies have not observed clinically significant differences (41). One randomized controlled trial by Bech et al. (42) found no effect of reducing caffeine consumption during pregnancy on mean birth weight or length of gestation. The authors speculated that previous nonexperimental studies may not have been able to adequately account for known association between caffeine intake and smoking and alcohol intake, both of which may influence birth weight (41).

A systematic review of studies examining the potential teratogenicity of caffeine concluded that there is no evidence that maternal caffeine exposure causes large increases in congenital anomalies, but the data are insufficient to rule out small risks for certain congenital anomalies (43). The few studies available on caffeine's effect on fertility have had varying results. One study found that high caffeine consumption may have had an effect on time to conception among women trying to conceive (44), although another found that caffeine consumption had no effect on the overall rates of conception (45). Regardless, more studies are needed to verify this link.

Caffeine does have several documented health benefits. Caffeine can be used as an ergogenic aid (46), improving performance and delaying fatigue in long-duration physical activity (47) (see Chapter 32).

Perhaps the most intriguing evidence to emerge in the past few years related to the potential health benefits of coffee stems from multiple prospective epidemiological studies demonstrating that long-term coffee consumption is associated with a statistically significant reduction of risk of type 2 diabetes mellitus (48,49). The systematic review of prospective cohort studies conducted by van Dam and Hu (50) found a relative risk of 0.65 (95% CI, 0.54 to 0.78) for type 2 diabetes in the highest group of coffee consumers (more than 6 or 7 cups per day) and a relative risk of 0.72 in the second-highest category of coffee consumption (4 to 6 cups per day), when compared to those consuming zero to 2 cups per day. This relationship held up regardless of sex, obesity, or geographic region.

The mechanisms by which coffee could potentially improve insulin sensitivity are not well understood, although several hypotheses exist. Coffee has been found to increase plasma adiponectin levels, leading to decreased insulin resistance (51). Caffeine has also recently been found to increase plasma levels of sex hormone binding globulin, a key modulator of sex hormones' effects on glucose homeostasis (52). Another interesting possibility is that long-term caffeine consumption has an upregulating effect on insulin-like growth factor 1 signaling, effectively increasing insulin sensitivity (53).

Of particular note, a modest inverse association between coffee and diabetes has also been found with decaffeinated coffee (54). Initially, these findings were surprising because caffeine and caffeinated coffee were known to impair glucose metabolism acutely following ingestion (55,56), primarily through impairment of glucose uptake by skeletal muscle (57). However, one randomized trial with crossover design found that intake of pure caffeine led to greater increases in plasma glucose than did equivalently caffeinated coffee (58), suggesting both that certain components in coffee may antagonize caffeine-induced glucose impairment and also that decaffeinated coffee may be most useful for diabetes prevention (59). Investigation has now turned to chlorogenic acid, an antioxidant present in coffee, to better understand the precise mechanisms underlying this association.

Coffee is the major dietary source of the antioxidant phenol chlorogenic acid, and it is a major contributor to the overall antioxidant capacity of the diet (60). Chlorogenic acid and other coffee-derived antioxidants may counter the oxidative forces that are thought to contribute to the development of insulin resistance and diabetes (61). In addition, chlorogenic acid has been shown to enhance intestinal glucose uptake (62), inhibit the glucose-6-phosphatase system (63), and stimulate glucose transport in skeletal muscles (64), all of which may represent potential mechanisms for enhanced glucose control (65).

Increasing evidence indicates that coffee consumption may offer protection against the development of Parkinson's disease in men (66). Ross et al. (67), examining data on more than 8,000 Japanese American men who completed 24-hour diet recalls and food frequency questionnaires were subsequently followed for up to 30 years, found that the age- and smoking-adjusted risk of Parkinson's disease for coffee abstainers was five-fold that of men reporting daily coffee consumption of 28 oz or more. It is unknown what mechanism accounts for the observed protective effects, but one probable mechanism involves the facilitation of dopamine D_2 receptor transmission by caffeine-induced blockage of adenosine receptors in the basal ganglia. A subsequent study of two large cohorts found similar results for men but not in women (68). In women, estrogen competes with caffeine for metabolism by the CYP1A2 isoenzyme of the P450 family and may inhibit its effects; one study addressing this hypothesis found that among postmenopausal women, those who used postmenopausal hormones and consumed coffee had an increased risk of Parkinson's disease compared to non-coffee drinkers, whereas those who never used hormones and drank coffee had a lower risk of Parkinson's disease than non-coffee drinkers (69). While caffeine's application as a therapeutic agent has undergone continued exploration, the current data do not support its use for treatment of the symptoms associated with Parkinson's disease (70).

Preliminary evidence has suggested a reduced risk of gallbladder disease in women who drink caffeinated coffee (71); however, data linking coffee consumption and reduced risk of gallstones in both men and women are mixed (72,73).

Recent cross-sectional studies by Choi et al. suggest an inverse association between coffee consumption and hyperuricemia (74,75) or risk of gout. Caffeine, a methyl xanthine, has been shown in animal models to competitively inhibit xanthine oxidase (76,77) and so might theoretically behave in humans in a manner similar to allopurinol; however, total caffeine or tea intake does not appear to be associated with hyperuricemia, raising the possibility that other non-caffeine components of coffee are contributing to this relationship (74).

Evidence to date does not support a relationship between coffee consumption and increased risk of cancer, including pancreatic, renal cell, colorectal, bladder, ovarian, breast, gastric, and prostate cancers (78–80). In fact, evidence from both case-control and prospective cohort studies has suggested an inverse association between coffee drinking and risk of hepatocellular carcinoma, particularly in those with preexisting cirrhosis or previously infected with hepatitis B or hepatitis C

virus (81). Inoue et al. (82) followed more than 90,000 Japanese men and women for 10 years and found that daily consumption of 5 or more cups of coffee was associated with a 76% lower risk of hepatocellular carcinoma when compared to coffee abstainers. Recent evidence suggests that caffeinated coffee may be necessary to acquire protective effects (83).

Coffee consumption has been inversely associated with the risk of cirrhosis (84) and with the risk of death from alcohol-related cirrhosis (85). Furthermore, a large study by Ruhl and Everhart (86) demonstrated an inverse association between coffee consumption and alanine aminotransferase (ALT), and the coffee-derived antioxidants cafestol and kahweol have also been implicated as contributing to the ability of coffee to prevent liver disease (87).

Another possible health benefit of coffee consumption is decreased risk of endometrial cancer. One case-control study found that consuming 1 to 2 cups and 3 or more cups of coffee per day was associated with an odds ratio for endometrial cancer of 0.64 (95% CI, 0.43 to 0.94) and 0.41 (95% CI, 0.19 to 0.87), respectively (88). Other studies, including a population-based cohort study with 15 years of follow-up, found similar relative risks (89).

Evidence from earlier case-control studies suggested an inverse association between coffee drinking and risk of colorectal cancer, although there was no consistent dose response (90). Data from prospective studies, however, have been contradictory. While earlier studies found no relationship (91), a more recent cohort study from Japan suggests a risk reduction for colorectal cancer in women but not in men (92). While evidence of preventative effect is weak at best, there is strong evidence of no harmful effect.

Coffee contains compounds shown to inhibit absorption of both iron (93,94) and zinc (95). Adequate intake of these nutrients to compensate for these effects in habitual coffee drinkers may assume some importance.

■ CLINICAL HIGHLIGHTS

Moderate amounts of coffee appear to be safe and may confer several health benefits. Concerns about potentially harmful cardiovascular effects of coffee or caffeine intake have been largely unsubstantiated. Pregnant women are advised to limit caffeine consumption to no more than 200 mg per day (roughly 1 cup of coffee) as a precautionary measure against the possibility of spontaneous abortion or impaired fetal growth. Coffee consumption may offer modest protection against type 2 diabetes. Coffee intake at high levels has long been associated with cigarette smoking, which of course poses diverse health threats and may have fostered an apparently fallacious impression of coffee-related harms. Coffee and caffeine-containing beverages may exacerbate symptoms of GERD; susceptible individuals are advised to reduce or eliminate intake for a trial of 3 to 6 months to see whether symptoms are alleviated. For most patients, moderate coffee consumption may certainly be sanctioned as part of a healthful dietary pattern.

REFERENCES

1. Higdon JV, Frei B. Coffee and health: a review of recent human research. *Crit Rev Food Sci Nutr* 2006;46101–46123.
2. US Department of Agriculture and Agricultural Research Service. *USDA nutrient database for standard reference.* Available at http://www.nal.usda.gov/fnic/foodcomp/search; accessed 11/7/07.
3. US Office of the Federal Register. 21 CFR 182.1180. US Code of Federal Regulations 462, April 1, 2003.
4. Fisone G, Borgkvist A, Usiello A. Caffeine as a psychomotor stimulant: mechanism of action. *Cell Mol Life Sci* 2004;61:857–872.
5. Cornelis MC, El-Sohemy A, Kabagambe EK, et al. Coffee, CYP1A2 genotype, and risk of myocardial infarction. *JAMA* 2006;295:1135.
6. Knight CA, Knight I, Mitchell DC, et al. Beverage caffeine intake in US consumers and subpopulations of interest: estimates from the Share of Intake Panel survey. *Food Chem Toxicol* 2004;42:1923–1930.
7. Nawrot P, Jordan S, Eastwood J, et al. Effects of caffeine on human health. *Food Addit Contam* 2003;20:1–30.
8. American Psychiatric Association. *Diagnostic and statistical manual of mental disorders,* 5th ed. Washington, DC: American Psychiatric Association, 2013.
9. Lohsiriwat S, Hirunsai M, Chaiyaprasithi B. Effect of caffeine on bladder function in patients with overactive bladder symptoms. *Urol Ann* 2011;3:14–18.
10. Jura YH, Townsend MK, Curhan GC, et al. Caffeine intake, and the risk of stress, urgency and mixed urinary incontinence. *J Urol* 2011;185(5):1775–1780.
11. Heaney RP. Effects of caffeine on bone and the calcium economy. *Food Chem Toxicol* 2002;40:1263–1270.
12. Massey LK. Is caffeine a risk factor for bone loss in the elderly? *Am J Clin Nutr* 2001;74:569–570.
13. Hannan MT, Felson DT, Dawson-Hughes B. Risk factors for longitudinal bone loss in elderly men and women: the Framingham Osteoporosis Study. *J Bone Miner Res* 2000;15:1119–1126.
14. Lloyd T, Johnson-Rollings N, Eggli DF. Bone status among postmenopausal women with different habitual caffeine intakes: a longitudinal investigation. *J Am Coll Nutr* 2000;19:256–261.
15. Horst K, Buxton RE, Robinson WD. The effect of the habitual use of coffee or decaffeinated coffee upon blood pressure and certain motor reactions of normal young men. *J Pharmacol Exp Ther* 1934;52:322–337.
16. Corti R, Binggeli C, Sudano I, et al. Coffee acutely increases sympathetic nerve activity and blood pressure independently of caffeine content: role of habitual versus nonhabitual drinking. *Circulation* 2002;106:2935–2940.
17. Hartley TR, Sung BH, Pincomb GA, et al. Hypertension risk status and effect of caffeine on blood pressure. *Hypertension* 2000;36:137–141.
18. Klag MJ, Wang N-Y, Meoni LA, et al. Coffee intake and risk of hypertension: the Johns Hopkins precursors study. *Arch Intern Med* 2002;162:657–662.
19. Winkelmayer WC, Stampfer MJ, Willett WC, et al. Habitual caffeine intake and the risk of hypertension in women. *JAMA* 2005;294:2330–2335.
20. Cannon ME, Cooke CT, McCarthy JS. Caffeine-induced cardiac arrhythmia: an unrecognized danger of healthfood products. *Med J Aust* 2001;174:520–521.
21. Burrows T, Pursey K, Neve M, et al. What are the health implications associated with the consumption of energy drinks? A systematic review. *Nutr Rev* 2013;71:135–148.
22. Frost L, Vestergaard P. Caffeine and risk of atrial fibrillation or flutter: the Danish Diet, Cancer, and Health Study. *Am J Clin Nutr* 2005;81:578–582.
23. Chelsky LB, Cutler JE, Griffith K, et al. Caffeine and ventricular arrhythmia. An electrophysiological approach. *JAMA* 1990;264:2236–2240.
24. Myers MG. Caffeine and cardiac arrhythmias. *Ann Intern Med* 1991;114:147–150.
25. Caldeira D, Martins C, Alves LB, et al. Caffeine does not increase the risk of atrial fibrillation: a systematic review and meta-analysis of observational studies. *Heart* 2013;99:1383–1389.
26. Lopez-Garcia E, van Dam RM, Willett WC, et al. Coffee consumption and coronary heart disease in men and women: a prospective cohort study. *Circulation* 2006;113:2045–2053.
27. Sofi F, Conti AA, Gori AM, et al. Coffee consumption and risk of coronary heart disease: a meta-analysis. *Nutr Metab Cardiovasc Dis* 2007;17:209–223.
28. Freedman ND, Park Y, Abnet CC, et al. Association of coffee drinking with total and cause-specific mortality. *N Engl J Med* 2012;366:1891–1904.
29. Lopez-Garcia E, van Dam RM, Li TY, et al. The relationship of coffee consumption with mortality. *Ann Intern Med* 2008;148:904.
30. Ricketts ML, Boekschoten MV, Kreeft AJ, et al. The cholesterol-raising factor from coffee beans, cafestol, as an agonist ligand for the farnesoid and pregnane X receptors. *Mol Endocrinol* 2007;21:1603–1616.
31. Urgert R, Meyboom S, Kuilman M, et al. Comparison of effect of cafetiere and filtered coffee on serum concentrations of liver aminotransferases and lipids: a six month randomized controlled trial. *BMJ* 1996;313:1362–1366.
32. Balat O, Balat A, Ugur MG, et al. The effect of smoking and caffeine on the fetus and placenta in pregnancy. *Clin Exp Obstet Gynecol* 2003;30:57–59.
33. Savitz DA, Chan RL, Herring AH, et al. Caffeine and miscarriage risk. *Epidemiology* 2008;19:55–62.

34. Bech BH, Nohr EA, Vaeth M, et al. Coffee and fetal death: a cohort study with prospective data. *Am J Epidemiol* 2005;162:983–990.

35. Cnattingius S, Signorello LB, Anneren G, et al. Caffeine intake and the risk of first-trimester spontaneous abortion. *N Engl J Med* 2000;343:1839–1845.

36. Signorello LB, McLaughlin JK. Maternal caffeine consumption and spontaneous abortion: a review of epidemiologic evidence. *Epidemiology* 2004;15:229–239.

37. Jahanfar S, Sharifah H. Effects of restricted caffeine intake by mother on fetal, neonatal and pregnancy outcome. *Cochrane Database Syst Rev* 2009;(2):CD006965.

38. American College of Obstetricians and Gynecologists. ACOG Committee Opinion No.462. Moderate caffeine consumption during pregnancy. *Obstet Gynecol* 2010;116(2 pt1):467–468.

39. Vik T, Bakketeig LS, Trygg KU, et al. High caffeine consumption in the third trimester of pregnancy: gender-specific effects on fetal growth. *Paediatr Perinat Epidemiol* 2003;17:324–331.

40. CARE Study Group. Maternal caffeine intake during pregnancy and risk of fetal growth restriction: a large prospective observational study. *BMJ* 2008;337:a2332.

41. Bracken MB, Triche EW, Belanger K, et al. Association of maternal caffeine consumption with decrements in fetal growth. *Am J Epidemiol* 2003;157:456–466.

42. Bech BH, Obel C, Henriksen TB, et al. Effect of reducing caffeine intake on birth weight and length of gestation: randomized controlled trial. *BMJ* 2007;334:409.

43. Browne M. Maternal exposure to caffeine and risk of congenital anomalies: a systematic review. *Epidemiology* 2006;17:324–331.

44. Bolumar F, Olsen J, Rebagliato M, et al. Caffeine intake and delayed conception: a European multicenter study on infertility and subfecundity. European Study Group on infertility subfecundity. *Am J Epidemiol* 1997;145:324–334.

45. Al-Saleh I, El-Doush I, Grisellhi B, et al. The effect of caffeine consumption on the success rate of pregnancy as well various performance parameters of in-vitro fertilization treatment. *Med Sci Monit* 2010;16:CR598.

46. Juhn MS. Ergogenic aids in aerobic activity. *Curr Sports Med Rep* 2002;1:233–238.

47. Davis JM, Zhao Z, Stock HS, et al. Central nervous system effects of caffeine and adenosine on fatigue. *Am J Physiol Regul Integr Comp Physiol* 2003;284:r399–r404.

48. van Dam RM, Feskens EJ. Coffee consumption and risk of type 2 diabetes mellitus. *Lancet* 2002;360:1477–1478.

49. Tuomilehto J, Hu G, Bidel S, et al. Coffee consumption and risk of type 2 diabetes mellitus among middle-aged Finnish men and women. *JAMA* 2004;291:1213–1219.

50. van Dam RM, Hu FB. Coffee consumption and risk of type 2 diabetes: a systematic review. *JAMA* 2005;294:97–104.

51. Williams CJ, Fargnoli JL, Hwang JJ, et al. Coffee consumption is associated with higher plasma adiponectin concentrations in women with or without type 2 diabetes: a prospective cohort study. *Diabetes Care* 2008;31:504.

52. Ding EL, Song Y, Manson JE, et al. Sex hormone-binding globulin and risk of type 2 diabetes in women and men. *N Engl J Med* 2009;361:1152.

53. Park S, Jang JS, Hong SM. Long-term consumption of caffeine improves glucose homeostasis by enhancing insulinotropic action through islet insulin/insulin-like growth factor 1 signaling in diabetic rats. *Metabolism* 2007;56:599.

54. Huxley R, Lee CM, Barzi F, et al. Coffee, decaffeinated coffee, and tea consumption in relation to incident type 2 diabetes mellitus: a systematic review with meta-analysis. *Arch Intern Med* 2009;169:2053.

55. Lane JD, Surwit RS, Barkauskas CE, et al. Caffeine impairs glucose metabolism in type 2 diabetes. *Diabetes Care* 2004;27:2047–2048.

56. Robinson LE, Savani S, Battram DS, et al. Caffeine ingestion before an oral glucose tolerance test impairs blood glucose management in men with type 2 diabetes. *J Nutr* 2004;134:2528–2533.

57. Thong FS, Derave W, Kiens B, et al. Caffeine-induced impairment of insulin action but not insulin signaling in human skeletal muscle is reduced by exercise. *Diabetes* 2002;51:583–590.

58. Battram DS, Arthur R, Weekes A, et al. The glucose intolerance induced by caffeinated coffee is less pronounced than that due to alkaloid caffeine in men. *J Nutr* 2006;136:1276–1280.

59. Greenberg JA, Boozer CN, Geliebter A. Coffee, diabetes, and weight control. *Am J Clin Nutr* 2006;84:682–693.

60. Clifford MN. Chlorogenic acid and other cinnamates—nature, occurrence, dietary burden, absorption and metabolism. *J Sci Food Agric* 2000;80:1033–1043.

61. Ceriello A, Motz E. Is oxidative stress the pathogenic mechanism underlying insulin resistance, diabetes, and cardiovascular disease? The common soil hypothesis revisited. *Arterioscler Thromb Vasc Biol* 2004;24:816–823.

62. Rodriguez de Sotillo DV, Hadley M. Chlorogenic acid modifies plasma and liver concentrations of: cholesterol, triacylglycerol, and minerals in (fa/fa) Zucker rats. *J Nutr Biochem* 2002;13:717–726.

63. Herling AW, Burger HJ, Schwab D. Pharmacodynamic profile of a novel inhibitor of the hepatic glucose-6-phosphatase system. *Am J Physiol* 1998;274:g1087–g1093.

64. Ong KW, Hsu A, Tan BK. Chlorogenic acid stimulates glucose transport in skeletal muscle via AMPK activation: a contributor to the beneficial effects of coffee on diabetes. *PLoS One* 2012;7(3):e32718.

65. Meng S, Cao J, Feng Q, et al. Roles of chlorogenic acid on regulating glucose and lipids metabolism: a review. *Evid Based Complement Alternat Med* 2013;2013:801457.

66. Ascherio A, Honglei C. Caffeinated clues for epidemiology of Parkinson's disease. *Neurology* 2003;s51–s54.

67. Ross GW, Abbott RD, Petrovich H, et al. Association of coffee and caffeine intake with the risk of Parkinson disease. *JAMA* 2000;283:2674–2679.

68. Ascherio A, Zhang SM, Hernan MA, et al. Prospective study of caffeine consumption and risk of Parkinson's disease in men and women. *Ann Neurol* 2001;50:56–63.

69. Ascherio A, Chen H, Schwarzschild MA, et al. Caffeine, postmenopausal estrogen, and risk of Parkinson's disease. *Neurology* 2003;60:790–795.

70. Postuma RB, Lang AE, Munhoz RP, et al. Caffeine for treatment of Parkinson disease: a randomized controlled trial. *Neurology* 2012;79(7):651–658.

71. Leitzmann MF, Stampfer MJ, Willett WC, et al. Coffee intake is associated with lower risk of symptomatic gallstone disease in women. *Gastroenterology* 2002;123:1823–1830.

72. Ruhl CE, Everhart JE. Association of coffee consumption with gallbladder disease. *Am J Epidemiol* 2000;152:1034–1038.

73. Ishizuk H, Eguchi H, Oda T, et al. Relation of coffee, green tea, and caffeine intake to gallstone disease in middle-aged Japanese men. *Eur J Epidemiol* 2003;18:401–405.

74. Choi HK, Curhan G. Coffee, tea, and caffeine consumption and serum uric acid level: the third national health and examination survey. *Arthritis Care and Research* 2007;57:816–821.

75. Choi HK, Willett W, Curhan G. Coffee consumption and risk of incident gout in men: a prospective study. *Arthritis Rheum* 2007;56:2049–2055.

76. Kela U, Vijzyvargiya R, Trivedi CP. Inhibitory effects of methylxanthines on the activity of xanthine oxidase. *Life Sci* 1980;27:2109–2119.

77. Miners JO, Birkett DJ. The use of caffeine as a metabolic probe for human drug metabolizing enzymes. *Gen Pharmacol* 1996;27:245–249.

78. Arab L. Epidemiologic evidence on coffee and cancer. *Nutr Cancer* 2010;62(3):271–283.

79. World Cancer Research Fund. *Food, nutrition, physical activity and the prevention of cancer: a global perspective.* 2007. Available from: http://www.dietandcancerreport.org/

80. Lee JE, Hunter DJ, Spiegelman D, et al. Intakes of coffee, tea, milk, soda, and juice and renal cell cancer in a pooled analysis of 13 prospective studies. *Int J Cancer* 2007;121:2246–2253.

81. Shimazu T, Tsubono Y, Kuriyama S, et al. Coffee consumption and the risk of primary liver cancer: pooled analysis of two prospective studies in Japan. *Int J Cancer* 2005;116:150–154.

82. Inoue M, Yoshimi I, Sobue T, et al. Influence of coffee drinking on subsequent risk of hepatocellular carcinoma: a prospective study in Japan. *J Natl Cancer Inst* 2005;97:293–300.

83. Montella M, Polesel J, La Vecchia C, et al. Coffee and tea consumption and risk of hepatocellular carcinoma in Italy. *Int J Cancer* 2007;120:1555–1559.

84. Corrao G, Zambon A, Bagnardi V. Coffee, caffeine, and the risk of liver cirrhosis. *Ann Epidemiol* 2001;11:458–465.

85. Tverdal A, Skurtveit S. Coffee intake and mortality from liver cirrhosis. *Ann Epidemiol* 2003;13:419–423.

86. Ruhl C, Everhart J. Coffee and caffeine consumption reduce the risk of elevated serum alanine aminotransferase activity in the United States. *Gastroenterology* 2005;128:24–32.

87. Homan DJ, Mobarhan S. Coffee: good, bad, or just fun? A critical review of coffee's effects on liver enzymes. *Nutr Rev* 2006;64:43–46.

88. Hirose K, Niwa Y, Wakai K, et al. Coffee consumption and the risk of endometrial cancer: evidence from a case-control study of female hormone-related cancers in Japan. *Cancer Sci* 2007;98:411–415.

89. Shimazu T, Inoue M, Sasazuki S, et al. Coffee consumption and risk of endometrial cancer: a prospective study in Japan. *Int J Cancer* 2008;123:2406–2410.

90. Michels KB, Willett WC, Fuchs CS, et al. Coffee, tea, and caffeine consumption and incidence of colon and rectal cancer. *J Natl Cancer Inst* 2005;97:282–292.

91. Tavani A, La Vecchia C. Coffee, decaffeinated coffee, tea and cancer of the colon and rectum: a review of epidemiological studies, 1990–2003. *Cancer Causes Control* 2004;15:743–757.

92. Lee KJ, Inoue M, Otani T, et al. Coffee consumption and risk of colorectal cancer in a population-based prospective cohort of Japanese men and women. *Int J Cancer* 2007;121:1312–1318.

93. Fairweather-Tait SJ. Iron nutrition in the UK: getting the balance right. *Proc Nutr Soc* 2004;63:519–528.

94. Morck TA, Lynch SR, Cook JD. Inhibition of food iron absorption by coffee. *Am J Clin Nutr* 1983;37:416–420.

95. Wen X, Enokizo A, Hattori H. Effect of roasting on properties of the zinc-chelating substance in coffee brews. *J Agric Food Chem* 2005;53:2684–2689.

CHAPTER 42

Macronutrient Food Substitutes

Macronutrient substitutes are generally used to replace either sugar or fat in the diet. The intent of such substitutions is to reduce caloric intake, dental caries, and chronic disease risk and to improve glucose and insulin metabolism and serum lipid levels. Carbohydrate substitutes may be used to replace starch as well as sugar. Fat is replaced with other macronutrients (protein or carbohydrate) modified to mimic the sensory characteristics of fat; synthetic substitutes that replace fat on a gram-for-gram basis but provide fewer or even no calories; or reduced-calorie fat molecules. Sugar substitutes are divided into nonnutritive intense sweeteners and nutritive bulk sweeteners.

OVERVIEW

Sweeteners/Sugar Substitutes

White sugar, usually in the form of granulated sugar, is purified sucrose, the crystals of which are naturally white. Brown sugar is less refined, containing some molasses from sugar cane. Alternatively, manufacturers may add back molasses to purified sucrose in order to control the ratio and the color.

Nutritionally, the differences between white and brown sugar are fairly trivial. When matched on the basis of volume, brown sugar has more calories because it tends to pack more densely; 1 cup of brown sugar provides 829 calories, while 1 cup of white granulated sugar provides 774 calories. However, when matched by weight, brown sugar has slightly fewer calories due to the presence of water in the molasses; 100 g of brown sugar contains 373 calories, as opposed to 396 calories in white sugar (1). Sugar crystals provide no nutrients other than sucrose, but molasses contains enough calcium, iron, and potassium to distinguish it from white sugar, although not enough to make it an important source.

Nonnutritive sweeteners are sugar substitutes that provide no, or virtually no, calories. To date, the Food and Drug Administration (FDA) has approved seven artificial, nonnutritive sweeteners: saccharin, acesulfame-K, aspartame, neotame, luo han guo fruit extract, sucralose, and one natural low-calorie sweetener, stevia. The safety and long-term health effects of these products have often come under scrutiny, fueling public controversy, health scares, and general distrust of regulatory oversight. It is difficult to quantify the usage of these products amongst the general population, and long-term studies on associated health outcomes are lacking. Much like food additives, these nonnutritive sweeteners are subject to a rigorous FDA approval process, which includes determination of probable intake, cumulative effect from all uses, and toxicology studies in animals. After examining the effects of sugar substitute consumption on overall health and specific medical conditions, such as diabetes, tooth decay, hyperlipidemia, and behavioral disorders, the American Dietetic Association concludes that consumers can safely enjoy these products in a diet guided by federal nutrition recommendations and individual health goals (2).

Saccharin is a synthetic compound with sweetness intensity up to 500 times that of sugar. It becomes bitter with heating, and for that reason, it can only be used in foods served cool. Animal studies with doses far beyond those expected in humans have raised concern about carcinogenicity, but there are no human epidemiological data to support an association. Saccharin is excreted unmetabolized in urine and egested in stool. Since 2001, the FDA has not had saccharin on its list of carcinogens, and saccharin-containing products are no longer required to carry a warning label (3).

Aspartame, marketed as Equal and Nutrasweet, is made by linking two amino acids, phenylalanine and aspartic acid. Aspartame does contain some calories, but it is used in small amounts due to its intense sweetness—it is roughly 200 times as sweet as sugar—so the calories it actually adds to the diet are negligible. (The intensity of sugar substitutes is assessed by tasters given varying dilutions in water.) Metabolism of aspartame yields phenylalanine and aspartic acid. Unlike saccharin, aspartame provides some nutrient energy, although very little, and it is the only nonnutritive sweetener that produces a glycemic response. Like saccharin, it does not tolerate heat and is limited to foods served cool. Aspartame is approximately 160 times as sweet as sugar. Because it contains phenylalanine, it is contraindicated in phenylketonuria. Because aspartame lacks bulk and is not heat stable, it cannot be used in baked goods.

There is ongoing controversy about health effects of aspartame, but claims that it can cause brain tumors or neurological disease are not considered credible by the FDA (4) and comprehensive review articles (5,6). The metabolism of phenylalanine to norepinephrine and epinephrine has raised concern that aspartame ingestion could alter neurotransmitter levels and result in neurotoxicity; no reliable data support this theoretical concern. However, numerous complaints have been filed on the FDA website (4).

Acesulfame-K is a synthetic compound nearly 200 times as sweet as sugar. It is often used in combination with other synthetic sweeteners in processed foods. Unlike saccharin and aspartame, acesulfame-K is stable when heated. Commercially prepared sugar substitutes are often combinations of natural sugar and an intense sweetener. Critics claim that acesulfame-K may be carcinogenic (7), but such concerns have been dismissed by both the FDA (8) and authorities in the European Union.

Neotame, a derivative of phenylalanine and aspartic acid, is approximately 7,000 to 13,000 times sweeter than sugar. Unlike aspartame, neotame does not release significant amounts of phenylalanine during metabolism, and it is therefore not contraindicated in phenylketonuria (9–11).

Sucralose, marketed as Splenda, is a disaccharide chlorocarbon compound that is up to 1,000 times as sweet as sugar. It is stable under heat and can be used in baking. Sucralose is poorly absorbed and provides virtually no energy; the majority of its caloric content is derived from dextrose bulking agents used to create a product that mimics the physical qualities of table sugar. Sucralose has no apparent effect on glucose homeostasis (12). Recent reports suggest that sucralose may trigger migraines in certain individuals (13). Concerns have been raised that Splenda, a commercial preparation containing sucralose, is potentially carcinogenic because of a chlorine atom incorporated into the molecule; the risk, if any, is likely small, and to date it is theoretical (14). Results from over 100 animal and clinical studies in the FDA approval process indicated a lack of risk associated with sucralose intake (15,16). Currently, only neotame and sucralose are deemed as "safe" by the consumer advocacy group Center for Science in the Public Interest (Comparison and Safety Ratings of Food Additives, CSPI).

Stevia is a sweetener made by purifying extracts from a group of herbs by the same name that grow in Central and South America. Due to some early controversy about the safety of the extracts, called stevioside and rebaudioside, stevia is available as a dietary supplement but not a food additive in the United States. Stevia has been widely used in foods in Japan for the past several decades, without any apparent adverse effects. Stevia has 30 to 300 times the sweetness of sugar, but it can produce a slightly bitter aftertaste. It does not raise blood glucose, and it may help stabilize blood insulin levels (17). Stevia was originally recognized as a dietary supplement in the U.S. and was not permitted as a food additive until 2008. The FDA granted to Generally Recognizable as Safe (GRAS) status rebaudioside A, one of the chemicals in stevia that makes it sweet. However, regarding the crude stevia plant, the FDA does not consider their use in food to be GRAS in light of reports raising concern about the metabolic, reproductive, cardiovascular, and renal effects of these substances. To date, comprehensive reviews on the health effects of stevia have not found concerning adverse effects (18–20). In fact, recent evidence suggests that stevia may have multiple health benefits, including positive effects on insulin secretion (21), reversal of hyperglycemia (22), and lowering of blood pressure (23). A summary of popular sugar substitutes is provided in Table 42.1.

Sugar substitution generally is intended either to reduce calorie intake or to avoid cariogenic

TABLE 42.1

Sugar Substitutes[a]

Category of Sugar Substitute	Chemical Name	Brand Name	Calorie Content (kcal/g)	Usable in Baking and Cooking	Effects on Blood Sugar Levels and Insulin Release
Nonnutritive intense Sweetners/nonbulking	Saccharine	Sweet 'N Low Sugar Twin Sweet Mate Sweet 10	0	Yes	None
	Aspartame[b]	Equal NutraSweet	Negligible	No, may lose sweetness when heated. May add after cooking	None
	Acesulfame-K	Sunnet Sweet One	0	Yes, but would not provide bulk as sugar does	None
	Sucralose	Splenda	0	Yes	None
Bulking agents	Sorbitol[c]		2	No	None
	Xylitol		2	No	None
	Mannitol		2	No	None
Natural alternatives to sucrose	Fructose[c] (also called levulose)	High-fructose corn syrup (HFCS) Crystalline fructose	4	In commercial products, although not routinely available for use in home baking	May result in less insulin release than sucrose

[a]Shown are the categories of substitutes, their calorie content, and their effects on blood sugar levels and insulin release. Standard table sugar is made up of sucrose. Sucrose provides approximately 4 kcal per g.

[b]Aspartame contains phenylalanine. Persons with the genetic disorder phenylketonuria (PKU) need to monitor their intake of phenylalanine.

[c]Sorbitol and fructose may have a laxative effect when eaten in large amounts.

Sources: American Diabetes Association, http://www.diabetes.org; American Dietetic Association, *Sweet talk: facts about sweeteners*; and Katz DL, Gonzalez MH, *The way to eat.* Naperville, IL: Sourcebooks, 2001.

exposures to sucrose. There is some available evidence to support the use of nonnutritive sweeteners in promoting weight loss (24), and such sweeteners do not appear to lead to the dysregulation of appetite control initiated by high intakes of sucrose, fructose, and other nutritive sweeteners (25). There is, however, evidence to suggest that calories removed from the diet through the use of noncaloric sugar substitutes may simply be added back elsewhere. Animal research suggests that the use of artificial sweeteners may confound the appetite center in a manner that contributes to overeating and weight gain (26). Nonnutritive sweeteners may prevent patients from associating sweetness with caloric intake; therefore, they may crave more sweets, tend to choose sweet over balanced nutrition, and gain weight (27,28). Alternatively, it has been suggested that such intense sweetness may in fact have an addictive property and trigger excessive sweet cravings (29).

Some studies suggest an adverse effect of artificial sweeteners on weight regulation in humans, although overall the literature is equivocal (30–32). Given the intense sweetness of popular sugar substitutes, they have the potential to raise the preference threshold for sweetness through a tolerance/habituation mechanism. This, in turn, might result in increased total dietary intake of sugar. This pathway is explored in more detail in Chapter 38.

Bulking Agents

In solid foods, sugar provides both sweetness and bulk and texture; therefore, substitution calls for both intense sweeteners and bulking agents. Polyols, or sugar alcohols, are hydrogenated simple sugar analogues. They tend to be used in candies and gum. Sugar alcohols are less bioavailable in the upper gastrointestinal tract than are the parent sugars. As a result, such sugars reach, and are fermented in, the large bowel. Sugar fermentation in the colon produces heat, gaseous waste such as methane, and short-chain fatty acids, thus releasing less usable energy than sugar absorption in the small bowel. Commonly used sugar alcohols include sorbitol, with an estimated energy content of 2.6 kcal per g; xylitol, with 2.4 kcal per g; and isomalt, with 2.0 kcal per g.

Sugar alcohols are less cariogenic than glucose or sucrose (see Chapter 37). Use of sorbitol and xylitol in chewing gum prevents the generation of cariogenic acid (33), primarily through stimulation of salivary flow (34). Xylitol has antibacterial effects, reducing colony counts of *Streptococcus mutans* (33,35). There is strong evidence that chewing xylitol-sweetened gum in the context of good oral hygiene can prevent cariogenesis (36); whether it can also exert an anticariogenic therapeutic effect is as yet undetermined.

Sorbitol is directly oxidized to fructose and does not appreciably raise serum glucose or insulin levels. At high doses, sorbitol and mannitol have a laxative effect due to their slow absorption. Erythritol is a bulking agent with no caloric value. Other bulking agent sugar substitutes include the sugar alcohols lactitol and maltitol, reduced starch hydrolysates, fructo-oligosaccharides, and polydextrose.

A potentially useful means of reducing the sugar content of baked items is to replace some portion of sugar with a roughly isovolemic portion of nonfat powdered milk. The texture and bulk of powdered milk are roughly comparable to those of the replaced sugar. Powdered milk adds calcium and protein, and it offers mild sweetness due to its lactose content. At equal volumes, powdered milk has just over half the calories of sugar (1,37).

A variety of natural fibers are used as bulking agents. Galactomannans derived from guar gum and locust bean gum are often used in reduced-fat or reduced-calorie foods to restore texture and consistency. Cellulose, derived from the cell walls of plants, is used as a noncaloric bulking agent. Some forms of starch are resistant to digestive enzymes and are of potential use as bulking agents. Resistant starch may offer health benefits comparable to those of dietary fiber. Guar, pectin, and inulin are commonly used carbohydrate bulking agents. Resistant starch in the large bowel increases bacterial mass, reduces transit time, and increases levels of butyrate, which is known to have antiproliferative properties. Resistant starches may reduce colon cancer risk by several mechanisms (38) (see Chapters 12 and 18).

Fat Substitutes

Availability, familiarity, and selectivity mediate food choice, as do anticipation and expectation based on taste, color, texture, and odor (39) (see Chapter 38). The use of macronutrient substitutes is directed at preserving the familiarity of traditional foods, a factor known to be a powerful determinant of dietary preference (see Chapter 44). The rate of introduction of fat-reduced foods by the food industry accelerated markedly during the 1990s, and thousands of products have been available since (40). By reducing the energy density of foods, macronutrient substitutes generally raise the nutrient density of the diet (i.e., the ratio of micronutrients to unit energy).

The principal rationale for fat substitution is to reduce an individual's fat intake and the energy density of food to help prevent obesity and the development of chronic diseases. Energy excess in the diet has differential effects on the metabolic processing of macronutrients. Oxidation of both carbohydrate and protein is augmented when energy is ingested in excess of need. In contrast, fat intake in excess of energy need does not lead to enhanced oxidation but rather to enhanced storage. Increasing adiposity promotes fat oxidation so that a new equilibrium state is established (41). Relatively high intake of dietary fat is associated with enhanced efficiency in fat metabolism so that fat is more readily stored in adipose tissue.

Although the use of fat substitutes to reduce dietary fat is based in part on the goal of reducing chronic disease, to date there is no direct evidence that fat substitution is associated with reduced disease risk or weight loss. The available evidence suggests that fat substitutes are generally effective at reducing fat intake but not necessarily at reducing calorie intake, as compensation may occur (42). The use of intense sweeteners may result in caloric compensation as well (43). There is some evidence that satiety may depend more on food mass than on calories, resulting in reduced energy consumption when food is made relatively dilute in calories (44). Whether fat substitutes might facilitate this effect remains uncertain. All in all, although fat substitutes can be safe and useful adjuncts in decreasing total dietary energy intake, consumers must be informed that fat- and calorie-reduced products cannot be consumed in unlimited amounts (45).

Population survey data from a decade ago indicated that nearly 90% of consumers were eating fat-reduced products, and nearly 80% within any 2-week period. Updated information on the topic since the advent of carbohydrate restriction is elusive. Modified foods apparently are used more often than exercise as a weight-loss strategy. Increased dietary fat consumption, as well as increased intake of animal protein, is consistently associated with the greater dietary variety that accompanies rising gross national product and per capita income. There is currently no evidence to indicate that a society can revert to a simpler, less varied, less energy-dense diet once the Western pattern has been assumed. Therefore, food modification as an attempt to modify the nutritional environment is seemingly justified, despite unproven benefit (44). Few concerns have been raised over the safety of fat substitutes. Excessive use may produce a laxative effect, but there is little supporting evidence to bolster claims that these substances are hazardous.

The three categories of fat replacers are fat mimetics, fat substitutes, and low-calorie fats. They may be derived from carbohydrates, proteins, fats, or combinations of macronutrients. Fat in foods confers many properties beyond energy density, including effects on flavor and palatability as well as creaminess and mouth feel (see Chapter 38). Ingredient substitutions in fat-reduced foods are often directed at restoring these characteristics to foods.

Fat mimetics are nonfat constituents of foods that replace fats, mimic the properties fats confer, and add fewer calories than the fats they replace. Examples include starches, cellulose, pectin, proteins, dextrins, polydextrose, and other products. Fat mimetics are often useful in desserts and spreads but generally of less use in foods that require frying or other high-temperature preparation. Fat mimetics range from 0 to 4 kcal per g.

Reduced-calorie fats are triglycerides modified to deliver less than the 9 kcal per g of most naturally occurring fats. Medium-chain triglycerides provide 7 to 8 kcal per g. Other commercially produced low-calorie fats are poorly absorbed because they are composed of fatty acids of varying chain lengths attached to glycerol. The calorie content of such products as Caprenin (Procter &

Gamble) and Salatrim (Nabisco) is approximately 5 kcal per g. Caprenin was withdrawn from the market in the mid-1990s.

Soluble fibers used as fat substitutes confer health benefits independent of fat replacement, such as cholesterol reduction and reduced postprandial insulin release (46–48). For some individuals, processed fat-reduced foods could represent a significant source of soluble fiber.

Limited evidence from dietary intervention trials of short duration and studies of consumer behavior reviewed several years ago by Mela (49) suggested that compensation for energy reduction resulting from macronutrient substitutions is consistent. Fat substitutes do not result in compensatory fat intake, however, and the reduced energy density of the diet is apparently associated with modest weight loss. Judicious dietary fat reduction may be helpful in long-term maintenance of weight loss (see Chapter 5), and fat substitutes may be useful in this context (50,51). Evidence that macronutrient substitutes adversely affect micronutrient intake is generally limited, with some evidence of beneficial effects. Consumption of fat-reduced products has historically been much less commonly reported by African Americans than by non-Hispanic whites (52). A recent study focusing on social and environmental factors influencing dietary intake found that individuals living in high-poverty, mixed-race, or African American areas had significantly less access to reduced-fat food options (53).

The substitution of skim milk for whole milk and of lean meats for beef reduces intake of fat and saturated fat but often not to recommended levels. Therefore, additional dietary modifications are required to achieve recommended dietary patterns. According to computer modeling, consistent substitution of fat-reduced or nonfat foods for their standard-fat counterparts would achieve fat intake goals (54). Evidence is fairly convincing that fat substitutes sustainably lower fat intake, but their effect on energy intake is as yet uncertain (45,55,). Children may be particularly adept at compensating for the calorie reductions associated with macronutrient substitutes, although the compensation may not be complete (56). As is true of adults, energy compensation in children is not specific to the macronutrient class being manipulated.

The most-studied fat substitute to date is the sucrose polyester olestra, developed by Procter and Gamble and marketed as Olean. Variations in the length of the fatty acids esterified can alter the melting point and other physical properties of the product. Because it is essentially indigestible, olestra passes through the gastrointestinal tract, carrying fat-soluble micronutrients with it. Approved by the FDA for use in snack foods, olestra is controversial because of the potential for gastrointestinal upset and the leaching of fat-soluble nutrients. A variety of products derived from alterations of fat molecules are being used commercially, and under development.

Studies of olestra have demonstrated significant short-term reductions in fat and energy intake (57,58). Longer-term studies have shown inconsistent results on weight loss (59,60). In a randomized, double-blind, placebo-controlled crossover trial of 51 adults, Hill et al. (57) demonstrated that use of olestra resulted in significant reductions in fat and energy intake over a 14-day period. Subjects compensated for 15% of the fat and 20% of the energy reduction. Cotton et al. (61) demonstrated that the degree of compensation is increased when the dietary fat reduction is more extreme. When fat intake was reduced by use of olestra from 32% to 20% of calories, subjects compensated for 74% of the energy deficit on the following day.

Olestra decreases absorption of vitamins A, D, E, and K, but this effect is at least partially compensated by the fortification of olestra-containing foods with fat-soluble vitamins and does not appear to be clinically significant (62). Concern had been expressed regarding the intensity of Procter and Gamble's campaign to win support for the product despite its potential to induce gastrointestinal distress (63). However, most evidence now suggests that olestra-containing snack foods, when consumed under ordinary circumstances, do not produce any more gastrointestinal symptoms than do standard products (64,65); since 2003, olestra-containing products have not been required to carry a warning about potential gastrointestinal symptoms.

Food substitutes based on unique chemical properties must generally be approved by the FDA through a process known as a food additive petition (FAP). Few concerns have been raised about the safety of fat substitutes. Carrageenan, olestra, and polydextrose have been approved by the U.S. FDA for use as food additives, a title that requires intensive testing over a wide demographic and the adherence to strict, predetermined, FDA criteria. Relatively minor modifications of natural foods may be approved through a less arduous process in which the product is labeled as GRAS (66).

■ CLINICAL HIGHLIGHTS

There is convincing evidence that judicious use of macronutrient substitutes can provide distinct, if limited, health benefits. Sugar substitutes are of principal value in reducing the risk of dental caries, although the use of sugar substitutes to reduce energy intake may also be of potential value. Sugar substitution is not of proven benefit for weight loss or management, although a beneficial effect is not ruled out by studies to date. However, incessant sweetness in the diet may increase one's sweet tolerance, and paradoxically, contributes to the consumption of even more sweet foods and hence excess weight. For now, it seems that alternatives to sugar are of greatest benefit for the management of diabetes and its antecedent states (see Chapter 6). Fat substitution is beneficial in reducing both the fat content of the diet and total energy intake. Evidence that macronutrient substitutions contribute to sustainable weight loss is suggestive at best; study outcomes are highly inconsistent. Thus, "diet" foods, particularly sodas, are popular despite the lack of evidence that such products confer the implied benefit of facilitating weight loss/control.

Recommendations to patients for health promotion should emphasize a dietary pattern based largely on minimally processed natural foods, particularly whole grains, vegetables, and fruits. In such a context, the use of macronutrient substitutes in processed foods may prove substantially irrelevant. That said, their use may help to further reduce fat and energy intake, to increase the nutrient density of the diet, to increase dietary fiber, and to attenuate the risk of dental caries. These potential benefits are offset by the possibility that intensely sweet alternatives to sugar may adversely affect taste preferences (see Chapter 38) and that fat substitutes may impair micronutrient absorption. The direct toxic effects of artificial sweeteners and other macronutrient substitutes are largely theoretical and of limited clinical concern. Indirect toxicity in the form of adverse influences on the overall dietary pattern is likely of far greater significance. Anecdotal reports of adverse reactions to various macronutrient substitutes are numerous, however, and may occur idiosyncratically (53). The use of nonfat powdered milk to replace some portion of sugar in baked goods represents an alternative approach—ingredient substitution—that may offer some of the theoretical benefits of macronutrient substitutes without the potential harms. Judicious and generally limited use of macronutrient substitutions may be recommended as an adjuvant, but certainly not an alternative, to efforts at achieving a salutary dietary pattern.

REFERENCES

1. US Department of Agriculture Research Service. *Nutrient data laboratory*. Available at http://www.nal.usda.gov/fnic/foodcomp/search; accessed 11/6/07.
2. Fitch C, Keim KS; Academy of Nutrition and Dietetics. Position of the Academy of Nutrition and Dietetics: use of nutritive and nonnutritive sweeteners. *J Acad Nutr Diet* 2012;112:739–758.
3. National Toxicology Program. *Availability of the report on carcinogens*, 9th ed. Washington, DC: Department of Health and Human Services, 2001.
4. US Food and Drug Administration. *Is aspartame safe?* Available at http://www.cfsan.fda.gov/~dms/qa-adf9.html; accessed 11/6/07.
5. Weihrauch MR, Diehl V. Artificial sweeteners—do they bear carcinogenic risk? *Ann Oncol* 2004;15:1460–1465.
6. Magnuson BA, Burdock GA, Doull J, et al. Aspartame: a safety evaluation based on current use levels, regulations, and toxicological and epidemiological studies. *Crit Rev Toxicol* 2007;37:629–727.
7. Karstadt ML. Testing needed for acesulfame potassium, an artificial sweetener. *Environ Health Perspect* 2006;114:A516; author reply A516–A517.
8. Kroger M, Meister K, Kava R. Low-calorie sweeteners and other sugar substitutes: a review of safety issues. *Compr Rev Food Sci Food Saf* 5:35–47.
9. Cui M, Jiang P, Maillet E, et al. The heterodimeric sweet taste receptor has multiple potential ligand binding sites. *Curr Pharm Des* 2006;12:4591–4600.
10. Mayhew DA, Comer CP, Stargel WW. Food consumption and body weight changes with neotame, a new sweetener with intense taste: differentiating effects of palatability from toxicity in dietary safety studies. *Regul Toxicol Pharmacol* 2003;38:124–143.
11. Walters DE, Prakash I, Desai N. Active conformations of neotame and other high-potency sweeteners. *J Med Chem* 2000;43:1242–1245.
12. Grotz VL, Henry RR, McGill JB, et al. Lack of effect of sucralose on glucose homeostasis in subjects with type 2 diabetes. *J Am Diet Assoc* 2003;103:1607–1612.
13. Patel RM, Sarma R, Grimsley E. Popular sweetener sucralose as a migraine trigger. *Headache* 2006;46:1303–1304.
14. Weihrauch MR, Diehl V. Artificial sweeteners—do they bear a carcinogenic risk? *Ann Oncol* 2004;15:1460–1465.
15. Grotz VL, Munro IC. An overview of the safety of sucralose. *Regul Toxicol Pharmacol* 2009;55:1–5.
16. Grice HC, Goldsmith LA. Sucralose—an overview of the toxicity data. *Food Chem Toxicol* 2000;38(suppl 2):S1–S6.
17. Lailerd N, Saengsirisuwan V, Sloniger JA, et al. Effects of stevioside on glucose transport activity in insulin-sensitive and insulin-resistant rat skeletal muscle. *Metabolism* 2004;53:101–107.
18. Benford D, Bolger PM, Carthew P, et al. Application of the margin of exposure (MOE) approach to substances in food that are genotoxic and carcinogenic. *Food Chem Toxicol* 2010;48(suppl 1):S2–S24.
19. Goyal SK, Goyal SRK. Stevia (*Stevia rebaudiana*) a biosweetener: a review. *Int J Food Sci Nutr* 2010;61(1):1–10.
20. Ulbricht C, Isaac R, Milkin T, et al. An evidence based systematic review of *Stevia* by the Natural Standard Research Collaboration. *Cardiovasc Hematol Agents Med Chem* 2010;8:113–127.
21. Jeppesen PB, Gregersen S, Poulson CR, et al. Stevioside acts directly on pancreatic beta cells to secrete insulin: actions independent of cyclic adenosine monophosphate and adenosine triphosphate-sensitive K$^+$-channel activity. *Metabolism* 2000;49:208–214.
22. Gregersen S, Jeppesen PB, Holst JJ, et al. Antihyperglycemic effects of stevioside in type 2 diabetic subjects. *Metabolism* 2004;53:73–76.
23. Chan P, Tomlinson B, Chen YJ, et al. A double-blind placebo-controlled study of the effectiveness and tolerability of oral stevioside in human hypertension. *Br J Clin Pharmacol* 2000;50:215–220.
24. Raben A, Vasilaras TH, Moller AC, et al. Sucrose compared with artificial sweeteners: different effects on ad libitum food intake and body weight after 10 weeks of supplementation in overweight subjects. *Am J Clin Nutr* 2002;76:721–729.
25. American Dietetic Association. Position of the American Dietetic Association: use of nutritive and nonnutritive sweeteners. *J Am Diet Assoc* 2004;104:255–275.
26. Davidson TL, Swithers SE. A Pavlovian approach to the problem of obesity. *Int J Obes Relat Metab Disord* 2004;28:933–935.
27. Fowler SP, Williams K, Resendez RG, et al. Fueling the obesity epidemic? Artificially sweetened beverage use and long term weight gain. *Obesity* (Silver Spring) 2008;16:1894–1900.
28. Swithers SE, Davidson TL. A role for sweet taste: calorie predictive relations in energy regulation by rats. *Behav Neurosci* 2008;122:161–173.
29. Lenoir M, Serre F, Cantin L, et al. Intense sweetness surpasses cocaine reward. *PLoS One* 2007;2:e698.
30. St-Onge MP, Heymsfield SB. Usefulness of artificial sweeteners for body weight control. *Nutr Rev* 2003;61:219–221.
31. Vermunt SH, Pasman WJ, Schaafsma G, et al. Effects of sugar intake on body weight: a review. *Obes Rev* 2003;4:91–99.
32. Mattes RD, Popkin BM. Nonnutritive sweetener consumption in humans: effects on appetite and food intake and their putative mechanisms. *Am J Clin Nutr* 2009;89:1–14.
33. Edgar W. Sugar substitutes, chewing gum and dental caries—a review. *Br Dent J* 1998;184:29–32.
34. Van Loveren C. Sugar alcohols: what is the evidence for caries-preventive and caries-therapeutic effects? *Caries Res* 2004;38:286–293.
35. Haresaku S, Hanioka T, Tsutsui A, et al. Long-term effect of xylitol gum use on mutans streptococci in adults. *Caries Res* 2007;41:198–203.

36. Burt BA. The use of sorbitol- and xylitol-sweetened chewing gum in caries control. *J Am Dent Assoc* 2006;137:190–196.

37. Katz DL, Katz CS. *The flavor point diet.* Emmaus, PA: Rodale, Inc., 2005.

38. Wollowski I, Rechkemmer G, Pool-Zobel BL. Protective role of probiotics and prebiotics in colon cancer. *Am J Clin Nutr* 2001;73:451s–455s.

39. Grivetti L. Social determinants of food intake. In: Anderson G, Rolls B, Steffen D, eds. *Nutritional implications of macronutrient substitutes. Annals of the New York Academy of Sciences.* New York, NY: New York Academy of Sciences, 1997:121–131.

40. Anderson G. Nutritional and health aspects of macronutrient substitution. In: Anderson G, Rolls B, Steffen D, eds. *Nutritional implications of macronutrient substitutes. Annals of the New York Academy of Sciences.* New York, NY: New York Academy of Sciences, 1997:1–10.

41. Tartaranni P, Ravussin E. Effect of fat intake on energy balance. In: Anderson G, Rolls B, Steffen D, eds. *Nutritional implications of macronutrient substitutes. Annals of the New York Academy of Sciences.* New York, NY: New York Academy of Sciences, 1997:37–43.

42. Wylie-Rosett J. Fat substitutes and health: an advisory from the Nutrition Committee of the American Heart Association. *Circulation* 2002;105:2800.

43. Anderson G, Rolls B, Steffen D, eds. *Nutritional implications of macronutrient substitutes. Annals of the New York Academy of Sciences.* New York, NY: New York Academy of Sciences, 1997.

44. Rolls BJ, Bell EA, Waugh BA. Increasing the volume of a food by incorporating air affects satiety in men. *Am J Clin Nutr* 2000;72:361–368.

45. American Dietetic association. Position of the American Dietetic association: fat replacers. *J Am Diet Assoc* 2005;105:266–275.

46. Behall K. Dietary fiber: nutritional lessons for macronutrient substitutes. In: Anderson G, Rolls B, Steffen D, eds. *Nutritional implications of macronutrient substitutes. Annals of the New York Academy of Sciences.* New York, NY: New York Academy of Sciences, 1997:142–154.

47. Howarth NC, Saltzman E, Roberts SB. Dietary fiber and weight regulation. *Nutr Rev* 2001;59:129–139.

48. Reyna NY, Cano C, Bermudez VJ, et al. Sweeteners and beta-glucans improve metabolic and anthropometrics variables in well-controlled type 2 diabetic patients. *Am J Ther* 2003;10:438–443.

49. Mela D. Impact of macronutrient-substituted foods on food choice and dietary intake. In: Anderson G, Rolls B, Steffen D, eds. *Nutritional implications of macronutrient substitutes. Annals of the New York Academy of Sciences.* New York, NY: New York Academy of Sciences, 1997:96–107.

50. Peters J. Nutritional aspects of macronutrient-substitute intake. In: Anderson G, Rolls B, Steffen D, eds. *Nutritional implications of macronutrient substitutes. Annals of the New York Academy of Sciences.* New York, NY: New York Academy of Sciences, 1997:169–179.

51. Bray GA, Lovejoy JC, Most-Windhauser M, et al. A nine-month randomized clinical trial comparing a fat-substituted and fat-reduced diet in healthy obese men: the Ole study. *Am J Clin Nutr* 2002;76:928–934.

52. Heimbach J, van der Riet B, Egan S. Impact of the use of reduced-fat foods on nutrient adequacy. In: Anderson G, Rolls

B, Steffen D, eds. *Nutritional implications of macronutrient substitutes. Annals of the New York Academy of Sciences.* New York, NY: New York Academy of Sciences, 1997:108–114.

53. Baker EA, Schootman M, Barnidge E, et al. The role of race and poverty in access to foods that enable individuals to adhere to dietary guidelines. *Prev Chronic Dis* 2006;3:A76.

54. Morgan R, Sigman-Grant M, Taylor D, et al. Impact of macronutrient substitutes on the composition of the diet and US food supply. In: Anderson G, Rolls B, Steffen D, eds. *Nutritional implications of macronutrient substitutes. Annals of the* New York Academy of Sciences. New York, NY: New York Academy of Sciences, 1997:70–95.

55. Lawton C, Blundell J. The role of reduced fat diets and fat substitutes in the regulation of energy and fat intake and body weight. *Curr Opin Lipidol* 1998;9:41–45.

56. Birch L, Fisher J. Food intake regulation in children. Fat and sugar substitutes and intake. In: Anderson G, Rolls B, Steffen D, eds. *Nutritional implications of macronutrient substitutes. Annals of the New York Academy of Sciences.* New York, NY: New York Academy of Sciences, 1997:194–220.

57. Hill J, Seagle H, Johnson S, et al. Effects of 14 d of covert substitution of olestra for conventional fat on spontaneous food intake. *Am J Clin Nutr* 1998;67:1178–1185.

58. Miller DL, Castellanos VH, Shide DJ, et al. Effect of fat-free potato chips with and without nutrition labels on fat and energy intakes. *Am J Clin Nutr* 1998;68:282.

59. Satia-Abouta J, Kristal AR, Patterson RE, et al. Is olestra consumption associated with changes in dietary intake, serum lipids, and body weight? *Nutrition* 2003;19:754–759.

60. Lovejoy JC, Bray GA, Lefevre M, et al. Consumption of a controlled low-fat diet containing olestra for 9 months improves health risk factors in conjunction with weight loss in obese men: the Ole' Study. *Int J Obes Relat Metab Disord* 2003;27:1242–1249.

61. Cotton J, Weststrate J, Blundell J. Replacement of dietary fat with sucrose polyester: effects on energy intake and appetite control in nonobese males. *Am J Clin Nutr* 1996;63:891–896.

62. Neuhouser ML, Rock CL, Kristal AR, et al. Olestra is associated with slight reductions in serum carotenoids but does not markedly influence serum fat-soluble vitamin concentrations. *Am J Clin Nutr* 2006;83:624–631.

63. Nestle M. The selling of Olestra. *Public Health* 1998; 113:508–520.

64. Sandler R, Zorich N, Filloon T, et al. Gastrointestinal symptoms in 3181 volunteers ingesting snack foods containing olestra or triglycerides. A 6-week randomized, placebo-controlled trial. *Ann Intern Med* 1999;130:253–261.

65. Thomson A, Hunt R, Zorich N. Review article: olestra and gastrointestinal safety. *Aliment Pharmacol Ther* 1998; 12:1185–1200.

66. Food and Drug Association. *GRAS Notification Program.* Available at http://www.fda.gov/~dms/opa-noti.html; accessed 11/6/07.

SUGGESTED READINGS

Blundell JE, Green SM. Effect of sucrose and sweeteners on appetite and energy intake. *Int J Obes Relat Metab Disord* 1996;20:s12.

Calorie Control Council website. Available at http://www.caloriecontrol.org; accessed 11/6/07.

Cohen S. Human relevance of animal carcinogenicity studies. *Regul Toxicol Pharmacol* 1995;21:75–80.

Drewnowski A. Intense sweeteners and energy density of foods: implications for weight control. *Eur J Clin Nutr* 1999;53:757.

Finley JW, Leveille GA. Macronutrient substitutes. In: Ziegler EE, Filer LJ, Jr, eds. *Present knowledge in nutrition*, 7th ed. Washington, DC: ILSI Press, 1996:581–595.

Hannah JS. Beyond calories: other benefits of macronutrient substitutes. effects on chronic disease. In: Anderson GH, Rolls BJ, Steffen DG, eds. *Nutritional implications of macronutrient substitutes. Annals of the New York Academy of Sciences*. New York, NY: New York Academy of Sciences, 1997:221–228.

Hathcock JN, Rader JI. Food additives, contaminants, and natural toxins. In: Shils ME, Olson JA, Shike M, eds. *Modern nutrition in health and disease*, 8th ed. Philadelphia, PA: Lea & Febiger, 1994:1593–1611.

Kinghorn AD, Kaneda N, Baek NI, et al. Noncariogenic intense natural sweeteners. *Med Res Rev* 1998;18:347.

Leveille GA, Finley JW. Macronutrient substitutes. Description and uses. In: Anderson GH, Rolls BJ, Steffen DG, eds. *Nutritional implications of macronutrient substitutes. Annals of the New York Academy of Sciences*. New York, NY: New York Academy of Sciences, 1997:11–21.

Rolls BJ. Fat and sugar substitutes and the control of food intake. In: Anderson GH, Rolls BJ, Steffen DG, eds. *Nutritional implications of macronutrient substitutes. Annals of the New York Academy of Sciences*. New York, NY: New York Academy of Sciences, 1997:180–193.

Scheie A, Fejerskov O. Xylitol in caries prevention: what is the evidence for clinical efficacy? *Oral Dis* 1998; 4:268–278.

Stubbs RJ, Prentice AM, James WPT. Carbohydrates and energy balance. In: Anderson GH, Rolls BJ, Steffen DG, eds. *Nutritional implications of macronutrient substitutes. Annals of the New York Academy of Sciences*. New York, NY: New York Academy of Sciences, 1997:44–69.

CHAPTER 43

Vegetarianism, Veganism, and Macrobiotic Diets

D ietary recommendations for health promotion and disease prevention consistently emphasize the importance of a diet relatively rich in fruits, vegetables, and whole grains. Thus, a vegetarian diet offers apparent health benefits, but the partial or complete exclusion of animal products from the diet does not ensure optimal or even balanced nutrition. Strict vegetarians are at potential risk of micronutrient or even protein deficiencies. A vegetarian diet based on processed rather than natural foods may combine the excesses of the Western diet with the risk of such deficiencies.

Vegetarianism is increasingly popular in Western countries. Although no conclusive estimates can be made, recent statistics suggest that between 5% and 13% of the US population follows a vegetarian diet (1,2). Whether resulting from personal ethics or health concerns, this is a marked increase from previous years and as such, the clinician should be well prepared to distinguish prudent from imprudent vegetarian diets and offer advice, as required, to promote dietary balance. The potential health benefits of a nutritionally adequate vegetarian diet appear to be considerable. A shift toward more plant-based dietary patterns at the population level offers considerable potential benefit to animals and the environment as well.

OVERVIEW

Vegetarianism is a generic term that encompasses a small variety of distinct dietary patterns. The term itself generally implies at least a relative avoidance of meat in the diet. *Veganism* is strict avoidance of all animal products, including eggs and dairy foods. *Lactovegetarianism* permits consumption of dairy products but not eggs. *Lactoovovegetarianism* permits consumption of dairy products and eggs. *Pescovegetarianism*, a

seldom-used term, refers to diets that permit fish but not other animal products. In common usage, *vegetarianism* may refer to any of these patterns or to the exclusion of only red meat. More restrictive patterns, such as macrobiotic diets, typically are bound by a religious or cultural belief system that stipulates the dietary exclusions.

Plant foods tend to be relatively high in fiber, and in the case of fruits and vegetables, water content, and consequently low in calories per unit volume. When caloric excess is more of a threat than caloric deficiency, this tends to be one of the benefits of vegetarianism, reducing the risk of obesity. Vegetarians are, on average, leaner than their omnivorous counterparts while vegans have been found to have the lowest body mass index levels (3,4,5). Energy may be deficient, however, when metabolic demand is high due to growth or activity. Thus, inclusion in the diets of vegetarian children of some calorically dense foods, such as nuts, peanut butter, avocados (one of only two "high-fat" fruits, the other being the olive), and vegetable oils, may be particularly important.

Nutritional Concerns of Vegetarian Diets

Protein is widely distributed in the food supply, and total protein deficiency is unlikely to be induced by a balanced vegetarian diet. A greater risk, when dairy products and eggs are excluded from the diet along with meat, is deficiency of one or more essential amino acids, which can be avoided through balanced selection of protein sources. Beans, peas, and lentils have an excellent amino acid profile, including lysine; grains are complementary, serving as a good source of methionine (see Chapters 3 and 4). Soybeans have been found to have an amino acid profile highly comparable to that of egg albumin. In addition, new research has suggested the amino acid profiles of quinoa (6), chia seeds (7), hemp seeds (8), hummus (6), cauliflower (6), and the microalgae chlorella (9) to be excellent as well. The consumption of these foods is therefore believed to be highly beneficial to those following a vegan diet.

Inclusion of cereals, as well as beans, peas, or lentils; nuts or seeds; and vegetables in the daily diet is likely to ensure adequate amino acid intake. Efficient use of essential amino acids can be achieved, provided that they are all consumed within the span of a day or two (see Chapter 3); therefore, balanced intake is important and must be consistent but need not occur at every meal.

The fat content of vegetarian diets tends to be lower than that of corresponding omnivorous diets, but not invariably so. When dairy is included in the diet, the substitution of cheese for meat can result in high intake of saturated fat. When fat intake is kept at moderate levels, the exclusion of fish from the diet may elevate the ratio of n-6 to n-3 fatty acids, with potentially adverse effects (see Chapter 2). The inclusion of sacha inchi (a Peruvian seed containing n-3 oils) (10), flaxseed, linseed, and their oils will add α-linolenic acid (ALA) to the diet and help prevent imbalance of essential fatty acids. Lactoovovegetarians may opt for chicken eggs while vegans may turn to kelp or other microalgae as an alternative.

Compared to vegetarian diets, the intake levels of arachidonic acid in omnivorous diets are high (11). Brain activity may be altered by these elevated levels in ways that promote mood disruption. The question therefore arose as to whether a restriction of meat, poultry, and fish would have any impact on mood. Through the use of two validated self-report mood scales, the Depression Anxiety Stress Scales (DASS) and the Profile of Mood States (POMS) questionnaire, a pilot randomized controlled trial found that after randomly assigning omnivores to an omnivore, pescovegetarian, or vegetarian groups for a two weeks positive mood changes occurred only in the vegetarian diet group (12). Supportive to these findings, and suggestive of biological adaptations to low intakes of long-chain fatty acids, are cross-sectional observations among Seventh Day Adventists. Followers of this sect of Christianity are well known for their meat abstinence and so their reports of having significantly less negative emotion than omnivores are noteworthy (13).

Several micronutrient deficiencies may result from vegetarian practices. Plant foods generally contain less concentrated sources of iron and zinc than meat, and the quantity present generally is less readily absorbed. Intake of both iron and zinc can be adequate when a balanced and diverse diet is maintained and absorption is enhanced by concomitant intake of vitamin C. A study among Australian men comparing nearly 50 vegetarians and 25 omnivores found higher iron intake among the vegetarians but significantly higher ferritin levels in the omnivores, suggesting the importance of dietary source and absorption (14). In tangent to these recommendations are the findings of tea's potential inhibitory effects on the absorption of iron. Its repressive qualities are due to the polyphenolic compounds present within tea, as well as coffee, and have been found to dramatically decrease absorption rates. A study in India comparing tea's effects on the amount of iron absorbed from rice meals with both native and added elemental iron found that when the meal was consumed alongside tea, dramatic reductions in iron absorption occurred among iron-deficient anemic, as well as healthy controls (15). The effect of tea consumption and iron absorption should be examined further, especially in vegetarians.

Diets excluding all animal products may lead to calcium deficiency. Although calcium is present in many vegetables, oxalate binding limits absorption and bioavailability. The association between dietary calcium and bone density, and the risk of osteoporosis, is complex and controversial. The World Health Organization (16) has generally advocated for lower calcium intake than the Institute of Medicine (17), a discrepancy apparently having had roots in transcultural lifestyle differences modifying the level of calcium intake required to prevent osteoporosis. Both bodies' advisements have since coalesced, each recommending 1,000 mg a day for healthy adults (18,19). Whether the previously viewed lifestyle differences relate to diet, physical activity, both, or other factors, remains unresolved.

Some evidence suggests that increased intake of fruits and vegetables mitigates the risk of osteoporosis by reducing the intake of protein and sodium and/or by increasing intake of beneficial micronutrients. Nonetheless, prior evidence suggests that increasing vegetable protein intake among meat-eaters, while in the presence of meat, may actually reverse roles and increase risk for osteoporosis (20). However, causality has not been established, and, as such, research on whole food and dietary pattern interactions is needed. A potentially adverse effect of high protein intake on bone health has been posited but is itself somewhat controversial (21). In the aggregate, some available data indicate the trend toward vegetarian diets, and in particular vegan diets, as being associated with lower bone mineral density, although the association is not significant (22). Other analyses, however, find that vegan diets do not have adverse effects on bone health (23) and, furthermore, have even suggested that a balanced vegetarian diet may be associated with reduced risk. Nonetheless, until understanding of the topic is further advanced, calcium supplementation should at least be considered for all vegetarians and should generally be encouraged for vegans. The influence of various nutrients and dietary patterns on bone health is addressed in more detail in Chapter 14.

Vitamin B_{12}, thought to be in abundance within animal foods, is technically not present naturally within plant or animal foods. It is the only vitamin currently known to be solely produced by microorganisms. Its saturation within organically raised animal flesh is a result of that animal having eaten other food containing B_{12}-producing bacteria. Recent studies of centenarian health have led to the Western world's discovery of a group of soybean-fermented foods, including *Doenjang, Chunggukjang,* and various seaweeds traditional to Korean fare, containing considerable amounts of B_{12} (24). There is evidence to suggest that the prevalence of B_{12} deficit is greater than once thought, impacting both vegetarians and nonvegetarians (25). However, due to the ease and convenience of obtaining animal derived foods, and subsequently an ample supply of daily B_{12}, strict vegans are faced with an increased risk for deficiency; supplementation is prudent.

The inclusion of dairy products or eggs in the diet will help maintain adequate B_{12} stores. Vitamin B_{12} and iron deficiency have been associated with veganism (26). Vitamin D is absent from plant foods, but needs can be met by synthesis in the skin with sufficient sun exposure. Additionally, there are food products currently available that are fortified with B_{12}, including nutritional yeast, hot and cold cereals, and various nondairy milks. Nonetheless, supplementation is prudent for vegans, particularly in temperate climates. The possibility of iodine deficiency has been raised (27,28), but it is an unlikely hazard if iodized salt is included in the diet.

When a vegetarian diet is based largely on processed foods, which apparently is a particular tendency among adolescents (see Chapter 30), the fiber content may be low, and the content of simple sugar may be high. Such a diet offers the potential hazards of animal food exclusions from the diet without the attendant benefits of well-practiced vegetarianism and generally should be discouraged.

Vegetarianism is increasingly popular among adolescents for reasons related to health and body image, as well as philosophy and ecology (29). There is some suggestion from survey research that vegetarianism in adolescents may be a means of masking an effort at dietary restraint (30,31) or even a tendency toward an eating disorder (32–34) (see Chapter 25).

Veganism potentially places young children at particular risk of nutrient deficiencies (see Chapter 29). Soy-based infant formulas can meet the nutrient needs of infants who are not breast-fed or who have been weaned. As vegan infants advance to solid foods, the principles outlined earlier provide some guidance. Particular effort should be made to ensure adequate intake of dietary fat. Cholesterol, which is found only in animal products, will be absent from the diet. The general practice of referring vegan families to a dietitian for tailored advice is appropriate.

States of high metabolic demand may expose adults to the same hazards of overly restrictive diets as children. Pregnancy, lactation, chronic disease, trauma, acute infection, and high levels of physical activity require heightened attention to ensure adequate intake of energy, protein, and micronutrients. Balanced approaches to vegetarianism appear to be supportive of even intense athletic activity (35).

The possibility of both clinical and subclinical disturbances in the menstrual cycle attributed to vegetarianism has been reported, but evidence is inconclusive (36). If such disturbances exist, low body fat percentage is one putative explanation, with resultant reduction in estradiol levels.

A vegetarian diet has been used in the context of a randomized pilot study in subjects with non-insulin-dependent diabetes mellitus (37). Compared with a conventional low-fat diet, the vegan diet used in the study produced significant reductions in weight, fasting glucose levels, and the need for medication over a 12-week period. Overall, findings from prior studies suggest that the vegetarian eating pattern, namely, an absence of red meat and processed meat products, may provide particular benefits in the management of diabetes and prediabetes (38,39). Postulated mechanisms include weight loss, changes in intramyocellular lipid content, reductions in saturated fat intake, reduced glycemic index, increased fiber intake, and a reduction in iron stores (40). Although generally associated with reduced risk of cardiovascular disease, vegetarianism is often associated with other lifestyle practices, such as the avoidance of smoking and physical activity, that complicate attribution. In a study that matched for other aspects of lifestyle between female Turkish vegetarians and omnivores, Karabudak et al. (41) reported elevated homocysteine and folate levels, as well as enhanced platelet aggregability in the vegetarians. A global perspective review investigating studies concerning the metabolism, biochemical assessment, and dietary intake of B_{12}, specifically among vegetarian and vegan populations, concluded with similar findings (42).

In order to assess how dietary habits may affect conversion of dietary ALA to essential long-chain n-3 PUFAs, 14,422 men and women...and vegans were observed to determine dietary ALA intake and circulating n-3 PUFA levels. Substantial differences in intakes and sources of n-3 PUFAs were found among the different groups; however, these differences were much smaller than expected, possibly because the product–precursor ratio may be greater and thus an increased estimated conversion of ALA in non-fish-eaters than in fish-eaters. These findings call for more investigation on the conversion of ALA among vegetarians (43).

Veganism and lactoovovegetarianism have been reported to produce a more favorable lipid profile than omnivorism (44). A review of 27 randomized controlled and observational trials revealed that vegetarian or vegan diets including nuts, soy, and/or fiber elicited reductions of plasma low-density lipoprotein cholesterol up to 35%, while interventions permitting small amount of lean meat demonstrated less dramatic reductions, both in total and low-density lipoprotein cholesterol (45). Thus, the clinical significance of the reported alterations of serum markers of cardiovascular risk seems to be in favor of vegetarian or vegan diets.

Observational data also suggest a benefit of vegetarianism on both cardiovascular and all-cause mortality (46,47). A study of elderly women in China, for example, found that vegetarianism was associated with a reduced rate of ischemic heart disease, although vegetarians were less likely than matched omnivores to smoke (48). The vegetarians in this study were subject to anemia due to deficiencies of vitamin B_{12} or iron, or both.

Of note, some health benefits are preferentially ascribed to ingestion of vegetables or fruits. It appears that different fruits and vegetables, as well as their method of intake, affect the likelihood of different cancer risks. For example, for protection against prostate cancer progression, only cruciferous vegetables were found to be efficacious; however, statistically significant benefits have only been reached when daily intake averages 5.7 servings (49). Additionally, the risks of both head and neck cancers have been found to be lower amongst those who consume more fruits and vegetables (50). Recent meta-analysis data suggest that a high intake of fruits, and of fruits and vegetables combined, may offer more meaningful protection against breast cancer than vegetable intake alone (51). Such data should be interpreted cautiously both because few if any studies of high methodologic quality have examined the isolated effects of fruit versus vegetable intake on health over time and because these classifications of foods may be rather arbitrary. While typically consumed as vegetables, olives, avocados, tomatoes, cucumbers, zucchini, and squash, for example, are technically (i.e., botanically) fruits.

Current Consensus

While the net health effects of strict vegetarianism invite debate, evidence for beneficial effects of more plant-based eating is in the aggregate both consistent and strong (52,53). Large prospective trials have demonstrated that populations following primarily plant-based diets, in particular vegetarian and vegan diets, face lower mortality risk from ischemic heart disease. The recent publication of the Adventist Health Study 2 brings with it persuasive evidence in support of meat-free diets' health advantages. A prospective cohort design analyzing mortality rates among 73,308 participants found that vegan men had the lowest rates for all-cause, ischemic heart disease, cardiovascular disease, and cancer mortality compared to pesco-, lacto-ovo-, semi- and non-vegetarian men (54). Among women however, pescovegetarianism was shown to be most protective against all-cause, ischemic heart, and cardiovascular disease mortality, while lacto-ovo was most protective against cancer (54). Another meta-analysis of data from cohort studies reveals an inverse association between fruit and vegetable intake and the risk of coronary heart disease (55,56) (see Chapter 7). Similar, albeit weaker, associations have been reported for cancer (57) (see Chapter 12).

Alternative Dieting

The macrobiotic diet, which was developed by a Japanese spiritualist, is actually a series of 10 increasingly restricted diets. According to its guidelines, the variations, timing, and necessity to enter each of these transitions vary from person to person. No food is prohibited in the macrobiotic diet; however, certain foods are encouraged or prohibited more than others. The philosophy is based on comprehensive approaches that take into account a wide variety of factors ranging from overall energy balance to family history and even climate (58).

There is an overarching tendency for adherents to follow these 10 phases and as such, a diverse and balanced diet is followed at the outset, progressing gradually into stages that exclude all but cereal grains, ostensibly in pursuit of spiritual purity. Vitamin B_{12} deficiency has been shown to persist following a macrobiotic diet, even after conversion to more mainstream dietary patterns. Strict adherence has been associated with deficiencies of protein, vitamin D, zinc, calcium, and iron; reduced bone mass has also been reported (59). The advanced levels of the diet have resulted in overt cases of nutritional deficiency and even death, and, from a health care perspective, are to be adamantly discouraged.

Recent Popular Diets

One dietary approach growing in popularity among Westerners is the raw food diet. With its principal rule being the avoidance of any foods heated over 115°F, the aims of the diet are to improve health, the environment, and very often to promote weight loss. There is no single definition for what comprises a raw food diet to date; however, the fundamental characteristics involve a high consumption of plant-based, uncooked, and unprocessed foods. Fruits, vegetables, nuts, and seeds form the bulk of the diet with inclusions of dairy and cereals being negligible within the raw-food community.

The theory behind the practice is centered on the preservation of nutrients and enzymes that may otherwise be destroyed through the application of heat. A well-known example of this can be seen with the anticarcinogen, sulforaphane, present in broccoli and other cruciferous vegetables. A study from the *Journal of Agricultural and Food Chemistry* found the sulforaphane within raw broccoli, when consumed with a warm meal, to have a bioavailability of 37% compared to 3.4% when the broccoli was cooked (60). Conversely, it has been observed that industrial heat processing of tomato increases lycopene's bioaccessibility (61). These findings may explain previously documented associations between strict, long-term adherence to a raw food diet and favorable β-carotene but low lycopene levels (62).

In 2005, findings from a 2-year study indicated that adherence to a strict raw food diet (95% raw and 97% plant-based) effectively lowered plasma total cholesterol levels and triglyceride concentrations while simultaneously lowering high-density lipoprotein cholesterol and increasing plasma homocysteine levels (63). Due to the lack of rigorous studies, the long-term beneficial effects of raw food diets remain to be seen.

Another diet that has gained popularity in recent days is the gluten-free diet. Gluten-free dieting (GFD) is an approach that is often grouped loosely with vegetarianism and raw food diets. It is most closely associated with celiac disease, an autoimmune disorder of the small intestine causing nutrient malabsorption through the destruction of villi triggered by the ingestion of foods containing gluten, a protein composite of gliadin and glutenin often found in wheat, barley, and rye. Also known as gluten-sensitive enteropathy, celiac disease can exhibit a variety of symptoms among different individuals, but digestive symptoms such as abdominal pain, vomiting, chronic diarrhea, and weight loss are more common among infants and young children. Adults are less likely to have such localized problems and may instead experience bone or joint pain, unexplained iron-deficiency anemia, dermatitis herpetiformis, or tingling sensations within the extremities (64).

The GFD is comparatively different from other well-known diets because of its intimate connection to one specific type of disease. As such, the primary institutive action involved in its fidelity is the exclusion of a one specific protein compound present in various foods and beverages, making the approach unique in that no inclusive food group or method of preparation is stressed upon. Within the United States, it is estimated that 1 out of every 141 people has celiac disease, similar to estimates observed in many European countries (65). While only a small percentage of the population may have true celiac disease, GFD has become a popular diet for those claiming "non-celiac gluten sensitivity". Followers report intestinal symptoms that resolve upon adoption of a GFD, despite testing negative for celiac disease. Thus far, neither gliadin-mediated mucosal inflammation nor basophil activation have been found among patients with non-celiac gluten sensitivity (66). Rather, recent evidence suggests that the offending agent may not be gluten per se, but rather fermentable oligo-, di-, and monosaccharides and polyols (FODMAPs), commonly found in gluten-containing foods (Biesiekierski JR, Peters SL, et al. No effects of gluten in patients with self-reported non-celiac gluten sensitivity after dietary reduction of fermentable, poorly absorbed, short-chain carbohydrates. Gastroenterology. 2013(145):320-328). These short-chain carbohydrates, when poorly absorbed in the intestines, may cause many of the symptoms of so-called gluten sensitivity. Further research is warranted.

Gene and Diet Interaction

No single dietary recommendation is conclusively known to positively affect all who follow it. Interindividual differences in response to diet and lifestyle changes are known to exist, with evidence for nutrition's positive effects on gene expression in the context of metabolic syndrome (67) and obesity (68). Additionally, beneficial decreases in potential oncogenes among men with low-risk prostate cancer have been detected after intensive nutrition and lifestyle interventions were followed (69). The value that such discoveries may hold is immense.

Vegetarianism and the Environment

While largely beyond the scope of this chapter, the potential benefits to other species and the planet of a population shift toward more plant-based eating are noteworthy (53). The Food and Agriculture Organization of the United Nations estimates that livestock are responsible for 18% of greenhouse gas emissions, a greater share than that of all transportation combined. Their report states that the livestock sector is without a doubt, the "single largest anthropogenic user of land," with grazing occupying over 26% of the Earth's terrestrial surface and feed crop production requiring approximately one-third of all arable land. It is estimated that the United States' meat, dairy, and egg industries are responsible for 37% of pesticide use, 50% of antibiotic use, and a third of the nitrogen and phosphorous loads in freshwater resources (70). With these statistics, and future generations in mind, it is strongly encouraged for patients and clinicians alike to reduce meat and poultry consumption, replacing lost calories and nutrients with those from plant-based foods.

CLINICAL HIGHLIGHTS

Observational data suggest that vegetarianism is associated with reduced risk of various chronic diseases and all-cause mortality. Such findings are potentially confounded by other health-promoting behaviors often associated with vegetarianism. The intrinsic nature of a vegetarian diet not only excludes meat products but by and large fosters an increase in the consumption of vegetables and fruits. This invariable adding and subtracting of food groups leaves the task of causal distinction highly complex. Studies of serum markers of cardiovascular risk are conflicting and inconclusive, although most suggest a benefit of plant-based diets. Judicious vegetarianism has been associated with improvement in anthropometric measures such as waist circumference (71), of particular interest at a time of epidemic obesity (see Chapter 5).

Whether vegetarianism is nutritionally optimal or simply superior to prevailing dietary patterns in the West is uncertain. Strict veganism poses some risk of micronutrient deficiencies, particularly of zinc, iron, calcium, and vitamins B_{12} and D. A diverse and balanced vegan diet that meets all nutrient needs, however, is readily achievable; useful guides have been published (72–74). Adolescents appear to be at particular risk of unbalanced vegetarian practices and should receive dietary counseling; routine referral to a dietitian is appropriate.

All vegetarian patients should be interviewed briefly to ascertain whether their diet is based on a balanced distribution of plant-based foods or on a preponderance of processed foods. In the latter instance, the patient is subject to the excesses of the Western diet and to nutrient deficiencies as well and should be counseled accordingly. For both reasons, if the patient is not well informed about the protein and nutrient content of plant foods, referring the patient to print and web-based sources of information (see Section VIIJ) and to a dietitian for detailed counseling is warranted. Vegetarianism adopted in adolescence should invite probing questions about the underlying motivations to ensure that body image is not distorted and to assess the possibility of an eating disorder.

The optimal distribution of nutrient intake for health promotion (see Chapter 45) is achievable with a vegetarian diet. Although a plant-based diet is rich in many micronutrients, certain deficiencies are particularly probable. A daily multivitamin/multimineral supplement is advisable, as is additional calcium supplementation (see Section VIIL) if dairy is excluded from the diet.

Whether or not they are inclined to renounce animal foods entirely, most patients should be encouraged to move toward more plant-based dietary patterns. Recent evidence suggests that the average intake of fruits and vegetables in the United States is well below recommended levels, with roughly 32.5% of the population said to consume fruit two or more times per day and only 26.3% consuming vegetables three or more times per day (75). Increased consumption of fruits and vegetables is strongly encouraged.

REFERENCES

1. http://www.publicpolicypolling.com/main/2013/02/food-issues-polarizing-america.html. May 26, 2014.
2. http://www.gallup.com/poll/156215/Consider-Themselves-Vegetarians.aspx?utm_source=alert&utm_medium=email&utm_campaign=syndication&utm_content=morelink&utm_term=USA%20-%20Wellbeing. May 26, 2014.
3. Rosell M, Appleby P, Spencer E, et al. Weight gain over 5 years in 21,966 meat-eating, fish-eating, vegetarian, and vegan men and women in EPIC-Oxford. Int J Obes (London) 2006;30:1389–1396.
4. Key TJ, Appleby PN, Rosell MS. Health effects of vegetarian and vegan diets. Proc Nutr Soc 2006;65:35–41.
5. Tonstad S, Butler T, Yan R, et al. Type of vegetarian diet, body weight, and prevalence of type 2 diabetes. Diabetes Care 2009;32(5):791–796.
6. Woolf PJ, Fu LL, Basu A. vProtein: identifying optimal amino acid complements from plant-based foods. PLoS One 2011;6(4):e18836. doi: 10.1371/journal.pone.0018836.
7. Liu S, Singh M. Amylose helical inclusion complexes for food and industrial applications: effect of chia seed meal on baking quality of cakes. October 19, 2011. Functional Foods Research Unit, Agricultural Research Service United States Department of Agriculture.
8. Rodriguez-Leyva D, Grant PN. The cardiac and haemostatic effects of dietary hempseed. Nutr Metab (Lond) 2010;7:32. doi:10.1186/1743-7075-7-32; <www.nutritionandmetabolism.com/content/7/1/3; accessed 5/19/13.
9. Becker EW. Microalgae as a protein source. Biotechnol Adv 2007;25(2):207–210.
10. Maurer NE, Hatta-Sakoda B, Pascual-Chagman G, et al. Characterization and authentication of a novel vegetable source of omega-3 fatty acids, sancha inchi (Plukenetia volubilis L.) oil. J Food Chem 2012;134:1173–1180.
11. Rosell MS, Lloyd-Wright Z, Appleby PN, et al. Long-chain n-3 polyunsaturated fatty acids in plasma in British meat-eating, vegetarian, and vegan men. Am J Clin Nutr 2005;82:327–334.
12. Beezhold BL, Johnston C. Restriction of meat, fish, and poultry in omnivores improves mood: a pilot randomized controlled trial. Nutr J 2012;11:9.
13. Beezhold BL, Johnston C, Diagle D. Vegetarian diets are associated with healthy mood states: a cross-sectional study in seventh day adventist adults. Nutr J 2010;9:26.
14. Wilson AK, Ball MJ. Nutrient intake and iron status of Australian male vegetarians. Eur J Clin Nutr 1999;53:189.
15. Thankachan P, Walczyk T, Muthayya S, et al. Iron absorption in young Indian women: the interaction of iron status with the influence of tea and ascorbic acid. Am J Clin Nutr 2008;87(4):881–886.
16. World Health Organization. Available at: http://whqlibdoc.who.int/publications/2004/9241546123_chap4.pdf. May 26, 2014.
17. Institute of Medicine. Available at: http://www.iom.edu/Object.File/Master/7/294/Webtableminerals.pdf.
18. FAO/World Health Organization Vitamin and Mineral Requirements in Human Nutrition 4. Calcium whqlibdoc.who.int/publications/2004/9241546123_chap4.pdf.
19. IOM Food and Nutrition Board, Dietary Reference Intakes for Calcium and Vitamin D. November 30, 2010; http://www.iom.edu/Reports/2010/Dietary-Reference-Intakes-for-Calcium-and-Vitamin-D/Report-Brief.aspx.
20. Thorpe D, Knutsen S, Beeson W, et al. Effects of meat consumption and vegetarian diet on risk of wrist fracture over 25 years in a cohort of peri and postmenopausal women. Public Health Nutr 2008;11(6):564–572.
21. Bonjour JP. Dietary protein: an essential nutrient for bone health. J Am Coll Nutr 2005;24:526s–536s.
22. Ho-Pam L, Nguyen T. Effect of vegetarian diets on bone mineral density: a bayesian meta-analysis. Am J Clin Nutr 2009;90(4):943–950.
23. Ho-Pham L, Vu B, Lai T, et al. Vegetarianism, bone loss, fracture and vitamin D: a longitudinal study in Asian vegans and non-vegans. Euro J Clin Nutr 2012;66(1):75–82.
24. Kwak CS, Lee MS, Oh SI, et al. Traditional Korean fermented foods found to be novel sources of B12. Curr Gerontol Geriatr Res 2010;2010:374897.
25. Tucker KL, Buranapin S. Nutrition and aging in developing countries. Am Soc Nutr Sci 2001;131(9):2417S–2423S.

26. Gilsing A, Crowe F, Key T, et al. Serum concentrations of vitamin B12 and folate in British male omnivores, vegetarians and vegans: results from a cross-sectional analysis of the EPIC-Oxford cohort study. *Eur J Clin Nutr* 2010;64(9):933–939.

27. Remer T, Neubert A, Manz F. Increased risk of iodine deficiency with vegetarian nutrition. *Br J Nutr* 1999;81:45–49.

28. Leung AM, LaMar A, He X, et al. Iodine status and thyroid function of Boston-area vegetarians and vegans. *J Clin Endocrinol Metab* 2011;96(8):E1303–E1307.

29. Johnston PK, Haddad E, Sabate J. The vegetarian adolescent. *Adolesc Med* 1992;3:417–438.

30. Perry CL, Mcguire MT, Neumark-Sztainer D, et al. Characteristics of vegetarian adolescents in a multiethnic urban population. *J Adolesc Health* 2001;29:406–416.

31. Martins Y, Pliner P, O'Connor R. Restrained eating among vegetarians: does a vegetarian eating style mask concerns about weight? *Appetite* 1999;32:145–154.

32. Greene-Finestone LS, Campbell MK, Evers SE, et al. Attitudes and health behaviours of young adolescent omnivores and vegetarians: a school-based study. *Appetite* 2008;51(1):104–110.

33. Robinson-O'Brien R, Perry CL, Wall MM, et al. Adolescent and young adult vegetarianism: better dietary intake and weight outcomes but increased risk of disordered eating behaviors. *J Am Diet Assoc* 2009;109(4):648–655.

34. Bas M, Karabudak E, Kiziltan G. Vegetarianism and eating disorders: association between eating attitudes and other psychological factors among Turkish adolescents. *Appetite* 2005;44:309–315.

35. Barr SI, Rideout CA. Nutritional considerations for vegetarian athletes. *Nutrition* 2004;20:696–703.

36. Baines S, Powers J, Brown W. How does the health and well-being of young Australian vegetarian and semi-vegetarian women compare with non-vegetarians? *Public Health Nutr* 2007;10(5):436–442.

37. Nicholson AS, Sklar M, Barnard ND, et al. Toward improved management of NIDDM: a randomized, controlled, pilot intervention using a lowfat, vegetarian diet. *Prev Med* 1999;29:87–91.

38. Marsh K, Brand-Miller J. Vegetarian diets and diabetes. *Am J Lifestyle Med* 2011;5(2):135–143.

39. White DL, Collinson A. Red meat, dietary heme iron, and risk of type 2 diabetes: the involvement of advanced lipoxidation endproducts. *Adv Nutr* 2013;4:403–411.

40. Barnard N, Katcher H, Jenkins D, et al. Vegetarian and vegan diets in type 2 diabetes management. *Nutr Rev* 2009;67(5):255–263.

41. Karabudak E, Kiziltan G, Cigerim N. A comparison of some of the cardiovascular risk factors in vegetarian and omnivorous Turkish females. *J Human Nutr Dietetics* 2008;21(1):13–22.

42. Elmadfa I, Singer I. Vitamin B-12 and homocysteine status among vegetarians: a global perspective. *Am J Clin Nutr* 2009;89(5):1693S–1698S.

43. Welch AA, Shakya-Shrestha S, Lentjes MA, et al. Dietary intake and status of n-3 polyunsaturated fatty acids in a population of fish-eating and non-fish-eating meat-eaters, vegetarians, and vegans and the product-precursor ratio [corrected] of α-linolenic acid to long-chain n-3 polyunsaturated fatty acids; results from the EPIC-Norfolk cohort. *Am J Clin Nutr* 2010;92(5):1040–1051.

44. Sambol S, Stimac D, Orlic Z, et al. Haematological, biochemical and bone density parameters in vegetarians and non-vegetarians. *West Indian Med J* 2009;58(6):512–517.

45. Ferdowsian HR, Barnard ND. Effects of plant-based diets on plasma lipids. *Am J Cardiol* 2009;104(7):947–956.

46. Yang S, Zhang H, Li X, et al. Relationship of carotid intima-media thickness and duration of vegetarian diet in Chinese male vegetarians. *Nutr Met* 2011;8(1):63.

47. Slavicek J, Kittnar O, Novak V, et al. Lifestyle decreases risk factors for cardiovascular diseases. *Central Eur J Public Health* 2008;16(4):161–164.

48. Woo J, Kwok T, Ho SC, et al. Nutritional status of elderly Chinese vegetarians. *Age Ageing* 1998;27:455–461.

49. Richman E, Carroll P, Chan J. Vegetable and fruit intake after diagnosis and risk of prostate cancer progression. *Int J Cancer* 2012;121(1):201–210.

50. Chuang S, Jenab M, Hashibe M, et al. Diet and the risk of head and neck cancer: a pooled analysis in the INHANCE consortium. *Cancer Causes & Control* 2012;23(1):L69–L88.

51. Aune D, Chan D, Norat T, et al. Fruits, vegetables and breast cancer risk: a systematic review and meta-analysis of prospective studies. *Breast Cancer Res Treat* 2012;134(2):479–493.

52. Sabate J. The contribution of vegetarian diets to health and disease: a paradigm shift? *Am J Clin Nutr* 2003;78:502s–507s.

53. Leitzmann C. Vegetarian diets: what are the advantages? *Forum Nutr* 2005;57:147–156.

54. Orlich M, Singh PN, Sabate J, et al. Vegetarian dietary patterns and mortality in adventist health study 2. *JAMA Intern Med* 2013;173:6473.

55. Crowe F, Roddam A, Riboli E, et al. Fruit and vegetable intake and mortality from ischaemic heart disease: results from the European Prospective Investigation into Cancer and Nutrition (EPIC) Heart Study. *Eur Heart J* 2011;32(10):1235–1243.

56. Winston CJ. Health effects of vegan diets. *Am J Clin Nutr* 2009;89:1627s–1633s.

57. Key T, Appleby P, Mann J, et al. Cancer incidence in British vegetarians. *Br J Cancer* 2009;101(1):192–197.

58. Kushi M, Jack A. The macrobiotic path to total health. *The Random House Publishing Group*, 2003:7. New York; Ballantine Books.

59. Weitzman S. Complementary and alternative (CAM) dietary therapies for cancer. *Pediatr Blood Cancer* 2008;50(2 Suppl):494–497.

60. Vermeulen M, Klopping-Ketelaars IW, van den Berg R. Bioavailability and kinetics of sulfurophane in humans after consumption of cooked versus raw broccoli. *J Agric Food Chem* 2008;56(22):10505–10509.

61. Page D, Van Stratum E, Degrou A. Kinetics of temperature increase during tomato processing modulate the bioaccessibility of Lycopene. *Food Chem* 2012;135(4): 2464–2469.

62. Garcia AL, Koebnick C, Dagnelie PC. Long-term strict raw food diet is associated with favourable plasma β carotene and low plasma lycopene concentrations. *Br J Nutr* 2008;99:1293–1300.

63. Koebnick C, Garcia AL, Dagnelie PC. Long-term consumption of a raw food diet is associated with favorable serum LDL cholesterol and triglycerides but also with elevated plasma homocysteine and low serum HDL cholesterol in humans. *J Nutr* 2005;135(10):2372–2378.

64. National Digestive Diseases Information Clearinghouse. A Service of the National Institute of Diabetes and Digestive and Kidney Diseases (NIDDK) January 2012, National Institutes of Health.

65. Rubio-Tapia A, Ludvigsson JF, Brantner TL. The prevalence of celiac disease in America. *Am J Gastroenterol* 2012; 107(10):1538–1544.

66. Bucci C, Zingone F, Russo I. Gliadin does not induce mucosal inflammation or basophil activation in patients with non-celiac gluten sensitivity. *Clin Gastroenterol Hepatol* 2013;11(10):1294–1299.

67. Kallio P, Kolehmainen M, Laaksonen DE, et al. Dietary carbohydrate modification induces alterations in gene expression in abdominal subcutaneous adipose tissue in persons with the metabolic syndrome: The FUNGNUT Study. *Am J Clin Nutr* 2007;85:1417–1427.

68. Dahlman I, Linder K, Arvidsson NE, et al. Changes in adipose tissue gene expression with energy-restricted diets in obese women. *Am J Clin Nutr* 2005;81:1275–1285.

69. Ornish D, Magbanua MJM, Weidner G, et al. Changes in prostate gene expression in men undergoing an intensive nutrition and lifestyle intervention. *Proc Natl Acad Sci USA* 2008;105(24):8369–8374.

70. Livestock Impacts on the Environment, Agriculture and Consumer Protection Department. Food and Agriculture Organization of the United Nations, 2006.

71. Phillips F, Hackett AF, Stratton G, et al. Effect of changing to a self-selected vegetarian diet on anthropometric measurements in UK adults. *J Hum Nutr Diet* 2004;17: 249–255.

72. Davis B, Melina V. *Becoming vegan*. Summertown, TN: Book Publishing Company, 2000.

73. Brazier B. *Thrive: the vegan nutrition guide to optimal performance in sports and life*. De Capo Press, 2008. Philadelphia; De Capo Press. Summertown, Tennessee; Healthy Living Publications.

74. Cheeke R, Abbott J. *Vegan bodybuilding and fitness*. Healthy Living Publications, 2010. Philadelphia; De Capo Press. Summertown, Tennessee; Healthy Living Publications.

75. State specific trends in fruit and vegetable consumption among adults-United States-2000-2009, Morbidity and Mortality Weekly Report. Centers For Disease Control and Prevention, September 10, 2010.

SUGGESTED READINGS

American Dietetic Association, Dietitians of Canada. Position of the American Dietetic Association and Dietitians of Canada: vegetarian diets. *J Am Diet Assoc* 2003;103:748–765.

Dwyer JT. Health aspects of vegetarian diets. *Am J Clin Nutr* 1988;48:712–738.

Hackett A, Nathan I, Burgess L. Is a vegetarian diet adequate for children? *Nutr Health* 1998;12:189–195.

Jacobson MF. *Six arguments for a greener diet*. Washington, DC: Center for Science in the Public Interest, 2006.

Johnston PK, Sabate J. Nutritional implications of vegetarian diets. In: Shils ME, Shike M, Ross AC, et al., eds. *Modern nutrition in health and disease*, 10th ed. Philadelphia: Lippincott Williams & Wilkins, 2006:1638–1654.

Robbins J. *The food revolution: how your diet can help save your life and the world*. Berkeley, CA: Conari Press, 2001.

Sanders TA. Vegetarian diets and children. *Pediatr Clin North Am* 1995;42:955–965.

Diet and Health Promotion: Establishing the Theme of Prudent Nutrition

CHAPTER 44

Culture, Evolutionary Biology, and the Determinants of Dietary Preference

If the presence of certain airborne toxins led researchers to conclude that human health would be promoted were we all to breathe underwater, we as clinicians would surely hesitate before offering that advice to our patients. The salient fact that we cannot breathe underwater would, and should, concern us more than the putative benefits of doing so. Even if a science developed that made it possible to distinguish—by virtue of depth, temperature, and content—optimal from less optimal water, the futility of such inquiry would impress us more than any such insights.

The fact is, we cannot breathe in water (while other species can) simply because we have not been designed to do so by the forces of evolution. Encouraging our patients to breathe in ways they cannot is not unlike encouraging them to eat in ways they cannot.

Among the environmental forces shaping the adaptation of species, diet, no less than air, has played a premier role (1–3). Only food, water, and air have been at work on our physiology from both without and within. Although the role of diet in evolution was clear to Darwin and seems self-evident now, much of dietary counseling and nutrition policy ignore its implications.

The conventional practice of nutrition counseling relies principally on an understanding of what patients should be advised to eat. That information becomes essential once we know why people eat as they do and understand what impediments must be overcome to change dietary behavior. But it is of decidedly less value with these questions unanswered. Limited success in the promotion of health and the amelioration of disease through the provision of dietary counseling (4–7) is cause not to renounce responsibilities in this area but rather to reconsider how they can be fulfilled.

The adaptations of our own species are less apparent to us than those of others and consequently are readily overlooked. Consider for a moment a polar bear in its natural habitat. Better still, consider 1,000 polar bears and transplant them all to Morocco. Let their perspicuous demise play itself briefly in your mind, as you consider its cause and obvious remedy. Now consider 1,000 people, or better still several hundred million, in their natural habitat. No particular scene springs readily to mind, for our apparent mastery of the environment has obscured our relationship with it. But although our ingenuity has largely allowed us to overcome the constraints of climate, we have fared less well in our excursions beyond the bounds of the native human diet (3). Much of the chronic disease burden and the majority of deaths in the industrialized world are directly or indirectly linked to a lifestyle and a diet at odds with human physiology (8–10).

For most species, the limits of tolerance are blatantly displayed in anatomic variation: the length of a coat, the presence of gills, the shape of a beak. If we generally overlook the limits of human environmental tolerance, it is because our frailties are concealed from view. We, less visibly but otherwise no less than any species, are well suited for a particular environment and ill-suited for others. To compensate for incompatibilities between human health and the prevailing environment, those incompatibilities must be understood. To modify human dietary behavior, we must know why we eat as we do (11).

Prehuman history, and consequently the origins of human dietary behavior, can be traced back reliably at least 4 to 6 million years (2). By examining fossilized teeth and fossilized human feces (coprolites) and by studying scanning electron microscopy of dental wear patterns, paleoanthropologists have gained considerable insight into prehuman nutrition.

The earliest identifiable human progenitors in the primate line were arboreal, and they were predominantly if not exclusively herbivorous (2,3). Over hundreds of thousands of years, prehuman primates increased in size and descended from the trees. As the cranial vault grew and intellect increased, our ancestors came together in cooperative groups, began to use first bone and then stone implements, and were able to scavenge successfully. Australopithecines began to use bone implements and were able to add meat to the diet through scavenging nearly 4 million years ago. Prehuman advances have been characterized by the nature of tools devised and used. Most of the 4-million-year-long human evolutionary period, characterized by the use of rough stone implements, is known as the Paleolithic era; the Neolithic period was ushered in by the manufacture of polished stone implements, little more than 10,000 years ago (12–16).

Advanced australopithecines ultimately were supplanted by *Homo erectus*, the first member of the genus *Homo*, which dates back approximately 2 million years; the genus included the species *habilis*, *erectus*, and *sapiens*. *Homo habilis* scavenged more successfully than its predecessors but had limited success in hunting. The greater cranial capacity of *H. erectus* permitted the planning and organizing necessary to ambush large game. Our ancestors became successful hunters in the time of *H. erectus* and continued to refine their skills thereafter. Cooking may have also played a key component in the evolution of human nutrition around the time of *H. erectus* as cooked food is easier to digest and more energy efficient, though of course it contributes to our current obesity epidemic by allowing us to consume a greater amount of calories in a shorter amount of time (15,16). Hunting and cooking became particularly important during the ascendancy of the species *sapiens*, in particular *Homo sapiens neanderthalensis*. The earliest members of *H. sapiens* date back some 300,000 years: *H. sapiens neanderthalensis* approximately

100,000 years, Cro-Magnon humans as much as 50,000 years ago, and modern *H. sapiens sapiens* approximately 30,000 years (17,18).

Although our ancestors became increasingly successful at hunting over time, studies of both the fossil record and modern-day hunter-gatherers suggest that early hominids obtained no more than 30% to 40% of total calories from hunting, with the remainder obtained through gathering. One of the more controversial topics in paleoanthropology is the extent to which we were hunters versus gatherers, with some experts espousing a larger role for hunting, and thus a greater prominence of meat in our native diet (19). There is widespread agreement, however, that the nutrient composition of animal foods consumed in the Stone Age differed substantially from that of domesticated feed animals predominant now.

Whatever the exact prominence of hunting, even a partial dependency on the hunt meant that as soon as prehumans began to eat more than vegetable matter, food supply was always in question. A large kill might supply an abundance of food for a brief period, but invariably it was followed by periods of potential famine. The cyclical redundancy of feast and famine, or at least the threat of that cycle, was among the salient characteristics of the nutritional environment to which our ancestors adapted, characterizing more than 99% of the hominid era on earth (20).

A pattern of eating in excess of caloric need and storing fat to endure periods of relative deprivation is observed in modern hunter-gatherers and is thought likely to have characterized the Paleolithic era as well (21). Because of the harsh survival demands of their world, including malnutrition, our ancestors lived a truncated life by modern standards; 19 of 20 Neanderthals (middle Paleolithic) were dead by the time they were 40; 10 of them by age 20 (2).

An increasing reliance on meat in the diet did not expose our ancestors to the type of dietary fat implicated in the chronic disease burden of developed countries. Although at times prehistoric hunters consumed a great deal of meat (19), accounting for up to 30% of calories (20), they consumed very different meat than we do today. Moreover, there is evidence to show that they had very favorable levels of serum cholesterol, blood pressure, and other cardiovascular risk factors, even with very high meat consumptions (22). Modern beef cattle are 25% to 30% fat by weight, whereas the average fat content of free-living African herbivores, thought to be representative of their ancestors, is 3.9% (3). Further, the flesh of wild game contains more than five times more polyunsaturated fat per gram than is found in modern meat, and it contains n-3 (omega-3) fatty acids, which are almost completely absent from domestic beef (3).

Paleolithic humans consumed far more fiber than we do (as much as 100 g per day), more calcium, one-sixth of the current US intake of sodium, and abundant vitamins from the variety of plant foods consumed (20). Of note, modern, cultivated plant foods are likely somewhat less nutrient dense than their wild Stone Age counterparts (21), contributing to the discrepancies between modern and ancestral human diets. In fact, yam, sweet potato, and taro were staple foods in many ancestral diets while grains, dairy, refined fats, and sugar were absent, suggesting that high carbohydrate intake in and of itself is not inherently bad. Fruit was also commonly consumed, which is a more salutary source of fructose than fructose in sucrose and high-fructose corn syrup as it is commonly found today (23).

Our ancestors generally ate less fat than we do, although the amount varied with time and place (19,20), and they may have even exceeded our intake of cholesterol from consumption of meat, eggs, organs, and bone marrow (2,3). Intake of saturated fat was low, and intake of naturally occurring trans fats was negligible. Western society, over the course of recent decades, has progressively consumed more fat (particularly saturated fat), less unrefined starch, more sugar, and less grain and fiber (24), further distancing us from the diet of our ancestry. There is some encouragement to be seen in a mean decrease in the intake of industrially produced trans fats in the United States following the 2003 U.S. Food and Drug Administration rules that established new labeling requirements (25), though individuals with certain dietary choices may still consume high levels of trans fats.

Also noteworthy is the dramatic decline in caloric expenditure since the Paleolithic, though physical energy expenditure itself has proven to have at times conflicting evidence in regard to weight loss (26). Our ancestors are estimated to have consumed more calories than we do but to have burned more than twice as many in the performance of work (3). Skeletal remains indicate that despite high caloric consumption, our ancestors were consistently lean. A discrepancy between caloric intake and expenditure, and the consequent advent of obesity, is fundamentally a modern phenomenon with origins in the Industrial Revolution (3). The impact of energy-saving devices on caloric expenditure has accelerated over the course of recent decades. Data in Great Britain reveal a 65% decline in work-related caloric expenditure since the 1950s (27); the proliferation of modern electronic devices has doubtless perpetuated this trend. A recent analysis of physical activity worldwide shows that 31% of adults 15 years and older worldwide are physically inactive, with a range of 17% in southeast Asia and 43% in the Americas and eastern Mediterranean (28).

Nonetheless, despite the important of physical activity for maintaining physical and mental health, there is also research that for the Hadza group in East Africa, which has a greater physical activity level than Westerners, total daily energy expenditure was in fact the same, suggesting that energy expenditure may be more consistent than previously thought across a range of lifestyles and cultures. Moreover, it points to overeating as a more important contributor to obesity than under-exercising, particularly given that the types of calories more widely available today are less healthy than those eaten by our ancestors (29).

The point of origin of human civilization is subject to debate, but the weight of evidence continues to favor Mesopotamia (2,30). Agriculture developed approximately 12,000 years ago in the delta of the Tigris and Euphrates rivers in what is now Iraq. Sumerians formalized agriculture based on irrigation, permitting the establishment of a reliable food supply for the first time in history.

A predictable food supply gave rise to unprecedented population density. Repeated cycles of irrigation caused salt to precipitate in the soil, destroying its fertility. For the first time, the nutritional needs of a human population exceeded the potential yield from hunting and gathering. The large, concentrated population that agriculture had sustained was compelled to spread out in search of adequate sustenance, giving rise to a human diaspora that ultimately colonized the planet and initiated trade, exploration, and conquest.

The notable nutritional consequence of human dispersion was dietary variation due largely to variations in climate and soil. Each new excursion resulted in the failure of certain established crops and the successful cultivation of new staples. Whereas barley was the principal grain in Mesopotamia, wheat flourished in Egypt, and bread was invented there (2,31).

Naturally, as humanity spread west, it also spread east. The reliance on millet and rice in the diets of eastern Asia reflects the early success of those crops there (32). Each interaction of human population and food supply left an indelible imprint on culture. The need to regulate the distribution of water in irrigation ditches along the banks of the Nile gave rise to centralized regulation that evolved into the pharaonic system of government. Legends developed around the public works of early Chinese leaders committed to producing more arable land to support a growing population.

In ancient Greece, a distinct culture by 1200 BC, olive trees were widely planted to replace trees felled to build houses and ships primarily because olive trees grew well over the superficial limestone characteristic of Greece. A demand for oil in cooking coupled with the increasing availability of olives resulted in reliance on the olive as a principal source because it happened to grow well. The now recognized health benefits of monounsaturated fatty acids (MUFAs) were introduced into the Mediterranean diet by agricultural happenstance. By the fourth century BC, a privileged class in Greece was enjoying a relatively rich diet; this group may have unknowingly benefited from the influence of MUFAs (33).

In ancient Rome, the need to feed a swelling population fostered conquest and further territorial expansion. Greater class distinctions encouraged a taste for the exotic among the wealthy. For the first time, dietary excess became a public health problem, albeit for a select group. The origins of "processing" are traced to Rome and may reflect a preference for heavily seasoned food as a result of nearly universal lead poisoning and a resultant blunting of taste (34).

Medieval Europe with its feudal system was profoundly influenced by food supply. Bread was a mainstay of the diet, and the word "lord" derives from the old English word "hlaford," meaning "keeper of the bread." Throughout the medieval period, shortages of food were frequent in late winter, and various pests decimated crops at regular intervals. The dense concentration of European populations, the lack of animal proteins in the diets of serfs, and widespread crop shortages were reflected in human stature. Human beings, both in the new world and old, were on average 6 inches shorter than their hunting ancestors (35). Average height reached the level of the earliest humans again only after the Industrial Revolution. In the Americas, corn thrived and became a staple, and as Michael Pollan has chronicled in *The Omnivore's Dilemma: A Natural History of Four Meals*, corn has come to dominate the American food system with growing concerns regarding "monoculture" agriculture and genetically modified organisms (GMOs). The tomato initially was discovered as a "weed" in the cornfields of ancient Central America (36).

The human diaspora has served largely to obscure the link between humanity and dietary adaptations about which generalizations can be made. The marked variations in diets around the globe in the modern era have concealed our common origins and our generally common dietary preferences. An obvious example is the Far East. Traditional Asian diets are quite different from American or European diets, and they have for years been invoked to explain marked differences in the epidemiology of chronic diseases, the most predominant examples of late being T. Colin Campbell and Thomas M. Campbell II's *The China Study* and Dan Buettner's *The Blue Zones* (37,38). Buettner argues that the longer, healthier lives of individuals in "Blue Zones" are largely a function of culture, environment, and lifestyle. These factors include a diet rich in beans, regular light exercise, supportive social interaction, a sense of purpose and belonging, and effective stress management, all of which in turn further support healthy eating patterns. But the differences between these populations and others around the world are narrowing in the age of a global economy; fast-food franchises serving hamburgers and French fries populate the planet from Baltimore, to Berlin, to Beijing (39–42). The current ascendancy of the Western or American dietary pattern as the global preference reveals our shared taste for sugar, salt, and fat and is a predictable consequence of our common origins (2,43). These tastes are exacerbated by growing trends toward away-from-home eating, snacking, and increased portion sizes, though of course heterogeneity in these patterns remains as for instance, away-from-home food intake and snacking are as high in the Philippines as in the United States but are rare in Russia and China (44).

The process of natural selection during the Paleolithic era remains an essential consideration in human dietary behavior, as the human genome has been essentially unchanged for thousands and perhaps tens of thousands of years (2,3,18,45). The current nutritional environment is one to which humanity has not had adequate time to adapt genetically (46). We are still characterized by the endowment of evolution, however irrelevant that legacy may now seem. The recent work of anthropologists reveals, for example, that men generally perform better than women in judging distance and throwing accurately and that this ability is genetically sex linked in a way that suggests it must have conferred an advantage that worked primarily through the male. Similarly, studies suggest that women see better in dim light and have sharper hearing. Such attributes would have served them well when they were searching for edible plants or tracking small game (2).

The prevailing diet of our distant ancestors remains the principal determinant of our nutritional physiology. The diet and the nutritional environment to which our ancestors adapted still dictate our preferences, tendencies, and aversions. That humanity adapted genetically to nutritional, environmental pressures may explain, in part, the prevalence of chronic disease in modern society. It is important to distinguish between the diet of our ancestors and pseudo "Paleolithic" diets popular today, including the facts that modern meat is not the same as Stone Age meat and that modern humans do not expend nearly as many calories through exercise as did our ancestors. Clearly a diet in the name of our meat-eating ancestors heavy in hamburgers, hot dogs, and bacon does not serve our health. There is also debate regarding the extent of meat consumption in the Paleolithic era, with recent evidence suggesting a greater proportion of plants and nuts in the Neanderthal diet than previously understood (47) as well as a significant amount of fiber (48). Ultimately the dietary details of the types of plant and animal foods consumed by our ancestors do matter. Thinking about our diet through an evolutionary lens is useful as a guide toward a well-practiced diet based on a variety of plants, nuts, seeds, eggs, fish, and lean meats.

In 1962, Neel (17) postulated that genes associated with type 2 diabetes mellitus were too prevalent in the gene pool to comply with conventional paradigms of genetic disease. Invoking the sickle cell gene as an analogy, Neel proposed that the "gene" for diabetes provided a survival advantage in the prevailing nutritional environment of human prehistory. The metabolically efficient individual, able to process and store energy optimally in times of plenty, almost certainly was best suited to endure periods of deprivation. The genotype, which under conditions of dietary excess manifests as obesity and type 2 diabetes, may have been the salvation of our nutritionally insecure ancestors.

This concept has since been embraced more broadly by some, although it remains controversial (see Chapter 6). As stated by Eaton and Konner (49) in an article on Paleolithic nutrition reported in the New England Journal of Medicine in 1985, "diets available to preagricultural human beings [determine] . . . the nutrition for which human beings are in essence genetically programmed." The authors contend that the divergence of humanity from the dietary pattern to which it adapted has significant implications for health, and a subsequent article by the authors 25 years later confirms and further supports this claim (50).

The imprint of evolution remains readily apparent in the idiosyncrasies of modern human dietary behavior and nutritional physiology. Perhaps the single most important example is the nearly universal tendency to gain weight easily and to lose it with considerably more difficulty. Vulnerability to weight gain may be mediated in part through elevated sensory preferences for calorie-dense food (see Chapters 5 and 38). Such a preference, which, like Neel's purported gene for diabetes, promotes obesity under conditions of sustained nutritional abundance, may have conveyed a survival advantage during millennia of subsistence and recurrent privation (17,51).

Recent studies have begun to elucidate the genetic basis for obesity (see Chapter 5). But genes responsible for a condition now affecting some two-thirds of the adult population in the United States, and lower but rising proportions in all developed countries, cannot simply be labeled "defective." The same metabolic thriftiness responsible for epidemic obesity was likely essential to the survival of our ancestors in a world of dietary deprivation. Jonathan Wells argues that adiposity is a "complex risk management system" for energy storage responding to multiple ecological stressors, including buffering famine, adaptation to cold, growth, energy for reproduction and immune function, buffering the brain, and aiding in sexual selection (52). This common susceptibility to weight gain has been dramatically revealed in the experience of the Pima Indians of the American Southwest. Adapted to a desert diet unusually low in fat and sugar and unusually high in soluble fiber derived from mesquite, the Pimas had, until the 1940s, a health profile typical of that of other indigent groups. After World War II, the government expanded support for Native Americans and provided the Pimas with, among other trappings of modern society, the typical American diet. Government support also resulted in a decrease in the caloric expenditure required for self-preservation, largely due to the advent of indoor plumbing.

In the ensuing decades, the Pimas have gone on to develop what were for some time the highest rates of obesity and type 2 diabetes of any population known. Although extensive study of this group has advanced our understanding of metabolic rate, the genetics of obesity, and the pathophysiology of the insulin-resistance syndrome, perhaps the most interesting finding is the most intuitive. When the Pimas resume consumption of their native diet, their health problems tend to dissipate (53).

The tendency to overeat calories may derive in part from the adaptive "feasting" of our ancestors when food was available. According to Dr. Jeffrey Flier and Sharman Apt Russell, we are programmed not only to overeat but also to fail to recognize immediately when we are too full so as to have more energy stores for the next time of famine (54). In rural Cameroon, one study showed the extraordinary rapidity with which weight can be gained through voluntary overfeeding for brief periods, as demonstrated by the Guru Walla ceremony where daily weight gains approaching 0.25 kg were observed in some individuals (55). Modern day overconsumption of calories may be not so much a problem of self-discipline as a problem of unprecedented access to calories. The problem of dietary excess is compounded by the variety of foods constantly available to modern consumers.

Sensory-specific satiety is the tendency to become satiated by consumption of a particular food and to consume more total calories when food is available in greater variety (see Chapter 38). Satiety is thought to derive from the interplay of characteristics inherent in food and the concurrent nutritional state of the body. The expression of satiety influences nutrient intake and energy balance.

The potential teleologic advantage of sensory-specific satiety, as posited by Rolls (56), is an incentive for the requisite dietary diversity to satisfy micronutrient requirements. Under current nutritional conditions of constant variety within and between meals, however, the tendency favors caloric overindulgence. Habitual consumption of high-energy foods may decrease sensory-specific satiety, which could lead to higher intake (57). Satiety thresholds are higher for sweets than for other foods, a fact that may account for the consumption of dessert at the end of the meal in most cultures: When satiety is attained, sugar remains desirable (58). Craving for sweetness may have had adaptive value as long as fruits and wild honey were the only available sweet foods, for they are a quick, convenient source of calories. In addition, naturally sweet foods are less apt to be toxic than are foods with a bland or bitter taste (2). The common use of nonsugar artificial sweeteners may further compound the craving for sweetness by dissociating sweetness from energy (59).

The incorporation of new foods into our ancestral diet was contingent on negotiation of the "omnivore's paradox": Although food sampling was essential to prevent nutrient deficiencies, any previously untried food represented potential danger. In reaction to these pressures, a natural curiosity developed toward new foods, whereas the degree of preference was associated with familiarity (60). Familiarity remains a profound influence on dietary preference, accounting for, in whole or part, the wide variations in dietary preferences among diverse cultures that are physiologically all but identical. Familiarity also influences expectations about fullness as one study found that children who ate certain foods more often expected those foods to give them greater satiation (61). Changes in dietary habits can establish new patterns of new familiar tastes and new preferences but require a commitment to work through a transitional period. The tendency for children to "dislike" food they have never tried, familiar to every parent, may reflect a deepseated tendency of the species rather than mere puerile obstinacy.

Sweet food may have more readily negotiated the omnivore's paradox than food associated with other flavors because of the consistency with which such food proved to be safe (2). The innate preference for sweet taste demonstrated by human infants (62) highlights an involuntary aspect of dietary selection. In addition to sweet foods, other reliable preferences among children include high-fat foods, energy-dense foods, and—at around 4 months of age—salty foods, and there is an innate tendency to reject sour or bitter foods (63).

The boundaries of individual control over dietary selection in an environment of constantly abundant food have not been established, though our primitive preference for sweets and fats goes beyond the allure of taste as opiate-blocking drugs have been shown to decrease sweet cravings, suggesting the potential (yet controversial) role of addictive qualities (64). These addictive qualities are not surprising given that our nervous system and endocrine system evolved to reward us for behaviors that require effort and are required for survival. Classic experiments by Clara Davis (65,66) revealed the ability of human infants to meet metabolic needs by self-selection of diet—but only when a variety of "simple, fresh, unsophisticated foods" was made readily available. Davis and reviewers of her work concur that were children exposed to less nutritious choices, the quality of their diets would suffer (65–67). Laboratory rats that were exposed to a "supermarket diet" in addition to standard chow become obese (67–69). There is evidence that neophobia/pickiness is a strongly heritable characteristic, while specific food preferences are modestly heritable and also influenced by the family environment (63). Unrestricted access to high-calorie, marginally nutritious foods may promote the development of obesity in children (68). Injudicious dietary patterns established early in life may contribute to the later development of heart disease, hypertension, and cancer (67,70). In contrast, promoting the restriction of certain types of foods (e.g., those high in sugar and/or fat) may decrease cravings and preferences for those foods (71).

Our fondness for dietary fat may derive from its prehistoric importance as a dense source of needed calories. As noted earlier, the fat available to our ancestors appears free of the ill effects of the fat we consume today. Preference for high-fat food apparently is mediated by metabolic, sensory, and sociocultural factors (see Chapter 38). There is evidence that ingestion of sugar and fat may stimulate pleasure by activation of the endogenous opioid peptide system. Consequently, there may be analogies between the intake of dietary fat and addiction (72).

Fats endow foods with a range of sensory characteristics and play a significant role in determining overall palatability. Improved socioeconomic status is associated with increased consumption of animal fats. Attempts to reduce the fat consumption of individuals or groups have been only partly successful, perhaps because of a failure to recognize that the regulation of fat consumption may have a physiologic as well as a psychological basis (72,73).

Studies in rats have demonstrated preferences for flavors coupled to the intragastric infusion of fat. Preference for fat was uncoupled from prior flavor preference, and the effect was enhanced by calorie deprivation (69). Generally, rats select high-fat (30% to 80%) diets when given a choice between low-fat and high-fat chow (74). The preference for high levels of dietary fat can be attributed to both the orosensory and nutritive properties of fat. Rats may have an innate attraction to the flavor of fat, but they also learn to prefer fat-associated flavors based on the postingestive effects of fat. Human studies support a similar affinity for dietary fat (see Chapter 38), and there may also be a genetic role explaining why some people have greater preferences for fat than others (75). Fat is less readily perceived in solid foods and, therefore, more readily accepted even by subjects educated to be fat averse (76). In a study of 30 human subjects conducted over 10 days' time, Mela and Sacchetti (77) found a correlation between fat preference and adiposity.

Innate and physiologically mediated food preferences are reinforced by environmental exposures. The convenient availability of a particular food has always been a significant determinant of its selection, and, as noted, familiarity is an important element in food preference (11,78). The innate predilection for sweet is modulated by experience. In an experimental setting, infants fed sweetened water exhibited a greater preference for sucrose solutions than others not previously exposed (62).

There is substantial animal evidence that familiarity is a principal determinant of dietary preferences. Geyer and Kare (79) studied young rats and mice and noted that the animals exhibit selective preference for the solid diet of the female from whom they received milk. The authors suggest that dietary selection by the nurturing female may be reflected in the taste of her milk.

Reed and Tordoff (80) fed nutritionally complete, isocaloric diets of differing fat composition to two groups of rats and reported that animals acclimated to the high-fat diet demonstrated greater acceptance of, and preference for, this preparation. In a similar study of weanling rats, Warwick et al. (81) demonstrated that 4 weeks of exposure to a high-fat diet engendered preference for high-fat preparations. In addition, rats that subsequently were crossed over to the control diet sustained the preferences for high fat generated during the earlier period. The authors suggest that sensory preferences acquired during early development may be more resistant to change than preferences acquired later. Another study showed that mice exposed to a high-fat diet during early life exhibited a significant preference for a diet high in fat as adults. This did not appear to be due to diet familiarity (as mice exposed to a novel high-carbohydrate diet during this same early period did not show differences in macronutrient preferences as adults), but rather may have been due to alterations in dopamine signaling in the nucleus accumbens (82).

In addition to the available research, there is the universally available empirical evidence that diverse human cultures have evolved preferences for a wide range of diets. That the palatability of such diets is often culturally limited and defined suggests that familiarity is significant. Human diets incorporate a spectrum of innately unpalatable tastes. Mechanisms responsible for the development of preference for an innately unpalatable substance remain largely unknown (62). One apparent mediator of preference for a particular taste is its association with a context of appropriate, or familiar, food. Preference for this context, itself, appears to be culturally mediated (62).

The differences between traditional dietary patterns in the United States and Japan, for example, have been ascribed to disparate tastes and preferences (72). As the standard of living among Japanese has risen, however, the popularity of meat and imported fast foods has increased in proportion to their accessibility (72). Nutritional differences between the Japanese and American diets, and among diets globally, are waning, as noted earlier. Universal dietary preferences evidently predominate over cultural patterns as nutrient-dilute, energy-dense foods

become available (83,84). For the most part, a lower socioeconomic status is associated with a lower-quality (energy-dense, nutrient-poor) diet (85), though similar to the Japanese and American example, higher education and occupation status is also associated with higher sugar and energy intake. Moreover, acculturation is associated with decreased dietary moderation and increased chronic disease risk among Asian Americans (86,87). Complications of these trends are found in many middle-income and low-income countries like South Africa, where there is a double burden of disease with increasing obesity coexisting alongside still-prevalent undernutrition (88).

Food and culture have always interacted, but whether functionally or dysfunctionally has been a matter of circumstance (58,89). Anthropologists believe that the acquisition of food may have shaped early religious beliefs, with late Neolithic period hunters/herders expressing their dependence on a variety of animals in the creation myth and early agricultural societies expressing their preoccupation with the seasonal demise and restoration of their food supply in resurrection myths (2). A preoccupation with the acquisition of food has clearly resounded through the ages. Success as a hunter was the principal means of gauging status in early tribal societies. In medieval Europe, control of land and the food it could produce gave rise to noble status. To this day, we link status to the acquisition of food, as evidenced by such words and phrases as "earning the dough," "breadwinner," and "bringing home the bacon" (58,90).

As food became equated with currency and success, holidays became times to rest and rejuvenate with mealtimes, and food became central to expressions of love, affection, and celebration. Finding joy in food—even sweets in limited quantities—and showing expressions of love are undeniably positive. However, using expressions of love as a way to continually turn food into unhealthy excess is not. Also prevalent is the belief that more food for less money is a bargain, as epitomized by the all-you-can-eat buffet, and technology has brought us more and more ways to lead sedentary lives.

Thus, genetic evolution and cultural history have cultivated human dietary preferences that are well suited for a world in which food is difficult to acquire. The endemic and epidemic health problems of modern societies are in large measure traceable

Loan Receipt
Liverpool John Moores University
Library Services

Borrower Name: Rechnio,Magda
Borrower ID: ********

Health Inequality :
3111 01504 1526
Due Date: 22/06/2017 23:59

The atlas of food :
3111 01366 0905
Due Date: 22/06/2017 23:59

Clinical nutrition /
3111 01490 3783
Due Date: 22/06/2017 23:59

Nutrition in clinical practice :
3111 01490 7677
Due Date: 22/06/2017 23:59

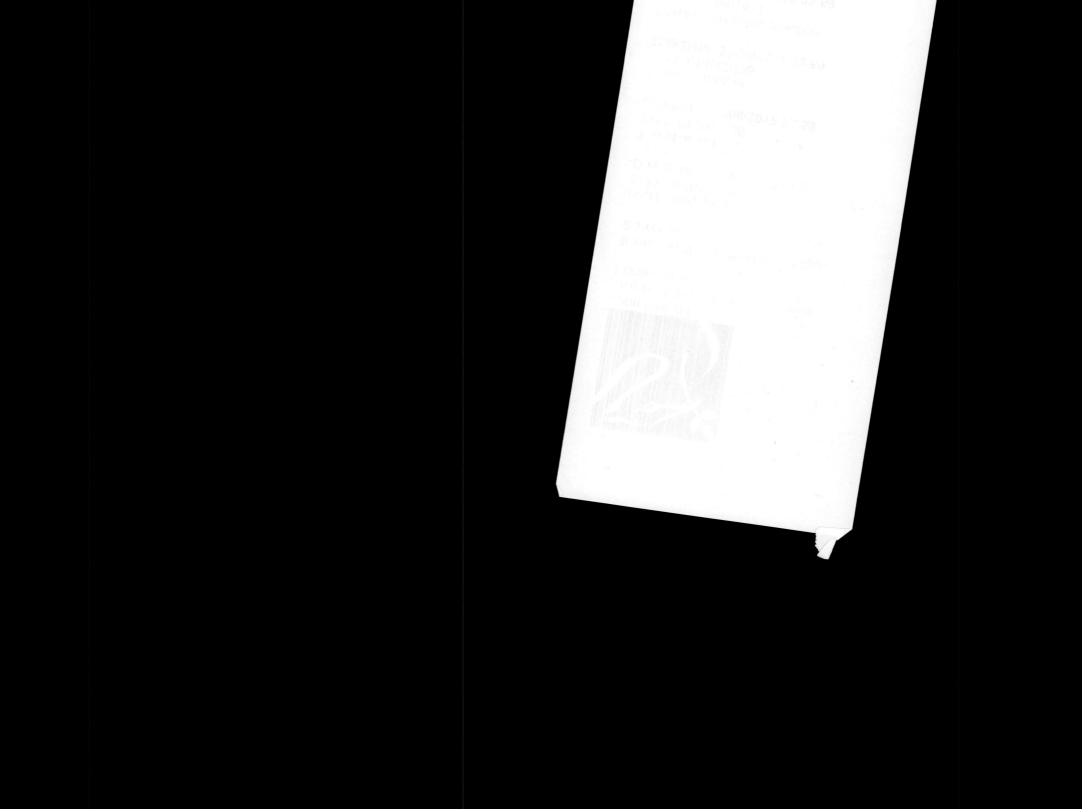

to our lack of defenses against dietary excess (91). Constant nutritional abundance, unknown to both human physiology and human culture for more than 4 million years, has become a modern vulnerability. Yet we usually wait until our health is "broken" to "fix" it, as opposed to considering—and attempting to change—the very cultural forces that have shaped our dietary behaviors.

The physiologic tendencies endowed by evolution, such as innate preferences for sugar and fat and sensory-specific satiety, are compounded by overt and covert activities of the food industry. Overtly, the food industry spends billions of dollars in advertisements promoting the taste and convenience of fast and processed foods, and it particularly targets children. Research on television advertising shows that exposure affects young people's consumption of the marketed products, and it influences their food and beverage purchasing patterns even 5 years after the initial exposure (92–94). The basis for preferring fat-dense, sweet, and salty food has already been addressed; other mediators of preference are familiarity and convenience (see Chapter 38). A destructive cycle is created as foods are produced that stimulate our shared preferences for sugar, salt, and fat and then familiarity with such foods is promoted through advertising. The role of healthful foods in the prevailing diet in the United States is increasingly threatened by their marginalization in the popular food culture (95).

In addition to advertising through the media, the food industry consistently presents information on food package labels to their maximal advantage and often to the detriment of the consumer, our patients. Bold lettering, for example, often implies that the absence of a certain ingredient, such as cholesterol, offers health benefits. Such labeling, however, often appears on products that are naturally free of cholesterol (i.e., all plant-based products) but rich in saturated or trans fat, sugar, or salt and limited in overall nutritional value. A study looking at 58 "Better-for-You"-labeled children's products found that 84% did not meet basic nutritional standards as derived from the U.S. Dietary Guidelines and National Academies of Science, with 95% with added sugar, and more than half low in fiber or not containing any fruits or vegetables (96).

Packages boasting an absence of the highly saturated tropical oils often contain products in which those oils have been replaced by partially hydrogenated fat. Fat-modified dairy products indicate how much fat they contain by weight (e.g., 2% milk) rather than how much fat was removed from the original product (e.g., 50% in the case of 2% milk). Whatever nutrient has most recently captured the public imagination as a means to promote health is named in bold letters on every package of processed foods. At present, front-of-package banner ads for "whole grain" content are in vogue. The marquee nutritional trait on a package generally makes a far more modest contribution to the actual composition of the food (the "contains oat bran" period is a good example) than to the marketing campaign. Many food companies try to promote a healthier image such as McDonald Happy Meals with apple slices instead of fries or Kraft's promotion of the Oreo as "milk's favorite cookie" and lower-calorie snack packs while simultaneously promoting even more decadent reformulations (63). A public preoccupation with the health-promoting properties of nature has resulted in widespread labeling of foods as "natural." Cheese, bacon, whole milk, cream, sugar, and butter may be "natural," but the benefits in promoting them as such accrue only to their producers, not to our patients.

The food industry exploits prevailing vulnerabilities of consumers in a more subtle or covert manner as well. The addition of sugar to such foods as tomato ketchup or processed meats, which would not generally fit into the cultural category of sweet foods, may exert subliminal pressure on the consumer to overindulge because of sensory-specific satiety and resultant undermining of self-restraint (58,97). The addition of salt to such foods as breakfast cereals, often in amounts comparable to those in salty snack foods, may exert a similar pressure, even though the taste of salt in such products is largely masked (98). Whereas an innate preference for sweet and a high associated satiety threshold are thought to have guided our ancestors toward such sources of readily available calories as fruits and wild honey, these traits have been rendered maladaptive by environmental change. With the proliferation of factory-sweetened foods and processed sugar, the guiding hand of evolution is misdirected toward temptation and overindulgence (58). This trend is exacerbated by the fact that more sugary, salty foods are also cheaper. One study showed that in Seattle-area supermarkets from 2004 to 2008, food prices overall rose about 25%, the most nutritious foods (red peppers, raw oysters, spinach, mustard greens, romaine lettuce) rose 29%, while the least nutritious foods (white sugar, hard candy, jelly beans, and cola) rose just 16% (99). However, even in supermarkets with reasonably priced healthy options, the average shopper lacks the skill set to reliably identify the more nutritious products (100). In modern Western society, therefore, cultural patterns, economic incentives, and socioeconomic disparities exacerbate physiologic tendencies, further undermining the capacity of our patients to select a health-promoting diet (58,90). These trends even extend to the athletic arena, where in the 2012 Olympics, for instance, the irony of sponsorships by major companies like Coca-Cola, McDonalds, and Cadbury create an unhelpful and unrealistic association between unhealthy eating and physical prowess.

There are clearly aspects of diet-related behavior that are predominantly nonvolitional with an increasing body of evidence pointing toward patterns of neural activation of reward circuitry and reduced activation of inhibitory regions in addictive-like eating behavior (101). Voluntary restriction of fat and sugar intake appears to be at odds with 6 million years of genetic adaptation and psychobehavioral conditioning. The same may be true for salt restriction. Kumanyika (102) reported that the intensity and cost of interventions necessary to achieve compliance with a sodium guideline of 3,000 mg per day are prohibitive given the prevailing US diet. Encouraging individual responsibility for diet without distinguishing volitional from nonvolitional factors is likely to be detrimental in two ways. First, frustration and duress will ensue as individuals fail in their efforts to master nonvolitional factors, often ironically predisposing many individuals to even more unhealthy eating as a coping mechanism for their emotional distress. The psychological consequences of obesity, the societal pressure against it, and the prevailing preoccupation with often unsuccessful dieting have been described by Brownell (103) and others (104) (see Chapter 5). Second, efforts to develop effective strategies for modifying diet, based on both individual counseling and alteration of the food supply, will receive insufficient emphasis as long as a "blame the victim" tendency prevails (see Chapter 47). This version of the personal responsibility argument is also reminiscent of the tobacco industry's efforts to thwart legislative and regulatory interventions.

A *Chicago Tribune* examination of tobacco-lawsuit documents found evidence of collaboration between food and tobacco brain scientists about issues of taste and smell, indicating the ways in which both products are designed to sway personal choices (64). More recent work in this area by the investigative journalist, Michael Moss, is consistent, highlighting the willful "engineering" of addictive junk foods (REFS).

Primary care providers must understand the diverse impediments to dietary modification and view that understanding as the basis for more artful counseling rather than as cause for pessimism. The public health stakes are simply too high for us to abandon our efforts at promoting nutritional health (8). Nutrition is of critical importance in the pathogenesis of the most prevalent chronic diseases in the United States, as well as obesity. National nutrition objectives in the United States for the year 2010 are predicated on the conviction that changes in diet and lifestyle can reduce or prevent prevalent causes of morbidity and mortality.

Dietary guidelines have been generated and disseminated with the presumption that individuals have both the will and capacity to modify dietary selection, independent of environmental constraints. There is ample cause to question this conviction (105), and there is evidence of an emerging shift toward a greater focus on societal solutions with a growing public discourse around the need for regulatory change to tackle the dietary environmental challenges individuals are faced with on a daily basis (106). There is an obvious conflict in a culture that exposes children to "junk food" and then encourages them to eat well (107). Fundamentally, our patients are threatened by a toxic nutritional environment (77,107–110). The constant temptations of dietary variety, sugar, salt, and fat are compounded by the conveniences of modern society and the resultant progressive decline in activity levels. These modern day conveniences also predispose us to expect food when and where we want it; in contrasting American versus European attitudes toward food, sociologists highlight the stereotypically American language of daily food allowances and personal food choices in contrast to the latter's emphasis on food as an enjoyable social experience and shared resource (111).

An understanding of the determinants of human dietary preference and selection is a prerequisite to dietary modification. Just as limited success in smoking cessation counseling has fostered greater efforts in this area, the limited successes of dietary counseling imply a need for greater efforts. Only an approach to dietary health that accommodates the physiologic characteristics and cultural predispositions with which humanity has been endowed has meaningful hope of success. As is the case for smoking, changing dietary behaviors likely will require multiple interventions and certainly will require an understanding of the obstacles to such change. Also similar to smoking, the role of stress with overeating is a significant obstacle, even in otherwise healthy eating environments (112).

Whereas admonishments to quit smoking are sufficient motivation for some patients, others require alternative interventions, such as nicotine replacement and pharmacotherapy. Advising nicotine-addicted patients to quit smoking was less successful before nicotine addiction was recognized. Similarly, means to reduce dietary fat intake have been devised on the basis of an understanding of dietary preferences; substitution of low-fat ingredients in the preparation of otherwise familiar food is one such method (113). Moreover, while these individual interventions are certainly critical, at least equally important was the cultural shift in smoking patterns that came with the fights against the tobacco companies, and that may likewise come with more changes in our food environment.

Participants in the Women's Health Trial, surveyed 1 year after the termination of the trial to assess maintenance of learned, low-fat dietary patterns, persisted in ingredient substitution and recipe modification, whereas efforts at avoiding fat and replacing high-fat food were less well maintained (113). Low-fat substitutions in food preparation may reduce fat intake while preserving the basic structure of the diet and its culturally important "meaning" (114). Further, establishing familiarity with a fat-reduced diet may be difficult but, once achieved, may substantially enhance acceptance and even preference. Participants in this study acclimated to a low-fat diet reported actual physical discomfort and aversion associated with high-fat meals (113). A similar effect has been seen with reducing salt in that simple exposure to the taste of no-added salt soup was sufficient to increase enjoyment of it to a level equivalent to the initially preferred salt level (115). In light of modern understanding, efforts to reduce dietary fat intake should be preferentially targeted to those classes of fat associated with adverse effects and/or customarily consumed in excess (see Chapters 2, 7, and 45).

Given the physiologic impulses with which millennia of evolution have endowed humanity, a prevailing preference for calorically dense food—refined sugar, processed carbohydrate, and fat—is what would be expected. To the extent that the nutritional environment accommodates these impulses, they are generally indulged. Recent studies investigating the impact of "food deserts" on obesity have challenged the link between food access and obesity, suggesting no relationship between the type of food sold in the neighborhood and childhood and adolescent obesity. However, it was found that poor neighborhoods do have more fast-food restaurants and convenience and corner stores, supporting the notion that it is not necessarily lack of access to better options that is the problem so much as greater availability of unhealthy options (116,117). Education and enhancement of individual motivation are most likely to achieve behavioral change when accompanied by environmental modification (78,118) that makes eating well less arduous. In fact, research on behavioral change more generally makes a similar argument about the necessity of effective change in three realms: directing the one's intellect, motivating one's emotions, and shaping the environment (119).

Although primary care providers can do little to modify the food supply, more effective dietary counseling will contribute to interim progress. There is evidence that the public receives most of its nutrition information from media sources (120–122) but that most people trust nutrition information from a personal physician or health care provider more than from any other source (121). There is also evidence, albeit limited, that dietary counseling by primary care providers meaningfully influences dietary behavior (7).

An approach to human nutrition based in part on evolutionary biology has certain limitations: We have at best imperfect knowledge of what/how our ancestors ate, our ancestors lived a relatively short lifespan, and we have limited knowledge of the nutrition-related health problems to which our ancestors may have been subject. The diet favored by natural selection for a 40-year lifespan is not necessarily optimal for a lifespan nearly twice as long. Yet our knowledge of our ancestors' diets is useful in explaining our dietary tendencies and preferences, even if it fails to identify the optimal diet for health promotion.

Zoo animals, by way of analogy, may live longer in captivity than their wild counterparts. But the wild condition is what explains the physiology of the captive animal. The native state, whether it is optimal in every way, is highly informative of appropriate environmental conditions, diet included. Consideration of evolutionary biology is valuable in emphasizing the relevance of our adaptation to a particular nutritional environment and our struggles in attempting to adapt to a very different one.

The adaptations of our ancestors, and the interplay of physiology, psychology, and culture, may thus explain our nutritional failings and inform our attempts to characterize the optimal diet for our patients. Whereas the health-promoting properties of the n-3 fatty acids have only recently begun to generate interest, the markedly higher intake of this fat by our ancestors may explain its compatibility with our metabolism.

An understanding of why we eat as we do and what impedes and promotes dietary change is an essential element in promoting nutritional health and discussed further in *Disease-Proof: The Remarkable Truth About What Makes Us Well* (Katz DL 2013). Such an understanding, shared with patients, alleviates feelings of personal failure in attempts to improve diet. Advising our patients what to eat without addressing the diverse impediments to dietary modification—our shared vulnerabilities, cravings, and aversions—may be comparable to encouraging polar bears in North Africa simply to stop retaining heat. By addressing the obstacles to nutritional health and working with our patients to circumvent them, we may hope to see our efforts at dietary counseling translate into appreciable improvements in the public health, one patient at a time. This practical application of this enterprise is addressed in Chapters 46 and 47.

REFERENCES

1. Darwin C. *Origin of species*. New York, NY: Avenel Books, 1979.
2. Tannahill R. *Food in history*. London, England: Penguin Books, 1988.
3. Eaton S, Konner M. Paleolithic nutrition revisited: a twelve-year retrospective on its nature and implications. *Eur J Clin Nutr* 1997;51:207–216.
4. Glanz K. Review of nutritional attitudes and counseling practices of primary care physicians. *Am J Clin Nutr* 1997;65:2016s–2019s.
5. Kushner R. Barriers to providing nutrition counseling by physicians: a survey of primary care practitioners. *Prev Med* 1995;24:546–552.
6. Lazarus K. Nutrition practices of family physicians after education by a physician nutrition specialist. *Am J Clin Nutr* 1997;65:2007s–2009s.
7. Nawaz H, Adams M, Katz DL. Weight loss counseling by health care providers. *Am J Public Health* 1999;89:764–767.
8. McGinnis J, Foege W. Actual causes of death in the United States. *JAMA* 1993;270:2207–2212.
9. US Department of Health and Human Services. *The Surgeon General's report on nutrition and health*. Washington, DC: US Government Printing Office, 1988.
10. US Department of Health and Human Services. *Healthy people 2000*. Washington, DC: US Government Printing Office, 1991.
11. Glanz K, Basil M, Maibach E, et al. Why Americans eat what they do: taste, nutrition, cost, convenience, and weight control concerns as influences on food consumption. *J Am Diet Assoc* 1998;98:1118–1126.
12. Eaton S, Konner M, Shostak M. Stone agers in the fast lane: chronic degenerative diseases in evolutionary perspective. *Am J Med* 1988;84:739–749.
13. Wrangham R. *Catching fire: how cooking made us human*. New York, Basic Books, 2009.
14. Carmody RN, Wrangham RW. Cooking and the human commitment to a high-quality diet. *Cold Spring Harb Symp Quant Biol* 2009;74:427–434.
15. Von Hippel A. *Human evolutionary biology: human anatomy and physiology from an evolutionary perspective*. Anchorage, AK: Stone Age Press, 1994.
16. Howell F. *Early man*. New York, NY: Time-Life Books, 1971.
17. Neel J. Diabetes mellitus: a "thrifty" genotype rendered detrimental by "progress?" *Am J Hum Genet* 1962;14:353–362.
18. Eaton SB, Eaton SB III, Konner MJ, et al. An evolutionary perspective enhances understanding of human nutritional requirements. *J Nutr* 1996;126:1732–1740.
19. Garn S. From the Miocene to olestra: a historical perspective on fat consumption. *J Am Diet Assoc* 1997;97:s54–s57.
20. Eaton SB. The ancestral human diet: what was it and should it be a paradigm for contemporary nutrition? *Proc Nutr Soc* 2006;65:1–6.
21. Arbor Communications. *Clinical nutrition update 270: is the nutrient content of our food falling?* January 29, 2007. Available at http://www.nutritionupdates.org; accessed 11/7/07.
22. Lindeberg S. *Food and Western disease: health and nutrition from an evolutional perspective*. Oxford, UK: Wiley-Blackwell, 2010.
23. Lindeberg S. Paleolithic diets as a model for prevention and treatment of western disease. *Am J Human Biol* 2012;24:110–115.
24. Gortner W. Nutrition in the United States, 1900 to 1974. *Cancer Res* 1975;35:3246–3253.
25. Doell D, Folmer D, Lee H, et al. Updated estimate of trans fat intake by the US population. *Food Addit Contam Part A Chem Anal Control Expo Risk Assess* 2012;29(6):861–874.
26. Rosenkilde M, Auerbach P, Reichkendler MH, et al. Body fat loss and compensatory mechanisms in response to different doses of aerobic exercise – a randomized controlled trial in overweight sedentary males. *Am J Physiol Regul Integr Comp Physiol* 2012;15:r571–r579.

27. Ministry of Agriculture, Fisheries and Foods. *Household food consumption and expenditure, with a study of trends over the period 1940–1990*. London, England: HMSO, 1990.

28. Hallal PC, Andersen LB, Bull FC, et al. Global physical activity levels: surveillance progress, pitfalls and prospects. *Lancet* 2012;380:247–257.

29. Pontzer H, Raichlen DA, Wood BM, et al. Hunter-gatherer energetics and human obesity. *PLoS ONE* 2012;7:e40503.

30. Kramer S. *Cradle of civilization*. New York, NY: Time-Life Books, 1967.

31. Casson L. Ancient Egypt. New York, NY: Time-Life Books, 1965.

32. Schafer E. *Ancient China*. New York:, NY Time-Life Books, 1967.

33. Bowra C. *Classical Greece*. New York, NY: Time-Life Books, 1965.

34. Hadas M. *Imperial Rome*. New York, NY: Time-Life Books, 1965.

35. Simons G. *Barbarian Europe*. New York, NY: Time-Life Books, 1968.

36. Leonard J. *Ancient America*. New York, NY: Time-Life Books, 1967.

37. T. Colin Campbell. *The China Study*. Dallas, TX: BenBella Books, 2006

38. Buettner D. *The Blue Zones*. Washington DC: National Geographic Society, 2008.

39. Hawks SR, Merrill RM, Madanat HN, et al. Intuitive eating and the nutrition transition in Asia. *Asia Pac J Clin Nutr* 2004;13:194–203.

40. Craven KL, Hawks SR. Cultural and western influences on the nutrition transition in Thailand. *Promot Educ* 2006;13:14–20.

41. Hawks SR, Madanat HN, Merrill RM, et al. A cross-cultural analysis of 'motivation for eating' as a potential factor in the emergence of global obesity: Japan and the United States. *Health Promot Int* 2003;18:153–162.

42. Popkin BM, Gordon-Larsen P. The nutrition transition: worldwide obesity dynamics and their determinants. *Int J Obes Relat Metab Disord* 2004;28:s2–s9.

43. Nestle M, Wing R, Birch L, et al. Behavioral and social influences on food choice. *Nutr Rev* 1998;56:s50–s74.

44. Popkin BM. Global nutrition dynamics: the World is shifting rapidly toward a diet linked with noncommunicable diseases. *Am J Clin* Nutr 2006;84:289–298.

45. Neel J. *Physician to the gene pool*. New York, NY: Wiley, 1994:302,315.

46. Cavalli-Sforza LL. Human evolution and nutrition. In: Walcher DN, Kretchmer N, eds. *Food, nutrition and evolution: food as an environmental factor in the genesis of human variability*. New York, NY: Masson Publishing USA, Inc., 1981:1–7.

47. Hardy K, Buckley S, MJ Collins, et al. Neanderthal medics? Evidence for food, cooking, and medicinal plants entrapped in dental calculus. *Naturwissenschaften* 2012;99: 617–626.

48. Boyd SB. The ancestral human diet: what was it and should it be a paradigm for contemporary nutrition. *Proc Nutr Soc* 2006;65:1–6.

49. Eaton S, Konner M. Paleolithic nutrition: a consideration of its nature and current implications. *N Engl J Med* 1985;312:283.

50. Konner M, Eaton B. Paleolithic nutrition: twenty-five years later. *Nutr Clin Prac* 2010;25:594–602.

51. Pettitt D, Lisse J, Knowler W, et al. Mortality as a function of obesity and diabetes mellitus. *Am J Epidemiol* 1982;115:359–366.

52. Wells JCK. The evolution of human adiposity and obesity: where did it all go wrong? *Dis Model Mech* 2012;5:595–607.

53. Fox C, Esparza J, Nicolson M, et al. Is a low leptin concentration, a low resting metabolic rate, or both the expression of the "thrifty genotype?" Results from Mexican Pima Indians. *Am J Clin Nutr* 1998;68:1053–1057.

54. Kluger J. The Science of Appetite. *Time*, June 11, 2007: 49–46.

55. Pasquet P, Brigant L, Froment A, et al. Massive overfeeding and energy balance in men: the Guru Walla model. *Am J Clin Nutr* 1992;56:483–490.

56. Rolls B. Sensory-specific satiety. *Nutr Rev* 1986;44:93–101.

57. Tey SL, Brown RC, Gray AR, et al. Long-term consumption of high energy-dense snack foods on sensory-specific satiety and intake. *Am J Clin Nutr* 2012;95:1038–1047.

58. Fischler C. Food preferences, nutritional wisdom, and sociocultural evolution. In: Walcher D, Kretchmer N, eds. *Food, nutrition and evolution: food as an environmental factor in the genesis of human variability*. New York, NY: Masson Publishing USA, 1981:59–67.

59. Mattes RD, Popkin BM. Nunnutritive sweetener consumption in humans: effects on appetite and food intake and their putative mechanisms. *Am J Clin Nutr* 2009;89:1–14.

60. Rozin P. The selection of foods by rats, humans and other animals. In: Rosenblatt J, Hinde R, Shaw E, et al., eds. *Advances in the study of behavior*. New York, NY: Academic Press, 1981.

61. Hardman CA. Children's familiarity with snack foods changes expectations about fullness. *Am J Clin Nutr* 2011;94: 1196–1201.

62. Beauchamp G. Ontogenesis of taste preferences. In: Walcher D, Kretchmer N, eds. *Food, nutrition and evolution: food as an environmental factor in the genesis of human variability*. New York, NY: Masson Publishing USA, 1981:49–57.

63. Wardle J, Cooke L. Genetic and environmental determinants of children's food preferences. *Br J Nutr* 2008;99: s15–s21.

64. "The Oreo, Obesity, and Us." *Chicago Tribune*. 2006; Available at http://www.chicagotribune.com/news/watchdog/chi-oreos-specialpackage,0,6758724.special. May 21 2014.

65. Davis C. Clara Davis revisited. *Nutr Rev* 1987;45.

66. Davis C. Self-selection of diet by newly weaned infants. *Am J Dis Child* 1992;36:651–679.

67. Story M, Brown J. Do young children instinctively know what to eat? *N Engl J Med* 1987;316:103–106.

68. Drewnowski A, Kirth C, Rahaim J. Taste preferences in human obesity: environmental and familial factors. *Am J Clin Nutr* 1991;54:635–641.

69. Lucas F, Sclafani A. Flavor preferences conditioned by intragastric fat infusions in rats. *Physiol Behav* 1989;46: 403–412.

70. Johnston F. Health implications of childhood obesity. *Ann Intern Med* 1985;103:1068–1072.

71. Martin CK, Rosenbaum D, Han H, et al. Changes in food cravings, food preferences, and appetite during a low-carbohydrate and low-fat diet. *Obesity* 2011;19:1963–1970.

72. Drewnowski A. Nutritional perspectives on biobehavioral models of dietary change. In: Henderson MM, Bowen DJ, DeRoos KK, et al., eds. *Promoting dietary change in communities: applying existing models of dietary change to*

population-based interventions. Seattle, WA: Cancer Prevention Research Program, Fred Hutchinson Cancer Research Center, 1992:96–109.

73. Davis JF. Exposure to elevated levels of dietary fat attenuates psychostimulant reward and mesolimbic dopamine turnover in the rat. *Behav Neurosci* 2008;122:1257–1263.

74. Sclafani A. Psychobiology of fat appetite. In: Henderson MM, Bowen DJ, DeRoos KK, et al., eds. *Promoting dietary change in communities: applying existing models of dietary change to population-based interventions.* Seattle, WA: Cancer Prevention Research Program, Fred Hutchinson Cancer Research Center, 1992:82–95.

75. Keller KL, Liang CH, Sakimura-McLean J, et al. Common variants in the CD36 gene are associated with oral fat perception, fat preferences, and obesity in African Americans. *Obesity* 2012;20:1066–1073.

76. Drewnowski A, Shrager E, Lipsky C, et al. Sugar and fat: sensory and hedonic evaluation of liquid and solid foods. *Physiol Behav* 1989;45:177–183.

77. Mela D, Sacchetti D. Sensory preferences for fats: relationships with diet and body composition. *Am J Clin Nutr* 1991;53:908–915.

78. Glanz K. Food supply modifications to promote population-based dietary change. In: Henderson MM, Bowen DJ, DeRoos KK, et al., eds. *Promoting dietary change in communities: applying existing models of dietary change to population-based interventions.* Seattle, WA: Cancer Prevention Research Program, Fred Hutchinson Cancer Research Center, 1992:195–204.

79. Geyer L, Kare M. Taste and food selection in the weaning on nonprimate mammals. In: Walcher D, Kretchmer N, eds. *Food, nutrition and evolution: food as an environmental factor in the genesis of human variability.* New York, NY: Masson Publishing, 1981:68–82.

80. Reed D, Tordoff M. Enhanced acceptance and metabolism of fats by rats fed a high-fat diet. *Am J Physiol* 1991;261:r1084–r1088.

81. Warwick Z, Schiffman S, Anderson J. Relationship of dietary fat content to food preferences in young rats. *Physiol Behav* 1990;48:581–586.

82. Teegarden SL, Scott AN, Bale TL. Early life exposure to a high fat diet promotes long-term changes in dietary preferences and central reward signaling. *Neuroscience* 2009;15:924–932.

83. Lands W, Hamazaki T, Yamazaki K, et al. Changing dietary patterns. *Am J Clin Nutr* 1990;51:991–993.

84. Drewnowski A, Popkin B. The nutrition transition: new trends in the global diet. *Nutr Rev* 1997;55:31–43.

85. Darmon N, Drewnowski A. Does social class predict diet quality? *Am J Clin Nutr* 2008;87:1107–1117.

86. Liu A, Berhane Z, Tseng M. Improved dietary variety and adequacy but lower dietary moderation with acculturation in Chinese women in the United Sates. *J Am Diet Assoc* 2010;110:457–462.

87. Tseng M, Fang CY. Socio-economic position and lower dietary moderation among Chinese immigrant women in the USA. *Public Health Nutr* 2012;15:415–423.

88. Rossouw HA, Grant CC, Viljoen M. Overweight and obesity in children and adolescents: The South African problem. *South African J Sci* 2012;5–6:2012.

89. Beidler L, Cantor S, Warren G, et al. *Sweeteners: issues and uncertainties.* Washington, DC: Academy Forum, National Academy of Sciences, 1979.

90. Axelson M. The impact of culture on food-related behavior. *Annu Rev Nutr* 1986;6:345–363.

91. Temple NJ, Burkitt DP. *Western diseases: their dietary prevention and reversibility.* Totowa, NJ: Humana Press, 1994.

92. Andreyeva T, Kelly IR. Exposure to food advertising on television, food choices and childhood obesity, 2010. Available at http://www.iza.org/conference_files/riskonomics2010/andreyeva_t5867.pdf. May 21 2014.

93. Harris JL, Bargh JA, Brownell KD. Priming effects of television food advertising on eating behavior. *Health Psychol* 2009;28(4):404–413.

94. Barr-Anderson DJ, Larson NI, Nelson MC, et al. Does television viewing predict dietary intake five years later in high school students and young adults? *Int J Behav Nutr Phys Act* 2009;6:7.

95. Pollan M. The age of nutritionism. *New York Times Magazine*, January 28, 2007.

96. Sims J, Mikkelsen L, Gibson P. *Claiming health: front-of-package labeling of children's food.* Prevention Institute, 2011. Available at http://www.preventioninstitute.org/component/jlibrary/article/id-293/127.html. May 21 2014.

97. Katz DL, Katz CS. *The flavor point diet.* Emmaus, PA: Rodale, 2005.

98. Callahan P, Manier J, Alexander D. Where there's smoke, there might be food research, too. Documents indicate Kraft, Philip Morris shared expertise on how the brain processes tastes, smells. *Chicago Tribune*, January 29, 2006.

99. Monsivais P, Mclain J, Drewnowski A. The rising disparity in the price of healthful foods: 2004-2008. *Food Policy* 2010;35:514–520.

100. Katz DL, Doughty K, Njike V, et al. A cost comparison of more and less nutritious food choices in the US supermarkets. *Public Health Nutr* 2011;14:1693–1699.

101. Gearhardt A, Yokum, S, Orr PT, et al. Neural correlates of food addiction. *Arch Gen Psychiatry.* 2011;68(8):808–816. Available at http://healthland.time.com/2012/04/05/yes-food-can-be-addictive-says-the-director-of-the-national-institute-on-drug-abuse/. May 21 2014.

102. Kumanyika S. Behavioral aspects of intervention strategies to reduce dietary sodium. *Hypertension* 1991;17:i90–i95.

103. Brownell K. The psychology and physiology of obesity: implications for screening and treatment. *J Am Diet Assoc* 1984;84:406–414.

104. Wadden TA, Stunkard AJ. Social and psychological consequences of obesity. *Ann Intern Med* 1985;103:1062–1067.

105. Institute of Medicine. *Improving America's diet and health: from recommendation to action.* Washington, DC: National Academy Press, 1991.

106. Hilton S, Patterson C, Teyhan A. Escalating coverage of obesity in UK newspapers. *Obesity* 2012;8:1688–1695.

107. Galanter R. To the victim belong the flaws. *Am J Public Health* 1977;67:1025–1026.

108. Milio N. Health, nutrition and public policy. *Nurs Outlook* 1991;39:6–9.

109. Becker M. The tyranny of health promotion. *Public Health Rev* 1986;14:15–25.

110. Cohen C, Cohen E. Health education: panacea, pernicious or pointless? *N Engl J Med* 1978;299:718–720.

111. Rozin P, Remick A, Fischler C. Broad themes of difference between French and Americans in attitudes to food and other life domains: personal versus communal

values, quantity versus quality, and comforts versus joys. *Front Psychol* 2011;2:177.

112. Michopoulos V, Toufexis D, Wilson ME. Social stress interacts with diet history to promote emotional feeding in females. *Psychoneuroendocrinology* 2012;37:1479–1490.

113. Kristal A. Public health implications of biobehavioral models. In: Henderson MM, Bowen DJ, DeRoos KK, et al., eds. *Promoting dietary change in communities: applying existing models of dietary change to population-based interventions*. Seattle, WA: Cancer Prevention Research Program, Fred Hutchinson Cancer Research Center, 1992:126–135.

114. Kinne S. Policy interventions on nutrition. In: Henderson MM, Bowen DJ, DeRoos KK, et al., eds. *Promoting dietary change in communities: applying existing models of dietary change to population-based interventions*. Seattle, WA: Cancer Prevention Research Program, Fred Hutchinson Cancer Research Center, 1992:205–213.

115. Methven L, Langreney E, Prescott J. Changes in liking for a no added salt soup as a function of exposure. *Food Quality Preference* 2012; 26:135–140.

116. Lee H. The role of local food availability in explaining obesity risk among young school-aged children. *Social Sci Med* 2012;74:1193–1203.

117. An R, Sturm R. School and residential neighborhood food environment and diet among California youth. *Am J Prev Med* 2012;42:129–135.

118. Glanz K. Environmental interventions to promote healthy eating: a review of models, programs and evidence. *Health Educ Q* 1988;15:395–415.

119. Heath D, Heath C. *Switch: how to change things when change is hard*. New York, NY: Broadway Books, 2010.

120. Achterberg C. Qualitative research: what do we know about teaching good nutritional habits? *J Nutr* 1994;124:1808s–1812s.

121. Hiddink G, Hautvast J, van Woerkum CM, et al. Consumers' expectations about nutrition guidance: the importance of the primary care physicians. *Am J Clin Nutr* 1997; 65:1974s–1979s.

122. Abusabha R, Peacock J, Achterberg C. How to make nutrition education more meaningful through facilitated group discussions. *J Am Diet Assoc* 1999;99:72–76.

SUGGESTED READINGS

Boaz NT, Almquist AJ. *Biological anthropology*. Upper Saddle River, NJ: Prentice Hall, 1997.

Dawkins R. *The ancestor's tale*. Boston, MA: Houghton Mifflin Company, 2004.

Diamond J. *Guns, germs, and steel*. New York, NY: W. W. Norton & Company, 1999.

Eaton SB. The ancestral human diet: what was it and should it be a paradigm for contemporary nutrition? *Proc Nutr Soc* 2006;65:1–6.

Katz DL, Brunner RL, St Jeor ST, et al. Dietary fat consumption in a cohort of American adults, 1985–1991: covariates, secular trends, and compliance with guidelines. *Am J Health Promot* 1998;12:382–390.

Katz DL, Colino S. *Disease-proof: the remarkable truth about what makes us well*. New York, NY: Hudson Street Press, 2013.

Kennedy E, Bowman S, Powell R. Dietary-fat intake in the US population. *J Am Coll Nutr* 1999;18:207–212.

McNamara K, Long J. *The evolution revolution*. Chichester, UK: Wiley, 1998.

Milton K. Nutritional characteristics of wild primate foods: do the diets of our closest living relatives have lessons for us? *Nutrition* 1999;15:488–498.

Relethford JH. *Reflections of our past*. Cambridge, MA: Westview Press, 2003.

Trevathan WR, Smith EO, McKenna JJ, eds. *Evolutionary medicine*. New York, NY: Oxford University Press, 1999.

CHAPTER 45

Dietary Recommendations for Health Promotion and Disease Prevention

F ood is the fuel on which the human body runs. It stands to reason that the quality of the diet has the potential to influence every aspect of our health. A high-performance body runs best on high-performance fuel. The content of this and other nutrition texts, as well as the primary literature, makes a strong case for this important linkage.

While much can be said about the universal fundamentals of healthful eating, it is equally important to note aspects of dietary quality that are context specific. In the context of subsistence living, for example, higher-energy-density foods (foods with the greatest amount of potential energy per unit of weight) may offer an advantage by helping to forestall potential caloric deficits when food is scarce. In the context of caloric excess and epidemic obesity, however, foods that provide nutrient density in conjunction with relatively few calories may offer an advantage. The quantity of dietary protein is of primary concern in populations subject to protein deficiency; associated nutrients (e.g., the mix of fats) take on primacy in populations with consistent access to more than sufficient protein. Given that overnutrition now afflicts more of the global population than undernutrition (1), the effects of dietary pattern on weight control are an obligatory consideration in attempting to characterize healthful eating.

Contextualizing the characteristics of a health-promoting diet need not end at the population level. The tantalizing promise of nutrigenomics—dietary guidance tailored to an individual on the basis of specific genetic variation—invites consideration of individualized recommendations for dietary health.

Regardless of whether the target is a population or an individual, the application of diet for health promotion follows two prerequisites. The first is the assertion of a healthful diet on the basis of a reliable and consistent base of evidence. The second is a reliable means of translating the evidence in support of a particular dietary pattern into behavior. There are, at present, certain controversies and uncertainties concerning the former; challenges to the latter are considerably more formidable. Nonetheless, the potential benefits of successful dietary health promotion justify a vigorous approach in clinical practice. Knowledge of diet, health, and effective behavioral counseling techniques (see Chapters 46 and 47) are both works in progress but sufficiently advanced to support constructive application. The influence of diet on health and the urgency of diet-related disease trends in modern society are sufficiently great to support the implementation of these practices.

Heart disease, the leading killer of adults in the United States, is amenable to dramatic risk reduction through diet by a variety of mechanisms (see Chapter 7). Similarly, obesity in the United States, increasingly a hybrid endemic and epidemic threat to both adults and children, is directly linked to diet and activity patterns (see Chapter 5). The estimate of Doll and Peto (2) that more than one-third of all cancers are potentially preventable through dietary manipulations is widely accepted, if not wholly substantiated (see Chapter 12). Stroke, hypertension, diabetes, pregnancy outcomes, degenerative arthritis, and innumerable other diseases, as well as general perceptions of well-being, are responsive to dietary influences.

There is currently considerably more consensus than controversy with regard to a health-promoting diet. Controversy persists and arises in areas such as the health effects of specific nutrients or the optimal diet for the prevention or reversal of specific diseases. Therefore, such controversies tend to be nutrient or disease specific. An extensive review of the diverse influences of diet on health serves to mitigate such controversies by providing contiguous lines of evidence that allow for clarification of overlapping recommendations. Elucidating that area of overlap is the principal aim of this chapter.

Behavior change is often facilitated in the context of established disease; individuals with disease perceive risk more acutely and therefore are more motivated to change behavior (see Chapters 46 and 47). Dietary recommendations in the setting of clinical disease are similar to those for health promotion, but they may be more extreme both in response to the greater acuity and in response to the patient's greater willingness to adhere to recommendations. The clustering of risk factors for various chronic diseases and of the diseases themselves requires that dietary manipulations for secondary and tertiary prevention not be overly disease specific. An obese patient with type II diabetes, for example, is at increased risk for heart disease, cancer, respiratory disease, and renal insufficiency. Therefore, although specific dietary intervention may be targeted to a single disease like diabetes, the dietary pattern usually remains consistent with recommendations for general chronic-disease prevention and health promotion. Exceptions arise only when disease-specific dietary modifications in the context of organ-system failure require departures from the basic pattern of healthful eating (e.g., protein restriction in liver or renal failure, see Chapters 16 and 17; carbohydrate restriction to reduce the respiratory quotient for pulmonary insufficiency, see Chapter 15).

This chapter characterizes the dietary recommendations that may be offered with confidence in the delivery of clinical care to virtually all patients.

DIETARY RECOMMENDATIONS FOR HEALTH PROMOTION

Consensus Recommendations

Diverse bodies of organizations and expert panels make general and disease-specific recommendations for healthy eating. The evidence base, rigorousness of review, and lens of interpretation vary considerably by organization, but there is a good deal of consensus in resultant recommendation statements. Selective recommendations, their commonalities, differences, and limitations are discussed below.

On the basis of its review of evidence linking dietary pattern to health outcomes, the U.S. Preventive Services Task Force recognizes that there is limited health benefit of initiating behavioral counseling regarding a healthy diet and physical activity in the primary care setting, except in selected individuals with cardiovascular risk factors (3). The *Dietary Guidelines for Americans, 2010* (4) and the corresponding U.S. Department of Agriculture food guide pyramid (5), now replaced by My Plate (http://www.choosemyplate. gov/), emphasize abundant intake of whole grains, vegetables, fruits, seafood, and low-fat or nonfat dairy, as well as restricted intake of simple sugars, saturated and trans fat, dietary cholesterol, and salt; however, these recommendations are limited by controversial results from the scientific literature, which are not reflected in the guidelines (6).

Important updates from the 2005 Dietary Guidelines for Americans include an emphasis on balancing calories to manage body weight and focusing on nutrient-dense foods and beverages. The 2010 guidelines focus on managing body weight through all life stages and on nutrition for children. They also incorporate eating patterns and behaviors, such as breakfast and snacking, for the first time and call greater attention to broader food-environment and food-systems issues to support healthy eating beyond the scope of this chapter.

The National Cancer Institute and the Centers for Disease Control and Prevention cosponsor the "5-a-day" program, encouraging fruit and vegetable intake and endorsing dietary guidelines that include 20 to 35 g of fiber per day, with less than 30% of calories from fat (7).

The American Heart Association offers dietary recommendations that call for efforts to balance caloric intake and physical activity to achieve and maintain a healthy body weight; consume a diet rich in vegetables and fruits; choose whole-grain, high-fiber foods; consume fish, especially oily fish, at least twice a week; limit intake of saturated fat to less than 7% of energy, trans fat to less than 1% of energy, and cholesterol to less than 300 mg per day by choosing lean meats and vegetable alternatives, fat-free (skim) or low-fat (1% fat) dairy products; minimize intake of partially hydrogenated fats; minimize intake of beverages and foods with added sugars; choose and prepare foods with little or no salt; if consuming alcohol at all, do so in moderation; and apply these recommendations when eating out as well as when eating at home (8).

The American Diabetes Association (ADA) recommends a generous intake of fruits and vegetables, beans, fish, whole grains, and nonfat dairy, along with judicious portion control and restriction of snack foods, sugar, and sweet consumption (9). The ADA supports the U.S. Department of Agriculture dietary guidelines and recommends a variety of grains, at least five servings of fruits and vegetables daily, restriction of saturated fat and cholesterol, and limited sugar and sweet consumption (10). Differing only in detail, all of these recommendations are substantially congruent.

In 2002, the National Academy of Sciences' Institute of Medicine (IOM) released dietary guidelines calling for 45% to 65% of calories from carbohydrate, 20% to 35% from fat, and 10% to 35% from protein, in conjunction with 60 minutes each day of moderately intense physical activity (11). The IOM guidelines further emphasize the restriction of saturated and trans fat and their replacement with monounsaturated and polyunsaturated fat. Also in 2002, on the basis of consensus opinion, the American College of Preventive Medicine formally adopted a position in support of dietary recommendations within the IOM ranges, and in opposition to carbohydrate restriction for purposes of weight control (12).

In its *Global Strategy on Diet, Physical Activity and Health*, the World Health Organization calls for an emphasis on energy balance and healthy weight: limiting total fat intake, attempting to eliminate trans fats, and shifting from saturated to unsaturated fats; increasing intake of fruits, vegetables, legumes, nuts, and whole grains; and limiting intake of sugar and salt (13). The concordance of these guidelines for global dietary health with those of leading organizations in the United States is noteworthy.

Most recommendations support the consumption of whole foods from plants (i.e., fruits, nuts, unprocessed grains, and vegetables including legumes and pulses). Recommendations generally advise moderating alcohol consumption

and limiting intake of processed foods and their usual components (e.g., added sugars, sodium, and trans fats). Where recommendations generally differ is in their advice around macronutrient distributions and types. It may be the case that there are both good and bad carbohydrates, fats, and proteins. Avoiding the bad types (e.g., refined sugars, trans fats, and possibly animal proteins) may be advisable, but the most optimal mix of macronutrients to advise for consumption remains uncertain. Table 45.1 provides a brief list of healthful modifications to the typical American diet supported by prevailing opinion.

Recommendations Supported by Confluent Evidence

Weight Control

Whereas dietary deficiencies have long been the predominant nutritional threat to health, caloric excess is especially prevalent globally (14). There are numerous reviews on the subject of diet for weight loss (see Chapter 5). In the aggregate, this literature lends strongest support to diets abundant in fruits, vegetables, and whole grains and relatively restricted in refined starches, added sugar, and total fat (15). Recent studies lend support to the Mediterranean dietary pattern and diets characterized by a low glycemic load (GL) (see Chapters 5 to 7). Strategies for the achievement of energy balance are beyond the scope of this discussion (see Chapters 5, 38, and 47), but given the increasing global significance of overweight and obesity, portion control and energy

---

TABLE 45.1

Steps to Improving the Typical American Diet That are Widely Supported in the Nutrition Community

- Reduce trans fat
- Reduce saturated fat
- Reduce sodium
- Increase fruits and vegetables
- Increase whole grains
- Reduce refined starches and simple sugars
- Replace "bad" fats with "good" fats
- Control portion size and total calories
- Increase physical activity

Source: From Katz DL. Presentation at *TIME Magazine*/ABC News summit on obesity. Williamsburg, VA, June 2004.

balance clearly figure among the key principles of healthful eating.

Dietary Fat

There is ongoing debate regarding the relative benefits of a diet restricted in total fat as compared to a diet with liberal fat intake but relatively rich in polyunsaturated and monounsaturated fatty acids (see Chapters 2 and 6). Studies by Ornish et al. (16) provide support for the extremely low-fat diet, at least for the prevention of cardiovascular events. Another study comparing a low-fat versus high-fat diet in obese people who had reduced energy intake by 25% showed that only the low-fat diet resulted in decreased waist circumference and fat mass, increased flow mediated dilation, and decreased leptin (17).

Estimates of our Paleolithic dietary intake suggest that we are adapted to a fat intake of as much as 30% to 40% of total calories (18), which is near the typical level in the United States today and below the liberal fat intake of some Mediterranean countries, and well above the intake advocated by Ornish and others. The benefits of a Paleolithic diet may include reductions in weight and cardiovascular risk factors. As reviewed by Kuipers et al., Osterdahl et al. showed that 3 weeks of a Paleolithic-like diet resulted in significant decreases in weight, body mass index, and waist circumference.

Based on the best available estimates, roughly one-third to one-half of the fat in Paleolithic diets derived from polyunsaturated fat, with an n-3 to n-6 ratio between 1:1 and 1:4. The remainder derived principally from monounsaturated fat. Although definitive evidence of n-3 fatty acid deficiency or of the benefits of supplementation may be lacking for any single disease, the weight of evidence overwhelmingly suggests a prevailing relative deficiency in the modern Western diet. There is preliminary evidence of a benefit of supplementing n-3 fatty acid intake in areas ranging from cognitive development (see Chapter 35) to the control of rheumatoid arthritis (see Chapter 20).

Unless consumption of wild fish or game is very consistent, n-3 fatty acid intake is sure to be lower than optimal, given the near-complete elimination of n-3 fatty acids from the flesh of farmed food animals. Consumption of nuts and seeds, particularly flaxseed, as a means of raising n-3 fatty acid intake is recommended. The use of flaxseed oil, totaling about 1 tablespoon per day for adults, is an easy way to increase n-3 consumption. Of note, n-3 fat from plant sources is generally α-linolenic acid, the conversion of which to eicosapentaenoic acid and docosahexaenoic acid (see Chapter 2 and Section VIIE) is variable.

A health-promoting diet may derive as little as 10% and as much as 45% of calories from fat, provided that fat is well chosen. The energy density and relatively low satiety index of fat suggest that intake toward the high end of this range may pose difficulties for those struggling with weight control (see Chapter 5).

Dietary Protein

The available evidence in the aggregate supports protein consumption in the range of 0.6 to 1 g per kg body weight in adults. Intakes up to approximately 2 g per kg may offer some advantages to vigorously active individuals, although this is uncertain (see Chapter 32). Higher intakes appear to be ill advised (see Chapters 3, 16, and 32). High-protein diets advocated for control of insulin resistance and weight loss are not supported by evidence of long-term health benefits and, in general, should be discouraged in favor of the pattern described (see Chapters 5 and 6). While there are studies to suggest cardiometabolic benefits of shifting calories from carbohydrate to protein, those benefits appear to be at least as great with high-carbohydrate but low-GL diets (19). Protein does offer the advantage of a high satiety index (see Table 45.2), and thus a modest increase in the percentage of calories from protein may offer weight control benefits to some (see Chapter 5).

The evidence that high intake of dietary protein is harmful in the context of impaired renal function and that protein consumption may accelerate the age-related decline in glomerular filtration rate is compelling; however, the harmful effects of protein independent of other lifestyle and dietary hazards are uncertain. There is some concern that high intake of protein may accelerate age-related osteopenia (see Chapter 14), but a recent study showed that diets higher in dietary dairy and protein led to favorable effects on bone biomarkers in exercising overweight women (20). If the overall dietary and lifestyle pattern are judicious, a relatively higher protein intake may be tolerated without sequelae. For example, regular, weight-bearing activity in particular attenuates the risk of osteopenia and

TABLE 45.2

A Comparison of the Energy Density and Satiety Indices of the Macronutrient Classes[a]

Macronutrient Class	Energy Density	Satiety Index	Comments
Fat	Highest; 9 kcal/g	Lowest	The notion seems to prevail that fat is filling, but on a calorie-for-calorie basis, it is the least satiating of the macronutrient classes.
Carbohydrate, simple[b]	4 kcal/g	Intermediate; lower than for complex carbohydrate	The satiety threshold for sugar is higher than that for other nutrients, thus making sugar an important contributor to caloric excess in most people.
Carbohydrate, complex[b]	<4 kcal/g	Intermediate; higher than for simple carbohydrate	Sources of complex carbohydrate—whole grains, fruits, and vegetables—are rich in water and fiber, both of which increase food volume and contribute to satiety yet provide no calories.
Protein	3–4 kcal/g	Highest	Protein is generally more filling, calorie-for-calorie, than other food classes, although this may not be true when compared to complex carbohydrate very high in fiber and/or water content.

[a]The satiety index is a measure of how filling a food is, based on comparison of isoenergetic servings (see Chapter 38).

[b]For purposes of this chart, *simple* and *complex* carbohydrate refer to the metabolic response to foods rather than their biochemical properties. For detailed discussion of this topic, see Chapter 1.

osteoporosis. Even in studies of competitive athletes, however, there is little evidence of benefit from very high protein intake.

Dietary Fiber

A diet consistent with consensus recommendations will result in considerably greater fiber intake than is typical in the United States (see Chapter 1 and Section VIIE). Although recommendations include a fiber intake of approximately 30 g per day, the weight of evidence also supports a specific effort to increase consumption of soluble, or viscous, fiber. Soluble fiber is found abundantly in beans and legumes and in a variety of fruits, vegetables, and oats and other grains. Consumption of soluble fiber tends to lower serum lipids and reduce the postprandial rise in both glucose and insulin via changes in intestinal viscosity, nutrient absorption, passage rate, and production of fatty acids and gut hormones (21). A specific recommendation to consume a variety of beans, lentils, apples, and oat-based products is supported by the available evidence. This is especially important for children as promoting the consumption of fiber-rich foods at a young age may prevent against carotid artery stiffening and related heart disease in adulthood (22).

Micronutrient Supplements

Nominal micronutrient deficiencies persist despite the abundance of the US diet. Supplements of vitamin B_6 and folate reduced elevated homocysteine levels, which may be a risk factor for cardiovascular disease; however, recent trials suggest that this effect may not translate into cardiovascular benefits as hoped (see Chapter 7). One recent meta-analysis does suggest some benefit for folate and other B vitamins with regards to stroke prevention (23). Folate supplementation before conception reduces the incidence among neonates of neural tube defects. Supplements of zinc appear to enhance immune function, and chromium supplements may improve insulin metabolism.

According to teleology, we may be adapted to a higher intake of micronutrients given the higher energy needs of our physically active ancestors and the calorie-dilute, nutrient-dense foods available to them (see Chapter 44). There is increasing evidence in support of vitamin D supplementation, and the combination of calcium and vitamin D (24) in supplement form may be of meaningful benefit in the prevention of osteoporosis (see Chapter 14). The role of calcium supplementation in the protection of bone is controversial, but other benefits of calcium supplementation are convincing (see Chapters 14, 28, and 34). Results from the Women's Health Initiative in 2010 suggest no benefit from calcium and vitamin D supplement on cardiovascular disease and blood pressure (25). Iron supplementation is probably not of universal benefit in the United States but is of potential importance for menstruating women with low intake of red meat.

There is insufficient evidence to support recommending a daily multivitamin for the prevention of chronic disease (26); however, there may be some evidence linking multivitamin/multimineral supplementation with improved cognition and mood (27). A recent study by Haskell et al. demonstrated that 9-week supplementation with a multivitamin in women aged 25 to 50 resulted in improved cognition and multi-tasking, as well as beneficial effects on mood and reduced homocysteine levels (28). Patients should be discouraged from using such a supplement as justification to comply less completely with dietary recommendations. The benefits of micronutrient supplementation are not nearly as well established as the benefits of a dietary pattern approximating recommendations. Inclusion of antioxidants in a supplement may offer specific benefits. Specific supplementation with high doses of single nutrients lacks supporting evidence for primary prevention but may be appropriate for more targeted disease prevention efforts. A fish oil supplement as a source of n-3 fatty acids may be generally advisable for both adults and children who do not routinely consume fatty fish. Dosing recommendations are offered in Section VIII.

Distribution of Meals

There is limited evidence that the consumption of frequent, small meals precipitates less insulin release than does the consumption of comparable calories in larger meals spaced further apart and that a "nibbling" pattern may offer other metabolic benefits (29,30). A recent study on diet records collected from over 2,300 girls in the National Heart, Lung, and Blood Institute Growth and Health study showed that lower eating frequency predicts greater gains in adiposity in adolescent girls independent from other contributing risk factors such as race, physical activity, and total energy intake (31). Other trials suggest that this apparent benefit may relate to dietary composition rather than distribution (32,33); but if meal and snack distribution influence composition, this distinction may be of

limited practical importance. For the majority of adults who would benefit from at least modest weight loss, frequent snacking may blunt appetite and help prevent bingeing, although this, too, is controversial. As discussed in Chapter 47, the psychological benefits of frequent eating may be considerable for patients working at weight loss or weight maintenance.

Energy Restriction

The evidence that total energy restriction may reduce all-cause morbidity and mortality is provocative although not definitive for humans. Long-term compliance with low-energy diets (i.e., calorie restriction) is unlikely in all but the most highly motivated individuals; given the obvious difficulty, most people have maintaining calorie intake at an appropriate level. Therefore, while of theoretical interest, a recommendation to patients to restrict calories to below normal levels as a health promotion strategy may be of limited practical value. In contrast, recent evidence shows that intermittent energy restriction (approximately 2 days per week) may be as effective as continuous energy restriction in producing weight loss and positive effects on health biomarkers. Intermittent energy restriction may be more feasible for most individuals (34).

Recommendations for Specific Food Groups

Meat

Whether meat consumption is beneficial, harmful, or neither for our health has been under debate. The most important point to understand is that contemporary meat consumption is strikingly different from that of our Stone Age ancestors. For example, there was no processed meat, pigs fed slop, or domesticated feed animals in the Stone Age. The flesh of grass-fed cattle may approximate the Paleolithic experience but imperfectly. The meats we consume today are higher in calories, harmful varieties of fat, and environmental contaminants that get concentrated as they move up the food chain. In addition, Paleolithic humans likely ate their meats raw so it stands to consider that contemporary food processing (i.e., curing with nitrites) and preparation (i.e., char grilling), both of which add carcinogens, are associated with poor health outcomes (35,36). There is also an environmental impact of factory farming, consolidation of feed lots, and confined animal feeding operations, which may relate back to human health directly (e.g., contaminating field crops and groundwater) and indirectly (e.g., through contributing to climate change) (37). Thus, it stands to reason that factory-farmed contemporary meat consumption should be limited, if not avoided.

Eggs

It is important to note that when discussing the impact of dietary fat on health, one must unbundle the effects of trans fat, saturated fat, and dietary cholesterol. In doing so, we see that the adverse effects of dietary cholesterol all but disappear. A recent study dissented the growing body of evidence supporting the nonmalignant nature of egg consumption and claimed that egg ingestion increases the risk of heart disease, indicated by the volume of atherosclerosis in the arteries of patients (38). This study, however, is severely flawed as it simply demonstrated an association rather than cause-and-effect, and was limited by investigator bias and predisposition. In contrast, we have conducted intervention studies, the results of which support the general evidence-based consensus that daily egg ingestion is not harmful. In fact, we found that egg consumption was nondetrimental in both healthy adults and those with high cholesterol. Notably, egg substitute ingestion was actually beneficial. Of course, one's overall dietary pattern is most important—and the processed sausage often accompanying eggs is almost certainly deleterious to your health.

Dairy

There is a growing body of evidence that dairy consumption is not only health promoting but also has the capability to lower the risk of cardiovascular disease. One recent meta-analysis showed that increasing dairy consumption to the recommended amount, i.e., three servings daily for people greater than 9 years of age, is associated with increased nutrient intake. Further, consuming greater than 3 servings daily leads to even better nutrient status, improved bone health, and lower risk of diabetes and hypertension (39). High intakes of milk, cheese, and yogurt do not appear to be associated with increased mortality, and substituting dairy saturated fat for meat may even lower one's cardiovascular risk by 25% (40,41).

Grains

Over the past 20 years, grains have been brought under attack (e.g., from low-carbohydrate advocates and those concerned about gluten sensitivities). Grains are made up of three parts: the bran or hull, the germ, and the endosperm. Whole grains contain all three while the principal component of refined grains is the least nutritious component, or the endosperm. In regards to paleoanthropology, grasses or grains are not native human foods but only entered the human diet with the advent of agriculture about 12,000 years ago, when their domestication led to increases in seed size. The question at hand is whether grains, whole or not, impact our health; and the answer is "most likely."

The recent National Health and Nutrition Examination Survey analyzed the impact of whole grain intake on various factors in just under 5,000 US adolescents. The study found that whole grain intake was not associated with body mass index but was related to positive nutrient profiles (i.e., lower fasting insulin levels and higher folate levels) and chronic disease risk factors (42). Further, other studies have demonstrated various sized reductions in risk of certain cancers, including colorectal cancer (43) and head and neck cancer (44) as well as better overall diet quality and nutrient intake associated with absolute intake of whole grains (45). The relationship between consumption of whole grains and weight is less clear as some studies have demonstrated an association with lower body weight; however, this may be confounded by increased fiber intake (45). Further exploration of carbohydrates is discussed below.

We cannot discuss grains without considering gluten intolerance (i.e., true celiac disease and reported gluten sensitivities), rising in prevalence in the United States in recent years. The reason for the increase is unknown but may have to do with genetic vulnerability or hereditability of disease, as well as new-age exposures to gluten (such as genetic modifications to gluten as well as nutrient combinations due to modern food processing) that may more likely trigger immune responses. Gluten, however, is not a poisonous toxin and is not related to weight gain or loss. While there is a small growing population of people truly intolerant or allergic to gluten who would benefit from eliminating it from their diets, the majority of the US population does not have such immune reactions. Eliminating gluten for most of us will not improve our health anymore than eliminating peanuts improves the health of people who are not allergic to them.

Sugar/Fructose

Firstly, sugar is not evil. We were born with a preference for sweet because that has fostered the survival of not only *Homo sapiens*, but mammals in generals. Even breast milk is a sweetened beverage so it cannot be all bad. Human breast milk is so sweet because we need a fairly concentrated dose of readily metabolizable fuel for our bodies and brains to grow. Our taste buds are geared to help us survive and they prefer sugar because we can safely digest it, and it supports our needs for cell growth and repair, hormone manufacture, and fight or flight from predators. Our brain connects sugar with pleasure rightfully so because this relationship has allowed our survival and procreation.

The problem ensues when we consume sugar in excess. Our Stone Age ancestors lived in a world scarce of food—while we live in an energy-rich environment. For us, sugar is addictive because the more there is (and there is a lot in our world), the more we habituate to it, and the more we desire. One of the reasons we eat too much sugar is because high-fructose corn syrup (HFCS) can be derived inexpensively from subsidized corn. An inexpensive sugar source makes it economical for food manufacturers to add copious amounts of sugar to our diets. Qualitatively, HFCS and table sugar (sucrose) are almost identical and consist of pairings of glucose and fructose in a 1:1 ratio. Thus, HFCS is bad for us because of the large quantities we consume.

Fructose, the component of many processed foods, is frequently attacked and while we do not condone eating candy and soda, we must emphasize that fructose is also the sugar of fruits. A diet can contain sugar, like fructose, and be optimal for health. A diet could be low in sugar but still be far from optimal (e.g., low in Ω-3 fat). Calories do count but it is the overall quality, and quantity of food consumption that is important—attacking one nutrient, such as fructose, is incorrect.

Organic Foods

Organic foods may be trendy, but it is unclear whether they are truly beneficial for health and even safe. For a food to be produced "organically," there can be no use of synthetic fertilizers, preventive antibiotics, irradiation, genetic modification etc. Contradicting reports compare the levels of vitamins and minerals and nitrates in organic versus conventionally prepared foods, and the jury is still out. It is difficult to make generalizations about organic foods because it is likely that nutritional content varies given differences in cultivation and production methods. Further, feeding trials in animals using organic versus conventional foods have been suggested as a means to assess the overall impact of organic food on health and apply that to humans. This system is inherently flawed, as we know that evaluating nutrition in health promotion requires consideration of the physiological network of an organism, human or animal. Simply looking at "health effects" of different diets in animals involves an overload of confounding variants. Measuring the effects of organic foods has thus been difficult and needs to be improved before we can include or exclude it as a dietary recommendation. Though many beliefs held regarding organic foods are likely unfounded, it does appear that organic foods result in lower consumption of pesticides; however, there are no studies establishing the causal relationship between consumption of conventionally grown foods and adverse health problems (46).

RECOMMENDATIONS FOR DISEASE PREVENTION

Cardiovascular Disease

Patients with established coronary artery disease are encouraged to comply with dietary recommendations offered by the American Heart Association (47,48) (see Chapter 7). However, the American Heart Association Step 1 guidelines, and even the more restrictive Step 2 guidelines, may not modify the prevailing US diet enough for the prevention of coronary events. Events have been prevented both with an extremely fat-restricted diet (16) and with a Mediterranean dietary pattern (49). Jenkins et al. (50) have demonstrated that a diet specifically designed to lower lipids can do so as effectively as statin drugs, but adherence to such a diet is difficult and unlikely.

McMillan-Price et al. (19) conducted a trial highlighting the importance of specific food choices as opposed to just macronutrient distribution in the mitigation of cardiovascular risk. Two diets relatively high in carbohydrate and two diets relatively high in protein (and lower in carbohydrate) were compared on the basis of differing GL. The GL, which considers both the glycemic index and the concentration of carbohydrate in a food source (see Chapter 6), has been shown in numerous trials to have potentially important implications for insulin metabolism, weight management, and cardiac risk. Simply, it means how fast a food makes your blood sugar rise and lead to an insulin surge. The study in question showed, as most do, that restricting calorie intake by any means led to roughly comparable weight loss in the short term, although trends hinted at a benefit of low GL. The percentage of subjects achieving an at least 5% weight reduction was significantly greater on the low-GL diets (irrespective of whether they were high carbohydrate or high protein) than on their higher-GL counterparts. Similarly, body fat loss was enhanced, at least among women, by the low-GL diets. Whereas low-density lipoprotein cholesterol decreased significantly with the high-carbohydrate, low-GL diet, it actually increased on the high-protein, low-GL diet. Importantly, a recent meta-analysis on prospective studies further concluded high glycemic load and index are associated with increased risk of cardiovascular disease, especially for women (51).

A low-GL diet can be achieved by minimizing carbohydrate intake, but this approach may toss out the baby with the bathwater. High-carbohydrate foods such as most whole grains, beans, legumes, vegetables, and even fruits can contribute to a low-GL dietary pattern. Such foods also provide a diversity of micronutrients of potential importance to overall health, and cardiovascular health specifically (antioxidants flavonoids and carotenoids noteworthy among them). It is most important to limit one's intake of refined grains, including white breads, pasta, and flour. It is easy to identify "bad" carbohydrates but increasingly more difficult to know what constitutes a "good" carbohydrate. Eating large amounts of whole grain carbohydrates may not be as health promoting as previously thought. It has been suggested that certain factors determine whether a carbohydrate is good and how good it is: the content of dietary fiber, glycemic index, whole grain content, and structure. Aiming for a ratio of total carbohydrate to fiber of less than 5:1 may be helpful (52).

By demonstrating that a high-carbohydrate, low-GL diet may offer particular cardiac benefit, the McMillan-Price et al. study points toward a diet in which choice within macronutrient categories is given at least as much consideration as choice among those categories. Cardiac health at the population level will likely be well served when dietary guidance is consistently cast in terms of healthful, wholesome foods rather than competition among the three macronutrient classes from which a diet is composed.

In light of all currently available evidence, patients at high risk for or with known coronary artery disease should be encouraged to adopt a basic dietary pattern matching that advocated for health promotion. Restriction of dietary cholesterol is of lesser importance and may not confer benefit (see Chapter 7). Frequent fish consumption, inclusion of flaxseed in baked goods, and use of flaxseed oil on salad should be encouraged.

Consumption of one alcoholic beverage per day is recommended; men may benefit from up to two drinks; however, the beneficial health effects observed with alcohol consumption may also be related to other chemicals in the drinks themselves as well as effects on eating behavior (53,54). Although the benefits of alcohol may pertain to all ethanol, polyphenols in the skins of grapes have antioxidant properties; therefore, red wine may offer additional benefits. Patients with hyperlipidemia should make a particular effort to increase intake of soluble fiber. They may do so by eating oatmeal, and particularly oat bran, consistently with breakfast; by eating oat-based breads and baked goods; and by eating beans, lentils, and apples. The use of spreads containing plant stanols and/or sterols at a dose of approximately 2 g per day may be advisable for such patients as well.

Cerebrovascular Disease

Cardiovascular disease and cerebrovascular disease share risk factors. Despite one study suggesting that high fat intake may reduce the risk of stroke (55), the weight of evidence favors comparable recommendations for the prevention of all sequelae of atherosclerotic disease (see Chapters 7, 10, and 20). There is insufficient basis to justify modifying the recommendations for prevention of cardiovascular disease in patients at risk for or with a history of cerebrovascular disease. The only caveat here pertains to patients with a history of intracranial bleeding, in whom fish oil and possibly vitamin E should be avoided depending on the etiology of the bleed, to avoid platelet inhibition.

The best-established means of preventing first or recurrent stroke is blood pressure control. The dietary recommendations for the control of blood pressure are provided in Chapter 8. In general, generous intake of calcium, magnesium, and potassium and restricted intake of sodium are recommended. A diet adhering to the pattern described for health promotion will offer these characteristics and facilitate control of blood pressure (56).

In addition, there may be a link between poor diet and neurodegenerative diseases, such as Alzheimer's dementia. A recent study found that greater adherence to the Mediterranean diet in elderly community-dwelling individuals is associated with reduced odds of having a stroke, or infarct, on magnetic resonance imaging (51).

Diabetes Mellitus

The Diabetes Prevention Program (57) provides convincing evidence that a diet conforming to basic guidance for overall health promotion, in combination with moderate physical activity, offers a powerful defense against diabetes in vulnerable patients. Specific benefits may be derived from a generous intake of soluble fiber from oats, beans, lentils, apples, and berries. A dietary pattern characterized by a low GL offers likely benefit as well, although this is readily achieved by adopting a healthful and substantially plant-based diet, with a relatively low intake of processed foods and refined grains. Additional details are addressed in Chapter 6.

Cancer

The maintenance of ideal body weight, low total energy consumption, and intake of a variety of fruits and vegetables appears to offer protection against many cancers, including but not limited to colorectal cancer, in which case a low-fiber diet is a known risk factor. Vitamins and minerals may also play a role, one such example being the association of high folate intake in postmenopausal women with a reduced incidence of breast cancer. These recommendations are consistent with those for health promotion and the prevention of other leading diseases. One departure is alcohol, which may reduce the risk of cardiovascular disease but appears to promote cancers of the breast, head, neck, pancreas, and other sites. Women at high risk of breast cancer, or individuals with a cancer history, are advised to abstain from alcohol. In such individuals also at risk for or suffering from heart disease, alternative means should be sought to provide the benefits of alcohol. Specifically, exercise and avoidance of refined carbohydrate may raise high-density lipoprotein, whereas aspirin and n-3 fatty acids may inhibit platelet aggregation. The antioxidants concentrated in red wine are readily obtained from fruits and vegetables, fruit juices (notably purple grape juice), green tea, and dark chocolate.

The benefits of energy restriction appear to pertain particularly to cancer prevention. Patients at high risk for or with a history of cancer should be encouraged to restrict calories to bring weight down to near ideal. In such situations, the use of micronutrient supplements is particularly important. In advanced cancer, nutritional goals should be shifted to weight maintenance, and energy restriction should be abandoned. See Chapter 12 for additional discussion.

Inflammatory Diseases

Although food intolerance may play a role for some individuals in the etiology of chronic inflammatory and autoimmune diseases, there is no evidence of such an association for the majority of patients. The most promising nutritional approach to chronic inflammation is improving the distribution of fats in the diet by reducing intake of saturated and trans fat, and reducing the intake of Ω-6 PUFAs and trying to consume more Ω-3 PUFAs (see Chapter 20). Fish containing a high concentration of n-3 fatty acids in particular may lower CRP and homocysteine levels, and these effects have been found to be clinically beneficial in patients with ulcerative colitis (58). A generous intake of fruits and vegetables is of likely benefit. Therefore, the dietary recommendations for health promotion need not be altered for patients at risk for or with chronic inflammatory conditions.

Infectious Disease

The principal effect of nutrition on the course of infectious disease is mediated through effects on immune system function. The one exception is in chronic infectious disease, such as HIV and AIDS, where cachexia may become an independent threat to health. A variety of micronutrients serve as cofactors in metabolic activities germane to immune function. Certain minerals important to the immune system, including zinc and magnesium, tend to be at nominal levels in the typical American diet.

A micronutrient supplement including minerals is reasonable, although of uncertain benefit, for the prevention of infectious disease and in all individuals with chronic infectious disease. The increased metabolic demands of infection, particularly when fever is present, require increased energy intake to maintain body mass. There is no evidence to suggest that the overall dietary pattern recommended for health promotion should be altered for purposes of preventing or managing infectious disease (see Chapter 11).

Renal Insufficiency

The most widely supported dietary manipulation for the management of renal insufficiency is restriction of protein to 0.6 g per kg (see Chapter 16). This intake level falls within the range recommended for health promotion and, therefore, may be advocated without concern of ill effects. The leading causes of renal failure in the United States are diabetes mellitus and hypertension, both of which are amenable to dietary management as described earlier and elsewhere (see Chapters 6 and 8). Notably, once a patient with chronic kidney disease begins dialysis, they must actually increase their protein intake to replace muscles and other tissues. According to the National Kidney Foundation Dietary Guidelines for Adults Starting on Hemodialysis, these people should eat 8 to 10 ounces (or 1.2 grams of protein per kilogram of body weight) of high-protein rich foods, such as poultry, fish, or eggs, each day (59).

Liver Disease

The principal dietary manipulations in patients with chronic liver disease are protein restriction and avoidance of alcohol. Moderate protein restriction relative to levels that prevail in the United States may be advisable for health promotion, whereas the optimal dose of dietary ethanol varies with individual circumstances. Thus, patients with liver disease should, for the most part, adhere to a diet consistent with recommendations for health promotion, while abstaining from alcohol. Supplementation with B vitamins generally is indicated and is provided if a multivitamin is taken daily. Preliminary evidence for nutriceuticals such as silymarin is discussed elsewhere (see Chapter 17).

Protein restriction is most important in the setting of overt hepatic encephalopathy; however though widely practiced, there is no existing evidence to support its implementation. In a recent review, Kachaamy et al. (60) ascertained that supplementation with branched-chain amino acids may be helpful for patients suffering from encephalopathy despite the usual pharmacologic treatments. They also stressed the importance of preventing starvation in cirrhotics, which can occur within hours of caloric deprivation versus days in healthy people. Patients with cirrhosis should always eat breakfast and have snacks, and may even benefit from probiotics.

Nutrigenomics

At present, dietary guidance for health promotion is based on principles of sound nutrition for the population at large. Recommendations are then further tailored on the basis of individual health and risk factor status. Family history may provide some insight regarding specific individual vulnerabilities before the advent of any overt manifestations.

There are in fact two new scientific fields: "nutrigenetics," which studies the effect of genetic variation on nutrient–gene interactions, and "nutrigenomics," which studies the impact of nutritional choices on health at the level of gene transcription and metabolism. Nutrigenomics is a nascent field devoted to linking dietary guidance to individual vulnerabilities discernible through genetic testing and the identification of specific polymorphisms (61,62). Genetic polymorphisms may account for variable susceptibility to adverse effects of dietary sodium or cholesterol, for example; for variable susceptibility to insulin resistance; and for variable micronutrient requirements. In other words, genetic polymorphisms explain why if two people who follow the exact same diet and exercise regimen, one may develop diabetes and the other may not.

Nutrient–gene interactions have been studied in patients with inflammatory bowel disease (63), as well as in breast and colon cancer prevention (64). Expanding the field of nutrigenomics will likely lead to the development of pharmaceuticals, with increasingly specific targets for individual people. To the extent that genomics may allow for more perfect dietary guidance, anticipation of that advance should not interfere with the good dietary guidance that can be offered right now.

Of note, *Homo sapiens* is a species with a native dietary habitat like other species (see below and Chapter 44). While there is doubtless genomic variation among, for example, lions, it is still self-evident that there is a basic dietary pattern suitable for lions—as there is for horses, koala bears, and tropical fish. While the pursuit of optimal health and cultural diversity complicate the formula for dietary health for humans, the principle that salutary dietary patterns are to some extent species relevant is still germane. The particular value of nutrigenomics may reside more in the motivational power of individualized health messaging (see Chapter 47) than in characterizing the dietary pattern conducive to health. While the relative importance of various aspects of diet may vary with alleles, in general, the fundamentals of nutrition that support health at the population level are apt to do so at the individual level as well. When available, the promise of nutrigenomics should be fully exploited. At present, however, the allure of that promise should not distract from dietary guidance that can and should be provided to virtually all patients with considerable confidence.

Evolutionary Biology

There is no denying that the evidence base for dietary recommendations for human health promotion is incomplete. There is, of course, substantially less scientific evidence to guide the development of dietary patterns for species other than our own, yet paradoxically, we seem to be far more confident when doing so. There is little controversy regarding the suitable diets for a wide range of domestic animals or, for that matter, wild animals held in zoos. The guiding principle on which that confidence is based is the "native" diet of each species. Lions in a zoo are not subjected to clinical trials to determine what they should be fed; they are fed something that approximates their diet in the wild. This approach, deemed reasonable and robust for diverse species, deserves application to humans as well. Consideration of our native diet is a useful construct for filling gaps in the science of human nutrition until or unless research advances fill those gaps.

Eaton (65) has made this very suggestion quite persuasively. The approach garners support from the fundamental confluence between dietary recommendations based on modern trials and epidemiological evidence and those based on methods of paleoanthropology to estimate our ancestral dietary pattern, which was rich in fruits and vegetables, high in fiber and micronutrients, low in salt and sugar, essentially free of trans fats, and low in saturated fat. The value of considering the dietary pattern to which our species is adapted in confronting the challenges of nutritional health today is addressed more fully in Chapter 44.

SUMMARY

The myriad effects of nutrition on health outcomes are documented in a vast literature of widely divergent quality. In certain vital areas, consensus has yet to develop. Sufficient evidence has been gathered, however, to permit the generation of dietary recommendations for health promotion and disease prevention with considerable confidence. There is overwhelming consensus in support of a diet characterized by a generous intake of vegetables and fruits, if choosing to eat grains, consuming the majority of them in the whole unprocessed form, beans, lentils, nuts, and seeds; an emphasis on fish and poultry or plant foods as protein sources; restriction of trans fat, saturated fat, refined starch, added sugar, and salt; a shift from animal and other saturated fats to unsaturated plant oils; and portion control conducive to energy balance and the maintenance of a healthy weight. Recommendations to include nonfat dairy in the diet are less universal but nonetheless predominant.

The same dietary pattern is appropriate for the prevention of most diseases. This has not always been evident and is worthy of note. Patients with cardiovascular disease often have diabetes, cerebrovascular disease, hypertension, or renal insufficiency, may have had or have cancer, and are constantly vulnerable to infectious disease. If each disease required a different diet, consistent recommendations could not be made to an individual, let alone to a population. The emergence of a "one diet" approach to nutritional health is a logical outgrowth of confluent lines of evidence and the clinical imperative for consistent and practicable advice. The benefits of a health-promoting diet should be combined with regular

physical activity for maximal benefit; a sedentary lifestyle may undermine many of the potential health benefits of an otherwise salutary dietary pattern.

All patients, with or without chronic disease or risk factors, should be encouraged to comply with a health-promoting diet. Patients with one or more predominant risk factors or diseases may benefit from modest disease- or factor-specific dietary adjustments. Although the advice may not change much with the development of disease, the conviction and frequency with which counseling is provided, and the willingness of the patient to change, should both increase.

An overview of dietary and related lifestyle recommendations for health promotion is provided in Tables 45.3, 45.4, and 45.5.

TABLE 45.3

Recommended Dietary Pattern for Optimal Health and Weight Control

Nutrient Class/Nutrient		Recommended Intake
Carbohydrate, predominately complex		Approximately 45% to 60% of total calories
Fiber, both soluble and insoluble		At least 25 g per day, with additional potential benefit from up to 50 g per day
Protein, predominantly plant-based sources		Up to 25% of total calories
Total fat		Up to 30%, and preferably approximately 25% of total calories
Types of fat	Monounsaturated fat	10% to 15% of total calories
	Polyunsaturated fat	Approximately 10% of total calories
	Ω-3 and Ω-6 fat	1:1 to 1:4 ratio
	Saturated fat and trans fat (partially hydrogenated fat)	Ideally, less than 5% of total calories; trans fat intake should be negligible
Sugar		Less than 10% of total calories
Sodium		Less than 2,300 mg per day
Water		8 glasses a day/64 oz/2 L, to vary with activity level, environmental conditions, and the fluid content of foods (e.g., fruits)
Alcohol, moderate intake if desired		Up to one drink per day for women, up to two drinks per day for men
Calorie level		Adequate to achieve and maintain a healthy weight
Physical activity/exercise		Daily moderate activity for 30 minutes or more Strength training twice weekly

Note: When absolute amounts are provided, they are referable to a prototypical 2,000 kcal/day diet.

Source: Adapted from Katz DL, Gonzalez MH. *The way to eat.* Naperville, IL: Sourcebooks, Inc., 2002:213.

TABLE 45.4

Recommended Foods and Overall Dietary Pattern to Meet Nutritional Objectives for Health Promotion

Food Group	Foods to Choose
Whole grains	At least seven to eight servings per day of whole grain breads, cereals, and grains with 2 g or more fiber per serving. Include oatmeal, oat bran, brown and wild rice varieties, semolina and whole wheat pasta, couscous, barley, and bulgur wheat.
Fruits	Four to five servings per day from a rainbow of colors, especially deep yellow, orange, and red: berries, apples, oranges, apricots, melons, mangos, and so on. Select from fresh, frozen, canned packed in juice, and dried varieties. Buy locally grown in season whenever possible.
Vegetables	Four to five servings per day from a rainbow of colors, especially deep yellow, orange, red, and leafy green: yellow, red, and green bell peppers; squash, carrots, tomatoes, spinach, sweet potatoes, broccoli, kale, Swiss chard, Brussels sprouts, eggplant, and so on. Select from fresh, frozen, and canned varieties but be mindful of the higher sodium content of canned. Buy locally grown in season whenever possible.
Beans and legumes	Include three to four times per week. Beans and legumes make a good alternative to meat. Include a variety of beans and legumes in your diet: black, red, kidney, white, cannelloni, garbanzo (chick pea), navy, pinto, lentils, split peas, black-eyed peas, and soy.
Fish[a] (and other seafood)	Include as often as three to four times per week. Fish is generally an excellent, lean source of high-quality protein, and several varieties (e.g., tuna, salmon, mackerel, halibut, and cod) are excellent sources of Ω-3 fatty acids. Seafood, such as shrimp and scallops, tends to be relatively high in cholesterol but is low in fat and also a good source of Ω-3 fatty acids.
Chicken and turkey[a]	Include up to one to two times per week. Skinless breast meat is preferred.
Lean beef, pork, lamb[a]	Moderate intake of meat, working toward a goal of roughly one to two meat-based meals per week, or four to eight per month, if desired. Select lean meats preferentially; the loin and round cuts are the leanest.
Milk and cheese[a]	Choose at least two servings per day from fat-free, skim, or low-fat versions.
Vegetable oils and other added fats	Choose monounsaturated and polyunsaturated sources daily, used in small amounts to avoid excess of calories: olive oil, canola oil, olives, avocados, almond butter, and peanut butter.
Nuts and seeds	Include four to five times per week in small amounts of unsalted raw or dry roasted types: almonds, walnuts, pistachios, peanuts, pecans, cashews, soy nuts, sunflower seeds, pumpkin seeds, and sesame seeds. Mix 1 tablespoon of ground flaxseed daily into other cooked foods.
Eggs[a]	Up to one egg per day on average (more egg white is fine). Preferably, choose an Ω-3 fatty acid-enriched brand.
Sweets	In moderation. Choose low-fat or nonfat varieties whenever reasonable. Dark chocolate (see Chapter 39) offers nutritional benefits.

[a] Optional items. Well-balanced vegetarian and vegan diets would omit these items. Note that fish is recommended for particular health benefits; flaxseed and/or an Ω-3 fatty acid supplement is especially recommended to those who do not eat fish.

Source: Adapted from Katz DL, Gonzalez MH. *The way to eat.* Naperville, IL: Sourcebooks, Inc., 2002.

TABLE 45.5

Portion Size Guide

Food Group	Standard Serving Size
Whole grains	■ 1 slice bread ■ 3/4–1 cup breakfast cereal ■ 1/2 cup cooked cereal, grains, or pasta
Fruits	■ 1 medium piece of fresh fruit ■ 4 oz 100% fruit juice ■ 1/2 cup canned, cooked, or chopped fruit ■ 1/4 cup dried fruit; about one small handful
Vegetables	■ 1/2 cup cooked vegetables (about the size of a tennis ball) ■ 1 cup raw vegetable or salad (about the size of your fist) ■ 6 oz vegetable juice
Vegetable oils and added fats	■ 1 teaspoon oil ■ 1/8 avocado ■ 1 tablespoon salad dressing ■ 1 teaspoon soft margarine
Nuts and seeds	■ 1 oz or 1/4 cup ■ 1 tablespoon peanut or almond butter (about the size of the tip of your thumb)
Beans and legumes	■ 1/2 cup cooked beans, lentils, or peas ■ 1/2 cup tofu ■ 1 cup soymilk
Fish, chicken, turkey, beef, pork, lamb	■ 3 oz cooked (about the size of a deck of cards)
Dairy	■ 1 cup milk or yogurt ■ 11/2 oz low-fat cheese (about the size of four stacked dice) ■ 1/2 cup ricotta cheese

REFERENCES

1. World Health Organization. *Obesity and overweight.* Available at http://www.who.int/mediacentre/factsheets/fs311/en/index.html; accessed 1/07/2011.
2. Doll R, Peto R. The causes of cancer: quantitative estimates of avoidable risks of cancer in the United States today. *J Natl Cancer Inst* 1981;66:1191–1308.
3. U.S. Preventive Services Task Force. *Behavioral counseling to promote a healthful diet and physical activity for cardiovascular disease prevention in adults,* Topic Page. Available at http://www.uspreventiveservicestaskforce.org/uspstf/uspsphys.htm; accessed 1/07/2011.
4. US Department of Health & Human Services. *Dietary guidelines for Americans.* Available at http://www.health.gov/dietaryguidelines/dga2005/document/; accessed 1/07/2005.
5. US Department of Agriculture. *Steps to a healthier you.* Available at http://www.choosemyplate.gov; accessed 1/07/2011.
6. Hite AH, Feinman RD, et al. In the face of contradictory evidence: report of the Dietary Guidelines for Americans Committee. *Nutrition* 2010;26(10):915–924.
7. Centers for Disease Control and Prevention, National Cancer Institute. *Introducing the next generation of 5 a day!* Available at http://www.5aday.gov; accessed 1/07/2011.

8. Lichtenstein AH, Appel LJ, Brands M, et al. Diet and lifestyle recommendations revision 2006: a scientific statement from the American Heart Association Nutrition Committee. *Circulation* 2006;114:82–96.
9. American Diabetes Association. *Making healthy food choices.* Available at http://www.diabetes.org/nutrition-and-recipes/nutrition/healthyfoodchoices.jsp; accessed 1/07/2011.
10. American Dietetic Association. Weight management—position of ADA. *J Am Diet Assoc* 2002;102:1145–1155.
11. Institute of Medicine. *Dietary reference intakes for energy, carbohydrate, fiber, fat, fatty acids, cholesterol, protein, and amino acids (macronutrients).* Washington, DC: National Academy Press, 2002.
12. American College of Preventive Medicine. *Diet in the prevention and control of obesity, insulin resistance, and type II diabetes.* Available at http://www.acpm.org/2002-057(F).htm; accessed 11/8/2007.
13. World Health Organization. *Global strategy on diet, physical activity and health.* Available at http://www.who.int/gb/ebwha/pdf_files/WHA57/A57_R17-en.pdf; accessed 1/07/2011.
14. USA Today. *Experts at International Congress on Obesity warn of deadly global pandemic.* Available at http://www.usatoday.com/news/health/2006-09-03-obesity-conference_x.htm; accessed 11/8/2007.

15. Katz DL. Competing dietary claims for weight loss: finding the forest through truculent trees. *Annu Rev Public Health* 2005;26:61–88.

16. Ornish D, Scherwitz L, Billings J, et al. Intensive lifestyle changes for reversal of coronary heart disease. *JAMA* 1998;280:2001–2007.

17. Varady KA, Bhutani S, et al. Improvements in vascular health by a low-fat diet, but not a high-fat diet, are mediated by changes in adipocyte biology [Results from the Lyons Heart Study offer similar support for the Mediterranean diet (17).]. *Nutr J* 2011;10:8.

18. Kuipers RS, Luxwolda MF, Dijck-Brouwer DA, et al. Estimated macronutrient and fatty acid intakes from an East African Paleolithic diet. *Br J Nutr* 2010;104(11):1666–1687.

19. McMillan-Price J, Petocz P, Atkinson F, et al. Comparison of 4 diets of varying glycemic load on weight loss and cardiovascular risk reduction in overweight and obese young adults: a randomized controlled trial. *Arch Intern Med* 2006;166:1466–1475.

20. Josse AR, Atkinson SA, Tarnopolsky MA, et al. Diets higher in dairy foods and dietary protein support bone health during diet- and exercise-induced weight loss in overweight and obese premenopausal women. *J Clin Endocrinol Metab* 2012;97(1):251–260.

21. Lattimer JM, Haub MD. Effects of dietary fiber and its components on metabolic health. *Nutrients* 2010;2(12):1266–1289.

22. van de Laar RJ, Stehouwer CD, van Bussel BC, et al. Lower lifetime dietary fiber intake is associated with carotid artery stiffness: the Amsterdam Growth and Health Longitudinal Study. *Am J Clin Nutr* 2012;96(1):14–23.

23. Ji Y, Tan S, Xu Y, et al. Vitamin B supplementation, homocysteine levels, and the risk of cerebrovascular disease: a meta-analysis. *Neurology* 2013;81:1298–1307.

24. Tenta R, Moschonis G, Koutsilieris M, et al. Calcium and vitamin D supplementation through fortified dairy products counterbalances seasonal variations of bone metabolism indices: the Postmenopausal Health Study. *Eur J Nutr* 2011;50(5):341–349.

25. Rajpathak SN, Xue X, Wassertheil-Smoller S, et al. Effect of 5 y of calcium plus vitamin D supplementation on change in circulating lipids: results from the Women's Health Initiative. *Am J Clin Nutr* 2010;91(4):894–899.

26. NIH State-of-the-Science Conference Statement on Multivitamin/Mineral Supplements and Chronic Disease Prevention. *NIH Consens State Sci Statements* 2006 May 15-17;23(2):1–30.

27. Grima NA, Pase MP, Macpherson H, et al. The effects of multivitamins on cognitive performance: a systematic review and meta-analysis. *J Alzheimer's Dis* 2012;29(3):561–569.

28. Haskell CF, Kennedy DO, Milne AL, et al. The effects of L-theanine, caffeine and their combination on cognition and mood. *Biol Psychol* 2008;77(2):113–122.

29. Jenkins DJ, Wolever TM, Vuksan V, et al. Nibbling versus gorging: metabolic advantages of increased meal frequency. *N Engl J Med* 1989;321:929–934.

30. Jenkins DJ, Khan A, Jenkins AL, et al. Effect of nibbling versus gorging on cardiovascular risk factors: serum uric acid and blood lipids. *Metabolism* 1995;44:549–555.

31. Ritchie LD. Less frequent eating predicts greater BMI and waist circumference in female adolescents. *Am J Clin Nutr* 2012;95(2):290–296.

32. Bellisle F, McDevitt R, Prentice AM. Meal frequency and energy balance. *Br J Nutr* 1997;77:s57–s70.

33. Murphy MC, Chapman C, Lovegrove JA, et al. Meal frequency; does it determine postprandial lipaemia? *Eur J Clin Nutr* 1996;50:491–497.

34. Harvie MN, Pegington M, et al. The effects of intermittent or continuous energy restriction on weight loss and metabolic disease risk markers: a randomized trial in young overweight women. *Int J Obes (Lond)* 2011;35(5):714–727.

35. Schulze Mb, Manson Je, Willett Wc, et al. Processed meat intake and incidence of type 2 diabetes in younger and middle-aged women. *Diabetologia* 2003;46:1465–1473.

36. Hu J, La Vecchia C, Morrison H, et al. Salt, processed meat and the risk of cancer. *Eur J Cancer Prev* 2011;20:132–139.

37. Barrett Ma, Osofsky SA. One health: the interdependence of people, other species, and the planet. In: Katz DL, Elmore JG, Wild DMG, Lucan SC, eds. *Epidemiology, biostatistics, preventive medicine, and public health*, 4th ed. Philadelphia, PA: Saunders/Elsevier, 2013.

38. Spence JD, Jenkins DJ, Davignon J. Egg yolk consumption and carotid plaque. *Atherosclerosis* 2012;224:469–473.

39. Rice BH, Quann EE, Miller GD. Meeting and exceeding dairy recommendations: effects of dairy consumption on nutrient intakes and risk of chronic disease. *Nutr Rev* 2013;71(4):209–223.

40. O'Sullivan TA, Hafekost K, Mitrou F, et al. Food sources of saturated fat and the association with mortality: a meta-analysis. *Am J Public Health* 2013;103(9):e31–e42.

41. de Oliveira Otto MC, Mozaffarian D, Kromhout D, et al. Dietary intake of saturated fat by food source and incident cardiovascular disease: the Multi-Ethnic Study of Atherosclerosis. *Am J Clin Nutr* 2012;96:397–404.

42. Hur Iy, Reicks M. Relationship between whole-grain intake, chronic disease risk indicators, and weight status among adolescents in the National Health And Nutrition Examination Survey, 1999-2004. *J Acad Nutr Diet* 2012;112(1):46–55.

43. Schatzkin A, Mouw T, Park Y, et al. Dietary fiber and whole-grain consumption in relation to colorectal cancer in the NIH-AARP Diet and Health Study. *Am J Clin Nutr* 2007;85(5):1353–1360.

44. Lam TK, Cross AJ, Freedman N, et al. Dietary fiber and grain consumption in relation to head and neck cancer in the NIH-AARP Diet and Health Study. *Cancer Causes & Control* 2011;22(10):1405–1414.

45. O'Neil CE, Nicklas TA, Zanovec M, et al. Whole-grain consumption is associated with diet quality and nutrient intake in adults: the National Health and Nutrition Examination Survey, 1999-2004. *J Am Diet Assoc* 2010;110(10):1461–1468.

46. Forman J, Silverstein J. Organic foods: health and environmental advantages and disadvantages. *Pediatrics* 2012;130(5):e1406–1415.

47. Geil P, Anderson J, Gustafson N. Women and men with hypercholesterolemia respond similarly to an American Heart Association Step 1 diet. *J Am Diet Assoc* 1995;95: 436–441.

48. Schaefer E, Lichtenstein A, Lamon-Fava S, et al. Efficacy of a National Cholesterol Education Program Step 2 diet in normolipidemic and hypercholesterolemic middle-aged and elderly men and women. *Arterioscler Thromb Vasc Biol* 1995;15:1079–1085.

49. deLorgeril M, Salen P, Martin J, et al. Mediterranean diet, traditional risk factors, and the rate of cardiovascular

complications after myocardial infarction: final report of the Lyon Diet Heart Study. *Circulation* 1999;99:779–785.

50. Jenkins DJ, Kendall CW, Marchie A, et al. Effects of a dietary portfolio of cholesterol-lowering foods vs lovastatin on serum lipids and C-reactive protein. *JAMA* 2003;290:502–510.

51. Ma XY, Liu JP, et al. Glycemic load, glycemic index and risk of cardiovascular diseases: meta-analyses of prospective studies. *Atherosclerosis* 2012;223(2):491–496.

52. Elejalde-Ruiz, Alexia. "Good Carb, Bad Carb." Chicago Tribune 25 Jan. 2012.

53. Corder R, Douthwaite JA, Lees DM, et al. Endothelin-1 synthesis reduced by red wine. *Nature* 2001;414(6866): 863-864.

54. Gruchow HW, Sobocinski KA, Barboriak JJ, et al. Alcohol consumption, nutrient intake and relative body weight among US adults. *Am J Clin Nutr* 1985;42(2):289–295.

55. Gillman M, Cupples L, Millen B, et al. Inverse association of dietary fat with development of ischemic stroke in men. *JAMA* 1997;278:2145–2150.

56. Moore T, Vollmer W, Appel L, et al. Effect of dietary patterns on ambulatory blood pressure: results from the Dietary Approaches to Stop Hypertension (DASH) Trial. DASH Collaborative Research Group. *Hypertension* 1999;34:472–477.

57. Knowler WC, Barrett-Connor E, Fowler SE, et al. Reduction in the incidence of type 2 diabetes with lifestyle intervention or metformin. *N Engl J Med* 2002;346:393–403.

58. Grimstad T, Berge RK, Bohov P, et al. Salmon diet in patients with active ulcerative colitis reduced the simple clinical colitis activity index and increased the anti-inflammatory fatty acid index–a pilot study. *Scand J Clin Lab Invest* 2011;71(1):68–73.

59. Kopple JD. The National Kidney Foundation K/DOQI clinical practice guidelines for dietary protein intake for chronic dialysis patients. *Am J Kidney Dis* 2001;38(4 Suppl 1): S68–S73.

60. Kachaamy T, Bajaj JS. Diet and cognition in chronic liver disease. *Curr Opin Gastroenterol* 2011;27(2):174–179.

61. Stover PJ. Influence of human genetic variation on nutritional requirements. *Am J Clin Nutr* 2006;83:436s–442s.

62. Mathers JC. Nutritional modulation of ageing: genomic and epigenetic approaches. *Mech Ageing Dev* 2006;127:584–589.

63. Gruber L, Lichti P, Rath E, et al. Nutrigenomics and nutrigenetics in inflammatory bowel diseases. *J Clin Gastroenterol* 2012;46(9):735–747.

64. Riscuta G, Dumitrescu RG. Nutrigenomics: implications for breast and colon cancer prevention. *Methods Mol Biol* 2012;863:343–358.

65. Eaton SB. The ancestral human diet: what was it and should it be a paradigm for contemporary nutrition? *Proc Nutr Soc* 2006;65:1–6.

SUGGESTED READINGS

Albert NM. We are what we eat: women and diet for cardiovascular health. *J Cardiovasc Nurs* 2005;20:451–460.

Alvarez-Leon EE, Roman-Vinas B, Serra-Majem L. Dairy products and health: a review of the epidemiological evidence. *Br J Nutr* 2006;96:s94–s99.

Bazzano LA, Serdula MK, Liu S. Dietary intake of fruits and vegetables and risk of cardiovascular disease. *Curr Atheroscler Rep* 2003;5:492–499.

Bengmark S. Impact of nutrition on ageing and disease. *Curr Opin Clin Nutr Metab Care* 2006;9:2–7.

Cassidy A. Diet and menopausal health. *Nurs Stand* 2005; 19:44–52.

Chahoud G, Aude YW, Mehta JL. Dietary recommendations in the prevention and treatment of coronary heart disease: do we have the ideal diet yet? *Am J Cardiol* 2004;94:1260–1267.

Cordain L, Eaton SB, Sebastian A, et al. Origins and evolution of the Western diet: health implications for the 21st century. *Am J Clin Nutr* 2005;81:341–354.

Ding EL, Mozaffarian D. Optimal dietary habits for the prevention of stroke. *Semin Neurol* 2006;26:11–23.

Ding EL, Mozaffarian D. Optimal dietary habits for the prevention of stroke. *Semin Neurol* 2006;26:11–23.

Dirks AJ, Leeuwenburgh C. Caloric restriction in humans: potential pitfalls and health concerns. *Mech Ageing Dev* 2006;127:1–7.

Dwyer J. Starting down the right path: nutrition connections with chronic diseases of later life. *Am J Clin Nutr* 2006;83:415s–420s.

Giugliano D, Ceriello A, Esposito K. The effects of diet on inflammation: emphasis on the metabolic syndrome. *J Am Coll Cardiol* 2006;48:677–685.

Halton TL, Willett WC, Liu S, et al. Low-carbohydrate-diet score and the risk of coronary heart disease in women. *N Engl J Med* 2006;355:1991–2002.

Heilbronn LK, de Jonge L, Frisard MI, et al; Pennington CALERIE Team. Effect of 6-month calorie restriction on biomarkers of longevity, metabolic adaptation, and oxidative stress in overweight individuals: a randomized controlled trial. *JAMA* 2006;295:1539–1548.

Holmes S. Nutrition and the prevention of cancer. *J Fam Health Care* 2006;16:43–46.

Howard BV, Van Horn L, Hsia J, et al. Low-fat dietary pattern and risk of cardiovascular disease: the Women's Health Initiative Randomized Controlled Dietary Modification Trial. JAMA 2006;295:655–666.

Hu FB, Willett WC. Diet and coronary heart disease: findings from the Nurses' Health Study and Health Professionals' Follow-up Study. *J Nutr Health Aging* 2001;5:132–138.

Hu FB, Willett WC. Optimal diets for prevention of coronary heart disease. *JAMA* 2002;288:2569–2578.

Jolly CA. Diet manipulation and prevention of aging, cancer and autoimmune disease. *Curr Opin Clin Nutr Metab Care* 2005;8:382–387.

Katz DL. Competing dietary claims for weight loss: finding the forest through truculent trees. *Annu Rev Public Health* 2005;26:61–88.

Katz DL. Pandemic obesity and the contagion of nutritional nonsense. *Public Health Rev* 2003;31:33–44.

Kennedy ET. Evidence for nutritional benefits in prolonging wellness. *Am J Clin Nutr* 2006;83:410s–414s.

Knowler WC. Optimal diet for glycemia and lipids. *Nestle Nutr Workshop Ser Clin Perform Programme* 2006;11:97–102.

McKevith B. Diet and healthy ageing. *J Br Menopause Soc* 2005;11:121–125.

Meyskens FL Jr, Szabo E. Diet and cancer: the disconnect be- tween epidemiology and randomized clinical trials. *Cancer Epidemiol Biomarkers Prev* 2005;14:1366–1369.

Moore VM, Davies MJ. Diet during pregnancy, neonatal out- comes and later health. *Reprod Fertil Dev* 2005;17:341–348.

Raatz S. Diet and nutrition—what should we eat? *Minn Med* 2003;86:28–33.

Ramaa CS, Shirode AR, Mundada AS, et al. Nutraceuticals— an emerging era in the treatment and prevention of cardio- vascular diseases. *Curr Pharm Biotechnol* 2006;7:15–23.

Schaefer EJ. Lipoproteins, nutrition, and heart disease. *Am J Clin Nutr* 2002;75:191–212.

Srinath Reddy K, Katan MB. Diet, nutrition and the preven- tion of hypertension and cardiovascular diseases. *Public Health Nutr* 2004;7:167–186.

Stoeckli R, Keller U. Nutritional fats and the risk of type 2 diabetes and cancer. *Physiol Behav* 2004 30;83:611–615.

Strychar I. Diet in the management of weight loss. *CMAJ* 2006;174:56–63.

Tapsell LC, Hemphill I, Cobiac L, et al. Health benefits of herbs and spices: the past, the present, the future. *Med J Aust* 2006;185:s4–s24.

Uauy R, Solomons N. Diet, nutrition, and the life-course approach to cancer prevention. *J Nutr* 2005;135: 2934s–2945s.

Walker AR, Walker BF, Adam F. Nutrition, diet, physical ac- tivity, smoking, and longevity: from primitive hunter- gatherer to present passive consumer—how far can we go? *Nutrition* 2003;19:169–173.

Willett WC, Sacks F, Trichopoulou A, et al. Mediterranean diet pyramid: a cultural model for healthy eating. *Am J Clin Nutr* 1995;61:1402s–1406s.

Willett WC, Stampfer MJ. Foundations of a healthy diet. In: Shils ME, Shike M, Ross AC, et al., eds. *Modern nutrition in health and disease*, 10th ed. Philadelphia, PA: Lippincott Williams & Wilkins, 2006:1625–1637.

Willett WC. Diet and health: what should we eat? *Science* 1994;264:532–537.

Williams MT, Hord NG. The role of dietary factors in cancer prevention: beyond fruits and vegetables. *Nutr Clin Pract* 2005;20:451–459.

World Health Organization. Diet, nutrition and the preven- tion of chronic diseases. *World Health Organ Tech Rep Ser* 2003;916:i–viii, 1–149, back cover.

Principles of Effective Dietary Counseling

Models of Behavior Modification for Diet and Activity Patterns and Weight Management

The health care setting offers nearly universal, if episodic, access to the population, and as such represents one of the best opportunities for providing nutrition and weight-loss counseling to the majority of people. Approximately 35 million Americans are hospitalized at least once each year (1,2). More than 70% of the US population visits a health care provider in any given year for a checkup (3). The utilization of hospital and physician services for diet and weight-related conditions increased substantially from 1992 to 2000. Office-based physician visits for diabetes care increased from 962 to 1,356 per 10,000 persons, while hospitalization rates for diabetes increased over 20% in this time period. Mention of anti-cholesterol medication and blood glucose regulators also increased dramatically during physician and hospital visits from 1994 to 2000 (4). When visits for all reasons are considered, the health care setting provides annual access to nearly the entire population; this access alone constitutes an important reason dietary and weight control counseling in the context of routine clinical care should be a priority.

BARRIERS TO COUNSELING BY PHYSICIANS

The potential contributions health care providers might make to improving diet and weight control efforts have historically been limited by an array of well-characterized barriers. These include: (1) lack of confidence in behavior change counseling due to insufficient provider training, (2) insufficient counseling tools and protocols, (3) lack of time,

(4) lack of reimbursement (5–10), (5) patient non-compliance, and (6) obesity bias. Unfortunately, most of these barriers persist today. Despite an increased awareness for the necessity of nutrition counseling by primary care physicians, the number of office visits that include dietary counseling for patients with cardiovascular disease (CVD), diabetes, or hypertension has actually decreased in recent years (11).

Lack of confidence and insufficient provider training may explain the reluctance of primary care physicians to incorporate behavioral counseling into their practice. A survey of 2,316 students at 16 US medical schools found that only 19% of students believed they had received extensive training in nutrition counseling and students reported infrequent counseling of patients about nutrition (12). A national survey conducted in 2005 found that 53% of physicians felt prepared to council patients on diet and exercise (13). Among internal medicine interns surveyed, only 14% felt adequately trained to provide nutrition counseling and a quiz of their nutrition knowledge showed notable deficits in their knowledge of nutrition assessment and obesity (14). Residents and attending physicians who counsel patients with cardiovascular disease reported that CVD risk factor counseling rates were lowest for diet and exercise; few physicians reported feeling confident in their counseling skills (15). Results of a survey of 509 physicians showed that 36% felt knowledgeable about weight management techniques but only 3% were confident that they could succeed in counseling effectively in their practice. Similar discrepancies in physician knowledge versus confidence were found for exercise (53% vs. 10%), and nutrition counseling (36% vs. 8%), as well as tobacco cessation (62% vs. 14%), alcohol reduction (46% vs. 7%), and stress management (35% vs. 5%). Although physicians realized the importance of healthy lifestyle practices in patient care, they felt that they lacked the training and counseling skills to advise patients about lifestyle behaviors and did not know how to implement these concepts in practice (16).

In another survey of 251 resident physicians, only 15.5% reported counseling more than 80% of their clinic patients about exercise. While over 93% understood the benefits of exercise and almost all (96%) felt that it was a physician's responsibility to counsel patients about exercise, only 29% felt successful at getting their patients to start exercising and only 28% felt confident in their skills to prescribe exercise for patients. Medical schools and postgraduate programs have only recently started emphasizing communication and counseling skills, and physicians still do not receive enough training in the essentials of counseling techniques (17,18).

In general, providers who feel effective at counseling are significantly more likely to provide extended counseling (≥3 min) than those who feel less effective (19). A survey of 418 primary care physicians in Massachusetts found a significant increase between 1981 and 1994 in the proportions of physicians who regularly gathered information about exercise (67% vs. 47%) and diet (56% vs. 47%) (20). The majority of physicians reported feeling "very prepared" to counsel patients about exercise, but less than half felt very prepared to counsel patients about diet. Only a small minority (4% to 13%) described themselves as currently "very successful" in helping with these behaviors. Even "given appropriate support," only a minority of physicians were optimistic about their potential to be "very successful" in helping patients change patients' behavior.

Physicians' confidence in lifestyle counseling is influenced both by the degree of counseling training they have received and by the physician's own weight status and exercise habits. A survey of 183 trainees and attending physicians found that physician confidence in counseling for exercise was greater for those who regularly exercised and who reported receiving adequate training in counseling. Interestingly, providers who reported being overweight themselves were more likely to counsel patients regarding exercise. Overall, up to 83% of the physicians felt limited by their lack of preventive care training (21). Counseling for diabetic patients may be particularly challenging for practitioners who feel inadequately prepared or trained. Internal medicine residents were more likely to provide diabetes patients with counseling on symptoms or medication adherence than dietary counseling. Residents with prior education in chronic disease counseling reported higher comfort with conducting diabetic dietary counseling with their patients (22).

This lack of confidence in counseling skills does not appear limited to American-trained physicians. Among physicians and nurses surveyed in Finland, only slightly more than half reported having sufficient skills in lifestyle counseling (23). General practitioners and nurses in Great Britain reported similar reluctance in addressing weight management when treating obese children (24). A survey of family physicians in British Columbia, Canada, found that 82.3% of respondents felt their medical school training in nutrition was inadequate and only 30% reported using nutrition-related services despite recognizing a need in more than 60% of their patients (25).

Insufficient counseling tools and protocols also contribute to physician reluctance. Currently there are few well-delineated counseling protocols or standardized office instruments designed to address lifestyle behaviors, and often physicians lack awareness of or access to these materials. Physicians do not have clear guidance on which behaviors to target, which counseling techniques to employ, or how to use their counseling time effectively (26). The results are often inappropriate assessment of the individual patient, long counseling sessions that conflict with provider time limitations, discussion of a large number of risk behaviors, lack of use of a behavioral change model approach, inappropriate method of advice delivery, poor follow-up, generic advice (as opposed to being tailored to the patient's gender, socioeconomic status, level of education, ethnicity, and readiness for change), and lack of specific recommendations for frequency, duration, and intensity of physical activity.

A review of studies relating to primary care physicians' knowledge, attitudes, beliefs, and practices regarding childhood obesity revealed a large heterogeneity in obesity assessment techniques, despite a promising increase in the use of body mass index (BMI) as an evaluation tool. The authors called for increased uniformity in assessment techniques in order to improve care and physicians' self-efficacy (27). A survey of pediatricians found that 96% chose better counseling tools as the most helpful clinical resource for treating obese children, suggesting that practice-based tool kits might improve pediatrician self-efficacy (28).

Lack of time is another major barrier in the primary care setting. The constraints and realities of a busy primary care practice make it difficult for health care providers to devote enough time and resources to counseling. Competing priorities in a limited office visit often preclude addressing nonacute conditions, leading to sporadic and unstructured lifestyle counseling (29). One study of physicians' attitudes toward counseling found that a majority of physicians believe that diet and weight-loss counseling require too much time as compared with smoking counseling and only 8% believed that patients would follow their advice if offered (30). The increasing number of services already recommended for preventive care place an unrealistic burden on physician time, as much as 7.4 hours per day. This competition for a physician's time is only expected to grow as we add genetic and other preventive screening tests to our medical arsenal. Already preventive visits are longer than chronic care visits, and physicians must prioritize which preventive counseling services to provide. Studies have shown physicians allot insufficient time to nutrition and exercise counseling, due to the competing need for cancer, cholesterol, and blood pressure screenings (31,32).

Lack of adequate reimbursement has been a major barrier to physician counseling in the past. Doctors have not always been reimbursed for their time spent counseling patients, and they have been reluctant to refer patients to other health professionals such as a dietician whose services would not be covered by insurance. Given that physicians were unlikely to be paid their anticipated hourly rate for counseling, preventive practices recommended by experts have been difficult to integrate into routine clinical practice (33).

In 2010, The Patient Protection and Affordable Care Act mandated that medical insurers must cover preventive care for beneficiaries. Under Title IV of the Affordable Care Act, private insurers are required to compensate physicians for providing weight loss and nutrition counseling, obesity screening, and counseling to promote sustained weight loss. Cost-sharing for these services is eliminated under this new law, meaning that insurers cannot charge a copay, coinsurance, or deductible to those who enrolled in a new insurance plan on or after September 23, 2010 (34,35). As of November 29, 2011, Medicare beneficiaries who qualify as obese (BMI ≥ 30 kg/m^2) are entitled to Intensive Behavioral Therapy (IBT) for Obesity in a primary care setting (36). A maximum of 22 IBT for obesity sessions are allowed in a 12-month period. Stipulations are outlined for weekly and monthly visits with a primary care physician, which the beneficiary is entitled to only if he or she meets the criteria of losing 3 kg (6.6 lbs) during the first 6 months. Those who fail to meet the weight-loss benchmark must wait 6 months to qualify for another round of counseling.

A key drawback to the regulations in the Affordable Care Act is the stipulation that the weight-loss counseling must be provided by a primary care doctor, nurse practitioner, clinical nurse specialist, or physician assistant. Given that doctors typically receive very little training in lifestyle behavioral changes such as nutrition and physical activity, and medical exams are often limited to brief encounters with little time for comprehensive counseling, patients might receive better results if referred to a certified health coach, registered dietician (RD), or a proven weight management program (37). Medicare will only reimburse obesity counseling that is provided by an MD and which takes place in a primary care setting; an RD is reimbursable only if an MD cosigns or if the counseling is specifically related to diabetes or renal disease.

Although the Affordable Care Act is federal law, each state and each private insurer within each state has different rules regarding what treatment is reimbursable, whether a referral is needed, how many visits are allowed, and the time frame allotted for treatment. The Healthcare Common Procedure Coding System (HCPCS) indicates that Code G0447 is used for billing "Face-to-face behavioral counseling for obesity, 15 minutes." According to the 2013 National Physician Fee Schedule Relative Value File, Code G0447 has a Work Relative Value Unit (RVU) of 0.45. The physician Work RVU indicates the relative level of time, skill, training, and intensity to provide a given service; therefore, the RVU codes can be compared for different physician services. For example, the RVU for over 10 minutes of tobacco counseling is 0.50. This indicates that physicians will be reimbursed slightly less for 15 minutes of obesity counseling than for over 10 minutes of tobacco-cessation counseling. However, the RVU codes are subject to review and revision every 5 years, so it is probable that physician compensation rates will be adjusted as the medical community's perception of obesity counseling changes (38,39).

Patient noncompliance is another barrier to lifestyle counseling. Provider perception that patients will not follow advice apparently deters many clinicians from delivering counseling messages (40). Family practitioners reported facing multiple challenges in discussing weight loss with obese patients, with a high percentage reporting that patients lack discipline or want an easy solution to weight loss. Despite their reported frustration with treating obese patients, practitioners gave high ratings to several strategies for improving care, including having nutrition and exercise therapists as well as community resources readily available (41). A survey conducted at The Children's Hospital of Philadelphia similarly found that over 90% of practitioners cited barriers for pediatric obesity prevention, including lack of parent and child motivation, overweight parents, and the prevalence of both fast food and a lack of exercise (42). Strategies required to remediate poor compliance (patient education, contracts, self-monitoring, social support, telephone follow-up, and tailoring of counseling messages) require extensive restructuring of primary care procedures and are often too resource intensive.

Lastly, obesity bias by physicians, and indeed society at large, may interfere with lifestyle counseling attitudes. Doctors have been shown to display less rapport with overweight and obese patients than with normal-weight patients (43), which may be due in part to physicians' feelings of frustrated intolerance in dealing with a problem they perceive as unfixable (44). The result may be a weakening of the patient–physician relationship, diminished patient adherence, and decreased effectiveness of lifestyle counseling (43).

OVERCOMING BARRIERS TO IMPROVE PHYSICIAN EFFECTIVENESS

There is hope, however, that these barriers can be overcome, through improved physician training and time management strategies. Physicians who receive training in counseling have a higher rate of success in obesity management (45). Among family practitioners in New Jersey, those with higher self-reported knowledge of weight-loss diets reported less dislike in discussing weight loss and were less likely to believe treatment is ineffective (41). Brief interventions to change diet and exercise patterns in primary care settings have demonstrated some success (46–49). There is evidence that physician training in nutrition enhances counseling (50). A study of 21 suburban physicians in the Midwestern United States found that when physicians were provided with educational outreach ("academic detailing"), their discomfort with obesity counseling dropped to zero and their patients' clinical outcomes for weight loss improved (51).

Time constraints can be addressed both with adjustment of the medical system that unburdens the physician and with counseling methods tailored to the primary care setting (52) (see Chapter 47). Limited, but nonetheless valuable, dietary (and physical activity) guidance can be offered in as little as 1.5 minutes. When more extensive counseling is required, the time commitment can be spread over a number of office visits, and much of the work can be delegated to a dietary consultant. Welty et al. (53) demonstrated that onsite dietician counseling, concurrent with the physician visit, can help achieve sustained weight loss in obese patients.

Perhaps the most important current strategy for improving physician effectiveness is to train physicians in the five A's—Ask, Advise, Assess, Assist, Arrange—as an organizational construct for clinical counseling. This strategy, promoted by the U.S. Public Health Service and the U.S. Preventive Services Task Force (USPSTF), helps physicians to organize their approach to behavioral counseling and is suitable for brief, primary care interventions (54,55). The five A's approach to counseling has taken on greater importance recently, as the Centers for Medicare and Medicaid Services (CMS) has stipulated that intensive behavioral intervention for obesity counseling of Medicare patients should follow the USPSTF's five A's framework (56). Each of the five techniques includes counseling practices aimed at helping patients meet goals such as tobacco cessation or weight loss. Physicians are trained in how to assess a patient's current behaviors, risks, and readiness to change, advise on a change of specific behaviors, agree on a collaborative effort to set goals, assist in addressing barriers and securing support for the patient, and lastly, arrange for follow-up treatment or evaluation (57). However, several studies have shown that physicians are often not utilizing the five A's adequately (58). In a pilot study in which physicians were trained in the five A's, the training intervention slightly improved the quality but not the quantity of the counseling. 72% of physicians counseled their obese patients, regardless of whether they received the training. Physicians who received the training failed to address most of the five A's when meeting with their patients (57). Jay et al. (59) found that although 85% of obese patients received counseling, physicians trained in the five A's focused mostly on assessment. Physicians who best adhered to the five A's model and who utilized more of the counseling techniques had better patient outcomes. Physicians who are trained in the five A's appear to have slightly greater success in helping their patients maintain weight loss 12-months posttreatment, possibly because the trained physicians were more likely to refer patients to weight-loss programs (60).

EFFECTIVENESS OF PHYSICIAN COUNSELING

Health care providers in general, and physicians in particular, remain the most trusted source of health-related information. A number of studies have shown that patients readily accept lifestyle counseling from their primary care providers. In a survey by Zogby, most respondents thought that their physicians should play a more active role in promoting a healthy lifestyle and two-thirds thought it important for a physician to focus on preventive measures, such as diet and physical activity, rather than just diagnosing and treating illnesses (61). In a national survey of nearly 13,000 obese adults who had seen their physicians for a routine visit during the previous year, Galuska et al. (62) found that patients who were advised to lose weight were nearly three times more likely to report an attempt to do so than those who did not receive such advice.

Physician nutrition counseling does influence patient behavior (63–66). An analysis of the 2005 to 2008 National Health and Nutritional Examination Survey (NHANES) found that adults with a BMI over 25 and those with BMI over 30

both perceived themselves as overweight and attempted to lose weight if they were identified as overweight by their physician. Yet only 45.2% of respondents with a BMI over 25, and 66.4% of those with a BMI of 30 or above, were told of their overweight status by a physician (67). A subsequent analysis of the NHANES data found that patients who reportedly discussed their weight status with their physician were more likely to report clinically significant weight loss (68). Similarly, data from the 2001 to 2003 Behavioral Risk Factor Surveillance System found that patients showed an increased probability of eating fewer calories and of using exercise to lose weight when advised to do so by their physician (69).

There is observational evidence that patients are more likely to lose weight when simply told by a physician that they are overweight (70). Overweight people tend to be more receptive to advice from health care professionals than from lay sources. One study reported that the odds of trying to lose weight were nearly three times greater for those receiving physician counseling than for patients receiving no such advice (71). In another study, 89% of obese patients who had been counseled to lose weight were attempting to lose weight compared to 52% of those who had not been counseled (72).

The utility of clinical counseling for behavior change is to date better established for various behaviors besides those related to diet and weight control, in particular smoking cessation. The importance of physician counseling for smoking cessation has been confirmed through randomized controlled clinical trials that show improved cessation rates when physicians are involved. More than 100 randomized controlled clinical trials have demonstrated modest but statistically significant improvements in tobacco-cessation rates for persons who receive physician counseling. In a meta-analysis of 56 studies, cessation rates of 10.7% were found for those receiving less than 3 minutes of counseling, 12.1% for those receiving between 3 and 10 minutes of counseling, and 18.7% for those receiving over 10 minutes of counseling (73–75). Intensive behavioral interventions have resulted in substantial increases in smoking cessation (76); however, less dramatic results are evident in trials utilizing low intensity interventions (77,78). Despite the importance of physician counseling, data from the 2002 National Ambulatory Medical Care Survey found that 78.6% of patients who smoke received no counseling regarding smoking cessation during their office visits (79).

Physician counseling is equally efficacious as part of routine primary care in reducing alcohol consumption. Whitlock et al. (80) systematically reviewed evidence for the efficacy of brief behavioral counseling interventions in primary care settings to reduce risky and harmful alcohol consumption. Six to 12 months after good-quality, brief, multi-contact behavioral counseling interventions, participants reduced the average number of drinks per week by 13% to 34% more than the controls, and the proportion of participants drinking at moderate or safe levels was 10% to 19% greater. Similarly, in a study by Garcia et al. (81) that followed 306 patients who reported excessive alcohol consumption, counseling provided by the family physician proved to be highly effective. Reiff-Hekking et al. (82) also determined that even brief, 5- to 10-minute counseling during a primary care visit significantly reduced alcohol consumption by high-risk drinkers.

Although physicians can be highly effective in promoting weight loss and good nutrition, they too often fail to broach the subject with their patients. While at least 80% of the population has contact with a medical provider each year, physician counseling in primary care settings remains limited. In a 1992 survey, 40% of internists reported assessing the activity status of patients, but only 25% of all the internists reported writing physical activity plans for patients (83,84). In another national survey of nearly 10,000 patients who had seen a physician during the previous year, Wee et al. (46) found that only 34% reported having received counseling about exercise. In a study by Anis et al. (85), trained students served as third-party observers of patient encounters with physicians. Their results showed that counseling about diet or physical activity occurred in only 20% to 25% of visits. Nawaz et al. (86) found that only 50% of adults surveyed reported discussing nutrition during their last routine checkup in the past year, and only 56% reported discussing exercise with their physician. Discussion of diet resulted in an increased likelihood of changes in fat or fiber intake as well as weight-loss success, particularly among overweight subjects.

Overall, it appears that the most common experience by patients of any weight is that their physician does not address the issue at all (87).

Multiple studies confirm this observation. The 2002 National Ambulatory Medical Care Survey found that for patients with type 2 diabetes, hyperlipidemia or hypertension, no diet or exercise counseling took place during more than half of all office visits (79). Among physicians, there appears to be a consistent rate of weight counseling: About one-fifth of overweight and one-third of obese patients are counseled (88). Several studies using data from the Behavioral Risk Factor Surveillance System have reported that anywhere from 29% to 43% of overweight and obese adults visiting their health care provider within the past year were advised to lose weight (89). Similar results have been found using patient surveys from outpatient primary care clinics. In a study of 267 patients who were overweight, based on a BMI greater than 27, only 29.6% had been instructed to lose weight (90). In another study, only 49% of those with a BMI over 30, 24% of those with BMI between 25 and 30, and 12% with BMI less than 25 had discussed their weight with their physicians.

Significant discrepancies exist in how physicians and patients view weight-loss counseling (91). Patients and their doctors view the necessity for weight loss and the likelihood for weight-loss success very differently. In one study of 28 primary care physicians, it was found that doctors assigned patients to higher weight categories and worse health outcomes than patients perceived for themselves. Moreover, patients were more optimistic about their weight loss potential and motivation than were their physicians (92). A survey conducted in an inner-city clinic in Bronx, NY, found that 86% of obese patients wanted to lose weight but only 17% received dietician referrals and 36% received a recommendation for weight loss by their physician. Only 21% of obese patients and 11% of overweight patients had this diagnosis documented on their charts (93). Patients and physicians frequently disagree on the weight-loss goals discussed during office visits. A survey of 29 rural, primary care practices in the Midwest found that physicians and patients even disagreed on whether weight loss, exercise, and physical activity were discussed at all during an office visit, indicating that physicians need to verify that patients have received their advice (94).

Gender of both the physician and the patient plays a significant role in how physicians address weight loss with their patients. There is evidence for gender bias in weight-loss counseling, as physicians are more likely to encourage women than men with a BMI of 25 kg/m^2 or more to lose weight, possibly due to the greater sociocultural stigma against overweight women. Yet an unexpected reverse gender effect was found for patients with a BMI of 32 kg/m^2. In this higher BMI category, physicians were more likely to counsel men to lose weight than women, possibly due to a greater concern about android body fat distribution in men (95). Physician gender appears to play a role as well, as female physicians are more likely to advise patients on weight loss, provide obesity counseling and refer patients for obesity treatment (96). One study found that physicians endorse greater weight loss for obese female patients than for their male patients, though female physicians were less stringent than male physicians in the weight-loss goals proposed for all patients (97). Patient–physician gender concordance appears to play a large role in whether diet/nutrition, exercise, and weight-loss counseling is provided to obese patients. An analysis of the 2005 to 2007 National Ambulatory Medical Care Survey revealed that obese patients were significantly more likely to receive diet/nutrition and exercise counseling when both the patient and physician were male (98). Locality, age, education level, and socioeconomic status play a role in whether physicians address weight loss with patients as well. Residents of the Northeast are more likely to be counseled than those living in other parts of the United States. After age 60, the likelihood of counseling declines for both men and women. Ironically, persons with a higher education level and socioeconomic status are more likely to receive advice about weight, but low-income patients are more likely to attempt to change their diet and exercise based on their physician's advice (99).

Whether or not patients receive an initial diagnosis of obesity also appears dependent upon gender, locality, and age, according to an analysis of the 2005 to 2007 National Ambulatory Medical Care Survey. Although only 28.9% of obese patients were given an obesity diagnosis, higher diagnosis rates were correlated with female gender, young age, living in the Midwest, and being severely/morbidly obese (100). The analysis found that one of the largest predictors for weight-related counseling was receipt of an obesity diagnosis. Thus, the low rate of obesity diagnosis for obese patients nationwide is a significant concern.

The most obvious means by which health care settings could make a meaningful contribution to obesity control efforts is through effective behavioral counseling. As noted previously, there is some contact between virtually the entire population and the health care setting during any given year. The near universality of health care system contact, the amenability of the health care setting to individualized guidance, and the unique influence of health care providers all argue for a dedicated effort to make high-quality dietary and weight management counseling a routine aspect of clinical care.

RECOMMENDATIONS FOR PRIMARY CARE COUNSELING

Several governmental agencies have provided guidelines for behavioral counseling in primary care. The USPSTF recommends intensive dietary and physical activity counseling for adult patients with hyperlipidemia and other known risk factors for cardiovascular and diet-related chronic disease (101,102) and intensive counseling for weight loss in obese patients (103), to be delivered in the primary care facility or by referral to nutritionists or dieticians (104). The USPSTF does not currently recommend that the general population receive behavioral counseling in the primary care setting to promote a healthy diet and exercise, as the health benefit of such brief behavioral counseling is small (105). The Academy of Nutrition and Dietetics (AND) recommends regular medical assessment of obesity by the primary care physician that should include measurement of height, weight, and waist circumference (106), as well as an estimate of energy needs based upon resting metabolic rate (107). The American Academy of Family Physicians similarly recommends that patients should be screened for obesity and offered intensive, multicomponent behavioral interventions (108). Physicians should also assess patients' knowledge of the relationship of their lifestyle to health and provide a clear and customized message about the importance of diet and exercise (109).

Translating such recommendations into counseling that actually influences behavior is a challenge best met through application of the science of behavior modification (110). Four broad categories of behavioral theories or models have contributed to the understanding of lifestyle change through counseling in medical practice (111): communication models, rational belief models, self-regulative systems models, and operant and social learning models.

Models of Behavior Modification

Communication Models highlight the importance of the generation of the health message, the reception of the message, message comprehension, and belief in the substance of the message. Carkhuff's Stems of Communication and Discrimination Index, for example, builds on the core conditions for good communication in any situation: empathy, warmth, and genuineness (112). Similarly, motivational interviewing (MI) techniques developed by Miller and Rollnick (113) from their work with problem drinkers emphasize the importance of working through ambivalence and developing self-efficacy. This counseling style combines warmth and empathy with reflective listening and elicits information by asking key questions. Physicians' use of MI techniques for weight loss has successfully resulted in both adult and pediatric patients attempting to lose weight and change their exercise patterns (114–116). A systematic review of trials in which MI was utilized by psychologists and physicians as an intervention method found an effect in 80% of the studies. Even one brief session of MI was sufficient to produce an effect in 64% of the cases reviewed (117). A review of studies focusing on nutrition-related behavior change similarly found that MI, in combination with cognitive behavioral therapy, was a highly effective counseling strategy (118). Although MI is patient centered, it is directive in nature, and the counselor has specific goals in mind and pursues systematic strategies to achieve those goals (119). The aim of MI is to help a patient work through his or her ambivalence; application of the approach is further explored in Chapter 47.

Green's Precede Model categorizes different external influences on behavior into predisposing, reinforcing, and enabling factors. By being attentive to these categories of external factors, the predictability of the behavior is increased, and there is a greater ability to communicate prescriptive information concerning intervention choices (120). More recently, a Precede-Proceed Model developed by Green proposes a patient counseling algorithm

for use in primary care (121). This approach helps determine a patient's needs within a given counseling context by assessing motivational characteristics; physical, manual, and economic barriers and facilitators; and specific circumstantial rewards and penalties. This helps the clinician avoid inappropriate techniques, such as trying to persuade an already motivated patient that change is necessary, and by skipping unnecessary steps it frees up time to focus on areas that require modification. PRECEDE-PROCEED has been successfully applied to developing an intuitive-eating weight management program, and as such can offer a holistic approach to long-term healthy behavioral change (122,123).

According to *rational belief models*, objective and logical thought processes determine behavior, provided that the clinician has appropriate information on both the risks and benefits. For example, the Health Beliefs Model emphasizes four perceived predictors: probability of threat, severity of threat, feasibility of benefits, and barriers to adopting the new pattern of behavior (124). This model has been very useful in identifying predictors of health behaviors and planning health promotion strategies. Another example is the Theory of Planned Behavior (TPB) developed by Azjen (125) to discern and predict determinants of volitional behavior: Intention to perform a behavior is viewed as a function of one's beliefs, attitude toward the behavior, and perceived social norms. TPB has been utilized to predict many health-related behaviors and can help explain intentions for physical activity and diet among populations ranging from diabetes patients to healthy adolescents (126,127).

Self-regulative Systems Models outline a three-part self-regulation process: self-monitoring, self-evaluation, and self-reinforcement. A basic assumption is that people will act in accordance with their interest, once they know it. These models highlight the impact of social and cultural values and norms of the surrounding environment (128). Prochaska's Transtheoretical Model of behavior change (TTM) assesses an individual's readiness to change according to four core constructs: stages of change (SOC), processes of change, decisional balance, and self-efficacy. The main construct, SOC, categorized as precontemplation, contemplation, preparation, action, and maintenance (129), have been applied to a variety of health modification interventions including those targeting physical activity (130). Tailoring of interventions to match a person's stage of change and the use of MI techniques are emphasized (131). Educational programs based on TTM have successfully increased the passing of subjects to higher stages of exercise behavior change (132). Application of this method is further explored in Chapter 47.

Operant and Social Learning Models focus on the stimuli that elicit or reinforce a specific behavior, such as Skinner's and Pavlov's conditioning approaches to behavior change. Bandura's Social Cognitive Theory emphasizes the immediate social reinforcing consequences related to attempting behavior change; three critical elements are self-efficacy, modeling, and self-management. The model attempts to link self-perception and individual action and assumes that individuals selectively heed information from four sources: active attainment of goal, vicarious experiences of others, persuasion, and physiological cues (133). New ways of behaving occur through imitation and modeling and through observation of the behavior of others (134–136). Social cognitive theory has been used as a basis for interventions aimed at weight gain prevention (137), dietary self-efficacy (138), and exercise adherence (139), among other health behaviors.

These and related behavioral modification constructs are largely products of psychology and do not readily lend themselves to application in primary care context. In order to meet the unique demands of a primary care setting, an effective behavioral counseling model must address the barriers to physician counseling outlined earlier in the chapter. Elements that can increase applicability and ease of implementation of a model include explicit guidance on counseling strategies; brevity of the counseling script; standardized, validated instruments to assess the patient; and clear delineation of provider response and responsibility.

Several counseling programs have focused exclusively on the primary care setting and have adapted constructs of the behavioral modification theories to fit the primary care context. Most of these programs use a general approach to assisting patients that includes the five A's: assess, advise, agree, assist, and arrange. A majority of these have adapted elements of various behavioral counseling models into a single counseling program.

PRIMARY CARE COUNSELING CONSTRUCTS

The efficacy of lifestyle counseling and lifestyle interventions has been well supported by such high-impact programs as the Diabetes Prevention Program (DPP) and the Increasing Motivation for Physical Activity Project (IMPACT). Diabetes incidence in the 10-year follow-up to the DPP program was lowest in the group randomly assigned to intensive lifestyle intervention, when compared to the metformin-treated group or the placebo (140). One-year results from the IMPACT study found that regular physical activity counseling for sedentary, low-income women resulted in significant increases in estimated total energy expenditure as compared to participants who did not receive telephone counseling (141). Both of these studies demonstrate the powerful impact of effective counseling, which can be successfully applied within a primary care counseling construct as well, as the studies below demonstrate.

The Worcester Area Trial for Counseling in Hyperlipidemia (WATCH)

Ockene et al. (142) examined the feasibility of a 3-hour training program that taught physicians skills to conduct a brief dietary risk assessment and provide patient-centered nutrition counseling. The counseling as taught in this program was grounded in social learning theory and emphasized the physician's use of a series of questions that focused on eliciting information and feelings from the patient to facilitate motivation and positive self-efficacy. A counseling algorithm was developed to guide the physician's efforts. After completion of the training, physicians' use of dietary counseling increased significantly ($p = 0.0001$). The same authors also tested the effectiveness of a physician-delivered nutrition counseling program in combination with an office support program. Forty-five primary care internists were randomized to three groups—usual care, a 3-hour physician nutrition counseling training, and physician nutrition counseling training plus an office support program that included in-office prompts, algorithms, and simple dietary assessment tools. Compared with patients in the first group, patients in the last group showed reduction in dietary fat intake, weight, and low-density lipoprotein levels (143).

Patient-Centered Assessment Counseling for Exercise and Nutrition

Patient-centered assessment counseling for exercise and nutrition (PACE) was designed by physicians, behavioral health scientists, and public health professionals to provide physical activity counseling to healthy adults within a limited time. The program was based on the SOC theory, which postulates that behavior moves along a continuum of change from precontemplation, to contemplation, to action. Accordingly, three distinct counseling strategies relevant to each stage were developed. The counseling strategies also employed principles of Social Cognitive Theory and took into account personal, interpersonal, social, and environmental factors. The PACE program was implemented in two stages, each lasting for 2 to 5 minutes. During the first stage, the receptionist administered the Physical Activity Readiness Questionnaire (PAR-Q) and the PACE questionnaire and then assigned the patient one of three physical activity counseling worksheets. In the second stage, the provider reviewed the documents and provided physical activity recommendations and scheduled a follow-up visit.

Norris et al. (144) studied the effectiveness of physician counseling to increase physical activity among inactive patients enrolled in a health maintenance organization. Physicians in 32 primary care practices received training in PACE, and 812 patients were randomized to usual care or to PACE counseling which consisted of a clinic visit followed by a reminder telephone call a month later. The study results showed that a one-time counseling session with PACE was not effective in increasing physical activity levels but did move the patients along the SOC continuum ($p = 0.03$).

An efficacy study by Calfas et al. (145) randomized 255 healthy, sedentary participants to an intervention group which consisted of two contacts with a health educator and a booster phone call. The control group received usual care. Results showed that patients receiving the PACE program reported 37 minutes per week in walking physical activity compared with 7 minutes per week in the control group. Green et al. (146) studied the effectiveness of using PACE in a 6-month telephone-based randomized clinical trial designed to increase physical activity in 316 inactive patients. The intervention group

received physical activity counseling and three 20 to 30 minute phone calls each month to assist in identifying strategies to increase physical activity. The control group did not receive the counseling or the phone calls. The intervention produced higher levels of exercise after the 6-month treatment period as compared with the control subjects (PACE score of 5.37 vs. 4.98, $p <0.05$). The authors concluded that telephone-based exercise counseling was an effective way to increase physical activity levels among patients.

Patrick et al. (147) conducted a PACE+ intervention designed to promote improved eating and physical activity behaviors among 878 adolescents, using a computer-supported intervention initiated in a primary care setting. The intervention was successful in reducing sedentary behaviors, increasing physical activity, and reducing saturated fat intake, although success rates varied by gender. Among female subjects, it was found that more frequent outreach and contacts were beneficial in promoting changes in multiple behaviors. Huang et al. (148) assessed the potential for adverse effects among adolescents in the PACE+ intervention and found no worsening of body satisfaction or self-esteem among adolescent participants, regardless of gender or change in weight status.

Activity Counseling Trial

The Writing Group for the Activity Counseling Trial (ACT) Research Group reported the results of a randomized controlled trial which compared the effects of two physical activity counseling interventions with standard care. The ACT interventions were based on Social Cognitive Theory, which was used to select key personal (self-efficacy), social (social support for exercise), and environmental (access to facilities and resources) constructs. Interventions consisted of advice (physician counseling plus educational materials), assistance (advice plus interactive mail), and behavioral counseling (advice and assistance plus regular phone calls and behavioral classes). At 24 months, VO_2 Max was significantly higher in the assistance and counseling groups compared to the advice group, but no significant differences were reported in physical activity. The 24-month effects of the ACT were also assessed for CVD risk factors (149), with substantial improvements found in both men and women who had high risk factors for CVD at baseline; no improvements were found for participants with normal baseline levels.

Step Test Exercise Prescription

Petrella et al. (150) compared two methods of exercise counseling by physicians—the first using only American College of Sports Medicine (ACSM) guidelines and the second using the ACSM guidelines along with an office-based assessment to determine fitness levels and prescribe an exercise training heart rate (Step test exercise prescription [STEP]). The assessment consisted of five questions to determine the patient's readiness to start a regular activity program, and fitness levels were determined by recording the heart rate after moderate exercise. Patients were offered pedometers as incentives to enhance fitness and increase adherence to the program. Participants in the STEP group reported significant ($p = 0.009$) improvement in the extent of physician counseling and knowledge compared to the control ACSM group. A study of 241 elderly, community-dwelling patients found that a STEP intervention consisting of exercise counseling and prescription of an exercise training heart rate improved aerobic fitness levels and exercise self-efficacy in participants (151). STEP benefits were maintained up to 12 months and may have contributed to improved exercise adherence.

Physically Active for Life

A feasibility study by Pinto et al. (152), called Physically Active for Life (PAL), integrated the constructs of the TTM into a patient-centered model of primary care. The study randomized 12 practices to the PAL intervention group and 12 to standard care. Physicians participating in the PAL program received a training manual, a desk prompt with summary information on counseling, and a poster on activity promotion, and they participated in a 1-hour training session. Patients enrolled in the PAL program received a five-section manual—one section for each stage of change. Cognitive, attitudinal, instrumental, behavioral, and social issues were addressed through a series of questions and statements by the counseling physician. Comparisons between the intervention and control groups showed significant improvements in confidence in the

intervention-group physicians, but no significant increase in frequency of exercise counseling provided to patients. Patients in the intervention group reported satisfaction with the exercise counseling and support materials. In a subsequent paper, Pinto et al. reported the effects of the PAL intervention on the underlying theoretical constructs used in the program. Motivational readiness for physical activity and related constructs of decisional balance (benefits and barriers; see Chapter 47), self-efficacy, and behavioral and cognitive processes of change were examined at baseline, 6 weeks, and 8 months. At 6 weeks, the intervention had significant effects on decisional balance, self-efficacy, and behavioral processes, but those effects were not maintained at 8 months (153).

Pressure System Model

The Pressure System Model (PSM) (154), developed by Katz, utilizes constructs of the TTM to separate the two fundamental goals of behavioral counseling: raising motivation and overcoming resistance. Traditionally, behavioral counseling has focused on raising motivation by apprising the patient of the risks associated with a particular behavior and highlighting the benefits of changing the behavior. PSM also takes into account impediments to behavior change and offers the patient and provider an opportunity to identify strategies to overcome these impediments. The utility of the model derives from its simplicity; while derived from elaborate behavior modification constructs, PSM relies on a two-question algorithm to identify the correct focus for counseling for any given patient. Clear guidance for counseling approaches to raise motivation or identify and troubleshoot barriers is incorporated. Chapter 47 details the salient features; it is intended to provide a specific counseling method for use in the primary care setting and resources that can be shared with patients to facilitate adoption of the behavioral changes recommended.

Katz et al. (154) assessed the effectiveness of the PSM in a randomized controlled trial in which six Yale University–affiliated internal medicine programs were randomly assigned to a PSM-based behavioral counseling training program (intervention) or standard curriculum (control) condition. Physicians at these sites received either PSM training or standard residency training. The PSM training program consisted of skill building in behavioral counseling, didactic sessions augmented by role-play exercises, use of a simple algorithmic approach to identify patients' counseling needs, a comprehensive list of commonly encountered barriers to physical activity and strategies to address them, and brief counseling scripts. Physical activity levels were measured in 195 patients who received physical activity counseling from a resident trained in PSM counseling methods, while 121 patients were similarly surveyed at the control sites. After 6 and 12 months of intervention, physical activity, as measured by the modified Yale Physical Activity Survey (YPAS), improved significantly from baseline in the intervention sites (1.77 ± 0.84; $p = 0.0376$ and 1.94 ± 0.98; $p = 0.0486$), with no change observed at the control sites (0.35 ± 1.00; $p = 0.7224$ and 0.99 ± 1.52; $p = 0.5160$).

Health Enhancement Through Lifestyle Practices

The Health Enhancement Through Lifestyle Practices (HELP) manual, developed by Katz et al. (155), built on previous work done with the PSM to offer streamlined nutrition and physical activity counseling protocols for primary care providers. The manual synthesized constructs from the SOC model and MI techniques to address both dietary and physical activity patterns. It used a brief questionnaire and simple algorithm to help the provider determine whether nutrition, physical activity, or both require attention, assess the patient's stage of change, and assign the appropriate counseling protocol. The manual included five counseling scripts, corresponding printed materials tailored to the patient's stage of change, and a clearly defined office implementation plan. Also the HELP manual targeted two distinct populations: pregnant women and families with children under age 5. The manual is thus equally applicable in pediatric, obstetrics, and family practices. Evaluation of the program (156) indicates enhanced provider self-efficacy for counseling and both patient and provider satisfaction. A study by Hwang on 253 community-dwelling older adults supported the clinical applicability and consistency of the HELP scores and confirmed the functioning of the 1- to 5-point rating scale used (157). Hwang concluded that HELP can assist in promoting healthy

lifestyles among older adults by monitoring risk factors and measuring the outcomes of healthy lifestyle interventions.

Impediment Profiling

In their work on smoking cessation, Katz et al. (158–160) have developed a novel behavior change approach called impediment profiling. As the name suggests, this technique involves a step in which each patient (or study subject) completes a survey designed to identify his or her personal barriers to a given behavior change. Intervention is then personalized to correspond to the personal profile of impediments revealed. The technique has resulted in very high rates of smoking cessation in early studies (158–160) and has been applied with good effect to the promotion of physical activity (161). The development of an online impediment profiler for dietary change is the focus of a National Institutes of Health-funded project called Nutrition Navigation on-Line Edge (NnoLEDGE) (162). The NnoLEDGE program currently serves the Princeton, NJ metropolitan area through its community wellness portal, www.princetonlivingwell.com, but with further funding may expand its features and the communities it serves (163).

The web-based, medical education program, "Online Weight Management Counseling for Healthcare Providers" (O.W.C.H.), developed by Dr. David L. Katz and the Yale-Griffin Prevention Resource Center (164), combines PSM and impediment profiling tools for both dietary change and physical activity. This educational program, which provides free CME credits, presents a counseling method tailored toward the time constraints of the primary care setting. This method offers incremental lifestyle counseling and behavior change, in a format manageable for both the patient and provider. This and other primary care counseling constructs are being made available to clinicians, with the understanding that compassionate, well-trained medical providers are critical contributors in solving the obesity-related health problems now reaching epidemic proportions in the United States and throughout the world.

CONCLUSIONS

Due to an increased emphasis on health promotion and disease prevention, the use of behavioral counseling strategies in primary care has become increasingly prevalent. The evolution of behavioral modification theories from the provenance of psychology to primary care can be traced in the adaptations and modifications described in this chapter. These revisions address a number of barriers to behavioral counseling commonly cited by primary care physicians. For example, behavioral counseling sessions by a psychologist can typically last 15 to 45 minutes, but primary care physicians are unable to devote that much time to counseling for health behavior change. All the programs discussed in this chapter provide brief, time-efficient behavioral counseling scripts for use by clinicians or other health care providers. Some of the programs also include instruments that allow the clinician to identify key risk behaviors efficiently and accurately, assess the patient's readiness to change, and track counseling activities. These instruments usually consist of a few questions to help the physician tailor a session to the needs of the patient, focus on the most important issues, and offer specific, personalized advice.

Clearly articulated strategies designed to address the impediments to a particular behavior change further serve to enhance effectiveness of primary care counseling. In contrast to other primary care counseling interventions, the HELP manual provides assessment tools that allow for behavioral assessment of the whole family as opposed to the individual patient (162). A majority of these models include a robust physician education component. These training curricula are typically based on principles of adult learning and build physician skills using interactive, sequential learning in workshops, group settings, or individual training sessions.

Even relatively brief physician training has led to improvements in physician self-efficacy for counseling (7). This was demonstrated in the PAL study in which physicians rated their confidence in performing a series of eight counseling activities. Physicians in the intervention group showed significant increases in their confidence to offer an individualized exercise plan to their patients, identify resources, and address issues associated with barriers (152). Similarly, physicians participating in the STEP program felt more knowledgeable and confident about the program compared to those in the control group (150).

Despite these advances, important limitations persist in the routine application of behavior modification techniques to primary care. Data to verify the efficacy of such efforts remain sparse, and follow-up periods are short. Even the behavior modification interventions designed for the primary care setting can be unclear about the frequency of counseling and/or the content of follow-up sessions after initial counseling. The frequency of encounters may be at odds with the recommended follow-up. Some of these interventions fail to articulate methods for systematic identification of patients most in need of behavioral counseling. While promising in many regards, the counseling advances to date warrant further evaluation in various practice settings and with diverse groups of patients before their general utility can be affirmed. That said, uptake of such methods into practice settings even as their evaluation proceeds is justified by the prevalence of obesity and attendant morbidity and the ineffectiveness of prevailing approaches. Of note, there is apt to be an important role for lifestyle counseling even when clinicians turn to pharmacotherapy (165) or bariatric surgery (166,167).

At the time of this writing, historic changes in how we view and treat obesity are being made on a national level in the United States. Obesity has traditionally been treated as a syndrome, not a disease, and as such has not been treated as a respected condition (44). However, the American Medical Association (AMA) voted for "Recognition of Obesity as a Disease" at their 2013 annual meeting by approving Resolution 420 "to recognize obesity as a disease state with multiple aspects requiring a range of interventions to advance obesity treatment and prevention" (168,169). The AMA further called for an improved measure of obesity than BMI alone, and better clinical and public health strategies for addressing obesity.

Immediately after the AMA's designation of obesity as a disease, new legislation was introduced into the Senate and House of Representatives called The Treat and Reduce Obesity Act (170). This bill (HR 2415) would require Medicare to cover more obesity treatment costs including prescription drugs for weight management, and to make it easier for almost 50 million elderly and disabled Medicare patients to receive weight-loss counseling. The bill would allow more providers to offer intensive behavioral counseling and would require the CMS to emphasize the behavioral counseling service to its beneficiaries.

The Affordable Care Act now mandates that medical insurers must provide free preventive care to beneficiaries. Under Title IV of the Affordable Care Act private insurers are required to compensate physicians for providing weight loss and nutrition counseling, obesity screening, and counseling to promote sustained weight loss. This new mandate could have far-reaching effects in how the medical community approaches obesity treatment and weight-loss counseling. It is likely that the AMA designation of obesity as a disease and the concurrent introduction of the Treat and Reduce Obesity Act will further influence how we prioritize and reimburse physician behavioral counseling in the future.

The health care setting provides annual access to nearly the entire population, allowing clinicians the unique opportunity to offer dietary and weight control counseling during routine clinical care. Yet the recent designation of obesity as a disease and the perception of weight loss as a medical procedure may have unintended repercussions. The disease designation implies that obesity warrants clinical treatments, including drugs and surgery, perhaps at the expense of societal solutions and prevention. In fact, obesity is a condition preventable by healthful eating and adequate physical exercise. Yet we seek medical and pharmaceutical remedies for a condition better treated or even avoided by adopting "lifestyle medicine" (171).

The fundamental question is whether obesity should be viewed as a cultural or a clinical problem. Our health care system is focused on disease care, rather than prevention, and this approach is exemplified by the classification of obesity as a disease. Katz and Colino (2013) argue that lifestyle changes alone can reduce our risk for heart disease, cancer, stroke, diabetes, dementia, and obesity by 80%, far surpassing the efficacy of any drug or medical intervention (172). Thus, it is prudent to shift our perspective to look at obesity as more of a cultural problem than a clinical one.

Clinician counseling should continue to play a vital role in curbing obesity, yet medical intervention can be complimented by structured, preventative programs aimed at helping people live healthier lives, including online weight-loss programs and even apps. For example, Weigh Forward, a lifelong approach to weight control by RediClinic (173), offers 10 visits with trained clinicians as well as online support. Popular apps that support personal fitness and weight management include MyFitnessPal (174), which allows users to track exercise and calories with its Calorie Counter and Diet Tracker applications. These online fitness and weight-loss tools can enhance the efficacy of clinical interventions, by empowering patients to manage their own preventive care.

The obesity epidemic calls for a comprehensive solution, based upon constructive, compassionate counseling by well-trained clinicians, coordinated with wellness programming available through community interventions as well as online and through apps. These measures, in turn, must be supported by structural, policy, and environmental changes that support healthy behaviors and lifestyles conducive to disease prevention, weight management, and wellness. The importance of clinician involvement in this critical area of public health cannot be overstated. Given the gravity of the current obesity crisis, it is unacceptable when clinicians fail to embrace this role, or perform ineffectively or with bias. Clinicians who are properly trained to provide effective and compassionate counseling are an integral part of the solution.

REFERENCES

1. Agency for Healthcare Research and Quality. *Hospitalization in the United States, 2002.* Available at www.ahrq.gov/data/hcup/factbk6/factbk6c.htm; accessed 6/18/07.
2. Centers for Disease Control and Prevention. National Center for Health Statistics. National Hospital Discharge Survey 2010. *Number, rate, and average length of stay for discharges from short-stay hospitals, by age, region, and sex: United States, 2010.* March 2012. Available online at http://www.cdc.gov/nchs/nhds.htm
3. National Center for Health Statistics. *Health, United States, 2004.* Available at http://www.cdc.gov/nchs/data/hus/hus04trend.pdf; accessed 6/18/07.
4. Centers for Disease Control and Prevention. National Center for Health Statistics. *Health care in America: trends in utilization.* DHHS Pub No. 2004-1031. Trends in utilization by selected condition, drug, procedure, outcome, and site of care. Available online at http://www.cdc.gov/nchs/data/misc/healthcare.pdf.
5. Petrella RJ, Lattanzio CN. Does counseling help patients get active? Systematic review of the literature. *Can Fam Physician* 2002;48:72–80.
6. Simons-Morton DG, Calfas KJ, Oldenburg B, et al. Effects of interventions in health care settings on physical activity or cardiorespiratory fitness. *Am J Prev Med* 1998; 15:413–430.
7. Whitlock EP, Orleans CT, Pender N, et al. Evaluating primary care behavioral counseling interventions. *Am J Prev Med* 2002;22:267–284.

8. Eakin E, Glasgow R, Riley K. Review of primary care-based physical activity intervention studies: effectiveness and implications for practice and future research. *J Fam Pract* 2000;49:158–168.

9. Eaton CB, Menard LM. A systematic review of physical activity promotion in primary care office settings. *Br J Sports Med* 1998;32:11–16.

10. Lawlor DA, Hanratty B. The effect of physical activity advice given in routine primary care consultations: a systematic review. *J Public Health Med* 2001;23:219–226.

11. Kolasa KM, Rickett K. Barriers to providing nutrition counseling cited by physicians. A survey of primary care practitioners. *Nutr Clin Pract* 2010;25:502–509.

12. Spencer EH, Frank E, Elon LK, et al. Predictors of nutrition counseling behaviors and attitudes in US medical students. *Am J Clin Nutr* 2006;84:655–662.

13. Park ER, Wolfe TJ, Rigotti NA. Perceived preparedness to provide preventive counseling. *J Gen Intern Med* 2005;20:386–391.

14. Vetter ML, Herring SJ, Sood M, et al. What do resident physicians know about nutrition? An evaluation of attitudes, self-perceived proficiency and knowledge. *J Am Coll Nutr* 2008;27:287–298.

15. Tsui JI, Dodson K, Jacobson TA. Cardiovascular disease prevention counseling in residency: resident and attending physician attitudes and practices. *J Natl Med Assn* 2004;96:1080–1091.

16. Castaldo J, Nester J, Wasser T, et al. Physician attitudes regarding cardiovascular risk reduction: the gaps between clinical importance, knowledge, and effectiveness. *Dis Manag* 2005;8:93–105.

17. Rogers LQ, Bailey JE, Gutin B, et al. Teaching resident physicians to provide exercise counseling: a needs assessment. *Acad Med* 2002;77:841–844.

18. Hauer KE, Carney PA, Chang A, et al. Behavior change counseling curricula for medical trainees: a systematic review. *Acad Med* 2012;87:956–968.

19. Lewis CE, Clancy C, Leake B, et al. The counseling practices of internists. *Ann Intern Med* 1991;114:54–58.

20. Wechsler H, Levine S, Idelson RK, et al. The physician's role in health promotion revisited—a survey of primary care practitioners. *N Engl J Med* 1996;334:996–998.

21. Howe M, Leidel A, Krishnan S M, et al. Patient-related diet and exercise counseling: do providers' own lifestyle habits matter? *Prev Cardiol* 2010;13:180–185.

22. Tang JW, Freed B, Arora VM. Internal medicine residents' comfort with and frequency of providing dietary counseling to diabetic patients. *J Gen Intern Med* 2009;24:1140–1143.

23. Jallinoja P, Absetz P, Kuronen R, et al. The dilemma of patient responsibility for lifestyle change: Perceptions among primary care physicians and nurses. *Scand J Prim Health* 2007;25:244–249.

24. Walker O, Strong M, Atchinson R, et al. A qualitative study of primary care clinicians' views of treating childhood obesity. *BMC Fam Pract* 2007;8:50.

25. Wynn K, Trudeau JD, Taunton K. Nutrition in primary care. Current practices, attitudes, and barriers. *Can Fam Physician* 2010;56:e109–e116.

26. Bass PF, Stetson BA, Rising W, et al. Development and evaluation of a nutrition and physical activity counseling module for first-year medical students. *Med Educ* 2004;9:23. Available at http://www.med-ed-online.org; accessed 6/18/07.

27. Van Gerwen M, Franc C, Rosman S, et al. Primary care physicians' knowledge, attitudes, beliefs and practices regarding childhood obesity: a systematic review. *Obes Rev* 2009; 10:227–236.

28. Perrin EM, Flower KB, Garrett J, et al. Preventing and treating obesity: pediatricians' self-efficacy, barriers, resources, and advocacy. *Ambul Pediatr* 2005;5:150–156.

29. Schnirring L. Survey suggests a decline in obesity counseling: physicians analyze reasons. *Phys Sports Med* 2004; 32(6):18–20.

30. Dolor RJ, Østbye T, Lyna P, et al. What are physicians' and patients' beliefs about diet, weight, exercise, and smoking cessation counseling? *Prev Med* 2010;51:440–442.

31. Yarnall KSH, Pollak KI, Michener JL. Primary care: is there enough time for prevention? *Am J Public Health* 2003;93:635–641.

32. Pollak KI, Krause KM, Yarnall KSH, et al. Estimated time spent on preventive services by primary care physicians. *BMC Health Svs Res* 2008;8:245.

33. Hudon E, Beaulieu MD, Roberge D. Canadian Task Force on preventive health care. Integration of the recommendations of the Canadian Task Force on preventive health care: obstacles perceived by a group of family physicians. *Fam Pract* 2004;21:11–17.

34. Healthcare.gov. *Where can I read the Affordable Care Act?* Available online at https://www.healthcare.gov/where-can-i-read-the-affordable-care-act/

35. Healthcare.gov. *What are my preventive care benefits?* Available online at https://www.healthcare.gov/what-are-my-preventive-care-benefits/.

36. Centers for Medicare and Medicaid Services. *National obesity determination (NCD) for intensive behavioral therapy for obesity (210.12).* Available online at http://www.cms.gov/medicare-coverage-database/details/ncd-details.aspx?NCDId=353&ncdver=1&CoverageSelection=Both&ArticleType=All&PolicyType=Final&s=All&KeyWord=obesity&KeyWordLookUp=Title&KeyWordSearchType=And&bc=gAAAABAAAAAA&.

37. Katz D. *Reimbursement for obesity counseling: so what?* Available online at http://www.huffingtonpost.com/david-katz-md/obesity-counseling-reimbursement_b_1127032.html.

38. Department of Health and Human Services. Centers for Medicare and Medicaid Services. Medicare Learning Network. *How to use the searchable Medicare Physician Fee Schedule* (MPFS). January 2012. Available online at http://www.cms.gov/Outreach-and-Education/Medicare-Learning-Network-MLN/MLNProducts/downloads/How_to_MPFS_Booklet_ICN901344.pdf.

39. Centers for Medicare and Medicaid Services. *Physician fee schedule.* Available online at http://www.cms.gov/Medicare/Medicare-Fee-for-Service-Payment/PhysicianFeeSched/index.html.

40. Thomas RJ, Kottke TE, Brekke MJ, et al. Attempts at changing dietary and exercise habits to reduce risk of cardiovascular disease: who's doing what in the community? *Prev Cardiol* 2002;5:102–108.

41. Ferrante JM, Piasecki AK, Crabtree BF. Family physicians' practices and attitudes regarding care of extremely obese patients. *Obesity* 2009;17:1710–1716.

42. Spivack JG, Swietlik M, Alessandrini E, et al. Primary care providers' knowledge, practices, and perceived barriers to

the treatment and prevention of childhood obesity. *Obesity* 2010;18:1341–1347.

43. Gudzune KA, Beach MC, Roter DL. Physicians build less rapport with obese patients. *Obesity* 21(20):2146–2152. doi:10.1002/oby.20384.

44. Katz DL. *Obesity, bias, and bedrock.* May 01, 2013. Available online at http://www.linkedin.com/today/post/article/20130501151527-23027997-obesity-bias-and-bedrock?trk=mp-edit-rr-posts.

45. Simkin-Silverman LR, Wing RR. Management of obesity in primary care. *Obes Res* 1997;6:603–612.

46. Wee C, McCarthy E, Davis R, et al. Physician counseling about exercise. *JAMA* 1999;282:1583–1588.

47. Cohen MD, D'Amico FJ, Merenstein JH. Weight reduction in obese hypertensive patients. *Fam Med* 1991;23:25–28.

48. Hiddink GJ, Hautvast JG, van Woerkum CM, et al. Information sources and strategies of nutrition guidance used by primary care physicians. *Am J Clin Nutr* 1997;65: 1974s–1979s.

49. Ettner SL. The relationship between behaviors of patients: does having a usual physician make a difference. *Med Care* 1999;37;6:547–555.

50. Mokdad AH, Ford ES, Bowman BA, et al. Diabetes trends in the US *Diabetes Care* 2000;23:1278–1283.

51. Schuster RJ, Tasosa J, Terwoord NA. Translational research – implementation of NHLBI obesity guidelines in a primary care community setting: the physician obesity awareness project. *J Nutr Health Aging* 2008;12:764–769.

52. Katz DL, Faridi Z. Health care system approaches to obesity prevention and control. In: Kumanyika S, Brownson RC, eds. *Handbook of obesity prevention.* New York, NY: Springer Publishing Co, 2007:285–316.

53. Welty FK, Nasca MM, Ruan Y. Effect of onsite dietician counseling on weight loss and lipid levels in an outpatient physician office. *Am J Cardiol* 2007;100:73–75.

54. U.S. Preventive Services Task Force. *Evidence-based methods for evaluating behavioral counseling interventions: the Five A's organizational construct for clinical counseling.* Available online at http://www.uspreventiveservicestaskforce.org/3rduspstf/behavior/behsum2.htm.

55. Whitlock EP, Orleans CT, Pender N, et al. Evaluating primary care behavioral counseling interventions: an evidence-based approach. *Am J Prev Med* 2002;22:267–284.

56. Centers for Medicare and Medicaid Services. *Decision memo for intensive behavioral therapy for obesity (CAG-00423N).* Available online at http://www.cms.gov/medicare-coverage-database/details/nca-decision-memo.aspx?&NcaName=Intensive%20Behavioral%20Therapy%20for%20Obesity&bc=ACAAAAAAIAAA&NCAId=253.

57. Jay M, Schlair S, Caldwell R, et al. From the patient's perspective: the impact of training on resident physician's obesity counseling. *J Gen Intern Med* 2010;25:415–422.

58. Gudzune KA, Clark JM, Appel LJ, et al. Primary care providers' communication with patients during weight counseling: a focus group study. *Patient Educ Couns* 2012;89:152–157.

59. Jay M, Gillespie C, Schlair S, et al. Physicians' use of the 5As in counseling obese patients: is the quality of counseling associated with patients' motivation and intention to lose weight? *BMC Health Serv Res* 2010;10:159.

60. Jay MR, Gillespie CC, Schlair SL, et al. The impact of primary care resident physician training on patient weight loss at 12 months. *Obesity* 2013;21:45–50.

61. *Associated Press Poll: Americans careful about eating habits*: http://www.msnbc.com/id/5953595/; 2004.

62. Galuska DA, Will JC, Serdula MK, et al. Are health care professionals advising obese patients to lose weight? [see comments] *JAMA* 1999;282:1576–1578.

63. Mokdad AH, Bowman BA, Ford ES, et al. The continuing epidemics of obesity and diabetes in the United States. *JAMA* 2001;286:1195–1200.

64. Mokdad AH, Ford ES, Bowman BA, et al. The continuing increase of diabetes in the US *Diabetes Care* 2001;24:412.

65. Centers for Disease Control and Prevention (CDC). *The burden of heart disease, stroke, cancer, and diabetes, United States.* Atlanta: CDC, 2002.

66. Engelgau MM, Geiss LS. The burden of diabetes mellitus. In: Leahy JL, Clark NG, Cefalu WT, eds. *Medical management of diabetes mellitus.* New York, NY: Marcel Dekker, Inc., 2000:1–17.

67. Post RE, Mainous AG 3rd, Gregorie SH, et al. The influence of physician acknowledgement of patients' weight status on patient perceptions of overweight and obesity in the United States. *Arch Intern Med* 2011;171:316–321.

68. Pool AC, Kraschnewski JL, Cover LA. The impact of physician weight discussion on weight loss in US adults. *Obes Res Clin Pract* 2013 in press; doi:10.1016/j.orcp.2013.03.003.

69. Loureiro ML, Nayga RM Jr. Obesity, weight loss, and physician's advise. *Soc Sci Med* 2006;62:2458–2468.

70. Levy BT, Williamson PS. Patient perceptions and weight loss of obese patients. *J Fam Pract* 1988;27:285–290.

71. Galuska DA, Will JC, Serdula MK, et al. Are health care professionals advising obese patients to lose weight? *JAMA* 1999;282:1576–1578.

72. Nawaz H, Adams ML, Katz DL. Weight loss counseling by health care providers. *Am J Public Health* 1999;89: 764–767.

73. US Preventive Services Task Force. *Counseling to prevent tobacco use and tobacco-caused disease.* http://www.ahrq.gov/clinic/3rduspstf/tobacccoun/tobcounrs.htm; 2005.

74. Fiore MC, Wetter DW, Bailey WC, et al. Smoking cessation clinical practice guideline. Rockville, MD: US Dept. of Health and Human Services, 1996.

75. Law M, Tang J. An analysis of the effectiveness of interventions intended to help people stop smoking. *Arch Intern Med* 1995;153:1933–1941.

76. Mottillo SM, Filion KB, Bélisle P, et al. Behavioural interventions for smoking cessation: a meta-analysis of randomized controlled trials. *Eur Heart J* 2009;30:718–730.

77. Stead LF, Bergson G, Lancaster T. *Physician advice for smoking cessation (review).* The Cochrane Collaboration. Available online at http://www.thecochranelibrary.com/SpringboardWebApp/userfiles/ccoch/file/World%20No%20Tobacco%20Day/CD000165.pdf.

78. Unrod M, Smith M, Winkel G. Randomized controlled trial of a computer-based, tailored intervention to increase smoking cessation counseling by primary care physicians. *J Gen Intern Med* 2007;22:478–484.

79. Heaton PC, Frede SM. Patients' need for more counseling on diet, exercise, and smoking cessation: results from the national ambulatory medical care survey. *J Am Pharm Assoc* 2006;46:364–369.

80. Whitlock EP, Polen MR, Green CA, et al. US Preventive Services Task Force. Behavioral counseling interventions

in primary care to reduce risky/harmful alcohol use by adults: a summary of the evidence for the US Preventive Services Task Force. *Ann Intern Med* 2004;140:557–568.

81. Fernandez Garcia JA, Ruiz Moral R, Perula de Torres LA, et al. Effectiveness of medical counseling for alcoholic patients and patients with excessive alcohol consumption seen in primary care. *Aten Primaria* 2003;31:146–153.

82. Reiff-Hekking S, Ockene JK, Reed GW. Brief physician and nurse practitioner-delivered counseling for high-risk drinking. *J Gen Intern Med* 2005;20:7–13.

83. Francis KT. Status of the year 2000 health goals for physical activity and fitness. *Phys Ther* 1999;79:405–414.

84. National Center for Health Statistics. *Healthy People 2000 Review 1997; DHHS Publication No. (PHS) 98-1256.* Hyattsville, MD: Public Health Service, 1997.

85. Anis NA, Lee RE, Ellerbeck EF, et al. Direct observation of physician counseling on dietary habits and exercise: patient, physician, and office correlates. *Prev Med* 2004; 38: 198–202.

86. Nawaz H, Adams ML, Katz DL. Physician-patient interactions regarding diet, exercise, and smoking. *Prev Med* 2000;31:652–657.

87. Potter MB, Vu JD, Croughan-Minihane M. Weight management: what patients want from their primary care physicians. *J Fam Pract* 2001;50:513–518.

88. Kristeller JL, Hoerr RA. Physician attitudes toward managing obesity: differences among six specialty groups. *Prev Med* 1997;26:542–549.

89. Friedman C, Brownson RC, Peterson DE, et al. Physician advice to reduce chronic disease risk factors. *Am J Prev Med* 1994;10:367–371.

90. Heath C, Grant W, Marcheni P, et al. Do family physicians treat obese patients? *Fam Med* 1993;25:401–402.

91. Heintze C, Metz U, Hahn D, et al. Counseling overweight in primary care: an analysis of patient-physician encounters. *Patient Educ Couns* 2010;80:71–75.

92. Befort CA, Greiner KA, Ahluwalia JS. Weight-related perceptions among patients and physicians. *J Gen Intern Med* 2006;21:1086–1090.

93. Davis NJ, Emerenini A, Wylie-Rosett J. Obesity management: physician practice patterns and patient preference. *Diabetes Educator* 2006;32:557–561.

94. Greiner KA, Born W, Ahluwalia JS. Discussing weight with obese primary care patients: physician and patient perceptions. *J Gen Intern Med* 2008;23:581–587.

95. Anderson C, Peterson CB, Fletcher L, et al. Weight loss and gender: an examination of physician attitudes. *Obes Res* 2001;9:257–263.

96. Dutton GR, Herman KG, Tan F, et al. Patient and physician characteristics associated with the provision of weight loss counseling in primary care. *Obes Res Clin Pract* 2013 in press; doi:10.1016/j.orcp.2012.12.004.

97. Dutton GR, Perri MG, Stine CC. Comparison of physician weight loss goals for obese male and female patients. *Prev Med* 2010;50:186–188.

98. Pickett-Blakely O, Bleich SN, Cooper LA. Patient-physician gender concordance and weight-related counseling of obese patients. *Am J Prev Med* 2011;40: 616–619.

99. Taira DA, Safran DG, Seto TB, et al. The relationship between patient income and physician discussion of health risk behaviors. *JAMA* 1997;278:1412–1417.

100. Bleich SN, Pickett-Blakely O, Cooper LA. Physician practice patterns of obesity diagnosis and weight-related counseling. *Patient Educ Couns* 2011;82:123–129.

101. US Preventive Services Task Force. Behavioral counseling in primary care to promote a healthy diet: recommendations and rationale. *Am J Prev Med* 2003;24:93–100.

102. US Preventive Services Task Force. Behavioral counseling in primary care to promote physical activity: recommendation and rationale. *Ann Intern Med* 2002;137:205–207.

103. US Preventive Services Task Force. *Screening and interventions to prevent obesity in adults.* Available at http://www.ahrq.gov/clinic/uspstf/uspsobes.htm; accessed 5/28/07.

104. U.S. Preventive Services Task Force. *Behavioral counseling in primary care to promote a healthy diet in adults at increased risk for cardiovascular disease.* Available online at http://www.uspreventiveservicestaskforce.org/uspstf/uspsdiet.htm.

105. U.S. Preventive Services Task Force. *Behavioral counseling in primary care to promote a healthy diet: recommendations and rationale.* Available online at http://www.uspreventiveservicestaskforce.org/3rduspstf/diet/dietrr.htm.

106. USOnlinerx.net. *Position of the American Dietetic Association: weight management.* http://www.usonlinerx.net/articles/position-of-american-dietetic-association-brief.html; 2005.

107. Seagle HM, Strain GW, Makris A et al. Position of the American Dietetic Association: weight management. *J Am Diet Assoc* 2009;109:330–346.

108. U.S. Preventive Services Task Force. Screening for and management of obesity in adults: recommendation statement. *Ann Intern Med* 2012;157:373–378.

109. Deen D. Metabolic syndrome: time for action. *Am Fam Physician.* 2004;69(12):2875–2882. http://www.aafp.org/afp/20040615/2875.html; 2005.

110. Spahn JM, Reeves RS, Keim KS, et al. State of the evidence regarding behavior change theories and strategies in nutrition counseling to facilitate health and food behavior change. *J Am Diet Assoc* 2010;110:879–891.

111. Leventhal H, Cameron L. Behavioural theories and the problem of compliance. *Patient Educ Couns* 1987;10:117–138.

112. Lewis CE, Wells KB, Ware J. A model for predicting the counseling practices of physicians. *J Gen Intern Med* 1986;1:14–19.

113. Miller MW, Rollnick S. *Motivational interviewing: preparing people to change addictive behavior.* New York, NY: The Guildford Press, 1991.

114. Pollak KI, Østbye T, Alexander SC, et al. Empathy goes a long way in weight loss discussions. *J Fam Pract* 2007;56:1031–1036.

115. Pollak KI, Alexander SC, Østbye T. Physician communication techniques and weight loss in adults. *Am J Prev Med* 2010;39:321–328.

116. Wong EM, Cheng MM. Effects of motivational interviewing to promote weight loss in obese children. *J Clin Nurs* 2013;22:2519–2530.

117. Rubak S, Sandbaek A, Christensen B. Motivational interviewing: a systematic review and meta-analysis. *Br J Gen Pract* 2005;55:305–312.

118. Spahn JM, Reeves RS, Keim KS, et al. State of the evidence regarding behavior change theories and strategies

in nutrition counseling to facilitate health and food behavior change. *J Am Diet Assoc* 2010:879–891.

119. Miller W. Motivational interviewing: research, practice, and puzzles. *Addict Behav* 1996;21:835–842.

120. Green L, Kreuter M. *Health promotion planning: an educational and environmental approach*, 2nd ed. Mountain View, CA: Mayfield Publishing Company, 1991.

121. Green LW. What can we generalize from research on patient education and clinical health promotion to physician counseling on diet? *Eur J Clin Nutr* 1999;53:s9–s18.

122. Cole RE, Horacek T. Applying PRECEDE-PROCEED to develop an intuitive eating nondieting approach to weight management pilot program. *J Nutr Educ Behav* 2009;41:120–126.

123. Cole RE, Horacek T. Effectiveness of the "My Body Knows When" intuitive-eating pilot program. *Am J Health Behav* 2010;34:286–297.

124. Becker MH. The health belief model and personal health behavior. *Health Educ Monogr* 1974;2:409–419.

125. Ajzen I. The theory of planned behavior. *Organ Behav Hum Dec Process* 1991;50:179–211.

126. Blue CL. Does the theory of planned behavior identify diabetes-related cognitions for intention to be physically active and eat a healthy diet? *Public Health Nurs* 2007;24:141–150.

127. Hamilton K, White KM. Extending the theory of planned behavior: the role of self and social influences in predicting adolescent regular moderate-to-vigorous physical activity. *J Sport Exercise Psy* 2008;30:56–74.

128. Leventhal H, Nerenz DR. *A model for stress research and some implications for control of the disorder. Stress prevention and management: a cognitive behavioural approach*. New York, NY: Plenum, 1983.

129. Prochaska J, DiClemente C, Norcross J. In search of how people change: applications to the addictive behaviors. *Am Psychol* 1992;47:1102–1114.

130. Hutchinson AJ. Physical activity behavior change interventions based on the transtheoretical model: a systematic review. *Health Educ Behav* 2009;36:829–845.

131. Elder J, Ayala G, Harris S. Theories and intervention approaches to health-behavior change in primary care. *Am J Prev Med* 1999;17:275–284.

132. Moeini B, Rahimi M, Hazaveie SMM, et al. Effect of education based on trans-theoretical model on promoting physical activity and increasing physical work capacity. *Iran J Military Med* 2010;12:123–130.

133. Henderson T, Hall J, Lipton T. Changing destructive behaviours. In: Stone GC, Cohen F, Adler NE, et al., eds. *Health psychology: a handbook: theories, applications, and challenges of a psychological approach to the health care system*. San Francisco, CA: Jossey-Bass Publishers; 1979:141–145.

134. Rudner HL, Bestvater D, Bader E. Evaluating family counseling skills training for family practice. *Med Educ* 1990;24:461–466.

135. Bandura A. Self-efficacy: toward a unifying theory of behavioral change. *Psychol Rev* 1977;84:191–215.

136. Bandura A. Social cognitive theory: an agentic perspective. *Annu Rev Psychol* 2001;52:1–26.

137. Dennis EA, Potter KL, Estabrooks PA, et al. Weight gain prevention for college freshmen: comparing two social cognitive theory-based interventions with and without explicit self-regulation training. *J Obes* 2012; 2012:803769. doi:10.1155/2012/803769.

138. Rinderknecht K, Smith C. Social cognitive theory in an after-school nutrition intervention for urban Native American youth. *J Nutr Educ Behav* 2004;36:298–304.

139. Hallam JS, Petosa R. The long-term impact of a four-session work-site intervention on selected social cognitive theory variables linked to adult exercise adherence. *Health Educ Behav* 2004;31:88–100.

140. Diabetes Prevention Program Research Group. 10-year follow-up of diabetes incidence and weight loss in the Diabetes Prevention Program Outcomes study. *Lancet* 2009;374:1677–1686.

141. Albright CL, Pruitt L, Castro C, et al. Modifying physical activity in a multiethnic sample of low-income women: one-year results from the IMPACT (Increasing Motivation for Physical ACTivity) project. *Ann Behav Med* 2005;30:191–200.

142. Ockene JK, Ockene IS, Quirk ME, et al. Physician training for patient-centered nutrition counseling in a lipid intervention trial. *Prev Med* 1995;24:563–570.

143. Ockene IS, Hebert JR, Ockene JK, et al. Effect of physician-delivered nutrition counseling training and an office-support program on saturated fat intake, weight, and serum lipid measurements in a hyperlipidemic population: Worcester Area Trial for Counseling in Hyperlipidemia (WATCH). *Arch Intern Med* 1999;159:725–731.

144. Norris SL, Grothaus LC, Buchner DM, et al. Effectiveness of physician-based assessment and counseling for exercise in a staff model HMO. *Prev Med* 2000;30:513–523.

145. Calfas K, Long B, Sallis J, et al. A controlled trial of physician counseling to promote the adoption of physical activity. *Prev Med* 1996;25:225–233.

146. Green BB, McAfee T, Hindmarsh M, et al. Effectiveness of telephone support in increasing physical activity levels in primary care patients. *Am J Prev Med* 2002;22:177–183.

147. Patrick K, Calfas KJ, Norman GJ. Randomized controlled trial of a primary care and home-based intervention for physical activity and nutrition behaviors: PACE+ for adolescents. *Arch Pediatr Adolesc Med* 2006;160:128–136.

148. Huang JS, Norman GJ, Patrick K. Body image and self-esteem among adolescents undergoing an intervention targeting dietary and physical activity behaviors. *J Adolesc Health* 2007;40:245–251.

149. Baruth M, Wilcox S, Sallis JF. Changes in CVD risk factors in the activity counseling trial. *Int J Gen Med* 2011;4:53–62.

150. Petrella R, Wight D. An office-based instrument for exercise counseling and prescription in primary care: the step test exercise prescription (STEP). *Arch Fam Med* 2000;9:339–344.

151. Petrella RJ, Koval JJ, Cunningham DA. Can primary care doctors prescribe exercise to improve fitness? The Step Test Exercise Prescription (STEP) project. *Am J Prev Med* 2003;24:316–322.

152. Pinto BM, Goldstein MG, DePue JD, et al. Acceptability and feasibility of physician-based activity counseling. The PAL project. *Am J Prev Med* 1998;15:95–102.

153. Pinto B, Lynn H, Marcus B, et al. Physician-based activity counseling: intervention effects on mediators of

motivational readiness for physical activity. *Ann Behav Med* 2001;23:2–10.

154. Katz DL. Behavior modification in primary care: the pressure system model. *Prev Med* 2001;32:66–72.

155. Katz DL, Shenson D, Williams A, et al. *Health Enhancement through Lifestyle Practices (HELP)* (training manual). New Haven, CT: Yale Prevention Research Center, 2004.

156. Faridi Z, Polascek M, Barth M, et al. Health Enhancement through Lifestyle Practices (HELP): a feasibility study. *Health Promot Pract* under review 1/08.

157. Hwang JE. Promoting healthy lifestyles with aging: development and validation of the Health Enhancement Lifestyle Profile (HELP) using the Rasch measurement model. *Am J Occup Ther* 2010;64:786–795.

158. O'Connell M, Comerford BP, Wall HK, et al. Impediment profiling for smoking cessation: application in the worksite. *Am J Health Promot* 2006;21:97–100.

159. Katz DL, Boukhalil J, Lucan SC, et al. Impediment profiling for smoking cessation. Preliminary experience. *Behav Modif* 2003;27:524–537.

160. O'Connell M, Lucan SC, Yeh MC, et al. Impediment profiling for smoking cessation: results of a pilot study. *Am J Health Promot* 2003;17:300–303.

161. Katz DL, Shuval K, Comerford BP, et al. Impact of an educational intervention on internal medicine residents' physical activity counseling: the pressure system model (Old name: using the pressure system model to promote physical activity in primary care: a randomized controlled trial). *J Eval Clin Pract* In Press; 2008;14(2):294–299.

162. Yale-Griffin Prevention Research Center, (7/05–8/07). *Nnoledge (nutrition navigation on-line edge) web portal.* National Institutes of Health, National Institute of Diabetes and Digestive and Kidney Diseases Grant #R43. DK070418.

163. Yale-Griffin Prevention Research Center. *Current and Completed Projects. Nutrition Navigation on-Line Edge* (NnoLEDGE). Available online at http://www.yalegriffin-prc.org/Research-Findings/Current-Completed-Projects .aspx?udt_1588_param_detail=1911.

164. O.W.C.H. *Online Weight Management Counseling for Healthcare Providers.* Available online at: http://www .turnthetidefoundation.org/OWCH/about.htm.

165. Wadden TA, Berkowitz RI, Womble LG, et al. Randomized trial of lifestyle modification and pharmacotherapy for obesity. *N Engl J Med* 2005;353:2111–2120.

166. Kushner RF, Noble CA. Long-term outcome of bariatric surgery: an interim analysis. *Mayo Clin Proc* 2006; 81:s46–s51.

167. McMahon MM, Sarr MG, Clark MM, et al. Clinical management after bariatric surgery: value of a multidisciplinary approach. *Mayo Clin Proc* 2006;81:s34–s45.

168. American Medical Association. *AMAWIRE.* June 19, 2013. Available online at http://www.ama-assn.org/ams/ pub/amawire/2013-june-19/2013-june-19.shtml.

169. *American Medical Association Resolution 420: Recognition of Obesity as a Disease. 2013.* Available online at http:// www.ama-assn.org/assets/meeting/2013a/a13-addendum-refcomm-d.pdf.

170. Abutaleb Y. *U.S. lawmakers float bill for Medicare to cover obesity treatment.* Reuters. June 19, 2013. Available online at http://www.reuters.com/article/2013/06/19/usa-senate-obesity-idUSL2N0EV1KD20130619.

171. Katz D. *Obesity as a disease: Why I vote no. Huffpost Healthy Living.* June 21, 2013. Available online at: http://www.huffingtonpost.com/david-katz-md/obesity-disease_b_3478322.html.

172. Katz DL, Colino S. *Disease Proof: The Remarkable Truth About What Makes Us Well.* USA: Hudson Street Press; 2013.

173. *Weigh Forward.* Available online at: http://www.rediclinic .com/weighforward/.

174. *MyFitnessPal.* Available online at: http://www.myfitnesspal .com/.

SUGGESTED READINGS

American Association of Diabetes Educators. Individualization of diabetes self-management education. *Diabetes Educ* 2002;28:741–745, 749.

American Association of Diabetes Educators. Intensive diabetes management: implications of the DCCT and UKPDS. *Diabetes Educ* 2002;28:735–740.

American Diabetes Association. Economic costs of diabetes in the US in 2002. *Diabetes Care* 2003;26:917–932.

American Diabetes Association. *National diabetes fact sheet.* Available at http://www.cdc.gov/diabetes/pubs/pdf/ndfs_ 2005.pdf; accessed 11/8/07.

American Diabetes Association. *Resources for professionals.* Available at http://www.diabetes.org/for-health-professionals-and-scientists/resources.jsp; accessed 11/8/07.

American Diabetes Association. Standards of medical care for patients with diabetes mellitus. *Diabetes Care* 2003;26: s33–s50.

American Healthways I. *American healthways reports third-quarter earnings per diluted share of $0.22 versus $0.14 for the third quarter last year.* Available at http://findarticles .com/p/articles/mi_m0EIN/is_2004_June_17/ai_n6083865; accessed 11/8/07.

Anderson RM, Funnell MM, Butler PM, et al. Patient empowerment. Results of a randomized controlled trial. *Diabetes Care* 1995;18:943–949.

Balinsky W, Muennig P. The costs and outcomes of multifaceted interventions designed to improve the care of congestive heart failure in the inpatient setting: a review of the literature. *Med Care Res Rev* 2003;60:275–293.

Banister NA, Jastrow ST, Hodges V, et al. Diabetes self-management training program in a community clinic improves patient outcomes at modest cost. *J Am Diet Assoc* 2004;104:807–810.

Baranowski P, Perry CL, Parcel GS. How individuals, environments, and health behavior interact: social cognitive theory. In: Glanz K, Rimer BK, eds. *Health behavior and health education: theory, research, and practice,* 2nd ed. San Francisco, CA: Jossey-Bass, 1997:165–184.

Bellazzi R, Arcelloni M, Bensa G, et al. Design, methods, and evaluation directions of a multi-access service for the management of diabetes mellitus patients. *Diabetes Technol Ther* 2003;5:621–629.

Bodenheimer T, Lorig K, Holman H, et al. Patient self-management of chronic disease in primary care. *JAMA* 2002;288:2469–2475.

Bonow RO, Gheorghiade M. The diabetes epidemic: a national and global crisis. *Am J Med* 2004;116:2s–10s.

Cagliero E, Levina EV, Nathan DM. Immediate feedback of HbA1c levels improves glycemic control in type i and insulin-treated type 2 diabetic patients. *Diabetes Care* 1999;22:1785–1989.

Centers for Disease Control and Prevention. *About chronic diseases*. Available at: http://www.cdc.gov/nccdphp; accessed 11/8/07.

Centers for Disease Control and Prevention. *Disability and health*. Available at: http://www.cdc.gov/ncbddd/dh/default.htm; accessed 11/8/07.

Centers for Disease Control and Prevention. *Health-related quality of life*. Available at: http://www.cdc.gov/hrqol; accessed 11/8/07.

Centers for Disease Control and Prevention (CDC). *National diabetes fact sheet: general information and national estimates on diabetes in the United States, 2003*. Atlanta: CDC.

Centers for Medicare & Medicaid Services. *Medicare preventive services*. Available at: http://www.cms.hhs.gov/MLNProducts/downloads/MPS_QuickReferenceChart_1.pdf; accessed 11/8/07.

Chapin RB, Williams DC, Adair RF. Diabetes control improved when inner-city patients received graphic feedback about glycosylated hemoglobin levels. *J Gen Intern Med* 2003;18:120–124.

Cranor CW, Bunting BA, Christensen DB. The Asheville Project: long-term clinical and economic outcomes of a community pharmacy diabetes care program. *J Am Pharm Assoc* (Wash DC) 2003;43:173–184.

Durso SC, Wendel I, Letzt AM, et al. Older adults using cellular telephones for diabetes management: a pilot study. *Medsurg Nurs* 2003;12:313–317.

Eliaszadeh P, Yarmohammadi H, Nawaz H, et al. Congestive heart failure case management: a fiscal analysis. *Dis Manag* 2001;4:25–32.

Gibson PG, Powell H, Coughlan J, et al. Self-management education and regular practitioner review for adults with asthma. *Cochrane Database Syst Rev* 2003;1:CD001117.

Gilbert GL, Christensen J, Conway ME. *Benefits of glycemic control*. Available at http://www.ceoncd.com/CD/CD0008/AB0052/ab0052.htm; accessed 11/8/07.

Gillespie G. Deploying an I.T. cure for chronic diseases. *Health Data Manag* 2000;8:68–70, 72, 74.

Glasgow RE, Boles SM, McKay HG, et al. The D-Net diabetes self-management program: long-term implementation, outcomes, and generalization results. *Prev Med* 2003;36:410–419.

Goldberg JH, Kiernan M. Innovative techniques to address retention in a behavioral weight-loss trial. *Health Educ Res* 2005;20:439–447.

Goldberg HI, Ralston JD, Hirsch IB, et al. Using an Internet comanagement module to improve the quality of chronic disease care. *Jt Comm J Qual Saf* 2003;29:443–451.

Janz NK, Champion VL, Strecher VJ. The health belief model. In: Glanz K, Lewis FM, Rimer BK, eds. *Health behavior and health education*. San Francisco, CA: Jossey-Bass Publishers; 1997:45–66.

Kavanagh DJ, Gooley S, Wilson PH. Prediction of adherence and control in diabetes. *J Behav Med* 1993;16:509–522.

Kreuter MW, Chheda SG, et al. How does physician advice influence patient behavior? Evidence for a priming effect. *Arch of Fam Med* 2000;9:426–433.

Kreuter MW, Wray RJ. Tailored and targeted health communication: strategies for enhancing information relevance. *Am J Health Behav* 2003;27:s227–s232.

Lazev A, Vidrine D, Arduino R, et al. Increasing access to smoking cessation treatment in a low-income, HIV-positive population: the feasibility of using cellular telephones. *Nicotine Tob Res* 2004;6:281–286.

Centers for Disease Control and Prevention. Levels of diabetes-related preventive care practices—United States, 1997–1999. *MMWR Morb Mortal Wkly Rep* 2000;49:954–958.

Lorig KR, Ritter P, Stewart AL, et al. Chronic disease self-management program: 2-year health status and health care utilization outcomes. *Med Care* 2001;39:1217–1223.

Mazzi CP. A framework for the evaluation of internet-based diabetes management. *J Med Internet Res* 2002;1:4:e1.

McCaul KD, Glasgow RE, Schafer LC. Diabetes regimen behaviors. Predicting adherence. *Med Care* 1987;25:868–881.

Miller CK, Edwards L, Kissling G, et al. Evaluation of a theory-based nutrition intervention for older adults with diabetes mellitus. *J Am Diet Assoc* 2002;102:1069–1081.

National Cancer Institute. *Health message tailoring*. Available at http://dccps.nci.nih.gov/messagetailoring/about.html; accessed 11/8/07.

Nicollerat JA. Implications of the United Kingdom Prospective Diabetes Study (UKPDS) results on patient management. *Diabetes Educ* 2000;26:8–10.

Nobel JJ, Norman GK. Emerging information management technologies and the future of disease management. *Dis Manag* 2003;6:219–231.

Petty R, Cacioppo J. *Attitudes and persuasion: classic and contemporary approaches*. Dubuque, IA: W. C. Brown Co, 1981.

Polonsky WH, Earles J, Smith S, et al. Integrating medical management with diabetes self-management training: a randomized control trial of the Diabetes Outpatient Intensive Treatment program. *Diabetes Care* 2003;26:3048–3053.

Ralston JD, Revere D, Robins LS, et al. Patients' experience with a diabetes support programme based on an interactive electronic medical record: qualitative study. *BMJ* 2004;328:1–4.

Rich MW. Management of heart failure in the elderly. *Heart Fail Rev* 2002;7:89–97.

Rich M, Beckham V, Leven C, et al. A multidisciplinary intervention to prevent the readmission of elderly patients with congestive heart failure. *N Eng J Med* 1995;333:1190–1195.

Rich M, Nease R. Cost-effectiveness analysis in clinical practice: the case of heart failure. *Arch Intern Med* 1999;159:1690–1700.

Ruggiero L, Glasgow RE, Dryfoos JM, et al. Diabetes self-management: self-reported recommendations and patterns in a large population. *Diabetes Care* 1997;20:568–576.

Schermer TR, Thoonen BP, van den Boom G, et al. Randomized controlled economic evaluation of asthma self-management in primary health care. *Am J Respir Crit Care Med* 2002;166:1062–1072.

Shea S, Starren J, Weinstock RS, et al. Columbia University's Informatics for Diabetes Education and Telemedicine

(IDEATel) Project: rationale and design. *J Am Med Inform Assoc* 2002;9:49–62.

Shore MF. Empowering individuals as carers of their own health. *World Hosp Health Serv* 2001;37:12–16, 33, 35.

Stam DM, Graham JP. Important aspects of self-management education in patients with diabetes. *Pharm Pract Manag Q* 1997;17:12–25.

Toobert DJ, Hampson SE, Glasgow RE. The summary of diabetes self-care activities measure: results from 7 studies and a revised scale. *Diabetes Care* 2000;23:943–950.

Tudor-Locke C, Bell RC, Myers AM, et al. Controlled outcome evaluation of the first step program: a daily physical activity intervention for individuals with type II diabetes. *Int J Obes Relat Metab Disord* 2004;28:113–119.

Whitlock EP, Orleans CT, Pender N, et al. Evaluating primary care behavioral counseling interventions. *Am J Prev Med* 2002;22:267–284.

Willett WC, Domolky S. *Strategic plan for the prevention and control of overweight and obesity in New England*. Available at http://www.neconinfo.org/02-11-2003_Strategic_Plan.pdf; accessed 11/8/07.

CHAPTER 47

Dietary Counseling in Clinical Practice

T he information in this and related books is just so much ink unless it is applied in clinical practice. Thus, dietary counseling is the medium of exchange that infuses significance into the study of clinical nutrition and renders nutrition a field directly relevant to health outcomes. But access to and knowledge and understanding of salient nutrition principles are by no means commensurate with the capacity to deliver those principles to patients effectively, persuasively, and productively. Effective dietary counseling requires astute consideration and handling of factors—some under the patient's control and some not—governing behavioral patterns (see Chapter 38); confrontation with traditional impediments to such counseling in the clinical setting; the avoidance of confrontation with a patient; identification of the particular assistance an individual patient needs and compassionate attention to it; the timely and judicious use of supporting materials and resources; an acceptance of the incremental nature of change and delayed gratification; and dedicated persistence. Few worthwhile endeavors are easy, and nutritional counseling is no exception.

But effective dietary counseling is of vital importance, given the impact of dietary pattern on health. The evidence to support the effectiveness of dietary counseling on modifying health outcomes is slowly accumulating, and there is more evidence now to support nutrition and lifestyle counseling than when the last edition of this book was published (1) (see Chapter 46). In line with this growing body of evidence, the Centers for Medicare and Medicaid Services have created new regulations that authorize reimbursement for obesity counseling (2) (see Chapter 46). However, the case is still far from ironclad that routine dietary counseling is beneficial. In 2012, the U.S. Preventive Services Task Force concluded that behavioral counseling has small-to-moderate

benefits in improving diet but recommended that behavioral counseling be used in selected patients rather than routinely (3). Similarly, the American Academy of Family Physicians recommends intensive behavioral lifestyle counseling specifically for patients with hyperlipidemia and other cardiovascular risk factors (4). In contrast, for pediatric patients, it is recommended that all children receive lifestyle counseling, with more intensive counseling for overweight and obese patients (5).

But with over 35% of US adults classified as obese (6), the argument for counseling is compelling. Diet is fundamental to the management and prevention of cardiovascular diseases, diabetes, cancer, and hypertension. Dietary practices divergent from recommendations, combined with lack of physical activity, are considered the second leading cause of preventable death in the United States, behind tobacco use (7). Because, however, everyone eats while only a minority of the population uses tobacco, in the aggregate, the health effects of nutrition are likely to be far greater. Even when not discernibly contributing to the development or prevention of a particular disease, nutrition plays a role in lifelong health, influencing appearance, functional status, self-esteem, socialization, energy level and vitality, athletic performance, susceptibility to infection, and possibly independent of morbidity, longevity. Therefore, the potential for dietary practices to modify health is tremendous and universally applicable.

When the importance of diet to health is acknowledged, we are duty bound to contend with it in practice, even if the success of our efforts is in question. We are, for instance, obligated to treat pain to the best of our ability, even if our best effort proves insufficient. In much of medical practice, our limitations are a goad to greater effort, not an invitation to abdicate. Dietary counseling deserves and demands its share of this pervasive clinical respect.

Thus, any controversies regarding dietary counseling in primary care should be devoted to how, not whether or why. There is reason to believe, on the basis of both judgment and empirical evidence, that greater commitment to nutrition counseling in clinical practice would lead to greater effectiveness. Once we are committed to dietary counseling as a matter of principle, the remaining choices are about how to make it work for our patients and ourselves. Laid out in this chapter is a framework that is equally respectful of the needs of both groups. Patients need advice that is sound, reliable, personally relevant, and compassionate rather than judgmental. Clinicians need a delivery system that is efficient, comfortable, replicable from encounter to encounter, and mindful of its place in the panoply of clinical obligations. That these disparate objectives can be met is the argument to which this chapter is dedicated.

INTRODUCTION OF THE COUNSELING CONSTRUCT

Chapter 46 provides an overview of behavior modification constructs relevant to dietary counseling and addresses some of the most salient barriers to that counseling. This chapter is principally devoted to the elaboration of a particular counseling approach predicated on that body of behavior change theory and designed to navigate around those barriers.

The Pressure System Model (PSM), developed by the author expressly to render elements of behavior change theory more amenable to application in the primary care setting, was first published in 2001 (8). Since that time, the model has been applied in a controlled trial of physical activity promotion (9); tailored for use by a large primary care group in Maine (10, unpublished data.); incorporated into a regional obesity control plan for the New England States (11); presented as an example of needed obesity control measures at the National Obesity Action Forum (12); been incorporated into a clinician-centered, skill-based weight management program (13); and adapted into an online module that has already had over 1,000 users as of Spring, 2013 (14). Additionally, training in the PSM is accessible online (15) and offers free Continuing Medical Education credits.

In brief, the PSM includes a two-question algorithm as the initiation of dietary counseling and then brief, targeted interventions directed to patient need, as determined by the algorithm. The PSM algorithm (see Figure 47.1) determines whether counseling should be focused primarily on raising motivation, lowering resistance, or both, by placing the patient into one of five categories (see Figure 47.2). The subsequent focus of counseling is category specific (see Table 47.1). The intent of the construct is to facilitate counseling that is productive in increments as brief as 90 seconds per encounter. When detailed and time-consuming dietary counseling is warranted, referral to a dietitian or another nutritionist with counseling expertise is generally advised.

Details of the Counseling Construct

Development of the PSM began with an effort to synthesize elements from various behavior modification models to characterize and influence the processes of change more effectively in the abbreviated context of primary care encounters (16). To that end, the governance of behavior

---

1. Are you currently eating a healthful diet (based mostly on vegetables, fruits, whole, grains, etc.) and/or engaging in regular physical activity?

YES:	Category **3**
NO, and I have never tried:	*Go to question 2*
NO, I have tried recently, but stopped temporarily:	Category **4**
NO, I have tried one or more times, and given up:	Category **5**

2. Are you ready to start eating a healthful diet/being physically active?

YES:	Category **2**
NO, and I have never tried:	Category **1**

FIGURE 47.1 PSM algorithm. The PSM counseling approach is predicated on just two basic questions that help determine whether a given patient primarily needs help in raising motivation or overcoming resistance/barriers. The categories are explained in Figure 47.2.

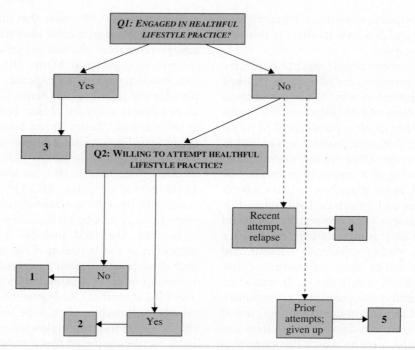

FIGURE 47.2 PSM categories. Solid lines indicate direct questioning; dashed lines indicate various potential patient responses to a given question.

TABLE 47.1

PSM Categories and Associated Counseling Approaches

Category	Algorithm Responses	Emphasis of Counseling	Special Considerations
1	No/No	Motivation	Patients in Category 1 are "precontemplative," not having thought about the behavior change in question. The goal of initial counseling is to raise awareness, interest, and motivation.
2	No/Yes	Motivation and resistance	Patients in Category 2 are considering behavior change and are thus "contemplative." This group will likely benefit from a primary focus on raising motivation to induce change but also some attention to the potential barriers that are fostering hesitation and ambivalence.
3	Yes	—	Patients in the "action" phase generally just need encouragement. However, as new barriers are encountered, troubleshooting assistance may be necessary.
4	No; relapse	Resistance	Patients in this group were motivated enough to attempt change; a relapse suggests that a barrier was encountered. Troubleshooting that barrier and attempting to identify and plan for others are warranted.
5	No; burnout	Resistance	Patients with multiple failed attempts at behavior change are apt to feel "burned out." This group needs to first understand why failure is not their fault—that it results from encountering barriers—and then needs assistance identifying and troubleshooting those barriers.

Source: Katz DL. Behavior modification in primary care: the pressure system model. *Prev Med* 2001;32:66–72.

maintenance and behavior change were distilled down into two fundamental and opposing forces: (17) the desire for change, or *motivation*, and (18) resistance to change, or *obstacles*. The potential utility of the model is closely allied to its simplicity: Facilitating behavior for any given patient begins merely by identifying which of these two forces warrants dedicated attention.

Believing in the importance of the condition to be avoided, in personal risk, and in the utility of the change are all components, or prerequisites, of motivation (19,20). A change believed to modify meaningfully a substantial, personal risk is desirable. Such a change, however, will occur only if the resultant motivation exceeds the aggregate resistance, whatever the nature or source of that resistance (see Figure 47.3).

In this regard, the established behavior change models discussed in Chapter 46 are informative. To effect a change, one must be capable of change. Individuals lacking self-efficacy cannot change their behavior until or unless they learn that they have the capacity to do so. The Stages of Change model represents sequential assessments of the balance between resistance and motivation.

When the difficulty is perceived to exceed the rewards of change, one is unwilling to change and fails to advance to the action stage. With new information or experience, motivation for change may rise as the perceived difficulty remains constant. As the gap between the two narrows, one perceives the potential for change and becomes contemplative. Change is attempted whenever motivation, at least temporarily, exceeds the recognized resistance. The behavior change is maintained until or unless difficulty overtakes motivation, at which time relapse occurs. A more realistic, or at least more practiced, assessment of both difficulty and motivation are the result of unsuccessful attempts at change. These attempts either serve as the necessary preparation for sustainable change or lead to frustration.

The complexities of diet make behavior change particularly difficult. The well-known slogan of drug control efforts in the United States, "Just say no," is clearly impertinent when it comes to diet. Diet cannot be avoided, but it must be managed. The need to struggle with the desired behavior change on a continuous basis is more than most people can manage successfully. Consequently,

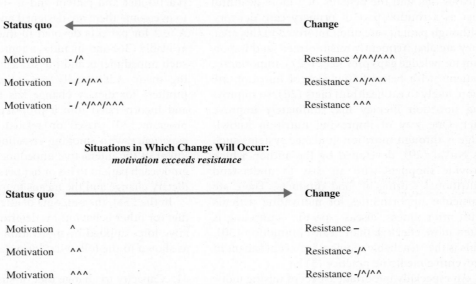

Situations in Which Change *Will Not* Occur:
resistance equals or exceeds motivation

Status quo	←	Change
Motivation	- /^	Resistance ^/^^/^^^
Motivation	- / ^/^^	Resistance ^^/^^^
Motivation	- / ^/^^/^^^	Resistance ^^^

Situations in Which Change Will Occur:
motivation exceeds resistance

Status quo	→	Change
Motivation	^	Resistance –
Motivation	^^	Resistance -/^
Motivation	^^^	Resistance -/^/^^

FIGURE 47.3 How gradients between motivation for change and barriers, or resistance to change, determine the outcome of behavior change efforts. The relative force of motivation and resistance, as represented by arrowheads, determines whether desired behavior change occurs or whether the status quo is maintained. A horizontal line represents neutrality, and increasing numbers of upward-pointing arrowheads represent increasing force, or "pressure."

the rate of compliance with dietary recommendations has historically been very low (21–23).

In primary care practice, most (but certainly not all) patients will be fairly motivated to select a health-promoting diet. This is true either because the patients are already sick and therefore motivated by the perception of personal risk, or they are seeking primary care despite being well, in which case they are seeking preventive and health-promotion services. The most common nutrition-related problem seen in primary care is obesity, and it is the problem most likely to have led to prior efforts to change diet. Obese adults seeking primary care are unlikely to need motivation for dietary change. Failure to change diet in most patients is the result not of inadequate motivation but of excessive resistance. The only ways to produce change under such circumstances are to reduce the difficulty and to increase motivation further.

Often, motivation can be raised, and specific methods of motivational interviewing have been developed (19,20). As noted by Botelho and Skinner (19), "advice giving," a relatively ineffective means of raising motivation, has tended to predominate in clinical practice. Minimally, motivation for dietary change requires knowledge of the link between diet and health. This is achieved by informing patients of the hazards of an injudicious diet and the benefits of a more healthful diet as a routine part of primary care delivery. Although patients are often informed in this area, they are also frequently misinformed, and important knowledge gaps prevail (24–27). Importantly, patients with better knowledge of nutrition are more likely to eat healthful diets (28), so improving nutrition literacy may ultimately improve diet. One way of improving nutrition knowledge is through nutrition guidance systems such as NuVal (29), developed by the author, which provide shoppers with an easy to understand nutritional scoring of food products. There are particular opportunities for motivating patients with prior illness; disease-specific counseling is often more effective than health promotion (30). This is the "teachable moment" concept salient in preventive medicine practice (31).

An especially important aspect of raising motivation to change is reestablishing self-esteem and self-efficacy when they have been lost. Paradoxically, one of the ways to reestablish a patient's self-efficacy may be to inform him or her how much of dietary behavior is beyond individual control.

This approach requires that the practitioner and patient distinguish between responsibility and blame and between factors subject to personal control and those beyond it, such as the built environment (32–35). Patients with repeated, unsuccessful efforts at changing diet (usually to lose weight) must be taught that factors beyond their control contrive to prevent such change. These factors include a litany of obesigenic influences from fast food to electronic devices, vending machines to video games, food processing to food marketing, and the fundamental mismatch between a Stone Age metabolism and a Space Age food supply (36) (see Chapter 44). Each of these and many related factors is either the direct product of physiologic adaptations to the forces of natural selection or the result of sociologic, psychological, religious, and cultural evolution.

There are two reasons a brief discussion of these exonerating factors is essential. First, by alleviating patients of their feelings of failure and futility, lost motivation for dietary change can be recaptured. Second, to prevent failure from recurring yet again, the balance between motivation and difficulty must be fundamentally altered. To do this, difficulty in changing diet must be reduced. This can be achieved only if the impediments to sustainable dietary change are recognized by both practitioner and patient and if strategies tailored to overcome them are designed and implemented. A text for patients devoted to this very matter is available (36) and includes a representative list of such impediments and the strategies for overcoming them. Additionally, an online "impediment profiler" for dietary change has been developed and incorporated into a proprietary weight-loss program (20), based on related and successful experience with smoking cessation (37–40). The intent of the interactive impediment profiler is to guide each patient to his or her personal barriers to dietary change and the means to overcome them.

In the PSM, the outcome of attempts to change diet (or other behaviors) is determined by the relative force applied by motivation and resistance, as shown in the following formulae:

1. Capacity to change diet or sustain change = Aggregate motivation − Aggregate resistance, where the difference must be positive
2. Inability to initiate or sustain dietary change = Aggregate resistance − Aggregate motivation, where the difference must be positive

3. Tendency to relapse after change varies directly with resistance and indirectly with motivation; relapse will occur when difficulty meets or exceeds motivation.

The conventional approach to behavioral counseling in primary care is to attempt to raise motivation (19), and motivational interviewing seems to enhance weight loss in obese and overweight patients (41) (see Chapter 46). Patients are apprised of the health risks associated with the maintenance of smoking, alcohol consumption, illicit drug use, and sedentary lifestyle and of the benefits of changing such behaviors. As shown in Figure 47.3, when motivation can be raised above resistance, behavior change will occur.

Generally unaddressed in counseling efforts, however, are the fixed impediments to behavior change. A schedule that does not readily accommodate exercise may overcome motivation for physical activity. A fellow household member's smoking may overcome an individual's motivation to quit. The convenience and familiarity of fast food, and uncertainty about how to change patterns of shopping and cooking, may overcome an individual's desire to improve his or her diet (42). As shown in Figure 47.3, even if motivation is fairly high, change cannot occur if resistance to change is higher still. While counseling may serve to raise motivation, the level may fail to exceed resistance.

The insidious danger in this traditional approach to counseling is the tendency to actually or at least apparently "blame the victim" of behavioral risk factors (43–48,48a). While an unmotivated patient may be encouraged by a clinician's efforts to motivate, an already motivated patient is apt to experience frustration when change does not occur. That frustration is generally shared by the practitioner, adversely affecting the relationship (49). The PSM serves as a reminder that motivation is not infinitely malleable and that when resistance is great enough, motivation alone cannot produce behavior change. This encourages both patient and provider to engage in the productive process of identifying impediments to change that may be surmountable instead of the unproductive process of self-recrimination.

The second contribution of the PSM is its capacity to define the appropriate focus of counseling efforts based on discrete and easily recognized clinical scenarios. This progression from theoretical construct to clinical algorithm renders the model practical under the constraints of primary care practice.

As shown in Table 47.1, each of the five categorical determinations facilitated by the PSM algorithm has specific implications for counseling. Patients for whom motivation is relevant should receive motivational interviewing. The salient principles of this method are shown in Table 47.2. A simple tool to expedite a patient's progress through his or her own ambivalence—the principal objective of motivational interviewing—is a decision balance, as shown in Figure 47.4. A decision balance enables a patient to map out the sources of ambivalence and modify them over time. The balance may be completed at an office visit or in between visits, and it may be productive for the patient when assessed in private as well as at a clinic visit. Apparent gaps in the balance are an opportunity for the practitioner to

TABLE 47.2	
Salient Principles of Motivational Interviewing	
Principle	Implications
Express empathy/acknowledge ambivalence	Legitimizes patient's feelings, shows respect
Develop discrepancy	Reveals disconnect between behavioral pattern and goals
Avoid argumentation	Conveys that patient is in charge; builds therapeutic alliance
Roll with resistance	Acknowledges that working through ambivalence is a process that may take time
Support self-efficacy	Conveys support for patient
Encourage social contracting	A confidante adds both support for change and a sense of accountability

Source: Miller WR. Motivational interviewing: research, practice, and puzzles. *Addict Behav* 1996;21:835–842.

	Change	Don't Change
Pros		
Cons		

FIGURE 47.4 A decision balance. Cells in the balance are filled in by a patient during or in between office visits. As the balance evolves over time, its implications for behavior change also evolve.

offer advice and information that might tip the balance in favor of desired behavior change. But the balance also pushes back and indicates to the practitioner and patient alike when an effort to change is likely to be premature and thus unsuccessful. At such times, continuing to work toward a more favorable balance is the prudent course.

When the patient's needs, as indicated by the PSM algorithm, relate more to barriers than to motivation, a focus on motivation may be counterproductive. In such encounters, an effort to identify and overcome barriers of personal relevance is most constructive. An online impediment profiler for dietary change (13) has been developed that allows a patient to navigate through a fairly comprehensive list of potential barriers to lifestyle change and identify those of personal relevance. The online system, modeled after an approach first tested for smoking cessation, and a related approach applied in one trial of physical activity promotion (9), includes strategies for contending successfully with each barrier encountered. As a surrogate for universal access to such systems online, a representative array of barriers and strategies is available to patients in book form (36).

To apply this model, the discrete components of motivation and difficulty must be identified so that they can be targeted as indicated in counseling efforts. Factors influencing motivation are summarized in the following relatively short list, although means of enhancing motivation are more subtle and complex:

■ Risks of not changing
■ Health benefits of changing
■ Body image benefits of change
■ Social/psychological benefits of change
■ Social support
■ Perceived self-efficacy

Whereas motivation may be inspired by a great many considerations but is ultimately composed of relatively few, the list of actual or potential barriers to dietary change is virtually endless. Only by working with an individual patient can the salient impediments to dietary modification be identified.

Structured Approach to ADEPT Dietary Counseling

One of the likely advantages of a nutrition text written by a primary care practitioner is the author's obligatory acceptance that nutrition in clinical practice will not, and should not, supplant other priorities. Just as clinical practice is deficient if it is inattentive to the profound influences of diet on health, so is clinical nutrition deficient if it is inattentive to the competing demands with which a provider must contend in all too little time.

With these considerations in mind, the approach to nutritional counseling laid out here is willfully streamlined. It is also applicable to the various lifestyle practices germane to health, notable among them being tobacco use and physical activity pattern, along with diet. In the context of this book, the guidance offered is cast in terms of dietary counseling preferentially, but it is a matter of clinical judgment that health-related behavior is most deserving of attention at any given time.

The recommended steps for structured dietary counseling, shown in Table 47.3, are:

1. Administer the PSM algorithm.
2. Determine the appropriate emphasis on motivation or resistance.
3. Provide tailored counseling.
4. Track behavior (e.g., dietary intake) over time.

TABLE 47.3

Steps in the Application of PSM in the Context of Primary Care Visits[a]

Counseling Step	Comment
Apply algorithm	Apply the two-question PSM algorithm to determine current lifestyle/dietary practices and willingness to alter them. (This can be about the individual patient or all members of a household if the patient manages the diets of others.)
Determine emphasis	Determine the appropriate emphasis on raising motivation, lowering resistance, or both, and providing encouragement if current dietary practices are healthful.
Provide tailored counseling	Use motivational interviewing techniques and a decision balance if the appropriate emphasis is on raising motivation. If the appropriate emphasis is on overcoming resistance, work with the patient to identify and troubleshoot barriers.
Track behavior	If patient reports a healthful diet, probe for particulars, such as information about a typical day, and offer guidance for any adjustments deemed important. Regardless of patient's PSM category, ask them to complete several days' worth of food intake diaries and either mail them in or bring them at follow-up to verify habitual dietary intake pattern, as warranted.

[a]The acronym to recall this sequence of steps is ADEPT.

The acronym ADEPT (Apply Algorithm; Determine Emphasis; Provide tailored counseling; and Track behavior) may be useful in remembering the sequence of steps. This acronym is, of course, tailored as a reminder specific to the PSM but is closely related in both its emphasis and sequence to the "five A's": assess, advise, agree, assist, and arrange follow-up (50,51).

The Medical Home and Lifestyle Counseling

The medical home is being promoted as a key component in the reform of primary care in the United States. The medical home is a patient-centered care model that involves the primary physician working with a multidisciplinary health care team to provide longitudinal care of the patient (52). Such models of care promote improved patient satisfaction and outcomes and decreased staff burnout (53). The medical home opens exciting avenues for the delivery of lifestyle counseling since it will be possible for the primary clinician to provide some lifestyle basic counseling and then refer the patient directly to an on-site dietician or nurse who can provide more intensive counseling.

Technological Innovations in Counseling

Advances in technology have allowed for novel and creative ways of enhancing lifestyle counseling through the use of internet-based platforms, smartphones, digital videos, and social networking. Technology can build on counseling efforts by allowing patients ways of self-monitoring (food and activity logs), providing reminders via phone, text, email, and serving as another source of peer support through chat rooms, online bulletin boards, and social networks (54). Smartphones may be a particularly useful tool for intervention since are increasingly more common and are dynamic and portable. However, though there an abundance of weight-loss apps available, formal testing of their efficacy in clinical trials remains scant. In a pilot trial comparing a weight-loss smartphone app to a website or paper diary, participants ranked the smartphone app highly and were more likely adhere to the intervention (55). More rigorous and extensive research is needed to figure out how best to optimize technological tools in counseling.

CONCLUSIONS

The combination of diet and physical activity pattern together constitute the second leading cause of premature death in the United States (7). Even this dominant role in health may be an underestimate; because everyone eats, the health of every patient seen is influenced, for good, bad, or both, by diet. Therefore, attention to dietary pattern in the course of clinical care is of universal importance.

Encouraging patients to eat well for the promotion of health and the prevention and/or amelioration of disease should be approached in the context of well-established principles of behavior modification. Some patients need to be motivated before they are willing to consider change, others need help strategizing to maintain change currently under way, and still others need help overcoming the sequelae of prior failed attempts. This latter group, perhaps predominant, may be harmed by counseling efforts focusing only on motivation. The PSM of behavior modification can be used to identify discrete clinical scenarios in which motivational counseling is needed and is likely to be productive. Much effort at dietary modification fails due to the diverse and challenging obstacles to a healthy diet in the modern "toxic" nutritional environment. The clinician committed to promoting the nutritional health of patients must commit to devising strategies, tailored to individual patients, over and around such obstacles.

Dietary and lifestyle patterns are predicated on many other considerations besides health (44). Given that human dietary metabolism and preferences are derivatives, largely, of the very different environment of prehistory (see Chapter 44) and that the modern nutritional environment has developed to satisfy preferences, health problems resulting from dietary excess are not surprising.

Given the multiple influences on dietary selection and the fact that health is generally not the dominant concern, professional guidance is clearly required to encourage and guide individual efforts to approximate a health-promoting dietary pattern. Such efforts must play out at the complex interface of medicine and lifestyle, physiology and sociology, anthropology and evolutionary biology, personal responsibility and environmental determinism, psychology, and metabolism. Of fundamental importance to such efforts is the understanding that any effort to change individual behavior requires talking individuals out of the behavioral pattern they have selected or into another they have not, along with respecting that many forces other than will or choice govern behavioral patterns. Thus, effective dietary counseling begins with identification of what is feasible for a given patient and then leans heavily on the power of persuasion. A therapeutic alliance is essential, as are patience and accommodation.

A limited assessment of dietary pattern should be routinely incorporated into every history and physical examination. A brief overview of a health-promoting diet should be provided on such occasions as well (see Chapter 45). Dietary counseling should always be linked to advice about physical activity, as the health benefits of each support those of the other; there is evidence that physician counseling effectively promotes physical activity (41,56,57) (see Chapter 46). Difficulties involved in making dietary and other lifestyle changes should be acknowledged.

When more involved dietary counseling is indicated as part of weight loss or disease management efforts, referral to a dietitian or another nutritional consultant is generally advisable. In such circumstances, the physician's role is to reinforce the detailed counseling provided by the dietitian, situate diet in the overall clinical plan, and encourage the patient's efforts by applying realistic behavior modification principles that distinguish between responsibility and blame, the reasons, and the methods.

No matter how refined clinical counseling techniques may become, it is rather implausible that they would ever represent a sufficient counterforce to the obesigenic modern environment (34,35,58–64). For the health care setting to contribute meaningfully to weight management will likely thus require fundamental adjustments to the systems of care delivery as well as coordination with resource allocations in other settings (32,65).

The evidence that dietary counseling in the context of clinical care can change behavior and/or outcomes is limited, but such evidence does exist and is increasing. The application of methods specifically tailored to the setting of clinical practice should lead to better outcomes than have been described to date. A concerted effort by clinicians to incorporate nonjudgmental dietary guidance into routine clinical care is clearly indicated by the importance, and universal relevance, of diet to health.

Though effective counseling and patient education is necessary to promote healthy lifestyles, it is not sufficient. In order to make effective lifestyle changes, in addition to knowing what choices to make, patients need to have the *means* and *abilities* to make those choices. For example, even if a patient of a low socioeconomic status wanted to increase her fruit and vegetable consumption, the price of fresh produce may be prohibitively expensive. Similarly, if she wanted to increase her physical activity, her neighborhood might not have a safe outdoor space for exercise. The very structure of the environment can make healthy eating a challenge and physical inactivity the norm (see Chapter 5). In order to curtail the obesity epidemic, lifestyle counseling needs to be coupled with broader changes to the environment that facilitate rather than hinder healthy living.

REFERENCES

1. Artinian NT, Fletcher GF, Mozaffarian D, et al. Interventions to promote physical activity and dietary lifestyle changes for cardiovascular risk factor reduction in adults a scientific statement from the American Heart Association. *Circulation* 2010;122(4):406–441.

2. http://www.cms.gov/medicare-coverage-database/details/nca-decision-memo.aspx?&NcaName=Intensive%20Behavioral%20Therapy%20for%20Obesity&bc=ACAAAAAAIAAA&NCANC=253&.

3. U.S. Preventive Services Task Force. *Behavioral counseling interventions to promote a healthful diet and physical activity for cardiovascular disease prevention in adults: U.S. Preventive Services Task Force Recommendation Statement.* AHRQ Publication No. 11-05149-EF-2, June 2012. Available at http://www.uspreventiveservicestaskforce.org/uspstf11/physactivity/physrs.htm. Last accessed 5/18/2014.

4. American Academy of Family Physicians. *Healthy diet.* Available at http://www.aafp.org/online/en/home/clinical/exam/healthydiet.html; accessed 3/22/13.

5. Barlow SE; the Expert Committee. Expert Committee Recommendations regarding the prevention, assessment, and treatment of child and adolescent overweight and obesity: summary report. *Pediatrics* 2007;120(Supplement): S164–S192.

6. Flegal KM, Carroll MD, Kit BK, et al. Prevalence of obesity and trends in the distribution of body mass index among US adults, 1999-2010. *JAMA* 2012;307(5):491–497.

7. Mokdad AHMJ. Actual causes of death in the United States, 2000. *JAMA* 2004;291(10):1238–1245.

8. Katz DL. Behavior modification in primary care: the Pressure System Model. *Prev Med* 2001;32:66–72.

9. Katz DL, Shuval K, Comerford BP, et al. Impact of an educational intervention on internal medicine residents' physical activity counseling: the Pressure System Model. *J Eval Clin Pract* 2008;14(2):294–299.

10. Faridi Z, Polasck M, Barth M, et al. Health enhancement through lifestyle practices (HELP): a feasibility study. *J Health Promot Pract.*

11. Willett WC, Domolky S. *Strategic plan for the prevention and control of overweight and obesity in New England.* Available at http://www.neconinfo.org/02-11-2003_Strategic_Plan.pdf; accessed 11/8/07.

12. Penn State University. *The National Obesity Action Forum.* Available at http://www.outreach.psu.edu/C&I/Obesity; accessed 11/8/07.

13. Weigh Forward. Available at http://www.rediclinic.com/weighforward/; accessed 3/22/13.

14. On-line Weight Management Counseling for Healthcare Providers. *OWCH: a painless process of lifestyle counseling.* Available at http://www.owch.net; accessed 11/8/07.

15. *Online Weight Management Counseling for Healthcare Providers.* Available at http://www.turnthetidefoundation.org/OWCH/index.htm; accessed 12/16/13.

16. Elder J, Ayala G, Harris S. Theories and intervention approaches to health-behavior change in primary care. *Am J Prev Med* 1999;17:275–284.

17. Agency for Healthcare Research and Quality. *Counseling for a healthy diet.* Available at http://www.ahrq.gov/clinic/uspstf/uspsdiet.htm; accessed 11/8/07.

18. Partnership for Prevention. *Priorities for America's health: capitalizing on life-saving, cost-effective preventive services.* Available at http://www.prevent.org/ncpp; accessed 11/8/07.

19. Botelho J, Skinner H. Motivating change in health behavior: implications for health promotion and disease prevention. *Primary Care* 1995;22:565–589.

20. Miller W. Motivational interviewing: research, practice, and puzzles. *Addict Behav* 1996;21:835–842.

21. Katz DL, Brunner RL, St Jeor ST, et al. Dietary fat consumption in a cohort of American adults, 1985–1991: covariates, secular trends, and compliance with guidelines. *Am J Health Promot* 1998;12:382–390.

22. Kennedy E, Bowman S, Powell R. Dietary-fat intake in the US population. *J Am Coll Nutr* 1999;18:207–212.

23. US Department of Agriculture, Center for Nutrition Policy and Promotion. *Diet quality of Americans in 2001-02 and 2007-09 as measured by the Healthy Eating Index-2010.* February, 2013. Available at http://www.cnpp.usda.gov/healthyeatingindex.htm; accessed 3/22/13.

24. Buttriss J. Food and nutrition: attitudes, beliefs, and knowledge in the United Kingdom. *Am J Clin Nutr* 1997;65:1985s–1995s.

25. Prabhu N, Duffy L, Stapleton F. Content analysis of prime-time television medical news: a pediatric perspective. *Arch Pediatr Adolesc Med* 1996;150:46–49.

26. Plous S, Chesne R, McDowell AR. Nutrition knowledge and attitudes of cardiac patients. *J Am Diet Assoc* 1995; 95:442–446.

27. Rothman RL, Housam R, Weiss H, et al. Patient understanding of food labels: the role of literacy and numeracy. *Am J Prev Med* 2006;31(5):391–398.

28. Wardle J, Parmenter K, Waller J. Nutrition knowledge and food intake. *Appetite* 2000;34(3):269–275.

29. Nuval: Nutrition made easy. Available at www.nuval.com; accessed 3/22/13. Last Accessed 5/18/2014.

30. Jekel J, Elmore J, Katz D. *Epidemiology, biostatistics, and preventive medicine.* Philadelphia, PA: WB Saunders, 1996.

31. Jekel JF, Katz DL, Elmore JG, et al. *Epidemiology, biostatistics, and preventive medicine,* 3rd ed. Philadelphia, PA: Saunders, Elsevier, 2007.

32. Katz DL. Obesity be dammed! What it will take to turn the tide. *Harv Health Policy Rev* 2006;7:135–151.

33. Fenton M. Battling America's epidemic of physical inactivity: building more walkable, livable communities. *J Nutr Educ Behav* 2005;37:s115–s120.

34. Lovasi GS, Hutson MA, Guerra M, et al. Built environments and obesity in disadvantaged populations. *Epidemiol Rev* 2009;31:7–20.

35. Singh GK, Siahpush M, Kogan MD. Neighborhood socioeconomic conditions, built environments, and childhood obesity. *Health Aff* 2010;29:503–512.

36. Katz DL, Gonzalez MH. *The way to eat.* Naperville, IL: Sourcebooks, Inc., 2002.

LIVERPOOL JOHN MOORES UNIVERSITY
LEARNING SERVICES

37. O'Connell M, Comerford BP, Wall HK, et al. Impediment profiling for smoking cessation: application in the worksite. *Am J Health Promot* 2006;21:97–100.

38. O'Connell ML, Freeman M, Jennings G, et al. Smoking cessation for high school students: impact evaluation of a novel program. *Behav Modif* 2004;28:133–146.

39. Katz DL, Boukhalil J, Lucan SC, et al. Impediment profiling for smoking cessation: preliminary experience. *Behav Modif* 2003;27:524–537.

40. O'Connell M, Lucan SC, Yeh MC, et al. Impediment profiling for smoking cessation: results of a pilot study. *Am J Health Promot* 2003;17:300–303.

41. Armstrong MJ, Mottershead TA, Ronksley PE, et al. Motivational interviewing to improve weight loss in overweight and/or obese patients: a systematic review and meta-analysis of randomized controlled trials. *Obesity Rev* 2011;12(9):709–723.

42. Glanz K, Basil M, Maibach E, et al. Why Americans eat what they do: taste, nutrition, cost, convenience, and weight control concerns as influences on food consumption. *J Am Diet Assoc* 1998;98:1118–1126.

43. Lowenberg J. Health promotion and the "ideology of choice." *Public Health Nurs* 1995;12:319–323.

44. Marantz P. Blaming the victim: the negative consequence of preventive medicine. *Am J Public Health* 1990;80:1186–1187.

45. Reiser S. Responsibility for personal health: a historical perspective. *J Med Philos* 1985;10:7–17.

46. Minkler M. Personal responsibility for health? A review of the arguments and the evidence at century's end. *Health Educ Behav* 1999;26(1):121–140.

47. Brownell K. Personal responsibility and control over our bodies: when expectation exceeds reality. *Health Psychol* 1991;10:303–310.

48. Steinbrook R. Imposing personal responsibility for health. *New England J Med* 2006;355(8):753–756;

48a. Wikler D. Personal and social responsibility for health. *Ethics Int Aff* 2002;16(2):47–55.

49. Butler C, Rollnick S, Scott N. The practitioner, the patient and resistance to change: recent ideas on compliance. *CMAJ* 1996;154:1357–1362.

50. Goldstein MG, Whitlock EP, DePue J. Multiple behavioral risk factor interventions in primary care: summary of research evidence. *Am J Prev Med* 2004;27:61–79.

51. Meriwether RA, Lee JA, Lafleur AS, et al. Physical activity counseling. *Am Fam Physician* 2008;77(8):1129–1136.

52. American College of Physicians. *The advanced medical home: a patient-centered, physician-guided model of health care.* Philadelphia: American College of Physicians; 2005: Position Paper. (Available from American College of Physicians, 190 N. Independence Mall West, Philadelphia, PA 19106.)

53. Reid RJ, Fishman PA, Yu O, et al. Patient-centered medical home demonstration: a prospective, quasi-experimental, before and after evaluation. *Am J Manag Care* 2009;15(9):e71–e87.

54. Blackburn DG, Spellman KD. The role of Internet technology in enhancing the effectiveness of lifestyle interventions for weight management. *Obesity Weight Manag* 2010;6(3):131–135.

55. Carter MC, Burley VJ, Nykjaer C, Cade JE. Adherence to a smartphone application for weight loss compared to website and paper diary: pilot randomized controlled trial. *J Med Internet Res* 2013;15(4):e32.

56. Calfas K, Long B, Sallis J, et al. A controlled trial of physician counseling to promote the adoption of physical activity. *Prev Med* 1996;25:225–233.

57. Morey MC, Peterson MJ, Pieper CF, et al. The veterans learning to improve fitness and function in elders study: a randomized trial of primary care-based physical activity counseling for older men. *J Am Geriatr Soc* 2009;57(7): 1166–1174.

58. Katz DL, O'Connell M, Yeh MC, et al. Public health strategies for preventing and controlling overweight and obesity in school and worksite settings: a report on recommendations of the Task Force on Community Preventive Services. *MMWR Recomm Rep* 2005;54:1–12.

59. Katz DL. Competing dietary claims for weight loss: finding the forest through truculent trees. *Annu Rev Public Health* 2005;26:61–88.

60. Katz DL. Pandemic obesity and the contagion of nutritional nonsense. *Public Health Rev* 2003;31:33–44.

61. Lowe MR. Self-regulation of energy intake in the prevention and treatment of obesity: is it feasible? *Obes Res* 2003;11:44s–59s.

62. Banwell C, Hinde S, Dixon J, et al. Reflections on expert consensus: a case study of the social trends contributing to obesity. *Eur J Public Health* 2005;15:564–568.

63. Booth KM, Pinkston MM, Poston WS. Obesity and the built environment. *J Am Diet Assoc* 2005;105:s110–s117.

64. Poston WS II, Foreyt JP. Obesity is an environmental issue. *Atherosclerosis* 1999;146:201–209.

65. Katz DL, Faridi Z. Healthcare system approaches to obesity prevention and control. In: Kumanyika S, Brownson R, eds. *Handbook on obesity epidemiology and prevention.* New York, NY: Springer; 2007:285–316.

▪ SUGGESTED READINGS

Abusabha R, Achterberg C. Review of self-efficacy and locus of control for nutrition- and health-related behavior. *J Am Diet Assoc* 1997;97:1122–1132.

Abusabha R, Achterberg C, Elder J, et al. Theories and intervention approaches to health-behavior change in primary care. *Am J Prev Med* 1999;17:275–284.

Achterberg C, McDonnel E, Bagny R. How to put the food guide pyramid into practice. *J Am Diet Assoc* 1994;94:1030–1035.

Ammerman AS, Lindquist CH, Lohr KN, et al. The efficacy of behavioral interventions to modify dietary fat and fruit and vegetable intake: a review of the evidence. *Prev Med* 2002;35:25–41.

Barr K. To eat, perchance to lie. *New York Times*, August 30, 1995.

Berg-Smith S, Stevens V, Brown K, et al. A brief motivational intervention to improve dietary adherence in adolescents: the Dietary Intervention Study in Children (DISC) Research Group. *Health Educ Res* 1999;14:399–410.

Bostik R. Diet and nutrition in the etiology and primary prevention of colon cancer. In: Bendich A, Deckelbaum RJ, eds. *Preventive nutrition: the comprehensive guide for health professionals.* Totowa, NJ: Humana Press, 1997.

Botelho R, Skinner H, Butler C, et al. The practitioner, the patient and resistance to change: recent ideas on compliance. *CMAJ* 1996;154:1357–1362.

Bradbury J, Thomason JM, Jepson NJ, et al. Nutrition counseling increases fruit and vegetable intake in the edentulous. *J Dent Res* 2006;85:463–468.

LIVERPOOL JOHN MOORES UNIVERSITY
LEARNING SERVICES

Bruer R, Schmidt R, Davis H. Nutrition counseling—should physicians guide their patients? *Am J Prev Med* 1994:308–311.

Brug J, Campbell M, Assema PV. The application and impact of computer-generated personalized nutrition education: a review of the literature. *Patient Educ Couns* 1999; 36:145–156.

Brunner E, White I, Thorogood M, et al. Can dietary interventions change diet and cardiovascular risk factors? A meta-analysis of controlled trials. *Am J Public Health* 1997; 87:1415–1422.

Burton L, Shapiro S, German P. Determinants of physical activity initiation and maintenance among community-dwelling older persons. *Prev Med* 1999;29:422–430.

Calfas KJ, Sallis JF, Zabinski MF, et al. Preliminary evaluation of a multicomponent program for nutrition and physical activity change in primary care: PACE+ for adults. *Prev Med* 2002;34:153–161.

Curry S, Kristal A, Bowen D. An application of the stage model of behavior change to dietary fat reduction. *Health Educ Res* 1992;7:319–325.

Damrosch S. General strategies for motivating people to change their behavior. *Nurs Clin North Am* 1991;26:833–843.

Davis C. The report to Congress on the appropriate federal role in assuring access by medical students, residents, and practicing physicians to adequate training in nutrition. *Public Health Rep* 1994;109:824–826.

Diabetes Prevention Program. Design and methods for a clinical trial in the prevention of type 2 diabetes. *Diabetes Care* 1999;22:623–634.

DiClemente C, Prochaska J. Self-change and therapy change of smoking behavior: a comparison of processes of change in cessation and maintenance. *Addict Behav* 1982;7:133–142.

Drewnowski A. Why do we like fat? *J Am Diet Assoc* 1997; 97:s58–s62.

Eaton S, Konner M. Paleolithic nutrition revisited: a twelve-year retrospective on its nature and implications. *Eur J Clin Nutr* 1997;51:207–216.

Evans AT, Rogers LQ, Peden JG Jr, et al. Teaching dietary counseling skills to residents: patient and physician outcomes. The CADRE Study Group. *Am J Prev Med* 1996;12:259–265.

Fallon EA, Wilcox S, Laken M. Health care provider advice for African American adults not meeting health behavior recommendations. *Prev Chronic Dis* 2006;3:A45.

Fleury J. The application of motivational theory to cardiovascular risk reduction. *Image J Nurs Sch* 1992;24:229–239.

Foreyt JP, Poston WS II. The role of the behavioral counselor in obesity treatment. *J Am Diet Assoc* 1998;98:s27–s30.

Galuska DA, Will JC, Serdula MK, et al. Are health care professionals advising obese patients to lose weight? *JAMA* 1999;282:1576–1578.

Glanz K. Review of nutritional attitudes and counseling practices of primary care physicians. *Am J Clin Nutr* 1997;65:2016s–2019s.

Green LW. What can we generalize from research on patient education and clinical health promotion to physician counseling on diet? *Eur J Clin Nutr* 1999;53:s9–s18.

Grimm J. Interaction of physical activity and diet: implications for insulin–glucose dynamics. *Public Health Nutr* 1999; 2:363–368.

Hark L, Deen D Jr. Taking a nutrition history: a practical approach for family physicians. *Am Fam Physician* 1999; 59:1521–1528, 1531–1532.

Hiddink G, Hautvast J, van Woerkum CM, et al. Consumers' expectations about nutrition guidance: the importance of the primary care physicians. *Am J Clin Nutr* 1997;65: 1974s–1979s.

Jha R. Thiazolidinediones—the new insulin enhancers. *Clin Exp Hypertens* 1999;21:157–166.

Katz DL. Behavior modification in primary care: the pressure system model. *Prev Med* 2001;32:66–72.

Kelly R, Zyzanski S, Alemagno S. Prediction of motivation and behavior change following health promotion: role of health beliefs, social support, and self-efficacy. *Soc Sci Med* 1991;32:311–320.

Kessler L, Jonas J, Gilham M. The status of nutrition education in ACHA college and university health centers. *J Am Coll Health* 1992;41:31–34.

Kreuter M, Scharff D, Brennan L, et al. Physician recommendations for diet and physical activity: which patients get advised to change? *Prev Med* 1997;26:825–833.

Kreuter M, Strecher V. Do tailored behavior change messages enhance the effectiveness of health risk appraisal? Results from a randomized trial. *Health Educ Res* 1996;11:97–105.

Kristal A, White E, Shattuck A, et al. Long-term maintenance of a low-fat diet: durability of fat-related dietary habits in the Women's Health Trial. *J Am Diet Assoc* 1992;92:553–559.

Kritchevsky D. Dietary guidelines—the rationale for intervention. *Cancer* 1993;72:1011–1114.

Kumanyika S. Behavioral aspects of intervention strategies to reduce dietary sodium. *Hypertension* 1991;17:i90–i95.

Kushner R. Barriers to providing nutrition counseling by physicians: a survey of primary care practitioners. *Prev Med* 1995;24:546–552.

Laforge RG, Greene GW, Prochaska JO. Psychosocial factors influencing low fruit and vegetable consumption. *J Behav Med* 1994;17:361–374.

Landsberg L. Insulin resistance and hypertension. *Clin Exp Hypertens* 1999;21:885–894.

Lazarus K. Nutrition practices of family physicians after education by a physician nutrition specialist. *Am J Clin Nutr* 1997;65:2007s–2009s.

Lichtman S, Pisarska K, Berman E, et al. Discrepancy between self-reported and actual caloric intake and exercise in obese subjects. *N Engl J Med* 1992;327:1893–1898.

Love M, Davoli G, Thurman Q. Normative beliefs of health behavior professionals regarding the psychosocial and environmental factors that influence health behavior change related to smoking cessation, regular exercise, and weight loss. *Am J Health Promot* 1996;10:371–379.

Lynch M, Cicchetti D. An ecological-transactional analysis of children and contexts: the longitudinal interplay among child maltreatment, community violence, and children's symptomatology. *Dev Psychopathol* 1998;10:235–257.

Mathers J, Daly M. Dietary carbohydrates and insulin sensitivity. *Curr Opin Clin Nutr Metab Care* 1998;1:553–557.

McInnis KJ. Diet, exercise, and the challenge of combating obesity in primary care. *J Cardiovasc Nurs* 2003;18:93–100.

Mhurchu C, Margetts B, Speller V. Applying the stages-of-change model to dietary change. *Nutr Rev* 1997;55:10–16.

Millen B, Quatromoni P, Gagnon D, et al. Dietary patterns of men and women suggest targets for health promotion: the Framingham Nutrition Studies. *Am J Health Promot* 1996;11:42–52.

National Cancer Institute. *Theory at a glance: a guide for health promotion practice.* Available at http://www.nci.nih.gov/aboutnci/oc/theory-at-a-glance; accessed 11/8/07.

Nawaz H, Adams M, Katz D. Weight loss counseling by health care providers. *Am J Public Health* 1999;89:764–767.

Neel J. Diabetes mellitus: A "thrifty" genotype rendered detrimental by "progress?" *Am J Hum Genet* 1962;14:353–362.

Nigg C, Burbank P, Padula C, et al. Stages of change across ten health risk behaviors for older adults. *Gerontologist* 1999; 39:473–482.

Nutrition Committee, American Heart Association. Dietary guidelines for healthy American adults. A statement for physicians and health professionals by the Nutrition Committee, American Heart Association. *Circulation* 1988;77:721A–724A.

Ockene I, Hebert J, Ockene J, et al. Effect of physician-delivered nutrition counseling training and an office-support program on saturated fat intake, weight, and serum lipid measurements in a hyperlipidemic population: Worcester Area Trial for Counseling in Hyperlipidemia (WATCH). *Arch Intern Med* 1999;159:725–731.

Parcel GS, Edmundson E, Perry CL, et al. Measurement of self-efficacy for diet-related behaviors among elementary school children. *J Sch Health* 1995;65:23–27.

Patrick K, Sallis JF, Prochaska JJ, et al. A multicomponent program for nutrition and physical activity change in primary care: PACE+ for adolescents. *Arch Pediatr Adolesc Med* 2001;155:940–946.

Pignone MP, Ammerman A, Fernandez L, et al. Counseling to promote a healthy diet in adults: a summary of the evidence for the US Preventive Services Task Force. *Am J Prev Med* 2003;24:75–92.

Plotnick GD, Corretti M, Vogel RA. Effect of antioxidant vitamins on the transient impairment of endothelium-dependent brachial artery vasoactivity following a single high-fat meal. *JAMA* 1997;278:1682–1686.

Poston WS II, Foreyt JP. Obesity is an environmental issue. *Atherosclerosis* 1999;146:201–209.

Prochaska J. Assessing how people change. *Cancer* 1991;67:805–807.

Prochaska J, Crimi P, Papsanski D, et al. Self-change processes, self-efficacy and self-concept in relapse and maintenance of cessation of smoking. *Psychol Rep* 1982;51:989–990.

Prochaska J, DiClemente C. Stages of change in the modification of problem behaviors. *Prog Behav Modif* 1992;28:183–218.

Rogers PJ. Eating habits and appetite control: a psychobiological perspective. *Proc Nutr Soc* 1999;58:59–67.

Rossi J, Prochaska J, DiClemente C. Processes of change in heavy and light smokers. *J Subst Abuse* 1988;1:1–9.

Rothman A, Salovey P. Shaping perceptions to motivate healthy behavior: the role of message framing. *Psychol Bull* 1997;121:3–19.

Ruggiero L, Rossi J, Prochaska J, et al. Smoking and diabetes: readiness for change and provider advice. *Addict Behav* 1999;24:573–578.

Saelens BE, Sallis JF, Wilfley DE, et al. Behavioral weight control for overweight adolescents initiated in primary care. *Obes Res* 2002;10:22–32.

Schectman J, Stoy D, Elinsky E. Association between physician counseling for hypercholesterolemia and patient dietary knowledge. *Am J Prev Med* 1994;10:136–139.

Sciamanna CN, DePue JD, Goldstein MG, et al. Nutrition counseling in the promoting cancer prevention in primary care study. *Prev Med* 2002;35:437–446.

Senekal M, Albertse EC, Momberg DJ, et al. A multidimensional weight-management program for women. *J Am Diet Assoc* 1999;99:1257–1264.

Shaw ME. Adolescent breakfast skipping: an Australian study. *Adolescence* 1998;33:851–861.

Smith D, Heckemeyer C, Kratt P, et al. Motivational interviewing to improve adherence to a behavioral weight-control program for older obese women with NIDDM. A pilot study. *Diabetes Care* 1997;20:52–54.

Somers E. *Food and mood*, 2nd ed. New York, NY: Henry Holt and Company, 1999.

Staten LK, Gregory-Mercado KY, Ranger-Moore J, et al. Provider counseling, health education, and community health workers: the Arizona Wisewoman Project. *J Womens Health (Larchmt)* 2004;13:547–556.

Stevens VJ, Glasgow RE, Toobert DJ, et al. Randomized trial of a brief dietary intervention to decrease consumption of fat and increase consumption of fruits and vegetables. *Am J Health Promot* 2002;16:129–134.

Strecher V, DeVellis B, Becker M, et al. The role of self-efficacy in achieving health behavior change. *Health Educ Q* 1986; 13:73–92.

Stunkard A, Sobal J. Psychosocial consequences of obesity. In: Brownell KD, Fairburn CF, eds. *Eating disorders and obesity: a comprehensive handbook*. New York, NY: Guilford Press, 1995:417–421.

Tannahill R. *Food in history*. London: Penguin Books, 1988.

Thomas B. *Nutrition in primary care*. Oxford, UK: Blackwell Science, 1996.

Thomas PR, ed. *Improving America's diet and health: from recommendations to action*. Washington, DC: National Academy Press, 1991.

US Department of Agriculture, Agricultural Research Service 1999. *USDA nutrient database for standard reference*. Available at http://www.nal.usda.gov/fnic/foodcomp/search/; accessed 11/8/07.

US Department of Agriculture, US Department of Health and Human Services. *Nutrition and your health: dietary guidelines for Americans*, 4th ed. Washington, DC: US Department of Agriculture and US Department of Health and Human Services, 1995.

US Food and Drug Administration. An FDA consumer special report: focus on food labeling. *FDA Consumer* 1993.

US Preventive Services Task Force. *Guide to Clinical Preventive Services*, 2nd ed. Alexandria, VA: International Medical Publishing, 1996.

van Weel C. Dietary advice in family medicine. *Am J Clin Nutr* 2003;77:1008s–1010s.

Velicer W, Hughes S, Fava J, et al. An empirical typology of subjects within stage of change. *Addict Behav* 1995;20:299–320.

Velicer W, Norman G, Fava J, et al. Testing 40 predictions from the transtheoretical model. *Addict Behav* 1999;24:455–469.

Wallston B, Wallston K. Locus of control and health: a review of the literature. *Health Educ Monogr* 1978;6:107–117.

Wong SY, Lau EM, Lau WW, et al. Is dietary counseling effective in increasing dietary calcium, protein and energy intake in patients with osteoporotic fractures? A randomized controlled clinical trial. *J Hum Nutr Diet* 2004;17:359–364.

Controversies in Contemporary Clinical Nutrition

This new section of *Nutrition in Clinical Practice* offers brief commentary and perspective on several topics in contemporary clinical nutrition both salient and controversial at the time of writing. Selective citations are included here, along with cross-references to the far more extensively referenced pertinent chapters elsewhere in the book.

CHAPTER 48

The Calorie

The refractory nature of the obesity epidemic has invited extensive reflection in the nutrition community, with almost all time-honored precepts subject to scrutiny and reconsideration. Included among these is the bedrock principle that weight regulation is ultimately a matter of energy balance, in turn a product of calories consumed versus calories expended. The question "is a calorie a calorie?" (1) has become a prominent refrain in both popular culture and the scientific literature.

The ostensible basis for the question is that a focus on calories has failed to produce an effective countermeasure to the obesigenic elements in modern society. An additional consideration is that a given incremental reduction in energy consumption or increase in energy expenditure does not translate into a standard change in weight or body composition. These and related observations have induced some writers to ask whether or not calories really matter (2), and others to go further and declare that they do not (3).

Fundamentally, the calorie is a standardized measure of stored energy, as is the joule, used routinely in Europe. The actual measure in common application to food in the United States is the kilocalorie. A kilocalorie is the energy required to raise the temperature of 1 L of water 1°C at sea level. From the perspective of a calorimeter, a calorie then is clearly a calorie, and exactly that.

But human beings are not calorimeters. Energy consumed as food is expended in support of basal metabolism; used for growth and repair; used to fuel physical exertion; wasted as heat; and/or converted into a storage reserve in the form of either glycogen (see Chapters 1 and 5) or fat (see Chapters 2 and 5). Energy demands for growth and repair vary with stage of the life cycle, and daily circumstance. The efficiency with which calories are utilized varies among people just as fuel efficiency varies among vehicles, with consequent variation in the degree to which calories

are wasted as heat (i.e., thermogenesis). Resting energy expenditure and basal metabolic rate vary in accord with genetic factors and body composition. Body composition in turn varies with genetic factors, dietary factors, and physical activity. Physical activity influences energy requirements both directly and indirectly via effects on lean body mass.

Such factors readily account for variable responses, in terms of weight and body composition, of different people to the same load of calories. The variation to account for this need not be vested in calories, for it is readily accounted for by known variations in human metabolism. The analogy to other vehicles is again apt. If two cars travel different distances or perform variably in other ways on identical gallons of fuel, it does not require hidden enigmas in the definition of a gallon. Rather, it invokes the far more evident explanation that not all cars are created equal (4).

The clinician is certainly well advised to acknowledge that two patients may eat and exercise much the same, yet wind up with very different weights. This is not testimony to flaws in the assertions about thermodynamics made by Sir Isaac Newton and others since, but simply a reflection on the well-established and in some cases quite marked (5) variance in human metabolic efficiency. New insights in this area derive both from studies of the genome and of the microbiome (see Chapter 5). There are some cases of quite marked vulnerability to weight gain, and/or resistance to weight loss, that are frustrating to patient and clinician alike, and likely multifactorial in origin. In addition, there is evolving understanding of the implications of changing body mass and composition for caloric requirements, with models elucidating the dynamic nature of energy balance (6–8).

Explanations for the disappointing performance of a calorie-centric view of weight management are no more elusive at the level of epidemiology. Despite a long-standing emphasis on portion control in official dietary guidance, the modern era has seen a consistent, and even accelerating, proliferation of energy-dense processed foods literally engineered to be as nearly irresistible as possible (9). Against this seemingly unstoppable force driven by profit motive, portion control has been an all too readily moveable object. Consequently, national nutrition surveys in the United States suggest that while there has been variation in the percentage of calories from specific macronutrient sources over recent decades, overall calorie intake has trended up, not down (see Chapter 5). The failure of the "calorie hypothesis" in public health is attributable not to flaws in the concept of the calorie, but egregious impairment in the execution of guidance due to the obesigenic influences of modern culture and modern environment.

Intervention studies of weight loss, reviewed extensively in Chapter 5, superficially imply differential effects of the macronutrient classes on weight. Reviewed thoroughly, however, the literature shows that diets achieve weight loss by restricting calories—some directly, and some indirectly by restricting choices—but all doing so. In addition, the weight-loss differences seen with competing diets tend to be nominal and devolve to insignificance over time. Any means to restricting calories, including a diet willfully comprised of "junk" foods, is conducive to weight loss in the short term (10), if not necessarily good health over time. Similarly, an intake of calories beyond requirement results in weight gain, regardless of the source of those calories (11).

There remains the contention that the same number of calories from different food sources will exert different effects on important aspects of metabolism, such as hormonal balance. Situated artfully in the context of argument, this point is leveraged to imply the inadequacy of the calorie concept and to justify the ruminations on the utility of the measure.

But this contention, stripped of its pretensions, is merely the assertion that the quality of foods matters along with the quantity. This does not rise above the level of self-evident. Of course a given number of calories from a sugar-sweetened beverage bereft of nutrient value is utilized quite differently by the body than the same number of calories from walnuts, or avocado, or wild salmon. In essence, a specious straw man

argument has been contrived so that it can be debunked: if calories count, then calories from diverse foods should all have the same effects. If all fixed quantities of food energy do not have the same effects, then calories must not count. Therefore, a calorie is "not" a calorie.

The argument is specious because the first clause is unfounded. The same amount of latent energy may be stored in foods of markedly varying nutritional quality. Nutritional quality, in turn, is a term defined on the basis of health effects: Foods vary in nutritional quality if they vary in their effects on health and metabolism. If, in fact, 100 kcal of apple, applesauce, apple cider, or apple strudel were metabolized identically, they would, ipso facto, be nutritionally identical. It is differential effects of food on measureable aspects of health and metabolic responses that justifies any relative ranking from less to more "nutritious" in the first place (12).

The effects of foods on endocrine responses vary, and this in turn has implications for the fate of calories. When insulin responses are brisk, the deposition of calories in fat may be facilitated (see Chapter 6), with preferential accumulation of fat centrally, including in the liver. Such visceral fat is an inciting element in the pathway leading to metabolic syndrome (see Chapter 6). That the quality of foods and their effects on metabolic responses matter was never in question. These factors can matter, and calories can matter, too. That both do matter is just what the weight of evidence suggests.

One final issue is of particular practical value. The quality of calories may provide the best means to controlling their quantity. As noted, portion control advice has tended to fail against the temptations of the modern food supply. Investigative journalists have revealed more than once the diligent and well-informed food industry efforts to maximize the number of calories it takes to achieve fullness (13,14). There is both reason to believe and evidence to suggest (see Chapter 5), that this process can be reverse engineered. Food formulations that raise energy density, increase glycemic load, and minimize satiety effects will result in both the adverse effects of poor quality and those of increased quantity. Foods with opposing properties—high nutrient density, relatively lower energy density, low glycemic load, and a high satiety index—will tend to exert favorable effects on health directly, and indirectly will facilitate portion control by reducing the calories required to achieve a satisfying feeling of fullness.

A calorie is a calorie. But soda pop is not salmon, or spinach. Both the quality and quantity of calories count. The best way to control the latter may well be a focus on the former. An unending debate about the implications of a measure of latent energy is unlikely to be conducive to either.

For additional commentary on the topic of calories by the author, see:

1. http://www.huffingtonpost.com/david-katz-md/what-are-calories_b_4170755.html
2. http://www.huffingtonpost.com/david-katz-md/calories_b_1369749.html
3. http://health.usnews.com/health-news/blogs/eat-run/2012/07/11/fathoming-the-calorie

REFERENCES

1. Buchholz AC, Schoeller DA. Is a calorie a calorie? *Am J Clin Nutr* 2004;79(5):899S–906S.
2. Bittman M. Is a calorie a calorie? *NY Times* On-line, Opionator. March 20, 2013. http://opinionator.blogs.nytimes.com/2012/03/20/is-a-calorie-a-calorie/
3. Diet Doctor. *A calorie is not a calorie.* June 29, 2012.http://www.dietdoctor.com/a-calorie-is-not-a-calorie
4. Katz DL. *Fathoming the Calorie.* US News & World Report, Eat and Run Blog. November 7, 2012. http://health.usnews.com/health-news/blogs/eat-run/2012/07/11/fathoming-the-calorie
5. Chamala S, Beckstead WA, Rowe MJ, et al. Evolutionary selective pressure on three mitochondrial SNPs is consistent with their influence on metabolic efficiency in Pima Indians. *Int J Bioinform Res Appl* 2007;3(4):504–522.
6. Hall KD. Metabolism of mice and men: mathematical modeling of body weight dynamics. *Curr Opin Clin Nutr Metab Care* 2012;15(5):418–423.
7. Hall KD. Modeling metabolic adaptations and energy regulation in humans. *Annu Rev Nutr* 2012;32:35–54.
8. Hall KD, Heymsfield SB, Kemnitz JW, et al. Energy balance and its components: implications for body weight regulation. *Am J Clin Nutr* 2012;95(4):989–994.
9. Moss M. *Salt sugar fat: how the food giants hooked us.* Random House, 2013.
10. Fell JS. A Twinkie diet? It comes down to calories. *Los Angeles Times.* December 6, 2010. http://articles.latimes.com/2010/dec/06/health/la-he-fitness-twinkie-diet-20101206
11. Bray GA, Smith SR, de Jonge L, et al. Effect of dietary protein content on weight gain, energy expenditure, and body composition during overeating: a randomized controlled trial. *JAMA* 2012;307(1):47–55.
12. Katz DL, Njike VY, Faridi Z, et al. The stratification of foods on the basis of overall nutritional quality: the overall nutritional quality index. *Am J Health Promot* 2009;24(2):133–143.
13. The Oreo, obesity, and us. *The Chicago Tribune.* http://www.chicagotribune.com/news/watchdog/chi-oreos-special package,0,6758724.special
14. Moss M. The extraordinary science of addictive junk food. *The New York Times.* February 20, 2013. http://www.nytimes.com/2013/02/24/magazine/the-extraordinary-science-of-junk-food.html

CHAPTER 49

The Search for Scapegoats and Silver Bullets

The modern era of nutrition guidance has propagated a focus on nutrient details to the relative exclusion of foods, and the overall dietary pattern. Michael Pollan has aptly characterized this preoccupation as "nutritionism" (1) and attributed much of what bedevils modern nutritional epidemiology to the tendency. To the extent that nutritionism does not fully account for prevailing dietary woes, the law of unintended consequences may explain the remainder (2). Nutrient-focused recommendations have created almost limitless opportunities for food industry elements to accentuate some particular positive part, with relative inattention to the whole.

We may thus hypothesize that the combination of nutritionism, and opportunistic exploitation of it, has done much to divert and forestall progress in public health nutrition (3). If that hypothesis is correct, many constituencies are complicit in the impasse, including clinicians.

Beginning with nutritional epidemiology, the modern era may be said to have begun with the work of Ancel Keys and the association of specific dietary patterns in developed and affluent countries, rich in animal foods, with cardiovascular disease (4). The era of nutritionism may be said to have begun then as well, as observations that were principally about overall dietary pattern and overall health pattern devolved into assertions about specific nutrients, specific chronic disease risk factors, and specific health outcomes—in this case, the implication of saturated fat and dietary cholesterol in dyslipidemia and the propagation of coronary atherosclerosis (see Chapter 7). The era of preoccupation with "low fat" eating ensued.

The complexities, subtleties, and fallacies of blaming atherosclerosis on saturated fat and/or dietary cholesterol are addressed at greater length in Chapter 7. Here, it suffices to note that dietary cholesterol appears to exert a weak or even negligible influence on serum cholesterol levels and cardiovascular risk; and saturated fat represents a whole class of nutrients with varying effects (see Chapters 2 and 7). Neglected in the initial focus on the daily dose of these nutrients was that they varied in accord with the overall dietary pattern. Of necessity, a diet deriving a greater proportion of its energy from foods rich in saturated fat and cholesterol was deriving less from plant foods intrinsically low in these constituents (5).

Even so, the advice that followed—to restrict dietary fat intake—may have led to improvements in health if it had been translated to mean: eat more foods naturally low in fat. That, in turn, could have led to higher intake of vegetables, fruits, beans, and lentils—prominent elements in many of the diets most decisively associated with good overall health (3) (see Chapter 45). Instead, the food industry took advantage of a "just cut fat" fixation by devising what is now a fixture in the food supply: Low-fat processed foods. Naturally, there was never any evidence that eating more low-fat cookies was going to promote health, nor did it do so.

The evolving historical perspective now tends toward an indictment of the "low fat" hypothesis, and era. But, in fact, naturally low-fat, plant-rich diets are among the contenders for best diet laurels (3) (see Chapter 45). The misstep was, as noted above, the conflation of a part of the diet (and indeed, parts of foods) for the whole, and food industry opportunism translating dietary guidance into unanticipated products.

This action in which researchers, epidemiologists, clinicians, policy makers, food manufacturers, and the public were all complicit induced, with Newtonian inevitability, a harsh reaction born of frustration and disgust as epidemics of obesity and chronic disease worsened rather than improved (see Chapters 5 and 6). If advice to reduce dietary fat had been so wrong, clearly the wrong nutrient class had been targeted. And so it was society moved on to its next scapegoat: Carbohydrate.

This topic, too, is addressed at considerable length elsewhere in these pages (see Chapters 1 and 5) and need not be belabored here. Suffice to say that foods as diverse as lentils and lollipops are carbohydrate sources, and the notion that all such foods could constructively meet with summary judgment was nonsensical from the start. But as with the low-fat dogma, "low-carb" admonishments had some potential to do good if they directed people away from starchy, sugary foods to wholesome foods relatively richer in protein and/or fat. Such a diet might have replaced bread and pastries with fish, seafood, nuts, seeds, avocado, and so on. Instead, the food industry once again saw opportunity in societal preoccupation with a rubric and gave us low-carb pasta, low-carb bread, and low-carb brownies. Again, there had never been a shred of evidence that consumption of more low-carb brownies would lead to health improvements. Whatever the flaws in the guidance, they were much confounded by misguided and unintended applications.

An adage famously asserts that failure to learn from the follies of history results in their repetition. This is ominously pertinent to modern public health nutrition.

Even as the effects of low-fat and low-carb preoccupation linger, inviting some degree of vitriol among competing factions, some loss of faith in so-called nutrition "experts," the tendency to seek isolated dietary scapegoats or silver bullets persists. Among the recent entries in this category is fructose (6), the vilification of which has resulted in the extreme assertion that sugar is "toxic" (7).

Without question, an excess of added sugar is among the salient liabilities of the modern diet. But this is a case of the dose making the poison. Fructose, per se, is almost never a stand-alone ingredient in processed food; it is found almost exclusively in fruit, and fruit juices (see Chapter 1). Overall, the weight of evidence supports fruit consumption even for the control of weight and prevention of diabetes (8), the particular harms of which fructose is accused. Thus, advice to restrict fructose intake, per se, is immediately encumbered by the need to clarify that the principal source of pure fructose in the diet is excluded.

Most fructose consumed in modern diets is constituent part of added sugar either as sucrose, or as high-fructose corn syrup. That an excess of added sugar is harmful in various ways is long established and codified in prevailing dietary guidance (see Chapters 5, 6, and 45). Acute harms of fructose per se are supported by research that tends to exaggerate and distort real-world exposures; thoughtful analysis of this literature suggests that under real-world conditions, sugar is sugar; and that sugar is not a toxin per se, but a prevailing excess is clearly injurious (9). Of note, using dose distortion to support alleged harm could quite handily allow for the designation of oxygen as a toxin. Little would be gained from such an exercise.

Even as the fructose hypothesis has maintained a large following and generated a best-selling book (6), competing contentions have done the same. Whereas concerns about the rising prevalence of gluten enteropathy and lesser forms of gluten sensitivity (see Chapters 18 and 24) are entirely legitimate, claims that the entire population should avoid wheat (10) are not. Evidence suggests that haphazard efforts to avoid gluten, or wheat, can reduce overall diet quality (11). Even so, the idea that gluten and/or wheat is "the" thing wrong with modern diets has captured the public's imagination.

Going a step further, another best-selling book argues that all grains are essentially toxic (12) despite their prominence in traditional diets associated with both exceptional longevity and vitality (13). Advice to avoid wheat or grains competes with long-standing advice to avoid animal products (14), which in some cases ascribes virtually all of the ills of modern epidemiology to that cause. Noteworthy is that each of these arguments is built on a selective sampling of the relevant literature, with each ignoring the evidence on which the claims of the others depend. Consequently, equally compelling, evidence-based indictments are built against wheat and meat, gluten, and fructose. The problem, of course, is that if any of the competing theories is right, all of the others are wrong, and thus millions of adherents have been perilously mislead.

The almost inevitable truth is far more probable: each such theory tells a partial but incomplete and exaggerated truth. The expanse and diversity of the nutrition literature are such that studies can almost invariably be found to substantiate an a priori hypothesis. The fact that such arguments readily substantiate mutually exclusive claims to truth, however, reveals their inherent inadequacies. A theory is robust not when carefully selected studies support it, but when the unselected weight of evidence tips in its favor.

Commenting on the challenges of natural selection and environmental adaptation, evolutionary biologist Richard Dawkins noted there are many more ways to be dead than alive (15). The statement indicates that most genetic mutations are useless or harmful, and only the rare among them confer a survival advantage. Similar thinking may be extended to public health nutrition: There are many more ways to eat badly than well. A low-fat diet may be composed of highly nutritious plant foods, or exclusively of cotton candy. A low-carb diet may be rich in salmon and walnuts, or bologna and brownies.

The perpetuation of efforts to identify a single dietary scapegoat or silver bullet represents a form of collusion. A public, frustrated with failed attempts to lose weight and find health, has subordinated common sense applied to other areas, such as money management, to gullibility and the perennial hope for a magical quick fix. Publishers and producers exploit this combination of hope and gullibility to profit from a seemingly endless parade of books and products. Clinicians have long contributed to the confusion, both as the expert sources behind competing claims and by offering dietary counseling subject to the "one nutrient at a time fallacy" (16). Dietary advice specific to medical specialty, health outcome, or organ system has long prevailed. Mainstream cardiologists have warned for years about the perils of atherogenic fats, even as diabetologists focused selectively on sugar and glycemic load.

A view from no great altitude reveals the obvious fallacy of any such construct. Diabetics are at particular risk for cardiovascular disease; should they then adhere to dietary guidance related to their diabetes or competing guidance to safeguard their coronaries? Similarly, cardiac patients generally have a constellation of risk factors, including inflammation, conducive to insulin resistance and type 2 diabetes; should they protect their hearts with a heart healthy diet or by defending themselves against the advent of diabetes?

Equal clarity ensues from viewing the situation in reverse. Dietary patterns associated with low rates of one chronic disease at the population level are almost invariably associated with low rates of all major chronic diseases (see Chapter 45). Adhering to the basic theme of healthful eating (3) is supportive of good health in general, and consequently protective against all chronic diseases by suppressing the common pathogenic elements: Inflammation, oxidation, glycation, etc. (3).

There is one final consideration with regard to dietary scapegoats and silver bullets. An isolated focus on the addition or exclusion of any given nutrient, nutrient category, or food is apt to be inattentive to a question the approach requires: If people exclude (or add) food "A," what food B will they add (or exclude) to compensate? A popular ad campaign suggests that the American population is fueled by the products of a national chain of donut shops (17); surely this was not the intended effect of advice to limit intake of eggs for breakfast.

One might argue that literal decades of opportunity in public health nutrition have been squandered in a repetition of the seminal folly of modern nutritional epidemiology: Facile, but ultimately fatuous, attempts to blame all of the challenges of eating well in the modern world on a single scapegoat. A focus on the overall nutritional quality of foods and of the dietary pattern was, and remains, far more consistent with the weight of evidence, and far more conducive to public health objectives (18).

Readers of this text are encouraged to renounce the hunt for either savior or scapegoat in any given nutrient or food, to adopt a more holistic view of nutrition, and to counsel patients accordingly.

REFERENCES

1. Pollan M. Unhappy meals. *The New York Times Magazine.* Available at http://www.nytimes.com/2007/01/28/magazine/28nutritionism.t.html?pagewanted=all; accessed 1/28/07.
2. Katz DL. Living and dying on a diet of unintended consequences. *The Huffington Post.* Available at http://www.huffingtonpost.com/david-katz-md/nutrition-advice_b_1874255.html; accessed 9/11/12.
3. Katz DL, Meller S. Can we say what diet is best for health? *Annu Rev Public Health* 2014;35:83–103.
4. Keys A. Centers for Disease Control and Prevention. *Morbidity and Mortality Weekly Report,* August 6, 1999.
5. Katz DL. *Eat and Run Blog: food and diet, pebble and pond.* US News & World Report, May 6, 2013. Available at http://health.usnews.com/health-news/blogs/eat-run/2013/05/06/health-hinges-on-the-whole-diet-not-just-one-food.

6. Lustig RH. Fat chance: beating the odds against sugar, processed food, obesity, and disease. New York, NY: Hudson Street Press; 2012.

7. Taubes G. Is sugar toxic? *The New York Times Magazine.* April 13, 2011. Available at http://www.nytimes.com/2011/04/17/magazine/mag-17Sugar-t.html?pagewanted=all.

8. Muraki I, Imamura F, Manson JE, et al. Fruit consumption and risk of type 2 diabetes: results from three prospective longitudinal cohort studies. *BMJ* 2013;347:f5001.

9. Ludwig DS. Examining the health effects of fructose. *JAMA* 2013;310(1):33–34.

10. Davis W. Wheat belly: lose the wheat, lose the Weight and find your path back to health. Emmaus, PA: Rodale Books;2011.

11. do Nascimento AB, Fiates GM, Dos Anjos A, et al. Analysis of ingredient lists of commercially available gluten-free and gluten-containing food products using the text mining technique. *Int J Food Sci Nutr* 2013;64(2): 217–222.

12. Perlmutter D. Grain brain: the surprising truth about wheat, carbs, and sugar- your brain's silent killers. Little Brown and Co. *Boston, MA* 2013.

13. Blue Zones: Live Longer, Better. http://www.bluezones.com/; accessed 5/19/14.

14. Campbell TC. *The China Study: the most comprehensive study of nutrition ever conducted.* Benbella Books. 2004.

15. Dawkins R. *Today in science history.* Available at http://www.todayinsci.com/D/Dawkins_Richard/Dawkins Richard-Quotations.htm.

16. Katz DL. Why holistic nutrition is the best approach. *The Huffington Post.* Available at http://www.huffingtonpost.com/david-katz-md/holistic-nutrition_b_842627.html; accessed 11/4/2009.

17. *Dunkin' Donuts YouTube Page.* Available at https://www.youtube.com/user/dunkindonuts.

18. Katz DL. Life and death, knowledge and power: why knowing what matters is not what's the matter. *Arch Intern Med* 2009;169(15):1362–1363.

CHAPTER 50

Obesity as Disease

The topic of obesity is covered extensively, perhaps even excruciatingly, in Chapter 5. Even so, the concept of obesity as a disease warrants independent, if brief, attention here.

In 2013, the American Medical Association (AMA) proclaimed obesity a disease (1), ostensibly in an effort to lend the condition medical legitimacy and encourage greater attention to it by clinicians, physicians in particular. The basis for an effort directed at legitimatization is clear and compelling. There have long been significant barriers to weight management counseling by physicians (2). The historical approach to obesity by physicians (and perhaps other clinicians, albeit to a lesser extent) has been either to ignore the problem entirely for want of comfort addressing it or to wag an admonishing finger. The latter approach has the distinct disadvantage of assaulting a patient's potentially fragile self-esteem, and to borrow an expression from the vernacular, making them feel "about an inch tall" (see Chapters 46 and 47). If clinical counseling reduces height but not weight, the effect on body mass index is counter-productive to say the least.

Compounding such challenges to counseling that is both constructive and compassionate is the problem of obesity bias, long noted to be prevalent in society at large and identified as a tendency among prospective physicians as well (3). While in some cases the admonishing wag of a finger may merely imply lack of competency, in other cases it may truly indicate the harsh judgment of a clinician "blaming" the victim based on preconceived notions about the causes of obesity.

To the extent that the AMA position is directed at rectifying such past transgressions, and encouraging both more attention to obesity by clinicians, and the acquisition of competencies to confront obesity compassionately and effectively, the measure is a welcome advance. Obesity as disease is preferable to obesity as character flaw.

But obesity as disease carries enormous potential liabilities (4). First among these is that with the great power to assert by fiat that obesity resides in the medical domain comes the great responsibility to fix it. Clinicians are obligated to shoulder a far greater share of the burden if obesity is medicalized, than is implied by the call for multidisciplinary action by such sources as the Institute of Medicine (5).

Second is the implied course of therapeutic action. If obesity is a disease, the standard approaches to disease presumably constitute the remedy, namely drugs and procedures. While there are FDA-approved drugs for obesity treatment (see Chapter 5), they are controversial with regard to both safety and efficacy. The history of pharmacotherapy for weight control has been singularly unencouraging to date. Bariatric surgery is effective, but comes with the human and monetary costs of operations, and with uncertainty about long-term effectiveness if the absence of robust, ancillary lifestyle coaching (see Chapter 5). Given the prevalence of obesity, if either drugs or surgery are the principal response, the capacity of our society to bear the economic burden of it is questionable at best.

Third, and most important, is the fact that the declaration of obesity as a disease may invite nonclinical entities to renounce their role in combating it. A medical problem with clinical solutions absolves the food industry, advertising, schools, businesses, and policy makers of any substantive commitment to remedial action. The AMA position invites our society, at least tacitly, to wait for the disease of obesity to manifest, and then let clinicians treat it as clinicians are wont to do.

The AMA position may thus derive partly from medical hubris (i.e., physicians can fix this), partly from the proverbial tendency to see nails when you hold a hammer, and partly from a failure to consider the breadth of medically legitimate conditions. Not all medically legitimate conditions are diseases. There are, of course, injuries and toxic exposures. And, perhaps most relevant of all, there is drowning.

Obesity as disease implies that the human body that gets fat is malfunctioning somehow;

maladaptive responses are intrinsic to the definition of disease. But, in fact, a human body that converts a surplus of food energy into a storage depot is functioning normally. The abnormality derives from an unending surplus of food energy so that the storage depot, once made, is only grown rather than being metabolized and replenished intermittently. Without question, disease can result from obesity; indeed, obesity is on the causal pathway to all prevalent chronic diseases that plague modern societies (see Chapter 5). But equally clear is that "fatness" can occur in the absence of either metabolic derangement or obvious morbidity. If obesity is a disease, then everyone with a body mass index above 30, however well they may feel, and however normal their metabolic profile, is accordingly "diseased" (6).

Drowning is a medically legitimate condition. Clinicians who deal in medical emergencies and intensive care must know how to treat it, and insurers are obligated to cover the costs of related care. But drowning is not misconstrued for disease, because it is self-evident that even the healthiest of human bodies is subject to drowning if under water for too long. Drowning denotes the harms of an interaction between a normal human body and an environment to which it lacks adequate adaptations.

The case might be made that exactly that description suits epidemic obesity. Normal human bodies gain weight as body fat in a context of constant food energy surplus. The obesigenic modern environment provides exactly that. Obesity may result from "drowning" in a constant surplus of willfully irresistible calories (see Chapters 5 and 49) and labor-saving technology because *Homo sapiens* has no native defenses against caloric excess or the lure of the couch. If the analogy is apt and extended to its limits, it suggests that the hunt for effective pharmacotherapy for weight control may be as likely to succeed as the effort to devise a pill to prevent drowning.

This, in turn, leads to considerations of how our society does address the peril of drowning. The emphasis is overwhelmingly society and preventive, rather than medical and therapeutic. Doctors treat drowning when it occurs, but other elements in our society take steps to ensure that drowning occurs as rarely as possible. There are laws regarding drinking and boating; public beaches provide lifeguards; pools are invariably fenced; and swimming lessons are encouraged and widely available. There are analogies to each of these in the realm of obesity control, from regulating food marketing; to ensuring access to wholesome foods and opportunities for physical activity; to imparting routinely the requisite skill set for selecting nutritious foods and fitting fitness into daily routines. The gravest danger in the AMA declaration is that it might dissuade our society from such comprehensive approaches to obesity prevention.

Obesity need not be a disease to be medically legitimate. Weight management counseling should be well informed, compassionate, and constructive (see Chapters 46 and 47). But the problem of obesity is culture wide; modern society is drowning in it. Clinicians are a part of the solution or a part of the problem. But an effort by the medical community to claim the whole problem and provide the whole solution misconstrues obesity as a by-product of pathophysiology. Obesity ensues from normal human physiology in an obesigenic environment for which it lacks adaptations. Culture-wide remedies directed at that interface undoubtedly constitute the most promising and cost-effective approach to this, as to any, form of drowning.

RECOMMENDED READINGS

For more real-time commentary by the author on topics in nutrition and preventive medicine, see the following sites:

1. LinkedIN: http://www.linkedin.com/influencer/23027997
2. Huffington Post: http://www.huffingtonpost.com/david-katz-md/
3. US News & World Report: http://health.usnews.com/topics/author/david_l_katz

REFERENCES

1. Pollack A. AMA Recognizes Obesity as a Disease. *The New York Times*. June 18, 2013.
2. Nawaz H, Katz DL. American College of Preventive Medicine Practice Policy statement. Weight management counseling of overweight adults. *Am J Prev Med* 2001;21(1):73–78.
3. Miller DP Jr, Spangler JG, Vitolins MZ, et al. Are medical students aware of their anti-obesity bias? *Acad Med* 2013;88(7):978–982.
4. Katz DL. Obesity as disease: why I vote No. *The Huffington Post*. Available at http://www.huffingtonpost.com/david-katz-md/obesity-disease_b_3478322.html; accessed 6/21/13.
5. Insitute of Medicine. Accelerating progress in obesity prevention: solving the weight of the Nation. Available at http://www.iom.edu/Reports/2012/Accelerating-Progress-in-Obesity-Prevention.aspx; accessed 5/8/12.
6. Katz DL. Are our children "diseased?" *Childhood Obesity* 2014;10(1):1–3.

Appendices and Resource Materials

SECTION VII

Appendices and Resource Materials

APPENDIX A   NUTRITION FORMULAS OF CLINICAL INTEREST

BIOLOGICAL VALUE OF PROTEIN

Biological value = Food N − (Fecal N + Urinary N)/(Food N − Fecal N), *where biological value of egg albumin is set at 100 as the reference standard*

PROTEIN CHEMICAL SCORE (TO MEASURE QUALITY)

Chemical score = (mg of limiting amino acid in 1 g of test protein/mg of amino acid in 1 g of reference protein) × 100, *where lysine, sulfur-containing amino acids, or tryptophan are generally the limiting amino acids*

CREATININE HEIGHT INDEX AS A MEASURE OF SOMATIC PROTEIN STATUS

(mg urinary creatinine in 24 hours in the study subject/mg urinary creatinine in 24 hours by normal subject of same height and sex) × 100

ENERGY UNITS

1 kilocalorie = 4.18 kilojoules

HAMWI EQUATION FOR IDEAL BODY WEIGHT

Men: 106 lb/5 ft + 6 lb/additional inch ± 10%
Women: 100 lb/5 ft + 5 lb/additional inch ± 10%

HARRIS-BENEDICT EQUATION FOR BASAL ENERGY EXPENDITURE

Men: BEE = [66 + (13.8 × W) + (5 × H) − (6.8 × A)] × SF
Women: BEE = [655 + (9.6 × W) + (1.8 × H) − (4.7 × A)] × SF
General: W × 30 kcal/kg/day × SF
BEE, basal energy expenditure; W, weight in kg; H, height in cm; A, age in years; SF = stress factor.
For weight gain of approximately 1 kg/week, an additional 100 kcal/day should be provided.

REPRESENTATIVE STRESS FACTORS

Alcoholism:	0.9
Burn (<40%):	2.0–2.5
Cancer:	1.10–1.45
Head trauma:	1.35
Long-bone fracture:	1.25–1.30
Mild starvation:	0.85–1.0
Multiple trauma:	1.30–1.55
Peritonitis:	1.05–1.25
Severe infection:	1.30–1.55
Uncomplicated postoperative recovery:	1.00–1.05

NITROGEN BALANCE

B = I − (U + F + S)
B, balance; I, intake; U, urine; F, feces; S, skin (desquamation)
Alternatively, Nitrogen balance = (Ni/6.25) − Ne + 4
Ni = dietary protein intake in g/24 hr, Ne = urinary urea nitrogen in g/24 hr, 4 estimates nonurea nitrogen losses

PERCENT IDEAL BODY WEIGHT

Percent ideal body weight = (Actual BW/Ideal BW) × 100
BW, body weight

(continued)

APPENDIX A   (Continued)

PERCENT USUAL BODY WEIGHT

Percent usual body weight = (Actual BW/Usual BW) × 100
BW, body weight

PROTEIN REQUIREMENT IN LACTATION

Additional protein required = [(750 ml × 0.011 g protein/ml)/0.70 efficiency] × 1.25 variance = 14.7 g/day

RESTING ENERGY EXPENDITURE BY OXIMETRY

Metabolic rate (kcal/hr) = $3.9 \times VO_2$(L/hr) + $1.1 \times VCO_2$(L/hr), VO_2 = oxygen consumption, VCO_2 = carbon dioxide generation

UNITS OF MEASURE

1 oz = 28.4 g
1 lb = 454 g
1 kg = 2.2 lb
1 pint (16 oz) = 568 ml
1 liter = 1.76 pints = 0.88 quarts
mg = mmol/atomic weight

Source: For additional information, see Frankenfield DC, Muth ER, Rowe WA. The Harris-Benedict studies of human basal metabolism: history and limitations. *J Am Diet Assoc* 1998;98:439–445; Boullata J, Williams J, Cottrell F, et al. Accurate determination of energy needs in hospitalized patients. *J Am Diet Assoc* 2007;107:393–401.

APPENDIX B   GROWTH AND BODY WEIGHT ASSESSMENT TABLES (PAGES 635–643)

WHO Growth Standards Are Recommended for Use in the U.S. for Infants and Children 0 to 2 Years of Age

The World Health Organization (WHO) released a new international growth standard statistical distribution in 2006, which describes the growth of children ages 0 to 59 months living in environments believed to support what WHO researchers view as optimal growth of children in six countries throughout the world, including the U.S. The distribution shows how infants and young children grow under these conditions, rather than how they grow in environments that may not support optimal growth.

The CDC recommends that health care providers:

Use the WHO growth charts to monitor growth for infants and children ages 0 to 2 years of age in the U.S. and use the CDC growth charts to monitor growth for children age 2 years and older in the U.S.

The CDC growth charts can be used continuously from ages 2–19. In contrast the WHO growth charts only provide information on children up to 5 years of age. For children 2–5 years, the methods used to create the CDC growth charts and the WHO growth charts are similar (http://www.cdc.gov/growthcharts/who_charts.htm; accessed 9/23/2013).

APPENDIX B1   BIRTH TO 24 MONTHS: BOYS WEIGHT-FOR-LENGTH PERCENTILES AND HEAD CIRCUMFERENCE-FOR-AGE PERCENTILES

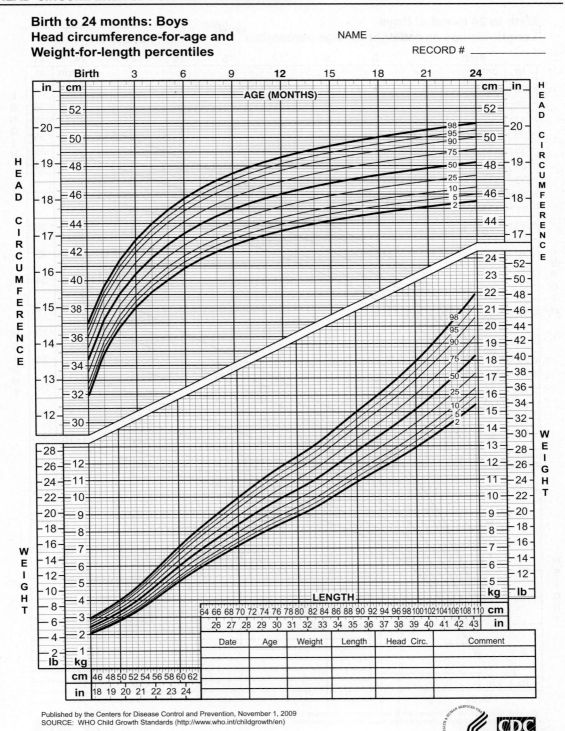

Birth to 24 months: Boys
Head circumference-for-age and
Weight-for-length percentiles

NAME _____

RECORD # _____

Published by the Centers for Disease Control and Prevention, November 1, 2009
SOURCE: WHO Child Growth Standards (http://www.who.int/childgrowth/en)

Source: http://www.cdc.gov/growthcharts/who_charts.htm; accessed 9/23/2013.

APPENDIX B2   BIRTH TO 24 MONTHS: BOYS LENGTH-FOR-AGE PERCENTILES AND WEIGHT-FOR-AGE PERCENTILES

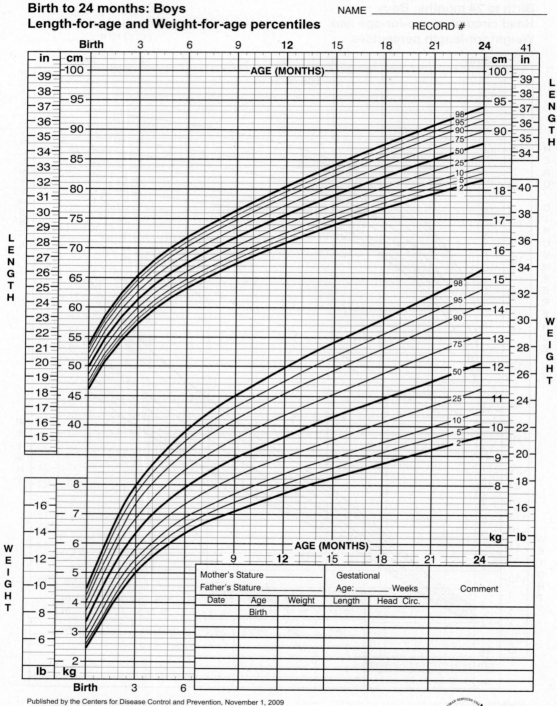

Birth to 24 months: Boys
Length-for-age and Weight-for-age percentiles

NAME _____

RECORD # _____

Published by the Centers for Disease Control and Prevention, November 1, 2009
SOURCE: WHO Child Growth Standards (http://www.who.int/childgrowth/en)

SAFER · HEALTHIER · PEOPLE™

Source: http://www.cdc.gov/growthcharts/who_charts.htm; accessed 9/23/2013.

APPENDIX B3 BIRTH TO 24 MONTHS: GIRLS WEIGHT-FOR-LENGTH PERCENTILES AND HEAD CIRCUMFERENCE-FOR-AGE PERCENTILES

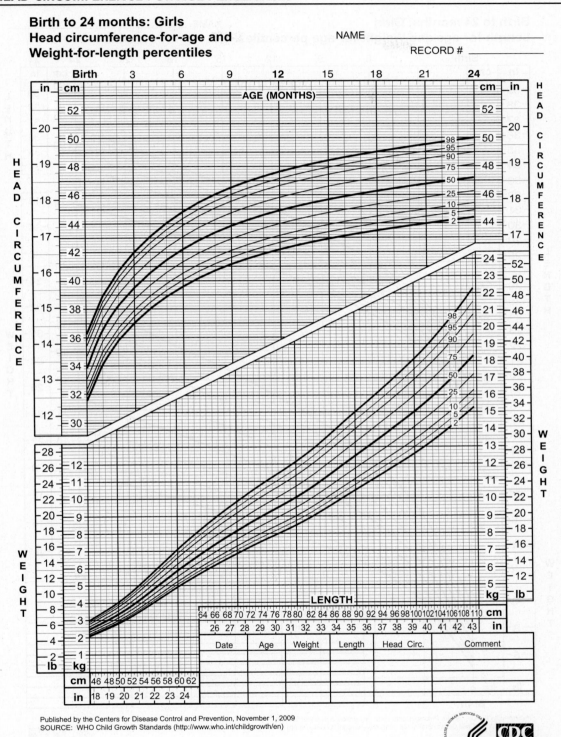

Birth to 24 months: Girls
Head circumference-for-age and
Weight-for-length percentiles

NAME _____

RECORD # _____

Published by the Centers for Disease Control and Prevention, November 1, 2009
SOURCE: WHO Child Growth Standards (http://www.who.int/childgrowth/en)

Source: http://www.cdc.gov/growthcharts/who_charts.htm; accessed 9/23/2013.

APPENDIX B4   BIRTH TO 24 MONTHS: GIRLS LENGTH-FOR-AGE PERCENTILES AND WEIGHT-FOR-AGE PERCENTILES

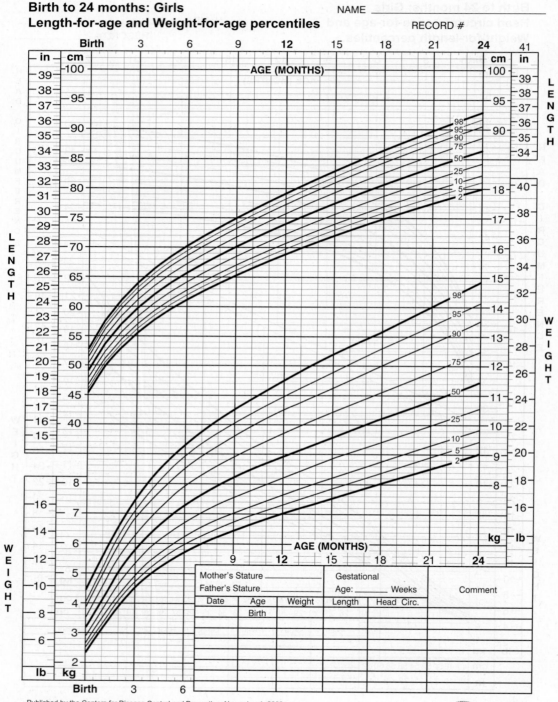

Birth to 24 months: Girls
Length-for-age and Weight-for-age percentiles

NAME _____

RECORD # _____

Published by the Centers for Disease Control and Prevention, November 1, 2009
SOURCE: WHO Child Growth Standards (http://www.who.int/childgrowth/en)

Source: http://www.cdc.gov/growthcharts/who_charts.htm; accessed 9/23/2013.

APPENDIX B5   GROWTH CHART, BIRTH TO 36 MONTHS, GIRLS

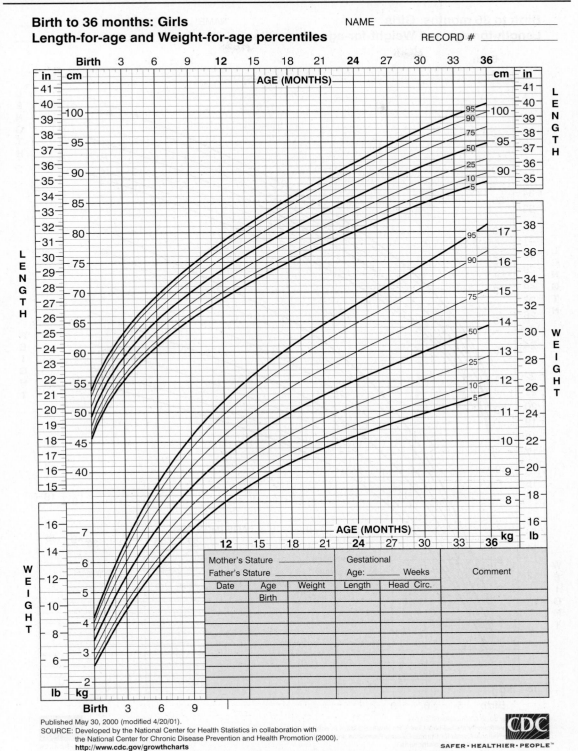

Birth to 36 months: Girls
Length-for-age and Weight-for-age percentiles

NAME _____

RECORD # _____

Published May 30, 2000 (modified 4/20/01).
SOURCE: Developed by the National Center for Health Statistics in collaboration with
the National Center for Chronic Disease Prevention and Health Promotion (2000).
http://www.cdc.gov/growthcharts

Source: Centers for Disease Control and Prevention, National Center for Health Statistics, National Center for Chronic Disease Prevention and Health Promotion. *2000 CDC growth charts: United States.* Available at http://www.cdc.gov/growthcharts; accessed 11/9/07.

APPENDIX B6   GROWTH CHART, BIRTH TO 36 MONTHS, BOYS

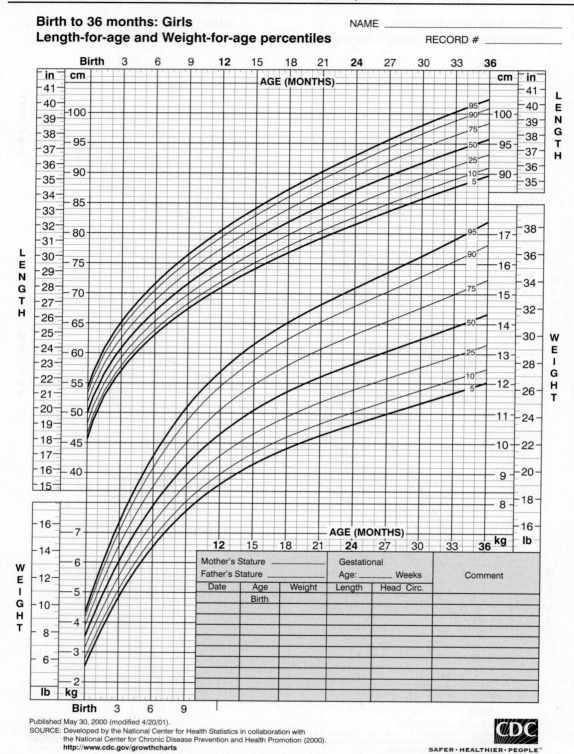

Birth to 36 months: Girls
Length-for-age and Weight-for-age percentiles

NAME _____

RECORD # _____

Published May 30, 2000 (modified 4/20/01).
SOURCE: Developed by the National Center for Health Statistics in collaboration with
the National Center for Chronic Disease Prevention and Health Promotion (2000).
http://www.cdc.gov/growthcharts

CDC
SAFER · HEALTHIER · PEOPLE™

Source: Centers for Disease Control and Prevention, National Center for Health Statistics, National Center for Chronic Disease Prevention and Health Promotion. *2000 CDC growth charts: United States.* Available at http://www.cdc.gov/growthcharts; accessed 11/9/07.

APPENDIX B7   GROWTH CHART, 2 TO 20 YEARS, GIRLS

2 to 20 years: Girls
Stature-for-age and Weight-for-age percentiles

NAME _____

RECORD # _____

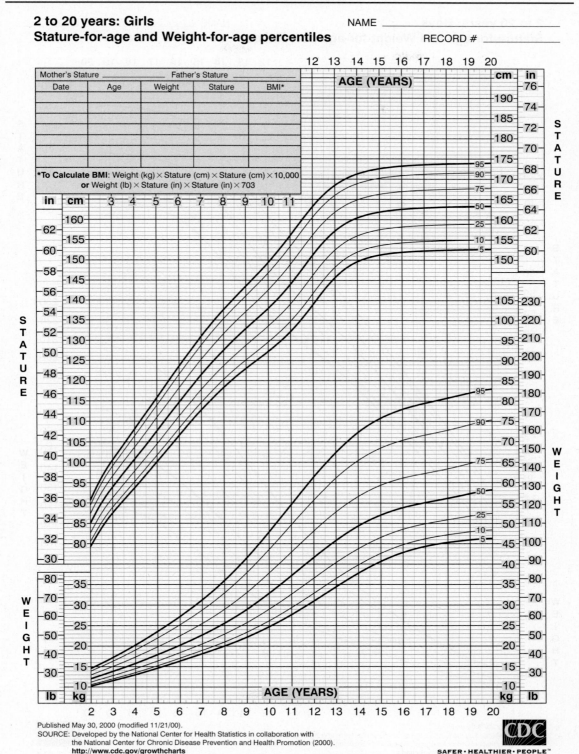

Mother's Stature _____		Father's Stature _____		
Date	Age	Weight	Stature	BMI*

*To Calculate BMI: Weight (kg) × Stature (cm) × Stature (cm) × 10,000
or Weight (lb) × Stature (in) × Stature (in) × 703

AGE (YEARS)

STATURE

WEIGHT

Published May 30, 2000 (modified 11/21/00).
SOURCE: Developed by the National Center for Health Statistics in collaboration with
the National Center for Chronic Disease Prevention and Health Promotion (2000).
http://www.cdc.gov/growthcharts

CDC
SAFER · HEALTHIER · PEOPLE™

Source: Centers for Disease Control and Prevention, National Center for Health Statistics, National Center for Chronic Disease Prevention and Health Promotion. *2000 CDC growth charts: United States.* Available at http://www.cdc.gov/growthcharts; accessed 11/9/07.

APPENDIX B8   GROWTH CHART, 2 TO 20 YEARS, BOYS

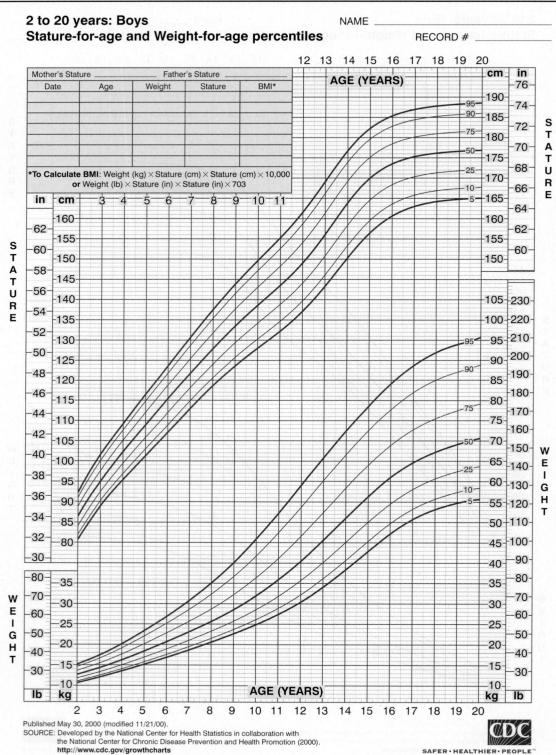

2 to 20 years: Boys
Stature-for-age and Weight-for-age percentiles

NAME _____

RECORD # _____

Published May 30, 2000 (modified 11/21/00).
SOURCE: Developed by the National Center for Health Statistics in collaboration with
the National Center for Chronic Disease Prevention and Health Promotion (2000).
http://www.cdc.gov/growthcharts

CDC
SAFER · HEALTHIER · PEOPLE™

Source: Centers for Disease Control and Prevention, National Center for Health Statistics, National Center for Chronic Disease Prevention and Health Promotion. *2000 CDC growth charts: United States.* Available at http://www.cdc.gov/growthcharts; accessed 11/9/07.

APPENDIX B9   BODY MASS INDEX NOMOGRAM: ADULTS

HEIGHT IN FEET AND INCHES[a]

Weight in Pounds	4'10"	5'	5' 2	5' 4"	5' 6"	5' 8"	5' 10"	6'	6' 2"	6' 4"
	2	20	18	<18	<18	<18	<18	<18	<18	<18
110	23	21.5	20	19	<18	<18	<18	<18	<18	<18
120	25	23.5	22	21	19	18	<18	<18	<18	<18
130	27	25	24	22	21	20	19	<18	<18	<18
140	29	27	26	24	23	21	20	19	18	<18
150	31	29	27.5	26	24	23	22	20	19	18
160	33.5	31	29	27.5	26	24	23	22	20.5	19.5
170	36	33	31	29	27.5	26	24	23	22	21
180	38	35	33	31	29	27	26	24.5	23	22
190	40	37	35	33	31	29	27	26	24.5	23
200	>40	39	37	34	32	30	29	27	26	24
210	>40	41	38	36	34	32	30	28.5	27	26
220	>40	>40	40	38	36	33	32	30	28	27
230	>40	>40	>40	40	37	35	33	31	30	28
240	>40	>40	>40	>40	39	37	34.5	33	31	29
250	>40	>40	>40	>40	40	38	36	34	32	30.5
260	>40	>40	>40	>40	>40	40	37	35	33	32
270	>40	>40	>40	>40	>40	>40	39	37	35	33
280	>40	>40	>40	>40	>40	>40	40	38	36	34
290	>40	>40	>40	>40	>40	>40	>40	39	37	35
300	>40	>40	>40	>40	>40	>40	>40	41	39	37

Evidence suggests the implications of body mass index (BMI) vary by race/ethnicity with South Asian, Chinese, and black subjects developing diabetes at a higher rate, at an earlier age, and at lower ranges of BMI than their white counterparts. (*Deriving ethnic-specific BMI cutoff points for assessing diabetes risk.* Available at http://care.diabetesjournals.org/content/34/8/1741.full; accessed 9/23/2013.)

As such, more specific BMI cut-offs have been considered (*Lancet—appropriate BMI for Asians.* Available at http://www.who.int/nutrition/publications/bmi_asia_strategies.pdf; accessed 9/23/2013.) and calculators have been developed for specific geographic populations: e.g., Asians and Asian Americans (*Asian American Diabetes Initiative—Joslin Diabetes Center.* Available at http://aadi.joslin.org/content/bmi-calculator; accessed 9/23/2013.) and South Asians (*South Asian BMI calculator.* Available at https://sites.google.com/site/southasianbmicalculator/; accessed 9/23/2013.).

[a]Height in feet and inches is shown across the top, and weight in pounds is shown in the left-hand column. Each entry in the table represents the body mass index (BMI) for a particular combination of height and weight. BMIs that represent the transition points from lean to overweight, from overweight to obese, and from one stage of obesity to the next are shown in bold. BMI values are close approximations due to rounding. BMI values in the recommended, or "healthiest," range are shaded in gray. Note that if a patient is very slight, or very muscular, that person's BMI might fall above or below the shaded area and still be consistent with excellent health. An online BMI calculator is available at http://www.nhlbisupport.com/bmi/bmicalc.htm. There is no adult "growth" curve as there is for children

Source: Katz DL, Gonzalez MH. *The way to eat.* Naperville, IL: Sourcebooks, 2002. An adult BMI calculator is available online at: http://www.cdc.gov/nccdphp/dnpa/bmi/adult_BMI/english_bmi_calculator/bmi_calculator.htm.
Centers for Disease Control and Prevention, National Center for Health Statistics, National Center for Chronic Disease Prevention and Health Promotion. *2000 CDC growth charts: United States.* Available at http://www.cdc.gov/growthcharts; accessed 11/9/07.

APPENDIX C   DIETARY INTAKE ASSESSMENT IN THE US POPULATION

Dietary intake patterns in the United States have been tracked with several surveys of nationally representative samples:

NATIONAL HEALTH AND NUTRITION EXAMINATION SURVEYS (NHANES)

These surveys are conducted by the National Center for Health Statistics of the Centers for Disease Control and Prevention (CDC). Probability samples of the US population are surveyed, using 24-hour recall and food-frequency questionnaire.

NHANES I:	1971–1974	N = 28,000
NHANES II:	1976–1980	N = 25,000
Hispanic HANES:	1982–1984	N = 14,000
NHANES III:	1988–1994	N = 35,000
Continuous NHANES:	1999–present	N = 5,000 per year*

*In 1999, the survey became a continuous program that examines a nationally representative sample of about 5,000 persons each year. These persons are located in counties across the country. (*National Health and Nutrition Examination Survey.* Available at http://www. cdc.gov/nchs/nhanes/about_nhanes.htm; accessed 9/23/2013.)

CONTINUING SURVEY OF FOOD INTAKES BY INDIVIDUALS (CFSII)

These surveys are conducted by the U.S. Department of Agriculture (USDA) at three-year intervals. Probability samples of the US population are surveyed, using one or more 24-hour recall surveys and a two-day food record.

CFSII:	1985–1986	N = 9,000
	1989–1991	N = 15,000
	1994–1996, 1998	N = 20,000

BEHAVIORAL RISK FACTOR SURVEILLANCE SYSTEM

This annual telephone survey (including cell phone extensions as of 2011) is conducted by the CDC and US States on a probability sample of >400,000 households in the 53 states and territories.[a] Limited information is provided on dietary intake.

[a]Available at http://www.cdc.gov/brfss/about/index.htm; accessed 9/23/2013 and http://www.cdc.gov/brfss/annual_data/2011/response_rates_11.htm; accessed 9/23/2013.

Source: For additional information, see Thompson FE, Byers T. Dietary assessment resource manual. *J Nutr* 1994;124:2245s–2317s; Kennedy ET, Bowman SA, Powell R. Dietary-fat intake in the US population. *J Am Coll Nutr* 1999;18:207–212; Munoz KA, Krebs-Smith SM, Ballard-Barbash R, et al. Food intakes of US children and adolescents compared with recommendations. *Pediatrics* 1997;100:323–329.

APPENDIX D   DIETARY INTAKE ASSESSMENT INSTRUMENTS

Various instruments are available for the assessment of individual dietary intake, each with particular advantages and disadvantages. Standard methods include 24-hour recall; food diaries of varying length, typically from 2 to 7 days; and semiquantitative food-frequency questionnaires. Useful resource materials for identifying and understanding the strengths and limitations of dietary-intake assessment instruments include:

■ Thompson FE, Byers T. Dietary assessment resource manual. *J Nutr* 1994;124:2245s–2317s.
■ US Department of Agriculture (USDA), Center for Nutrition Policy and Promotion. *The healthy eating index.* Washington, DC: USDA Office of Communications, 2005.
■ Olendzki B, Hurley TG, Hebert JR, et al. Comparing food intake using the Dietary Risk Assessment with multiple 24-hour dietary recalls and the 7-day dietary recall. *J Am Diet Assoc* 1999;99:1433–1439.
■ Bingham SA, Gill C, Welch A. Comparison of dietary assessment methods in nutritional epidemiology: weighed records v. 24 h recalls, food-frequency questionnaires and estimated-diet records. *Br J Nutr* 1994;72(4):619–643. http://www.ncbi.nlm.nih.gov/pubmed/7986792.
■ Willett, W. *Nutritional epidemiology*, 3rd ed. 2012. http://www.barnesandnoble.com/listing/2687416744070?r=1&cm_mmca2=pla&cm_mmc=GooglePLA-_-TextBook_NotInStock_26To75-_-Q000000633-_-2687416744070.
■ *USDA Food and nutrition information center. Dietary assessment.* Available at http://fnic.nal.usda.gov/dietary-guidance/dietary-assessment; accessed 23/2013.

There are also several instruments and methodologies for measuring food environments to which individuals are exposed. Standard methods include: geographic analysis, menu analysis, nutrient analysis, sales analysis, and food supply analysis with instruments to measure food stores, public facilities, restaurants, schools, worksites, and homes.

■ NCI Applied Research Cancer Control and Population Sciences. *Measures of the food environment.* Available at http://appliedresearch.cancer.gov/mfe/defining-measures-instruments-and-methodologies; accessed 23, 2013.

On the following page is a form patients can use for compiling a diet diary. The form is supportive of the counseling goals provided in Chapter 47. The patient should be given one copy of the form for each day of intake assessment.

DIETARY INTAKE FORM (Page 645)

To the patient: Use the following table to record your dietary intake *during a single day* (indicate the date and day of the week at the top of the table). Make an effort to eat as you usually do and to record everything in detail. Provide information on what you ate, an estimate of the portion size, when you ate (time), where you ate or the source of the food (e.g., home, car, restaurant, office, vending machine), and why (e.g., for hunger, boredom, stress relief, or some other reason). You will be able to review this diary with your doctor, dietitian, or other professional nutrition counselor to identify both what you should change to improve your diet and how you can implement recommended changes successfully.

MEAL/SNACK	DESCRIPTORS	DAY OF THE WEEK	DATE	WORK DAY? Y/N
Prebreakfast	What			
	How much			
	When			
	Where			
	Why			
Breakfast	What			
	How much			
	When			
	Where			
	Why			
A.M. snack(s)	What			
	How much			
	When			
	Where			
	Why			
Lunch	What			
	How much			
	When			
	Where			
	Why			
P.M. snack(s)	What			
	How much			
	When			
	Where			
	Why			
Dinner	What			
	How much			
	When			
	Where			
	Why			
Evening	What			
	Snack(s)			
	How much			
	When			
	Where			
	Why			
Other				

APPENDIX E   NUTRIENT/NUTRICEUTICAL REFERENCE TABLES: INTAKE RANGE AND DIETARY SOURCES

The following tables provide detailed information for a representative sample of micronutrients for which there are both current interest in supplementation beyond the traditionally recommended range and a body of pertinent and controversial research evidence in the literature.

ARGININE

BIOLOGICAL FUNCTION(S) IN HUMANS/KEY PROPERTIES: Amino acid essential in infants but not in healthy adults who can synthesize it endogenously. May become essential in stress conditions when demand increases. Plays an important role in cell division, wound healing, and immune function. Immediate precursor of nitric oxide (NO), necessary for synthesis of creatine and other vital proteins. Synthesized primarily in the kidney.

ABSORPTION/SOLUBILITY/STORAGE/PHARMACOKINETICS: Water soluble. Intestinal absorption is active. Arginine is rapidly transported into enterocytes and then transported to the liver for metabolism before distribution to the systemic circulation.

RATIONALE FOR SUPPLEMENTATION: Enhanced vascular function; hypotensive effect; potential contributions to immune function, wound healing, and preservation of lean body mass.[a]

EVIDENCE IN SUPPORT OF SUPPLEMENTATION TO AND ABOVE THE DRI: No RDA or AI set for arginine.

Recommended Intake Ranges (US RDA): None established.

AVERAGE INTAKE, US ADULTS:	3.5–5.0 g
ESTIMATED MEAN PALEOLITHIC INTAKE (ADULT):	Not available
COMMON DOSE RANGE FOR USE AS SUPPLEMENT:	2–30 g
DO DIETARY PATTERNS MEETING GUIDELINES PERMIT INTAKE IN THE SUPPLEMENT RANGE?	Yes
INCLUDED IN TYPICAL MULTIVITAMIN/MULTIMINERAL TABLET?	No

DEFICIENCY

Intake Level:	Variable.
Syndromes:	Impaired insulin production, muscle weakness, possible hair loss. Decreased sperm function in men.

TOXICITY

Intake Level:	The maximum dose considered to be safe is 400–6,000 mg, although doses as high a 24 g have been given daily for 8 weeks in the treatment of peripheral vascular disease and claudication, for example, without apparent adverse effect.[b] There are no known signs of toxicity in doses up to 30 g/day. Adverse symptoms may occur at higher doses (>30 g) or if administered rapidly.
Syndromes:	Nausea, abdominal cramps, diarrhea, skin thickening, weakness, may increase activity of some viruses (e.g., herpes).

Dietary Sources[c]: Whole wheat, chocolate, nuts, dairy products, meat, peanuts, brown rice, corn/popcorn, soy products, raisins, sesame and sunflower seeds, coconut, gelatin, buckwheat, barley, chicken, meats, oats.[d]

[a] May PE, Barber A, D'Olimpio JT, et al. Reversal of cancer-related wasting using oral supplementation with a combination of beta-hydroxy-beta-methylbutyrate, arginine, and glutamine. *Am J Surg* 2002;183:471–479.
[b] Available at http://www.mayoclinic.com/health/l-arginine/NS_patient-arginine/DSECTION=safety; accessed 9/23/2013.
[c] The nutrient composition of most foods can be checked by accessing the U.S. Department of Agriculture nutrient database, at http://www.nal.usda.gov/fnic/foodcomp/search.
[d] Available at http://www.mayoclinic.com/health/l-arginine/NS_patient-arginine/DSECTION=safety; accessed 9/23/2013.

Additional details, evidence, and references for dosing and safety for many nutrients and substances individuals might choose to ingest can be found at http://www.mayoclinic.com/health/search/search, http://ods.od.nih.gov/, and http://www.nlm.nih.gov/medlineplus/.

Sources: DRI tables for macronutrients, including protein and amino acids. http://www.iom.edu/Object.File/Master/7/300/Webtable macro.pdf.
Ensminger AH, Ensminger ME, Konlande JE, et al. *The concise encyclopedia of foods and nutrition.* Boca Raton, FL: CRC Press, Inc., 1995.
Margen S. *The wellness nutrition counter.* New York, NY: Health Letter Associates, 1997.
Murray MT. *Encyclopedia of nutritional supplements.* Rocklin, CA: Prima Publishing, 1996.
National Research Council. *Recommended dietary allowances*, 10th ed. Washington, DC: National Academy Press, 1989.
Otten JJ, Hellwig JP, Meyers LD, eds. *Dietary reference intakes. The essential guide to nutrient requirements.* Washington, DC: National Academies Press, 2006.
Pizzorno JE, Murray MT. *Textbook of natural medicine*, 3rd ed. St. Louis, MO: Church Livingstone Elsevier, 2006.
Shils ME, Shike M, Ross AC, et al., eds. *Modern nutrition in health and disease*, 10th ed. Philadelphia, PA: Lippincott Williams & Wilkins, 2005.
U.S. Department of Agriculture. *USDA nutrient database for standard reference.* Release 19. 2006.
U.S. Department of Agriculture. *USDA nutrient intake from NHANES 2001–2002 data.*
Ziegler EE, Filer LJ Jr, eds. *Present knowledge in nutrition*, 7th ed. Washington, DC: ILSI Press, 1996.

BIOTIN/VITAMIN B₇

BIOLOGICAL FUNCTION(S) IN HUMANS/KEY PROPERTIES: Functions in the transport of carboxyl groups. Essential in carbohydrate and lipid metabolism and is a cofactor in the metabolic pathways of certain amino acids. Exists in both protein-bound and free forms in diet; free form is functional.

ABSORPTION/SOLUBILITY/STORAGE/PHARMACOKINETICS: Water soluble. Absorption is thought to occur primarily in the jejunum. Produced by intestinal flora. There is some egestion of biotin in feces; excretion in urine rises with dietary intake. Avidin, a protein found in uncooked egg albumin, binds biotin and prevents absorption.

RATIONALE FOR SUPPLEMENTATION: Advocated to improve insulin sensitivity in diabetes mellitus, to strengthen nails and hair, and for treatment of seborrheic dermatitis.

EVIDENCE IN SUPPORT OF SUPPLEMENTATION TO AND ABOVE THE DRI: Studies of biotin supplementation in humans are limited; animal literature is far more extensive.

Recommended Intake Range (US RDA): Intake in the range of 30–35 μg/day is considered safe and adequate.

BIOTIN RECOMMENDED INTAKE RANGE (US AI)[a]:

	Infancy (age 0–6 mo)	Infancy (age 7–12 mo)	Childhood (age 1–3 y)	Childhood (age 4–8 y)	Adolescence (age 9–13 y)	Adolescence (age 14–18 y)	Adult (age ≥19 y)	Pregnancy	Lactation
Male	7 μg	7 μg	8 μg	12 μg	20 μg	25 μg	30 μg	—	—
Female	7 μg	7 μg	8 μg	12 μg	20 μg	25 μg	30 μg	30 μg	35 μg

AVERAGE INTAKE, US ADULTS:	30–70 μg/day
ESTIMATED MEAN PALEOLITHIC INTAKE (ADULT)[b]:	Not available
COMMON DOSE RANGE FOR USE AS SUPPLEMENT:	1,000–10,000 μg/day
DO DIETARY PATTERNS MEETING GUIDELINES PERMIT ADEQUATE INTAKE?	No
INCLUDED IN TYPICAL MULTIVITAMIN/MULTIMINERAL TABLET?	Yes (dose: 45 μg)

DEFICIENCY

Intake Level: Intake threshold for deficiency not established in healthy individuals. Deficiency may be induced after intestinal resection or with ingestion of large amounts of raw egg whites. Raw egg white contains a substance (avidin) that binds biotin in the intestine and keeps it from being absorbed. Eating two or more uncooked egg whites daily for several months has caused biotin deficiency that is serious enough to produce symptoms.[a] Deficiency may also be induced by protracted antibiotic use and eradication of normal intestinal flora. Long-term anticonvulsant drug use affects absorption and may result in a deficiency.

Syndromes: Anorexia, nausea, vomiting, glossitis, seborrheic dermatitis, depression, lethargy, alopecia.

TOXICITY

Intake Level: Not established; no toxicity demonstrated at doses up to 10 mg/day.
Syndromes: None known.

Dietary Sources[c]: Cereal grains contain biotin in amounts in the range 3–30 μg/100 g but with varying bioavailability: Most of the biotin in wheat, for example, is bound and not bioavailable. Fruits and meats contain negligible amounts of biotin. Peanut butter and mushrooms are sources.

Food	Serving Size (g)	Energy (kcal)	Biotin (μg)	Food	Serving Size (g)	Energy (kcal)	Biotin (μg)
Liver	100	161	100–200	Yeast	100	295	100–200
Soy flour	100	436	60–70	Egg yolk	100	358	16

Effects of Food Preparation and Storage: Not reported to be a generally important determinant of dietary intake levels.

Additional details, evidence, and references for dosing and safety for many nutrients and substances individuals might choose to ingest can be found at http://www.mayoclinic.com/health/search/search, http://ods.od.nih.gov/, and http://www.nlm.nih.gov/medlineplus/.

[a]Biotin MedlinePlus. Available at http://www.nlm.nih.gov/medlineplus/druginfo/natural/313.html; accessed 9/23/13.
[b]Eaton SB, Eaton SB III, Konner MJ. Paleolithic nutrition revisited: a twelve-year retrospective on its nature and implications. *Eur J Clin Nutr* 1997;51:207–216; Eaton SB, Eaton SB. Paleolithic vs. modern diets–selected pathophysiological implications. *Eur J Nutr* 2000;39:67–70.
[c]The nutrient composition of most foods can be checked by accessing the US Department of Agriculture nutrient database, at http://www.nal.usda.gov/fnic/foodcomp/search.

Sources: Ensminger AH, Ensminger ME, Konlande JE, et al. *The concise encyclopedia of foods and nutrition.* Boca Raton, FL: CRC Press, Inc., 1995.

(continued)

APPENDIX E (Continued)

Margen S. *The wellness nutrition counter*. New York, NY: Health Letter Associates, 1997.

Murray MT. *Encyclopedia of nutritional supplements*. Rocklin, CA: Prima Publishing, 1996.

National Research Council. *Recommended dietary allowances*, 10th ed. Washington, DC: National Academy Press, 1989.

Otten JJ, Hellwig JP, Meyers LD, eds. *Dietary reference intakes. The essential guide to nutrient requirements*. Washington, DC: National Academies Press, 2006.

Pizzorno JE, Murray MT. *Textbook of natural medicine*, 3rd ed. St. Louis, MO: Church Livingstone Elsevier, 2006.

Shils ME, Shike M, Ross AC, et al., eds. *Modern nutrition in health and disease*, 10th ed. Philadelphia, PA: Lippincott Williams & Wilkins, 2005.

US Department of Agriculture. *USDA nutrient database for standard reference*. Release 19. 2006.

US Department of Agriculture. *USDA nutrient intake from NHANES 2001–2002 data*.

Ziegler EE, Filer LJ Jr. eds. *Present knowledge in nutrition*, 7th ed. Washington, DC: ILSI Press, 1996.

BORON

BIOLOGICAL FUNCTION(S) IN HUMANS/KEY PROPERTIES: May play a role in the metabolism of calcium, phosphorous, magnesium, steroid hormones, and vitamin D. May play a role in the regulation of cell membrane function. Boron may enhance the effects of estrogen on bone density.

ABSORPTION/SOLUBILITY/STORAGE/PHARMACOKINETICS: Boron in food is rapidly absorbed and excreted predominantly in urine. Boron is distributed throughout the body compartments but most concentrated in bone, teeth hair, nails, spleen, and thyroid tissue.

RATIONALE FOR SUPPLEMENTATION: Prevention and treatment of osteoporosis and arthritis. Possibly prevention of urolithiasis and prostate cancer. May lower cardiovascular risks as a result of increasing endogenous estrogen.

EVIDENCE IN SUPPORT OF SUPPLEMENTATION TO AND ABOVE THE DRI: No RDA or AI established. The study of therapeutic effects of supplemental boron is in its infancy. Small human studies, including few randomized, double-blind pilot studies, show beneficial effects on bone metabolism and symptoms of osteoarthritis (see Chapter 14).

Recommended Intake Range (US RDA): No RDA has been established; no essential biological role for it has been identified. Approximately 0.25 and 3.25 mg of boron daily per 2,000 kcal are considered high and low intake, respectively.[a]

AVERAGE INTAKE, US ADULTS:	0.33–2.74 mg/day
ESTIMATED MEAN PALEOLITHIC INTAKE (ADULT)[b]:	Not available
COMMON DOSE RANGE FOR USE AS SUPPLEMENT:	3 mg/day
DO DIETARY PATTERNS MEETING GUIDELINES PERMIT INTAKE IN THE SUPPLEMENT RANGE?	Yes
INCLUDED IN TYPICAL MULTIVITAMIN/MULTIMINERAL TABLET?	No

DEFICIENCY

Intake Level: Below 0.3 mg/day; possibly, below 1 mg/day.
Syndromes: Uncertain; may contribute to osteoporosis and may depress both muscle and cognitive function.

TOXICITY

Intake Level[a]: Boron Tolerable Upper Intake Levels (UL):

	Infancy (age 0–6 mo)	Infancy (age 7–12 mo)	Childhood (age 1–3 y)	Childhood (age 4–8 y)	Adolescence (age 9–13 y)	Adolescence (age 14–18 y)	Adult (age ≥19 y)	Pregnancy (age 19–50 y)*	Lactation (age 19–50 y)
Male	—	—	3 mg	6 mg	11 mg	17 mg	20 mg	—	—
Female	—	—	3 mg	6 mg	11 mg	17 mg	20 mg	20 mg	20 mg

Syndromes: Nausea, vomiting, diarrhea, dermatitis, lethargy.

Dietary Sources[c]: The boron content of foods is not included in the U.S. Department of Agriculture database and is not readily available from other published sources. Boron is abundant in noncitrus fruits, green leafy vegetables, nuts, legumes, beer, wine, and cider. Meat, fish, and dairy products are poor sources.

Effects of Food Preparation and Storage: Not available.

---

*Pregnant or breastfeeding women 14–18 years of age, the UL is 17 mg/day.

Additional details, evidence, and references for dosing and safety for many nutrients and substances individuals might choose to ingest can be found at http://www.mayoclinic.com/health/search/search, http://ods.od.nih.gov/, and http://www.nlm.nih.gov/medlineplus/.

[a] Boron MedlinePlus. Available at http://www.nlm.nih.gov/medlineplus/druginfo/natural/894.html; accessed 9/24/2013.
[b] Eaton SB, Eaton SB. Paleolithic vs. modern diets—selected pathophysiological implications. Eur J Nutr 2000;39:67–70.
[c] The nutrient composition of most foods can be checked by accessing the U.S. Department of Agriculture nutrient database, at http://www.nal.usda.gov/fnic/foodcomp/search.

Sources: Ensminger AH, Ensminger ME, Konlande JE, et al. *The concise encyclopedia of foods and nutrition.* Boca Raton, FL: CRC Press, Inc., 1995.
Margen S. *The wellness nutrition counter.* New York, NY: Health Letter Associates, 1997.
Murray MT. *Encyclopedia of nutritional supplements.* Rocklin, CA: Prima Publishing, 1996.
National Research Council. *Recommended dietary allowances,* 10th ed. Washington, DC: National Academy Press, 1989.
Otten JJ, Hellwig JP, Meyers LD, eds. *Dietary reference intakes. The essential guide to nutrient requirements.* Washington, DC: National Academies Press, 2006.
Pizzorno JE, Murray MT. *Textbook of natural medicine,* 3rd ed. St. Louis, MO: Church Livingstone Elsevier, 2006.
Shils ME, Shike M, Ross AC, et al., eds. *Modern nutrition in health and disease,* 10th ed. Philadelphia, PA: Lippincott Williams & Wilkins, 2005.
US Department of Agriculture. *USDA nutrient database for standard reference.* Release 19. 2006.
US Department of Agriculture. *USDA nutrient intake from NHANES 2001–2002 data.*
Ziegler EE, Filer LJ Jr, eds. *Present knowledge in nutrition,* 7th ed. Washington, DC: ILSI Press, 1996.

CAFFEINE

BIOLOGICAL FUNCTION(S) IN HUMANS/KEY PROPERTIES: Stimulates central nervous system through antagonism of adenosine receptors, enhancing dopamine activity and leading to increased alertness. Can also acutely raise serotonin levels, leading to enhanced mood. Caffeine is a xanthine alkaloid compound, and while not necessary for health, it constitutes the world's most commonly used psychoactive substance and may have health benefits when used in moderation (see Chapter 41).

ABSORPTION/SOLUBILITY/STORAGE/PHARMACOKINETICS: Slightly water soluble. Stomach and intestinal absorption is rapid following ingestion. Caffeine is metabolized by the liver by the cytochrome P450 oxidase enzyme system, generating three active metabolites: paraxanthine (84%), theobromine (12%), and theophylline (4%). Crosses the blood–brain barrier.

RATIONALE FOR SUPPLEMENTATION: Enhanced cognitive or physical performance; combating drowsiness.

EVIDENCE IN SUPPORT OF SUPPLEMENTATION TO AND ABOVE THE DRI: No RDA or DRI established for caffeine. Caffeine supplementation has been shown to improve speed in cycling and rowing events, (Kovacs EM, Stegen JH, Brouns F. Effect of caffeinated drinks on substrate metabolism, caffeine excretion, and performance. *J Appl Physiol*. 1998;85(2):709–715. Bruce CR, Anderson ME, Fraser SF, et al. Enhancement of 2000-m rowing performance after caffeine ingestion. *Med Sci Sports Exerc*. 2000;32(11):1958–1963), reduce perceived exertion during exercise (*Scand J Med Sci Sports*. 2005 Apr;15(2):69–78. Effects of caffeine ingestion on rating of perceived exertion during and after exercise: a meta-analysis. Doherty M, Smith PM.) an enhance endurance in sports activities at doses of 2-5 mg/kg (*J Sports Sci*. 2006 Jul;24(7):749–61. Dietary supplements for football. Hespel P, Maughan RJ, Greenhaff PL.) Caffeine has also demonstrated efficacy as an adjuvant treatment for acute pain (*Cochrane Database Syst Rev*. 2012 Mar 14;3:CD009281. doi: 10.1002/14651858.CD009281.pub2. Caffeine as an analgesic adjuvant for acute pain in adults. Derry CJ, Derry S, Moore RA.) and may be useful in enhancing performance in shift workers (*Cochrane Database Syst Rev*. 2010 May 12;(5):CD008508. doi: 10.1002/14651858.CD008508. Caffeine for the prevention of injuries and errors in shift workers. Ker K, Edwards PJ, Felix LM, Blackhall K, Roberts I.) In people with asthma, caffeine may modestly improve airway function (*Cochrane Database Syst Rev*. 2010 Jan 20;(1):CD001112. doi: 10.1002/14651858.CD001112. pub2. Caffeine for asthma. Welsh EJ, Bara A, Barley E, Cates CJ).

Recommended Intake Range (US RDA): None established. Two to four 8-oz cups of coffee (about 200–300 mg of caffeine) per day and 5 servings of caffeinated soft drinks or tea are considered an average or moderate amount of caffeine.[a]

AVERAGE INTAKE, US ADULTS[b]:	300 mg/day
ESTIMATED MEAN PALEOLITHIC INTAKE (ADULT):	Not available
COMMON DOSE RANGE FOR USE AS SUPPLEMENT:	100–200 mg
DO DIETARY PATTERNS MEETING GUIDELINES PROVIDE ADEQUATE INTAKE?	N/A
INCLUDED IN TYPICAL MULTIVITAMIN/MULTIMINERAL TABLET?	No

DEFICIENCY

Intake Level: Not required for health; therefore, no deficiency syndrome exists. However, regular usage may induce tolerance and produce a withdrawal syndrome if intake is stopped abruptly.

Syndromes: Withdrawal symptoms include headache, nausea, fatigue, drowsiness, inability to concentrate, irritability, depression.

TOXICITY

Intake Level: Caffeine intake in excess of 500–600 mg may cause unpleasant symptoms,[c] and hospitalization from toxicity may be required at 2 g of ingestion. Lethal doses are possible, but very rare, usually only from overdose of caffeine pills.

Syndromes: Restlessness, insomnia, facial flushing, polyuria, gastrointestinal disturbance, tremors, irritability, irregular or rapid heartbeat, psychomotor agitation.

Dietary Sources: Coffee, tea, chocolate, and cola (unless they are labeled "caffeine-free") are the main sources in the diet.

Additional details, evidence, and references for dosing and safety for many nutrients and substances individuals might choose to ingest can be found at http://www.mayoclinic.com/health/search/search, http://ods.od.nih.gov/, and http://www.nlm.nih.gov/medlineplus/.

[a]MedlinePlus. *Caffeine in the diet*. Available at http://www.nlm.nih.gov/medlineplus/ency/article/002445.htm; accessed 9/23/2013 and Mayo Clinic. *Nutrition and healthy eating: Caffeine*. Available at http://www.mayoclinic.com/health/caffeine/NU00600; accessed 9/23/2013.

[b] FDA. *Caffeine intake for US population*. Available at http://www.fda.gov/downloads/AboutFDA/CentersOffices/OfficeofFoods/ CFSAN/CFSANFOIAElectronicReadingRoom/UCM333191.pdf; accessed 9/24/2013.

[c]Mayo Clinic. *Nutrition and healthy eating: Caffeine*. Available at http://www.mayoclinic.com/health/caffeine/NU00600; accessed 9/23/2013.

CALCIUM

BIOLOGICAL FUNCTION(S) IN HUMANS/KEY PROPERTIES: Calcium is the most abundant mineral in the body. It is the principal mineral of bone and teeth. Extraskeletal calcium functions in nerve conduction muscle, contraction, coagulation and hemostasis, and cell membrane permeability.

ABSORPTION/SOLUBILITY/STORAGE/PHARMACOKINETICS: When daily calcium intake is at or near the mean for adults in the United States (750 mg), approximately 25%–50% is absorbed. Calcium absorption is enhanced when it is ingested with food; gastric acid appears to be a factor. Absorption in the duodenum and proximal jejunum is saturable and vitamin D dependent. Passive nonsaturable absorption occurs throughout the small bowel especially in the ileum. Approximately 4% of ingested calcium is absorbed in the large bowel. Calcium in serum is about 8%–10% ionized and 40%–45% protein bound; 45%–50% is found as free ions disassociated. Ionized calcium is the metabolically active moiety. Serum levels are maintained at or near 10 mg/dL by the actions of parathyroid hormone calcitonin and vitamin D. Body stores are 99% skeletal and 1% exchangeable pool. Calcium regulation is influenced by the actions of glucocorticoids, thyroid hormone, growth hormone, insulin, and estrogen. Renal filtration in the adult is approximately 8.6 g/day of which all but 100–200 mg is reabsorbed. Daily fecal losses include approximately 150 mg of calcium in intestinal secretions as well as unabsorbed dietary calcium; losses therefore vary with intake and approximate 300–600 mg. Small losses in sweat (i.e., 15 mg/day) occur as well. Dietary protein potentiates loss of calcium in urine: for every 50 g increment in daily protein ingestion, an additional 60 mg of calcium is excreted. Increased sodium and caffeine intake also increases urinary calcium excretion. Absorption is enhanced by lactose mainly in infants, pregnancy, and calcium deficiency. Plants with oxalates (e.g., spinach, rhubarb, beets) interfere with calcium absorption by forming indigestible salts with calcium, and calcium absorption is likewise reduced when foods contain high amounts of phytates (e.g., soy).[a] Calcium competes for absorption with certain other mineral cations (e.g., magnesium).[b] Vitamin D helps promote calcium absorption.[c]

RATIONALE FOR SUPPLEMENTATION: Women in the United states consistently ingest less calcium than the RDA. Intake in males generally approximates recommended levels. Supplementation is particularly advocated for the prevention of osteoporosis in women. Supplemental calcium may lower blood pressure and may confer some protection against colon cancer. Oyster shell calcium, dolomite calcium, and bone meal calcium supplements should generally be avoided due to the possibility of lead contamination. Preferred supplements include chelated calcium citrate, gluconate, lactate, and fumarate. Calcium carbonate may be slightly less well absorbed although this appears to be insignificant if ingested with food.

EVIDENCE IN SUPPORT OF SUPPLEMENTATION TO AND ABOVE THE DRI: The literature on both dietary and supplemental calcium is extensive. There is strong evidence that supplemental calcium contributes to bone density, but not bone fracture risk. Evidence of a modest beneficial effect on blood pressure, particularly systolic blood pressure, as well as on blood pressure in pregnancy is well substantiated. There is supportive evidence for preventive efficacy against colon cancer. Evidence for other benefits is preliminary.

Recommended Intake Range (US RDA): An intake of 1,000–1,300 g/day of calcium is recommended for adults.

CALCIUM RECOMMENDED INTAKE RANGE (US AI)[d]:

	Infancy (age 0–6 mo)	Infancy (age 7–12 mo)	Childhood (age 1–3 y)	Childhood (age 4–8 y)
Male	200 mg	260 mg	700 mg	1,000 mg
Female	200 mg	260 mg	700 mg	1,000 mg
	Adolescence (age 9–13 y)	Adolescence (age 14–18 y)	Adult (age 19–50 y)	Adult (age ≥ 51 y)
Male	1,300 mg	1,300 mg	1,000 mg	1,000 mg
Female	1,300 mg	1,300 mg	1,000 mg	1,000 mg
	Pregnancy (age ≤ 18 y)	Pregnancy (age 19–50 y)	Lactation (age 18 ≤ y)	Lactation (age 19–50 y)
Male	—	—	—	—
Female	1,300 mg	1,000 mg	1,300 mg	1,000 mg

(continued)

APPENDIX E   (Continued)

Recommended Intake Range (NIH Consensus Statement[e]):

	Infancy (age 0–6 mo)	Infancy (age 6 m–1 y)	Childhood (age 1–5 y)	Childhood (age 6–10 y)	Puberty/ Adolescence/ Early Adulthood (age 11–24 y)
Male	400 mg	600 mg	800 mg	800–1,200 mg	1,200–1,500 mg
Female	400 mg	600 mg	800 mg	800–1,200 mg	1,200–1,500 mg

	Adulthood (age 25–50 y)	Postmenopause	Senescence	Pregnancy	Lactation
Male	1,000 mg	—	1,500 mg	—	—
Female	1,000 mg	On estrogen: 1,000 mg; Not on estrogen: 1,500 mg	1,500 mg	1,200–1,500 mg	1,200–1,500 mg

AVERAGE INTAKE, US ADULTS: 746–982 mg/day

ESTIMATED MEAN PALEOLITHIC INTAKE (ADULT)[f]: 1,622 mg/day

COMMON DOSE RANGE FOR USE AS SUPPLEMENT: Up to 1,200 mg/day

DO DIETARY PATTERNS MEETING GUIDELINES PROVIDE THE RDA Yes

INCLUDED IN TYPICAL MULTIVITAMIN/MULTIMINERAL TABLET? Yes (dose: 175 mg)

DEFICIENCY

Intake Level: Approximately 550 mg/day

Syndromes: Accelerated osteoporosis, hypocalcemia

TOXICITY

Intake Level:	Safe Upper Limits[d]
Life Stage	**Upper Safe Limit**
Birth to 6 mo	1,000 mg
Infants 7–12 mo	1,500 mg
Children 1–8 y	2,500 mg
Children 9–18 y	3,000 mg
Adults 19–50 y	2,500 mg
Adults 51 y and older	2,000 mg
Pregnant and breastfeeding teens	3,000 mg
Pregnant and breastfeeding adults	2,500 mg

Syndromes: Hypercalcemia; constipation; impaired absorption of iron, zinc, and other micronutrients. While foods rich in calcium appear to decrease risk for symptomatic kidney stones, supplemental calcium may increase risk.[g] Similarly, there is evidence that calcium supplementation, but not dietary intake, particularly in excess of 500 mg daily, may increase the risk of cardiovascular events (myocardial infarction, coronary revascularization, death from coronary heart disease, and stroke).[h] The most recent meta-analysis did not find that increased cardiovascular disease (CVD) risk was statistically significant[i]; however, randomized controlled trials of 800–1,600 mg of supplemental calcium daily do suggest a statistically significant increased risk of hip fracture with calcium supplementation.[j]

Dietary Sources:[k] Abundant in dairy products, tofu, sardines, and green leafy vegetables. However for calcium, as for other nutrients, the nutrient content of specific foods may overestimate the amount of nutrient available to consumer (due to various interactions and absorption issues like those noted above).

Food	Serving Size	Energy (kcal)	Calcium (mg)	Food	Serving Size	Energy (kcal)	Calcium (mg)
Sardines	1 can (370 g)	770	1,413	Ricotta cheese	1 cup	339	669
Yogurt, nonfat, plain	1 cup	137	488	Skim milk	1 cup	86	301

Food	Serving Size	Energy (kcal)	Calcium (mg)	Food	Serving Size	Energy (kcal)	Calcium (mg)
Whole milk	1 cup	146	276	Tofu, fried	1/4 block (81 g)	220	301
Buttermilk, low fat	1 cup	98	284	Collard greens, boiled	1 cup (190 g)	49	266
Sesame seeds, roasted and toasted	1 oz	158	277	Amaranth	100 g	374	153
				Soybeans	1 cup (172 g)	253	339
Swiss cheese	1 slice (1 oz)	106	221	Almonds	1 oz	164	70
Oatmeal with water	100 g	55	56	Onions	1 medium (110 g)	44	25
				Peas, frozen	1/2 cup (72 g)	55	16
Provolone cheese	1 slice (1 oz)	98	212	Figs, dried	1 fig	21	14
Cheddar cheese	1 slice (1 oz)	114	300	Celery	1 stalk (40 g)	6	16

Effects of Food Preparation and Storage: Generally unimportant.

Additional details, evidence, and references for dosing and safety for many nutrients and substances individuals might choose to ingest can be found at http://www.mayoclinic.com/health/search/search, http://ods.od.nih.gov/, and http://www.nlm.nih.gov/medlineplus/.

[a]Heaney RP, Weaver CM, Fitzsimmons ML. Soybean phytate content: effect on calcium absorption. *AJCN* 1991;53(3):745–747. Available at http://ajcn.nutrition.org/content/53/3/745.short; accessed 9/27/2013.

[b]Hendrix JZ, Alcock NW, Archibald RM. Competition between calcium, strontium, and magnesium for absorption in the isolated rat intestine. *Clin Chem* 1963;9(6):734–744. Available at http://www.clinchem.org/content/9/6/734.short; accessed 9/27/2013.

[c]MedlinePlus. *Calcium in the diet.* Available at http://www.nlm.nih.gov/medlineplus/ency/article/002412.htm; accessed 9/27/2013.

[d]Office of Dietary Supplements. *Calcium.* Available at http://ods.od.nih.gov/factsheets/Calcium-QuickFacts/; accessed 9/27/2013.

[e]Optimal calcium intake. NIH Consens Statement 1994;12:1–31.

[f]Eaton SB, Eaton SB. Paleolithic vs. modern diets—selected pathophysiological implications. *Eur J Nutr* 2000;39:67–70.

[g]Curhan GC, Willett WC, Speizer FE, et al. Comparison of dietary calcium with supplemental calcium and other nutrients as factors affecting the risk for kidney stones in women. *Ann Intern Med* 1997;126(7):497–504. http://annals.org/article.aspx?articleid=710409.

[h]Bolland M, Avenell A, Baron JA, et al. Effect of calcium supplements on risk of myocardial infarction and cardiovascular events: meta-analysis. *BMJ* 2010;341:c3691. http://www.ncbi.nlm.nih.gov/pmc/articles/PMC2912459/; and Bolland M, Grey A, Avenell A, et al. Calcium supplements with or without vitamin D and risk of cardiovascular events: reanalysis of the Women's Health Initiative limited access dataset and meta-analysis. *BMJ* 2011;342:d2040. http://www.ncbi.nlm.nih.gov/pmc/articles/PMC3079822/.

[i]Mao PJ, Zhang C, Tang L, et al. Effect of calcium or vitamin D supplementation on vascular outcomes: a meta-analysis of randomized controlled trials. *Int J Cardiol* 2013;169(2):106–111. doi:10.1016/j.ijcard.2013.08.055. http://www.ncbi.nlm.nih.gov/pubmed/24035175.

[j]Bischoff-Ferrari HA, Dawson-Hughes B, Baron JA et al. Calcium intake and hip fracture risk in men and women: a meta-analysis of prospective cohort studies and randomized controlled trials. *Am J Clin Nutr* 2007;86(6):1780–1790. http://ajcn.nutrition.org/content/86/6/1780.short.

[k]The nutrient composition of most foods can be checked by accessing the U.S. Department of Agriculture nutrient database, at http://www.nal.usda.gov/fnic/foodcomp/search. A more extensive list of food sources of calcium is available in Margen S. *The wellness nutrition counter.* New York, NY: Health Letter Associates, 1997.

Sources: Ensminger AH, Ensminger ME, Konlande JE, et al. *The concise encyclopedia of foods and nutrition.* Boca Raton, FL: CRC Press, Inc., 1995.

Margen S. *The wellness nutrition counter.* New York, NY: Health Letter Associates, 1997.

Murray MT. *Encyclopedia of nutritional supplements.* Rocklin, CA: Prima Publishing, 1996.

National Research Council. *Recommended dietary allowances,* 10th ed. Washington, DC: National Academy Press, 1989.

Otten JJ, Hellwig JP, Meyers LD, eds. *Dietary reference intakes. The essential guide to nutrient requirements.* Washington, DC: National Academies Press, 2006.

Pizzorno JE, Murray MT. *Textbook of natural medicine,* 3rd ed. St. Louis, MO: Church Livingstone Elsevier, 2006.

Shils ME, Shike M, Ross AC, et al., eds. *Modern nutrition in health and disease,* 10th ed. Philadelphia, PA: Lippincott Williams & Wilkins, 2005.

US Department of Agriculture. *USDA nutrient database for standard reference.* Release 19. 2006.

US Department of Agriculture. *USDA nutrient intake from NHANES 2001–2002 data.*

Ziegler EE, Filer LJ Jr, eds. *Present knowledge in nutrition,* 7th ed. Washington, DC: ILSI Press, 1996.

CARNITINE/LEVOCARNITINE

BIOLOGICAL FUNCTION(S) IN HUMANS/KEY PROPERTIES: Transports long-chain fatty acids into mitochondria. Carnitine may function in fatty acid synthesis and ketone body metabolism. Carnitine is synthesized in the liver and kidney from lysine and methionine; vitamins C, B_6, and niacin are cofactors in carnitine biosynthesis. Carnitine may be an essential nutrient for newborns, who have limited ability to synthesize carnitine. It is present in breast milk at a concentration of 28–95 μmol/L.

ABSORPTION/SOLUBILITY/STORAGE/PHARMACOKINETICS: Water soluble. Intestinal absorption is both active and passive. Carnitine is rapidly transported into cells, and intracellular stores greatly exceed levels in circulation. Approximately 97% of body stores are in skeletal muscle. Carnitine is filtered in the kidney, and approximately 95% is reabsorbed. With elevated serum levels, reabsorption declines.

RATIONALE FOR SUPPLEMENTATION: Enhancement of exercise tolerance in healthy individuals and performance athletes. Improvement in oxidation metabolism with reduced symptoms in angina and peripheral vascular disease. Improved cardiac function in congestive heart failure (CHF). Improved cognitive function in Alzheimer's and other forms of senile dementia. Anemia management in end-stage renal disease. Relief of diabetic neuropathy. May slow the death of lymphocytes/HIV progression, reduce neuropathy, and favorably affect blood lipid levels in HIV-infected individuals.[a]

EVIDENCE IN SUPPORT OF SUPPLEMENTATION TO AND ABOVE THE DRI: No established RDA or AI. But an extensive literature on carnitine dates back to the 1970s. Evidence of some benefit in cardiac ischemia, hemodialysis, cardiomyopathy, dementia, and male infertility is supported by randomized, placebo-controlled trials. There is also trial evidence for improved walking distance and perceived quality of life in those with peripheral vascular disease, reduced nerve pain and improved vibration perception in those with diabetic neuropathy,[a] and reduced all-cause mortality in those with established cardiovascular disease.[b]

Recommended Intake Range (US RDA): None established. Carnitine is considered a conditionally essential nutrient; dietary deficiency may cause adverse effects under predisposing conditions. The liver and kidneys produce sufficient amounts of carnitine from the amino acids lysine and methionine to meet daily needs.[a]

AVERAGE INTAKE, US ADULTS:	100–300 mg/day
ESTIMATED MEAN PALEOLITHIC INTAKE (ADULT)[c]:	Not available; likely higher than current levels due to importance of red meat in the Paleolithic diet.
COMMON DOSE RANGE FOR USE AS SUPPLEMENT:	1,500–4,000 mg/day
DO DIETARY PATTERNS MEETING GUIDELINES PERMIT INTAKE IN THE SUPPLEMENT RANGE?	No
INCLUDED IN TYPICAL MULTIVITAMIN/MULTIMINERAL TABLET?	No

DEFICIENCY

Intake Level: No intake level has been specified for healthy adults; deficiency generally results from a genetic defect. Deficiency may occur in newborns, especially premature, on formula not containing carnitine. May be induced by hemodialysis, total parenteral nutrition, or use of valproic acid. Strict vegetarian diets are likely to be low in carnitine but have not been decisively linked to relevant carnitine deficiencies.

Syndromes: Progressive muscle weakness, impaired ketogenesis, and cardiomyopathy.

TOXICITY

Intake Level: Supplementation with the naturally occurring L-stereoisomer is apparently safe; use of the D isomer should be avoided as it can lead to functional carnitine deficiency. At doses of approximately 3 g/day, carnitine supplements can cause symptoms.[a]

Syndromes: Nausea, vomiting, abdominal cramps, diarrhea, and a "fishy" body odor. Rarer side effects include muscle weakness in uremic patients and seizures in those with seizure disorders. Supplementation with the D-isomer may result in deficiency symptoms, particularly muscle pain and reduced exercise tolerance.[a] Emerging evidence suggests intestinal bacteria metabolize carnitine to TMAO (trimethylamine-N-oxide), a substance that might increase the risk of CVD. This effect appears to be less pronounced in vegetarians than in those who consume meat, who seem to have different gut flora[d,e,f,g]

Dietary Sources[h]: Red meat, dairy to a lesser extent.

Food	Serving Size (g)	Energy (kcal)	Carnitine (mg)	Food	Serving Size (g)	Energy (kcal)	Carnitine (mg)
Beef steak	100	321	95	Pork	100	226	28
Ground beef	100	282	94	Bacon	100	576	23

Food	Serving Size (g)	Energy (kcal)	Carnitine (mg)	Food	Serving Size (g)	Energy (kcal)	Carnitine (mg)
Cod fish	100	82	5.6	Ice cream	100	201	3.7
Chicken breast	100	172	3.9	Whole milk	100	60	3.3
American cheese	100	331	3.7				

Effects of Food Preparation and Storage: Not reported to be a generally important determinant of dietary intake levels.

Additional details, evidence, and references for dosing and safety for many nutrients and substances individuals might choose to ingest can be found at http://www.mayoclinic.com/health/search/search, http://ods.od.nih.gov/, and http://www.nlm.nih.gov/medlineplus/.

[a]Office of Dietary Supplements. *Carnitine.* Available at http://ods.od.nih.gov/factsheets/Carnitine-HealthProfessional/;accessed 9/27/2013.
[b]DiNicolantonio JJ, Lavie JC, Fares H, et al. L-carnitine in the secondary prevention of cardiovascular disease: systematic review and meta-analysis. *Mayo Clinic Proceedings* 2013;88(6):544–551. http://www.mayoclinicproceedings.org/article/S0025-6196%2813%2900127-4/abstract.
[c]Eaton SB, Eaton SB. Paleolithic vs. modern diets—selected pathophysiological implications. *Eur J Nutr* 2000;39:67–70.
[d]Tang WHW, Wang Z, Levison BS, et al. Intestinal microbial metabolism of phosphatidylcholine and cardiovascular risk. *N Engl J Med* 2013;368:1575. http://dx.doi.org/10.1056/NEJMoa1109400; Loscalzo J. Gut microbiota, the genome, and diet in atherogenesis. *N Engl J Med* 2013;368:1647. http://dx.doi.org/10.1056/NEJMe1302154; Koeth RA, Wang Z, Bruse S, et al. Intestinal microbiota metabolism of L-carnitine, a nutrient in red meat, promotes atherosclerosis. *Nat Med* 2013;19:576. http://dx.doi.org/10.1038/nm.3145; Bäckhed F. Meat-metabolizing bacteria in atherosclerosis. *Nat Med* 2013;19:533. http://dx.doi.org/10.1038/nm.3178; Koeth RA, Wang Z, Levison BS, et al. Intestinal microbiota metabolism of L-carnitine, a nutrient in red meat, promotes atherosclerosis. *Nat Med* 2013;19:576–585. doi:10.1038/nm.3145. http://www.nature.com/nm/journal/v19/n5/full/nm.3145.html.
[e]Loscalzo J. Gut microbiota, the genome, and diet in atherogenesis. *N Engl J Med* 2013 Apr 25; 368:1647. (http://dx.doi.org/10.1056/NEJMe1302154)
[f]Koeth RA et al. Intestinal microbiota metabolism of l-carnitine, a nutrient in red meat, promotes atherosclerosis. *Nat Med* 2013 May; 19:576. (http://dx.doi.org/10.1038/nm.3145)
[g]Bäckhed F. Meat-metabolizing bacteria in atherosclerosis. *Nat Med* 2013 May; 19:533. (http://dx.doi.org/10.1038/nm.3178)
[h]The carnitine content of foods is not currently included in the USDA nutrient database. As a general rule, carnitine is abundant in meat and more abundant the redder the meat. Carnitine is present in dairy products; levels in plant foods are negligible. The table is adapted from Broquist HP. Carnitine. In: Shils ME, Shike M, Ross AC, et al., eds. *Modern nutrition in health and disease,* 10th ed. Philadelphia, PA: Lippincott Williams & Wilkins, 2005:540. Energy content of foods listed is from the USDA nutrient database, at http://www.nal.usda.gov/fnic/foodcomp/search.

Sources: Ensminger AH, Ensminger ME, Konlande JE, et al. *The concise encyclopedia of foods and nutrition.* Boca Raton, FL: CRC Press, Inc., 1995.
Margen S. *The wellness nutrition counter.* New York, NY: Health Letter Associates, 1997.
Murray MT. *Encyclopedia of nutritional supplements.* Rocklin, CA: Prima Publishing, 1996.
National Research Council. *Recommended dietary allowances,* 10th ed. Washington, DC: National Academy Press, 1989.
Otten JJ, Hellwig JP, Meyers LD, eds. *Dietary reference intakes. The essential guide to nutrient requirements.* Washington, DC: National Academies Press, 2006.
Pizzorno JE, Murray MT. *Textbook of natural medicine,* 3rd ed. St. Louis, MO: Church Livingstone Elsevier, 2006.
Shils ME, Shike M, Ross AC, et al., eds. *Modern nutrition in health and disease,* 10th ed. Philadelphia, PA: Lippincott Williams & Wilkins, 2005.
US Department of Agriculture. *USDA nutrient database for standard reference.* Release 19. 2006.
US Department of Agriculture. *USDA nutrient intake from NHANES 2001–2002 data.*
Ziegler EE, Filer LJ Jr, eds. *Present knowledge in nutrition,* 7th ed. Washington, DC: ILSI Press, 1996.

CAROTENOIDS/VITAMIN A

BIOLOGICAL FUNCTION(S) IN HUMANS/KEY PROPERTIES: The essential role of carotenoids in human health as precursors of vitamin A has long been recognized; potential health effects of their antioxidant properties have come under investigation more recently. Vitamin A is essential in cell proliferation and growth, immune function, and vision. There are more than 600 carotenoids known, of which approximately 50 are known to serve as precursors of retinol, the biologically active form of vitamin A. These carotenoid precursors of retinol are said to have provitamin A activity. Of the many, only a few are considered important sources of vitamin A: α-carotene, β-carotene, and β-cryptoxanthin. Of these, all-trans-β-carotene is the most active. Carotenoids are responsible for the bright pigments in many plants and are essential to photosynthesis. They apparently act as antioxidants in both plants and animals. The functions of carotenoids other than as antioxidants and vitamin A precursors remain to be elucidated.

ABSORPTION/SOLUBILITY/STORAGE/PHARMACOKINETICS: Carotenoids are fat soluble. Retinol is 70%–90% absorbed in the small intestine, while carotenoids are generally 9%–22% absorbed. Carotenoid absorption is downregulated by high intake. Absorption is dependent on the activity of pancreatic enzymes and bile acids and is enhanced by dietary fat, protein, and vitamin E. Ingested provitamin A carotenoids and preformed vitamin A (retinyl esters) are directly absorbed from the intestine. Carotenoids are widely distributed in tissues, while β-carotene and ingested retinol are stored in the liver as retinyl esters in subject with adequate vitamin A stores. Inactive metabolites of retinol are 70% egested in stool, 30% excreted in urine. Retinol is slowly released from liver stores to meet metabolic requirements and it circulates in conjunction with a binding protein. Due to hepatic storage capacity, large, intermittent doses of vitamin A or its precursors can prevent deficiency as effectively as consistent dietary intake.

RATIONALE FOR SUPPLEMENTATION: There is no specific RDA for carotenoids, other than as vitamin A precursors. Carotenoid intake from dietary sources will be high if the diet is rich in dark green and other brightly colored vegetables and fruits (see "Dietary Sources," below). For individuals with limited intake of vegetables and individuals with limited intake of dietary provitamin A, provitamin A carotenoid supplementation may be indicated to assure adequate vitamin A status. The use of carotenoid supplements has been recommended to enhance immune function and to treat photosensitivity. Other carotenoids, such as lutein, are recommended to prevent age-related eye diseases. In those who are deficient, supplementation may be helpful for preventing cardiovascular disease and cancer, but the evidence is thus far inconclusive.

EVIDENCE IN SUPPORT OF SUPPLEMENTATION TO AND ABOVE THE DRI: Epidemiologic evidence is consistent that high dietary intake and high serum levels of carotenoids are associated with reduced risk of certain cancers[a] and mortality.[b] However, only β-carotene has been studied as a supplement in randomized trials, with consistently negative results. In such trials, β-carotene has been associated with lack of effect on angina or cardiovascular events[c,d] and either no effect[e] or an adverse effect[c] on cancer incidence in smokers. Proponents of carotenoid supplementation argue that antioxidant effects require combination supplements, but evidence of benefit is lacking to data. Preliminary studies of other carotenoids, including lycopene and lutein, are promising.

Recommended Intake Range (US RDA[f]):

VITAMIN A RECOMMENDED INTAKE RANGE (US RDA)[g]:
RAE = retinol activity equivalents, IU = International Units

- 1 IU RETINOL = 0.3 μg RAE
- 1 IU β-CAROTENE FROM DIETARY SUPPLEMENTS = 0.15 μg RAE
- 1 IU β-CAROTENE FROM FOOD = 0.05 μg RAE
- 1 IU α-CAROTENE or β-cryptoxanthin = 0.025 μg RAE
- 1 μg RAE RETINOL = 3.33 IU
- 1 μg RAE β-CAROTENE FROM DIETARY SUPPLEMENTS = 6.67 IU
- 1 μg RAE β-CAROTENE FROM FOOD = 20 IU
- 1 μg RAE α-CAROTENE OR β-CRYPTOXANTHIN = 40 IU

	Infancy (age 0–6 mo)	Infancy (age 7–12 mo)	Childhood (age 1–3 y)	Childhood (age 4–8 y)
Male	400 μg RAE	500 μg RAE	300 μg RAE	400 μg RAE
Female	400 μg RAE	500 μg RAE	300 μg RAE	400 μg RAE

	Adolescence (age 9–13 y)	Adolescence (age 14–18 y)	Adult (age $\geq$ 19 y)	Pregnancy (age $\leq$ 18 y)
Male	600 μg RAE	900 μg RAE	900 μg RAE	—
Female	600 μg RAE	700 μg RAE	700 μg RAE	750 μg RAE

	Pregnancy (age 19–50 y)	Lactation (age 18 $\leq$ y)	Lactation (age 19–50 y)
Male	—	—	—
Female	770 μg RAE	1,200 μg RAE	1,300 μg RAE

APPENDIX E   (Continued)

AVERAGE INTAKE, US ADULTS:	570–661 μg RAE
ESTIMATED MEAN PALEOLITHIC INTAKE (ADULT)[h]:	2,870 μg RE
COMMON DOSE RANGE FOR USE AS SUPPLEMENT:	A daily dose of 900 μg RAE for men and 700 μg RAE for women; acute doses up to 50,000 μg RAE are proposed for use during acute viral illness.
DO DIETARY PATTERNS MEETING GUIDELINES PERMIT ADEQUATE INTAKE?	Yes
INCLUDED IN TYPICAL MULTIVITAMIN/MULTIMINERAL TABLET?	Yes (dose: 1,375 μg RAE)

DEFICIENCY (CAROTENOIDS/VITAMIN A)

Intake Level: Below 390 μg RAE (when vitamin A blood levels dip below 0.7 μmol/L).

Syndromes: Xerophthalmia, anorexia, hyperkeratosis, immunosuppression, increased risk of morbidity and mortality through symptoms such as diarrhea.

TOXICITY (CAROTENOIDS)

Intake Level: None for carotenoids; 3,000 μg/day vitamin A.

VITAMIN A TOLERABLE UPPER INTAKE LEVEL (UL): Safe upper limits for β-carotene and other forms of provitamin A have not been established. The safe upper limits for preformed vitamin A in IU[h]:

	Infancy (age 0–6 mo)	Infancy (age 7–12 mo)	Childhood (age 1–3 y)	Childhood (age 4–8 y)
Male	2,000 IU	2,000 IU	2,000 IU	3,000 IU
Female	2,000 IU	2,000 IU	2,000 IU	3,000 IU

	Adolescence (age 9–13 y)	Adolescence (age 14–18 y)	Adult (age ≥19 y)	Pregnancy (age 14–18 y)
Male	5,667 IU	9,333 IU	10,000 IU	—
Female	5,667 IU	9,333 IU	10,000 IU	—

	Pregnancy (age 19–50 y)	Lactation (age 14–18 y)	Lactation (age 19–50 y)
Male	—	—	—
Female	—	—	—

Syndromes: **Carotenoids:** None; with extreme doses, harmless and reversible skin discoloration may occur; in smokers, high doses of β-carotene—with or without vitamin A—may increase the risk of lung and other cancers, and the combination of β-carotene and vitamin A may be associated with greater risk of cardiovascular events.[i]

Vitamin A: Hepatotoxicity; bone abnormalities; in pregnancy, birth defects.

Dietary Sources: Vitamin A is found abundantly in animal-based foods, such as liver, dairy products, and fish liver oils. Dietary carotenoids are found primarily in specific oils, dark green and other brightly colored vegetables, and fruits. The following chart uses RAE units to equate carotenoids and vitamin A.[g]

Food	Serving Size	Energy (kcal)	Carotenoid (μg RAE)	Food	Serving Size	Energy (kcal)	Carotenoid (μg RAE)
Apricot, dried	1 cup (130 g)	309	941	Pumpkin, cooked	1 cup (245 g)	49	265
Sweet potato, cooked	1 medium (114 g)	117	2,487	Peppers, yellow	1 large (186 g)	50	45
Tomato juice	1 cup (243 g)	41	136	Peppers, red	1 medium (119 g)	32	678
Carrots	1 medium (61 g)	26	1,716	Collard greens, cooked	1 cup (190 g)	49	595
Kale, raw	1 cup (67 g)	33.5	596	Saffron	1 table spoon (2.1 g)	6.5	1.1

APPENDIX E (Continued)

Food	Serving Size	Energy (kcal)	Carotenoid (μg RAE)	Food	Serving Size	Energy (kcal)	Carotenoid (μg RAE)
Paprika	1 table spoon (6.9 g)	20	418	Broccoli, cooked	1 medium stalk (180 g)	50	250
Apricots, fresh	1 medium (35 g)	17	91	Cantaloupe	1 medium wedge (69 g)	24	222
Swiss chard, cooked	1 cup (175 g)	35	550	Corn, cooked	1 ear (77 g)	83	17
Spinach, raw	10 oz (284 g)	62	1,908	Tangerines	1 medium (84 g)	37	77
Parsley, raw	1 cup (60 g)	22	312	Orange	1 medium (131 g)	62	28
Tomato paste	1 can (170 g)	139	415	Watermelon	1 wedge (286 g)	92	106
Romaine lettuce	1/2 cup (28 g)	4	73	Tomato, fresh	1 medium (123 g)	26	76

Distribution of Carotenoids of Potential Clinical Importance in the Food Supply (Leading Sources):

β-carotene:	Apricots, carrots, sweet potato, collard greens, spinach, kale
Lycopene:	Tomato juice, tomato paste, guava, watermelon, grapefruit (pink)
Lutein:	Kale, collard greens, spinach, endive, watercress, Swiss chard, romaine lettuce
α-carotene:	Pumpkin, carrots, squash, corn, apples, peaches
β-cryptoxanthin:	Tangerine, papaya, lemons, oranges, persimmons, corn, green peppers
Zeaxanthin:	Spinach, paprika, corn

Effects of Food Preparation and Storage: The bioavailability tends to increase somewhat with lower-temperature cooking (e.g., steaming or sautéing in oil), whereas bioavailability decreases with higher-temperature methods, such as boiling. The addition of dietary fiber, inadequate dietary fat, and use of nondigestible fat substitutes can decrease carotenoid bioavailability. Some carotenoid tends to be lost with freezing.

Additional details, evidence, and references for dosing and safety for many nutrients and substances individuals might choose to ingest can be found at http://www.mayoclinic.com/health/search/search, http://ods.od.nih.gov/, and http://www.nlm.nih.gov/medlineplus/.

[a]Sun SY, Lotan R. Retinoids and their receptors in cancer development and chemoprevention. *Crit Rev Oncol Hematol* 2002;41:41–55.

[b]Darlow BA, Grahm PJ. Vitamin A supplementation for preventing morbidity and mortality in very low birthweight infants. *Cochrane Database Syst Rev* 2002;4:CD000501.

[c]Rappola JM, Virtamo J, Haukka JK, et al. Effect of vitamin E and beta carotene on the incidence of angina pectoris. *JAMA* 1996;275:693–698. Alpha-tocopherol, Beta Carotene Cancer Prevention Study Group. The effect of vitamin E and beta carotene on the incidence of lung cancer and other cancers in male smokers. *N Engl J Med* 1994;330:1029–1035. Omenn GS, Goodman G, Thornquist M, et al. The -carotene and Retinol Efficacy Trial (CARET) for chemoprevention of lung cancer in high risk populations: smokers and asbestos-exposed workers. *Cancer Res* 1994;54:2038s–2043s.

[d]Hennekens CH, Buring JE, Manson JE, et al. Lack of effect of long-term supplementation with beta carotene on the incidence of malignant neoplasms and cardiovascular disease. *N Engl J Med* 1996;334:1145–1149.

[e]Greenberg ER, Baron JA, Tosteson TD, et al. A clinical trial of antioxidant vitamins to prevent colorectal adenoma. *N Engl J Med* 1994:331:141–147.

[f]There is no RDA for carotenoids per se, other than as vitamin A precursors. Recommended intake is therefore expressed as μg RAE. One μg RAE is equal to 1 μg all-trans-retinol, 12 μg β-carotene, and 24 μg α-carotene or β-cryptoxanthin. An intake of 700–1,300 μg RAE/day of vitamin A is recommended for adults.

[g]Office of Dietary Supplements. *Vitamin A.* Available at http://ods.od.nih.gov/factsheets/VitaminA-QuickFacts/; accessed 9/27/2013.

[h]Eaton SB, Eaton SB. Paleolithic vs. modern diets—selected pathophysiological implications. *Eur J Nutr* 2000;39:67–70.

N.B: Vitamin A supplementation should be avoided during pregnancy; see vitamin A table.

[i]Blomhoff R. Vitamin A and carotenoid toxicity. *Food Nutr Bull* 2001;22(3):320–334. http://www.ingentaconnect.com/content/nsinf/fnb/2001/00000022/00000003/art00009.

Sources: Ensminger AH, Ensminger ME, Konlande JE, et al. *The concise encyclopedia of foods and nutrition.* Boca Raton, FL: CRC Press, Inc., 1995.

Margen S. *The wellness nutrition counter.* New York, NY: Health Letter Associates, 1997.

Murray MT. *Encyclopedia of nutritional supplements.* Rocklin, CA: Prima Publishing, 1996.

National Research Council. *Recommended dietary allowances*, 10th ed. Washington, DC: National Academy Press, 1989.

Otten JJ, Hellwig JP, Meyers LD, eds. *Dietary reference intakes. The essential guide to nutrient requirements*. Washington, DC: National Academies Press, 2006.

Pizzorno JE, Murray MT. *Textbook of natural medicine*, 3rd ed. St. Louis, MO: Church Livingstone Elsevier, 2006.

Shils ME, Shike M, Ross AC, et al., eds. *Modern nutrition in health and disease*, 10th ed. Philadelphia, PA: Lippincott Williams & Wilkins, 2005.

The nutrient composition of most foods can be checked by accessing the U.S. Department of Agriculture nutrient database, at http://www.nal.usda.gov/fric/foodcomp/search.

US Department of Agriculture. *USDA nutrient database for standard reference*. Release 19. 2006.

US Department of Agriculture. *USDA nutrient intake from NHANES 2001–2002 data*.

Ziegler EE, Filer LJ Jr, eds. *Present knowledge in nutrition*, 7th ed. Washington, DC: ILSI Press, 1996.

CHROMIUM

Biological Function(s) in Humans/key Properties: The principal role of chromium is as an insulin cofactor, improving glucose tolerance.

Absorption/Solubility/Storage/Pharmacokinetics: Chromium absorption is limited and varies with intake level from a low of 0.4% to a high of 2.5% of the portion ingested. Chromium is stored in bone, spleen, kidney, and liver. Chromium accumulates in the lungs with advancing age, while levels in others tissues decline; the significance of this is unclear. Ingested chromium that remains unabsorbed is excreted in the feces; absorbed chromium is excreted in urine. Evidence suggests a correlation between the ingestion of certain substances and an effect on chromium bioavailability. Vitamin C has been shown to increase absorption of chromium, while phytate and some antacid drugs have been shown to decrease chromium absorption. A diet excessive in simple sugars has been shown to increase urinary excretion of chromium.

Rationale for Supplementation: Usual intake in the United States is below the recommended intake range of 50–200 μg/day. Chromium deficiency may contribute to insulin resistance. Doses higher than the RDA show promise for ameliorating insulin resistance or impairments of glucose metabolism.[a] Up to 1,000 μg/day is recommended by some practitioners for treatment of insulin resistance or diabetes and as an aid in weight loss.

Evidence in Support of Supplementation to and Above the DRI: The literature on chromium supplementation is fairly extensive, but evidence of therapeutic effect in any condition is not definitive. There is evidence of benefit in some groups of diabetics and in the preferential loss of fat during weight reduction efforts.[b] Arguments against routine supplementation for primary prevention have been raised.[c] Trow et al.[d] found no evidence of benefit from chromium supplementation in a small group of type 2 diabetics. Chromium also failed to enhance the beneficial effects of exercise on glucose tolerance in overweight adults.[e] However, corticosteroid-induced diabetes mellitus has been reported to respond to chromium supplementation.[f] High-dose supplementation apparently has some potential toxicity,[g] although this is generally considered to be limited. Overall, chromium supplementation is considered promising in diabetes and insulin resistance,[h,i] less so for weight management.[j] A meta-analysis of 15 trials of chromium supplementation on markers of diabetes failed to show an effect on glucose or insulin concentrations in non-diabetic subjects or in those with diabetes, except in one trial in China in which study subjects were likely chromium deficient.[k] Thus far, chromium does not appear to be effective at reducing body fat or building lean muscle mass to a degree that is clinically meaningful.[l,m]

Recommended Intake Range (US RDA): Estimated safe and adequate daily dietary intake is provided rather than RDA. An intake of 25–45 μg/day of chromium is recommended for adults.

CHROMIUM RECOMMENDED INTAKE RANGE (US AI):

	Infancy (age 0–6 mo)	Infancy (age 7–12 mo)	Childhood (age 1–3 y)	Childhood (age 4–8 y)
Male	0.2 μg	5.5 μg	11 μg	15 μg
Female	0.2 μg	5.5 μg	11 μg	15 μg
	Adolescence (age 9–13 y)	**Adolescence (age 14–18 y)**	**Adult (age 19–50 y)**	**Adult (age ≥ 51 y)**
Male	25 μg	35 μg	35 μg	30 μg
Female	21 μg	24 μg	25 μg	20 μg
	Pregnancy (age ≤ 18 y)	**Pregnancy (age 19–50 y)**	**Lactation (age ≤ 18 y)**	**Lactation (age 19–50 y)**
Male	—	—	—	—
Female	29 μg	30 μg	44 μg	45 μg

Average Intake, US Adults:	30–80 μg
Estimated Mean Paleolithic Intake (Adult)[n]:	Not available
Common Dose Range for Use as Supplement:	50–1,000 μg/day
Do dietary patterns meeting guidelines permit Adequate intake?	Yes
Included in typical multivitamin/multimineral tablet?	Yes (25 μg)

DEFICIENCY

Intake Level: Below 50 μg/day
Syndromes: Insulin resistance, glucose intolerance

Toxicity

Intake Level: Uncertain
Syndromes: None known

Dietary Sources[o]: Chromium is found abundantly in whole foods like meats, liver, eggs, whole-grain products, brewer's yeast, seafood, nuts, and some fruits, vegetables, and spices.

Effects of Food Preparation and Storage: Processing of food may directly affect the chromium content. Processing of refined sugars, grains, and flours tends to reduce the chromium content, while acidic foods have been shown to increase chromium content if processing involves stainless steel.

Additional details, evidence, and references for dosing and safety for many nutrients and substances individuals might choose to ingest can be found at http://www.mayoclinic.com/health/search/search, http://ods.od.nih.gov/, and http://www.nlm.nih.gov/medlineplus/.

[a]Martin J, Wang ZQ, Zhang XH, et al. Chromium picolinate supplementation attenuates body weight gain and increases insulin sensitivity in subjects with type 2 diabetes. *Diabetes Care* 2006;29:1826–1832; Wang ZQ, Zhang XH, Russell JC, et al. Chromium picolinate enhances skeletal muscle cellular insulin signaling in vivo in obese, insulin-resistant JCR:LA-cp rats. *J Nutr* 2006;136:415–420; Cefalu WT, Hu FB. Role of chromium in human health and in diabetes. *Diabetes Care* 2004;27:2741–2751; Cefalu WT, Wang ZQ, Zhang XH, et al. Oral chromium picolinate improves carbohydrate and lipid metabolism and enhances skeletal muscle Glut-4 translocation in obese, hyperinsulinemic (JCR-LA corpulent) rats. *J Nutr* 2002;132:1107–1114.

[b]Preuss HG, Anderson RA. Chromium update: examining recent literature 1997–1998. *Curr Opin Clin Nutr Metab Care* 1998;1:509–512.

[c]Porter DJ, Raymond LW, Anastasio GD. Chromium: friend or foe? *Ann Fam Med* 1999;8:386–390.

[d]Trow LG, Lewis J, Greenwood RH, et al. Lack of effect of dietary chromium supplementation on glucose tolerance, plasma insulin and lipoprotein levels in patients with type 2 diabetes. *Int J Vitam Nutr Res* 2000;70:14–18.

[e]Joseph LJ, Farrell PA, Davey SL, et al. Effect of resistance training with or without chromium picolinate supplementation on glucose metabolism in older men and women. *Metabolism* 1999;48:546–553.

[f]Ravina A, Slezak L, Mirsky N, et al. Reversal of corticosteroid-induced diabetes mellitus with supplemental chromium. *Diabet Med* 1999;16:164–167.

[g]Young PC, Turiansky GW, Bonner MW, et al. Acute generalized exanthematous pustulosis induced by chromium picolinate. *J Am Acad Dermatol* 1999;41:820–823.

[h]Lukaski HC. Chromium as a supplement. *Annu Rev Nutr* 1999;19:279–302.

[i]Anderson RA. Chromium, glucose intolerance and diabetes. *J Am Coll Nutr* 1998;17:548–555.

[j]Vincent JB. The potential value and toxicity of chromium picolinate as a nutritional supplement, weight loss agent and muscle development agent. *Sports Med* 2003;33:213–230.

[k]Althuis MD, Jordan NE, Ludington EA, et al. Glucose and insulin responses to dietary chromium supplements: a meta-analysis. *Am J Clin Nutr* 2002;76:148–155.

[l]Clarkson PM, Rawson ES. Nutritional supplements to increase muscle mass. *Crit Rev Food Sci Nutr* 1999;39:317–328.

[m]Vincent JB. The potential value and toxicity of chromium picolinate as a nutritional supplement, weight loss agent and muscle development agent. *Sports Med* 2003;33:213–230; Pittler MH, Stevinson C, Ernst E. Chromium picolinate for reducing body weight: meta-analysis of randomized trials. *Int J Obes Relat Metab Disord* 2003;27:522–529.

[n]Eaton SB, Eaton SB. Paleolithic vs. modern diets—selected pathophysiological implications. *Eur J Nutr* 2000;39:67–70.

[o]Chromium content is not routinely listed in the USDA nutrient database (http://www.nal.usda.gov/fnic/foodcomp/search).

Sources: Ensminger AH, Ensminger ME, Konlande JE, et al. *The concise encyclopedia of foods and nutrition.* Boca Raton, FL: CRC Press, Inc., 1995.

Margen S. *The wellness nutrition counter.* New York, NY: Health Letter Associates, 1997.

Murray MT. *Encyclopedia of nutritional supplements.* Rocklin, CA: Prima Publishing, 1996.

National Research Council. *Recommended dietary allowances*, 10th ed. Washington, DC: National Academy Press, 1989.

Otten JJ, Hellwig JP, Meyers LD, eds. *Dietary reference intakes. The essential guide to nutrient requirements.* Washington, DC: National Academies Press, 2006.

Pizzorno JE, Murray MT. *Textbook of natural medicine*, 3rd ed. St. Louis, MO: Church Livingstone Elsevier, 2006.

Shils ME, Shike M, Ross AC, et al., eds. *Modern nutrition in health and disease*, 10th ed. Philadelphia, PA: Lippincott Williams & Wilkins, 2005.

US Department of Agriculture. *USDA nutrient database for standard reference.* Release 19. 2006.

US Department of Agriculture. *USDA nutrient intake from NHANES 2001–2002 data.*

Ziegler EE, Filer LJ Jr, eds. *Present knowledge in nutrition*, 7th ed. Washington, DC: ILSI Press, 1996.

COENZYME Q$_{10}$/UBIQUINONE

BIOLOGICAL FUNCTION(S) IN HUMANS/KEY PROPERTIES: Functions in electron transport and as an antioxidant, quenching free radicals. Involved in the generation of adenosine triphosphate (ATP) in mitochondria. May contribute to exercise capacity. Can be synthesized endogenously.

ABSORPTION/SOLUBILITY/STORAGE/PHARMACOKINETICS: Coenzyme Q$_{10}$ absorption is limited in the small intestine because of its lipid-soluble nature. Higher absorption is therefore observed when coenzyme Q$_{10}$ is taken with meals in combination with a higher lipid load. Upon absorption, coenzyme Q$_{10}$ is packaged inside chylomicrons for transport to the liver. The nutrient is later released into circulation in a combination of lipoproteins to reach its target tissues. Coenzyme Q$_{10}$ is a benzoquinone, also known as ubiquinone because of its remarkably widespread distribution in nature and in virtually every cell in the human body. Metabolically active tissues and cells (e.g., heart, liver, kidney, muscle) have the highest coenzyme Q$_{10}$ requirements and concentrations. The major excretory pathway is through biliary and fecal passing, with smaller amounts seen in urine excretion.[a]

RATIONALE FOR SUPPLEMENTATION: Generation of ATP in myocardium; antioxidant effects. Recommended for CHF and coronary disease. Because coenzyme Q$_{10}$ shares a common metabolic pathway with the production of cholesterol, HMG-CoA reductase inhibitors (statins) are shown to cause a depletion of coenzyme Q$_{10}$.[b] May be beneficial in a wide range of disease states associated with oxidative injury. Preserves vitamin E and vitamin C levels.

EVIDENCE IN SUPPORT OF SUPPLEMENTATION TO AND ABOVE THE DRI: No RDA or AI established. There have been numerous animal and observational studies. There are positive results from double-blind, placebo-controlled studies in humans, in particular for use in CHF (see Chapter 7); a meta-analysis suggests improved ejection fraction with coenzyme Q10 supplementation in CHF.[c] Coenzyme Q$_{10}$ may also improve endothelial function[d] and ameliorate myalgia associated with use of statins, although a systematic review showed insufficient evidence for coenzyme Q$_{10}$ deficiency leading to statin-associated myopathy and concluded that the routine use of coenzyme Q$_{10}$ cannot be recommended in statin-treated patients.[e] Solubilized forms of coenzyme Q$_{10}$ tend to show the most benefit. Coenzyme Q10 helps protect the heart from the damaging side effects of the cancer drug, doxorubicin.[f] More widespread use of coenzyme Q$_{10}$ in cardiology and primary care practice appears to warrant consideration, although definitive evidence of benefit is for the most part lacking. Randomized controlled trials (RCTs) have shown no evidence of benefit for fatigue, arterial stiffness, metabolic parameters, inflammatory markers, or blood pressure.[g] The usual doses in trials range from 100–300 mg/day (1–2 mg/kg/day). Such doses appear safe, with virtually no reports of significant toxicity.[h]

Recommended Intake Range (US RDA): None established.

AVERAGE INTAKE, US ADULTS:	Unknown
ESTIMATED MEAN PALEOLITHIC INTAKE (ADULT)[i]:	Unknown
COMMON DOSE RANGE FOR USE AS SUPPLEMENT:	30–1,200 mg/day; 1–2 mg/kg/day
DO DIETARY PATTERNS MEETING GUIDELINES PERMIT INTAKE IN THE SUPPLEMENT RANGE?	No
INCLUDED IN TYPICAL MULTIVITAMIN/MULTIMINERAL TABLET?	No

DEFICIENCY

Intake Level: Unknown.
Syndromes: Unknown.

TOXICITY

Intake Level: Unknown.
Syndromes: Unknown.

Dietary Sources[j]: Coenzyme Q$_{10}$ is known as ubiquinone due to its ubiquitous distribution in nature. While widely distributed in both plant and animal foods, however, dietary sources do not allow for intake in the supplement range. The concentration of ubiquinone in various foods has been studied, but not systematically reported. Foods such as meats, fish, vegetables, and fruits appear to contain decent sources for replenishment of coenzyme Q$_{10}$.[k]

Effects of Food Preparation and Storage: Not reported to be a generally important determinant of dietary intake levels.

Additional details, evidence, and references for dosing and safety for many nutrients and substances individuals might choose to ingest can be found at http://www.mayoclinic.com/health/search/search, http://ods.od.nih.gov/, and http://www.nlm.nih.gov/medlineplus/.

[a]Bhagavan HN, Chopra RK. Coenzyme Q$_{10}$: absorption, tissue uptake, metabolism and pharmacokinetics. *Free Radic Res* 2006;40:445–453.

[b]Nawarskas JJ. HMG-CoA reductase inhibitors and coenzyme Q$_{10}$. *Cardiol Rev* 2005;13:76–79.

[c]Fotino AD, Thompson-Paul AM, Bazzano LA. Effect of coenzyme Q$_{10}$ supplementation on heart failure: a meta-analysis. *Am J Clin Nutr* 2013;97(2):268–275. doi:10.3945/ajcn.112.040741.

[d]Gao L, Mao Q, Cao J, et al. Effects of coenzyme Q_{10} on vascular endothelial function in humans: a meta-analysis of randomized controlled trials. *Atherosclerosis* 2012;221(2):311–316. doi:10.1016/j.atherosclerosis.2011.10.027.

[e]Marcoff L, Thompson, PD. The role of coenzyme Q_{10} in statin-associated myopathy: a systematic review. *J Am Coll Cardiol* 2007;49:2231–2237.

[f]NCI—*Coenzyme Q10*. Available at http://www.cancer.gov/cancertopics/pdq/cam/coenzymeQ10/patient; accessed 9/27/2013.

[g]Lee YJ, Cho WJ, Kim JK, et al. Effects of coenzyme Q_{10} on arterial stiffness, metabolic parameters, and fatigue in obese subjects: a double-blind randomized controlled study. *J Med Food* 2011;14:386–390; Ho MJ, Bellusci A, Wright JM. Blood pressure lowering efficacy of coenzyme Q10 for primary hypertension (review). *Cochrane Database Syst Rev* 2009:CD007435.

[h]Hathcock JN, Shao A. Risk assessment for coenzyme Q_{10} (ubiquinone). *Regul Toxicol Pharmacol* 2006;45:282–288.

[i]Eaton SB, Eaton SB. Paleolithic vs. modern diets—selected pathophysiological implications. *Eur J Nutr* 2000;39:67–70.

[j]The USDA nutrient database does not currently report ubiquinone content.

[k]Weant KA, Smith KM. The role of coenzyme Q_{10} in heart failure. *Ann Pharmacother* 2005;39:1522–1526.

Sources: Ensminger AH, Ensminger ME, Konlande JE, et al. *The concise encyclopedia of foods and nutrition.* Boca Raton, FL: CRC Press, Inc., 1995.

Margen S. *The wellness nutrition counter.* New York, NY: Health Letter Associates, 1997.

Murray MT. *Encyclopedia of nutritional supplements.* Rocklin, CA: Prima Publishing, 1996.

Otten JJ, Hellwig JP, Meyers LD, eds. *Dietary reference intakes. The essential guide to nutrient requirements.* Washington, DC: National Academies Press, 2006.

Pizzorno JE, Murray MT. *Textbook of natural medicine,* 3rd ed. St. Louis, MO: Church Livingstone Elsevier, 2006.

Shils ME, Shike M, Ross AC, et al., eds. *Modern nutrition in health and disease,* 10th ed. Philadelphia, PA: Lippincott Williams & Wilkins, 2005.

US Department of Agriculture. *USDA nutrient database for standard reference.* Release 19. 2006.

US Department of Agriculture. *USDA nutrient intake from NHANES 2001–2002 data.*

Ziegler EE, Filer LJ, Jr, eds. *Present knowledge in nutrition,* 7th ed. Washington, DC: ILSI Press, 1996.

CREATINE

BIOLOGICAL FUNCTION(S) IN HUMANS/KEY PROPERTIES: Creatine is synthesized endogenously from the amino acids glycine and arginine and available methyl groups. Concentrated in skeletal muscle and brain, creatine functions in energy metabolism, supplying energy to muscle cells and neurons.

ABSORPTION/SOLUBILITY/STORAGE/PHARMACOKINETICS: Creatine is a water-soluble molecule synthesized from amino acids in the kidney and liver and transported for use to skeletal muscles.[a] Its absorptions, storage, and pharmacokinetics are largely unknown. Muscle creatine rises with supplementation, apparently to a maximum level of approximately 20% above baseline with supplementation in the range of 3 g/day.[b] Urinary excretion of creatinine rises with creatine loading. Ingesting carbohydrates with creatine can increase muscle creatine levels more than ingesting creatine alone.[c]

RATIONALE FOR SUPPLEMENTATION: Enhanced athletic performance. Possible improved endurance in patients with heart failure and improved muscle strength in people with muscular dystrophies.

EVIDENCE IN SUPPORT OF SUPPLEMENTATION TO AND ABOVE THE DRI: No RDA or AI established. Numerous double-blind, randomized, and crossover studies showing improved work output with creatine supplementation. Most studies have been small and of short duration.[d] Evidence of benefit for sustained activity appears less convincing than evidence for an effect on short-burst activity. The available literature includes both positive and negative studies (see Chapter 32). Creatinine appears to enhance select athletic performance, lean muscle mass, and peak muscle strength but provides no statistically significant improvements in swimming, running, peak torque, or acceleration times.[e] Meta-analyses support the benefits of creatine supplementation in people with muscular dystrophies and neuromuscular disorders.[f]

Recommended Intake Range (US RDA): Unknown.

AVERAGE INTAKE, US ADULTS:	Unknown; daily turnover in an adult male is estimated at 2 g/day[g]
ESTIMATED MEAN PALEOLITHIC INTAKE (ADULT)[h]:	Unknown; Paleolithic dietary patterns likely resulted in higher intake than do current patterns.
COMMON DOSE RANGE FOR USE AS SUPPLEMENT:	Approximately 2–10 g/day.
DO DIETARY PATTERNS MEETING GUIDELINES PERMIT INTAKE IN THE SUPPLEMENT RANGE?	No
INCLUDED IN TYPICAL MULTIVITAMIN/MULTIMINERAL TABLET?	No

DEFICIENCY

Intake Level: None; creatine can by synthesized endogenously. Genetic deficiencies in synthesizing creatine lead to severe neurological defects

Syndromes: None known

TOXICITY

Intake Level: Unknown

TOLERABLE UPPER INTAKE LEVEL (UL): Creatine has been used in doses as high as 20 g/day in heart failure and as loading doses for athletic performance with apparently no adverse effects.[c]

Syndromes: Unknown; side effects with common dosing are limited largely to gastrointestinal cramping and weight gain.

Dietary Sources: Dietary sources of creatine are not systematically reported. Creatine is abundant in red meat and fish.

Effects of Food Preparation and Storage: Not available.

Additional details, evidence, and references for dosing and safety for many nutrients and substances individuals might choose to ingest can be found at http://www.mayoclinic.com/health/search/search, http://ods.od.nih.gov/, and http://www.nlm.nih.gov/medlineplus/.

[a]MayoClinic. *Creatinine.* Available at http://www.mayoclinic.com/health/creatine/NS_patient-creatine; accessed 9/27/2013.

[b]Hultman E. Soderlund K, Timmons JA, et al. Muscle creatine loading in men. *J Appl Physiol* 1996;81:232–237.

[c]MedlinePlus. *Creatinine.* Available at http://www.nlm.nih.gov/medlineplus/druginfo/natural/873.html; accessed 9/27/2013.

[d]Mujika I, Padilla S. Creatine supplementation as an ergogenic acid for sports performance in highly trained athletes: a critical review. *Int J Sports Med* 1997;18:491–496; Jones AM, Carter H, Pringle JSM, et al. Effect of creatine supplementation on oxygen uptake kinetics during submaximal cycle exercise. *J Appl Physiol* 2002;92:2571–2577.

[e]Branch JD. Effect of creatine supplementation on body composition and performance: a meta-analysis. *Int J Sport Nutr Exerc Metab* 2003;13(2):198–226; Cramer JT, Stout JR, Culbertson JY, et al. Effects of creatine supplementation and three days of resistance training on muscle strength, power output, and neuromuscular function. *J Strength Cond Res* 2007;21(3):668–677; Dempsey RL, Mazzone MF, Meurer LN. Does oral creatine supplementation improve strength? A meta-analysis. *J Fam Pract* 2002;51(11):945–951.

[f]Kley RA, Vorgerd M, Tarnopolsky MA. Creatine for treating muscle disorders. *Cochrane Database Syst Rev* 2007;1:CD004760.

[g]Balsom PD, Soderlund K, Ekblom B. Creatine in humans with special reference to creatine supplementation. *Sports Med* 1994;18:268–280.

[h]Eaton SB, Eaton SB. Paleolithic vs. modern diets—selected pathophysiological implications. *Eur J Nutr* 2000;39:67–70.

Sources: Ensminger AH, Ensminger ME, Konlande JE, et al. *The concise encyclopedia of foods and nutrition.* Boca Raton, FL: CRC Press, Inc., 1995.

Margen S. *The wellness nutrition counter.* New York, NY: Health Letter Associates, 1997.

Murray MT. *Encyclopedia of nutritional supplements.* Rocklin, CA: Prima Publishing, 1996.

Otten JJ, Hellwig JP, Meyers LD, eds. *Dietary reference intakes. The essential guide to nutrient requirements.* Washington, DC: National Academies Press, 2006.

Pizzorno JE, Murray MT. *Textbook of natural medicine,* 3rd ed. St. Louis, MO: Church Livingstone Elsevier, 2006.

Shils ME, Shike M, Ross AC, et al., eds. *Modern nutrition in health and disease,* 10th ed. Philadelphia, PA: Lippincott Williams & Wilkins, 2005.

US Department of Agriculture. *USDA nutrient database for standard reference.* Release 19. 2006.

US Department of Agriculture. *USDA nutrient intake from NHANES 2001–2002 data.*

Ziegler EE, Filer LJ Jr, eds. *Present knowledge in nutrition,* 7th ed. Washington, DC: ILSI Press, 1996.

ESSENTIAL FATTY ACIDS

BIOLOGICAL FUNCTION(S) IN HUMANS/KEY PROPERTIES: Essential fatty acids (EFAs) are those polyunsaturated fatty acids (PUFAs) required in metabolism that cannot be synthesized endogenously. The two classes of EFAs are n-6 and n-3. Linoleic acid is an essential n-6 fatty acid (C_{18}; i.e., 18 carbons in its chain) that is a precursor to arachidonic acid (C_{20}); when linoleic acid intake is deficient, arachidonic acid becomes an essential nutrient as well. The other EFA is [a]-linolenic (ALA) acid, a n-3 with 18 carbons. Linolenic acid is a precursor to eicosapentaenoic acid (EPA; C_{20}) and docosahexaenoic acid (DHA; C_{22}). However, the efficiency of EPA, and particularly DHA, synthesis from linolenic acid is in question. Animal evidence suggests that supplementation with DHA more effectively raises tissue levels of DHA than does supplementation with ALA.[a,b] EFAs in phospholipids are key structural components of cellular and subcellular membranes. They are metabolic precursors of eicosanoids with a wide range of effects, from inflammatory reactions and immunity to platelet aggregation. DHA is concentrated in the brain and retina.

ABSORPTION/SOLUBILITY/STORAGE/PHARMACOKINETICS: The absorption of ingested fatty acids is highly efficient, ranging from 95% to nearly 100%. Ingested fat releases fatty acids (see Chapter 2) that can be utilized immediately as a fuel source, stored as triglyceride in adipose tissue, or used in anabolism. Changes in dietary intake of EFAs are reflected in tissue stores over a period of days to weeks. Animal data suggest that PUFAs, including EFAs, may be preferentially released from adipose tissue in response to catabolic stimuli.[c] A predominance of n-6 over n-3 fatty acids in the diet fosters preferential synthesis of the products of n-6 FA metabolism, as EFAs of both classes utilize the same enzyme systems. With the exception of γ-linolenic acid (GLA), the products of n-6 fatty acid metabolism tend to be proinflammatory leukotrienes and prostaglandins that promote platelet aggregation, while the products of n-3 fatty acid metabolism generally have opposite effects. Thus, an imbalance in EFA intake in favor of the n-6 class may contribute to inflammation and a prothrombotic tendency. GLA, although of the n-6 class, uniquely bypasses the rate-limiting enzyme (Δ6 desaturase) in EFA metabolism and, as a result, preferentially leads to the synthesis of prostaglandins in the 1 series, which have anti-inflammatory and antiplatelet effects, as well as the suppression of proinflammatory cytokine synthesis.[d–g]

RATIONALE FOR SUPPLEMENTATION: There is no RDA per se for EFAs, and overt deficiency syndromes are exceedingly rare when dietary intake is basically adequate; EFA deficiency is generally associated with abnormal nurture (e.g., parenteral nutrition, starvation). However, n-6 fatty acid intake in the United States is considerably greater than n-3 fatty acid intake due to the wide distribution of linoleic acid in commonly used vegetable oils. Approximately 7% of the energy in a typical diet in the United States is derived from linoleic acid. In contrast, the distribution of linolenic acid is narrow, and intake levels are low. Unlike most other nutrients with nutriceutical applications, fatty acids are ingested at a macro level, contributing appreciably to energy intake. Therefore, there is no rationale per se for megadosing of any fatty acid, and such a practice would carry with it the risk of excess energy intake or displacement of other vital nutrients from the diet. The underlying rationale for supplementation of either n-3 fatty acids or GLA is to reduce the synthesis of inflammatory cytokines and platelet-stimulating prostaglandins and preferentially support the synthesis of anti-inflammatory cytokines by shifting the distribution of fatty acids in the diet.

EVIDENCE IN SUPPORT OF SUPPLEMENTATION TO AND ABOVE THE DRI: There is no RDA for EFAs per se, but the adequate intake level established by the Institute of Medicine in 2002 is 1.1 g/day and 1.6 g/day of α-linolenic acid for adult women and men, respectively. There is no reference intake for the other EFAs. There is suggestive evidence for the therapeutic use of supplemental EFAs in a wide range of inflammatory conditions and convincing evidence in the aggregate for shifting the distribution of EFAs from the now prevailing pattern in the United States to a more balanced distribution of n-3s and n-6s to promote health. The typical diet in the United States provides n-6 to n-3 fatty acids in a ratio of at least 10:1, with roughly 7% of calories derived from EFAs. An intake ratio of n-6 to n-3 of between 4:1 and 1:1 is thought to be preferable and health promoting, although conclusive evidence is not available. There is no clear evidence that total EFA intake should be increased, and there is at least suggestive evidence that substituting dietary linoleic acid for saturated fats increases the rates of death from cardiovascular disease and all causes.[h] Total PUFA intake in the range of 10%–15% of calories is consistent with recommendations for diet and general health promotion (see Chapter 45). Relatively greater intake of n-3 fatty acids is supported by studies of cognitive development and visual acuity in infants (see Chapters 27 and 29); by studies of chronic inflammatory conditions (see Chapters 11, 20, 22–24); by studies of cardiovascular disease (see Chapter 7); and , to a lesser extent, by the cancer prevention literature (see Chapter 12). Studies of prostate cancer specifically have produced inconsistent results, with some studies suggesting an increased risk of prostate cancer with ALA.[i] Convincing evidence is available of benefit from n-3 fatty acid supplementation at a daily dose of 3 g of EPA and DHA in combination in rheumatoid arthritis.[j] A similar benefit has been suggested in inflammatory bowel disease, but the evidence is less consistent and therefore must be considered preliminary.[k] Supplementation of the maternal diet with DHA during pregnancy has theoretical support and is unlikely to be harmful but is as yet not supported by conclusive outcome studies.[l,m] Evidence of benefit of DHA in infant nutrition is convincing with regard to visual acuity[n] and suggestive in the area of cognitive development.[o,p] In the aggregate, evidence of cardiovascular benefit from fish oil supplementation is convincing[q] (see Chapter 7). The immunologic effects of n-3 fatty acids are convincingly favorable in inflammatory states but may be disadvantageous in relatively immunocompromised individuals; concurrent vitamin E supplementation may prevent attendant immunosuppression.[r] A potential beneficial role in inflammatory diseases of the lung (e.g., asthma, bronchitis) has been suggested[s] (see Chapter 15).

There is some evidence that n-6 fatty acids may act as promoters in carcinogenesis, while n-3 fatty acids have the opposite effect. Therapeutic applications of GLA are supported by diverse sources of evidence as well. A 2000 study demonstrated an accelerated clinical response in patients with endocrine receptor-positive breast cancer treated with GLA (2.8 g/day) in addition to tamoxifen as compared to tamoxifen alone.[t] Inhibition of atherogenesis with GLA has been demonstrated *in vitro* and in animal studies.[u] A therapeutic role for GLA in atopic eczema is convincingly supported by available evidence.[v] A benefit of GLA in rheumatologic conditions[w] and diabetic neuropathy[x] is suggested.

Recommended Intake Range (US RDA): There is much uncertainty about the optimal percentage of daily calories that should come from fat, the percentage of this total that should derive from PUFAs, and the percentage of PUFAs that should be ALA, EPA, or DHA. The Food and Agriculture Organization of the United Nations and World Health Organization (FAO/WHO), based on varying levels of imperfect evidence, recommend that for adults, 15%–35% of total daily energy comes from dietary fat and 6%–11% of total daily energy comes from PUFAs. Somewhere between 2.5% and 9% of total daily energy should be from n-6 PUFAs and 0.5%–2% of total daily energy from n-3 PUFAs, with >0.5% of total daily energy form ALA and 0.25%–2% of total daily energy from DHA+EPA specifically. Recommended percentages for fat and PUFAs are higher for children and adolescents[y].

ESSENTIAL FATTY ACIDS RECOMMENDED INTAKE RANGE (US AI): n-6, LINOLEIC ACID/AI

	Infancy (age 0–6 mo)	Infancy (age 7–12 mo)	Childhood (age 1–3 y)	Childhood (age 4–8 y)
Male	4.4 g	4.6 g	7 g	10 g
Female	4.4 g	4.6 g	7 g	10 g

	Adolescence (age 9–13 y)	Adolescence (age 14–18 y)	Adult (age 19–50 y)	Adult (age ≥ 51 y)
Male	12 g	16 g	17 g	14 g
Female	10 g	11 g	12 g	11 g

	Pregnancy (all ages)	Lactation (all ages)		
Male	—	—		
Female	13 g	13 g		

N-3, α-LINOLENIC ACID/AI

	Infancy (age 0–6 mo)	Infancy (age 7–12 mo)	Childhood (age 1–3 y)	Childhood (age 4–8 y)
Male	0.5 g	0.5 g	0.7 g	0.9 g
Female	0.5 g	0.5 g	0.7 g	0.9 g

	Adolescence (age 9–13 y)	Adolescence (age 14–18 y)	Adult (age 19–50 y)	Adult (age ≥ 51 y)
Male	1.2 g	1.6 g	1.6 g	1.6 g
Female	1.0 g	1.6 g	1.1 g	1.1 g
Male	—	—		
Female	1.4 g	1.3 g		

AVERAGE INTAKE, US ADULTS:	Total EFA: approximately 7%–10% of calories; n-6 to n-3 ratio: between 10:1 and 20:1
ESTIMATED MEAN PALEOLITHIC INTAKE (ADULT)[z]:	Total EFA: approximately 7%–10% of calories; n-6 to n-3 ratio: between 4:1 and 1:1

Paleolithic intake of n-3 fatty acids is thought to have been considerably greater than that in most industrialized countries in part because the meat of wild ungulates is rich in n-3 fatty acids. Thus, the Paleolithic diet is thought to have provided n-3 fatty acids from sources other than marine animals.

COMMON DOSE RANGE FOR USE AS SUPPLEMENT:	Fish oil: 5–15 g/day (generally a combination of EPA and DHA) ALA: approximately 10 g/day GLA: approximately 1.5–3 g/day

(continued)

APPENDIX E   (Continued)

DO DIETARY PATTERNS MEETING GUIDELINES PERMIT INTAKE IN THE SUPPLEMENT RANGE? Generally no; possibly, if intake of certain fish (e.g., salmon, mackerel), other marine animals, or wild game is unusually high. Of note, the n-3 fatty acid content of fish is derived from the algae and phytoplankton the fish ingest. Fish raised commercially tend to have a much reduced n-3 fatty acid content in their diet and therefore a much lower n-3 content in their flesh (much like what has occurred with the domestication of cattle). While the efficiency of conversion of ALA to EPA and especially DHA is questionable, dietary supplementation with ALA appears to provide most of the health benefit of directly ingesting the longer-chain n-3s. Given the potential importance of EFAs in health promotion, and the disproportionate representation of n-6 PUFAs in the Western diet, a general recommendation for increasing ALA in the diet is reasonable. The recommended dose of approximately 10 g/day can be obtained by using 1–2 tablespoons of flaxseed (flax) oil daily. Flaxseed oil is available in health food stores. It can be used on salads and in cold dishes but is not suitable for cooking (which changes the oil and its chemical and health properties). Vitamin E requirements rise with intake of PUFAs, and therefore vitamin E supplementation in conjunction with regular EFA ingestion is not unreasonable (see "Vitamin E"). Flaxseed oil might be used to displace other less-healthy or less-needed fats from the diet (particularly *trans* fats, and n-6 PUFAs).

INCLUDED IN TYPICAL MULTIVITAMIN/MULTIMINERAL TABLET? No

DEFICIENCY

Intake Level:	EFAs <1% of calories
Syndromes:	Dry skin; hair loss; immunosuppression

Toxicity

Intake Level:	Variable; dependent in part on the ratio of n-6 to n-3
Syndromes:	Pro-oxidant effects; cancer promotion; bleeding diathesis/platelet dysfunction

α-linolenic Acid (ALA) Dietary Sources[b]

Food	Serving Size	Energy (kcal)	ALA (g)
Canola oil	1 tablespoon (14 g)	124	1.3
Flax (flaxseed) oil	1 tablespoon (13.6 g)	110	7.2
Kale	1 cup (67 g)	3	0.1
Soybean oil	1 tablespoon (13.6 g)	120	0.9
Spinach	2 cups (30 g)	14	0.1

Docosahexaenoic Acid (DHA) Dietary Sources:

Food	Serving Size	Energy (kcal)	DHA (g)
Mackerel (Atlantic)	1 fillet (112 g)	230	1.6
Oysters (cooked)	6 medium (150 g)	244	0.8
Salmon (Atlantic)	1/2 fillet (198 g)	281	2.2
Sardines (canned in oil)	1 can (92 g)	191	0.5
Scallops (raw)	3 oz. (85 g)	75	0.1

Eicosapentaenoic Acid (EPA) Dietary Sources:

Food	Serving Size	Energy (kcal)	EPA (g)
Mackerel (Atlantic)	1 fillet (112 g)	230	1.0
Oysters (cooked)	6 medium (150 g)	244	1.3
Salmon (Atlantic)	1/2 fillet (198 g)	281	0.6
Sardines (canned in oil)	1 can (92 g)	191	0.4
Scallops (raw)	3 oz. (85 g)	75	0.08

δ-linolenic Acid (GLA) (Medicinal Oils):

Food	Dose	Energy (kcal)	GLA (g)
Black currant seed oil	1 tablespoon (13.6 g)	120	2.3
Borage seed oil	1 tablespoon (13.6 g)	102	3.0
Evening primrose oil	1 tablespoon (13.6 g)	120	1.2

Linoleic Acid Dietary Sources[a1]:

Food	Serving Size	Energy (kcal)	Linoleic Acid (g)
Corn oil	1 tablespoon (13.6 g)	120	7.2
Flax (flaxseed) oil	1 tablespoon (13.6 g)	120	1.7
Safflower oil	1 tablespoon (13.6 g)	120	10.1
Sunflower oil	1 tablespoon (13.6 g)	120	8.9

Effects of Food Preparation and Storage: Expeller-pressing is the preferred extraction method for oil. Hydrogenation enhances the commercial properties of PUFAs at the expense of their health effects; "partial hydrogenation" produces trans stereoisomers (i.e., *trans* fats). PUFAs are susceptible to degradation when exposed to light and/or heat; opaque, plastic packaging is preferred. Oils rich in n-3 fatty acids are particularly heat intolerant and generally cannot be used for cooking.

Additional details, evidence, and references for dosing and safety for many nutrients and substances individuals might choose to ingest can be found at http://www.mayoclinic.com/health/search/search, http://ods.od.nih.gov/, and http://www.nlm.nih.gov/medlineplus/.

[a]Abedin L, Lien EL, Vingrys AJ, et al. The effects of dietary α-linolenic acid compared with docosahexaenoic acid on brain, retina, liver, and heart in the guinea pig. *Lipids* 1999;34:475–482.

[b]Su HM, Bernardo L, Mirmiran M, et al. Bioequivalence of dietary α-linolenic and docosahexaenoic acids as sources of docosahexaeno-ate accretion in brain and associated organs of neonatal baboons. *Pediatr Res* 1999;45:87–93.

[c]Conner WE, Lin DS, Colvis C. Differential mobilization of fatty acids from adipose tissue. *J Lipid Res* 1996;37:290–298.

[d]Dirks J, van Aswegen CH, du Plessis DJ. Cytokine levels affected by gamma-linolenic acid. *Prostaglandins Leukot Essent Fatty Acids* 1998;59:273–277.

[e]Villalobos MA, De La Cruz JP, Martin-Romero M, et al. Effect of dietary supplementation with evening primrose oil on vascular throm-bogenesis in hyperlipemic rabbits. *Thromb Haemost* 1998;80:696–701.

[f]Wu D, Meydani M, Leka LS, et al. Effect of dietary supplementation with black currant seed oil on the immune response of healthy elderly subjects. *Am J Clin Nutr* 1999;70:536–543.

[g]Fan YY, Chapkin RS. Importance of dietary gamma-linolenic acid in human health and nutrition. *J Nutr* 1998;128:1411–1414.

[h]Ramsden CE, Zamora D, Leelarthaepin B, et al. Use of dietary linoleic acid for secondary prevention of coronary heart disease and death: evaluation of recovered data from the Sydney Diet Heart Study and updated meta-analysis. *BMJ* 2013;346:e8707

[i]Simon JA, Chen YH, Bent S. The relation of alpha-linolenic acid to the risk of prostate cancer: a systematic review and meta-analysis. *Am J Clin Nutr* 2009;89(5):1558S–1564S. doi: 10.3945/ajcn.2009.26736E; Carayol M, Grosclaude P, Delpierre C. Prospective studies of dietary alpha-linolenic acid intake and prostate cancer risk: a meta-analysis. *Cancer Causes Control* 2010;21(3):347–355. doi:10.1007/s10552-009-9465-1.

[j]Kremer JM. n-3 Fatty acid supplements in rheumatoid arthritis. *Am J Clin Nutr* 2000;71:349s–351s.

[k]Belluzzi A, Boschi S, Brignola C, et al. Polyunsaturated fatty acids and inflammatory bowel disease. *Am J Clin Nutr* 2000;71:339s–342s.

[l]Al MD, van Houwelingen AC, Hornstra G. Long-chain polyunsaturated fatty acids, pregnancy, and pregnancy outcome. *Am J Clin Nutr* 2000;71:285s–291s.

[m]Makrides M, Gibson RA. Long-chain polyunsaturated fatty acid requirements during pregnancy and lactation. *Am J Clin Nutr* 2000;71:307s–311s.

[n]Neuringer M. Infant vision and retinal function in studies of dietary long-chain polyunsaturated fatty acids: methods, results, and impli-cations. *Am J Clin Nutr* 2000;71:256s–267s.

[o]Morley R. Nutrition and cognitive development. *Nutrition* 1998;14:752–754.

[p]Innis SM. Essential fatty acids in infant nutrition: lessons and limitations from animal studies in relation to studies on infant fatty acid requirements. *Am J Clin Nutr* 2000;71:238s–244s.

[q]Nestel PJ. Fish oil and cardiovascular disease: lipids and arterial function. *Am J Clin Nutr* 2000;71:228s–231s.

[r]Wu D, Meydani SN. n-3 polyunsaturated fatty acids and immune function. *Proc Nutr Soc* 1998;57:503–509.

[s]Schwartz J. Role of polyunsaturated fatty acids in lung disease. *Am J Clin Nutr* 2000;71:393s–296s.

[t]Kenny FS, Pinder SE, Ellis IO, et al. Gamma linolenic acid with tamoxifen as primary therapy in breast cancer. *Int J Cancer* 2000;85:643–648.

[u]Fan YY, Ramos KS, Chapkin RS. Modulation of atherogenesis by dietary gamma-linolenic acid. *Adv Exp Med Biol* 1999;469:485–491.

[v]Horrobin DF. Essential fatty acid metabolism and its modification in atopic eczema. *Am J Clin Nutr* 2000;71:367s–372s.

[w]Belch JJ, Hill A. Evening primrose oil and borage oil in rheumatologic conditions. *Am J Clin Nutr* 2000;71:352s–356s.

[x]Vinik AI. Diabetic neuropathy: pathogenesis and therapy. *Am J Med* 1999;107:17s–26s.

[y]FOA/WHO 2008. *Interim Summary of Conclusions and Dietary Recommendations on Total Fat & Fatty Acids.* http://www.who.int/nutrition/topics/FFA_summary_rec_conclusion.pdf

(continued)

APPENDIX E   (Continued)

[z]Eaton SB, Eaton SB III, Konner MJ. Paleolithic nutrition revisited: a twelve-year retrospective on its nature and implications. *Eur J Clin Nutr* 1997;51:207–216.

[a1]The nutrient composition of most foods can be checked by accessing the US Department of Agriculture nutrient database, at http://www.nal.usda.gov/fnic/foodcomp/search; For more information, see Goodman J.*The omega solution*. Rocklin, CA: Prima Publishing, 2001.

Sources: Ensminger AH, Ensminger ME, Konlande JE, et al. *The concise encyclopedia of foods and nutrition*. Boca Raton, FL: CRC Press, Inc., 1995.

Margen S. *The wellness nutrition counter*. New York, NY: Health Letter Associates, 1997.

Murray MT. *Encyclopedia of nutritional supplements*. Rocklin, CA: Prima Publishing, 1996.

Otten JJ, Hellwig JP, Meyers LD, eds. *Dietary reference intakes. The essential guide to nutrient requirements*. Washington, DC: National Academies Press, 2006.

Pizzorno JE, Murray MT. *Textbook of natural medicine*, 3rd ed. St. Louis, MO: Church Livingstone Elsevier, 2006.

Sardesai VM. *Introduction to clinical nutrition*. New York, NY: Marcel Dekker, Inc., 1998.

Shils ME, Shike M, Ross AC, et al., eds. *Modern nutrition in health and disease*, 10th ed. Philadelphia, PA: Lippincott Williams & Wilkins, 2005.

US Department of Agriculture. *USDA nutrient database for standard reference*. Release 19. 2006.

US Department of Agriculture. *USDA nutrient intake from NHANES 2001–2002 data*.

Ziegler EE, Filer LJ Jr, eds. *Present knowledge in nutrition*, 7th ed. Washington, DC: ILSI Press, 1996.

FIBER

BIOLOGICAL FUNCTION(S) IN HUMANS/KEY PROPERTIES: Fiber is, by definition, indigestible plant material, generally categorized along with carbohydrate. Soluble fiber dissolves in water. Dissolution of soluble fiber in the gastrointestinal tract causes delayed absorption of glucose and fatty acids, blunting postprandial rises. Soluble fiber has lipid-lowering properties and attenuates postprandial insulin release. Soluble fibers of relative importance include guar gum, psyllium, pectin, and β-glucan. Insoluble fibers, such as lignins, celluloses, and hemicelluloses, reduce GI transit time and increase fecal bulk. Both categories of fiber may increase the satiating capacity of food. Certain fibers differentially support the growth of various gut bacteria, alternating the intestinal microbiome,[a] which is emerging as a key consideration for overall health promotion and disease prevention in humans. Some of the beneficial effects of fiber through gut bacteria and their metabolites may be mediated through systemic and local anti-inflammatory activites.[a] Still, some fibers may promote gastrointestinal sensitivity. Fibers like fructans and galactans are part of a heterogeneous group of compounds collectively knows as FODMAPs (Fermentable, Oligo-, Di-, Monosaccharides, And Polyols), which may produce symptoms similar to those of gluten-sensitivity/celiac disease, irrespective of gluten intake or actual bowel inflammation. Because many gluten-containing foods also are high in FODMAPs, improved symptoms with gluten-free diets in individuals reporting gluten sensitivity might actually reflect simultaneous reduction in FODMAP intake.[b]

ABSORPTION/SOLUBILITY/STORAGE/PHARMACOKINETICS: By definition, fiber is not digested and therefore neither absorbed nor stored. However, various species of bacteria in the human colon do ferment certain dietary fibers, producing short-chain fatty acids, which are absorbed. The exact role of these fatty acids in human energy balance remains uncertain, but it is clear that fibers contribute some calories to diets in man.[c]

RATIONALE FOR SUPPLEMENTATION: There is no RDA for dietary fiber.

Intake of soluble fiber at levels above the prevailing average in the United States is associated with reductions in lipid and insulin levels. Intake of insoluble fiber at levels above the prevailing average in the United States is generally associated with reduced risk of diverticular disease and colon cancer. However, gastrointestinal intolerance tends to be dose limiting so that megadosing of fiber is not practical.

EVIDENCE IN SUPPORT OF SUPPLEMENTATION TO AND ABOVE THE DRI: No RDA or AI established. Soluble fiber supplementation is effective in lowering serum lipids even when the diet is already fat restricted.[d] Soluble fiber can also improve glycemic control in diabetes.[e] Increased intake of insoluble fiber is effective in the management of constipation, and relatively high intake of insoluble fiber is associated with reduced risk of diseases of the large bowel, from diverticulosis to cancer (see Chapters 12 and 18).

Recommended Intake Range (US RDA): There is no RDA for either total or soluble fiber.[f]

FIBER RECOMMENDED INTAKE RANGE (US AI): g/1,000 kcal (g/day)

	Infancy (age 0–6 mo)	Infancy (age 7–12 mo)	Childhood (age 1–3 y)	Childhood (age 4–8 y)
Male	—	—	14 (19)	14 (25)
Female	—	—	14 (19)	14 (25)

	Adolescence (age 9–13 y)	Adolescence (age 14–18 y)	Adult (age 19–50 y)	Adult (age ≥ 51 y)
Male	14 (31)	14 (38)	14 (38)	14 (30)
Female	14 (26)	14 (26)	14 (25)	14 (21)

	Pregnancy (all ages)	Lactation (all ages)
Male	—	—
Female	14 (28)	14 (29)

AVERAGE INTAKE, US ADULTS:	12 g/day total fiber
ESTIMATED MEAN PALEOLITHIC INTAKE (ADULT)[g]:	104 g/day total fiber
COMMON DOSE RANGE FOR USE AS SUPPLEMENT:	3–20 g/day soluble fiber
DO DIETARY PATTERNS MEETING GUIDELINES PERMIT INTAKE IN THE SUPPLEMENT RANGE?	Yes
INCLUDED IN TYPICAL MULTIVITAMIN/MULTIMINERAL TABLET?	No

DEFICIENCY

Intake Level: Variable.
Syndromes: Constipation.

TOXICITY

Intake Level: Variable.
Syndromes: Gastrointestinal intolerance; micronutrient malabsorption

(continued)

APPENDIX E   (Continued)

Dietary Sources[h]: Insoluble fiber is abundant in whole grains, especially wheat, nuts, beans, vegetables; soluble fiber is abundant in fruits, oats, lentils, peas, and beans, carrots, barley, and psyllium.

Food[i]	Serving Size	Energy (kcal)	Fiber (g)	Food[j]	Serving Size	Energy (kcal)	Fiber (g)
Wheat bran (raw)	1 cup (58 g)	125	25	Raspberries Lentils	1 cup (123 g)	64	8
Bulgur wheat (cooked)	1 cup (182 g)	151	8.2	Lentils (cooked)	1 cup (198 g)	230	15.6
Barley, pearled (cooked)	1 cup (157 g)	193	6	Chick peas	1 cup (164 g)	269	12.5
Bread, whole wheat	1 slice (28 g)	69	2	Apples	1 medium (138 g)	72	3.3
Brown rice (cooked)	1 cup (195 g)	218	3.5	Carrots	1 medium (61 g)	25	1.7
Pasta (fiber content not listed)	1 cup (140 g)	197	2.4				
Oat bran (raw)	1 cup (94 g)	231	14.5				

Effects of Food Preparation and Storage: Health effects of fiber are generally unaffected by food preparation and storage under normal conditions.

Additional details, evidence, and references for dosing and safety for many nutrients and substances individuals might choose to ingest can be found at http://www.mayoclinic.com/health/search/search, http://ods.od.nih.gov/, and http://www.nlm.nih.gov/medlineplus/.

[a]Kuo SM. The interplay between fiber and the intestinal microbiome in the inflammatory response. *Adv Nutr* 2013;4(1):16–28. doi:10.3945/an.112.003046.

[b]Biesiekierski JR, Peters SL, Newnham ED, et al. No effects of gluten in patients with self-reported non-celiac gluten sensitivity after dietary reduction of fermentable, poorly absorbed, short-chain carbohydrates. *Gastroenterology* 2013;145:320.

[c]Salyers AA, West SE, Vercellotti JR, et al. Fermentation of mucins and plant polysaccharides by anaerobic bacteria from the human colon. *Appl Environ Microbiol* 1977;34(5):529–533; Cummings JH. Short chain fatty acids in the human colon. *Gut* 1981;22:763–770. doi:10.1136/gut.22.9.763.

[d]Jenkins DJ, Kendall CW, Vidgen E, et al. The effect on serum lipids and oxidized low-density lipoprotein of supplementing self-selected low-fat diets with soluble fiber, soy, and vegetable protein foods. *Metabolism* 2000;49:67–72.

[e]Wursch P, Pi-Sunyer FX. The role of viscous soluble fiber in the metabolic control of diabetes. A review with special emphasis on cereals rich in beta-glucan. *Diabetes Care* 1997;20:1774–1780.

[f]Dietary reference intakes for energy, carbohydrate. fiber, fat, fatty acids, cholesterol, protein, and amino acids. http://fnic.nal.usda.gov/dietary-guidance/dietary-reference-intakes/dri-tables; Available at http://www.iom.edu/Global/News%20Announcements/~/media/C5CD2DD7840544979A549EC47E56A02B.ashx; accessed 9/28/2013.

[g]Eaton SB, Eaton SB III, Konner MJ. Paleolithic nutrition revisited: a twelve-year retrospective on its nature and implications. *Eur J Clin Nutr* 1997;51:207–216.

[h]The nutrient composition of most foods can be checked by accessing the US Department of Agriculture nutrient database, at http://www.nal.usda.gov/fnic/foodcomp/search.

[i]Good sources of insoluble fiber. Values for all grains are reported for cooked portions unless otherwise stated.

[j]Good sources of soluble fiber.

Sources: Ensminger AH, Ensminger ME, Konlande JE, et al. *The concise encyclopedia of foods and nutrition.* Boca Raton, FL: CRC Press, Inc., 1995.

Margen S. *The wellness nutrition counter.* New York, NY: Health Letter Associates, 1997.

Murray MT. *Encyclopedia of nutritional supplements.* Rocklin, CA: Prima Publishing, 1996.

Otten JJ, Hellwig JP, Meyers LD, eds. *Dietary reference intakes. The essential guide to nutrient requirements.* Washington, DC: National Academies Press, 2006.

Pizzorno JE, Murray MT. *Textbook of natural medicine,* 3rd ed. St. Louis, MO: Church Livingstone Elsevier, 2006.

Shils ME, Shike M, Ross AC, et al., eds. *Modern nutrition in health and disease,* 10th ed. Philadelphia, PA: Lippincott Williams & Wilkins, 2005.

US Department of Agriculture. *USDA nutrient database for standard reference.* Release 19. 2006.

US Department of Agriculture. *USDA nutrient intake from NHANES 2001–2002 data.*

Ziegler EE, Filer LJ Jr, eds. *Present knowledge in nutrition,* 7th ed. Washington, DC: ILSI Press, 1996.

FLAVONOIDS

BIOLOGICAL FUNCTION(S) IN HUMANS/KEY PROPERTIES: Flavonoids are brightly colored phenolic compounds in plants. While the class contains more than 4,000 known compounds, interest to date has focused on proanthocyanidins (procyanidolic oligomers [PCOs]), quercetin, a group of bioflavonoids in citrus (hydroxyethylrutosides [HER]), polyphenolic compounds in tea, and isoflavones in soy (see Chapter 33). Some proprietary products, such as Pycnogenol, are patented combinations of purified bioflavonoids. Flavonoids are not known as essential nutrients in humans; however, their deficiency may contribute to the manifestations of scurvy; some consider them semi-essential. Flavonoids play an important role as antioxidants. They chelate divalent cations and by doing so may preserve levels of ascorbate (vitamin C). An effect on capillary permeability under experimental conditions may be direct, or may be mediated via ascorbate.

ABSORPTION/SOLUBILITY/STORAGE/PHARMACOKINETICS: Flavonoids are water soluble; their metabolism is similar to that of ascorbate. They are in general efficiently absorbed in the upper small bowel; however, absorption may vary between food sources and supplements. Excretion is in the urine, and storage is limited. The typical American diet provides 0.15–1 g of mixed flavonoids daily.

RATIONALE FOR SUPPLEMENTATION: Supplements of various flavonoids in varying doses are used by naturopathic practitioners for health promotion and for the treatment of venous insufficiency and inflammatory conditions. PCO is advocated for its antioxidant effects at a dose of approximately 50 mg/day and for therapy of venous insufficiency or retinopathy at a dose of up to 300 mg/day. A dose of 100 mg quercetin daily is advocated for chronic inflammatory conditions such as asthma, rheumatoid arthritis, or atopy. HER is recommended at a dose in the range of 1 g/day for conditions of venous insufficiency. Up to 400 mg/day of green tea polyphenols is recommended for cancer prevention.

EVIDENCE IN SUPPORT OF SUPPLEMENTATION TO AND ABOVE THE DRI: No RDA or AI established. Flavonoids may contribute to the health benefits of various plant-based foods, but most of the evidence in support of flavonoid supplementation remains preliminary and based mostly on observations studies. RCTs of flavonoid-rich foods have shown reduced blood pressure with chocolate, reduced low-density lipoprotein (LDL) with green tea, and reduced blood pressure and LDL with soy.[a] Related to diabetes, green tea may reduce fasting blood glucose, although an RCT showed no effect on fasting blood insulin or glycosylated hemoglobin (A1c).[b] An isolated isoflavone supplement resulted in a lower incidence of prostate cancer in an RCT among Japanese men taking, but only for those 65 years of age or older.[c] Soy isoflavone might also be safe and effective for vasomotor symptoms in postmenopsual women[d] and may result in lower LDL in both sexes.[e] Semi synthetic hydroxyethylrutosides, closely related to the natural flavoid, rutin, are of clear benefit in venous insufficiency, consistently producing greater improvements in pain, cramping, swelling, and tired and restless legs than placebo.[f]

Recommended Intake Range (US RDA): There is no RDA for flavonoids, nor is there an obvious source for a generalizable recommendation for an intake range for all adults. On the basis of various lines of evidence from diverse sources, an argument could be made that total flavonoid intake in the range 1–2 g/1,000 kcal would likely offer health benefits without any appreciable risk relative to the typical American intake of <500 mg/1,000 kcal.

AVERAGE INTAKE, US ADULTS:	<1 g/day
ESTIMATED MEAN PALEOLITHIC INTAKE (ADULT)[g]:	Uncertain; likely in the range of 3–6 g/day
COMMON DOSE RANGE FOR USE AS SUPPLEMENT:	Varies with particular compound; from 50 mg to 1 g
DO DIETARY PATTERNS MEETING GUIDELINES PERMIT INTAKE IN THE SUPPLEMENT RANGE?	Yes
INCLUDED IN TYPICAL MULTIVITAMIN/MULTIMINERAL TABLET?	No

DEFICIENCY

Intake Level:	None known with certainty
Syndromes:	Vascular permeability

TOXICITY

Intake Level:	None known with certainty
Syndromes:	Pro-oxidant effects. Consuming black tea may increase blood pressure.[a]

Flavonoids Dietary Sources[h]**:** The flavonoid content of specific foods is available via the USDA database for the flavonoid content of selected foods, created in 2003 (http://www.nal.usda.gov/fnic/foodcomp/Data/Flav/flav.html).[i] Flavonoids are concentrated in the brightly colored outer layers, skin, or peel of many fruits and vegetables. Concentrated sources include citrus fruits, berries, grapes, peaches, tomatoes, red cabbage, onion, peppers, beans, sage, soy, dark chocolate, green tea, and red wine.

Effects of Food Preparation and Storage: Flavonoids are relatively heat resistant. Food processing is not thought to substantially alter flavonoid content or activity.

Additional details, evidence, and references for dosing and safety for many nutrients and substances individuals might choose to ingest can be found at http://www.mayoclinic.com/health/search/search, http://ods.od.nih.gov/, and http://www.nlm.nih.gov/medlineplus/.

[a]Hooper L, Kroon PA, Rimm EB, et al. Flavonoids, flavonoid-rich foods, and cardiovascular risk: a meta-analysis of randomized controlled trials. *Am J Clin Nutr* 2008;88(1):38–50.

(continued)

APPENDIX E   (Continued)

[b]Zheng XX, Xu YL, Li SH, et al. Effects of green tea catechins with or without caffeine on glycemic control in adults: a meta-analysis of randomized controlled trials. *Am J Clin Nutr* 2013;97(4):750–762. doi:10.3945/ajcn.111.032573.

[c]Miyanaga N, Akaza H, Hinotsu S, et al. Prostate cancer chemoprevention study: an investigative randomized control study using purified isoflavones in men with rising prostate-specific antigen. *Cancer Sci* 2012;103(1):125–130. doi: 10.1111/j.1349-7006.2011.02120.x.

[d]Nahas EA, Nahas-Neto J, Orsatti FL, et al. Efficacy and safety of a soy isoflavone extract in postmenopausal women: a randomized, double-blind, and placebo-controlled study. *Maturitas* 2007;58(3):249–258.

[e]Zhuo XG, Melby MK, Watanabe S. Soy isoflavone intake lowers serum LDL cholesterol: a meta-analysis of 8 randomized controlled trials in humans. *J Nutr* 2004;134(9):2395–400.

[f]Poynard T, Valterio C. Meta-analysis of hydroxyethylrutosides in the treatment of chronic venous insufficiency. *Vasa* 1994;23(3):244–250.

[g]Eaton SB, Eaton SB. Paleolithic vs. modern diets—selected pathophysiological implications. *Eur J Nutr* 2000;39:67–70.

[h]The nutrient composition of most foods can be checked by accessing the US Department of Agriculture nutrient database, at http://www.nal.usda.gov/fnic/foodcomp/search. Flavonoid data are available for a limited food list. See: http://www.nal.usda.gov/fnic/foodcomp/Data/Flav/flav.html.

[i] Kuhnau J. The flavonoids: A class of semi-essential food components. *World Rev Nutr Diet* 1976;24:117–191.

Sources: Ensminger AH, Ensminger ME, Konlande JE, et al. *The concise encyclopedia of foods and nutrition.* Boca Raton, FL: CRC Press, Inc., 1995.

Margen S. *The wellness nutrition counter.* New York, NY: Health Letter Associates, 1997.

Murray MT. *Encyclopedia of nutritional supplements.* Rocklin, CA: Prima Publishing, 1996.

National Research Council. *Recommended dietary allowances,* 10th ed. Washington, DC: National Academy Press, 1989.

Otten JJ, Hellwig JP, Meyers LD, eds. *Dietary reference intakes. The essential guide to nutrient requirements.* Washington, DC: National Academies Press, 2006.

Pizzorno JE, Murray MT. *Textbook of natural medicine,* 3rd ed. St. Louis, MO: Church Livingstone Elsevier, 2006.

Shils ME, Shike M, Ross AC, et al., eds. *Modern nutrition in health and disease,* 10th ed. Philadelphia, PA: Lippincott Williams & Wilkins, 2005.

US Department of Agriculture. *USDA nutrient database for standard reference.* Release 19. 2006.

US Department of Agriculture. *USDA nutrient intake from NHANES 2001–2002 data.*

Ziegler EE, Filer LJ Jr, eds. *Present knowledge in nutrition,* 7th ed. Washington, DC: ILSI Press, 1996.

FOLATE/VITAMIN B₉

BIOLOGICAL FUNCTION(S) IN HUMANS/KEY PROPERTIES: Folate, also referred to as folic acid or folacin, is a part of the B vitamin complex, and it functions in the transfer of single carbon units in metabolic processes. Folate is an essential cofactor in amino acid and nucleic acid synthesis and is thus fundamental to all cell replication.

ABSORPTION/SOLUBILITY/STORAGE/PHARMACOKINETICS: Folate is water soluble and absorbed efficiently with saturation kinetics in the jejunum. Approximately 5–10 mg is stored in the average adult, half of which is in the liver. Excretion occurs through both urine and bile.

RATIONALE FOR SUPPLEMENTATION: There is now widespread consensus that folate intake should be at least 400 μg/day to prevent neural tube defects in infants (see Chapters 27 and 29) and vascular injury due to elevated homocysteine levels in older adults (see Chapter 7).[a] While compliance with guidelines for fruit and vegetable intake could lead to the recommended level of folate from the diet, there is evidence that between 80% and 90% of adults in the United States consume less than the recommended level of folate. The usual intake of folate in the United States is thought to be approximately 280–300 μg/day in men and less in women. Nominal folate deficiency is considered the most common nutritional deficiency in the United States. Although greater folate intake could be achieved with simple dietary modification (e.g., choosing whole wheat bread over enriched white bread for >50% more folate),[b] absorption of folate in supplement form is more complete than absorption from food. Routine use of 400 μg of supplemental folate by at least women of child-bearing age and older adults may be appropriate.

A very limited literature suggests that megadoses of folate, in the range of 10 mg/day (25 times the current recommended intake level), may be beneficial in cervical dysplasia and that a dose of 15 mg/day may be beneficial in depression. In neither case is the literature adequate to support routine clinical application.

EVIDENCE IN SUPPORT OF SUPPLEMENTATION TO AND ABOVE THE DRI: The evidence that intake of at least 400 μg of folate/day around the time of conception can reduce the risk of neural tube defects is strong and is the basis for fortification of the US food supply.[c] Prenatal vitamins typically contain 1,000 μg of folate. Evidence that folate intake can influence the risk of cardiovascular disease via effects on serum homocysteine (see Chapter 7) is also strong[d,e] with some suggestive evidence for a modest benefit in stroke prevention[f] but not other vascular outcomes or mortality.[g] Baseline homocysteine level may matter.[h] Other effects on homocysteine, related to diabetes, suggest modest benefit for glycemic control with folate supplementation.[i] Beneficial effects of folate supplementation on vascular reactivity (endothelial function) have been demonstrated.[j]

Recommended Intake Range (US RDA): An intake of 400 μg/day of total folate is recommended for all adults and women of reproductive age. All women and teen girls who could become pregnant should consume 400 μg of folic acid daily from supplements, fortified foods, or both in addition to the folate they get naturally from foods.[k]

FOLATE RECOMMENDED INTAKE RANGE (US RDA):

	Infancy (age 0–6 mo)	Infancy (age 7–12 mo)	Childhood (age 1–3 y)	Childhood (age 4–8 y)	Adolescence (age 9–13 y)
Male	65 μg	80 μg	150 μg	200 μg	300 μg
Female	65 μg	80 μg	150 μg	200 μg	300 μg

	Adolescence (age 14–18 y)	Adult (age ≥ 19 y)	Pregnancy (all ages)	Lactation (all ages)
Male	400 μg	400 μg	—	—
Female	400 μg	400 μg	600 μg	500 μg

AVERAGE INTAKE, US ADULTS: 194–250 μg/day

ESTIMATED MEAN PALEOLITHIC INTAKE (ADULT)[l]: 360 μg/day

COMMON DOSE RANGE FOR USE AS SUPPLEMENT: 400–1,000 μg/day

DO DIETARY PATTERNS MEETING GUIDELINES PERMIT ADEQUATE INTAKE? Yes

INCLUDED IN TYPICAL MULTIVITAMIN/MULTIMINERAL TABLET? Yes (dose: 600 μg; prenatal vitamin dose: 1,000 μg)

DEFICIENCY

Intake Level: 100 μg/day to prevent overt deficiency; 400 μg/day to prevent nominal deficiency
Syndromes: Megaloblastic anemia; neural tube defects; hyperhomocysteinemia

TOXICITY

Intake Level: Intake at the RDA can mask vitamin B₁₂ deficiency; doses in excess of 10 mg/day (25 times DRI) may be toxic

(continued)

APPENDIX E   (Continued)

FOLATE TOLERABLE UPPER INTAKE LEVELS (UL)[m]:

	Infancy (age 0–6 mo)	Infancy (age 7–12 mo)	Childhood (age 1–3 y)	Childhood (age 4–8 y)
Male	—	—	300 μg	400 μg
Female	—	—	300 μg	400 μg

	Adolescence (age 9–13 y)	Adolescence (age 14–18 y)	Adult (age ≥ 19 y)	Pregnancy (age 14–18 y)
Male	600 μg	800 μg	1,000 μg	—
Female	600 μg	800 μg	1,000 μg	800 μg

	Pregnancy (age 19–50 y)	Lactation (age 14–18 y)	Lactation (age 19–50 y)
Male	—	—	—
Female	1,000 μg	800 μg	1,000 μg

Syndromes: Masking vitamin B_{12} deficiency with resultant neurologic sequelae; seizures in susceptible individuals with megadosing. Meta-analyses of RCTs have come to conflicting conclusions about whether folic acid supplementation increases cancer incidence;[n] if there is a true effect, it is likely modest

Folate Dietary Sources[o]: Green vegetables, beans, legumes, and whole grains; to a lesser extent, fruit and fruit juice.

Food	Serving Size	Energy (kcal)	Folate (μg)	Food	Serving Size	Energy (kcal)	Folate (μg)
Lentils	1 cup (198 g)	230	358	Radishes (raw)	1 medium (4.5 g)	1	1
Kidney beans	1 cup (177 g)	225	230	Peas	1 cup (160 g)	134	101
Asparagus	4 spears (60 g)	11	81	White beans	1 cup (179 g)	249	145
Avocado	1 whole (201 g)	322	163	Wild rice	1 cup (164 g)	166	43
Wheat germ	1 cup (115 g)	414	323	Banana	1 medium (118 g)	105	24
Pinto beans	1 cup (171 g)	245	294	Endive	1 head (513 g)	87	728
Chickpeas	1 cup (164 g)	269	282	Broccoli, 1 medium stalk	(180 g)	63	194
Lima beans	1 cup (188 g)	216	156	Brussels sprouts	1/2 cup (78 g)	28	47
Spinach	1 cup (180 g)	41	263	Lettuce (butterhead)	1 head (163 g)	21	119
Oatmeal with water	100 g	55	43				
Orange juice	1 cup (248 g)	112	74				

Effects of Food Preparation and Storage: Not reported to be a generally important determinant of dietary intake levels.

Additional details, evidence, and references for dosing and safety for many nutrients and substances individuals might choose to ingest can be found at http://www.mayoclinic.com/health/search/search, http://ods.od.nih.gov/, and http://www.nlm.nih.gov/medlineplus/.

[a]Standing Committee on the Scientific Evaluation of Dietary Reference Intakes, Institute of Medicine. Dietary Reference Intakes for thiamin, riboflavin, niacin, vitamin B_6, folate, vitamin B_{12}, pantothenic acid, biotin, and choline. Washington, DC: National Academy Press, 2000. Available at http://www.iom.edu/Object.File/Master/7/296/webtablevitamins.pdf.

[b]Whitney EN, Rolfes SR. *Understanding nutrition*, 7th ed. St. Paul, MN: West Pub.; 1996.

[c]Toriello HV; Policy and Practice Guideline Committee of the American College of Medical Genetics. Policy statement on folic acid and neural tube defects. *Genet Med* 2011;13(6):593–596. doi:10.1097/GIM.0b013e31821d4188; Blencowe H, Cousens S, Modell B, et al. Folic acid to reduce neonatal mortality from neural tube disorders. *Int J Epidemiol* 2010;39(suppl 1):i110–i121. doi:10.1093/ije/dyq028.

[d]Christensen B, Landaas S, Stensvold I, et al. Whole blood folate, homocysteine in serum, and risk of first acute myocardial infarction. *Atherosclerosis* 1999;147:317–326.

[e]Bunout D, Garrido A, Suazo M, et al. Effects of supplementation with folic acid and antioxidant vitamins on homocysteine levels and LDL oxidation in coronary patients. *Nutrition* 2000;16:107–110.

[f]Yang HT, Lee M, Hong KS, et al. Efficacy of folic acid supplementation in cardiovascular disease prevention: an updated meta-analysis of randomized controlled trials. *Eur J Intern Med* 2012;23(8):745–754. doi:10.1016/j.ejim.2012.07.004; Huo Y, Qin X, Wang J, et al. Efficacy of folic acid supplementation in stroke prevention: new insight from a meta-analysis. *Int J Clin Pract* 2012;66(6):544–551. doi:10.1111/j.1742-1241.2012.02929.x.

[g]Zhou YH, Tang JY, Wu MJ, et al. Effect of folic acid supplementation on cardiovascular outcomes: a systematic review and meta-analysis. *PLoS One* 2011;6(9):e25142. doi:10.1371/journal.pone.0025142.

[h]Miller ER 3rd, Juraschek S, Pastor-Barriuso R, et al. Meta-analysis of folic acid supplementation trials on risk of cardiovascular disease and risk interaction with baseline homocysteine levels. *Am J Cardiol* 2010;106(4):517–527. doi:10.1016/j.amjcard.2010.03.064.

[i]Sudchada P, Saokaew S, Sridetch S, et al. Effect of folic acid supplementation on plasma total homocysteine levels and glycemic control in patients with type 2 diabetes: a systematic review and meta-analysis. *Diabetes Res Clin Pract* 2012;98(1):151–158. doi:10.1016/j.diabres.2012.05.027.

[j]Woo KS, Chook P, Lolin YI, et al. Folic acid improves arterial endothelial function in adults with hyperhomocystinemia. *J Am Coll Cardiol* 1999;34:2002–2006.

[k]Office of Dietary Supplements. *Folate*. Available at http://ods.od.nih.gov/factsheets/Folate-QuickFacts/; accessed 9/29/2013.

[l]Eaton SB, Eaton SB. Paleolithic vs. modern diets—selected pathophysiological implications. *Eur J Nutr* 2000;39:67–70.

[m]Office of Dietary Supplements. *Folate (for health professionals)*. Available at http://ods.od.nih.gov/factsheets/Folate-HealthProfessional/; accessed 9/29/2013.

[n]Vollset SE, Clarke R, Lewington S. Effects of folic acid supplementation on overall and site-specific cancer incidence during the randomised trials: meta-analyses of data on 50,000 individuals. *Lancet* 2013;381(9871):1029–1036; Baggott JE, Oster RA, Tamura T. Meta-analysis of cancer risk in folic acid supplementation trials. *Cancer Epidemiol* 2012;36(1):78–81. doi:10.1016/j.canep.2011.05.003.

[o]The nutrient composition of most foods can be checked by accessing the US Department of Agriculture nutrient database, at http://www.nal.usda.gov/fnic/foodcomp/search.

Sources: Ensminger AH, Ensminger ME, Konlande JE, et al. *The concise encyclopedia of foods and nutrition*. Boca Raton, FL: CRC Press, Inc., 1995.

Margen S. *The wellness nutrition counter*. New York, NY: Health Letter Associates, 1997.

Murray MT. *Encyclopedia of nutritional supplements*. Rocklin, CA: Prima Publishing, 1996.

National Research Council. *Recommended dietary allowances*, 10th ed. Washington, DC: National Academy Press, 1989.

Otten JJ, Hellwig JP, Meyers LD, eds. *Dietary reference intakes. The essential guide to nutrient requirements*. Washington, DC: National Academies Press, 2006.

Pizzorno JE, Murray MT. *Textbook of natural medicine*, 3rd ed. St. Louis, MO: Church Livingstone Elsevier, 2006.

Shils ME, Shike M, Ross AC, et al., eds. *Modern nutrition in health and disease*, 10th ed. Philadelphia, PA: Lippincott Williams & Wilkins, 2005.

US Department of Agriculture. *USDA nutrient database for standard reference*. Release 19. 2006.

US Department of Agriculture. *USDA nutrient intake from NHANES 2001–2002 data*.

Ziegler EE, Filer LJ, Jr, eds. *Present knowledge in nutrition*, 7th ed. Washington, DC: ILSI Press, 1996.

LYCOPENE

BIOLOGICAL FUNCTION(S) IN HUMANS/KEY PROPERTIES: Lycopene is a non-provitamin A carotenoid with 11 carbons arranged linearly in conjugated double bonds and no ionone ring. The antioxidant capacity of carotenoids is related to the number of conjugated double bonds; the antioxidant capacity of lycopene is the greatest of known carotenoids and exceeds that of β-carotene by a factor of 2. Lycopene is thought to serve as a potent quencher of oxygen-free radicals within cells and on the inner surfaces of cell membranes; other functions in human physiology remain to be elucidated. Lycopene is not known to be an essential nutrient.

ABSORPTION/SOLUBILITY/STORAGE/PHARMACOKINETICS: In general, carotenoids are protein bound and lipid soluble. Heating foods can cause dissociation of such complexes and enhance carotenoid bioavailability. Carotenoids in general and lycopene in particular are more efficiently absorbed when ingested with a lipid source, such as oil. Nonabsorbable lipid mimics, such as olestra, are likely to decrease lycopene absorption. Lycopene is hydrophobic and transported predominantly near the core of lipoprotein particles, in particular LDL; levels are lower in small, dense LDL particles than in normal LDL particles. Serum concentrations vary over a wide range, from 50–900 nM/L. Serum lycopene changes gradually in response to varied intake, with a plasma depletion half-life of between 12 and 33 days; levels in chylomicrons are a better marker of short-term change. Lycopene is prominently stored in the adrenal glands, testes, liver, and prostate. Storage in adipose tissue varies with as yet undetermined factors.

RATIONALE FOR SUPPLEMENTATION: None known. The rationale for increasing lycopene intake is enhanced antioxidant activity and possible protection against gastrointestinal and prostate cancers. Protection against myocardial infarction has also been suggested.[a]

EVIDENCE IN SUPPORT OF SUPPLEMENTATION TO AND ABOVE THE DRI: No RDA or AI established. The latest of at least three meta-analyses of prostate-related trials concluded "Given the limited number of RCTs published, and the varying quality of existing studies, it is not possible to support, or refute, the use of lycopene for the prevention or treatment of BPH or prostate cancer."[b] Nonetheless, supplemental lycopene may improve high-density lipoprotein and reduce systemic inflammation, relevant to cardiovascular disease.[c] Lycopene also seems to improve lichen planus, a dermatologic condition rooted in oxidative stress[d] and may have some benefit for male infertility.[e]

Recommended Intake Range (US RDA): None.

AVERAGE INTAKE, US ADULTS: 5.2–7.9 mg/day

ESTIMATED MEAN PALEOLITHIC INTAKE (ADULT)[f]: Not known. Paleolithic intake may have been low, given that tomatoes are the predominant source of lycopene and tomatoes entered the human diet only recently; the tomato plant was originally discovered as a weed in fields of maize and beans in Central America.[g]

COMMON DOSE RANGE FOR USE AS SUPPLEMENT: Internet sites advertise supplements providing between 5 and 10 mg lycopene.

DO DIETARY PATTERNS MEETING GUIDELINES PERMIT INTAKE IN THE SUPPLEMENT RANGE? Yes, provided that tomato and tomato-product intake is high.

INCLUDED IN TYPICAL MULTIVITAMIN/MULTIMINERAL TABLET? Not consistently but included in some products

Deficiency

Intake Level: None known

Syndromes: None known

Toxicity

Intake Level: None known.

Syndromes: None known. A trial of supplemental lycopene given to first-time pregnant women to prevent preeclampsia resulted in worse outcomes: higher rates of preterm birth and low birth weight than with placebo (and no benefit for preeclampsia).[h]

Lycopene Dietary Sources[i]:

Food	Serving Size (g)	Energy (kcal)	Lycopene (μg)	Food	Serving Size (g)	Energy (kcal)	Lycopene (μg)
Tomatoes, raw	100	18	2,573	Tomato juice, canned	100	17	9,037
Tomatoes, fresh, cooked	100	18	3,041	Tomato catsup (not in data)	100	104	9,900
Tomato sauce, canned	100	37	15,111	Grapefruit, pink	100	42	1,419

Food	Serving Size (g)	Energy (kcal)	Lycopene (μg)	Food	Serving Size (g)	Energy (kcal)	Lycopene (μg)
Guava	100	68	5,204	Watermelon	100	30	4,532
Tomato paste, canned	100	82	28,764	Papaya	100	39	2,000–5,300 indicates 0 in data

Effects of Food Preparation and Storage: Heating foods, particularly in the presence of oil, enhances the absorption and bioavailability of lycopene. Freezing preserves lycopene content.

Additional details, evidence, and references for dosing and safety for many nutrients and substances individuals might choose to ingest can be found at http://www.mayoclinic.com/health/search/search, http://ods.od.nih.gov/, and http://www.nlm.nih.gov/medlineplus/.

[a]Kohlmeier L, Kark JD, Gomez-Garcia E, et al. Lycopene and myocardial infarction risk in the EURAMIC Study. *Am J Epidemiol* 1997;146:618–626.

[b]Ilic D, Misso M. Lycopene for the prevention and treatment of benign prostatic hyperplasia and prostate cancer: a systematic review. *Maturitas* 2012;72(4):269–276. doi:10.1016/j.maturitas.2012.04.014.

[c]McEneny J, Wade L, Young IS, et al. Lycopene intervention reduces inflammation and improves HDL functionality in moderately overweight middle-aged individuals. *J Nutr Biochem* 2013;24(1):163–168. doi:10.1016/j.jnutbio.2012.03.015.

[d]Saawarn N. Lycopene in the management of oral lichen planus: a placebo-controlled study. *Indian J Dent Res* 2011;22(5):639–643. doi:10.4103/0970-9290.93448.

[e]Gupta NP, Kumar R. Lycopene therapy in idiopathic male infertility—a preliminary report. *Int Urol Nephrol* 2002;34(3):369–372.

[f]Eaton SB, Eaton SB. Paleolithic vs. modern diets—selected pathophysiological implications. *Eur J Nutr* 2000;39:67–70.

[g]Tannahill R. *Food in history*. New York, NY: Three Rivers Press, 1988.

[h]Banerjee S, Jeyaseelan S, Guleria RJ. Trial of lycopene to prevent pre-eclampsia in healthy primigravidas: results show some adverse effects. *Obstet Gynaecol Res* 2009;35(3):477–482. doi:10.1111/j.1447-0756.2008.00983.x.

[i]Lycopene content is derived from Gerster H. The potential role of lycopene for human health. *J Am College Nutr* 1997;16:109–126. The nutrient composition of most foods can be checked by accessing the US Department of Agriculture nutrient database, at http://www.nal.usda.gov/fnic/foodcomp/search. However, at present, the lycopene content of foods is not reported in the nutrient database.

Sources: Clinton SK. Lycopene: chemistry, biology, and implications for human health and disease. *Nutr Rev* 1998;56:35–51.

Ensminger AH, Ensminger ME, Konlande JE, et al. *The concise encyclopedia of foods and nutrition*. Boca Raton, FL: CRC Press, Inc., 1995.

Gerster H. The potential role of lycopene for human health. *J Am College Nutr* 1997;16:109–126.

Margen S. *The wellness nutrition counter*. New York, NY: Health Letter Associates, 1997.

Murray MT. *Encyclopedia of nutritional supplements*. Rocklin, CA: Prima Publishing, 1996.

National Research Council. *Recommended dietary allowances*, 10th ed. Washington, DC: National Academy Press, 1989.

Otten JJ, Hellwig JP, Meyers LD, eds. *Dietary reference intakes. The essential guide to nutrient requirements*. Washington, DC: National Academies Press, 2006.

Pizzorno JE, Murray MT. *Textbook of natural medicine*, 3rd ed. St. Louis, MO: Church Livingstone Elsevier, 2006.

Shils ME, Shike M, Ross AC, et al., eds. *Modern nutrition in health and disease*, 10th ed. Philadelphia, PA: Lippincott Williams & Wilkins, 2005.

Stahl W, Sies H. Lycopene: a biologically important carotenoid for humans? *Arch Biochem Biophys* 1996;336:1–9.

US Department of Agriculture. *USDA nutrient database for standard reference*. Release 19. 2006.

US Department of Agriculture. *USDA nutrient intake from NHANES 2001–2002 data*.

Ziegler EE, Filer LJ Jr, eds. *Present knowledge in nutrition*, 7th ed. Washington, DC: ILSI Press, 1996.

MAGNESIUM

BIOLOGICAL FUNCTION(S) IN HUMANS/KEY PROPERTIES: Magnesium is known to function in more than 300 enzyme systems in the human body, impacting virtually all aspects of metabolism.

ABSORPTION/SOLUBILITY/STORAGE/PHARMACOKINETICS: Roughly 33% of ingested magnesium is absorbed in the upper small bowel. Poorly understood homeostatic mechanisms generally maintain a plasma magnesium concentration of 1.4–2.4 mg/dL (0.65–1.0 mM/L). Excretion occurs through the urine; when serum magnesium begins to fall, the kidney compensates by reabsorbing most filtered magnesium. Approximately 20–28 g of magnesium is stored in the body of an adult, with slightly more than half (60%) in the skeleton and slightly less than half in muscles and soft tissue; 1% of body stores are distributed in extracellular fluid. Thiazide diuretics and alcohol increase urinary losses. Long-term use of proton pump inhibitors (PPIs) may cause hypomagnesemia.[a]

RATIONALE FOR SUPPLEMENTATION: Average intake in the United States is estimated to be below the RDA level. Therefore, the risk of nominal magnesium deficiency exists with typical American dietary patterns. Supplementation is a reasonable means of precluding such deficiency.

Doses up to approximately twice the RDA are advocated for the treatment of myocardial ischemia, cardiac dysrhythmia, CHF, hypertension, claudication, osteoporosis, fibromyalgia, osteoporosis, and premenstrual syndrome. Supplementation during pregnancy has been advocated to reduce the risk of preeclampsia.

EVIDENCE IN SUPPORT OF SUPPLEMENTATION TO AND ABOVE THE DRI: Evidence supporting intake of magnesium at approximately the RDA is considerable, and in the aggregate represents the rationale for the particular recommendations made. To the extent that supplementation is required to achieve the RDA, supplementation is therefore of likely benefit. Evidence of benefit from supplementation beyond the RDA is generally suggestive at best. Magnesium depletion may accompany diuretic use in CHF, and there is some evidence of acute[b] and sustained[c] suppression of ventricular dysrhythmias in such patients. Magnesium supplementation may improve cardiac function in those with coronary artery disease, improving exercise tolerance and LVEF[d] There is inconsistent evidence of increased bone density with magnesium supplementation,[e,f] although a randomized trial in healthy girls showed benefit for bone mineral content of the hip (not other sites) with supplementation.[g] Supplemental magnesium may produce small reductions in blood pressure (3–4 mm Hg systolic, 2–3 mm Hg diastolic) with greater effect at greater doses.[h] Evidence does not support magnesium supplementation in pregnancy for maternal or neonatal outcomes.[i,j] Magnesium deficiency is associated with insulin resistance; magnesium supplementation past sufficiency may reduce c-peptide concentration and possibly fasting insulin, with improvement with some metabolic parameters[k] but no improvement in glycemic control or lipid profiles.[l]

Recommended Intake Range (US RDA): An intake of 310–420 mg/day of total magnesium is recommended for adults.

MAGNESIUM RECOMMENDED INTAKE RANGE (US RDA)[m]

	Infancy (age 0–6 mo)	Infancy (age 7–12 mo)	Childhood (age 1–3 y)	Childhood (age 4–8 y)	Adolescence (age 9–13 y)
Male	30 mg*	75 mg*	80 mg	130 mg	240 mg
Female	30 mg*	75 mg*	80 mg	130 mg	240 mg

	Adolescence (age 14–18 y)	Adult (age ≥ 19 y)	Pregnancy (age ≤ 18 y)	Pregnancy (age 19–30 y)	Pregnancy (age 31–50 y)
Male	410 mg	400–420 mg**	—	—	—
Female	360 mg	310–320 mg**	400 mg	350 mg	360 mg

	Lactation (age ≤ 18 y)	Lactation (age 19–30 y)	Lactation (age 31–50 y)
Male	—	—	—
Female	360 mg	310 mg	320 mg

AVERAGE INTAKE, US ADULTS:	242–324 mg/day
ESTIMATED MEAN PALEOLITHIC INTAKE (ADULT)[n]:	1,223 mg/day
COMMON DOSE RANGE FOR USE AS SUPPLEMENT:	100–1,000 mg/day
DO DIETARY PATTERNS MEETING GUIDELINES PERMIT ADEQUATE INTAKE?	Yes
INCLUDED IN TYPICAL MULTIVITAMIN/MULTIMINERAL TABLET?	Yes (dose: 50 mg)

* = AI. All other values in table are for RDA.
** Lower values are for 19–30 years, higher values are for >=31 years.

DEFICIENCY

Intake Level: Variable; deficiency is often due to malabsorption, alcoholism, or use of diuretics.

Syndromes: Weakness, muscle tremors, tetany, cardiac dysrhythmia, mental status changes, effects on vitamin D metabolism, seizures.

TOXICITY

Intake Level: Variable, depending on renal function; toxicity of oral magnesium is limited. Children 1–3 and 4–8 years of age have a tolerable upper limit at 65 mg/day and 110 mg/day, respectively. However, individuals above 9 years of age have an upper limit up to 350 mg/day.

Syndromes: Diarrhea, nausea, vomiting, hypotension; if extreme, respiratory depression and asystole.

Magnesium Dietary Sources[o]: Magnesium is abundant in leafy green vegetables, grains, legumes, certain fish, nuts, seeds, and chocolate.

Food	Serving Size	Energy (kcal)	Magnesium (μg)	Food	Serving Size	Energy (kcal)	Magnesium (μg)
Sunflower seeds	1 oz (28 g)	165	52	Cashews	1 oz (28 g)	157	83
Wild rice	1 cup (164 g)	166	52	Soybeans	1 cup (172 g)	298	148
Wheat germ Halibut	1 cup (115 g)	414	275	White beans	1 cup (179 g)	249	113
				Peaches	1 medium (150 g)	58	14
Halibut	1/2 fillet (159 g)	379	53	Bulgur wheat	1 cup (182 g)	151	58
Avocado	1 medium (201 g)	322	58	Navy beans	1 cup (182 g)	255	96
				Oatmeal	100 g	55	23
Mackerel	1 fillet (112 g)	230	85	Lettuce (butterhead)	1 head (163 g)	21	21
Almonds	1 oz (28 g)	164	78	Banana	1 medium (118 g)	105	32
Chocolate (semi-sweet)	1 oz (28 g)	136	33	Buckwheat	1 cup (168 g)	155	86
Spinach	1 cup (180 g)	41	157	Swiss chard	1 cup (175 g)	35	150

Effects of Food Preparation and Storage: Not reported to be a generally important determinant of dietary intake levels.

Additional details, evidence, and references for dosing and safety for many nutrients and substances individuals might choose to ingest can be found at http://www.mayoclinic.com/health/search/search, http://ods.od.nih.gov/, and http://www.nlm.nih.gov/medlineplus/.

[a]FDA. *Proton Pump Inhibitor drugs (PPIs): Drug Safety Communication—low magnesium levels can be associated with long-term use.* Available at http://www.fda.gov/Safety/MedWatch/SafetyInformation/SafetyAlertsforHumanMedicalProducts/ucm245275.htm.

[b]Ceremuzynski L, Gebalska J, Wolk R, et al. Hypomagnesemia in heart failure with ventricular arrhythmias. Beneficial effects of magnesium supplementation. *J Intern Med* 2000;247:78–86.

[c]Bashir Y, Sneddon JF, Staunton HA, et al. Effects of long-term oral magnesium chloride replacement in congestive heart failure secondary to coronary artery disease. *Am J Cardiol* 1993;72:1156–1162.

[d]Pokan R, Hofmann P, von Duvillard SP, et al. Oral magnesium therapy, exercise heart rate, exercise tolerance, and myocardial function in coronary artery disease patients. *Br J Sports Med* 2006;40(9):773–778.

[e]Martini LA. Magnesium supplementation and bone turnover. *Nutr Rev* 1999;57:227–229.

[f]Doyle L, Flynn A, Cashman K. The effect of magnesium supplementation on biochemical markers of bone metabolism or blood pressure in healthy young adult females. *Eur J Clin Nutr* 1999;53:255–261.

[g]Carpenter TO, DeLucia MC, Zhang JH, et al. A randomized controlled study of effects of dietary magnesium oxide supplementation on bone mineral content in healthy girls. *J Clin Endocrinol Metab* 2006;91(12):4866–4872.

[h]Kass L, Weekes J, Carpenter L. Effect of magnesium supplementation on blood pressure: a meta-analysis. *Eur J Clin Nutr* 2012;66(4):411–418. doi:10.1038/ejcn.2012.4. Epub 2012 Feb 8.

[i]Mattar F, Sibai BM. Prevention of preeclampsia. *Semin Perinatol* 1999;23:58–64.

[j]Makrides M, Crowther CA. Magnesium supplementation in pregnancy. *Cochrane Database Syst Rev* 2001;(4):CD000937.

[k]Chacko SA, Sul J, Song Y, et al. Magnesium supplementation, metabolic and inflammatory markers, and global genomic and proteomic profiling: a randomized, double-blind, controlled, crossover trial in overweight individuals. *Am J Clin Nutr* 2011;93(2):463–473. doi:10.3945/ajcn.110.002949.

(continued)

APPENDIX E   (Continued)

[l]de Valk HW, Verkaaik R, van Rijn HJ, et al. Oral magnesium supplementation in insulin-requiring type 2 diabetic patients. *Diabet Med* 1998;15(6):503–507.

[m]Office of Dietary Supplements. *Magnesium.* Available at http://ods.od.nih.gov/factsheets/Magnesium-HealthProfessional/; accessed 9/30/2013.

[n]Eaton SB, Eaton SB. Paleolithic vs. modern diets—selected pathophysiological implications. *Eur J Nutr* 2000;39:67–70.

[o]The nutrient composition of most foods can be checked by accessing the US Department of Agriculture nutrient database, at http://www.nal.usda.gov/fnic/foodcomp/search.

Sources: Ensminger AH, Ensminger ME, Konlande JE, et al. *The concise encyclopedia of foods and nutrition.* Boca Raton, FL: CRC Press, Inc., 1995.

Margen S. *The wellness nutrition counter.* New York, NY: Health Letter Associates, 1997.

Murray MT. *Encyclopedia of nutritional supplements.* Rocklin, CA: Prima Publishing, 1996.

National Research Council. *Recommended dietary allowances,* 10th ed. Washington, DC: National Academy Press, 1989.

Otten JJ, Hellwig JP, Meyers LD, eds. *Dietary reference intakes. The essential guide to nutrient requirements.* Washington, DC: National Academies Press, 2006.

Pizzorno JE, Murray MT. *Textbook of natural medicine,* 3rd ed. St. Louis, MO: Church Livingstone Elsevier, 2006.

Shils ME, Shike M, Ross AC, et al., eds. *Modern nutrition in health and disease,* 10th ed. Philadelphia, PA: Lippincott Williams & Wilkins, 2005.

US Department of Agriculture. *USDA nutrient database for standard reference.* Release 19. 2006.

US Department of Agriculture. *USDA nutrient intake from NHANES 2001–2002 data.*

Ziegler EE, Filer LJ Jr, eds. *Present knowledge in nutrition,* 7th ed. Washington, DC: ILSI Press, 1996.

PHOSPHOROUS

BIOLOGICAL FUNCTION(S) IN HUMANS/KEY PROPERTIES: Phosphorous is an essential dietary mineral. Most (85%) of the 800–850 g stored in the body of an adult is incorporated in the hydroxyapatite matrix of bone in a ratio of 1:2 with calcium. Phosphorous is essential to the hardening of both bone and tooth mineral. Phosphorous participates in the regulation of blood pH. It is present as a component of lipid particles (phospholipids). Phosphorous is a key component of many chemical messengers, including cyclic-AMP (adenosine monophosphate), cyclic GMP (guanine monophosphate), and 2,3-diphosphoglyecerate. Renal calcitriol production is in part mediated by serum phosphate levels. Phosphorous also plays a role in the transport of many nutrients into cells, and is required for the synthesis of DNA and RNA. Phosphate bonds in adenosine triphosphate are the principal source of energy for metabolism.

ABSORPTION/SOLUBILITY/STORAGE/PHARMACOKINETICS: Phosphorous absorption takes place in the small intestine by a mechanism independent of calcium and vitamin D; by a mechanism dependent on both calcium and vitamin D; and by a mechanism dependent on vitamin D but independent of calcium. Nearly 90% of phosphorous in human milk is absorbed by infants. Adults absorb more than 50% of ingested phosphorous, with absorption rising as habitual intake falls. The skeleton is the principal storage depot for phosphorous. Virtually all phosphorous lost from the body is excreted in the urine.

RATIONALE FOR SUPPLEMENTATION: Phosphorous deficiency does not normally occur but can be seen with extensive use of phosphate-binding antacids (i.e., aluminum based) by adults or in premature infants. In infants, phosphorous deficiency leads to hypophosphatemic rickets, while in adults it induces bone loss, weakness, and malaise.

There appears to be no rationale for megadosing of phosphorous.

EVIDENCE IN SUPPORT OF SUPPLEMENTATION TO AND ABOVE THE DRI: None.

Recommended Intake Range (US RDA)[a]

PHOSPHORUS RECOMMENDED INTAKE RANGE (US RDA):

	Infancy (age 0–6 mo)	Infancy (age 7–12 mo)	Childhood (age 1–3 y)	Childhood (age 4–8 y)
Male	100 mg*	275 mg*	460 mg	500 mg
Female	100 mg*	275 mg*	460 mg	500 mg

	Adolescence (age 9–13 y)	Adolescence (age 14–18 y)	Adult (age ≥ 19 y)	Pregnancy (age ≤ 18 y)
Male	1,250 mg	1,250 mg	700 mg	—
Female	1,250 mg	1,250 mg	700 mg	1,250 mg

	Pregnancy (age 19–50 y)	Lactation (age ≤ 18 y)	Lactation (age 19–50 y)
Male	—	—	—
Female	700 mg	1,250 mg	700 mg

AVERAGE INTAKE, US ADULTS:	Approximately 1,126–1,565 mg/day for adult men, 313–395 mg/day for women.
ESTIMATED MEAN PALEOLITHIC INTAKE (ADULT)[b]:	3,200 mg/day
COMMON DOSE RANGE FOR USE AS SUPPLEMENT:	N/A
DO DIETARY PATTERNS MEETING GUIDELINES PERMIT ADEQUATE INTAKE?	Yes (dose: 120 mg)
INCLUDED IN TYPICAL MULTIVITAMIN/MULTIMINERAL TABLET?	Yes (approximately 125 mg)

DEFICIENCY

    Intake Level: Uncertain; a 1:1 ratio with ingested calcium is the recommended minimum.

    Syndromes: Hypophosphatemic rickets in neonates; osteopenia and malaise in adults. Acute hypophosphatmia can cause myopathy, cardiomyopathy, and rhabdomyolysis. When the product of calcium ion and phosphate ion (the double product) is less than 0.7 mmol/L, there is likely to be a bone mineralization defect.

TOXICITY

    Intake Level: More than twice the intake level of calcium

* = AI. Other values = RDA.

(continued)

APPENDIX E   (Continued)

PHOSPHORUS TOLERABLE UPPER INTAKE LEVELS (UL)[a]:

	Infancy (age 0–6 mo)	Infancy (age 7–12 mo)	Childhood (age 1–3 y)	Childhood (age 4–8 y)	Adolescence (age 9–13 y)
Male	—	—	3,000 mg	4,000 mg	4,000 mg
Female	—	—	3,000 mg	4,000 mg	4,000 mg

	Adolescence (age 14–18 y)	Adult (age 19–70 y)	Adult (age ≥ 70 y)	Pregnancy (all ages)	Lactation (all ages)
Male	4,000 mg	4,000 mg	3,000 mg	—	—
Female	4,000 mg	4,000 mg	3,000 mg	3,500 mg	4,000 mg

Syndromes: High intake of phosphorous does not appear to be toxic when calcium and vitamin D intake are adequate. When either calcium or vitamin D intake is marginal, high phosphorous intake may induce hypocalcemia. Neither this nor the hyperparathyroidism induced in laboratory animals is a clinical entity that ordinarily occurs. Acute hyperphosphatemia can cause hypocalcemic tetany. When the calcium phosphate ion double product is greater than 2.2 mmol/L, soft tissue calcification is likely.

Phosphorous Dietary Sources[c]: Phosphorous is particularly abundant in fish, poultry, meat, and dairy products.

Food	Serving Size	Energy (kcal)	Phosphorous (μg)
Wheat germ	1 cup (115 g)	414	968
Sunflower seeds	1 cup (128 g)	745	1,478
Sardines	1 can (92 g)	191	451
Wild rice	1 cup (164 g)	166	134
Pumpkin seeds	1 cup (64 g)	285	59
Salmon	1/2 fillet (154 g)	280	394
Tuna, white, canned	1 can (172 g)	220	373
Flounder/sole	1 fillet (127 g)	149	367
Skim milk	1 cup (247 g)	86	249
Yogurt, nonfat	1 cup (245 g)	137	385

Effects of Food Preparation and Storage: Phosphorous is relatively unaffected by food processing.

Additional details, evidence, and references for dosing and safety for many nutrients and substances individuals might choose to ingest can be found at http://www.mayoclinic.com/health/search/search, http://ods.od.nih.gov/, and http://www.nlm.nih.gov/medlineplus/.

[a]Dietary reference intakes for calcium, phosphorous, magnesium, vitamin d, and fluoride (1997). Available at http://www.iom.edu/Global/News%20Announcements/~/media/48FAAA2FD9E74D95BBDA2236E7387B49.ashx; accessed 9/30/2013.

[b]Eaton SB, Eaton SB 3rd, Konner MJ. Paleolithic nutrition revisited: a twelve-year retrospective on its nature and implications. *Eur J Clin Nutr* 1997;51:207–216.

[c]The nutrient composition of most foods can be checked by accessing the US Department of Agriculture nutrient database, at http://www.nal.usda.gov/fnic/foodcomp/search.

Sources: Ensminger AH, Ensminger ME, Konlande JE, et al. *The concise encyclopedia of foods and nutrition.* Boca Raton, FL: CRC Press, Inc., 1995.

Margen S. *The wellness nutrition counter.* New York, NY: Health Letter Associates, 1997.

Murray MT. *Encyclopedia of nutritional supplements.* Rocklin, CA: Prima Publishing, 1996.

National Research Council. *Recommended dietary allowances,* 10th ed. Washington, DC: National Academy Press, 1989.

Otten JJ, Hellwig JP, Meyers LD, eds. *Dietary reference intakes. The essential guide to nutrient requirements.* Washington, DC: National Academies Press, 2006.

Pizzorno JE, Murray MT. *Textbook of natural medicine,* 3rd ed. St. Louis, MO: Church Livingstone Elsevier, 2006.

Shils ME, Shike M, Ross AC, et al., eds. *Modern nutrition in health and disease,* 10th ed. Philadelphia, PA: Lippincott Williams & Wilkins, 2005.

Standing Committee on the Scientific Evaluation of Dietary Reference Intakes, Food and Nutrition Board, Institute of Medicine. *Dietary Reference Intakes for calcium, phosphorous, magnesium, vitamin D, and fluoride.* Washington, DC: National Academy Press, 1997.

US Department of Agriculture. *USDA nutrient database for standard reference.* Release 19. 2006.

US Department of Agriculture. *USDA nutrient intake from NHANES 2001–2002 data.*

Ziegler EE, Filer LJ Jr, eds. *Present knowledge in nutrition,* 7th ed. Washington, DC: ILSI Press, 1996.

SELENIUM

BIOLOGICAL FUNCTION(S) IN HUMANS/KEY PROPERTIES: Selenium is a mineral that functions as a component of glutathione peroxidase, an essential antioxidant system. It is involved in the metabolism of vitamin E and in thyroid function.

ABSORPTION/SOLUBILITY/STORAGE/PHARMACOKINETICS: Selenium is generally well absorbed in the small bowel and is transported in circulation bound to protein. The mineral is concentrated in liver and kidney, and to a lesser extent myocardium. Excretion is primarily in the urine, secondarily in stool. An adult of average size stores approximately 15 mg of selenium.

RATIONALE FOR SUPPLEMENTATION: The typical diet in the United States provides well in excess of the RDA for selenium. Supplementation is indicated to prevent deficiency syndromes in parts of the world where the soil is selenium deficient. Selenium deficiency has been most extensively evaluated in rural areas of China with selenium-poor soil and little access to outside food sources. Under such conditions, selenium supplementation in the range of the RDA is indicated to prevent overt deficiency, manifested as Keshan disease, a cardiomyopathy,[a,b] and Kashin-Beck syndrome, a form of arthritis,[c] as well as to reduce cancer risk.[d,e]

Selenium supplementation beyond the RDA is advocated for putative benefits in cancer prevention, cardiovascular disease prevention (especially the prevention of events in those with established coronary artery disease), immune enhancement, rheumatoid arthritis, cataract prevention, and the prevention of sudden infant death syndrome (SIDS). However, the evidence for most of these effects is either limited to conditions of selenium deficiency or is highly speculative. As selenium toxicity is well established at a dose of 1 mg (1,000 μg) per day, there is no rationale for megadosing.

EVIDENCE IN SUPPORT OF SUPPLEMENTATION TO AND ABOVE THE DRI: Some evidence suggests a reduced risk of prostate cancer with selenium supplementation.[f] More general reductions in cancer risk may be most pronounced among those having low selenium levels at baseline,[g] but the totality of evidence for selenium supplementation preventing cancer in general remains overall inconsistent and unconvincing.[h] Selenium supplementation may be of benefit to select individuals with Hashimoto's thyroiditis, based on baseline antibody levels,[i] and as an adjunct to medication for patients with chronic asthma.[j] Evidence does not support selenium supplementation for cardiovascular disease,[k] or Alzheimer's disease [l]

Recommended Intake Range (US RDA): An intake of 45–70 μg/day of total selenium is recommended for adults.

SELENIUM RECOMMENDED INTAKE RANGE (US RDA)[m]:

	Infancy (age 0–6 mo)	Infancy (age 7–12 mo)	Childhood (age 1–3 y)	Childhood (age 4–8 y)	Adolescence (age 9–13 y)
Male	15 μg*	20 μg*	20 μg	30 μg	40 μg
Female	15 μg*	20 μg*	20 μg	30 μg	40 μg

	Adolescence (age 14–18 y)	Adult (age ≥ 19 y)	Pregnancy (all ages)	Lactation (all ages)
Male	55 μg	55 μg	—	—
Female	55 μg	55 μg	60 μg	70 μg

AVERAGE INTAKE, US ADULTS:	90.9–127.1 μg/day
ESTIMATED MEAN PALEOLITHIC INTAKE (ADULT)[n]:	Not available
COMMON DOSE RANGE FOR USE AS SUPPLEMENT:	50–200 μg/day
DO DIETARY PATTERNS MEETING GUIDELINES PERMIT ADEQUATE INTAKE?	Yes
INCLUDED IN TYPICAL MULTIVITAMIN/MULTIMINERAL TABLET?	Yes (dose: 25 μg)

DEFICIENCY
Intake Level: <10–20 μg/day.
Syndromes: Cardiomyopathy (Keshan disease), arthritis (Kashin-Beck syndrome), immunosuppression, increased susceptibility to cancer.

TOXICITY
Intake Level: <1,000 μg/day.[m]

* = AI. Other values = RDA.

(continued)

APPENDIX E   (Continued)

SELENIUM TOLERABLE UPPER INTAKE LEVELS (UL):

	Infancy (age 0–6 mo)	Infancy (age 7–12 mo)	Childhood (age 1–3 y)	Childhood (age 4–8 y)	Adolescence (age 9–13 y)
Male	45 μg	60 μg	90 μg	150 μg	280 μg
Female	45 μg	60 μg	90 μg	150 μg	280 μg

	Adolescence (age 14–18 y)	Adult (age ≥ 19 y)	Pregnancy (all ages)	Lactation (all ages)
Male	400 μg	400 μg	—	—
Female	400 μg	400 μg	400 μg	400 μg

Syndromes: Hair and nail brittleness and loss, nausea and vomiting, neuropathy.

Selenium Dietary Sources[o]: Organ meats, fish, and shellfish are generally selenium rich. The selenium content of grains and other plant-based foods varies with the soil content.

Food	Serving Size	Energy (kcal)	Selenium (μg)	Food	Serving Size	Energy (kcal)	Selenium (μg)
Tuna	1 can (172 g)	220	113	Yogurt (nonfat)	1 cup (245 g)	137	9
Oysters	6 medium (42 g)	58	30	Skim milk	1 cup (247 g)	86	5
Flounder (or sole)	1 fillet (127 g)	149	74	Peanut butter	2 tablespoons (32 g)	188	2
Wheat germ	1 cup (115 g)	414	91	Pecans	1 oz (28 g)	196	1
Turkey	1 lb. (112 g)	212	32.6	White bread	1 slice (25 g)	67	6
Chicken	1/2 breast (98 g)	193	24	Egg	1 large (50 g)	78	15
				Almonds	1 oz (28 g)	164	1
Farina	1 cup (233 g)	112	21	Walnuts, English	1 oz (28 g)	185	1
Shrimp	4 large (22 g)	22	9	Mozzarella (part skim)	1 slice (28 g)	72	4
Mushrooms	1/2 cup (78 g)	22	9				
Barley, pearled	1 cup (157 g)	193	14	Swiss cheese	1 slice (28 g)	106	5

Effects of Food Preparation and Storage: Not known to be a significant factor.

Additional details, evidence, and references for dosing and safety for many nutrients and substances individuals might choose to ingest can be found at http://www.mayoclinic.com/health/search/search, http://ods.od.nih.gov/, and http://www.nlm.nih.gov/medlineplus/.

[a]Neve J. Selenium as a risk factor for cardiovascular diseases. *J Cardiovascu Risk* 1996;3:42–47.

[b]Hensrud DD, Heimburger DC, Chen J, et al. Antioxidant status, erythrocyte fatty acids, and mortality from cardiovascular disease and Keshan disease in China. *Eur J Clin Nutr* 1994;48:455–464.

[c]Moreno-Reyes R, Suetens C, Mathieu F, et al. Kashin-Beck osteoarthropathy in rural Tibet in relation to selenium and iodine status. *N Engl J Med* 1998;339:1112–1120.

[d]Blot WJ, Li JY, Taylor PR, et al. The Linxian trials: mortality rates by vitamin-mineral intervention group. *Am J Clin Nutr* 1995;62:1424s–1426s.

[e]Taylor PR, Li B, Dawsey SM, et al. Prevention of esophageal cancer: the nutrition intervention trials in Linxian, China. Linxian Nutrition Intervention Trials Study Group. *Cancer Res* 1994;54:2029s–2031s.

[f]Hurst R, Hooper L, Norat T, et al. Selenium and prostate cancer: systematic review and meta-analysis. *Am J Clin Nutr* 2012;96(1): 111–122. doi:10.3945/ajcn.111.033373.

[g]Lee EH, Myung SK, Jeon YJ, et al. Effects of selenium supplements on cancer prevention: meta-analysis of randomized controlled trials. *Nutr Cancer* 2011;63(8):1185–1195. doi:10.1080/01635581.2011.607544.

[h]Dennert G. Selenium for preventing cancer. *Cochrane Database Syst Rev* 2011;(5):CD005195. doi:10.1002/14651858.CD005195.pub2.

[i]Toulis KA, Anastasilakis AD, Tzellos TG, et al. Selenium supplementation in the treatment of Hashimoto's thyroiditis: a systematic review and a meta-analysis. *Thyroid* 2010;20(10):1163–1173. doi:10.1089/thy.2009.0351.

[j]Allam MF, Lucane RA. Selenium supplementation for asthma. *Cochrane Database Syst Rev* 2004;(2):CD003538.

[k]Rees K, Hartley L, Day C, et al. Selenium supplementation for the primary prevention of cardiovascular disease. *Cochrane Database Syst Rev* 2013;1:CD009671. doi:10.1002/14651858.CD009671.

[l]Loef M, Schrauzer GN, Walach H. Selenium and Alzheimer's disease: a systematic review. *J Alzheimers Dis* 2011;26(1):81–104. doi:10.3233/JAD-2011-110414.

[m]Office of Dietary Supplements. *Selenium.* Available at http://ods.od.nih.gov/factsheets/Selenium-HealthProfessional/; accessed 9/30/2013.

[n]Eaton SB, Eaton SB. Paleolithic vs. modern diets—selected pathophysiological implications. *Eur J Nutr* 2000; 39:67–70.

[o]The nutrient composition of most foods can be checked by accessing the US Department of Agriculture nutrient database, at http://www.nal.usda.gov/fnic/foodcomp/search.

Sources: Ensminger AH, Ensminger ME, Konlande JE, et al. *The concise encyclopedia of foods and nutrition.* Boca Raton, FL: CRC Press, Inc., 1995.

Margen S. *The wellness nutrition counter.* New York, NY: Health Letter Associates, 1997.

Murray MT. *Encyclopedia of nutritional supplements.* Rocklin, CA: Prima Publishing, 1996.

National Research Council. *Recommended dietary allowances,* 10th ed. Washington, DC: National Academy Press, 1989.

Otten JJ, Hellwig JP, Meyers LD, eds. *Dietary reference intakes. The essential guide to nutrient requirements.* Washington, DC: National Academies Press, 2006.

Pizzorno JE, Murray MT. *Textbook of natural medicine,* 3rd ed. St. Louis, MO: Church Livingstone Elsevier, 2006.

Shils ME, Shike M, Ross AC, et al., eds. *Modern nutrition in health and disease,* 10th ed. Philadelphia, PA: Lippincott Williams & Wilkins, 2005.

US Department of Agriculture. *USDA nutrient database for standard reference.* Release 19. 2006.

US Department of Agriculture. *USDA nutrient intake from NHANES 2001–2002 data.*

Ziegler EE, Filer LJ Jr, eds. *Present knowledge in nutrition,* 7th ed. Washington, DC: ILSI Press, 1996.

PYRIDOXINE/VITAMIN B$_6$

BIOLOGICAL FUNCTION(S) IN HUMANS/KEY PROPERTIES: Several forms of vitamin B$_6$, pyridoxine, pyridoxal, and pyridoxamine, function in a variety of metabolic pathways, especially transamination, decarboxylation, and racemization of amino acids. Vitamin B$_6$ is vital to protein metabolism, the manufacture of neurotransmitter production, gluconeogenesis, and glycogenolysis. Vitamin B$_6$ requirements vary directly with protein intake.

ABSORPTION/SOLUBILITY/STORAGE/PHARMACOKINETICS: Water soluble. Intestinal absorption is nonsaturable. Storage occurs primarily in plasma in a complex with albumin and in erythrocytes.

RATIONALE FOR SUPPLEMENTATION: Intake below the RDA is apparently widespread, especially among the elderly and both pregnant and lactating women. Low vitamin B$_6$ intake is associated with elevated plasma homocysteine, a risk factor for cardiovascular disease.

Claims for megadoses of vitamin B$_6$ have been made for therapeutic roles in asthma, immunodepression, carpal tunnel syndrome, pregnancy-induced nausea, and premenstrual syndrome, among other conditions.

EVIDENCE IN SUPPORT OF SUPPLEMENTATION TO AND ABOVE THE DRI: There is consensus that supplementation to meet the RDA is appropriate among groups at risk of deficiency. In addition, low levels are widespread among smokers, women taking oral contraceptives, during pregnancy and lactation, and among individuals taking isoniazid and other drugs that alter vitamin B$_6$ status; supplementation is recommended for these groups. Supplementation in the form of a multivitamin tablet generally provides up to 150% of the RDA for adults. The use of supplements for certain conditions is supported by randomized trials,[a,b] but these are mostly small, and there is lack of consensus. The evidence does not support a benefit for cognitive function,[c] pregnancy/labor outcomes,[d] cardiovascular events,[e] incident cancer,[f] or depression in cardiovascular-disease survivors.[g] Doses of up to 250 mg/day are considered safe.

Recommended Intake Range (US RDA):

VITAMIN B$_6$ RECOMMENDED INTAKE RANGE (US RDA)[h]:

	Infancy (age 0–6 mo)	Infancy (age 7–12 mo)	Childhood (age 1–3 y)	Childhood (age 4–8 y)
Male	0.1 mg*	0.3 mg*	0.5 mg	0.6 mg
Female	0.1 mg*	0.3 mg*	0.5 mg	0.6 mg

	Adolescence (age 9–13 y)	Adolescence (age 14–18 y)	Adult (age 19–30 y)	Adult (age ≥ 31 y)
Male	1.0 mg	1.3 mg	1.3 mg	1.7 mg
Female	1.0 mg	1.2 mg	1.3 mg	1.5 mg

	Pregnancy (all ages)	Lactation (all ages)
Male	—	—
Female	1.9 mg	2.0 mg

AVERAGE INTAKE, US ADULTS:	1.53–2.24 mg
ESTIMATED MEAN PALEOLITHIC INTAKE (ADULT)[i]:	Unknown
COMMON DOSE RANGE FOR USE AS SUPPLEMENT:	50–100 mg/day
DO DIETARY PATTERNS MEETING GUIDELINES PERMIT ADEQUATE INTAKE?	Yes
INCLUDED IN TYPICAL MULTIVITAMIN/MULTIMINERAL TABLET?	Yes (dose: 5.0 mg)

DEFICIENCY
Intake Level: Below 0.016 mg vitamin B$_6$/g dietary protein.
Syndromes: Dermatitis, cheilosis (scaling on the lips and cracks at the corners of the mouth) and glossitis (swollen tongue), anemia, depression, seizures.

TOXICITY
Intake Level: Above 200 mg/day for extended periods (months).

* = AI. All other values in table represent RDA.

VITAMIN B$_6$ TOLERABLE UPPER INTAKE LEVELS (UL)[h]:

	Infancy (age 0–6 mo)	Infancy (age 7–12 mo)	Childhood (age 1–3 y)	Childhood (age 4–8 y)
Male	—	—	30 mg	40 mg
Female	—	—	30 mg	40 mg

	Adolescence (age 9–13 y)	Adolescence (age 14–18 y)	Adult (age ≥ 19 y)	Pregnancy (age 14–18 y)
Male	60 mg	80 mg	100 mg	—
Female	60 mg	80 mg	100 mg	80 mg

	Pregnancy (age 19–50 y)	Lactation (age 14–18 y)	Lactation (age 19–50 y)	
Male	—	—	—	—
Female	100 mg	80 mg	100 mg	

Syndromes: Ataxia, myalgia, peripheral neuropathy, irritability, dermatological lesions.

Vitamin B$_6$ Dietary Sources[b:] B$_6$ is widespread in the food supply; especially abundant in poultry, bananas, avocados, and organ meats.

Food	Serving Size	Energy (kcal)	Vitamin B$_6$ (mg)	Food	Serving Size	Energy (kcal)	Vitamin B$_6$ (mg)
Tuna, yellowfin, cooked	3 oz (85 g)	118	0.88	Carrot juice	1 cup (236 g)	94	0.51
Avocado, Florida	One (304 g)	365	0.24	Snapper	3 oz (85 g)	109	0.39
Potato, with skin	One (173 g)	115	0.36	Beef, sirloin	3 oz (85 g)	211	0.36
Banana	1 medium (118 g)	105	0.43	Sweet potato	One (medium); 114 g	103	0.33
Salmon	3 oz (85 g)	127	0.2	Halibut	3 oz (85 g)	119	0.34
Chicken	1/2 breast (98 g)	193	0.55	Swordfish	3 oz (85 g)	132	0.32
Chickpeas	1 cup (164 g)	269	0.23	Tuna, white, canned	3 oz (85 g)	109	0.18
Turkey	1 lb (112 g)	212	0.54	Pepper (green)	1 medium (119 g)	24	0.27
Prune juice	1 cup (256 g)	182	0.56	Sunflower seeds	1 oz (28 g)	165	0.23
Lentils	1 cup (198 g)	230	0.35	Walnuts, English	1 oz (28 g)	185	0.15

Effects of Food Preparation and Storage: Freezing and processing of meats, grains, fruits, and vegetables can result in losses of up to 70% of native Vitamin B$_6$.

Additional details, evidence, and references for dosing and safety for many nutrients and substances individuals might choose to ingest can be found at http://www.mayoclinic.com/health/search/search, http://ods.od.nih.gov/, and http://www.nlm.nih.gov/medlineplus/.

[a]Vutyavanich T, Wongrangan S, Ruangsri R. Pyridoxine for nausea and vomiting of pregnancy: a randomized, double-blind, placebo-controlled trial. *Am J Obstet Gynecol* 1995;173:881–884.

[b]The nutrient composition of most foods can be checked by accessing the US Department of Agriculture nutrient database, at http://www.nal.usda.gov/fnic/foodcomp/search. A more extensive list of food sources of vitamin C is available in Margen S. *The wellness nutrition counter.* New York, NY: Health Letter Associates, 1997.

[c]Balk EM, Raman G, Tatsioni A, et al. Vitamin B$_6$, B$_{12}$, and folic acid supplementation and cognitive function: a systematic review of randomized trials. *Arch Intern Med* 2007;167(1):21–30.

[d]Thaver D, Saeed MA, Bhutta ZA. Pyridoxine (vitamin B$_6$) supplementation in pregnancy. *Cochrane Database Syst Rev* 2006;(2):CD000179

[e]Albert CM, Cook NR, Gaziano JM, et al. Effect of folic acid and B vitamins on risk of cardiovascular events and total mortality among women at high risk for cardiovascular disease: a randomized trial. *JAMA* 2008;299(17):2027–2036. doi:10.1001/jama.299.17.2027.

(continued)

APPENDIX E   (Continued)

[f]Andreeva VA, Touvier M, Kesse-Guyot E, et al. B vitamin and/or ω-3 fatty acid supplementation and cancer: ancillary findings from the supplementation with folate, vitamins B6 and B12, and/or omega-3 fatty acids (SU.FOL.OM3) randomized trial. *Arch Intern Med* 2012;172(7):540–547. doi:10.1001/archinternmed.2011.1450.

[g]Andreeva VA, Galan P, Torrès M, et al. Supplementation with B vitamins or n-3 fatty acids and depressive symptoms in cardiovascular disease survivors: ancillary findings from the Supplementation with Folate, vitamins B-6 and B-12 and/or OMega-3 fatty acids (SU.FOL.OM3) randomized trial. *Am J Clin Nutr* 2012;96(1):208–214. doi:10.3945/ajcn.112.035253.

[h]Office of Dietary Supplements. *Vitamin B_6.* Available at http://ods.od.nih.gov/factsheets/VitaminB6-HealthProfessional/; accessed 9/30/2013.

[i]Eaton SB, Eaton SB III, Konner MJ. Paleolithic nutrition revisited: a twelve-year retrospective on its nature and implications. *Eur J Clin Nutr* 1997;51:207–216.

Sources: Ensminger AH, Ensminger ME, Konlande JE, et al. *The concise encyclopedia of foods and nutrition.* Boca Raton, FL: CRC Press, Inc., 1995.

Margen S. *The wellness nutrition counter.* New York, NY: Health Letter Associates, 1997.

Murray MT. *Encyclopedia of nutritional supplements.* Rocklin, CA: Prima Publishing, 1996.

National Research Council. *Recommended dietary allowances*, 10th ed. Washington, DC: National Academy Press, 1989.

Otten JJ, Hellwig JP, Meyers LD, eds. *Dietary reference intakes. The essential guide to nutrient requirements.* Washington, DC: National Academies Press, 2006.

Pizzorno JE, Murray MT. *Textbook of natural medicine*, 3rd ed. St. Louis, MO: Church Livingstone Elsevier, 2006.

Shils ME, Shike M, Ross AC, et al., eds. *Modern nutrition in health and disease*, 10th ed. Philadelphia, PA: Lippincott Williams & Wilkins, 2005.

US Department of Agriculture. *USDA nutrient database for standard reference.* Release 19. 2006.

US Department of Agriculture. *USDA nutrient intake from NHANES 2001–2002 data.*

Ziegler EE, Filer LJ Jr, eds. *Present knowledge in nutrition*, 7th ed. Washington, DC: ILSI Press, 1996.

ASCORBIC ACID/VITAMIN C

BIOLOGICAL FUNCTION(S) IN HUMANS/KEY PROPERTIES: An essential cofactor for eight known enzymes; functions as an electron donor. Facilitates hydroxylation reactions. Vital for a range of metabolic pathways. Required for the biosynthesis of collagen, L-carnitine, and certain neurotransmitters. Involved in protein metabolism. Cannot be synthesized by humans.

ABSORPTION/SOLUBILITY/STORAGE/PHARMACOKINETICS: Water soluble. Absorbed via sodium-dependent transport mechanism in small intestine. Body stores are largely intracellular and saturate in adults at a level of approximately 3 g. Steady-state levels rise minimally with intakes exceeding 200 mg/day and are maximized at an intake level of 500 mg/day.[a]

RATIONALE FOR SUPPLEMENTATION: Vitamin C is a potent water-soluble antioxidant. Megadosing is touted to prevent cancers, heart disease, respiratory infections, and a wide range of other health problems. Doses up to 10 g/day have been advocated to the public.

EVIDENCE IN SUPPORT OF SUPPLEMENTATION TO AND ABOVE THE DRI: Available evidence derives predominantly from observational studies and is based primarily on vitamin C in whole foods rather than supplement form. In short-term trials, vitamins C has been shown to produce modest reductions in systolic and diastolic blood pressure, about 3.8 mm Hg and about 1.5 mm Hg, respectively.[b] Some vitamin C trials conducted in those living in crowded lodgings (e.g., military recruits and marathon runners) have demonstrated reductions in the incidence of respiratory infections,[c] but evidence does not support vitamin C supplementation for respiratory conditions like asthma[d] except possibly in the case of exercise-induced bronchospasm.[e] Evidence also does not support vitamin C supplementation to prevent atrial fibrillation after coronary artery bypass grafting[f] or to prevent preeclampsia or other adverse pregnancy outcomes.[g]

Recommended Intake Range (US RDA)[h]:

VITAMIN C (ASCORBIC ACID) RECOMMENDED INTAKE RANGE (US RDA):

	Infancy (age 0–6 mo)	Infancy (age 7–12 mo)	Childhood (age 1–3 y)	Childhood (age 4–8 y)
Male	40 mg*	50 mg*	15 mg	25 mg
Female	40 mg*	50 mg*	15 mg	25 mg

* = AI

	Adolescence (age 9–13 y)	Adolescence (age 14–18 y)	Adult (age ≥ 19 y)	Pregnancy (age ≤ 18 y)
Male	45 mg	75 mg	90 mg	—
Female	45 mg	65 mg	75 mg	80 mg

	Pregnancy (age 19–50 y)	Lactation (age ≤ 18 y)	Lactation (age 19–50 y)
Male	—	—	—
Female	85 mg	115 mg	120 mg

AVERAGE INTAKE, US ADULTS:	85.7–103.7 mg
ESTIMATED MEAN PALEOLITHIC INTAKE (ADULT)[i]:	604 mg
COMMON DOSE RANGE FOR USE AS SUPPLEMENT:	100 mg to several grams
DO DIETARY PATTERNS MEETING GUIDELINES PERMIT ADEQUATE INTAKE?	Yes
INCLUDED IN TYPICAL MULTIVITAMIN/MULTIMINERAL TABLET?	Yes (dose: 90 mg)

DEFICIENCY

Intake Level:	Below 10 mg/day in adults.
Syndromes:	Scurvy, dyspnea, edema, fatigue, depression.

TOXICITY

Intake Level:	Above 3,000 mg/day in adults.

* = AI. All other values in table represent RDA.

(continued)

APPENDIX E   (Continued)

VITAMIN C TOLERABLE UPPER INTAKE LEVELS (UL)[h]:

	Infancy (age 0–6 mo)	Infancy (age 7–12 mo)	Childhood (age 1–3 y)	Childhood (age 4–8 y)
Male	—	—	400 mg	650 mg
Female	—	—	400 mg	650 mg

	Adolescence (age 9–13 y)	Adolescence (age 14–18 y)	Adult (age ≥ 19 y)	Pregnancy (age 14–18 y)
Male	1,200 mg	1,800 mg	2,000 mg	—
Female	1,200 mg	1,800 mg	2,000 mg	1,800 mg

	Pregnancy (age 19–50 y)	Lactation (age 14–18 y)	Lactation (age 19–50 y)
Male	—	—	—
Female	2,000 mg	1,800 mg	2,000 mg

Syndromes: diarrhea, nausea, abdominal cramps, and other gastrointestinal disturbances due to the osmotic effect of unabsorbed vitamin C in the gastrointestinal tract; pro-oxidant effects

VITAMIN C (ASCORBIC ACID) DIETARY SOURCES[j]: VITAMIN C IS ABUNDANT IN A VARIETY OF FRUITS AND VEGETABLES.

Food	Serving Size	Energy (kcal)	Vitamin C (mg)	Food	Serving Size	Energy (kcal)	Vitamin C (mg)
Acerola (West Indian cherry)	1 cup (98 g)	31	1644	Kiwi	One (76 g)	46	71
				Cantaloupe	1 cup (156 g)	53	57
Sweet red peppers, raw	1 cup (149 g)	39	190	Red cabbage, raw	1 cup (70 g)	22	40
Sweet green peppers, raw	1 cup (149 g)	30	120	Peas, boiled	1/2 cup (80 g)	34	38
Orange juice, fresh	1 cup (248 g)	112	124	Tomatoes, raw	1 medium (123 g)	22	16
				Raspberries	1 cup (123 g)	64	32
Orange juice, frozen concentrate	1 cup (249 g)	112	97	Sweet potato, baked	1 medium (114 g)	103	22
Grapefruit juice, pink	1 cup (247 g)	96	94	Potato with skin, baked	1 medium (173 g)	161	17
Strawberries	1 cup (152 g)	49	89	Salsa	1/2 cup (130 g)	35	3
Broccoli	1 cup (91 g)	31	81	Avocado, Florida	One (304 g)	365	53
Oranges, navel	One (140 g)	69	83	Onions, raw	1 cup (160 g)	64	12

Effects of Food Preparation and Storage: Not reported to be a generally important determinant of dietary intake levels.

Additional details, evidence, and references for dosing and safety for many nutrients and substances individuals might choose to ingest can be found at http://www.mayoclinic.com/health/search/search, http://ods.od.nih.gov/, and http://www.nlm.nih.gov/medlineplus/.
[a]Blanchard J, Tozer TN, Rowland M. Pharmacokinetic perspectives on megadoses of ascorbic acid. *Am J Clin Nutr* 1997;66:1165–1171.
[b]Juraschek SP, Guallar E, Appel LJ, et al. Effects of vitamin C supplementation on blood pressure: a meta-analysis of randomized controlled trials. *Am J Clin Nutr* 2012;95(5):1079–1088. doi:10.3945/ajcn.111.027995.
[c]Hemilä H. Vitamin C supplementation and respiratory infections: a systematic review. *Mil Med* 2004;169(11):920–925.
[d]Kaur B, Rowe BH, Arnold E. Vitamin C supplementation for asthma. *Cochrane Database Syst Rev* 2009;(1):CD000993. doi:10.1002/14651858.CD000993.
[e]Tecklenburg SL, Mickleborough TD, Fly AD, et al. Ascorbic acid supplementation attenuates exercise-induced bronchoconstriction in patients with asthma. *Respir Med* 2007;101(8):1770–1778.

[f]Bjordahl PM, Helmer SD, Gosnell DJ, et al. Perioperative supplementation with ascorbic acid does not prevent atrial fibrillation in coronary artery bypass graft patients. *Am J Surg* 2012;204(6):862–867; discussion 867. doi:10.1016/j.amjsurg.2012.03.012.

[g]Dror DK, Allen LH. Interventions with vitamins B6, B12 and C in pregnancy. *Paediatr Perinat Epidemiol* 2012;26(suppl 1):55–74. doi:10.1111/j.1365-3016.2012.01277.x; Conde-Agudelo A, Romero R, Kusanovic JP. Supplementation with vitamins C and E during pregnancy for the prevention of preeclampsia and other adverse maternal and perinatal outcomes: a systematic review and meta-analysis. *Am J Obstet Gynecol* 2011;204(6):503.e1–12. doi:10.1016/j.ajog.2011.02.020; Steyn PS, Odendaal HJ, Schoeman J. A randomised, double-blind placebo-controlled trial of ascorbic acid supplementation for the prevention of preterm labour. *J Obstet Gynaecol* 2003;23(2):150–155.

[h]Office of Dietary Supplements. *Vitamin C.* http://ods.od.nih.gov/factsheets/VitaminC-HealthProfessional/; accessed 10/1/2013.

[i]Eaton SB, Eaton SB III, Konner MJ. Paleolithic nutrition revisited: a twelve-year retrospective on its nature and implications. *Eur J Clin Nutr* 1997;51:207–216.

[j]The nutrient composition of most foods can be checked by accessing the US Department of Agriculture nutrient database. http://www.nal.usda.gov/fnic/foodcomp/search. A more extensive list of food sources of vitamin C is available in Margen S. *The wellness nutrition counter.* New York, NY: Health Letter Associates, 1997.

Sources: Ensminger AH, Ensminger ME, Konlande JE, et al. *The concise encyclopedia of foods and nutrition.* Boca Raton, FL: CRC Press, Inc., 1995.

Margen S. *The wellness nutrition counter.* New York, NY: Health Letter Associates, 1997.

Murray MT. *Encyclopedia of nutritional supplements.* Rocklin, CA: Prima Publishing, 1996.

National Research Council. *Recommended dietary allowances,* 10th ed. Washington, DC: National Academy Press, 1989.

Otten JJ, Hellwig JP, Meyers LD, eds. *Dietary reference intakes. The essential guide to nutrient requirements.* Washington, DC: National Academies Press, 2006.

Pizzorno JE, Murray MT. *Textbook of natural medicine,* 3rd ed. St. Louis, MO: Church Livingstone Elsevier, 2006.

Shils ME, Shike M, Ross AC, et al., eds. *Modern nutrition in health and disease,* 10th ed. Philadelphia, PA: Lippincott Williams & Wilkins, 2005.

US Department of Agriculture. *USDA nutrient database for standard reference.* Release 19. 2006.

US Department of Agriculture. *USDA nutrient intake from NHANES 2001–2002 data.*

Ziegler EE, Filer LJ, Jr, eds. *Present knowledge in nutrition,* 7th ed. Washington, DC: ILSI Press, 1996.

CHOLECALCIFEROL/VITAMIN D

BIOLOGICAL FUNCTION(S) IN HUMANS/KEY PROPERTIES: Refers to calciferol and related chemical compounds. Essential if inadequate skin exposure to ultraviolet light. Vitamin D functions as a hormone, regulating the metabolism of calcium and phosphorus via promotion of intestinal absorption. Promotes bone formation, inhibits parathyroid hormone secretion, and promotes immunosuppression and phagocytosis.

ABSORPTION/SOLUBILITY/STORAGE/PHARMACOKINETICS: Fat soluble. Once ingested, vitamin D is hydrolyzed in the liver and kidney to its biologically active form, 1,25-dihydroxyvitamin D. Breast milk provides approximately 25 IU vitamin D/L. Vitamin D is stored in adipose tissue, making it less bioavailable to obese individuals with increased body fat.

RATIONALE FOR SUPPLEMENTATION: Bone health, defense against osteoporosis; defense against cancer; enhanced immunity.

EVIDENCE IN SUPPORT OF SUPPLEMENTATION TO AND ABOVE THE DRI: In some populations (e.g., darker skin, little outdoor exposure, living in northern latitudes, malabsorption conditions), vitamin D deficiency is common and the benefits of supplementation may depend to a large extent on baseline vitamin D status. For instance, it is unlikely that vitamin D supplements are beneficial for bone health in children and in adolescents with normal vitamin D levels[a] or for muscle strength in nondeficient adults.[b] For older adults, however, supplementation with vitamin D seems to improve strength, gait, and balance, regardless of vitamin D status.[c] Vitamin D supplementation may also reduce the risk of fractures in older women, but is most effective when combined with calcium supplementation.[d] Vitamin D supplements do not seem to reduce cardiovascular risk, except in perhaps for those who are vitamin D deficient (e.g., those with renal disease).[e] Data on vitamin D related to cardiometabolic outcomes are uncertain; some trials show improved insulin resistance but do not show consistent or significant effects on glycemic control, diabetes incidence, blood pressure, or cardiovascular outcomes.[f] Data on cancer prevention are mixed, for cancer overall and for specific malignancies; some studies suggest vitamin D supplementation increases cancer incidence, some that it decreases it.[g] Data on total mortality is clear though. Vitamin D supplementation reduces mortality rates in those who are vitamin D deficient: 8 of 9 trials included in a meta-analysis showing a mortality benefit were in populations with baseline vitamin-D levels that were deficient (serum level ≤20 ng/mL) and the ninth trial was in a population that was vitamin D insufficient (serum level ≤30 ng/mL).[h] Whether vitamin D supplementation confers a mortality benefit in individuals with baseline blood levels >30 ng/mL (considered by most experts to be the level of sufficiency) is an open question.

Recommended Intake Range (US RDA)[i:]

Age	Male	Female	Pregnancy	Lactation
0–12 mo*	400 IU (10 μg)	400 IU (10 μg)		
1–13 y	600 IU (15 μg)	600 IU (15 μg)	600 IU (15 μg)	600 IU (15 μg)
14–18 y	600 IU (15 μg)	600 IU (15 μg)	600 IU (15 μg)	600 IU (15 μg)
19–50 y	600 IU (15 μg)	600 IU (15 μg)		
51–70 y	600 IU (15 μg)	600 IU (15 μg)		
≥70 y	800 IU (20 μg)	800 IU (20 μg)		

AVERAGE INTAKE, US ADULTS[j:]	144–288 IU/d
ESTIMATED MEAN PALEOLITHIC INTAKE (ADULT):	Unavailable
COMMON DOSE RANGE FOR USE AS SUPPLEMENT:	200–400 IU
DO DIETARY PATTERNS MEETING GUIDELINES PERMIT ADEQUATE INTAKE?	Yes (provided fortified foods like dairy products are included, although most vitamin D comes from sun exposure rather than from dietary sources)
INCLUDED IN TYPICAL MULTIVITAMIN/MULTIMINERAL TABLET?	Yes

DEFICIENCY

Intake Level: Serum 25(OH)D values <20–25 mmol/L, or <200 IU/day.
Syndromes: Rickets in children, osteomalacia in adults, possibly decreased muscle strength and coordination, and earlier mortality.

TOXICITY

Intake Level[i]:

---

* Adequate Intake (AI)

Age	Male	Female	Pregnancy	Lactation
0–6 months	1,000 IU (25 μg)	1,000 IU (25 μg)		
7–12 months	1,500 IU (38 μg)	1,500 IU (38 μg)		
1–3 y	2,500 IU (63 μg)	2,500 IU (63 μg)		
4–8 y	3,000 IU (75 μg)	3,000 IU (75 μg)		
≥9 y	4,000 IU (100 μg)	4,000 IU (100 μg)	4,000 IU (100 μg)	4,000 IU (100 μg)

Syndromes: Soft tissue calcification, kidney stones, hypercalcemia. Nausea, vomiting, constipation, anorexia, weight loss, polyuria, and heart arrhythmias. Possibly greater risk of cancer at some sites like the pancreas, greater risk of cardiovascular events, and more falls and fractures among the elderly. Possibly greater all-cause mortality.

VITAMIN D DIETARY SOURCES[k]:

Food	Serving Size	Energy (kcal)	Vitamin D (IU)
Cod liver oil	1 tablespoon (15 mL)	123	1,360
Sardines	1 can (92 g)	191	250
Tuna, canned in oil	1 can (3 oz)	158	200
Milk, fortified	1 cup	146	100
Salmon, cooked	3.5 oz	181	360
Egg	1 whole	78	20
Mushrooms	½ cup (3 oz)	22	2,700 (if UV exposed)
Margarine, fortified	1 tablespoon	101	60

Additional details, evidence, and references for dosing and safety for many nutrients and substances individuals might choose to ingest can be found at http://www.mayoclinic.com/health/search/search, http://ods.od.nih.gov/, and http://www.nlm.nih.gov/medlineplus/.

[a]Winzenberg T, Powell S, Shaw KA, et al. Effects of vitamin D supplementation on bone density in healthy children: systematic review and meta-analysis. *BMJ* 2011;342:c7254. doi:10.1136/bmj.c7254.

[b]Stockton KA, Mengersen K, Paratz JD. Effect of vitamin D supplementation on muscle strength: a systematic review and meta-analysis. *Osteoporos Int* 2011;22(3):859–871. doi:10.1007/s00198-010-1407-y.

[c]Muir SW, Montero-Odasso M. Effect of vitamin D supplementation on muscle strength, gait and balance in older adults: a systematic review and meta-analysis. *J Am Geriatr Soc* 2011;59(12):2291–2300. doi:10.1111/j.1532-5415.2011.03733.x.

[d]Bergman GJ, Fan T, McFetridge JT. Efficacy of vitamin D3 supplementation in preventing fractures in elderly women: a meta-analysis. *Curr Med Res Opin* 2010;26(5):1193–1201. doi:10.1185/03007991003659814.

[e]Wang L, Manson JE, Song Y. Systematic review: Vitamin D and calcium supplementation in prevention of cardiovascular events. *Ann Intern Med* 2010;152(5):315–323. doi:10.7326/0003-4819-152-5-201003020-00010;

[f]Mitri J, Muraru MD, Pittas AG. Vitamin D and type 2 diabetes: a systematic review. *Eur J Clin Nutr* 2011;65(9):1005–1015. doi:10.1038/ejcn.2011.118; Pittas AG, Chung M, Trikalinos T, Systematic review: Vitamin D and cardiometabolic outcomes. *Ann Intern Med* 2010;152(5):307–314. doi:10.7326/0003-4819-152-5-201003020-00009.

[g]Chung M, Lee J, Terasawa T. Vitamin D with or without calcium supplementation for prevention of cancer and fractures: an updated meta-analysis for the U.S. Preventive Services Task Force. *Ann Intern Med* 2011;155(12):827–838. doi:10.7326/0003-4819-155-12-201112200-00005.

[h]Autier P, Gandini S. Vitamin D supplementation and total mortality: a meta-analysis of randomized controlled trials. *Arch Intern Med* 2007;167(16):1730–1737.

[i]Office of Dietary Supplements. *Vitamin D.* Available at http://ods.od.nih.gov/factsheets/VitaminD-HealthProfessional/; accessed 10/1/2013.

[j]NHANES. Available at http://ods.od.nih.gov/factsheets/VitaminD-HealthProfessional/; accessed 10/1/2013.

[k]The nutrient composition of most foods can be checked by accessing the US Department of Agriculture nutrient database at http://www.nal.usda.gov/fnic/foodcomp/search. A more extensive list of food sources of vitamin D is available in Margen S. *The wellness nutrition counter.* New York, NY: Health Letter Associates, 1997.

Sources: Ensminger AH, Ensminger ME, Konlande JE, et al. *The concise encyclopedia of foods and nutrition.* Boca Raton, FL: CRC Press, Inc., 1995.

Margen S. *The wellness nutrition counter.* New York, NY: Health Letter Associates, 1997.

Murray MT. *Encyclopedia of nutritional supplements.* Rocklin, CA: Prima Publishing, 1996.

National Research Council. *Recommended dietary allowances*, 10th ed. Washington, DC: National Academy Press, 1989.

Otten JJ, Hellwig JP, Meyers LD, eds. *Dietary Reference Intakes. The essential guide to nutrient requirements.* Washington, DC: National Academies Press, 2006.

(continued)

APPENDIX E   (Continued)

Pizzorno JE, Murray MT. *Textbook of natural medicine*, 3rd ed. St. Louis, MO: Church Livingstone Elsevier, 2006.

Shils ME, Shike M, Ross AC, et al., eds. *Modern nutrition in health and disease*, 10th ed. Philadelphia, PA: Lippincott Williams & Wilkins, 2005.

US Department of Agriculture. *USDA nutrient database for standard reference*. Release 19. 2006.

US Department of Agriculture. *USDA nutrient intake from NHANES 2001–2002 data*.

Ziegler EE, Filer LJ Jr, eds. *Present knowledge in nutrition*, 7th ed. Washington, DC: ILSI Press, 1996.

TOCOPHEROL/VITAMIN E

BIOLOGICAL FUNCTION(S) IN HUMANS/KEY PROPERTIES: Vitamin E refers to a group of compounds, collectively known as tocopherols and tocotrienols. The most abundant and biologically active is α-tocopherol (α-TE). Vitamin E functions as a lipid antioxidant, protecting and preserving the integrity of cellular and subcellular membranes.

ABSORPTION/SOLUBILITY/STORAGE/PHARMACOKINETICS: Absorption of vitamin E is relatively inefficient, ranging from 20%–80% of the amount ingested. Vitamin E is lipid soluble and transported along with lipoprotein particles. It is stored preferentially in liver and organs with high lipid content, such as the adrenal glands.

RATIONALE FOR SUPPLEMENTATION: Many individuals, particularly those with low intakes of vegetable oils, nuts, and seeds (that may both contain vitamin E and support its absorption through accompanying fat), may have intake below the recommended level.

The antioxidant effects of vitamin E are thought to be of benefit in the prevention of a variety of chronic diseases, including cardiovascular disease and cancer. Antioxidants are thought to have an antiaging effect as well. Increasingly, evidence suggests that antioxidant benefit is greatest when lipid-soluble antioxidants (such as vitamin E) and water-soluble antioxidants (such as vitamin C) are combined. However, recent trial evidence mitigates consistently against such benefits and against the use of supplemental vitamin E for disease prevention.

EVIDENCE IN SUPPORT OF SUPPLEMENTATION TO AND ABOVE THE DRI: Data from the Cambridge Heart Antioxidant Study suggest a benefit of supplemental vitamin E in the prevention of second myocardial infarction, although evidence of a mortality benefit was not found.[a] Beneficial effects of acute vitamin E supplementation on endothelial function have been reported. However, in the GISSI–Prevenzione trial, patients with recent myocardial infarction (n = 11,324) randomly assigned to vitamin E supplementation (300 mg) did not do better than those assigned to placebo with regard to myocardial infarction or death.[b] Similarly, the HOPE trial demonstrated no significant benefit of vitamin E supplementation (400 IU) with regard to both myocardial infarction and death in high-risk coronary patients.[c] Recent trial data and meta-analyses mitigate against use of supplemental vitamin E for the prevention of cancer or cardiovascular disease.[d–j] Likewise, meta-analyses demonstrate no benefit for vitamin E + vitamin C in pregnancy to prevent preeclampsia[k] or for vitamin E alone with regard to glycemic control.[l] Most importantly, vitamin E supplementation does not appear to have an overall mortality benefit,[m] and may actually increase mortality at high doses (>400 IU/d).[n]

Recommended Intake Range (US RDA)[o]:

VITAMIN E RECOMMENDED INTAKE RANGE (US RDA):

	Infancy (age 0–6 mo)	Infancy (age 7–12 mo)	Childhood (age 1–3 y)	Childhood (age 4–8 y)	Adolescence (age 9–13 y)
Male	4 mg (6 IU)*	5 mg (7.5 IU)*	6 mg (9 IU)	7 mg (10.4 IU)	11 mg (16.4 IU)
Female	4 mg (6 IU)*	5 mg (7.5 IU)*	6 mg (9 IU)	7 mg (10.4 IU)	11 mg (16.4 IU)

	Adolescence (age 14–18 y)	Adult (age ≥ 19 y)	Pregnancy (all ages)	Lactation (all ages)
Male	15 mg (22.4 IU)	15 mg (22.4 IU)	—	—
Female	15 mg (22.4 IU)	15 mg (22.4 IU)	15 mg (22.4 IU)	19 mg (28.4 IU)

AVERAGE INTAKE, US ADULTS:	6.3–8 mg α-TE
ESTIMATED MEAN PALEOLITHIC INTAKE (ADULT)[p]:	33 mg α-TE
COMMON DOSE RANGE FOR USE AS SUPPLEMENT:	133–533 mg α-TE (200–800 IU)
DO DIETARY PATTERNS MEETING GUIDELINES PERMIT ADEQUATE INTAKE?	Yes
INCLUDED IN TYPICAL MULTIVITAMIN/MULTIMINERAL TABLET?	Yes (dose: 20.3 mg)

DEFICIENCY

    Intake Level: Intake below RDA and/or fat malabsorption for years.

    Syndromes: Neurologic dysfunction/neuropathy, ataxia, muscle weakness, hemolysis, impaired vision, myopathy, retinopathy, and impairment of the immune response

TOXICITY

    Intake Level: Uncertain; in excess of 1,200 IU/day (although risk of death begins to increase at a dose almost 10 times lower)[n]

---

* = AI. All other values in table are for RDA.

(continued)

APPENDIX E   (Continued)

VITAMIN E TOLERABLE UPPER INTAKE LEVELS (UL)°:

	Infancy (age 0–6 mo)	Infancy (age 7–12 mo)	Childhood (age 1–3 y)	Childhood (age 4–8 y)
Male	—	—	200 mg (300 IU)	300 mg (450 IU)
Female	—	—	200 mg (300 IU)	300 mg (450 IU)

	Adolescence (age 9–13 y)	Adolescence (age 14–18 y)	Adult (age ≥ 19 y)	Pregnancy (age 14–18 y)
Male	600 mg (900 IU)	800 mg (1,200 IU)	1,000 mg (1,500 IU)	—
Female	600 mg (900 IU)	800 mg (1,200 IU)	1,000 mg (1,500 IU)	800 mg (1,200 IU)

	Pregnancy (age 19–50 y)	Lactation (age 14–18 y)	Lactation (age 19–50 y)
Male	—	—	—
Female	1,000 mg (1,500 IU)	800 mg (1,200 IU)	1,000 mg (1,500 IU)

Syndromes: Diarrhea, headache, coagulopathy, increased risk of hemorrhagic stroke, and possibly earlier mortality.

Vitamin E Dietary Sources[q]: Vitamin E is relatively abundant in vegetable oils, nuts, seeds, and whole grains

Food	Serving Size	Energy (kcal)	Vitamin E (mg α-TE)	Food	Serving Size	Energy (kcal)	Vitamin E (mg α-TE)
Wheat germ oil	1 tablespoon (13.6 g)	120	20.3	Corn oil	1 tablespoon (13.6 g)	120	1.9
Sardines	1 can (92 g)	191	1.9	Avocado	1 medium (201 g)	322	4.2
Almonds	1 oz (28 g)	164	7.3	Flounder	1 fillet (127 g)	149	0.8
Peanut butter	2 tablespoons (32 g)	188	2.9	Swiss chard (boiled)	1 cup (175 g)	35	3.3
Blueberries	1 cup (148 g)	84	0.8	Broccoli	1 spear (37 g)	13	0.5
Tomato puree	1 cup (250 g)	95	4.9	Nectarines	1 medium (142 g)	62	1.1
Canola oil	1 tablespoon (14 g)	124	2.4				

Effects of Food Preparation and Storage: Vitamin E will be lost if fat or oil is removed during cooking or preparation.

Additional details, evidence, and references for dosing and safety for many nutrients and substances individuals might choose to ingest can be found at http://www.mayoclinic.com/health/search/search, http://ods.od.nih.gov/, and http://www.nlm.nih.gov/medlineplus/.

[a]Stephens NG, Parsons A, Schofield PM, et al. Randomized controlled trial of vitamin E in patients with coronary disease: Cambridge Heart Antioxidant Study (CHAOS). *Lancet* 1996;347:781–786.

[b]GISSI–Prevenzione Investigators. Dietary supplementation with n-3 polyunsaturated fatty acids and vitamin E after myocardial infarction: results of the GISSI-Prevenzione trial. *Lancet* 1999;354:447–455.

[c]The Heart Outcomes Prevention Evaluation Study Investigators. Vitamin E supplementation and cardiovascular events in high-risk patients. *N Engl J Med* 2000:342:154–160.

[d]Bjelakovic G, Nikolova D, Gluud LL, et al. Mortality in randomized trials of antioxidant supplements for primary and secondary prevention: systematic review and meta-analysis. *JAMA* 2007;297:842–857.

[e]Bjelakovic G, Nagorni A, Nikolova D, et al. Meta-analysis: antioxidant supplements for primary and secondary prevention of colorectal adenoma. *Aliment Pharmacol Ther* 2006;24:281–291.

[f]Bjelakovic G, Nikolova D, Simonetti RG, et al. Antioxidant supplements for preventing gastrointestinal cancers. *Cochrane Database Syst Rev* 2004;4:CD004183.

[g]Bleys J, Miller ER 3rd, Pastor-Barriuso R, et al. Vitamin-mineral supplementation and the progression of atherosclerosis: a meta-analysis of randomized controlled trials. *Am J Clin Nutr* 2006;84:880–887.

[h]Lee IM, Cook NR, Gaziano JM, et al. Vitamin E in the primary prevention of cardiovascular disease and cancer: the Women's Health Study: a randomized controlled trial. *JAMA* 2005;294:56–65.

[i]Shekelle PG, Morton SC, Jungvig LK, et al. Effect of supplemental vitamin E for the prevention and treatment of cardiovascular disease. *J Gen Intern Med* 2004;19(4):380–389.

[j]Pham DQ, Plakogiannis R. Vitamin E supplementation in cardiovascular disease and cancer prevention: part 1. *Ann Pharmacother* 2005;39(11):1870–1878.

[k]Conde-Agudelo A, Romero R, Kusanovic JP, et al. Supplementation with vitamins C and E during pregnancy for the prevention of preeclampsia and other adverse maternal and perinatal outcomes: a systematic review and meta-analysis. *Am J Obstet Gynecol* 2011;204(6):503.e1–12. doi:10.1016/j.ajog.2011.02.020.

[l]Suksomboon N, Poolsup N, Sinprasert S. Effects of vitamin E supplementation on glycaemic control in type 2 diabetes: systematic review of randomized controlled trials. *J Clin Pharm Ther* 2011;36(1):53–63. doi:10.1111/j.1365-2710.2009.01154.x.

[m]Schmitt FA, Mendiondo MS, Marcum JL, et al. Vitamin E and all-cause mortality: a meta-analysis. *Curr Aging Sci* 2011;4(2):158–170; Berry D, Wathen JK, Newell M. Bayesian model averaging in meta-analysis: vitamin E supplementation and mortality. *Clin Trials* 2009;6(1):28–41. doi:10.1177/1740774508101279.

[n]Miller ER 3rd, Pastor-Barriuso R, Dalal D, et al. Meta-analysis: high-dosage vitamin E supplementation may increase all-cause mortality. *Ann Intern Med* 2005;142(1):37–46.

[o]Office of Dietary Supplements.*Vitamin E*. Available http://ods.od.nih.gov/factsheets/VitaminE-HealthProfessional/; accessed 10/1/13.

[p]Eaton SB, Eaton SB 3rd, Konner MJ. Paleolithic nutrition revisited: a twelve-year retrospective on its nature and implications. *Eur J Clin Nutr* 1997;51:207–216.

[q]The nutrient composition of most foods can be checked by accessing the US Department of Agriculture nutrient database. http://www.nal.usda.gov/fnic/foodcomp/search.

Sources: Ensminger AH, Ensminger ME, Konlande JE, et al. *The concise encyclopedia of foods and nutrition.* Boca Raton, FL: CRC Press, Inc., 1995.

Margen S. *The wellness nutrition counter.* New York, NY: Health Letter Associates, 1997.

Murray MT. *Encyclopedia of nutritional supplements.* Rocklin, CA: Prima Publishing, 1996.

National Research Council. *Recommended dietary allowances*, 10th ed. Washington, DC: National Academy Press, 1989.

Otten JJ, Hellwig JP, Meyers LD, eds. *Dietary reference intakes. The essential guide to nutrient requirements.* Washington, DC: National Academies Press, 2006.

Pizzorno JE, Murray MT. *Textbook of natural medicine*, 3rd ed. St. Louis, MO: Church Livingstone Elsevier, 2006.

Shils ME, Shike M, Ross AC, et al., eds. *Modern nutrition in health and disease*, 10th ed. Philadelphia, PA: Lippincott Williams & Wilkins, 2005.

US Department of Agriculture. *USDA nutrient database for standard reference.* Release 19. 2006.

US Department of Agriculture. *USDA nutrient intake from NHANES 2001–2002 data.*

Ziegler EE, Filer LJ Jr, eds. *Present knowledge in nutrition*, 7th ed. Washington, DC: ILSI Press, 1996.

ZINC

BIOLOGICAL FUNCTION(S) IN HUMANS/KEY PROPERTIES: Zinc functions in nearly 100 enzyme systems with prominent roles in CO_2 transport and digestion. Zinc also influences DNA and RNA synthesis, immune function, collagen synthesis, olfaction, and taste. Recent interest in zinc has focused on its role in immune function. Zinc lozenges and sprays have been studied for the treatment of upper respiratory infection, and zinc has been found to confer some benefit in lower respiratory infections.[a,b] Evidence of benefit is inconsistent, however, and refuted by the results of some trials.[c,d]

ABSORPTION/SOLUBILITY/STORAGE/PHARMACOKINETICS: The efficiency of zinc absorption varies inversely with body stores. The absorption of zinc is impeded by fiber phytates, and influenced by the stores and dietary intake of other minerals. Zinc is stored in bone and muscle, but these stores do not readily exchange with the circulation, and therefore cannot compensate rapidly for dietary deficiency.

RATIONALE FOR SUPPLEMENTATION: The typical American diet provides approximately 5 mg of zinc/1,000 kcal. An intake of 15 mg/day is recommended for men, 12 mg/day for women. Older adults in particular are unlikely to take in sufficient calories to meet the RDA for zinc without supplementation.

Supplementation in the range 15–60 mg/day is advocated to enhance immune function; improve pregnancy outcomes; improve male sexual function and fertility; and provide a therapeutic effect in rheumatoid arthritis, acne, Alzheimer's dementia, and macular degeneration. Zinc supplementation may be beneficial in Wilson's disease, a state of copper overload, because zinc interferes with copper absorption.

EVIDENCE IN SUPPORT OF SUPPLEMENTATION TO AND ABOVE THE DRI: Mechanistic studies suggest that zinc plays a role in cell-mediated immune function. Targeted dosing of zinc to the upper airway has shown benefit in some studies of viral infections but not in others.[d] In zinc-deficient populations, zinc supplementation is of benefit against infectious diseases. For HIV-infected individuals (who are commonly zinc deficient), supplementation may help boost CD4 counts, protect against opportunistic infections, and prevent diarrhea.[e] In developing countries, supplementation helps prevent pediatric pneumonia and infectious diarrhea,[f] but does not seem to prevent malaria or malarial deaths.[g] In nondeficient populations, zinc supplementation appears to be of no benefit in pediatric pneumonia,[h] or as a measure to prevent childhood diarrhea.[i] However, zinc supplementation does show a weak relationship with lower risk of preterm birth, which, if causal, might reflect a reduction in maternal infection (a primary cause of prematurity).[j] Beyond infectious considerations, randomized controlled trials demonstrate no benefit of zinc supplementation for ADHD in children[k] or for Alzheimer's disease or cognitive decline in the elderly.[l] Other trials suggest a modest effect of zinc supplementation in reducing glucose concentration in diabetics, but without statistically significant reductions in A1c.[m] Zinc supplementation does not appear to prevent the incidence of diabetes in those with baseline insulin resistance.[n]

Recommended Intake Range (US RDA): An intake of 8–13 mg/day of total zinc is recommended for adults.

ZINC RECOMMENDED INTAKE RANGE (US RDA)[o]:

	Infancy (age 0–6 mo)	Infancy (age 7–12 mo)	Childhood (age 1–3 y)	Childhood (age 4–8 y)
Male	2 mg*	3 mg	3 mg	5 mg
Female	2 mg*	3 mg	3 mg	5 mg
	Adolescence (age 9–13 y)	Adolescence (age 14–18 y)	Adult (age ≥ 19 y)	Pregnancy (age 14–18 y)
Male	8 mg	11 mg	11 mg	—
Female	8 mg	9 mg	8 mg	12 mg
	Pregnancy (age 19–50 y)	Lactation (age 14–18 y)	Lactation (age 19–50 y)	
Male	—	—	—	
Female	11 mg	13 mg	12 mg	

AVERAGE INTAKE, US ADULTS:	9.9–14.4 mg/day
ESTIMATED MEAN PALEOLITHIC INTAKE (ADULT)[o]:	43.4 mg/day
COMMON DOSE RANGE FOR USE AS SUPPLEMENT:	15–60 mg/day
DO DIETARY PATTERNS MEETING GUIDELINES PERMIT ADEQUATE INTAKE?	Yes
INCLUDED IN TYPICAL MULTIVITAMIN/MULTIMINERAL TABLET?	Yes (dose: 15.0 mg)

* = AI. All other values in table represent RDA.

DEFICIENCY

Intake Level: Below RDA.

Syndromes: Impaired taste and smell; impaired immune function and wound healing; deficiency may lead to eye and skin lesions, alopecia, growth retardation and delayed sexual maturation, impotence, hypogonadism, and mental lethargy.

TOXICITY

Intake Level: ≥50 mg/day.

ZINC TOLERABLE UPPER INTAKE LEVELS (UL)[o]:

	Infancy (age 0–6 mo)	Infancy (age 7–12 mo)	Childhood (age 1–3 y)	Childhood (age 4–8 y)
Male	4 mg	5 mg	7 mg	12 mg
Female	4 mg	5 mg	7 mg	12 mg
	Adolescence (age 9–13 y)	Adolescence (age 14–18 y)	Adult (age ≥ 19 y)	Pregnancy (age 14–18 y)
Male	23 mg	34 mg	40 mg	—
Female	23 mg	34 mg	40 mg	34 mg
	Pregnancy (age 19–50 y)	Lactation (age 14–18 y)	Lactation (age 19–50 y)	
Male	—	—	—	
Female	40 mg	34 mg	40 mg	

Syndromes: Nausea, vomiting, loss of appetite, abdominal cramps, diarrhea, and headaches; impaired copper status; at higher intake levels, reduced high-density lipoprotein and impaired hematopoiesis.

Zinc Dietary Sources[q]: Zinc is found abundantly in shellfish, red meat, legumes, and nuts.

Food	Serving Size	Energy (kcal)	Zinc	Food	Serving Size	Energy (kcal)	Zinc
Oysters	6 medium (42 g)	58	76	White beans	1 cup (179 g)	249	2.5
King crab	1 leg (134 g)	130	10.2	Almonds	1 oz (28.3 g)	164	1
Wheat germ	1 cup (115 g)	414	14.1	Avocado	1 medium (201 g)	322	1.3
Sardines	1 can (92 g)	191	1.2	Barley, pearled	1 cup (157 g)	193	1.3
Lamb	3 oz (85 g)	219	3.7	Chick peas	1 cup (164 g)	269	2.5
Turkey breast	1 lb (112 g)	212	2.3	Lentils	1 cup (198 g)	230	2.5
Cashews	1 oz (28 g)	157	1.6	Chicken breast	1/2 breast (98 g)	193	1
Swordfish	1 piece (106 g)	164	1.6	Oat bran	1 cup (219 g)	88	1.2
Tofu	1/2 cup (126 g)	85	1.1	Oatmeal	100 g	55	0.5

Effects of Food Preparation and Storage: Not reported to be a generally important determinant of dietary intake levels.

Additional details, evidence, and references for dosing and safety for many nutrients and substances individuals might choose to ingest can be found at http://www.mayoclinic.com/health/search/search, http://ods.od.nih.gov/, and http://www.nlm.nih.gov/medlineplus/.

[a]Sazawal S, Black RE, Jalla S, et al. Zinc supplementation reduces the incidence of acute lower respiratory infections in infants and pre-school children: a double-blind, controlled trial. *Pediatrics* 1998;102:1–5.

[b]Marshall S. Zinc gluconate and the common cold. Review of randomized controlled trials. *Can Fam Physician* 1998;44:1037–1042.

[c]Macknin ML, Piedmonte M, Calendine C, et al. Zinc gluconate lozenges for treating the common cold in children: a randomized controlled trial. *JAMA* 1998;279:1962–1967.

[d]Macknin ML. Zinc lozenges for the common cold. *Cleve Clin J Med* 1999;66:27–32.

[e]Zeng L, Zhang L. Efficacy and safety of zinc supplementation for adults, children and pregnant women with HIV infection: systematic review. *Trop Med Int Health* 2011;16(12):1474–1482. doi:10.1111/j.1365-3156.2011.02871.x; Baum MK, Lai S, Sales S, et al. Randomized, controlled clinical trial of zinc supplementation to prevent immunological failure in HIV-infected adults. *Clin Infect Dis* 2010;50(12):1653–60. doi:10.1086/652864.

(continued)

APPENDIX E (Continued)

[f]Bhutta ZA, Black RE, Brown KH, et al; Prevention of diarrhea and pneumonia by zinc supplementation in children in developing countries: pooled analysis of randomized controlled trials. Zinc Investigators' Collaborative Group. *J Pediatr* 1999;135(6):689–697; Müller O, Becher H, van Zweeden AB, et al. Effect of zinc supplementation on malaria and other causes of morbidity in west African children: randomised double blind placebo controlled trial. *BMJ* 2001;322(7302):1567.

[g]Müller O, Becher H, van Zweeden AB, et al. Effect of zinc supplementation on malaria and other causes of morbidity in west African children: randomised double blind placebo controlled trial. *BMJ* 2001;322(7302):1567.

[h]Haider BA, Lassi ZS, Ahmed A, et al. Zinc supplementation as an adjunct to antibiotics in the treatment of pneumonia in children 2 to 59 months of age. *Cochrane Database Syst Rev* 2011;(10):CD007368. doi:10.1002/14651858.CD007368.

[i]Patel AB, Mamtani M, Badhoniya N, et al. What zinc supplementation does and does not achieve in diarrhea prevention: a systematic review and meta-analysis. *BMC Infect Dis* 2011;11:122. doi:10.1186/1471-2334-11-122.

[j]Chaffee BW, King JC. Effect of zinc supplementation on pregnancy and infant outcomes: a systematic review. *Paediatr Perinat Epidemiol* 2012;26(suppl 1):118–137. doi:10.1111/j.1365-3016.2012.01289.x.

[k]Ghanizadeh A, Berk M. Zinc for treating of children and adolescents with attention-deficit hyperactivity disorder: a systematic review of randomized controlled clinical trials. *Eur J Clin Nutr* 2013;67(1):122–124. doi:10.1038/ejcn.2012.177.

[l]Loef M, von Stillfried N, Walach H. Zinc diet and Alzheimer's disease: a systematic review. *Nutr Neurosci* 2012;15(5):2–12. doi:10.1179/1476830512Y.0000000010.

[m]Capdor J, Foster M, Petocz P, et al. Zinc and glycemic control: a meta-analysis of randomised placebo controlled supplementation trials in humans. *J Trace Elem Med Biol* 2013;27(2):137–142. doi:10.1016/j.jtemb.2012.08.001.

[n]Beletate V, El Dib RP, Atallah AN. Zinc supplementation for the prevention of type 2 diabetes mellitus. *Cochrane Database Syst Rev* 2007;(1):CD005525.

[o]Office of Dietary Supplements. *Zinc.* Available at http://ods.od.nih.gov/factsheets/Zinc-HealthProfessional/; accessed 10/1/2013.

[p]Eaton SB, Eaton SB 3rd, Konner MJ. Paleolithic nutrition revisited: a twelve-year retrospective on its nature and implications. *Eur J Clin Nutr* 1997;51:207–216.

[q]The nutrient composition of most foods can be checked by accessing the US Department of Agriculture nutrient database, at http://www.nal.usda.gov/fnic/foodcomp/search.

Sources: Ensminger AH, Ensminger ME, Konlande JE, et al. *The concise encyclopedia of foods and nutrition.* Boca Raton, FL: CRC Press, Inc., 1995.

Margen S. *The wellness nutrition counter.* New York, NY: Health Letter Associates, 1997.

Murray MT. *Encyclopedia of nutritional supplements.* Rocklin, CA: Prima Publishing, 1996.

National Research Council. *Recommended dietary allowances,* 10th ed. Washington, DC: National Academy Press, 1989.

Otten JJ, Hellwig JP, Meyers LD, eds. *Dietary reference intakes. The essential guide to nutrient requirements.* Washington, DC: National Academies Press, 2006.

Pizzorno JE, Murray MT. *Textbook of natural medicine,* 3rd ed. St. Louis, MO: Church Livingstone Elsevier, 2006.

Shils ME, Shike M, Ross AC, et al., eds. *Modern nutrition in health and disease,* 10th ed. Philadelphia, PA: Lippincott Williams & Wilkins, 2005.

US Department of Agriculture. *USDA nutrient database for standard reference.* Release 19. 2006.

US Department of Agriculture. *USDA nutrient intake from NHANES 2001–2002 data.*

Ziegler EE, Filer LJ Jr, eds. *Present knowledge in nutrition,* 7th ed. Washington, DC: ILSI Press, 1996.

APPENDIX F   RESOURCES FOR NUTRIENT COMPOSITION OF FOODS

RESOURCE MATERIAL

ONLINE RESOURCES

The nutrient composition of most foods can be checked by accessing the U.S. Department of Agriculture nutrient database, at http://www.nal.usda.gov/fnic/foodcomp/search. At this address, simply enter the name of the food of interest. A list of food choices within the pertinent category will be displayed. Once a specific food is chosen, portion size options are displayed. Once the portion is selected, a table of nutrient composition is displayed.

Some nutrient content can now also be checked using Google (www.google.com). On the main search page, simply type:

"How many/how much [A] in [B] of [C]?" and get an instantaneous answer.

[A] can be any information on a Nutrition Facts label (i.e., calories, total fat, saturated fat, polyunsaturated fat, monounsaturated fat, cholesterol, sodium, potassium, total carbohydrate, dietary fiber, sugar, protein, vitamin A, calcium, vitamin B_6, vitamin B_{12}, vitamin C, Iron, or magnesium).

[B] can be any units in terms of numerical quantity (e.g., "3"), volume (e.g., "oz" or "ounces", "c" or "cups"), or weight (e.g., "g" or "grams").

[C] can be just about any whole food (fruit, vegetable, nut, meat, dairy), nonproprietary processed food (e.g., potato chips, pretzels, crackers, ice cream), or nonproprietary mixed food (e.g., lasagna, hamburger, chicken fingers, pizza).

As of the time of this writing, the Google search allows limited ability to distinguish different preparations (e.g., baked vs. fried) and varieties (e.g., low-fat vs. regular) using dropdown menus

PRINT RESOURCES

Margen S. *The wellness nutrition counter.* New York, NY: Health Letter Associates, 1997. Produced by the University of California at Berkeley, this text provides detailed nutritional information for more than 6,000 foods.

Morrill JS, Bakun S, Murphy SP. *Are you eating right? Analyze your diet using the nutrient content of more than 5,000 foods,* 4th ed. Menlo Park, CA: Orange Grove Publishers, 1997. A user-friendly guide to the nutrient composition of more than 5,000 foods. Nutrient content is displayed in measures comparable to those appearing on food labels.

APPENDIX G   DIET–DRUG INTERACTIONS

EXAMPLES OF DIET–DRUG INTERACTIONS

Alcohol: Alcohol increases the potential hepatotoxicity of many drugs, acetaminophen being a noteworthy example.[a]

Folate: Phenytoin depletes folate, and folate facilitates the maintenance of steady-state phenytoin levels. Folate (500 mg/day) should be supplemented when phenytoin is prescribed.[b]

Grapefruit Juice: Grapefruit juice inhibits the cytochrome P450 enzyme CYP3A4, thereby potentially affecting the levels of the many drugs metabolized in the P450 system.[c]

Vitamin K: Warfarin (Coumadin) is opposed by dietary vitamin K. Dark green vegetables are rich sources of vitamin K, but distribution in the food supply is wide. If anticoagulation is difficult, a dietary assessment is indicated [d]

REFERENCE MATERIAL

ONLINE SOURCES

An online brochure on food and drug interactions is available from the FDA at: http://www.cfsan.fda.gov/~lrd/fdinter.html.

An online food–drug interaction guide from the University of Florida: http://www.druginteractioncenter.org/.

An online guide to nutrient interactions with cancer drugs from the University of Texas MD Anderson Cancer Center http://www.mdanderson.org/departments/nutrition/dIndex.cfm?pn=67CA5DD8-7BA0-11D5-812D00508B603A14.

Mayo Clinic http://www.mayoclinic.com/health-information (search for specific nutrients and find drug–nutrient interactions)

Medline Plus http://www.nlm.nih.gov/medlineplus/medlineplus.html (search for specific nutrients and find drug–nutrient interactions)

(continued)

APPENDIX G   (Continued)

National Institutes of Health—Office of Dietary Supplements http://ods.od.nih.gov/factsheets/list-all/ (search for specific nutrients and find drug–nutrient interactions)

Safety information on herbs and supplements from the National Institutes of Health is available at: http://www.nlm.nih.gov/medlineplus/druginformation.html.

BOOKS

Boullata JI, Armenti VT. *Handbook of drug–nutrient interactions.* Totowa, NJ: Humana Press, 2004.

Holt GA, ed. *Food and drug interactions: a guide for consumers.* Chicago, IL: Bonus Books, 1998.

Lininger SW, ed. *The A–Z guide to drug–herb and vitamin interactions.* Rocklin, CA: Prima Publishing, 1999.

McCabe-Sellers BJ, Wolfe JJ, Frankel EH, eds. *Handbook of food-drug interactions.* Boca Raton, FL: CRC Press, 2003.

OTHER PRINT SOURCES

Brazier NC, Levine MA. Drug-herb interaction among commonly used conventional medicines: a compendium for health care professionals. *Am J Ther* 2003;10:163–169.

Cupp MJ. Herbal remedies: adverse effects and drug interactions. *Am Fam Physician* 1999;59:1239–1245.

Harris RZ, Jang GR, Tsunoda S. Dietary effects on drug metabolism and transport. *Clin Pharmacokinet* 2003;42:1071–1088.

Jefferson JW. Drug and diet interactions: avoiding therapeutic paralysis. *J Clin Psychiatr* 1998;59:31–39. (*Review article of drug–diet interactions in psychiatry, particularly the treatment of depression.*)

Santos CA, Boullata JI. An approach to evaluating drug–nutrient interactions. *Pharmacotherapy* 2005;25:1789–1800.

Singh BN. Effects of food on clinical pharmacokinetics. *Clin Pharmacokinet* 1999;37:213–255.

William L, Holl DP Jr, Davis JA, et al. The influence of food on the absorption and metabolism of drugs: an update. *Eur J Drug Metab Pharmacokinet* 1996;21:201–211.

[a]Holtzman JL. The effect of alcohol on acetaminophen hepatotoxicity. *Arch Intern Med* 2002;162:1193.

[b]Seligmann H, Potasman I, Weller B, et al. Phenytoin–folic acid interaction: a lesson to be learned. *Clin Neuropharmacol* 1999;22:268–72.

[c]Kirby BJ, Unadkat JD. Grapefruit juice, a glass full of drug interactions? *Clin Pharmacol Ther* 2007;81:631–633.

[d]Booth SL, Centurelli MA. Vitamin K: a practical guide to the dietary management of patients on Coumadin. *Nutr Rev* 1999;57:288–296.

APPENDIX H   NUTRIENT REMEDIES FOR COMMON CONDITIONS: PATIENT RESOURCES

ESOURCE MATERIAL

ONLINE RESOURCES

HTTP://WWW.DRKOOP.COM/NATURALMEDICINE.HTML (provides condition-specific nutrition information) A site that exposes false and legitimate claims about dietary supplements: http://www.supplementwatch.com/.

Guidance on use of supplements from the US Government: http://www.nutrition.gov/index.php?mode=subject&subject=ng_supplements&d_subject=Dietary%20Supplements.

English translation of German Commission E Monographs through American Botanical Council: http://cms.herbalgram.org/commissione/index.html

Natural Medicines Comprehensive Database (Requires Fee): http://naturaldatabase.therapeuticresearch.com/home.aspx?cs=&s=ND

PRINT RESOURCES

Craig SY, Haigh J, Harrar S, eds. *The complete book of alternative nutrition.* Emmaus, PA: Rodale Press, Inc., 1997.

Lininger SW, ed. *The natural pharmacy: from the top experts in the field, your essential guide to vitamins, herbs, minerals and homeopathic remedies.* Rocklin, CA: Prima Publishing, 1998.

Murray MT. *Encyclopedia of nutritional supplements.* Rocklin, CA: Prima Publishing, 1996.

Tyler VE. *The doctor's book of herbal home remedies: cure yourself with nature's most powerful healing agents: advice from 200 experts for more than 150 conditions.* Emmaus, PA: Rodale Press, 2000.

APPENDIX I   PRINT AND WEB-BASED RESOURCE MATERIALS FOR PROFESSIONALS

RESOURCE MATERIAL

Readers are referred to the books included under "Suggested Readings" in the bibliographies provided at the end of each chapter.

NEWSLETTERS

Arbor Nutrition Updates. Summaries of latest research findings on diverse nutrition topics of clinical interest; free subscription.

HTTP://WWW.OVID.COM/SITE/CATALOG/JOURNAL/1881.JSP?TOP2&MID=3&BOTTOM=7&SUBECTION=12.

WEB-BASED RESOURCES

HTTP://WWW.HEALTHFINDER.GOV

This site, useful to both professional and lay users, is maintained by the U.S. Department of Health and Human Services and serves as a directory to credible sources of health information on the web. A search engine allows for easy identification of nutrition sites of interest.

HTTP://WWW.ARS.USDA.GOV/BA/BHNRC/NDL

This site provides access to the U.S. Department of Agriculture Nutrient Data Laboratory. The nutrient composition of virtually any food can be found in the database. To determine the nutrient composition of a food, click "Search" and enter the name of the food.

HTTP://WWW.AOA.GOV/PRESS/FACT/ALPHA/FACT_ELDERLY_NUTRITION.ASP

The Administration on Aging maintains this website, which details the Elderly Nutrition Program, an assistance program for older adults. The information is of use in efforts to provide nutrition to older patients with limited ability to maintain a balanced diet.

HTTP://WWW.FNS.USDA.GOV/CND/CONTACTS/STATEDIRECTORY.HTM

The US Department of Agriculture maintains this site, which indexes food assistance program offices for children by state.

HTTP://WWW.CDC.GOV/NCHS/NHANES.HTM

This site, maintained by the National Center for Health Statistics at the Centers for Disease Control and Prevention, provides access to dietary intake data from the National Health and Nutrition Examination Survey.

HTTP://WWW.EATRIGHT.ORG

This site, maintained by the American Dietetic Association, provides information about the services of dietitians as well as a search engine to find a local dietitian listed with the association.

HTTP://WWW.NIDDK.NIH.GOV/HEALTH/NUTRIT/NUTRIT.HTM

This site, which provides updated information on diet and obesity, is maintained by the National Institute of Diabetes, Digestive and Kidney Disease (NIDDK) at the National Institutes of Health.

HTTP://FNIC.NAL.USDA.GOV

This site, maintained by the US Department of Agriculture, provides updated dietary guidelines.

HTTP://WWW.NHLBI.NIH.GOV/HEALTH/PROF/HEART/INDEX.HTM

This site, maintained by the National Heart, Lung, and Blood Institute at the National Institutes of Health, provides professional links to information on the management of cardiovascular risk factors, including hypertension, obesity, and hyperlipidemia.

HTTP://ODS.OD.NIH.GOV/

The National Institutes of Health Office of Dietary Supplements website, which provides overviews of individual vitamins, minerals and other dietary supplements with links (e.g., to nutrient recommendations and Dietary Reference Intakes), "QuickFacts", and detailed "Fact Sheets"

APPENDIX J   PRINT AND WEB-BASED RESOURCE MATERIALS FOR PATIENTS

RESOURCE MATERIAL

NEWSLETTERS/MAGAZINES/ARTICLES

Eating well. Where good taste meats good health. Charlotte, VT. [Subscriptions: (802)425-5700; http://www.eatingwell.com]

A magazine about both food and health, with excellent recipes.

Kostas G. Low-fat and delicious: can we break the taste barrier? *J Am Diet Assoc* 1997;97:s88–s92.

A discussion of methods for translating nutrition guidelines into actual cooking and eating; appropriate reading for patients as well as providers.

Tufts University Health & Nutrition Letter [Phone: (800)274-7581; http://www.healthletter.tufts.edu]

Sound nutrition advice for the layperson from a leading school of nutrition.

University of California, Berkeley Wellness Letter [Phone: (800)829-9170]

Excellent and credible advice on health promotion, including nutrition, fitness, and lifestyle.

BOOKS

COOKBOOKS

Books listed below are considered particularly helpful but are a representative sample only; books to guide nutritious cooking are available by virtually every category of cuisine and health condition. The patient with a specific interest not addressed below should be referred to an actual or online bookstore.

Goldfarb A. *The six o'clock scramble.* New York, NY: St. Martin's Press, 2006.

Hagman B. *The gluten-free gourmet cooks fast and healthy: wheat-free with less fuss and fat.* New York, NY: Henry Holt, 1997.

Pannell M, ed. *Allergy free cookbook (healthy eating).* New York, NY: Lorenz Books, 1999.

Pascal C. *The whole foods allergy cookbook: two hundred gourmet & homestyle recipes for the food allergic family.* Ridgefield, CT: Vital Health Publishing, 2005.

Ponichtera BJ. *Quick & healthy volume II.* Dalles, OR: Scale Down Publishing, 1995.

DIET AND HEALTH

Castelli WP, Griffin GC. *Good fat, bad fat: how to lower your cholesterol and reduce the odds of a heart attack.* Tucson, AZ: Fisher Books, 1997.

D'Agostino J. *Convertible cooking for a healthy heart.* Easton, PA: Healthy Heart, 1991.

Editors of the Wellness Cooking School, University of California at Berkeley. *The simply healthy lowfat cookbook.* New York, NY: Rebus, Inc., 1995.

Editors of the Wellness Cooking School, University of California at Berkeley. *The Wellness lowfat cookbook.* New York, NY: Rebus, Inc., 1993.

Katz DL, Gonzalez MH. *The way to eat.* Naperville, IL: Sourcebooks, Inc., 2002.

Katz DL, Katz CS. *The flavor full diet.* Emmaus, PA: Rodale, Inc., 2007.

Katzen M, Willett WC. *Eat, drink, & weigh less.* New York, NY: Hyperion, 2006.

Lund JM, Alpert B. *Cooking healthy with the kids in mind: a healthy exchanges cookbook.* New York, NY: Putnam Publishing Group, 1998.

Lund JM. *The diabetic's healthy exchanges cookbook (healthy exchanges cookbooks).* New York, NY: Perigee, 1996.

Mateljan G. *The world's healthiest foods.* Seattle, WA: George Mateljan Foundation, 2007.

Melina V, Forest J, Picarski R. *Cooking vegetarian: healthy, delicious, and easy vegetarian cuisine.* New York, NY: Wiley, 1998.

Nestle M. *What to eat.* New York, NY: North Point Press, 2007.

Nigro N, Nigro S. *Companion guide to healthy cooking: a practical introduction to natural ingredients.* Charlottesville, VA: Featherstone Inc., 1996.

Nixon DW, Zanca JA, DeVita VT. *The cancer recovery eating plan: the right foods to help fuel your recovery.* New York, NY: Times Books, 1996.

Pensiero L, Olivieria S, Osborne M. *The Strang cookbook for cancer prevention.* New York, NY: Dutton, 1998.

Ponichtera BJ. *Quick & healthy recipes and ideas: for people who say they don't have time to cook healthy meals.* Dalles, OR: Scaledown, 1991.

Ponichtera BJ. *Quick & healthy volume II: more help for people who say they don't have time to cook healthy meals.* Dalles, OR: Scaledown, 1995.

Rolls B. *The volumetrics eating plan: techniques and recipes for feeling full on fewer calories.* New York, NY: Harper Paperbacks, 2007.

Rosso J. *Great good food.* New York, NY: Crown/Turtle Bay Books, 1993.

Starke RD, Winston M, eds. *American Heart Association low-salt cookbook: a complete guide to reducing sodium and fat in the diet.* New York, NY: Times Books, 1990.

Willett WC. *Eat, drink and be healthy.* New York, NY: Simon and Schuster Source, 2001.

Wood R. *The new whole foods encyclopedia: a comprehensive resource for healthy eating.* New York, NY: Penguin Books, 1999.

WEB-BASED RESOURCES

HTTP://WWW.HEALTHFINDER.GOV

This site, useful to both professional and lay users, is maintained by the U.S. Department of Health and Human Services and serves as a directory to credible sources of health information on the web. A search engine allows for easy identification of nutrition sites of interest.

www.choosemyplate.gov/

These sites provide images of the U.S. Department of Agriculture's My Plate meal planning guide

HTTP://WWW.ARS.USDA.GOV/BA/BHNRC/NDL

This site provides access to the U.S. Department of Agriculture Nutrient Data Laboratory. The nutrient composition of virtually any food can be found in the database. To determine the nutrient composition of a food, click "Search" and enter the name of the food.

HTTP://WWW.DELICIOUSDECISIONS.ORG

This site, maintained by the American Heart Association, provides a wealth of information about heart-healthy eating and cooking, including detailed recipes.

HTTP://WWW.NOAH-HEALTH.ORG/EN/HEALTHY/NUTRITION

The New York Online Access to Health (NOAH) website provides health information in both English and Spanish. The nutrition index is extensive and very user friendly.

HTTP://VM.CFSAN.FDA.GOV/~DMS/WH-NUTR.HTML

This site provides essays on topics in nutrition and health by the U.S. Food and Drug Administration's Center for Food Safety and Applied Nutrition.

HTTP://WWW.AOA.GOV/ELDFAM/HEALTHY_LIFESTYLES/HEALTHY_LIFESTYLES.ASP

Maintained by the Administration on Aging, this site provides advice on diet and physical activity for health promotion that is tailored to older adults.

HTTP://WWW.IFIC.ORG/FOOD/SAFETY/INDEX.CFM

This site, maintained by the International Food Information Council, provides consumer-oriented information on food safety.

HTTP://VM.CFSAN.FDA.GOV/LABEL.HTML

This site, maintained by U.S. Food and Drug Administration Center for Food Safety and Applied Nutrition, provides detailed information on the interpretation of food labels, including their use for specific health goals.

HTTP://WWW.EATRIGHT.ORG

This site, maintained by the American Dietetic Association, provides information about the services of dietitians as well as a search engine to find a local dietitian listed with the association.

HTTP://WWW.KIDSHEALTH.ORG/PARENT/NUTRITION_FIT

A private foundation, the Nemours Center for Children's Health Media, maintains this website, which offers detailed information on nutrition for the newborn. Information on diet and nutrition for older children, through adolescence, is easily accessible from this site.

HTTP://WWW.NIDDK.NIH.GOV/HEALTH/NUTRITION.HTM

This site, maintained by the National Center for Diabetes, Digestive and Kidney Diseases (NIDDK) at the National Institutes of Health, provides extensive references on cooking and nutrition in the management of diabetes.

HTTP://WWW.MAYOCLINIC.COM/HEALTH/HEALTHY-RECIPES/RE99999

This site provides a virtual cookbook maintained by the Mayo Foundation for Medical Education and Research of the Mayo Clinic. Patients can select from a variety of recipes and see the nutritional composition for standard and modified recipes side-by-side.

HTTP://WIN.NIDDK.NIH.GOV/PUBLICATIONS/SMOKING.HTM

This site, maintained by the National Center for Diabetes, Digestive and Kidney Diseases (NIDDK) at the National Institutes of Health, provides information to patients on how to avoid weight gain during smoking cessation.

HTTP://CANCERNET.NCI.NIH.GOV/CANCERTOPICS

This site, maintained by the National Cancer Institute at the National Institutes of Health, provides detailed information on diet tailored for patients with cancer.

HTTP://VM.CFSAN.FDA.GOV/~LRD/ADVICE.HTML

This site, maintained by the Food and Drug Administration Center for Food Safety and Applied Nutrition, provides the consumer information on safe food handling and preparation.

HTTP://WWW.TOPS.ORG

This is the home page for Take Off Pounds Sensibly, an international club that provides information and support for sensible weight loss.

HTTP://WWW.NHLBI.NIH.GOV/HEALTH/PUBLIC/HEART/OBESITY/LOSE_WT/WTL_PROG.HTM

This site, maintained by the National Heart, Lung, and Blood Institute at the National Institutes of Health, provides guidance in choosing a safe and reasonable weight-loss program.

HTTP://WIN.NIDDK.NIH.GOV/PUBLICATIONS/CHOOSING.HTM

This site, maintained by the National Institute of Diabetes, Digestive and Kidney Diseases (NIDDK) at the National Institutes of Health, provides guidance in choosing a safe and reasonable weight loss program.

HTTP://WWW.HEALTHYDININGFINDER.COM

This site provides a guide to better-for-you chain restaurant meals.

HTTP://WWW.THEWAYTOEAT.NET

This site is an online meal plan by the author.

ODS.OD.NIH.GOV/FACTSHEETS/

The National Institutes of Health Office of Dietary Supplements website, which provides overviews of individual vitamins, minerals and other dietary supplements with links (e.g., to nutrient recommendations and Dietary Reference Intakes) and "QuickFacts"

APPENDIX K   PATIENT-SPECIFIC MEAL PLANNERS

As this text goes to press, plans are in place to develop meal plans based on the Overall Nutritional Quality Index (ONQI) (www.onqi.com) that are tailored to a wide variety of personal preferences and medical conditions. Check www.onqi.com for update information.

An online, subscription-service, meal plan, developed by the author, is available at:

WWW.THEWAYTOEAT.NET

For patients with or at risk for high blood pressure, see:

HTTP://WWW.NHLBI.NIH.GOV/HEALTH/PUBLIC/HEART/HBP/HBP_LOW/HBP_LOW.PDF

HTTP://WWW.MAYOCLINIC.COM/HEALTH/DASH-DIET/HI00047

For patients with, or at risk for, heart disease, heart-healthy recipes are available from the National Heart, Lung, and Blood Institute:

HTTP://WWW.NHLBI.NIH.GOV/HEALTH/PUBLIC/HEART/OTHER/KTB_RECIPEBK/

A portal to meal plans and recipes for diabetes management and prevention is provided by the American Diabetes Association at:

HTTP://WWW.DIABETES.ORG/NUTRITION-AND-RECIPES/NUTRITION/DIABETES-MEAL-PLAN.JSP

Meal plans for a variety of health conditions may be developed at:

HTTP://WWW.SPARKPEOPLE.COM/

APPENDIX L   GENERAL SUPPLEMENT GUIDELINES

Nutrient supplementation to redress overt deficiencies and recognized gaps in dietary intake is generally advisable for obvious reasons. Nutrient supplementation to achieve levels above mere sufficiency may offer advantages or disadvantages depending on the clinical context, nutrient preparation, nutrient combinations, and other factors. Decisions should be informed by a consideration of potential risks as well as benefits, and should be goal-oriented.

In general, an omega-3 fatty acid supplement might be a good idea for most people (i.e., those not regularly consuming fatty fish, other marine animals, flax seed oil, or wild game). Other supplements are most appropriate in certain populations; for instance folic acid taken by women prior to pregnancy to prevent neural tube defects. Still other supplements are specifically ill-advised in certain populations; for instance, beta carotene in smokers may increase the risk of lung and other cancers. The U.S. Preventive Services Task Force has recently determined that there is not enough evidence to recommend for or against most vitamin and mineral supplements—alone or in combination — for preventing cardiovascular disease or cancer, (http://www.uspreventiveservicestaskforce.org/draftrec2.htm Accessed 11/12/13) but the Task Force does not comment on supplements for other reasons. Individual supplements might best be used in a manner that is tailored to the health and risk factor profile of the given patient. The clinician is referred to the sections entitled "Nutrients, Nutriceuticals, and Functional Foods" and "Clinical Highlights" of the chapter pertaining to the condition of interest for further guidance. Information on the quality of some common supplements may be obtained at www.consumerlab.com.

As for multivitamins (or more precisely, multinutrient vitamin/mineral combinations), evidence in support of a daily usage is considered inconclusive by the National Institutes of Health (NIH State-of-the-Science Conference Statement on Multivitamin/Mineral Supplements and Chronic Disease Prevention. *Ann Intern Med* 2006;145:364–371; http://consensus.nih.gov/2006/MVMFINAL080106.pdf). Some research suggests small reductions in cancer risk with multivitamin supplementation, (Gaziano JM, Sesso HD, Christen WG, et al. Multivitamins in the prevention of cancer in men: the Physicians' Health Study II randomized controlled trial. *JAMA: the Journal of the American Medical Association.* Nov 14 2012;308(18):1871–1880.) although without effect on cancer mortality, or vascular or all-cause mortality (*Am J Clin Nutr.* 2013 Feb;97(2):437–44. doi: 10.3945/ajcn.112.049304. Epub 2012 Dec 19. Multivitamin-multimineral supplementation and mortality: a meta-analysis of randomized controlled trials. Macpherson H, Pipingas A, Pase MP.) Some studies also suggest no benefit of multivitamins, specifically for primary prevention of cancer, (Ann Pharmacother. 2011 Apr;45(4):476–84. doi: 10.1345/aph.1P445. Epub 2011 Apr 12. Multivitamin supplement use and risk of breast cancer: a meta-analysis. Chan AL, Leung HW, Wang SF.) or secondary prevention of heart attacks, stroke, or early death after previous myocardial infarction. (Lamas GA, Boineau R, Goertz C, et al. Oral High-Dose Multivitamins and Minerals After Myocardial Infarction. Annals of Internal Medicine. 2013;159(12)). Multivitamins may help enhance immediate free-recall memory, as one isolated aspect of cognition, (Ann Pharmacother. 2011 Apr;45(4):476–84. doi: 10.1345/aph.1P445. Epub 2011 Apr 12. Multivitamin supplement use and risk of breast cancer: a meta-analysis. Chan AL, Leung HW, Wang SF) but do not seem to protect against dementia. (Grodstein F, O'Brien J, Kang JH, et al. Long-Term Multivitamin Supplementation and Cognitive Function in Men: The Physicians' Health Study II. *Annals of Internal Medicine.* 2013;159(12)) They may lead to fewer sick days in eldery people, *BMJ.* 2005 Apr 16;330(7496):871. Epub 2005 Mar 31. Role of multivitamins and mineral supplements in preventing infections in elderly people: systematic review and meta-analysis of randomised controlled trials. El-Kadiki A, Sutton AJ.) and other potential benefits of a daily multinutrient supplement cannot be ruled out (especially in the undernourished and those who consume a typical Western diet). Nonetheless, multivitamins are typically consumed the most by those who need them the least and vice versa. For most people, there is currently no compelling reason to take a multivitamin. By the same token, there is no compelling reason not to.

INDEX

Figures are indicated by page numbers followed by *f*. Tables are indicated by page numbers followed by *t*.